RECEIVED

0 6 MAR 2012

Moreton Morrell Site

£45.99

KT-556-354

4
POW
(023)

EXERCISE PHYSIOLOGY

Theory and Application to Fitness and Performance

EIGHTH EDITION

Scott K. Powers
University of Florida

Edward T. Howley
University of Tennessee, Knoxville

WARWICKSHIRE
COLLEGE
LIBRARY

WITHDRAWN

Mc
Graw
Hill

Connect
Learn
Succeed™

Warwickshire College

00675739

The McGraw·Hill Companies

Mc Graw Hill) Connect Learn Succeed™

EXERCISE PHYSIOLOGY: THEORY AND APPLICATION TO FITNESS AND PERFORMANCE,
EIGHTH EDITION

Published by McGraw-Hill, an imprint of The McGraw-Hill Companies, Inc., 1221 Avenue of the Americas,
New York, NY 10020. Copyright © 2012 by The McGraw-Hill Companies, Inc. All rights reserved. No part of
this publication may be reproduced or distributed in any form or by any means, or stored in a database or retrieval
system, without the prior written consent of The McGraw-Hill Companies, Inc., including, but not limited to,
in any network or other electronic storage or transmission, or broadcast for distance learning.

Some ancillaries, including electronic and print components, may not be available to customers outside
the United States.

This book is printed on acid-free paper.

1 2 3 4 5 6 7 8 9 0 DOW/DOW 10 9 8 7 6 5 4 3 2 1

ISBN 978-0-07-131626-2

MHID: 0-07-131626-4

WARWICKSHIRE COLLEGE
LIBRARY

Class No
612.044

Acc No
00675739

Price & Loan Type
45.99

Dedicated to Lou and Ann
for their love, patience, and support.

Warwickshire College
Library
Vacation Market Centre

Brief Contents

Contents

Class No: 612.044
Acc No: 00675739

Preface

As with all previous editions, the eighth edition of *Exercise Physiology: Theory and Application to Fitness and Performane* is intended for students interested in exercise physiology, clinical exercise physiology, human performance, kinesiology/exercise science, physical therapy, and physical education. The overall objective of this text is to provide the student with an up-to-date understanding of the physiology of exercise. Moreover, the book contains numerous clinical applications, including exercise tests to evaluate cardiorespiratory fitness and information on exercise training for improvements in health-related physical fitness and sports performance.

This book is intended for a one-semester, upper-level undergraduate or beginning graduate exercise physiology course. Clearly, the text contains more material than can be covered in a fifteen-week semester. This is by design. The book was written to be comprehensive to afford instructors the freedom to select the material that they consider to be the most important for the composition of their class.

NEW TO THIS EDITION

The eighth edition of our book has undergone *major* revisions and highlights the latest research in exercise physiology. Indeed, every chapter contains new and expanded discussions, new text boxes, new figures, updated references, and contemporary suggested readings. Furthermore, we have added an additional chapter to this book that focuses on exercise and the immune system. Also in this eighth edition, students are exposed to new information on the cell signaling events leading to skeletal muscle adaptation to both resistance and endurance exercise training.

New Topics and Updated Content

The content of this new edition has been expanded and updated. The following list describes some of the major changes that have made the eighth edition more complete and up to date:

- The central theme of the book remains regulation of homeostasis during exercise, and the revised text now contains a detailed discussion of how signaling pathways regulate cellular homeostasis and lead to exercise-induced muscle adaptation to exercise.
- Numerous new and revised box features added to chapters throughout the book
- A new chapter to discuss the impact of exercise on the immune system.
- New information on the size principle of motor unit recruitment.
- Updated and new information on the causes of exercise-induced muscle fatigue.
- Expanded and revised chapter on endocrine function during exercise along with a new and detailed discussion of muscle as an endocrine organ.
- New information on the cause of exercise-induced muscle cramps.
- Updated material on heart rate variability during exercise.
- New information on the age-related changes in skeletal muscle.
- Updated information on the regulation of the cardiovascular and ventilatory responses to exercise.

- Updated information on the role of inflammation related to atherosclerosis and other chronic diseases

- Expanded discussion of the new U.S. Physical Activity Guidelines, including the link of physical activity to reduction in chronic disease risk and death from all causes.

- Update on guidelines related to exercise testing and prescription for specific diseases (e.g., diabetes, COPD) and populations (older individuals, pregnant women).

- Expanded discussion of nutritional factors related to managing exercise-induced asthma.

- Update on the new Dietary Guidelines for Americans; expanded discussion of possible role of high fructose corn syrup on obesity; latest information on the prevalence of overweight and obesity in children and adults; update on drugs, exercise, and weight loss.

- Contemporary information on the laboratory testing of athletes.

- New information on training for performance in both young and masters athletes.

- Up-to-date material on the impact of aging on performance.

- New discussion of carbohydrate loading in female athletes; expanded debate of water and carbohydrate intake prior to and immediately following performance; and expanded discussion of hyponatremia.

- Expanded discussion of how altitude natives acclimatize to altitude exposure over generations, with clear differences between Andean and Tibetan populations.

McGraw Hill create

CREATE, BECAUSE CUSTOMIZATION MATTERS

Design your ideal course materials with McGraw-Hill's *Create*: www.mcgrawhillcreate.com. Rearrange or omit chapters, combine material from other sources, and/or upload your syllabus or any other content you have written to make the perfect resource for your students. Search thousands of leading McGraw-Hill textbooks to find the best content for your students, then arrange it to fit your teaching style. You can even personalize your book's appearance by selecting the cover and adding your name, school, and course information. When you order a *Create* book, you receive a complimentary review copy. Get a printed copy in three to five business days or an electronic copy (eComp) via e-mail in about an hour.

Register today at **www.mcgrawhillcreate.com,** and craft your course resources to match the way you teach.

INSTRUCTOR AND STUDENT ONLINE RESOURCES

www.mhhe.com/powers8e

The Online Learning Center at **www.mhhe.com/powers8e** includes valuable teaching and learning tools including assessment tools, classroom presentations, practice quizzes, and updated reference materials.

ACKNOWLEDGEMENTS

A text such as *Exercise Physiology: Theory and Application to Fitness and Performance* is not the effort of only two authors, but represents the contributions of hundreds of scientists from around the world. Although it is not possible to acknowledge every contributor to this work, we would like to recognize the following scientists who have greatly influenced our thinking, careers, and lives in general: Drs. Bruno Balke, Ronald Byrd, Jerome Dempsey, Stephen Dodd, H. V. Forster, B. D. Franks, Steven Horvath, Henry Montoye, Francis Nagle, and Hugh G. Welch.

Moreover, we would like to thank Erin Talbert and Brian Parr for their assistance in providing suggestions for revisions to this book. Indeed, both of these individuals provided numerous contributions to the improvement of the eighth edition of this book. Finally, we would like to thank the following reviewers who provided helpful comments about the sixth edition of *Exercise Physiology*:

Tom Ball
De Pauw University

Burch Oglesby
University of Tennessee, Chattanooga

Justus Ortega
Humboldt State University

Linda Romaine
Raritan Valley Community College

Hank Williford
Auburn University, Montgomery

Robert Chapman
Indiana University, Bloomington

Charles Darracott
Augusta State University

Steven Hawkins
California Lutheran University

Robert Lehnhard
University of Maine

Brian McFarlin
University of Houston

Clay Nicks
Columbus State University

Engaging Presentation of Key Concepts Supported by the Latest Research

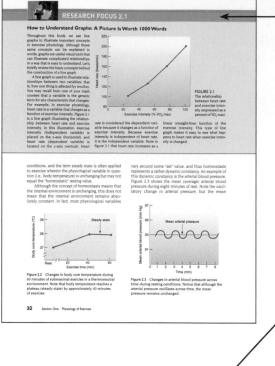

Research Focus

No matter what their career direction, students must learn how to read and think about the latest research. Research Focus presents new research and explains why it's relevant.

A Closer Look

A Closer Look offers an in-depth view of topics that are of special interest to students. This feature encourages students to dig deeper about key concepts.

Ask the Expert

This question-and-answer feature lets you find out what leading scientists have to say about topics such as the effect of space flight on skeletal muscle and the effect of exercise on bone health.

Practical Applications of Exercise Physiology

New Chapter

A new Chapter 6 presents the growing body of research on exercise-induced changes in the immune system and its significance for applied exercise physiology.

Clinical Applications

Learn how exercise physiology is used in the clinical setting.

The Winning Edge

How do athletes find the "extra edge" that can make the difference between victory and defeat? These features explain the science behind a winning performance.

Physiology of Exercise

0

Introduction to Exercise Physiology

Does one have to have a "genetic gift" of speed to be a world-class runner, or is it all due to training? What happens to your heart rate when you take an exercise test that increases in intensity each minute? What changes occur in your muscles as a result of an endurance-training program that allows you to run at faster speeds over longer distances? What fuel—carbohydrate or fat—is most important when running the marathon? Research in exercise physiology provides answers to these and similar questions.

Physiology is the study of the function of tissues (e.g., muscle, nerve), organs (e.g., heart, lungs), and systems (e.g., cardiovascular system). Exercise physiology extends this to evaluate the effect of a single bout of exercise (acute exercise) and repeated bouts of exercise (i.e., training programs) on these tissues, organs, and systems. In addition, the responses to acute exercise and training may be studied at high altitude or in extremes of heat and humidity to determine the impact of these environmental factors on our ability to respond and adapt to exercise. Finally, studies are conducted on young and old individuals, both healthy and those with disease, to understand the role of exercise in the prevention of or rehabilitation from various chronic diseases.

Consistent with this perspective, we go beyond simple statements of fact to show how information about the physiology of exercise is applied to the prevention of and rehabilitation from coronary heart disease, the performances of elite athletes, and the ability of a person to work in adverse environments such as high altitudes. The acceptance of terms such as *sports physiology*, *sports nutrition*, and *sports medicine* is evidence of the growth of interest in the application of physiology of exercise to real-world problems. Careers in athletic training, personal-fitness training, cardiac rehabilitation, and strength and conditioning, as well as the traditional fields of physical therapy and medicine, are of interest to students studying exercise physiology. We will expand on career opportunities later in the chapter.

In this chapter we provide a brief history of exercise physiology to help you understand where we have been and where we are going. In addition, throughout the text a variety of scientists and clinicians are highlighted in a historical context as subject matter is presented (i.e., muscle, cardiovascular responses, altitude). We hope that by linking a person to a major accomplishment within the context of a chapter, history will come alive and be of interest to you.

BRIEF HISTORY OF EXERCISE PHYSIOLOGY

The history of exercise physiology represents a global perspective involving scientists from many different countries. In this section we begin with the impact European scientists have had on the development of exercise physiology. We then describe the role of the Harvard Fatigue Lab in the growth of exercise physiology in this country.

European Heritage

A good starting place to discuss the history of exercise physiology in the United States is in Europe. Three scientists, A. V. Hill of Britain, August Krogh of Denmark, and Otto Meyerhof of Germany, received Nobel Prizes for research on muscle or muscular exercise (12). Hill and Meyerhof shared the Nobel Prize in Physiology or Medicine in 1922. Hill was recognized for his precise measurements of heat production during muscle contraction and recovery, and Meyerhof for his discovery of the relationship between the consumption of oxygen and the measurement of lactic acid in muscle. Hill was trained as a mathematician before becoming interested in physiology. In addition to his work cited for the Nobel Prize, his studies on humans led to the development of a framework around which we understand the physiological factors related to distance-running performance (6) (see chapter 19).

A. Archibald V. Hill, B. August Krogh, C. Otto F. Meyerhof

Chapter Zero   Introduction to Exercise Physiology   **3**

Although Krogh received his Nobel Prize for his research on the function of capillary circulation, he had a major impact on numerous areas of investigation. Further, like many productive investigators, his influence was not due only to his own work, but to that of his students and colleagues as well. Krogh's collaboration with Johannes Lindhard resulted in classic studies dealing with carbohydrate and fat metabolism during exercise, and how the cardiovascular and respiratory systems' responses are controlled during exercise (4). Three of Krogh's students, Erling Asmussen, Erik Hohwü-Christensen, and Marius Nielsen (called the three musketeers by Krogh), had a major impact on exercise physiology research throughout the middle of the twentieth century. These investigators, in turn, trained a number of outstanding physiologists, several of whom you will meet throughout this text. The August Krogh Institute in Denmark contains some of the most prominent exercise physiology laboratories in the world. Marie Krogh, his wife, was a noted scientist in her own right and was recognized for her innovative work on measuring the diffusing capacity of the lung. We recommend the biography of the Kroghs written by their daughter, Bodil Schmidt-Nielsen (see Suggested Readings), for those interested in the history of the physiology of exercise.

Several other European scientists must also be mentioned, not only because of their contributions to the physiology of exercise, but because their names are commonly used in a discussion of exercise physiology. J. S. Haldane did some of the original work on the role of CO_2 in the control of breathing. Haldane also developed the respiratory gas analyzer that bears his name (15). C. G. Douglas did pioneering work with Haldane in the role of O_2 and lactic acid in the control of breathing during exercise, including some work conducted at various altitudes. The canvas-and-rubber gas collection bag used for many years in exercise physiology laboratories around the world carries Douglas's name. A contemporary of Douglas, Christian Bohr of Denmark, did the classic work on how O_2 binds to hemoglobin. The "shift" in the oxygen-hemoglobin dissociation curve due to the addition of CO_2 bears his name (see chapter 10). Interestingly, it was Krogh who did the actual experiments that enabled Bohr to describe his famous "shift." (4, 15).

IN SUMMARY

- A. V. Hill, August Krogh, and Otto Meyerhof received the Nobel Prize for work related to muscle or muscular exercise.
- Numerous European scientists have had a major impact on the field of exercise physiology.

Harvard Fatigue Laboratory

A focal point in the history of exercise physiology in the United States is the Harvard Fatigue Laboratory. Professor L. J. Henderson organized the laboratory within the Business School to conduct physiological research on industrial hazards. Dr. David Bruce Dill was the research director from the time the laboratory opened in 1927 until it closed in 1947 (18). Table 0.1 shows that the scientists conducted research in numerous areas, in the laboratory and in the field, and the results of those early studies have been supported by recent investigations. Dill's classic text, *Life, Heat, and Altitude* (14), is recommended reading for any student of exercise and environmental physiology. Much of the careful and precise work of the laboratory was conducted using the now-classic Haldane analyzer for respiratory gas analysis and the van Slyke apparatus for blood-gas analysis. The advent of computer-controlled equipment in the 1980s has made data collection easier but has not improved on the accuracy of measurement (see figure 0.1).

The "three musketeers": From left to right: Erling Asmussen, Erik Hohwü-Christensen, and Marius Nielsen

David Bruce Dill

TABLE 0.1	Active Research Areas in the Harvard Fatigue Laboratory

Metabolism
 Maximal oxygen uptake
 Oxygen debt
 Carbohydrate and fat metabolism during
  long-term work
Environmental physiology
 Altitude
 Dry and moist heat
 Cold
Clinical physiology
 Gout
 Schizophrenia
 Diabetes
Aging
 Basal metabolic rate
 Maximal oxygen uptake
 Maximal heart rate
Blood
 Acid-base balance
 O_2 saturation: role of PO_2, PCO_2, and carbon
  monoxide
 Nutrition assessment techniques
 Vitamins
 Foods
Physical fitness
 Harvard Step Test

The Harvard Fatigue Laboratory attracted doctoral students as well as scientists from other countries. Many of the alumni from the laboratory are recognized in their own right for excellence in research in the physiology of exercise. Two doctoral students, Steven Horvath and Sid Robinson, went on to distinguished careers at the Institute of Environmental Stress in Santa Barbara and Indiana University, respectively.

Foreign "Fellows" included the "three musketeers" mentioned in the previous section (E. Asmussen, E. Hohwü-Christensen, and M. Nielsen), and the Nobel Prize winner August Krogh. These scientists brought new ideas and technology to the lab, participated in laboratory and field studies with other staff members, and published some of the most important work in the physiology of exercise between 1930 and 1980. Rudolpho Margaria, from Italy, went on to extend his classic work on oxygen debt and described the energetics of locomotion. Peter F. Scholander, from Norway, gave us his chemical gas analyzer that is a primary method of calibrating tank gas used to standardize electronic gas analyzers (18).

In summary, under the leadership of Dr. D. B. Dill, the Harvard Fatigue Laboratory became a model for research investigations into exercise and environmental physiology, especially as it relates to humans. When the laboratory closed and the staff dispersed, the ideas, techniques, and approaches to scientific inquiry were distributed throughout the world, and with them, Dill's influence in the area of environmental and exercise physiology. Dr. Dill continued his research outside Boulder City, Nevada, into the 1980s. He died in 1986 at the age of 93.

Progress toward understanding any issue in exercise physiology transcends time, national origin, and scientific training. Solutions to difficult questions require the interaction of scientists from diverse disciplines and professions such as physiology, biochemistry, molecular biology, and medicine. We recommend *Exercise Physiology—People and Ideas* (see the Suggested Readings) to further your understanding of important historical connections. In this book, internationally known scientists provide a historical treatment of a number of important issues in exercise physiology with an emphasis on the cross-continent flow of energy and ideas. We highlight several scientists and clinicians with our Ask the Expert boxes throughout the text, both to introduce them to you

Figure 0.1 Comparison of old and new technology used to measure oxygen consumption and carbon dioxide production during exercise. (*Left*: The Carnegie Institute of Washington, D.C.; *Right*: COSMED.)

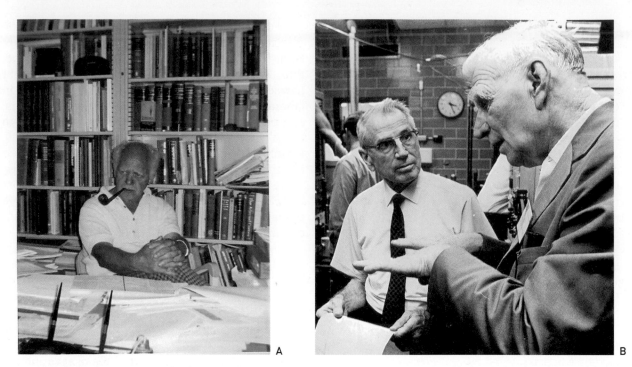

A. Steven Horvath, B. Sid Robinson (left) in his lab, talking with A. C. Burton

and for them to share their current ideas. In addition, A Look Back—Important People in Science, is used to recognize well-known scientists who have influenced our understanding of exercise physiology. In this context you will get to know those who have gone before and those who are currently leading the charge.

IN SUMMARY

■ The Harvard Fatigue Laboratory was a focal point in the development of exercise physiology in the United States. Dr. D. B. Dill directed the laboratory from its opening in 1927 until its closing in 1947. The body of research in exercise and environmental physiology produced by the scientists in that laboratory formed the foundation for new ideas and experimental methods that still influence us today.

PHYSIOLOGY, PHYSICAL FITNESS, AND HEALTH

Physical fitness is a popular topic today, and its popularity has been a major factor in motivating college students to pursue careers in physical education, physiology of exercise, health education, nutrition, physical therapy, and medicine. In 1980, the Public Health Service listed "physical fitness and exercise" as one of fifteen areas of concern related to improving the country's overall health (30). Although this might appear to be an unprecedented event, similar interests and concerns about physical fitness existed in this country more than one hundred years ago. Between the Civil War and the First World War (WWI), physical education was primarily concerned with the development and maintenance of fitness, and many of the leaders in physical education were trained in medicine (13) (p. 5). For example, Dr. Dudley Sargent, hired by Harvard University in 1879, set up a physical training program with individual exercise prescriptions to improve a person's structure and function to achieve "that prime physical condition called fitness—fitness for work, fitness for play, fitness for anything a man may be called upon to do" (33) (p. 297).

Dudley Sargent

Sargent was clearly ahead of his time in promoting health-related fitness. Later, war became a primary force driving this country's interest in physical fitness. Concerns about health and fitness were raised during WW I and WW II when large numbers of draftees failed the induction exams due to mental and physical defects (17) (p. 407). These concerns influenced the type of physical education programs in the schools during these years, making them resemble premilitary training programs (37) (p. 484). Interestingly, whereas stunted growth and being underweight were major reasons for rejecting military recruits in WW II, obesity is the major cause for rejecting recruits today (see "Too Fat to Fight" at http://cdn.missionreadiness.org/MR_Too_Fat_to_Fight-1.pdf).

The present interest in physical activity and health was stimulated in the early 1950s by two major findings: (1) autopsies of young soldiers killed during the Korean War showed that significant coronary artery disease had already developed, and (2) Hans Kraus showed that American children performed poorly on a minimal muscular fitness test compared to European children (37) (p. 516). Due to the latter finding, President Eisenhower initiated a conference in 1955 that resulted in the formation of the President's Council on Youth Fitness. The American Association for Health, Physical Education, and Recreation (AAHPER) supported these activities and in 1957 developed the AAHPER Youth Fitness Test with national norms to be used in physical education programs throughout the country. Before he was inaugurated, President Kennedy expressed his concerns about the nation's fitness in an article published in *Sports Illustrated*, called "The Soft American" (22):

> For the physical vigor of our citizens is one of America's most precious resources. If we waste and neglect this resource, if we allow it to dwindle and grow soft, then we will destroy much of our ability to meet the great and vital challenges which confront our people. We will be unable to realize our full potential as a nation.

During Kennedy's term, the council's name was changed to the "President's Council on Physical Fitness" to highlight the concern for fitness. The name was changed again in the Nixon administration to the "President's Council on Physical Fitness and Sports," which supported fitness not only in schools but in business, industry, and for the general public (see **www.fitness.gov**). The name was most recently changed by President Obama to the "President's Council on Fitness, Sports, & Nutrition" to focus more attention on the obesity epidemic. Items in the Youth Fitness Test were changed over the years, and in 1980 the American Alliance for Health, Physical Education, Recreation, and Dance (AAHPERD) published a sepa-

rate *Health-Related Physical Fitness Test Manual* (1) to distinguish between "performance testing" (e.g., 50-yard dash) and "fitness testing" (e.g., skinfold thickness). This health-related test battery is consistent with the direction of lifetime fitness programs, being concerned with obesity, cardiorespiratory fitness, and low-back function. A parallel fitness test, Fitness-Gram®, was developed by The Cooper Institute in 1982, including software to support the scoring and printing of reports (see **http://www.fitnessgram.net/home/**). For readers interested in the history of fitness testing in schools, we recommend Park's monograph in the Suggested Readings.

Paralleling this interest in the physical fitness of youth was the rising concern about the death rate from coronary heart disease in the middle-aged American male population. Epidemiological studies of the health status of the population underscored the fact that degenerative diseases related to poor health habits (e.g., high-fat diet, smoking, inactivity) were responsible for more deaths than the classic infectious and contagious diseases. In 1966, a major symposium highlighted the need for more research in the area of physical activity and health (31). In the 1970s, there was an increase in the use of exercise tests to diagnose heart disease and to aid in the prescription of exercise programs to improve cardiovascular health. Large corporations developed "executive" fitness programs to improve the health status of that high-risk group. While most Americans are now familiar with such programs, and some students of exercise physiology seek careers in "Corporate Fitness," such programs are not new. The photo in figure 0.2, taken from the 1923 edition of McKenzie's *Exercise in Education and Medicine* (25), show a group of businessmen in costume doing dance exercises. In short, the

Figure 0.2 A group of businessmen in a dancing class under the direction of Oliver E. Hebbert.

By the early to mid-1980s, it had become clear that physical inactivity was a major public health concern (30). In 1992, the American Heart Association made physical inactivity a major risk factor for cardiovascular diseases, just like smoking, high blood pressure, and high serum cholesterol (3). In 1995, the Centers for Disease Control and Prevention (CDC) and the American College of Sports Medicine published a public health physical activity recommendation that "Every U.S. adult should accumulate 30 minutes or more of moderate-intensity physical activity on most, preferably all, days of the week" (28). A year later, the *Surgeon General's Report on Physical Activity and Health* was published (36).

This report highlighted the fact that physical inactivity was killing U.S. adults, and the problem was a big one—60% of U.S. adults did not engage in the recommended amount of physical activity, and 25% were not active at all. This report was based on the large body of evidence available from epidemiological studies, small-group training studies, and clinical investigations showing the positive effects of an active lifestyle. For example, physical activity was shown to:

- lower the risk of dying prematurely and from heart disease
- reduce the risk of developing diabetes and high blood pressure
- help maintain weight and healthy bones, muscles, and joints
- help lower blood pressure in those with high blood pressure n promote psychological well-being

In 2008 the first edition of the *U.S. Physical Activity Guidelines* was published (http://www.health.gov/paguidelines/guidelines/default.aspx). This document was developed on the basis of an Advisory Committee's comprehensive review of the research since the publication of the Surgeon General's Report in 1996 (for the Advisory Committee Report, see http://www.health.gov/paguidelines/Report/Default.aspx). The *U.S. Physical Activity Guidelines*, along with the *Dietary Guidelines for Americans 2010* (http://www.health.gov/dietaryguidelines/), provide important information on how to address our problems of inactivity and obesity. (We discuss this in more detail in chapters 16, 17, and 18.)

---

idea that regular physical activity is an important part of a healthy lifestyle was "rediscovered." If any questions remained about the importance of physical activity to health, the publication of the Surgeon General's Report in 1996 and the appearance of the first U.S. Physical Activity Guidelines in 2008 put them to rest (see A Closer Look 0.1).

IN SUMMARY

- Fitness has been an issue in this country from the latter part of the nineteenth century until the present. War, or the threat of war, exerted a strong influence on fitness programs in the public schools. In WW II, being underweight and small of stature were major reasons for rejecting military recruits; today, obesity is a major cause for rejection.
- Recent interest in fitness is related to the growing concern over the high death rates from disease processes that are attributable to preventable factors, such as poor diet, lack of exercise, and smoking. Government and professional organizations have responded to this need by educating the public about these problems.
- Schools use health-related fitness tests, such as the skinfold estimation of body fatness, rather than the more traditional performance tests, to evaluate a child's physical fitness.

PHYSICAL EDUCATION TO EXERCISE SCIENCE AND KINESIOLOGY

Undergraduate academic preparation in physical education has changed over the past five decades to reflect the explosion in the knowledge base related to the physiology of exercise, biomechanics, and exercise prescription. This occurred at a time of a perceived reduced need for school-based physical education teachers and an increased need for exercise professionals in the preventive and clinical settings. These factors, as well as others, led some college and university departments to change their names from Physical Education to Exercise Science or Kinesiology. This trend is likely to continue as programs move further away from traditional roots in education and become integrated within colleges of Arts and Sciences or Allied Health Professions (35). There has been an increase in the number of programs requiring undergraduates to take one year of calculus, chemistry, and physics, and courses in organic chemistry, biochemistry, anatomy, physiology, and nutrition. In many colleges and universities, little difference now exists between the first two years of requirements in a pre-physical therapy or pre-medical track and the track associated with fitness professions. The differences among these tracks lie in the "application" courses that follow. Biomechanics, physiology of exercise, fitness assessment, exercise prescription, strength and conditioning, and so on belong to the physical education/exercise science track. However, it must again be pointed out that this new trend is but another example of a rediscovery of old roots rather than a revolutionary change. Kroll describes two 4-year professional physical education programs in the 1890s, one at Stanford and the other at Harvard, that were the forerunners of today's programs (23) (pp. 51–64). They included the detailed scientific work and application courses with clear prerequisites cited. Finally, considerable time was allotted for laboratory work. No doubt, Lagrange's 1890 text, *Physiology of Bodily Exercise* (24), served as an important reference source for these students. The expectations and goals of those programs were almost identical to those specified for current exercise physiology undergraduate tracks. In fact, one of the aims of the Harvard program was to allow a student to pursue the study of medicine after completing two years of study (23) (p. 61).

GRADUATE STUDY AND RESEARCH IN THE PHYSIOLOGY OF EXERCISE

While the Harvard Fatigue Laboratory was closing in 1947, the country was on the verge of a tremendous expansion in the number of universities offering graduate study and research opportunities in exercise physiology. A 1950 survey showed that only 16 colleges or universities had research laboratories in departments of physical education (19). By 1966, 151 institutions had research facilities, 58 of them in exercise physiology (37) (p. 526). This expansion was due to the availability of more scientists trained in the research methodology of exercise physiology, the increased number of students attending college due to the GI Bill and student loans, and the increase in federal dollars to improve the research capabilities of universities (11, 35).

"The scholar's work will be multiplied many fold through the contribution of his students." This quote, taken from Montoye and Washburn (26, 27), expresses a view that has helped attract researchers and scholars to universities. Evidence to support this quote was presented in the form of genealogical charts of contributors to the *Research Quarterly* (27). These charts showed the tremendous influence a few people had through their students in the expansion of research in physical education. Probably the best example of this is Thomas K. Cureton, Jr., of the University of Illinois, a central figure in the training of productive researchers in exercise physiology and

fitness (see A Look Back—Important People in Science).

An example of a major university program that can trace its lineage to the Harvard Fatigue Laboratory is found at Pennsylvania State University. Dr. Ancel Keys, a staff member at the Harvard Fatigue Laboratory, brought Henry Longstreet Taylor back to the Laboratory for Physiological Hygiene at the University of Minnesota, where he received his Ph.D. in 1941 (10). Taylor subsequently advised the research work of Elsworth R. Buskirk, who designed and directed the Laboratory for Human Performance Research (Noll Laboratory) at Pennsylvania State University. Noll Laboratory continues in the tradition of the Harvard Fatigue Laboratory with a comprehensive research program of laboratory and field research into basic exercise, environmental, and industrial research questions (9). However, it is clear that excellent research in exercise and environmental physiology is conducted in laboratories other than those that have a tie to the Harvard Fatigue Lab. Laboratories are found in physical education departments, physiology departments in medical schools, clinical medicine programs at hospitals, and in independent facilities such as the Cooper Institute for Aerobics Research. The proliferation and specialization of research involving exercise is discussed in the next section.

It should be no surprise that the major issues studied by researchers in exercise physiology have changed over the years. Table 0.2, from Tipton's look at the fifty years following the closing of the Harvard Fatigue Lab, shows the subject matter areas that were studied in considerable detail between 1954 and 1994 (35). A great number of these topics fit into the broad area of systemic physiology or were truly applied physiology issues. Although research continues to take place in most of these areas, Tipton believes that many of the most important questions to be addressed in the future will be answered by those with special training in molecular biology. Baldwin (5) supported Tipton's viewpoint and provided a summary of important questions dealing with exercise and chronic disease whose answers are linked to functional genomics and proteomics, important new tools for the molecular biologist. However, he also noted the need for increased research to address physical activity and chronic diseases at the lifestyle and behavioral levels. This "integrated" approach, crossing disciplines and technologies, should be reflected in the academic programs educating the next generation of exercise science students. We recommend the chapters by Tipton (35) and Buskirk and Tipton (11) for those interested in a detailed look at the development of exercise physiology in the United States.

A LOOK BACK—IMPORTANT PEOPLE IN SCIENCE

Thomas K. Cureton, Jr., Ph.D.

Dr. Thomas K. Cureton, Jr., was born in Florida in 1901. He studied electrical engineering for two years at Georgia Tech and completed his undergraduate degree in that area at Yale University in 1925. During his childhood and throughout his college career he was very interested in sports, becoming a champion runner and swimmer along the way. This stimulated his interest in exercise and training, and he completed elective coursework in anatomy, physiology, and biology at Yale as a part of his undergraduate degree. After graduation, and while working full time, he completed coursework for a B.S. in physical education in 1929 at Springfield College, one of the best-known schools for training in that area. He was appointed as an instructor in mathematics and chemistry at that college and eventually became director of its Biophysics, Anthropometry, and Kinesiology Laboratory. Over the course of the next 10 years, he completed his M.S. (Springfield College) and Ph.D. (Columbia University) degrees (7).

The focus of Dr. Cureton's research was on physical fitness. In 1941 he was hired by the University of Illinois, and three years later he opened the Physical Fitness Research Laboratory, one of the few laboratories in the world dedicated to studying the impact of exercise on fitness and health. The laboratory developed and validated fitness tests, established norms for those tests, developed methods to prescribe exercise to improve fitness, and provided opportunities for graduate students to do research projects (7, 23) (pp. 177–83).

Dr. Cureton was an incredibly productive writer and speaker, not just for science-related publications and conferences, but also for public consumption, especially through the YMCA. He was a strong voice for using physical activity to help patients recover from various medical problems. The fact that this was a time when physicians were recommending bed rest, it is no surprise that he had an uphill battle. However, Dr. Cureton made his point by showing, through his research, the importance of having patients become physically active in order to return to a productive life. In addition, he was an early advocate of preventing problems in the first place; his "Run for Your Life" program at the University of Illinois was put in place long before jogging became a popular activity. He became a well-known public figure appearing on TV, was interviewed by numerous papers, and became a focus of a special Time-Life book, *The Healthy Life: How Diet and Exercise Affect Your Heart and Vigor* (7). If you were to read that book today, within the context of our current epidemics of obesity and physical inactivity, you would realize how far ahead Dr. Cureton was in the promotion of physical activity and fitness.

As mentioned earlier, one of the primary purposes of Dr. Cureton's Physical Fitness Research Laboratory was to provide opportunities for graduate students to become trained in doing research on physical fitness. The proceedings from a symposium honoring Dr. Cureton in 1969 listed sixty-eight Ph.D. students who completed their work under his direction (16). Although Dr. Cureton's scholarly record includes hundreds of research articles and dozens of books dealing with physical fitness, the publications of his students in the areas of epidemiology, fitness, cardiac rehabilitation, and exercise physiology represent the "multiplying effect" that students have on a scholar's productivity. For those who would like to read more about Dr. Cureton, see Berryman's article (7).

TABLE 0.2	Significant Exercise Physiology Subject Matter Areas That Were Investigated Between 1954 and 1994

A. Basic Exercise Physiology	
Exercise Specificity	Plasticity of Muscle Fibers
Exercise Prescription	Motor Functions of the Spinal Cord
Central and Peripheral Responses and Adaptations	Hormonal Responses
Responses of Diseased Populations	The Hypoxemia of Severe Exercise
Action of Transmitters	Cellular and Molecular Adaptive Responses
Regulation of Receptors	**B. Applied Exercise Physiology**
Cardiovascular and Metabolic Feed Forward and Feedback Mechanisms	Performance of Elite Athletes
	Performance and Heat Stress
Substrate Utilization Profiles	Exercise at Altitude
Matching Mechanisms for Oxygen Delivery and Demand	Nutritional Aspects of Exercise
	Fluid Balance During Exercise
Mechanisms of Signal Transduction	Performance and Ergogenic Aids
Intracellular Lactate Mechanisms	Training for Physical Fitness

From: C. M. Tipton, Contemporary exercise physiology: Fifty years after the closure of Harvard Fatigue Laboratory. In *Exercise and Sport Sciences Reviews*, vol. 26, pp. 315–39, 1998. Edited by J. O. Holloszy. Baltimore: Williams & Wilkins.

10 Section One Physiology of Exercise

- The increase in research in exercise physiology was a catalyst that propelled the transformation of physical education departments into exercise science and kinesiology departments. The number of exercise physiology laboratories increased dramatically between the 1950s and 1970s, with many dealing with problems in systemic and applied physiology and the biochemistry of exercise.
- In the future, the emphasis will be on molecular biology and its developing technologies as the essential ingredients needed to solve basic science issues related to physical activity and health.
- However, there is no question about the need for additional research to better understand how to permanently change the physical activity and eating behaviors of individuals in order to realize health-related goals.

PROFESSIONAL AND SCIENTIFIC SOCIETIES AND RESEARCH JOURNALS

The expansion of interest in exercise physiology and its application to fitness and rehabilitation resulted in an increase in the number of professional societies in which scientists and clinicians could present their work. Prior to 1950, the two major societies concerned with physiology of exercise and its application were the American Physiological Society (APS) and the American Association of Health, Physical Education, and Recreation (AAHPER). The need to bring together physicians, physical educators, and physiologists interested in physical activity and health into one professional society resulted in the founding of the American College of Sports Medicine (ACSM) in 1954 (see Berryman's history of the ACSM in the Suggested Readings). The ACSM now has more than 20,000 members, with twelve regional chapters throughout the country, each holding its own annual meeting to present research, sponsor symposiums, and promote sports medicine.

The explosion in exercise physiology research over the past 60 years has been accompanied by a dramatic increase in the number of professional and scientific societies and research journals communicating research findings. Table 0.3 provides a brief summary of research journals that publish research in exercise physiology.

Training in Research

One of the clear consequences of this increase in research activity is the degree to which scientists

TABLE 0.3 Sample of Research Journals for Exercise Physiology Research

Acta Physiologica (Scandinavica)
Adapted Physical Activity Quarterly
American Journal of Physiology
Aviation, Space and Environmental Medicine
Canadian Journal of Physiology and Pharmacology
European Journal of Occupational and Applied Physiology
International Journal of Sports Medicine
International Journal of Sport Nutrition
Journal of Aging and Physical Activity
Journal of Applied Physiology
Journal of Cardiopulmonary Rehabilitation
Journal of Clinical Investigation
Journal of Nutrition
Journal of Physical Activity and Health
Journal of Physiology
Journal of Sport Science
Journal of Strength and Conditioning Research
Medicine and Science in Sports and Exercise
Pediatric Exercise Physiology
Research Quarterly for Exercise and Sport

must specialize to compete for research grants and to manage the research literature. Laboratories may focus on neuromuscular physiology, cardiac rehabilitation, or the influence of exercise on bone structure. Graduate students need to specialize earlier in their careers as researchers, and undergraduates must investigate graduate programs very carefully to make sure they meet their career goals (21).

This specialization in research has generated comments about the need to emphasize "basic" research examining the mechanisms underlying a physiological issue rather than "applied" research, which might describe responses of persons to exercise, environmental, or nutritional factors. It would appear that both types of research are needed and, to some extent, such a separation is arbitrary. For example, one scientist might study the interaction of exercise intensity and diet on muscle hypertrophy, another may characterize the changes in muscle cell size and contractile protein, a third might study changes in the energetics of muscle contraction relative to cytoplasmic enzyme activities, and a fourth might study the gene expression needed to synthesize that contractile protein. Where does "applied" research begin and "basic" research end? In the introduction to his text *Human Circulation* (32), Loring Rowell provided a quote from T. H. Huxley that bears on this issue:

I often wish that this phrase "applied science," had never been invented. For it suggests that there is a sort of scientific knowledge of direct practical use, which can be studied apart from another sort of scientific knowledge, which is of no practical utility, and which is termed "pure science." But there is no more complete fallacy than this. What people call applied science is nothing but the application of pure science to particular classes of problems. It consists of deductions from those principles, established by reasoning and observation, which constitute pure science. No one can safely make these deductions until he has a firm grasp of the principles; and he can obtain that grasp only by personal experience of the operations of observation and of reasoning on which they are found (20).

Solutions to chronic disease problems related to physical inactivity (e.g., type 2 diabetes, obesity) will come from a range of scientific disciplines—from epidemiologists on the one hand (36) to cell biologists on the other (8). We hope that all forms of inquiry are supported by fellow scientists so that present theories related to exercise physiology are continually questioned and modified. Last, we completely agree with the sentiments expressed in a statement ascribed to Arthur B. Otis: "Physiology is a good way to make a living and still have fun" (34).

IN SUMMARY

- The growth and development of exercise physiology over the past 60 years has resulted in dramatic increases in the number of organizations and research journals. These journals and professional meetings provide additional opportunities for research findings to be disseminated.
- A greater need exists for graduate students to identify and specialize in a particular area of research earlier in their careers in order to find the best mentor and university program to realize career goals.

CAREERS IN EXERCISE SCIENCE AND KINESIOLOGY

Over the past 30 years there has been a sustained growth in career opportunities for those with academic training in exercise science and kinesiology. Currently, students pursue careers in personal-fitness training in private, commercial, work-site, and hospital settings; strength and conditioning in commercial, rehabilitative, and sport-related environments; cardiac rehabilitation; athletic training; massage therapy; and the traditional allied health professions (e.g., physical or occupational therapy) and medicine (e.g., physician assistant, physician). For those interested in careers in fitness and cardiac rehabilitation, coursework is not enough—students must develop the requisite skills needed to perform the job. That means that students should be completing practicum and internship experiences under the direction of a professional who can pass along what cannot be taught in a classroom or laboratory. Students should make contact with their advisors early in the program to maximize what can be gained from these experiences. Interested students should read the article by Pierce and Nagle on the internship experience (29). However, more may be needed to realize your career goal.

Those interested in cardiac rehabilitation and athletic training usually pursue graduate study (though there are exceptions) to realize their goals. If that is the case for you, apply early because there are limited spaces in most graduate programs. It is important to note that passing an appropriate certification exam is a normal part of the process to being welcomed into the community of professionals. This is simple within athletic training because there is only one official exam (offered by the National Athletic Training Association's Board of Certification). In the fitness area, it is much more complicated given the number of certification exams available. If a certification exam requires a one-day workshop with little or no formal coursework and results in a high pass rate, the certification is worthless from a professional's point of view. It is important to pass the most rigorous and respected certification exams that have, at a minimum, a formal education requirement in an appropriate field. Check out the American College of Sports Medicine **(www.acsm.org)** and the National Strength and Conditioning Association websites for additional information **(www.nsca-lift.org)** for certifications that are recognized as being of high quality.

Over the past few years a special initiative, Exercise is Medicine™ **(http://exerciseismedicine.org),** was developed by the American College of Sports Medicine and the American Medical Association to encourage those working in the medical and the allied health professions to routinely promote physical activity to their patients. In addition to that goal, these health professionals need to know where to refer patients when they need more formal support for their physical activity program. For example, physical therapists need to know where to direct their patients after the mandated maximum number of rehabilitation sessions has been completed. This emphasizes the need for good communication between the allied health and fitness professionals. This text provides the essential information to help all of you be more effective in that regard.

Last, but not least, if you are interested in pursuing a career in research so that you can teach and do research at a college or university, you should become involved in research while you are an undergraduate. You might volunteer as a subject for another student's research project, take course credit to assist your professor in his or her research, or use a summer break to work in a researcher's lab at another institution. If a particular area of research interests you, do a PubMed search to see who is currently active in the area; that will help you narrow down potential graduate programs. Finally, you also need to get online and determine what the requirements are for admission to the graduate programs you are interested in; this will give you time to take appropriate coursework to meet those requirements.

IN SUMMARY

- A variety of career paths exist for undergraduates majoring in exercise science and kinesiology. Get some practical experience while you are an undergraduate to help you make a decision about your future, and facilitate entry to a profession or graduate school.
- Organizations such as the American College of Sports Medicine and the National Strength and Conditioning Association have developed certification programs to establish a standard of knowledge and skill to be achieved by those who lead exercise programs.

STUDY QUESTIONS

1. Identify two of the most prolific scientists in your personal area of interest in exercise physiology and briefly describe what they have done. Use a research database at the library to find your references.
2. Pick a topic of interest in exercise physiology and describe how a molecular biologist might approach it compared to a scientist interested in doing studies with humans.
3. Identify one potential career that you are interested in and find out the current expectations for growth in that profession, what a typical salary is in your part of the country, and what additional degrees (if any) are needed to realize your goal.
4. Identify the primary scientific meeting your professors attend. Find out if the organization that sponsors that meeting has a membership category for students, how much it costs, and what you would receive (e.g., journals) if you joined.

SUGGESTED READINGS

Berryman, J. W. 1995. *Out of Many, One: A History of the American College of Sports Medicine.* Champaign, IL: Human Kinetics

Park, R. S. 1989. *Measurement of Physical Fitness: A Historical Perspective.* Washington, DC: ODPHP National Health Information Center.

Schmidt-Nielsen, B. 1995. *August & Marie Krogh—Lives in Science.* New York, NY: Oxford University Press.

Tipton, C. M. 2003. *Exercise Physiology—People and Ideas.* New York, NY: Oxford University Press.

REFERENCES

1. **American Alliance for Health, Physical Education, Recreation and Dance.** *Lifetime Health Related Physical Fitness: Test Manual.* Reston, VA: 1980.
2. **American College of Sports Medicine.** *ACSM's Guidelines for Exercise Testing and Prescription.* Baltimore: Lippincott, Williams & Wilkins, 2006.
3. **American Heart Association.** Statement on exercise. *Circulation* 86: 340–344, 1992.
4. **Åstrand P-O.** Influence of Scandinavian scientists in exercise physiology. *Scand J Med Sci Sports* 1: 3–9, 1991.
5. **Baldwin K.** Research in the exercise sciences: where do we go from here? *J Appl Physiol* 88: 332–336, 2000.
6. **Bassett D, Jr., and Howley E.** Maximal oxygen uptake: "classical" versus "contemporary" viewpoints. *Med Sci Sports Exerc* 29: 591–603, 1997.
7. **Berryman J. Thomas K. Cureton, Jr.:** pioneer researcher, proselytizer, and proponent for physical fitness. *Res Q Exerc Sport* 67: 1–12, 1996.
8. **Booth F, Chakravarthy M, Gordon S, and Spangenburg E.** Waging war on physical inactivity: using modern molecular ammunition against an ancient enemy. *J Appl Physiol* 93: 3–30, 2002.
9. **Buskirk E.** *From Harvard to Minnesota: Keys to Our History.* Baltimore: Williams & Wilkins, 1992, p. 1–26.
10. **Buskirk E.** Personal communication based on "Our extended family: graduates from the Noll Lab for Human Performance Research." Noll Laboratory, Pennsylvania State University. University Park, PA: 1987.
11. **Buskirk E, and Tipton C.** *Exercise Physiology.* Champaign: Human Kinetics, 1977, p. 367–438.
12. **Chapman C, and Mitchell J.** The physiology of exercise. *Sci Am* 212: 88–96, 1965.
13. **Clarke H, and Clark D.** *Developmental and Adapted Physical Education.* Englewood Cliffs: Prentice-Hall, 1978.
14. **Dill D.** *Life, Heat, and Altitude.* Cambridge: Harvard University Press, 1938.
15. **Fenn W, and Rahn H.** *Handbook of Physiology: Respiration.* Washington, D.C.: American Physiological Society, 1964.
16. **Franks B.** *Exercise and Fitness.* Chicago: The Athletic Institute, 1969.
17. **Hackensmith C.** *History of Physical Education.* New York: Harper & Row, 1966.
18. **Horvath S, and Horvath E.** *The Harvard Fatigue Laboratory: Its History and Contributions.* Englewood Cliffs: Prentice-Hall, 1973.
19. **Hunsicker P.** A survey of laboratory facilities in college physical education departments. *Res Q Exerc Sport* 21: 1950.

20. **Huxley T.** *Selection from Essays.* New York: Appleton-Century-Crofts, 1948.

21. **Ianuzzo D, and Hutton R.** A prospectus for graduate students in muscle physiology and biochemistry. *Sports Medicine Bulletin* 22: 17–18, 1987.

22. **Kennedy J.** The soft American. *Sports Illustrated* 13: 14–17, 1960.

23. **Kroll W.** *Perspectives in Physical Education.* New York: Academic Press, 1971.

24. **Lagrange F.** *Physiology of Bodily Exercise.* New York: D. Appleton and Company, 1890.

25. **McKenzie R.** *Exercise in Education and Medicine.* Philadelphia: W. B. Saunders, 1923.

26. **Montoye H, and Washburn R.** Genealogy of scholarship among academy members. *The Academy Papers* 13: 94–101, 1980.

27. **Montoye H, and Washburn R.** Research quarterly contributors: An academic genealogy. *Res Q Exerc Sport* 51: 261–266, 1980.

28. **Pate R, Pratt M, Blair S, Haskell W, Macera C, Bouchard C, Buchner D, Ettinger W, Heath G, and King A.** Physical activity and public health. A recommendation from the Centers for Disease Control and Prevention and the American College of Sports Medicine. JAMA 273: 402–407, 1995.

29. **Pierce P, and Nagle E.** Uncommon sense for the apprentice! Important steps for interns. ACSM's *Health & Fitness Journal* 9: 18–23, 2005.

30. **Powell K, and Paffenbarger R.** Workshop on epidimiologic and public health aspects of physical activity and exercise: a summary. *Public Health Reports* 100: 118–126, 1985.

31. **Proceedings of the International Symposium on Physical Activity and Cardiovascular Health.** *Canadian Medical Association Journal* 96: 695–915, 1967.

32. **Rowell L.** *Human Circulation: Regulation During Physical Stress.* New York: Oxford University Press, 1986.

33. **Sargent D.** *Physical Education.* Boston: Ginn and Company, 1906.

34. **Stainsby W.** Part two: "For what is a man profited?" *Sports Medicine Bulletin* 22: 15, 1987.

35. **Tipton C.** Contemporary exercise physiology: Fifty years after the closure of Harvard Fatigue Laboratory. *Exercise and Sport Sciences Review* 26: 315–339, 1998.

36. **US Department of Health and Human Services.** *Physical Activity and Health: A Report of the Surgeon General.* Atlanta: U.S. Department of Health and Human Services, 1996.

37. **Van Dalen D, and Bennett B.** A *World History of Physical Education: Cultural, Philosophical, Comparative.* Englewood Cliffs: Prentice-Hall, 1971.

1

Measurement of Work, Power, and Energy Expenditure

■ Objectives

By studying this chapter, you should be able to do the following:

1. Define the terms *work*, *power*, *energy*, and *net efficiency*.
2. Give a brief explanation of the procedure used to calculate work performed during (a) cycle ergometer exercise and (b) treadmill exercise.
3. Describe the concept behind the measurement of energy expenditure using (a) direct calorimetry and (b) indirect calorimetry.
4. Discuss the procedure used to estimate energy expenditure during horizontal treadmill walking and running.
5. Define the following terms: (a) kilogram-meter, (b) relative $\dot{V}O_2$, (c) MET, and (d) open-circuit spirometry.
6. Describe the procedure used to calculate net efficiency during steady-state exercise.

■ Outline

■ Key Terms

cycle ergometer
direct calorimetry
ergometer
ergometry
indirect calorimetry
kilocalorie (kcal)
metabolic equivalent (MET)
net efficiency
open-circuit spirometry
percent grade
power
relative $\dot{V}O_2$
System International (SI) units
work

To study exercise physiology, we need to share a common understanding of the equipment used, the measurements made during exercise tests, and how work, power, and energy expenditure are expressed. For example, adequate knowledge of the energy requirements of physical activities (e.g., running at different speeds) is important to a coach planning a training program for athletes, an exercise specialist prescribing exercise for adults in a fitness program, and a researcher who wants subjects to exercise at a fixed rate of energy expenditure. Therefore, an understanding of human energy expenditure, how it is measured, and its practical significance is critical for the physical therapist, coach, physical educator, exercise specialist, or exercise physiologist. The purpose of this chapter is to describe the common pieces of equipment used in exercising testing, to discuss how energy expenditure is measured, and show how the units for work, power, and energy expenditure can be expressed in different ways.

UNITS OF MEASURE

Metric System

In the United States, the English system of measurement remains in common use. In contrast, the metric system, which is used in many other countries, is the standard system of measurement for scientists and is used by almost all scientific journals. In the metric system, the basic units of length, volume, and mass are the meter, the liter, and the gram, respectively. The main advantage of the metric system is that subdivisions or multiples of its basic units are expressed in factors of 10 using prefixes attached to the basic unit. Students not familiar with the metric system should refer to table 1.1 for a list of the basic prefixes used in metric measurements.

SI Units

An ongoing problem in exercise science is the failure of scientists to standardize units of measurement employed in presenting research data. In an effort to

TABLE 1.1	Common Metric Prefixes

mega: one million (1,000,000)
kilo: one thousand (1,000)
centi: one-hundredth (0.01)
milli: one-thousandth (0.001)
micro: one-millionth (0.000001)
nano: one-billionth (0.000000001)
pico: one-trillionth (0.000000000001)

TABLE 1.2	SI Units of Importance in the Measurement of Human Exercise Performance
Units for Quantifying Human Exercise	**SI Unit**
Mass	kilogram (kg)
Distance	meter (m)
Time	second (s)
Force	Newton (N)
Work	joule (J)
Energy	joule (J)
Power	watt (W)
Velocity	meters per second $(m \cdot s^{-1})$
Torque	newton-meter (N $\cdot$ m)

eliminate this problem, a uniform system of reporting scientific measurement has been developed through international cooperation. This system, known as **System International units,** or SI units, has been endorsed by almost all exercise and sports medicine journals for the publication of research data (24, 25). The SI system ensures standardization in the reporting of scientific data and makes comparison of published values easy. Table 1.2 contains SI units of importance in the measurement of exercise performance.

IN SUMMARY

- The metric system is the system of measurement used by scientists to express mass, length, and volume.
- In an effort to standardize terms for the measurement of energy, force, work, and power, scientists have developed a common system of terminology called System International (SI) units.

WORK AND POWER DEFINED

Work

Work is defined as the product of force and the distance through which that force acts:

$$\text{Work} = \text{force} \times \text{distance}$$

The SI unit for force is Newtons (N), whereas the SI unit for distance is meters (m). Consider the following example to compute work during a weight-lifting

Term	Abbreviation	Conversion Table
Kilogram-meter	kgm	1 kgm = 9.81 joules (J)
Kilopond-meter	kpm	1 kpm = 1 kgm
Kilocalorie	kcal	1 kcal = 4186 J or 4.186 kJ
		1 kcal = 426.8 kgm
Joule*	J	1 J = 1 Newton-meter (N · m)
		1 J = 2.39 × 10^{-4} kcal
		1 J = 0.102 kgm

*The joule is the basic unit adopted by the System International (called SI unit) for expression of energy expenditure or work.

exercise. If you lifted a 10-kilogram (kg) weight upward over the distance of two meters (m), the work performed can be calculated as follows:

Convert kg to N, where 1 kg = 9.81 N,
so 10 kg = 98.1 N

Work = 98.1 N × 2 m
= 196.2 Newton-meters (N · m) or 196.2 joules (J)

Therefore, the work performed was computed by multiplying the force (expressed in N) times the distance traveled (expressed in m) with the resulting work being expressed in joules, which is the SI unit for work (where 1 joule = 1 N · m; table 1.3).

Although the SI units are the preferred units for quantifying exercise performance and energy expenditure, you will encounter situations in which a number of traditional units are used to express both work and energy. Using the preceding example, work may be expressed in kilogram-meters (kgm) or kilopond-meters (kpm). In the preceding example, the 10-kg weight is considered 10-kg force (or 10 kiloponds), which when moved through 2 m, results in work of 20 kgm or 20 kpm. Since 1 kgm is equal to 9.81 J (see table 1.3), the work performed is 196.2 J (20 kgm × 9.81 J/kgm). Table 1.3 contains a list of terms that are in common use today to express work and energy—remember that the SI unit for both work and energy is the joule. For example, the energy content of commercial food products is often listed on the label in kilocalories. However, the

SI unit for energy content and expenditure is joules, where 1 kilocalorie is equal to 4186 joules (J) or 4.186 kilojoules (kJ).

Power

Power is the term used to describe how much work is accomplished per unit of time. The SI unit for power is the watt (W) and is defined as 1 joule per second (table 1.4). Power can be calculated as:

Power = Work ÷ time

The concept of power is important because it describes the rate at which work is being performed (work rate). It is the work rate or power output that describes the intensity of exercise. Given enough time, any healthy adult could perform a total work output of 20,000 J. However, only a few highly trained athletes could perform this amount of work in 60 seconds (s). The power output of these athletes can be calculated as follows:

Power = 20,000 joules/60 seconds
= 333.3 watts (W)

Note that the SI unit for power is the watt. Table 1.4 contains a list of both the SI and more traditional terms and units used to express power. The ability to convert from one expression of work, energy, or power to another is important, as we will see later in the chapter when we calculate mechanical efficiency.

TABLE 1.4 | Common Terms and Units Used to Express Power

Term	Abbreviation	Conversion Table
Watt*	W	1 W = 1 J · s^{-1}
		1 W = 6.12 kgm · min^{-1}
Horsepower	hp	1 hp = 745.7 W or J · s^{-1}
		1 hp = 10.69 kcal · min^{-1}
Kilogram-meter · min^{-1}	kgm · min^{-1}	1 kgm · min^{-1} = 0.163 W

*The watt is the basic unit adopted by the System International (called SI unit) for expression of power.

MEASUREMENT OF WORK AND POWER

Bench Step

The term **ergometry** refers to the measurement of work output. The word **ergometer** refers to the apparatus or device used to measure a specific type of work. Many types of ergometers are in use today in exercise physiology laboratories (figure 1.1). A brief introduction to commonly used ergometers follows.

One of the earliest ergometers used to measure work capacity in humans was the bench step. This ergometer is still in use today and simply involves the subject stepping up and down on a bench at a specified rate. Calculation of the work performed during bench stepping is very easy. Suppose a 70-kg man steps up and down on a 30-centimeter (0.3 meter) bench for 10 minutes at a rate of thirty steps per minute. The amount of work performed during this 10-minute task can be computed as follows:

$$\text{Force} = 686.7 \text{ N (i.e., 70 kg} \times 9.81 \text{ N/kg)}$$

$$\text{Distance} = 0.3 \text{ m} \cdot \text{step}^{-1} \times 30 \text{ steps} \cdot \text{min}^{-1} \times 10 \text{ min}$$
$$= 90 \text{ m}$$

Therefore, the total work performed is:

$$686.7 \text{ N} \times 90 \text{ m} = 61,803 \text{ joules or } 61.8 \text{ kilojoules (kJ)}$$
(rounded to nearest 0.1)

(a)

(b)

(c)

(d)

Figure 1.1 Illustrations of four different ergometers used in the measurement of human work output and power. (*a*) A bench step. (*b*) Friction-braked cycle ergometer. (*c*) Motor-driven treadmill. Both the treadmill elevation and the horizontal speed can be adjusted by electronic controls. (*d*) Arm crank ergometer. Arm crank ergometry can be used to measure work output with the arms and is based on the same principle as cycle ergometry.

A LOOK BACK—IMPORTANT PEOPLE IN SCIENCE

August Krogh: Nobel Prize Winner and Inventor

As mentioned in the previous chapter, **August Krogh** (1872–1949) received the Nobel Prize for Physiology or Medicine in 1920 for his research on regulation of blood flow through capillaries in skeletal muscle. Krogh was born in Grenaa, Denmark, in 1874. After entering the University of Copenhagen in 1893, he began to study medicine, but developed a strong interest in research and decided to leave his medical studies to devote himself to the study of physiology. Krogh began his research career at the University of Copenhagen in the medical physiology laboratory of the famous Danish physiologist Christian Bohr.

Krogh completed his Ph.D. studies in 1903 and two years later married Marie Jørgensen, a renowned physiologist. August Krogh was a dedicated physiologist with extreme curiosity. He devoted his entire life to understanding physiology, and he worked both day and night in his laboratory to achieve his research goals. In fact, Krogh even performed physiology experiments on his wedding day!

During his distinguished research career, Dr. Krogh made many important contributions to physiology. For example, Dr. Krogh's work greatly advanced our understanding of respiratory gas exchange in both mammals and insects. Further, he studied water and electrolyte homeostasis in animals and published an important book titled *Osmotic Regulation* in 1939. Nonetheless, Krogh is best known for his work on the regulation of blood flow in the capillaries of skeletal muscle. He was the first physiologist to describe the changes in blood flow to muscle in accordance with the metabolic demands of the tissue. Indeed, his research demonstrated that the increase in muscle

blood flow during contractions was achieved by the opening of arterioles and capillaries. This is the work that earned him the Nobel Prize.

In addition to physiology research, August Krogh invented many important scientific instruments. For instance, he developed both the spirometer (a device used to measure pulmonary volumes) and an apparatus for measuring metabolic rate (an instrument used to measure oxygen consumption). Although Krogh did not invent the first cycle ergometer, he is credited with developing an automatically controlled cycle ergometer in 1913. This ergometer was a large improvement in the cycle ergometers of the day and permitted Krogh and his colleagues to accurately measure the amount of work performed during exercise physiology experiments. Cycle ergometers similar to the one developed by August Krogh are still in use today in exercise physiology laboratories.

The power output during this 10 minutes (600 seconds) of exercise can be calculated as:

$$\text{Power} = 61{,}803 \text{ J}/600 \text{ seconds}$$
$$= 103 \text{ J} \cdot \text{s}^{-1} \text{ or } 103 \text{ watts (W)}$$

Using a more traditional unit of work, the kilogrammeter (kgm), power can be calculated as follows:

$$\text{Work} = 70 \text{ kg} \times 0.3 \text{ m} \times 30 \text{ steps} \cdot \text{min}^{-1} \times 10 \text{ min}$$
$$= 6300 \text{ kgm}$$

$$\text{Power} = 6300 \text{ kgm} \div 10 \text{ min} = 630 \text{ kgm min}^{-1} \text{ or}$$
$$103 \text{ watts (See table 1.4 for conversions)}$$

Cycle Ergometer

The **cycle ergometer** was developed more than 100 years ago and remains a popular ergometer in exercise physiology laboratories today (see A Look Back—Important People in Science). This type of ergometer is a stationary exercise bicycle that per-

mits accurate measurement of the amount of work performed. A common type of cycle ergometer is the Monark friction-braked cycle, which incorporates a belt wrapped around the wheel (called a flywheel) (figure 1.1b). The belt can be loosened or tightened to provide a change in resistance. The distance the wheel travels can be determined by computing the distance covered per revolution of the pedals (6 meters per revolution on a standard Monark cycle) times the number of pedal revolutions. Consider the following example for the computation of work and power using the cycle ergometer. Calculate work given:

Duration of exercise = 10 min
Resistance against flywheel = 1.5 kg or 14.7 N
Distance traveled per pedal revolution = 6 m
Pedaling speed = 60 rev · min^{-1}
Therefore, the total revolutions in 10 min
= 10 min × 60 rev · min^{-1} = 600 rev

Hence, total work = 14.7 N × (6 m · rev^{-1} × 600 rev)
= 52,920 J or 52.9 kJ

The power output in this example is computed by dividing the total work performed by time:

Power = 52,920 joules ÷ 600 seconds
= 88.2 watts

The following steps show how to do the calculations using alternate units:

Work = 1.5 kg × 6 m · rev^{-1} × 60 rev · min^{-1} × 10 min
= 5400 kgm or kpm
Power = 5400 kgm ÷ 10 min = 540 kgm · min^{-1}
= 88.2 watts (See table 1.4 for conversions)

Treadmill

Calculation of the work performed while a subject runs or walks on a treadmill is not generally possible when the treadmill is horizontal. Although running horizontally on a treadmill requires energy, the vertical displacement of the body's center of gravity is not easily measured. Therefore, the measurement of work performed during horizontal walking or running is complicated. However, quantifiable work is being performed when walking or running up a slope, and calculating the amount of work done is a simple task. The incline of the treadmill is expressed in units called "percent grade." **Percent grade** is defined as the amount of vertical rise per 100 units of belt travel. For instance, a subject walking on a treadmill at a 10% grade travels 10 meters vertically for every 100 meters of the belt travel. Percent grade is calculated by multiplying the sine of the treadmill angle by 100. In practice, the treadmill angle (expressed in degrees) can be determined by simple trigonometric computations (figure 1.2) or by using a measurement device called an inclinometer (9).

To calculate the work output during treadmill exercise, you must know both the subject's body weight and the distance traveled vertically. Vertical travel can be computed by multiplying the distance the belt travels by the percent grade. This can be written as:

Vertical displacement = % grade × distance

where percent grade is expressed as a fraction and the total distance traveled is calculated by multiplying the treadmill speed (m · min^{-1}) by the total minutes of exercise. Consider the following sample calculation of work output during treadmill exercise:

Subject's body weight = 60 kg (i.e., force = 588.6 N)
Treadmill speed = 200 m · min^{-1}
Treadmill angle = 7.5% grade (7.5% ÷ 100
= 0.075 as fractional grade)
Exercise time = 10 min
Total vertical distance traveled = 200 m · min^{-1}
× 0.075
× 10 min
= 150 m
Therefore, total work performed = 588.6 N × 150 m
= 88,290 J or 88.3 kJ

Using more traditional units, the following calculations can be made:

Work = 60 kg × 0.075 × 200 m · min^{-1} × 10 min
= 9000 kgm or 88,290 J (88.3 kJ)

IN SUMMARY

- An understanding of the terms *work* and *power* is necessary to compute human work output and the associated exercise efficiency.
- Work is defined as the product of force times distance:

Work = Force × distance

- Power is defined as work divided by time:

Power = Work ÷ time

Fixed rear-axle treadmill
Grade = Sine θ = Rise ÷ Hypotenuse

Figure 1.2 Determination of the "percent grade" on an inclined treadmill. Theta (θ) represents the angle of inclination. Percent grade is computed as the sine of angle θ × 100.

MEASUREMENT OF ENERGY EXPENDITURE

Measurement of an individual's energy expenditure at rest or during a particular activity has many practical applications. One direct application applies to exercise-assisted weight-loss programs. Clearly, knowledge of the energy cost of walking, running, or swimming at various speeds is useful to individuals who use these modes of exercise as an aid in weight loss. Further, an industrial engineer might measure the energy cost of various tasks around a job site and use this information in making the appropriate job assignments to workers (17, 35). In this regard, the engineer might recommend that the supervisor assign those jobs that demand large energy requirements to workers who are physically fit and possess high work capacities. In general, two techniques are employed in the measurement of human energy expenditure: (1) direct calorimetry and (2) indirect calorimetry.

Direct Calorimetry

When the body uses energy to do work, heat is liberated. This production of heat by cells occurs via both cellular respiration (bioenergetics) and cell work. The general process can be drawn schematically as (5, 36, 37):

$$\text{Foodstuff} + O_2 \rightarrow \text{ATP} + \text{heat}$$
$$\downarrow \text{cell work}$$
$$\text{Heat}$$

The process of cellular respiration is discussed in detail in chapter 3. Note that the rate of heat production in an individual is directly proportional to the metabolic rate. Therefore, measuring heat production (calorimetry) of a person gives a direct measurement of metabolic rate.

The SI unit to measure heat energy is the joule (the same as for work). However, a common unit employed to measure heat energy is the calorie (see table 1.3). A calorie is defined as the amount of heat required to raise the temperature of one gram of water by one degree Celsius. Because the calorie is very small, the term **kilocalorie (kcal)** is commonly used to express energy expenditure and the energy value of foods. One kcal is equal to 1000 calories. In converting kcals to SI units, 1 kcal is equal to 4186 joules or 4.186 kilojoules (kJ) (see table 1.3 for conversions). The process of measuring a person's metabolic rate via the measurement of heat production is called **direct calorimetry,** and it has been used by scientists since the eighteenth century. This technique involves placing the person in a tight chamber (called a calorimeter), which is insulated from the environment (usually by a jacket of water surrounding the chamber), and allowance is made for the free exchange of O_2 and CO_2 from the chamber (figure 1.3). The person's body heat raises the temperature of the water circulating around the chamber. Therefore, by measuring the temperature change per unit of time, the amount of heat production can be computed. In addition, heat is lost from the person by evaporation of water from the skin and respiratory passages. This heat loss is measured and is added to the total heat picked up by the water to yield an estimate of the rate of energy utilization by the person (5, 9).

Figure 1.3 Diagram of a simple calorimeter used to measure metabolic rate by measuring the production of body heat. This method of determining metabolic rate is called direct calorimetry.

Indirect Calorimetry

Although direct calorimetry is considered to be a precise technique for the measurement of metabolic rate, construction of a chamber that is large enough for doing exercise physiology research on humans is expensive. Also, the use of direct calorimetry to measure metabolic rate during exercise is complicated because the ergometer itself may produce heat. Fortunately, another procedure can be used to measure metabolic rate. This technique is termed **indirect calorimetry** because it does not involve the direct measurement of heat production. The principle of indirect calorimetry can be explained by the following relationship:

$$\underset{\text{(Indirect calorimetry)}}{\text{Foodstuffs} + O_2} \rightarrow \underset{\text{(Direct calorimetry)}}{\text{Heat} + CO_2 + H_2O}$$

Because a direct relationship exists between O_2 consumed and the amount of heat produced in the body, measuring O_2 consumption provides an estimate of metabolic rate (3, 5, 15). To convert the amount of O_2 consumed into heat equivalents, it is necessary to know the type of nutrient (i.e., carbohydrate, fat, or protein) that was metabolized. The energy liberated when fat is the only foodstuff metabolized is 4.7 kcal (or 19.7 kJ) $\cdot$ L O_2^{-1}, whereas the energy released when only carbohydrates are used is 5.05 kcal (or 21.13 kJ) $\cdot$ L O_2^{-1}. Although it is not exact, the caloric expenditure of exercise is often estimated to be approximately 5 kcal (or 21 kJ) per liter of O_2 consumed (19). Therefore, a person exercising at an oxygen consumption of 2.0 L $\cdot$ min^{-1} would expend approximately 10 kcal (or 42 kJ) of energy per minute.

The most common technique used to measure oxygen consumption today is termed **open-circuit spirometry.** In the classic technique the subject wore a nose clip (to prevent nasal breathing) and a respiratory valve that allowed room air to be breathed in while the exhaled gas was directed to a collection bag (Douglas bag) that was later analyzed for gas volume and percent of O_2 and CO_2. Gas volume was measured in a gasometer, and the O_2 and CO_2 were either analyzed chemically or with the aid of calibrated gas analyzers. The steps provided in Appendix A were followed to calculate O_2 consumption and CO_2 production. (See all appendices online at www.mhhe.com/powers8e.) Modern-day, open-circuit spirometry (see figure 1.4) employs computer technology that measures the volume of the exhaled gas on a breath-by-breath basis, which is then directed to a mixing chamber where samples are taken for continuous gas analysis. The calculations of O_2 consumption and CO_2 production are done automatically. Although the computer-based system certainly makes the process of measuring oxygen consumption easier, the traditional method is used as the "gold standard" to make sure the automated system is working correctly (4).

IN SUMMARY

- Measurement of energy expenditure at rest or during exercise is possible using either direct or indirect calorimetry.
- Direct calorimetry uses the measurement of heat production as an indication of metabolic rate.
- Indirect calorimetry estimates metabolic rate via the measurement of oxygen consumption.

Figure 1.4 The TrueOne metabolic measurement system utilizes eletronic flow sensors, gas analyzers, and computer technology. These devices are used to measure oxyzen uptake and carbon dioxide production at rest and during exercise.

COMMON EXPRESSIONS OF ENERGY EXPENDITURE

The oxygen consumption can be used to express energy expenditure in different ways (21).

$\dot{V}O_2$ (L · min^{-1}) By following the steps outlined in Appendix A, oxygen consumption ($\dot{V}O_2$) can be calculated in liters of oxygen used per minute (L/min). (See all appendices online at www.mhhe.com/powers8e.) For example, the following data were collected on a 60-kg trained woman during a submaximal run on a treadmill:

$$\text{ventilation (STPD)} = 60 \text{ L} \cdot \text{min}^{-1}; \text{inspired } O_2 = 20.93\%; \text{expired } O_2 = 16.93\%.$$

$$\dot{V}O_2 \text{ (L} \cdot \text{min}^{-1}\text{)}. = 60 \text{ L} \cdot \text{min}^{-1} \times (20.93\% \; O_2 - 16.93 \;\% O_2) = 2.4 \text{ L} \cdot \text{min}^{-1}$$

kcal · min^{-1} Oxygen uptake can also be expressed in kilocalories used per minute. The caloric equivalent of 1 L of O_2 varies from 4.7 kcal · L^{-1} for fats to 5.05 kcal · L^{-1} for carbohydrates. However, for practical reasons, and with little error, 5 kcal per liter of O_2 is used to convert the $\dot{V}O_2$ to kilocalories per minute. Total energy expenditure is calculated by multiplying the kilocalories expended per minute (kcal · min^{-1}) by the duration of the activity in minutes. For example, if the 60-kg woman mentioned previously runs on the treadmill for 30 minutes at a $\dot{V}O_2 = 2.4$ L · min^{-1}, the total energy expenditure can be calculated as follows:

$$2.4 \text{ L} \cdot \text{min}^{-1} \times 5 \text{ kcal} \cdot \text{L}^{-1} \; O_2 = 12 \text{ kcal} \cdot \text{min}^{-1}$$
$$12 \text{ kcal} \cdot \text{min}^{-1} \times 30 \text{ min} = 360 \text{ kcal} \cdot \text{min}^{-1}$$

$\dot{V}O_2$ (ml · kg^{-1} · min^{-1}) When the measured oxygen uptake, expressed in liters per minute, is multiplied by 1000 to yield milliliters per minute and then divided by the subject's body weight in kilograms, the value is expressed in milliliters of O_2 per kilogram of body weight per minute, or ml · kg^{-1} · min^{-1}. This allows comparisons among people of different body sizes. For example, for the 60-kg woman with a $\dot{V}O_2 = 2.4$ L · min^{-1}:

$$2.4 \text{ L} \cdot \text{min}^{-1} \times 1000 \text{ ml} \cdot \text{L}^{-1} \div 60 \text{ kg}$$
$$= 40 \text{ ml} \cdot \text{kg}^{-1} \cdot \text{min}^{-1}$$

METs The resting metabolic rate is usually measured with an individual at quiet supine rest, after a period of fasting and not participating in exercise. The resting metabolic rate varies with age and gender, being less in females than males, and decreases with age (23). The **MET (metabolic equivalent)** is a term used to represent resting metabolism and is taken, by convention, to be 3.5 ml · kg^{-1} · min^{-1}. This is called 1 MET. In essence, the energy cost of activities can be expressed in terms of multiples of the MET unit. Using the preceding information:

$$40 \text{ ml} \cdot \text{kg}^{-1} \cdot \text{min}^{-1} \div 3.5 \text{ ml} \cdot \text{kg}^{-1} \cdot \text{min}^{-1} = 11.4 \text{ METs}$$

kcal · kg⁻¹ · hr⁻¹ The MET expression can also be used to express the number of calories the subject uses per kilogram of body weight per hour. In the example mentioned previously, the subject is working at 11.4 METs, or 40 ml · kg⁻¹ min⁻¹. When this value is multiplied by 60 min · hr⁻¹, it equals 2400 ml · kg⁻¹ · hr⁻¹, or 2.4 L · kg⁻¹ · hr⁻¹. If the person is using a mixture of carbohydrates and fats as the fuel, the $\dot{V}O_2$ is multiplied by 4.85 kcal per liter of O_2 (average between 4.7 and 5.05 kcal/L O_2) to give 11.6 kcal · kg⁻¹ · hr⁻¹. The following steps show the detail.

$$11.4 \text{ METs} \times 3.5 \text{ ml} \cdot \text{kg}^{-1} \cdot \text{min}^{-1} = 40 \text{ ml} \cdot \text{kg}^{-1} \cdot \text{min}^{-1}$$

$$40 \text{ ml} \cdot \text{kg}^{-1} \cdot \text{min}^{-1} \times 60 \text{ min} \cdot \text{hr}^{-1}$$
$$= 2400 \text{ ml} \cdot \text{kg}^{-1} \cdot \text{hr}^{-1} = 2.4 \text{ L} \cdot \text{kg}^{-1} \cdot \text{hr}^{-1}$$

$$2.4 \text{ L} \cdot \text{kg}^{-1} \cdot \text{hr}^{-1} \times 4.85 \text{ kcal} \cdot \text{L}^{-1} O_2$$
$$= 11.6 \text{ kcal} \cdot \text{kg}^{-1} \cdot \text{hr}^{-1}$$

IN SUMMARY

- Energy expenditure can be expressed in L · min⁻¹, kcal · min⁻¹, ml · kg⁻¹ · min⁻¹, METs, and kcal · kg⁻¹ · hr⁻¹. To convert L · min⁻¹ to kcal · min⁻¹, multiply by 5.0 kcal · L⁻¹. To convert L · min⁻¹ to ml · kg⁻¹ · min⁻¹, multiply by 1000 and divide by body weight in kilograms. To convert ml · kg⁻¹ · min⁻¹ to METs or kcal · kg⁻¹ · hr⁻¹, divide by 3.5 ml · kg⁻¹ · min⁻¹.

ESTIMATION OF ENERGY EXPENDITURE

Researchers studying the oxygen cost (O_2 cost = $\dot{V}O_2$ at steady state) of exercise have demonstrated that it is possible to estimate the energy expended during physical activity with reasonable precision (8, 10, 11, 19, 31). Walking, running, and cycling are activities that have been studied in detail. The O_2 requirements of walking and running graphed as a function of speed are presented in figure 1.5. Note that the relationships between the relative O_2 requirement (ml · kg⁻¹ · min⁻¹) and walking/running speed are straight lines (2, 19). A similar relationship exists for cycling, up to a power output of about 200 W. (see figure 1.6). The fact that this relationship is linear over a wide range of speeds and power outputs is convenient and makes the calculation of the O_2 cost (or energy cost) very easy (see A Closer Look 1.1, 1.2, and 1.3 for examples). Estimation of the energy expenditure of other types of activities is more complex. For example, estimation of energy expenditure during tennis is dependent on whether the match is singles or doubles, and is also influenced by the participants' skill

Figure 1.5 The relationship between speed and $\dot{V}O_2$ cost is linear for both walking and running. Note that x equals the walking/running speed in meters · min⁻¹.

level. Nonetheless, an estimate of the energy expended during a tennis match is possible. See the Compendium of Physical Activities (**http://sites.google.com/ site/compendiumofphysicalactivities/**) for a detailed list of the oxygen cost (MET values) of numerous physical activities (1).

IN SUMMARY

- The energy cost of horizontal treadmill walking or running and cycling can be estimated with reasonable accuracy because the O_2 requirements increase as a linear function of speed and power, respectively.

CALCULATION OF EXERCISE EFFICIENCY

Efficiency describes the capacity to convert energy expenditure into work; it is expressed as the ratio of the work done to the energy put in to do the work. A more efficient individual uses less energy to do the same amount of work. Exercise physiologists have long searched for ways to mathematically describe the efficiency of human movement. Although measurements of gross, net, delta, and instantaneous efficiency have been used to describe exercise efficiency, one of the most common and simple expressions is **net efficiency** (6, 7, 10, 13, 16, 30, 31, 38, 39). Net efficiency is defined as the mathematical ratio of work output divided by the energy expended above rest:

$$\% \text{ net efficiency} = \frac{\textbf{Work Output}}{\textbf{Energy Expended}} \times 100$$

No machine is 100% efficient, because some energy is lost due to friction of the moving parts.

A CLOSER LOOK 1.1

Estimation of the O_2 Requirement of Treadmill Walking

The O_2 requirement of horizontal treadmill walking can be estimated with reasonable accuracy for speeds between 50 and 100 m $\cdot$ min^{-1} using the following formula:

$$\dot{V}O_2 \text{ (ml} \cdot \text{kg}^{-1} \cdot \text{min}^{-1}) = 0.1 \text{ ml} \cdot \text{kg}^{-1} \cdot \text{min}^{-1}/(\text{m} \cdot \text{min}^{-1}) \times \text{speed (m} \cdot \text{min}^{-1}) + 3.5 \text{ ml} \cdot \text{kg}^{-1} \cdot \text{min}^{-1} \text{ (resting } \dot{V}O_2)$$

This equation tells us that the O_2 requirement of walking increases as a linear function of walking speed. The slope of the line is 0.1 and the Y intercept is 3.5 ml $\cdot$ kg^{-1} $\cdot$ min^{-1} (resting $\dot{V}O_2$). The O_2 cost of grade walking is:

$$\dot{V}O_2 \text{ (ml} \cdot \text{kg}^{-1} \cdot \text{min}^{-1}) = 1.8 \text{ ml} \cdot \text{kg}^{-1} \cdot \text{min}^{-1} \times \text{speed (m} \cdot \text{min}^{-1}) \times \% \text{ grade (expressed as a fraction)}$$

The total O_2 requirement of graded treadmill walking is the sum of the horizontal O_2 cost and the vertical O_2 cost. For example, the O_2 cost of walking at 80 m $\cdot$ min^{-1} at 5% grade would be:

$$\text{Horizontal } O_2 \text{ cost} = 0.1 \text{ ml} \cdot \text{kg}^{-1} \cdot \text{min}^{-1} \times 80 \text{ m} \cdot \text{min}^{-1} + 3.5 \text{ ml} \cdot \text{kg}^{-1} \cdot \text{min}^{-1}$$
$$= 11.5 \text{ ml} \cdot \text{kg}^{-1} \cdot \text{min}^{-1}$$
$$\text{Vertical } O_2 \text{ cost} = 1.8 \text{ ml} \cdot \text{kg}^{-1} \cdot \text{min}^{-1} \times (0.05 \times 80) = 7.2 \text{ ml} \cdot \text{kg}^{-1} \cdot \text{min}^{-1}$$

Hence, the total O_2 requirement of walking would amount to:

$$11.5 \text{ ml} \cdot \text{kg}^{-1} \cdot \text{min}^{-1} + 7.2 \text{ ml} \cdot \text{kg}^{-1} \cdot \text{min}^{-1} = 18.7 \text{ ml} \cdot \text{kg}^{-1} \cdot \text{min}^{-1}$$

This O_2 requirement can be expressed in METs by dividing the measured (or estimated) $\dot{V}O_2$ (ml $\cdot$ kg^{-1} $\cdot$ min^{-1}) by 3.5 ml $\cdot$ kg^{-1} $\cdot$ min^{-1} per MET:

$$18.7 \text{ ml} \cdot \text{kg}^{-1} \cdot \text{min}^{-1} \div 3.5 \text{ ml} \cdot \text{kg}^{-1} \cdot \text{min}^{-1} \text{ per MET} = 5.3 \text{ METs}$$

Formulas are taken from reference (2).

A CLOSER LOOK 1.2

Estimation of the O_2 Requirement of Treadmill Running

The O_2 requirements of horizontal treadmill running for speeds greater than 134 m $\cdot$ min^{-1} can be estimated in a manner similar to the procedure used to estimate the O_2 requirement for treadmill walking. The O_2 cost of the horizontal component is calculated using the following formula:

$$\dot{V}O_2 \text{ (ml} \cdot \text{kg}^{-1} \cdot \text{min}^{-1}) = 0.2 \text{ ml} \cdot \text{kg}^{-1} \cdot \text{min}^{-1}/\text{m} \cdot \text{min}^{-1} \times \text{speed (m} \cdot \text{min}^{-1}) + 3.5 \text{ ml} \cdot \text{kg}^{-1} \cdot \text{min}^{-1} \text{ (resting } \dot{V}O_2)$$

What is the oxygen cost of a person running at 6 mph (161 m/min or 9.7 km/hr)?

$$\dot{V}O_2 \text{ (ml} \cdot \text{kg}^{-1} \cdot \text{min}^{-1}) = 0.2 \text{ ml} \cdot \text{kg}^{-1} \cdot \text{min}^{-1}/\text{m} \cdot \text{min}^{-1} \times 161 \text{ m} \cdot \text{min}^{-1} + 3.5 \text{ ml} \cdot \text{kg}^{-1} \cdot \text{min}^{-1} = 35.7 \text{ ml} \cdot \text{kg}^{-1} \cdot \text{min}^{-1} \text{ or}$$
$$10.2 \text{ METs } (35.7 \div 3.5)$$

Formulas are taken from reference (2).

Likewise, the human machine is not 100% efficient because energy is lost as heat. It is estimated that the gasoline automobile engine operates with an efficiency of approximately 20% to 25%. Similarly, net efficiency for humans exercising on a cycle ergometer ranges from 15% to 27%, depending on work rate (13, 16, 31, 34, 39).

To compute net efficiency during cycle ergometer or treadmill exercise requires measurement of work output and the subject's energy expenditure during the exercise and at rest. It should be emphasized that $\dot{V}O_2$ measurements must be made during steady-state conditions. The work rate on the cycle ergometer or treadmill is calculated as discussed earlier and is generally expressed in kgm $\cdot$ min^{-1}. The energy expenditure during these types of exercise is usually estimated by first measuring $\dot{V}O_2$ (L $\cdot$ min^{-1}) using open-circuit spirometry, and then converting it to either kcal or kJ

A CLOSER LOOK 1.3

Estimation of the O₂ Requirement of Cycling

Similar to the energy cost of walking and running, the oxygen requirement of cycling is also linear (straight line) over a range of work rates up to about 200 W (figure 1.6). Because of this linear relationship, the O₂ requirement of cycling can be easily estimated for power outputs between 50 and 200 watts (i.e., ~300 and 1,200 kgm · min⁻¹). The total O₂ cost of cycling on a cycle ergometer is comprised of three components. These include the resting O₂ consumption, the O₂ demand associated with unloaded cycling (i.e., energy cost of moving the legs), and the O₂ requirement that is directly proportional to the external load on the cycle.

An explanation of how the O₂ cost of these components is computed follows.

First, the resting O₂ consumption is estimated at 3.5 ml · kg⁻¹ · min⁻¹. Second, at a cranking speed of 50–60 rpm, the oxygen cost of unloaded cycling is also approximately 3.5 ml · kg⁻¹ · min⁻¹. Finally, the relative O₂ cost of cycling against an external load is 1.8 ml · kgm⁻¹ × work rate × body mass⁻¹. Putting these three components together, the collective formula to compute the O₂ of cycling is:

$\dot{V}O_2$ (ml · kg⁻¹ · min⁻¹) = 1.8 ml · kgm⁻¹ (work rate) × M⁻¹ + 7 ml · kg⁻¹ · min⁻¹

Where:

work rate on the cycle ergometer is expressed in kgm · min⁻¹

M is body mass in kilograms

7 ml · kg⁻¹ · min⁻¹ is the sum of resting O₂ consumption (3.5) and the O₂ cost of unloaded cycling (3.5).

For example, the O₂ cost of cycling at 600 kgm/min (~ 100 W) for a 70-kg man is:

1.8 ml · kgm⁻¹ (600 kgm · min⁻¹) × 70 kg⁻¹ + 7 ml · kg⁻¹ · min⁻¹ = 22.4 ml · kg⁻¹ · min⁻¹

Formulas are from reference (2).

FIGURE 1.6 The relationship between work rate and $\dot{V}O_2$ cost is linear for cycling over a wide range of workloads. This figure illustrates the relative oxygen cost (i.e., $\dot{V}O_2$ per kilogram of body mass) of cycling for a 70-kg individual.

using the exact conversion based on the types of foodstuff being used as fuel (see chapter 4 for details). In the following example we will use 5 kcal · L⁻¹ O₂ to show how to do this calculation. To do the computation using the net-efficiency formula, both numerator and denominator must be expressed in similar terms. Because the numerator (work rate) is expressed in kgm · min⁻¹ and energy expenditure is expressed in kcal · min⁻¹, we have to convert one unit to match the other. Consider the following sample calculation of net efficiency during submaximal, steady-state cycle ergometer exercise. Given:

Resistance against the cycle flywheel = 2 kg
Cranking speed = 50 rpm

Steady-state resting $\dot{V}O_2$ = 0.25 L · min⁻¹
Steady-state exercise $\dot{V}O_2$ = 1.5 L · min⁻¹
Distance traveled per revolution = 6 m · rev⁻¹
Therefore:
Work rate = [2 kg × (50 m · rev⁻¹ × 6 m · rev⁻¹)]
       = 600 kgm · min⁻¹
Net energy expenditure = [1.5 L · min⁻¹ − 0.25 L · min⁻¹]
       × 5 kcal · L⁻¹ = 6.25 kcal · min⁻¹

To convert kgm to kcal: 600 kgm · min⁻¹ ÷ 426.8 kgm · kcal⁻¹ = 1.41 kcal · min⁻¹

Hence, net efficiency $= \dfrac{1.41 \text{ kcal} \cdot \text{min}^{-1}}{6.25 \text{ kcal} \cdot \text{min}^{-1}} \times 100\%$

$= 22.6\%$

Figure 1.7 Changes in net efficiency during arm crank ergometry as a function of work rate.

Factors That Influence Exercise Efficiency

The efficiency of exercise is influenced by several factors: (1) the exercise work rate, (2) the speed of movement, and (3) the fiber composition of the muscles performing the exercise. A brief discussion of each of these factors follows.

Work Rate and Exercise Efficiency Figure 1.7 depicts the changes in net efficiency during cycle ergometry exercise as a function of work rate. Note that efficiency decreases as the work rate increases (13, 31). This is because the relationship between energy expenditure and work rate is curvilinear rather than linear over a broad range of power outputs (see figure 1.8) (16, 31). This may appear to be at odds with the previous section in which we stated that oxygen

consumption could be estimated from power outputs because of the linear relationship between work rate and energy expenditure. However, at low-to-moderate work rates (<200 W), the relationship is close to linear and little error is introduced into the estimation of $\dot{V}O_2$. In contrast, when we look at this relationship across the full range of power outputs, it is clearly curvilinear. The result is that as work rate increases, total body energy expenditure increases out of proportion to the work rate; this results in a lower efficiency at higher power outputs.

Movement Speed and Efficiency Research has shown that there is an "optimum" speed of movement for any given work rate. Evidence suggests that the optimum speed of movement increases as the power output increases (8). In other words, at higher power outputs, a greater speed of movement is required to obtain optimum efficiency. At low-to-moderate work rates, a pedaling speed of 40 to 60 rpm is generally considered optimum during arm or cycle ergometry (12, 14, 16, 28, 31, 33). Note that any change in the speed of movement away from the optimum results in a decrease in efficiency (figure 1.9). This decline in efficiency at low speeds of movement is probably due to inertia (31). That is, there may be an increased energy cost of performing work when movements are slow and the limbs involved must repeatedly stop and start. The decline in efficiency associated with high-speed movement (low work rates) may be because increasing speeds might augment muscular friction and thus increase internal work (6, 31).

Fiber Type and Efficiency People differ in their net efficiency during cycle ergometer exercise. Why? Recent evidence suggests that subjects with a high percentage of slow muscle fibers display a higher

Figure 1.8 Relationship between energy expenditure and work rate. Note that energy expenditure increases as a curvilinear function of work rate.

Figure 1.9 Effects of decreasing or increasing speed of movement on exercise efficiency. Note an optimum speed of movement for maximum efficiency at any given work rate.

exercise efficiency compared to subjects with a high percentage of fast muscle fibers (see chapter 8 for a discussion of muscle fiber types) (20, 22, 26, 32). The physiological explanation for this observation is that slow muscle fibers are more efficient than fast fibers. That is, slow fibers require less ATP per unit of work performed compared to fast fibers.

A superior efficiency can improve exercise performance. For example, compared to subjects with a relatively low efficiency, subjects with high efficiency can generate a greater power output at any rate of energy expenditure. Therefore, it is not surprising that studies have shown that endurance performance is improved by a high exercise efficiency (20).

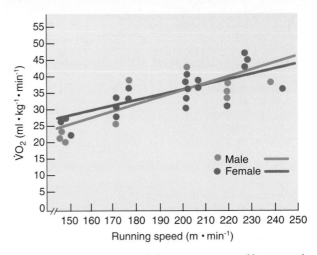

Figure 1.10 Comparison of the oxygen cost of horizontal treadmill running between highly trained men and women distance runners.

IN SUMMARY

- Net efficiency is defined as the mathematical ratio of work performed divided by the energy expenditure above rest, and is expressed as a percentage:

$$\% \text{ Net efficiency} = \frac{\textbf{Work Output}}{\textbf{Energy Expenditure}} \times 100$$

- The efficiency of exercise decreases as the exercise work rate increases. This occurs because the relationship between work rate and energy expenditure is curvilinear.
- To achieve maximal efficiency at any work rate, there is an optimal speed of movement.
- Exercise efficiency is greater in subjects who possess a high percentage of slow muscle fibers compared to subjects with a high percentage of fast fibers. This occurs because slow muscle fibers are more efficient than fast fibers.

RUNNING ECONOMY

As discussed previously, the computation of work is not generally possible during horizontal treadmill running, and thus a calculation of exercise efficiency cannot be performed. However, the measurement of the steady-state $\dot{V}O_2$ requirement (O_2 cost) of running at various speeds offers a means of comparing running economy (not efficiency) between two runners or groups of runners (18, 19, 27). Figure 1.10 compares the O_2 cost of running between a group of highly trained male and female distance runners at slow running speeds (i.e., slower than race pace). A runner who exhibits poor running economy would require a higher $\dot{V}O_2$ (ml · kg^{-1} · min^{-1}) at any given running speed than an economical runner. Notice that the O_2 cost of running labeled on the ordinate (y-axis) is

expressed as $\dot{V}O_2$ in ml · kg^{-1} · min^{-1}. Expressing $\dot{V}O_2$ as a function of the body weight is referred to as **relative $\dot{V}O_2$,** and it is appropriate when describing the O_2 cost of weight-bearing activities such as running, climbing steps, walking, or ice skating.

Do gender differences exist in running economy? This issue has been studied by numerous investigators, with mixed findings. Figure 1.10 illustrates the results of one of these studies (19). This study compared the oxygen cost of running between highly trained men and women distance runners. The runners were matched for maximal aerobic power and the number of years of training experience. The similar slopes of the two lines suggests that running economy is comparable for highly trained men and women distance runners at slow running speeds (19). However, evidence suggests that at fast "race pace" speeds, male runners may be more economical than females (10). The reason for this apparent gender variation in running economy is unclear and requires further study (29).

IN SUMMARY

- Although it is not easy to compute efficiency during horizontal running, the measurement of the O_2 cost of running (ml · kg^{-1} · min^{-1}) at any given speed offers a measure of running economy.
- Running economy does not differ between highly trained men and women distance runners at slow running speeds. However, at fast "race pace" speeds, male runners may be more economical than females. The reasons for these differences are unclear.

STUDY QUESTIONS

1. Define the following terms:
   a. work
   b. power
   c. percent grade
   d. relative $\dot{V}O_2$
   e. net efficiency
   f. metric system
   g. SI units

2. Calculate the total amount of work performed in 5 minutes of exercise on the cycle ergometer, given the following:

   Resistance on the flywheel = 25 N
   Cranking speed = 60 rpm
   Distance traveled per revolution = 6 meters

3. Compute total work and power output per minute for 10 minutes of treadmill exercise, given the following:

   Treadmill grade = 15%
   Horizontal speed = 90 m · min^{-1}
   Subject's weight = 70 kg

4. Briefly, describe the procedure used to estimate energy expenditure using (a) direct calorimetry and (b) indirect calorimetry.

5. Compute the estimated energy expenditure (ml · kg^{-1} · min^{-1}) during horizontal treadmill walking for the following examples:
   a. Treadmill speed = 50 m · min^{-1}
      Subject's weight = 62 kg
   b. Treadmill speed = 100 m · min^{-1}
      Subject's weight = 75 kg

6. Calculate the estimated O_2 cost of horizontal treadmill running (ml · kg^{-1} · min^{-1}) for a 70-kg subject at 150, 200, and 235 m · min^{-1}.

7. Calculate the power output (kgm · min^{-1}, and watts) during 1 minute of cycle ergometer exercise, given the following:

   Resistance on the flywheel = 3.0 kg
   Cranking speed = 50 rpm
   Distance traveled per revolution = 6 meters

8. Calculate net efficiency, given the following:
   Resting $\dot{V}O_2$ = 0.3 L · min^{-1}
   Exercise $\dot{V}O_2$ = 2.1 L · min^{-1}
   Work rate = 150 W
   Distance traveled per revolution = 6 meters

9. Compute the oxygen cost of cycling (ml · kg^{-1} · min^{-1}) at work rates of 50, 75, 100, 125 W for a 60-kg person.

SUGGESTED READINGS

American College of Sports Medicine. 2010. *Guidelines for Exercise Testing and Prescription*. Baltimore, MD: Lippincott, Williams & Wilkins.

American College of Sports Medicine Metabolic Calculations Tutorial (CD-ROM). 2001. L. Kaminisky.

Bentley, D., J. Newell, and D. Bishop. 2007. Incremental exercise test design and analysis: Implications for performance diagnostics in endurance athletes. *Sports Medicine* 37:575–86.

Brooks, G., T. Fahey, and K. Baldwin. 2005. *Exercise Physiology: Human Bioenergetics and Its Applications* (4th ed.). New York, NY: McGraw-Hill Companies.

Gore, C. (Ed.). 2000. *Physiological Tests for Elite Athletes*. Champaign, IL: Human Kinetics Publishers.

Morrow, J. et al. 2005. *Measurement and Evaluation of Human Performance*. Champaign, IL: Human Kinetics Publishers.

Powers, S., and S. Dodd. 2009. *Total Fitness and Wellness*. San Francisco, CA: Benjamin Cummings.

Van Praagh, E. 2007. Anaerobic fitness tests: What are we measuring? *Medicine and Sport Science* 50:26–45.

REFERENCES

1. **Ainsworth BE, Haskell WL, Herrmann SD, Meckes N, Bassett Jr DR, Tudor-Locke C, Greer JL, Vezina J, Whitt-Glover MC, and Leon AS.** Compendium of Physical Activities: a second update of codes and MET values. *Medicine and Science in Sports and Exercise* 43: 1575–1581, 2011.

2. **American College of Sports Medicine.** *Guidelines for Exercise Testing and Prescription*. Baltimore: Lippincott, Williams & Wilkins, 2010.

3. **Åstrand P.** *Textbook of Work Physiology*. Champaign: Human Kinetics, 2003.

4. **Bassett DRJ, Howley ET, Thompson DL, King GA, Strath SJ, McLaughlin JE, and Parr BB.** Validity of inspiratory and expiratory methods of measuring gas exchange with a computerized system. *J Appl Physiol* 91: 218–224, 2001.

5. **Brooks G, Fahey T, and Baldwin K.** *Exercise Physiology: Human Bioenergetics and Its Applications*. New York: McGraw-Hill, 2005.

6. **Cavanagh PR, and Kram R.** Mechanical and muscular factors affecting the efficiency of human movement. *Med Sci Sports Exerc* 17: 326–331, 1985.

7. **Cavanagh PR, and Kram R.** The efficiency of human movement—a statement of the problem. *Med Sci Sports Exerc* 17: 304–308, 1985.

8. **Coast JR, and Welch HG.** Linear increase in optimal pedal rate with increased power output in cycle ergometry. *Eur J Appl Physiol Occup Physiol* 53: 339–342, 1985.

9. **Consolazio C, Johnson R, and Pecora L.** *Physiological Measurements of Metabolic Function in Man*. New York: McGraw-Hill, 1963.

10. **Daniels J, and Daniels N.** Running economy of elite male and elite female runners. *Med Sci Sports Exerc* 24: 483–489, 1992.

11. **Daniels JT.** A physiologist's view of running economy. *Med Sci Sports Exerc* 17: 332–338, 1985.

12. **Deschenes MR, Kraemer WJ, McCoy RW, Volek JS, Turner BM, and Weinlein JC.** Muscle recruitment patterns regulate physiological responses during exercise of the same intensity. *Am J Physiol Regul Integr Comp Physiol* 279: R2229–2236, 2000.

13. **Donovan CM, and Brooks GA.** Muscular efficiency during steady-rate exercise. II. Effects of walking speed and work rate. *J Appl Physiol* 43: 431–439, 1977.

14. **Ferguson RA, Ball D, Krustrup P, Aagaard P, Kjaer M, Sargeant AJ, Hellsten Y, and Bangsbo J.** Muscle oxygen uptake and energy turnover during dynamic exercise at different contraction frequencies in humans. *J Physiol* 536: 261–271, 2001.

15. **Fox E, Foss M, and Keteyian S.** *Fox's Physiological Basis for Exercise and Sport.* New York: McGraw-Hill, 1998.

16. **Gaesser GA, and Brooks GA.** Muscular efficiency during steady-rate exercise: effects of speed and work rate. *J Appl Physiol* 38: 1132–1139, 1975.

17. **Grandjean E.** *Fitting the Task to the Man: An Ergonomic Approach.* New York: International Publications Service, 1982.

18. **Hagan RD, Strathman T, Strathman L, and Gettman LR.** Oxygen uptake and energy expenditure during horizontal treadmill running. *J Appl Physiol* 49: 571–575, 1980.

19. **Hopkins P, and Powers SK.** Oxygen uptake during submaximal running in highly trained men and women. *Am Correct Ther J* 36: 130–132, 1982.

20. **Horowitz JF, Sidossis LS, and Coyle EF.** High efficiency of type I muscle fibers improves performance. *Int J Sports Med* 15: 152–157, 1994.

21. **Howley E, and Franks B.** *Health Fitness Instructor's Handbook.* Champaign: Human Kinetics, 2007.

22. **Hunter GR, Newcomer BR, Larson-Meyer DE, Bamman MM, and Weinsier RL.** Muscle metabolic economy is inversely related to exercise intensity and type II myofiber distribution. *Muscle Nerve* 24: 654–661, 2001.

23. **Knoebel LK.** Energy metabolism. In: *Physiology*, edited by Selkurt E. Boston: Little Brown & Co., 1984, p. 635–650.

24. **Knuttgen H, and Komi P.** Basic definitions for exercise. In: *Strength and Power in Sport*, edited by Komi P. Oxford: Blackwell Scientific Publications, 1992.

25. **Knuttgen HG.** Force, work, power, and exercise. *Med Sci Sports* 10: 227–228, 1978.

26. **Lucia A, Rivero JL, Perez M, Serrano AL, Calbet JA, Santalla A, and Chicharro JL.** Determinants of $\dot{V}O_{(2)}$ kinetics at high power outputs during a ramp exercise protocol. *Med Sci Sports Exerc* 34: 326–331, 2002.

27. **Margaria R, Cerretelli P, Aghemo P, and Sassi G.** Energy cost of running. *J Appl Physiol* 18: 367–370, 1963.

28. **Michielli DW, and Stricevic M.** Various pedaling frequencies at equivalent power outputs. Effect on heart-rate response. *N Y State J Med* 77: 744–746, 1977.

29. **Morgan DW, and Craib M.** Physiological aspects of running economy. *Med Sci Sports Exerc* 24: 456–461, 1992.

30. **Moseley L, and Jeukendrup AE.** The reliability of cycling efficiency. *Med Sci Sports Exerc* 33: 621–627, 2001.

31. **Powers SK, Beadle RE, and Mangum M.** Exercise efficiency during arm ergometry: effects of speed and work rate. *J Appl Physiol* 56: 495–499, 1984.

32. **Scheuermann BW, Tripse McConnell JH, and Barstow TJ.** EMG and oxygen uptake responses during slow and fast ramp exercise in humans. *Exp Physiol* 87: 91–100, 2002.

33. **Seabury JJ, Adams WC, and Ramey MR.** Influence of pedalling rate and power output on energy expenditure during bicycle ergometry. *Ergonomics* 20: 491–498, 1977.

34. **Shephard R.** *Physiology and Biochemistry of Exercise.* New York: Praeger, 1982.

35. **Singleton W.** *The Body at Work.* London: Cambridge University Press, 1982.

36. **Spence A, and Mason E.** *Human Anatomy and Physiology.* Menlo Park: Benjamin-Cummings, 1992.

37. **Stegeman J.** *Exercise Physiology: Physiological Bases of Work and Sport.* Chicago: Year Book Publishers, 1981.

38. **Stuart MK, Howley ET, Gladden LB, and Cox RH.** Efficiency of trained subjects differing in maximal oxygen uptake and type of training. *J Appl Physiol* 50: 444–449, 1981.

39. **Whipp BJ, and Wasserman K.** Efficiency of muscular work. *J Appl Physiol* 26: 644–648, 1969.

2

Control of the Internal Environment

■ Objectives

By studying this chapter, you should be able to do the following:

1. Define the terms *homeostasis* and *steady state*.
2. Diagram and discuss a biological control system.
3. Give an example of a biological control system.
4. Explain the term *negative feedback*.
5. Define what is meant by the gain of a control system.

■ Outline

■ Key Terms

acclimation
adaptation
autocrine signaling
biological control system
cell signaling
control center
effector
endocrine signaling
endocrine system
gain
heat shock proteins
homeostasis
intracrine signaling
juxtracrine signaling
negative feedback
paracrine signaling
sensor
steady state
stress proteins

A LOOK BACK—IMPORTANT PEOPLE IN SCIENCE

Claude Bernard—A Founding Father of Physiology

Claude Bernard (1813–1878) was a French physician and physiologist who is considered one of the founding "fathers of physiology." Indeed, Dr. Bernard's research and writings greatly improved our understanding of physiology during the nineteenth century, and he is credited with recognizing the importance of a constant internal environment. A brief overview of Dr. Bernard's life and contributions to physiology follows.

Claude Bernard was born in the French village of Saint-Julien and received his early education at the local Jesuit school. He attended Lyon College briefly but left college to devote his efforts toward becoming a successful

writer. At the age of 21, Mr. Bernard went to Paris to formally launch his writing career. However, following discussions with literature critics, Mr. Bernard abandoned writing and decided to study medicine as a career. As a medical intern at a Paris hospital, Dr. Bernard began to work with a senior French physician/physiologist, Francois Magendie, who was involved in research and teaching medical students. Dr. Bernard quickly became Magendie's deputy professor and later succeeded him as a professor.

During his research and medical career, Claude Bernard made many important contributions to physiology and medicine. One of his first important studies was aimed at understanding the role of the pancreas in digestion. He also discovered that the liver was capable of synthesizing glucose from prod-

ucts (e.g., lactate, etc.) removed from the blood. Additionally, Dr. Bernard discovered the vasomotor system, and this important discovery led to our understanding that the nervous system can act to both dilate and constrict blood vessels. Finally, although Dr. Bernard proposed the idea that maintaining a stable internal environment is a requirement for the body to remain healthy, he is not responsible for the concept of homeostasis. Indeed, the maintenance of a relatively stable internal environment was termed "homeostasis" by Walter Cannon in 1932. The word *homeostasis* comes from the Greek words *homoios* (meaning the same) and *stasis* (meaning to stay or stand). For more details on the work of Walter Cannon, see A Look Back—Important People in Science, in chapter 5.

If you had a body temperature of 104° F (40° C) while sitting at rest, you would know that something is wrong. As children we learned that normal body temperature is 98.6° F (37° C) and that values above or below normal signify a problem. How does the body manage to maintain core temperature within a narrow range? Further, how is it that during exercise, when the body is producing great amounts of heat, we generally do not experience overheating problems?

More than 100 years ago, the French physiologist Claude Bernard observed that the "milieu interior" (internal environment) of the body remained remarkably constant despite a changing external environment (see A Look Back—Important People in Science). The fact that the body manages to maintain a relatively constant internal environment in spite of various stressors such as exercise, heat, cold, or fasting is not an accident but the result of many complex control systems (15). Control mechanisms that are responsible for maintaining a stable internal environment constitute a major chapter in exercise physiology, and it is helpful to examine their function in light of simple control theory. Therefore, the purpose of this chapter is to introduce the concept of "control systems" and to discuss how the body maintains a rather constant internal environment during periods of stress. However, before you begin to read this chapter, take time to review Research Focus 2.1. This box provides an overview of how to interpret graphs and gain useful information from these important tools of science.

HOMEOSTASIS: DYNAMIC CONSTANCY

The term **homeostasis** is defined as the maintenance of a relatively constant internal environment. A similar term, **steady state,** is often used to denote a steady and unchanging level of some physiological variable (e.g., heart rate). Although the terms homeostasis and steady state are similar, they differ in the following way. The term homeostasis is commonly used to denote a relatively constant and normal internal environment during resting conditions (8, 16). In contrast, a steady state does not mean that a physiological variable is at resting values but that the physiological variable is constant and unchanging.

An example that is useful in distinguishing between these two terms is the case of body temperature during exercise. Figure 2.2 illustrates the changes in body core temperature during 60 minutes of constant-load submaximal exercise in a thermoneutral environment (i.e., low humidity and low temperature). Note that core temperature reaches a new and steady level within 40 minutes after commencement of exercise. This plateau of core temperature represents a steady state because temperature is constant; however, this constant temperature is above the normal resting body temperature and thus does not represent a true homeostatic condition. Therefore, the term homeostasis is generally reserved for describing normal resting

How to Understand Graphs: A Picture Is Worth 1000 Words

Throughout this book, we use line graphs to illustrate important concepts in exercise physiology. Although these same concepts can be explained in words, graphs are useful visual tools that can illustrate complicated relationships in a way that is easy to understand. Let's briefly review the basic concepts behind the construction of a line graph.

A line graph is used to illustrate relationships between two variables; that is, how one thing is affected by another. You may recall from one of your math courses that a variable is the generic term for any characteristic that changes. For example, in exercise physiology, heart rate is a variable that changes as a function of exercise intensity. Figure 2.1 is a line graph illustrating the relationship between heart rate and exercise intensity. In this illustration, exercise intensity (independent variable) is placed on the x-axis (horizontal), and heart rate (dependent variable) is located on the y-axis (vertical). Heart rate is considered the dependent variable because it changes as a function of exercise intensity. Because exercise intensity is independent of heart rate, it is the independent variable. Note in figure 2.1 that heart rate increases as a linear (straight-line) function of the exercise intensity. This type of line graph makes it easy to see what happens to heart rate when exercise intensity is changed.

FIGURE 2.1
The relationship between heart rate and exercise intensity (expressed as a percent of $\dot{V}O_2$ max).

conditions, and the term steady state is often applied to exercise wherein the physiological variable in question (i.e., body temperature) is unchanging but may not equal the "homeostatic" resting value.

Although the concept of homeostasis means that the internal environment is unchanging, this does not mean that the internal environment remains absolutely constant. In fact, most physiological variables vary around some "set" value, and thus homeostasis represents a rather dynamic constancy. An example of this dynamic constancy is the arterial blood pressure. Figure 2.3 shows the mean (average) arterial blood pressure during eight minutes of rest. Note the oscillatory change in arterial pressure, but the mean

Figure 2.2   Changes in body core temperature during 60 minutes of submaximal exercise in a thermoneutral environment. Note that body temperature reaches a plateau (steady state) by approximately 40 minutes of exercise.

Figure 2.3   Changes in arterial blood pressure across time during resting conditions. Notice that although the arterial pressure oscillates across time, the mean pressure remains unchanged.

(average) arterial pressure remains around 93 mm Hg. The reason such an oscillation occurs in physiological variables is related to the "feedback" nature of biological control systems (16). This is discussed later in the chapter in the "Negative Feedback" section.

IN SUMMARY

■ Homeostasis is defined as the maintenance of a constant or unchanging "normal" internal environment during unstressed conditions.
■ The term steady state is also defined as a constant internal environment, but this does not necessarily mean that the internal environment is at rest and normal. When the body is in a steady state, a balance has been achieved between the demands placed on the body and the body's response to those demands.

CONTROL SYSTEMS OF THE BODY

The body has literally hundreds of different control systems, and the overall goal of most is to regulate some physiological variable at or near a constant value (16). The most intricate of these control systems reside inside the cell itself. These cellular control systems regulate cell activities such as protein breakdown and synthesis, energy production, and maintenance of the appropriate amounts of stored nutrients. Almost all organ systems of the body work to help maintain homeostasis (14). For example, the lungs (pulmonary system) and heart (circulatory system) work together to replenish oxygen and to remove carbon dioxide from the extracellular fluid. The fact that the cardiopulmonary system is usually able to maintain normal levels of oxygen and carbon dioxide even during periods of strenuous exercise is not an accident but the end result of a good control system.

Although much is known about how specific control systems of the body operate, the details of how many control systems work to maintain homeostasis remain a mystery. This remains an active area of research in exercise physiology.

NATURE OF THE CONTROL SYSTEMS

To develop a better understanding of how the body maintains a stable internal environment, let's begin with the analogy of a simple, nonbiological control system, such as a thermostat-regulated heating and cooling system in a home. Suppose the thermostat is

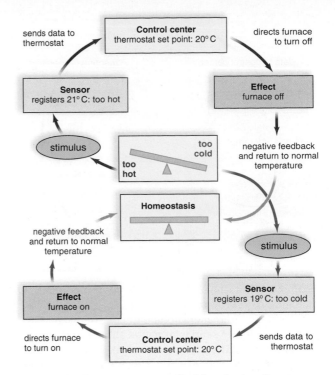

Figure 2.4 A thermostat-controlled heating/cooling system is an example of a nonbiological (mechanical) control system that uses negative feedback to regulate room temperature. An increase in room temperature above the set point (i.e., 20°C) directs the furnace to turn off and therefore reduce the temperature in the room (top). In contrast, a decrease in room temperature below the set point results in turning on the furnace to release warm air into the room (bottom)

set at 20° C. Any change in room temperature away from the 20° C "set point" results in the appropriate response by the temperature "control center" to return the room temperature to 20° C. If the room temperature rises above the set point, the thermostat signals the control center to turn off the furnace, which gradually returns the room temperature to 20° C. In contrast, a decrease in temperature below the set point results in the thermostat signaling the furnace to begin operation (figure 2.4). In both cases the response by the control center was to correct the condition—low or high temperature—that initially turned it on.

Similar to the example of a mechanical control system, a **biological control system** is a series of interconnected components that maintain a chemical or physical parameter of the body near a constant value (16). Biological control systems are composed of three elements: (1) a sensor (or receptor); (2) a control center (i.e., center to integrate response); and (3) effectors (i.e., organs that produce the desired effect) (figure 2.5). The signal to begin the operation of a control system is the stimulus that represents a change in the internal environment (i.e., too much or too little of a regulated variable). The stimulus excites a **sensor**

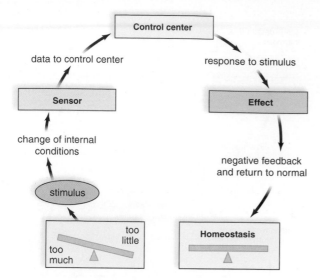

Figure 2.5 This schematic illustrates the components of a biological control system. The process begins with change in the internal environment (i.e., stimulus), which excites a sensor to send information about the change to a control center. The control center makes an assessment of the amount of response that is needed to correct the problem and sends the appropriate message to the appropriate organs to bring about the desired effect. This effect is responsible for correcting the disturbance, and thus the stimulus is removed.

that is a receptor in the body capable of detecting change in the variable in question. The excited sensor then sends a message to the control center. The **control center** integrates the strength of the incoming signal from the sensor and sends an appropriate message to the **effectors** to bring about the appropriate response to correct the disturbance (i.e., desired effect). The return of the internal environment to normal results in a decrease in the original stimulus that triggered the control system into action. This type of feedback loop is termed *negative feedback* and is the primary method responsible for maintaining homeostasis in the body (16) (figure 2.5).

Negative Feedback

Most control systems of the body operate via **negative feedback** (16). Negative feedback is an important class of biological control systems in the body that serves to restore normal values of a variable to maintain homeostasis. An example of negative feedback can be seen in the respiratory system's regulation of the CO_2 concentration in extracellular fluid. In this case, an increase in extracellular CO_2 above normal levels triggers a receptor, which sends information to the respiratory control center (integrating center) to increase breathing. The effectors in this example are the respiratory muscles. This increase in breathing will reduce extracellular CO_2 concentrations back to normal,

thus reestablishing homeostasis. This type of feedback is termed *negative* because the response of the control system is negative (opposite) to the stimulus.

Positive Feedback

Although negative feedback is the primary type of feedback used to maintain homeostasis in the body, positive feedback control loops also exist. Positive feedback control mechanisms act to increase the original stimulus. This type of feedback is termed *positive* because the response is in the same direction as the stimulus.

A classic example of a positive feedback mechanism involves the enhancement of labor contractions when a woman gives birth. For example, when the head of the baby moves into the birth canal, the increased pressure on the cervix (narrow end of the uterus) stimulates sensory receptors. These excited sensors then send a neural message to the brain (i.e., control center), which responds by triggering the release of the hormone oxytocin from the pituitary gland. Oxytocin then travels via the blood to the uterus and promotes increased contractions. As labor continues, the cervix becomes more stimulated and uterine contractions become even stronger until birth occurs. At this point, the stimulus (i.e., the pressure) for oxytocin release stops and thus shuts off the positive feedback mechanism.

Gain of a Control System

The precision with which a control system maintains homeostasis is called the **gain** of the system. Gain can be thought of as the "capability" of the control system. This means that a control system with a large gain is more capable of correcting a disturbance in homeostasis than a control system with a low gain. As you might predict, the most important control systems of the body have large gains. For example, control systems that regulate body temperature, breathing (i.e., pulmonary system), and delivery of blood (i.e., cardiovascular system) all have large gains. The fact that these systems have large gains is not surprising, given that these control systems all deal with life-and-death issues.

IN SUMMARY

- A biological control system is composed of a receptor, a control center, and an effector.
- Most control systems act by way of negative feedback.
- The degree to which a control system maintains homeostasis is termed the *gain of the system*. A control system with a large gain is more capable of maintaining homeostasis than a system with a low gain.

EXAMPLES OF HOMEOSTATIC CONTROL

To better understand biological control systems, consider a few examples of homeostatic control.

Regulation of Body Temperature

An excellent example of a homeostatic control system that uses negative feedback is the regulation of body temperature (15). The sensors in this system are thermal receptors located in several body locations. The control center for temperature regulation is located in the brain, and when body temperature increases above normal, temperature sensors send a neural message to the control center that temperature is above normal (top portion of figure 2.6). The control center responds to this stimulus by directing a response to promote heat loss (i.e., skin blood vessels dilate and sweating occurs). When body temperature returns to normal, the control center is inactivated.

When body temperature falls below normal, temperature sensors send these data to the control center in the brain, which responds by preventing the loss of body heat (e.g., blood vessels in the skin constrict); this action serves to conserve heat (bottom portion of figure 2.6). Again, when body temperature returns to normal, the control center becomes inactive. Complete details about how the body regulates temperature during exercise are presented in chapter 12.

Regulation of Blood Glucose

Homeostasis is also a function of the **endocrine system** (see chapter 5). The body contains eight major endocrine glands, which synthesize and secrete blood-borne chemical substances called *hormones*. Hormones are transported via the circulatory system throughout the body as an aid to regulate circulatory and metabolic functions (4, 16). An example of the endocrine system's role in the maintenance of homeostasis is the control of blood glucose levels. Indeed, in health, the blood glucose concentration is carefully regulated by the endocrine system. For example, the hormone insulin regulates cellular uptake and the metabolism of glucose and is therefore important in the regulation of the blood glucose concentration. After a large carbohydrate meal, the blood glucose level increases above normal (figure 2.7). The rise in blood glucose signals the pancreas to release insulin, which then lowers blood glucose by increasing cellular uptake. Failure of the blood glucose control system results in disease (diabetes) and is discussed in Clinical Applications 2.1.

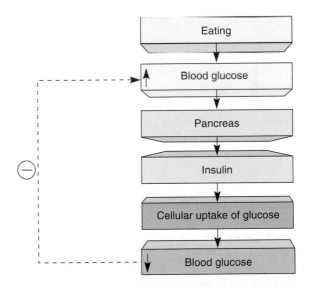

Figure 2.7 Illustration of the regulation of blood glucose concentration. Changes in blood glucose concentration from the normal range regulate insulin secretion. Insulin, in turn, acts to regulate blood glucose levels (completing the negative feedback loop) and to maintain homeostasis. In this system the pancreas is both the sensor and the effector organ. It senses the change in blood glucose from normal and releases insulin appropriately.

Figure 2.6 Illustration of the negative feedback that is used to regulate body temperature. See text for details of how this system operates.

CLINICAL APPLICATIONS 2.1

Failure of a Biological Control System Results in Disease

Failure of any component of a biological control system results in a disturbance in homeostasis. A classic illustration of the failure of a biological control system is the disease diabetes. Although there are two forms of diabetes (type 1 and type 2), both types are characterized by abnormally high blood glucose levels

(called hyperglycemia). In type 1 diabetes, the beta cells in the pancreas (beta cells produce insulin) become damaged. Hence, insulin is no longer produced and released into the blood to promote the transport of glucose into tissues. Therefore, damage to the pancreatic beta cells represents a failure of

the "effector" component of this control system. If insulin cannot be released in response to an increase in blood glucose following a high-carbohydrate meal, glucose cannot be transported into body cells and the end result is hyperglycemia and diabetes.

EXERCISE: A TEST OF HOMEOSTATIC CONTROL

Muscular exercise presents a dramatic test of the body's homeostatic control systems because exercise has the potential to disrupt many homeostatic variables. For example, during heavy exercise, skeletal muscle produces large amounts of heat, which poses a challenge for the body to prevent overheating. Additionally, heavy exercise results in large increases in muscle O_2 requirements, and large amounts of CO_2 are produced. These changes must be countered by increases in breathing (pulmonary ventilation) and blood flow to increase O_2 delivery to the exercising muscle and remove metabolically produced CO_2. The body's control systems must respond rapidly to prevent drastic alterations in the internal environment.

In a strict sense, the body rarely maintains true homeostasis while performing intense exercise or during prolonged exercise in a hot or humid environment. Heavy exercise or prolonged work results in disturbances in the internal environment that are generally too great for even the highest gain control systems to overcome, and thus a steady state is not possible. Severe disturbances in homeostasis result in fatigue and, ultimately, cessation of exercise (7, 13, 3). Understanding how various body control systems minimize exercise-induced disturbances in homeostasis is extremely important to the exercise physiology student and is thus a major theme of this textbook. Specific details about individual control systems (e.g., circulatory, respiratory) that affect the internal environment during exercise are discussed in chapters 4 through 12. Further, improved exercise performance following exercise training is largely due to training adaptations that result in a better maintenance of homeostasis; this is discussed in chapter 13. In the

next segment we highlight the processes that promote exercise-induced improvements in the body's homeostatic control mechanisms.

EXERCISE IMPROVES HOMEOSTATIC CONTROL VIA CELLULAR ADAPTATION

The term **adaptation** refers to a change in the structure and function of a cell or organ system that results in an improved ability to maintain homeostasis during stressful conditions. Indeed, a cell's ability to respond to a challenge is not fixed and can be improved by prolonged exposure to a specific stress (e.g., regular bouts of exercise). Also, cells can adapt to environmental stresses, such as heat stress due to a hot environment. This type of environmental adaptation—the improved function of an existing homeostatic system—is known as **acclimation (16)**.

It is well known that regular bouts of exercise promote cellular changes that result in an improved ability to preserve homeostasis during the "stress" of exercise. This improved ability of cells and organ systems to maintain homeostasis occurs via a variety of cell signaling mechanisms. The term **cell signaling** refers to a system of communication between cells that coordinates cellular activities. The ability of cells to detect changes in their internal environment and correctly respond to this change is essential in the maintenance of homeostasis. It should be no surprise that a variety of cell signaling mechanisms coordinate all the different functions of the body. As you read this text, you will encounter five cell signaling mechanisms. These signaling mechanisms are illustrated in figure 2.8 and are briefly defined below.

■ **Intracrine signaling.** Intracrine signaling occurs when a chemical messenger is produced

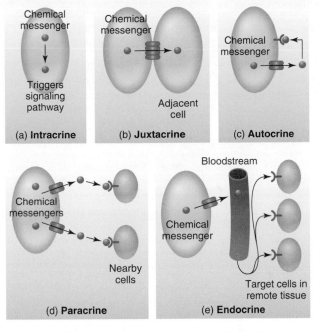

Figure 2.8 Illustration of the five major cell signaling mechanisms that participate in the control of homeostasis and cellular adaptation. (a) Intracrine signaling occurs when a chemical messenger is produced inside a cell and triggers an intracellular signaling pathway that leads to a specific cellular response. (b) Juxtacrine signaling occurs when the cytoplasm of one cell is in contact with the cytoplasm of another cell through small junctions that bridge the two cell membranes. This permits a chemical messenger from one cell to move into the neighboring cell. (c) Autocrine signaling occurs when a cell produces and releases a chemical messenger into the extracellular fluid that acts upon the cell producing the signal. (d) Paracrine signaling occurs when one cell produces a chemical messenger that acts on nearby cells to bring about a coordinated response. (e) Endocrine signaling occurs when a cell releases a chemical messenger (hormone) into the blood and this hormone is then carried by the blood stream throughout the body to target cells.

inside a cell that triggers a signaling pathway within the same cell that leads to a specific cellular response. Examples of intracrine signaling are provided in chapter 13, where we discuss the cell signaling mechanisms responsible for skeletal muscle adaptation to exercise training.

■ **Juxtacrine signaling.** Some cells communicate by cell-to-cell contact, in which the cytoplasm of one cell is in contact with the cytoplasm of another through small junctions that connect the two cell membranes. This type of cell signaling is called juxtacrine signaling. You will see this in chapter 9 as the method by which one heart cell signals the next one to contract so that the heart contracts in a smooth and effective manner.

■ **Autocrine signaling.** Autocrine signaling occurs when a cell produces and releases a chemical messenger into the extracellular fluid that acts upon the cell producing the signal. For example, during resistance training, autocrine signaling within the muscle cell triggers the DNA in the nucleus to produce more contractile protein, which in turn increases the size of that muscle cell. This type of cell signaling is discussed in chapter 13. A Closer Look 2.1 presents an overview of how cell signaling can promote protein synthesis in cells.

■ **Paracrine signaling.** Some cells produce signals that act locally on nearby cells (paracrine signals) to bring about a coordinated response. For example, we will see in chapter 6 how immune cells communicate with each other to generate a coordinated attack to protect the body from infection and injury. Further, synaptic signaling is another type of paracrine signaling that occurs in the nervous system (chapter 7).

■ **Endocrine signaling.** Finally, some cells release chemical signals (hormones) into the blood and these hormones are then carried throughout the body. However, the cells that respond to the hormone are only cells with a receptor specific to this hormone. This is called endocrine signaling and is covered in chapter 5.

STRESS PROTEINS ASSIST IN THE REGULATION OF CELLULAR HOMEOSTASIS

A disturbance in cellular homeostasis occurs when a cell is faced with a "stress" that surpasses its ability to defend against this particular type of disturbance. A classic illustration of how cells use control systems to combat stress (i.e., disturbances in homeostasis) is termed the *cellular stress response*. The cellular stress response is a biological control system in cells that battles homeostatic disturbances by manufacturing proteins designed to defend against stress. A brief overview of the cellular stress response system and how it protects cells against homeostatic disturbances follows.

At the cellular level, proteins are important in maintaining homeostasis. For example, proteins play critical roles in normal cell function by serving as intracellular transporters or as enzymes that

A CLOSER LOOK 2.1

An Overview of Cellular Protein Synthesis

Often, the exercise-induced improved ability of cells to maintain homeostasis results from increased synthesis of the specific proteins that participate in maintaining cellular balance. Exercise-induced protein synthesis occurs via cell signaling events that ultimately lead to the activation of genes and, subsequently, protein synthesis (1, 2). A brief overview of how cell signaling results in protein synthesis follows.

Human cells contain between 20,000–25,000 genes, and each gene is responsible for the synthesis of a specific protein (6). Cellular signals regulate protein synthesis by "turning on" or "turning off" specific genes. Figure 2.9 illustrates the process of exercise-induced protein synthesis in a muscle fiber. The process begins with the "stress" of exercise stimulating a specific cell signaling pathway that results in the activation of a molecule called a transcriptional activator. Transcriptional activators are responsible for "turning on" specific genes to syn-

thesize new proteins. Once activated in the sarcoplasm, the transcriptional activator moves into the nucleus and binds to the promoter region of the gene. Activation of the gene's promoter provides the stimulus for transcription. Transcription results in the formation of a message called messenger RNA (mRNA), which contains the genetic information for a specific protein's amino acid sequence. The message (i.e., mRNA) leaves the nucleus and travels through the sarcoplasm to the ribosome, which is the site of protein synthesis. At the ribosome, the mRNA is translated into a specific protein. Individual proteins differ in structure and function; this is important because the types of proteins contained in a muscle fiber determine the fiber characteristic and its ability to perform specific types of exercise. Therefore, understanding the cellular signaling pathways that promote or inhibit gene activation in skeletal muscle is of major importance to exercise

physiologists. Details of how exercise promotes skeletal muscle adaptation by altering gene expression are discussed in chapter 13.

Note that dissimilar modes of exercise promote the expression of different genes in the active muscle fibers. For example, resistance exercise and endurance exercise promote the activation of different cell signaling pathways; therefore, different genes are activated resulting in the expression of diverse proteins. However, you will also learn that resistance exercise and endurance exercise activate several common genes, such as the genes that express stress proteins. Numerous stress proteins exist in cells and play an important role in maintaining cellular homeostasis. A brief introduction to stress proteins and their role in the control of cellular homeostasis is discussed in the section titled "Stress Proteins Assist in the Regulation of Cellular Homeostasis."

FIGURE 2.9 Illustration of how exercise promotes the activation of cell signaling pathways in muscle fibers that lead to increased gene expression and the synthesis of new proteins.

catalyze chemical reactions. Damage to cellular proteins by stress (e.g., low pH, free radicals, etc.) can result in cell damage and a disturbance in homeostasis. To combat this type of disruption in homeostasis, cells respond by rapidly manufacturing protective proteins called **stress proteins** (5, 9, 10). The term stress protein refers to a family of proteins that are manufactured in cells in response to a variety of stresses (e.g., high temperature). One of the most important families of stress proteins is called **heat shock proteins.** It is well known that exercise training results in significant increases in the production of numerous heat shock proteins within the trained skeletal muscle (10).

After synthesis, heat shock proteins go to work to protect the cell by repairing damaged proteins and restoring homeostasis. Figure 2.10 illustrates how this control system regulates protein homeostasis in cells. The process starts with a stressor that promotes protein damage. Stresses associated with exercise that are known to produce cellular protein damage include high temperatures, reduced cellular oxygen, low pH, and the production of free radicals (11, 12). Damaged proteins become signals for the cell to produce stress proteins. After synthesis, these stress proteins work to repair damaged proteins and restore homeostasis (9). See Noble et al. (2008) and Morton et al. (2009) in Suggested Readings for a detailed discussion of exercise and heat shock proteins.

IN SUMMARY

- Exercise represents a challenge to the body's control systems to maintain homeostasis. In general, the body's many control systems are capable of maintaining a steady state during most types of submaximal exercise in a cool environment. However, intense exercise or prolonged work in a hostile environment (i.e., high temperature/humidity) may exceed the ability of a control system to maintain a steady state, and severe disturbances in homeostasis may occur.
- Acclimation is the change that occurs in response to repeated stresses and results in the improved function of an existing homeostatic system.
- Cell signaling is defined as a system of communication that governs cellular activities and coordinates cell actions.
- A variety of cell signaling mechanisms participate in the regulation of homeostasis and are required to regulate cellular adaptation. The major cell signaling mechanisms include: 1) intracrine signaling, 2) juxtracrine signaling, 3) autocrine signaling, 4) paracrine signaling, and 5) endocrine signaling.
- Exercise-induced protein synthesis occurs via cell signaling events that lead to the activation of genes, which leads to protein synthesis and to an improved ability to maintain homeostasis during the "stress" of exercise.

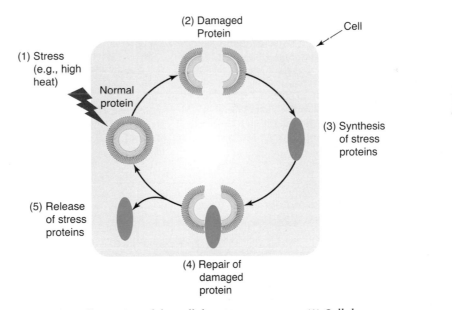

Figure 2.10 Illustration of the cellular stress response. (1) Cellular stressors (e.g., high temperature) can damage normal protein and produce (2) damaged protein. These damaged proteins signal the (3) synthesis of stress proteins. (4) These stress proteins can then repair the damaged protein to restore homeostasis in the cell.

STUDY QUESTIONS

1. Define the term *homeostasis*. How does it differ from the term *steady state*?
2. Cite an example of a biological homeostatic control system.
3. Draw a simple diagram that demonstrates the relationships between the components of a biological control system.
4. Briefly explain the role of the receptor, the integrating center, and the effector organ in a biological control system.
5. Explain the term *negative feedback*. Give a biological example of negative feedback.
6. Discuss the concept of gain associated with a biological control system.
7. Define cell signaling and outline the five types of cell signaling mechanisms that participate in the regulation of homeostasis and cellular adaptation.
8. List the steps that lead to exercise-induced increases in protein synthesis in skeletal muscles.

SUGGESTED READINGS

Karp, G. 2009. *Cell and Molecular Biology: Concepts and Experiments*. Hoboken, NJ. Wiley Publishers.

Morton, J. P., A. C. Kayani, A. McArdle, and B. Drust. 2009. The exercise-induced stress response of skeletal muscle, with specific emphasis on humans. *Sports Medicine* 39: 643–62.

Noble E. G., K. J. Milne, and C. W. Melling. 2008. Heat shock proteins and exercise: a primer. *Applied Physiology, Nutrition, and Metabolism = Physiologie Appliquee, Nutrition et Metabolisme* 33:1050–65.

Widmaier, E., H. Raff, and K. Strang. 2008. *Vander's Human Physiology*. New York, NY: McGraw-Hill.

REFERENCES

1. **Alberts B, Johnson A., Raff J.** *Molecular Biology of the Cell*. New York: Garland Science, 2007.
2. **Berk H, Kaiser C, and Krieger M.** *Molecular Cell Biology*. New York: W. H. Freeman, 2007.
3. **Fitts RH.** The cross-bridge cycle and skeletal muscle fatigue. *J Appl Physiol* 104: 551–558, 2008.
4. **Fox S.** *Human Physiology*. New York: McGraw-Hill, 2011.
5. **Harkins MS.** Exercise regulates heat shock proteins and nitric oxide. *Exercise and Sport Sciences Reviews* 37: 73–77, 2009.
6. **Karp G.** *Cell and Molecular Biology: Concepts and Experiments*. Hoboken, NJ: Wiley, 2009.
7. **Lamb GD.** Mechanisms of excitation-contraction uncoupling relevant to activity-induced muscle fatigue. *Applied Physiology, Nutrition, and Metabolism (Physiologie appliquee, nutrition et metabolisme)* 34: 368–372, 2009.
8. **Marieb E, and Hoehn K.** *Human Anatomy and Physiology*. Menlo Park, CA: Benjamin-Cummings, 2007.
9. **Morton JP, Kayani AC, McArdle A, and Drust B.** The exercise-induced stress response of skeletal muscle, with specific emphasis on humans. *Sports Medicine (Auckland, NZ)* 39: 643–662, 2009.
10. **Noble EG, Milne KJ, and Melling CW.** Heat shock proteins and exercise: a primer. *Applied physiology, nutrition, and metabolism (Physiologie appliquee, nutrition et metabolisme)* 33: 1050–1065, 2008.
11. **Powers SK, and Jackson MJ.** Exercise-induced oxidative stress: cellular mechanisms and impact on muscle force production. *Physiological Reviews* 88: 1243–1276, 2008.
12. **Powers SK, Quindry JC, and Kavazis AN.** Exercise-induced cardioprotection against myocardial ischemia-reperfusion injury. *Free Radical Biology & Medicine* 44: 193–201, 2008.
13. **Reid MB.** Free radicals and muscle fatigue: of ROS, canaries, and the IOC. *Free Radical Biology & Medicine* 44: 169–179, 2008.
14. **Saladin K.** *Anatomy and Physiology*. Boston: McGraw-Hill, 2010.
15. **Schlader ZJ, Stannard SR, and Mundel T.** Human thermoregulatory behavior during rest and exercise—a prospective review. *Physiology & Behavior* 99: 269–275, 2010.
16. **Widmaier E, Raff H, and Strang K.** *Vander's Human Physiology*. Boston: McGraw-Hill, 2008.

3

Bioenergetics

■ Objectives

By studying this chapter, you should be able to do the following:

1. Discuss the function of the cell membrane, nucleus, and mitochondria.
2. Define the following terms: (1) *endergonic reactions*, (2) *exergonic reactions*, (3) *coupled reactions*, and (4) *bioenergetics*.
3. Describe the role of enzymes as catalysts in cellular chemical reactions.
4. List and discuss the nutrients that are used as fuels during exercise.
5. Identify the high-energy phosphates.

6. Discuss the biochemical pathways involved in anaerobic ATP production.
7. Discuss the aerobic production of ATP.
8. Describe the general scheme used to regulate metabolic pathways involved in bioenergetics.
9. Discuss the interaction between aerobic and anaerobic ATP production during exercise.
10. Identify the enzymes that are considered rate limiting in glycolysis and the Krebs cycle.

■ Outline

■ Key Terms

acetyl-CoA
activation energy
adenosine diphosphate
   (ADP)
adenosine triphosphate
   (ATP)
aerobic
anaerobic
ATPase
ATP-PC system
beta oxidation
bioenergetics
cell membrane
chemiosmotic hypothesis
coupled reactions
cytoplasm
electron transport chain
endergonic reactions
energy of activation
enzymes
exergonic reactions
flavin adenine
   dinucleotide (FAD)

glucose
glycogen
glycogenolysis
glycolysis
inorganic
inorganic phosphate (P_i)
isocitrate dehydrogenase
Krebs cycle
lactate
metabolism
mitochondrion
molecular biology
nicotinamide adenine
   dinucleotide (NAD^+)
nucleus
organic
oxidation
oxidative phosphorylation
phosphocreatine (PC)
phosphofructokinase (PFK)
reduction

Thousands of chemical reactions occur throughout the body during each minute of the day. Collectively, these reactions are called **metabolism.** Metabolism is broadly defined as the total of all cellular reactions and includes chemical pathways that result in the synthesis of molecules (anabolic reactions) as well as the breakdown of molecules (catabolic reactions).

Because energy is required by all cells, it is not surprising that cells possess chemical pathways that are capable of converting foodstuffs (i.e., fats, proteins, carbohydrates) into a biologically usable form of energy. This metabolic process is termed **bioenergetics.** For you to run, jump, or swim, skeletal muscle cells must be able to continuously extract energy from food nutrients. In fact, the inability to transform energy contained in foodstuffs into usable biological energy would limit performance in endurance activities. The explanation for this is simple. To continue to contract, muscle cells must have a continuous source of energy. When energy is not readily available, muscular contraction is not possible, and thus work must stop. Therefore, given the importance of cellular energy production during exercise, it is critical that students of exercise physiology develop a thorough understanding of bioenergetics. It is the purpose of this chapter to introduce both general and specific concepts associated with bioenergetics.

CELL STRUCTURE

Cells were discovered in the seventeenth century by the English scientist Robert Hooke. Advancements in the microscope over the past 300 years have led to improvements in our understanding of cell structure and function. To understand bioenergetics, it is important to have some appreciation of cell structure and function. Four elements (an element is a basic chemical substance) compose over 95% of the human body. These include oxygen (65%), carbon (18%), hydrogen (10%), and nitrogen (3%) (10). Additional elements found in rather small amounts in the body include sodium, iron, zinc, potassium, magnesium, chloride, and calcium. These various elements are linked by chemical bonds to form molecules or compounds. Compounds that contain carbon are called **organic** compounds, whereas those that do not contain carbon are termed **inorganic.** For example, water (H_2O) lacks carbon and is thus inorganic. In contrast, proteins, fats, and carbohydrates contain carbon and are organic compounds.

As the basic functional unit of the body, the cell is a highly organized factory capable of synthesizing the large number of compounds necessary for normal cellular function. Figure 3.1 illustrates the structure of a muscle cell (muscle cells are typically called muscle fibers). Note that not all cells are alike, nor do they all

Figure 3.1 A muscle cell (fiber) and its major organelles.

perform the same functions. Nonetheless, in general, cell structure can be divided into three major parts:

1. **Cell membrane** The cell membrane (also called the *sarcolemma* in skeletal muscle fibers) is a semipermeable barrier that separates the cell from the extracellular environment. The two most important functions of the cell membrane are to enclose the components of the cell and to regulate the passage of various types of substances in and out of the cell (1, 10, 21).
2. **Nucleus** The nucleus is a large, round body within the cell that contains the cellular genetic components (genes). Genes are composed of double strands of deoxyribonucleic acids (DNA), which serve as the basis for the genetic code. In short, genes regulate protein synthesis, which determines cell composition and controls cellular activity. The field of **molecular biology** is concerned with understanding the composition and regulation of genes and is introduced in A Closer Look 3.1. Note that although most cells have only one nucleus, skeletal muscle cells have many nuclei along the entire length of the muscle fiber.
3. **Cytoplasm** (called *sarcoplasm* in muscle cells) This is the fluid portion of the cell between the nucleus and the cell membrane. Contained within the cytoplasm are various organelles (minute structures) that are concerned with specific cellular functions. One such organelle, the **mitochondrion,** is often called the powerhouse of the cell and is involved in the oxidative conversion of foodstuffs into usable cellular energy. Also contained in the cytoplasm are the enzymes that regulate the breakdown of glucose (i.e., glycolysis).

BIOLOGICAL ENERGY TRANSFORMATION

All energy on earth comes from the sun. Plants use light energy from the sun to drive chemical reactions to form carbohydrates, fats, and proteins. Animals (including

A CLOSER LOOK 3.1

Molecular Biology and Exercise Physiology

Molecular biology is defined as the study of biology at the molecular level. That is, molecular biology is the study of molecular structures and events underlying biological processes. Moreover, molecular biology is concerned with understanding the relationship between genes and the cellular characteristics that they determine. The field of molecular biology overlaps with other areas of biology, including physiology, biochemistry, and genetics (figure 3.2).

Recall from chapter 2 that each gene is responsible for the synthesis of a specific cellular protein. Cellular signals regulate protein synthesis by "turning on" or "turning off" specific genes. Therefore, understanding those factors that act as signals to promote or inhibit protein synthesis is of importance to exercise physiologists.

The technical revolution in the field of molecular biology offers another opportunity to make use of scientific information for the improvement of

FIGURE 3.2   The different fields of biology have overlapping areas of study.

human performance. For example, exercise training results in modifications in the amounts and types of proteins synthesized in the exercised muscles (see chapter 13 for details). Indeed, it is well known that regular strength training results in an increase in muscle size due to an increase in contractile proteins. The techniques of molecular biology provide the exercise physiologist with the "tools" to understand how exercise controls gene function and the synthesis of new proteins. Ultimately, understanding how exercise promotes the synthesis of specific proteins in muscles will allow the exercise scientist to design the most effective training program to achieve the desired training effects.

---

humans) then eat plants and other animals to obtain the energy required to maintain cellular activities.

Energy exists in several forms (e.g., electrical, mechanical, chemical), and all forms of energy are interchangeable (21). For example, muscle fibers convert chemical energy obtained from carbohydrates, fats, or proteins into mechanical energy to perform movement. The bioenergetic process of converting chemical energy to mechanical energy requires a series of tightly controlled chemical reactions. Before discussing the specific reactions involved, we provide an overview of cellular chemical reactions.

Cellular Chemical Reactions

Energy transfer in the body occurs via the releasing of energy trapped within chemical bonds of various molecules. Chemical bonds that contain relatively large amounts of potential energy are often referred to as "high-energy bonds." As mentioned previously, bioenergetics is concerned with the transfer of energy from foodstuffs into a biologically usable form. This energy transfer in the cell occurs as a result of a series of chemical reactions. Many of these reactions require that energy be added to the reactants (**endergonic reactions**) before the reaction will "proceed." However, because energy is added to the reaction, the products contain more free energy than the original reactants.

Reactions that give off energy as a result of chemical process are known as **exergonic reactions.** Note that the words *endergonic* and *endothermic* can be used interchangeably. The same applies for the words *exergonic* and *exothermic*. Figure 3.3 illustrates that the amount of total energy released via exergonic reactions is the same whether the energy is released in one single reaction (combustion) or many small, controlled steps that usually occur in cells (cellular oxidation).

Coupled Reactions   Many of the chemical reactions that occur within the cell are called **coupled reactions.** Coupled reactions are reactions that are linked, with the liberation of free energy in one reaction being used to "drive" a second reaction. Figure 3.4 illustrates this point. In this example, energy released by an exergonic reaction is used to drive an energy-requiring reaction

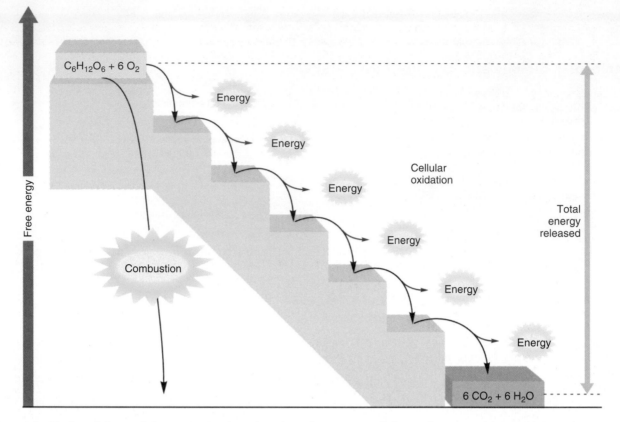

Figure 3.3 The breakdown of glucose into carbon dioxide and water via cellular oxidation results in a release of energy. Reactions that result in a release of free energy are termed exergonic.

Exergonic reactions   Endergonic reactions

Figure 3.4 Model showing the coupling of exergonic and endergonic reactions. Note that the energy given off by the exergonic reaction (drive shaft) powers the endergonic reactions (smaller gear).

(endergonic reaction) in the cell. This is like two meshed gears in which the turning of one (energy-releasing, exergonic gear) causes the movement of the second (endergonic gear). In other words, energy-liberating reactions are "coupled" to energy-requiring reactions. Oxidation-reduction reactions are an important type of coupled reaction and are discussed in the next section.

IN SUMMARY

■ Metabolism is defined as the total of all cellular reactions that occur in cells of the body; this includes both the synthesis of molecules and the breakdown of molecules. Cell structure includes the following three major parts: (1) cell membrane, (2) nucleus, and (3) cytoplasm (called *sarcoplasm* in muscle).
■ The cell membrane provides a protective barrier between the interior of the cell and the extracellular fluid.
■ Genes (located within the nucleus) regulate protein synthesis within the cell.
■ The cytoplasm is the fluid portion of the cell and contains numerous organelles.

Oxidation-Reduction Reactions

The process of removing an electron from an atom or molecule is called **oxidation.** The addition of an electron to an atom or molecule is referred to as **reduction.** Oxidation and reduction are always coupled reactions because a molecule cannot be oxidized unless it donates electrons to another atom. The molecule that donates the electron is known as the *reducing agent,* whereas the one that accepts the electrons is called an *oxidizing agent*. Note that a molecule can act as both an oxidizing agent and a reducing agent. For example, when molecules play both roles, they can gain electrons in one reaction and then pass these electrons to another molecule to produce an oxidation-reduction reaction. Hence, coupled oxidation-reduction reactions are analogous to a bucket brigade, with electrons being passed along in the buckets.

Note that the term *oxidation* does not mean that oxygen participates in the reaction. This term is derived from the fact that oxygen tends to accept electrons and therefore acts as an oxidizing agent. This important property of oxygen is used by cells to produce a usable form of energy and is discussed in detail in the section "Electron Transport Chain."

Keep in mind that oxidation-reduction reactions in cells often involve the transfer of hydrogen atoms (with their electrons) rather than free electrons. This occurs because a hydrogen atom contains one electron and one proton in the nucleus. Therefore, a molecule that loses a hydrogen atom also loses an electron and therefore is oxidized; the molecule that gains the hydrogen (and electron) is reduced. In many biological oxidation-reduction reactions, pairs of electrons are passed along between molecules as free electrons or as pairs of hydrogen atoms.

Two molecules that play important roles in the transfer of electrons are 1) **nicotinamide adenine dinucleotide** and 2) **flavin adenine dinucleotide.** Nicotinamide adenine dinucleotide is derived from the vitamin niacin (vitamin B_3), whereas flavin adenine dinucleotide comes from the vitamin riboflavin (B_2). The oxidized form of nicotinamide adenine dinucleotide is written as NAD^+, whereas the reduced form is written as NADH. Similarly, the oxidized form of flavin adenine dinucleotide is written as FAD, and the reduced form is abbreviated as FADH. Note that FADH can also accept a second hydrogen, forming $FADH_2$. Therefore, FADH and $FADH_2$ can be thought of as the same molecule because they undergo the same reactions. An illustration of how NADH is formed from the reduction of NAD^+ during a coupled oxidation-reduction reaction is shown in figure 3.5. Details of how NAD^+ and FAD function as "carrier molecules" during bioenergetic reactions are discussed later in this chapter in the section "Electron Transport Chain."

Enzymes

The speed of cellular chemical reactions is regulated by catalysts called **enzymes.** Enzymes are proteins that play a major role in the regulation of metabolic pathways in the cell. Enzymes do not cause a reaction

(a)

NAD$^+$ — Oxidized state   NADH — Reduced state

(b)

FAD — Oxidized state   FADH$_2$ — Reduced state

Figure 3.5 Structural formulas for NAD^+, NADH, FAD, and $FADH_2$. (a) When NAD^+ reacts with two hydrogen atoms, it binds to one of them and accepts the electron from the other. This is shown by two dots above the nitrogen ($\ddot{N}$) in the formula for NADH. (b) When FAD reacts with two hydrogen atoms to form $FADH_2$, it binds each of them to a nitrogen atom at the reaction sites.

Figure 3.6 Enzymes catalyze reactions by lowering the energy of activation. That is, the energy required to start the reaction is reduced. Note the difference in the energy of activation in the catalyzed reaction versus the noncatalyzed reaction.

Figure 3.7 The lock-and-key model of enzyme action: (a) The substrate (i.e., sucrose) approaches a pocket on the enzyme called the active site. (b) The substrate fits into the active site in the enzyme, forming an enzyme-substrate complex. (c) The enzyme then breaks the bond between the two sugars in sucrose and releases glucose and fructose (i.e., reaction products). The enzyme remains unchanged and is free to be used again.

to occur, but simply regulate the rate or speed at which the reaction takes place. Further, the enzyme does not change the nature of the reaction nor its final result.

Chemical reactions occur when the reactants have sufficient energy to proceed. The energy required to initiate chemical reactions is called the **activation energy** (8, 31). Enzymes work as catalysts by lowering the activation energy. The end result is to increase the rate at which these reactions take place. Figure 3.6 illustrates this concept. Note that the activation energy is greater in the noncatalyzed reaction on the left when compared to the enzyme-catalyzed reaction pictured on the right. By reducing the activation energy, enzymes increase the speed of chemical reactions and therefore increase the rate of product formation.

The ability of enzymes to lower the activation energy results from unique structural characteristics. In general, enzymes are large protein molecules with a three-dimensional shape. Each type of enzyme has characteristic ridges and grooves. The pockets that are formed from the ridges or grooves located on the enzyme are called active sites. These active sites are important because it is the unique shape of the active site that causes a specific enzyme to adhere to a particular reactant molecule (called a *substrate*). The concept of how enzymes fit with a particular substrate molecule is analogous to the idea of a lock and key (figure 3.7). The shape of the enzyme's active site is specific for the shape of a particular substrate, which allows the two molecules (enzyme + substrate) to form a complex known as the enzyme-substrate complex. After the formation of the enzyme-substrate complex, the energy of activation needed for the reaction to occur is lowered, and the reaction is more easily brought to completion. This is followed by the dissociation of the enzyme and the product. The ability of an enzyme to work as a catalyst is not constant and can be modified by several factors; this will be discussed shortly.

Note that cellular enzymes can often play a key role in diagnosing specific illnesses. For example, when tissues become damaged as a result of diseases, dead cells within these tissues can release enzymes into the blood. Many of these enzymes are not normally found in blood and therefore provide a clinical "clue" to diagnose the source of the illness. Details about the use of blood enzyme levels in the diagnosis of diseases are contained in Clinical Applications 3.1.

Classification of Enzymes In the early days of biochemistry, enzymes were named by the scientist who discovered the enzyme. Often these names did not provide a clue to the function of the enzyme. Therefore, to reduce confusion, an international committee developed a systematic naming system that names the enzyme according to the type of chemical reaction it catalyzes. In this scheme, enzymes are provided a systematic name and a numerical identification. In addition, a shorter version of the systematic name, called the recommended name, was provided for everyday use. With the exception of some older

Diagnostic Value of Measuring Enzyme Activity in the Blood

When tissues become diseased, dead cells often break open and release their enzymes into the blood. Because many of these intracellular enzymes are not normally found in blood, the presence of a specific enzyme in blood provides important diagnostic information regarding the source of the medical problem. In practice, the diagnostic test proceeds as follows. A doctor obtains a blood sample from the patient and forwards the sample to a clinical laboratory for analysis. The laboratory then determines the activity of a specific enzyme in a test tube by addition of the blood sample and appropriate substrates for the enzyme. The results of this test can often assist in making a diagnosis. For example, the finding that the blood sample contains high levels of the enzyme lactate dehydrogenase would suggest that the patient experienced a myocardial infarction (i.e., heart attack). Similarly, elevated blood levels of the enzyme creatine kinase would also indicate cardiac injury and would provide additional evidence that the patient suffered a heart attack. See table 3.1 for additional examples of the diagnostic usage for specific enzymes found in blood.

TABLE 3.1	Examples of the Diagnostic Value of Enzymes Found in Blood
Enzyme	**Diseases Associated with High Blood Levels of Enzyme**
Lactate dehydrogenase (cardiac-specific isoform)	Myocardial infarction
Creatine kinase	Myocardial infarction, muscular dystrophy
Alkaline phosphatase	Carcinoma of bone, Paget's disease, obstructive jaundice
Amylase	Pancreatitis, perforated peptic ulcer
Aldolase	Muscular dystrophy

enzyme names (e.g., pepsin, trysin, and rennin) all enzyme names end with the suffix "ase" and reflect both the job category of the enzyme and the reaction it catalyzes. For example, enzymes called kinases add a phosphate group (i.e., phosphorylate), a specific molecule. Other enzyme categories include dehydrogenases, which remove hydrogen atoms from their substrates, and oxidases, which catalyze oxidation-reduction reactions involving molecular oxygen. Enzymes called isomerases rearrange atoms within their substrate molecules to form structural isomers (i.e., molecules with the same molecular formula but with a different structural formula).

Factors That Alter Enzyme Activity The activity of an enzyme, as measured by the rate at which its substrates are converted into products, is influenced by several factors. Two of the more important factors include temperature and pH (pH is a measure of acidity or alkalinity) of the solution.

Individual enzymes have an optimum temperature at which they are most active. In general, a small rise in body temperature above normal (i.e., 37° C) increases the activity of most enzymes. This is useful during exercise because muscular work results in an increase in body temperature. The resulting elevation in enzyme activity would enhance bioenergetics (ATP production)

by speeding up the rate of reactions involved in the production of biologically useful energy. This point is illustrated in figure 3.8. Notice that enzyme activity is less than maximum at normal body temperature (37° C). Also, note that an exercise-induced increase in body temperature (e.g., 40° C) results in a temperature-induced increase in enzyme activity.

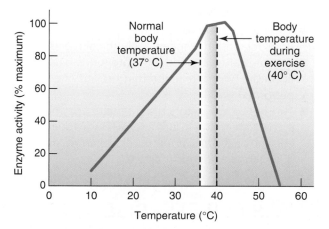

Figure 3.8 The effect of body temperature on enzyme activity. Notice that an optimal range of temperatures exists for enzyme activity. An increase or decrease in temperature away from the optimal temperature range results in diminished enzyme activity.

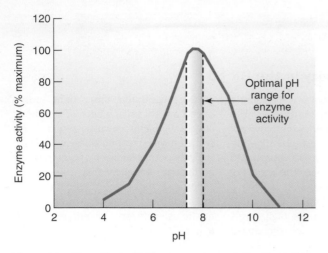

Figure 3.9 The effect of pH on enzyme activity. Note that every enzyme has a narrow range of optimal pH. An increase or decrease of pH away from this optimum range results in a decrease in enzyme activity.

The pH of body fluids also has a large effect on enzyme activity. The relationship between pH and enzyme activity is similar to the temperature/enzyme activity relationship; that is, individual enzymes have a pH optimum. If the pH is altered from the optimum, the enzyme activity is reduced (figure 3.9). This has important implications during exercise. For example, during intense exercise, skeletal muscles can produce large amounts of hydrogen ions (34). Accumulation of large quantities of hydrogen ions results in a decrease in the pH of body fluids below the optimum pH of important bioenergetic enzymes. The end result is a decreased ability to provide the energy (i.e., ATP) required for muscular contraction. In fact, extreme acidity is an important limiting factor in various types of intense exercise. This will be discussed again in chapters 10 and 19.

> ### IN SUMMARY
>
> - Enzymes that serve as catalysts for these reactions regulate the speed of chemical reactions.
> - Enzymes are classified into categories based upon the type of reaction that the enzyme performs.
> - Two important factors that regulate enzyme activity are temperature and pH. Individual enzymes have an optimum temperature and pH at which they are most active.

FUELS FOR EXERCISE

The body uses carbohydrate, fat, and protein nutrients consumed daily to provide the necessary energy to maintain cellular activities both at rest and during exercise. During exercise, the primary nutrients used for energy are fats and carbohydrates, with protein contributing a small amount of the total energy used (3).

Carbohydrates

Carbohydrates are composed of atoms of carbon, hydrogen, and oxygen. Stored carbohydrates provide the body with a rapidly available form of energy, with 1 gram of carbohydrate yielding approximately 4 kcal of energy (36). As mentioned earlier, plants synthesize carbohydrates from the interaction of CO_2, water, and solar energy in a process called photosynthesis. Carbohydrates exist in three forms (36): (1) monosaccharides, (2) disaccharides, and (3) polysaccharides. Monosaccharides are simple sugars such as glucose and fructose. **Glucose** is familiar to most of us and is often referred to as "blood sugar." It can be found in foods or can be formed in the digestive tract as a result of cleavage of more complex carbohydrates. Fructose is contained in fruits or honey and is considered to be the sweetest of the simple carbohydrates (33).

Disaccharides are formed by combining two monosaccharides. For example, table sugar is called sucrose and is composed of glucose and fructose. Maltose, also a disaccharide, is composed of two glucose molecules. Sucrose is considered to be the most common dietary disaccharide in the United States and constitutes approximately 25% of the total caloric intake of most Americans (28). It occurs naturally in many carbohydrates, such as cane sugar, beets, honey, and maple syrup.

Polysaccharides are complex carbohydrates that contain three or more monosaccharides. Polysaccharides may be rather small molecules (i.e., three monosaccharides) or relatively large molecules containing hundreds of monosaccharides. In general, polysaccharides are classified as either plant or animal polysaccharides. The two most common forms of plant polysaccharides are cellulose and starch. Humans lack the digestive enzymes necessary to digest cellulose, and thus cellulose is discarded as waste in the fecal material. On the other hand, starch—found in corn, grains, beans, potatoes, and peas—is easily digested by humans and is an important source of carbohydrate in the American diet (28). After ingestion, starch is broken down to form monosaccharides and may be used as energy immediately by cells or stored in another form within cells for future energy needs.

Glycogen is the term used for the polysaccharide stored in animal tissue. It is synthesized within cells by linking glucose molecules using the action of the enzyme glycogen synthase. Glycogen molecules are generally large and may consist of hundreds to thousands of glucose molecules. Cells store glycogen as a means of supplying carbohydrates as an energy source. For example, during exercise, individual muscle cells break down glycogen into glucose (this process is called **glycogenolysis**) and use the glucose as a source of energy for contraction. On the other hand, glycogenolysis also occurs in the liver, with the free glucose being released into the bloodstream and transported to tissues throughout the body.

Important to exercise metabolism is that glycogen is stored in both muscle fibers and the liver. However, total glycogen stores in the body are relatively small and can be depleted within a few hours as a result of prolonged exercise. Therefore, glycogen synthesis is an ongoing process within cells. Diets low in carbohydrates tend to hamper glycogen synthesis, whereas high-carbohydrate diets enhance glycogen synthesis (see chapter 23).

Fats

Although fats contain the same chemical elements as carbohydrates, the ratio of carbon to oxygen in fats is much greater than that found in carbohydrates. Stored body fat is an ideal fuel for prolonged exercise because fat molecules contain large quantities of energy per unit of weight. One gram of fat contains about 9 kcal of energy, which is more than twice the energy content of either carbohydrates or protein (33). Fats are insoluble in water and can be found in both plants and animals. In general, fats can be classified into four general groups: (1) fatty acids, (2) triglycerides, (3) phospholipids, and (4) steroids. Fatty acids consist of long chains of carbon atoms linked to a carboxyl group at one end (a carboxyl group contains a carbon, oxygen, and hydrogen group) Importantly, fatty acids are the primary type of fat used by muscle cells for energy.

Fatty acids are stored in the body as triglycerides. Triglycerides are composed of three molecules of fatty acids and one molecule of glycerol (not a fat but a type of alcohol). Although the largest storage site for triglycerides is fat cells, these molecules are also stored in many cell types, including skeletal muscle. In times of need, they can be broken down into their component parts, with fatty acids being used as energy substrates by muscle and other tissues. The process of breaking down triglycerides into fatty acids and glycerol is termed *lipolysis* and is regulated by a family of enzymes called *lipases*. The glycerol released by lipolysis is not a direct energy source for muscle, but can be used by the liver to synthesize glucose. Therefore, the entire triglyceride molecule is a useful source of energy for the body.

Phospholipids are not used as an energy source by skeletal muscle during exercise (17). Phospholipids are lipids combined with phosphoric acid and are synthesized in virtually every cell in the body. The biological roles of phospholipids vary from providing the structural integrity of cell membranes to providing an insulating sheath around nerve fibers (10).

The final classification of fats is the steroids. Again, these fats are not used as energy sources during exercise, but will be mentioned briefly to provide a clearer understanding of the nature of biological fats. The most common steroid is cholesterol. Cholesterol is a component of all cell membranes. It can be synthesized in every cell in the body and, of course, can be consumed in foods. In addition to its role in membrane structure, cholesterol is needed for the synthesis of the sex hormones estrogen, progesterone, and testosterone (10). Although cholesterol has many "useful" biological functions, high blood cholesterol levels have been implicated in the development of coronary artery disease (38) (see chapter 18).

Proteins

Proteins are composed of many tiny subunits called amino acids. At least twenty types of amino acids are needed by the body to form various tissues, enzymes, blood proteins, and so on. Nine amino acids, called essential amino acids, cannot be synthesized by the body and therefore must be consumed in foods. Proteins are formed by linking amino acids by chemical bonds called peptide bonds. As a potential fuel source, proteins contain approximately 4 kcal per gram (8). For proteins to be used as substrates for the formation of high-energy compounds, they must be broken down into their constituent amino acids. Proteins can contribute energy for exercise in two ways. First, the amino acid alanine can be converted in the liver to glucose, which can then be used to synthesize glycogen. Liver glycogen can be degraded into glucose and transported to working skeletal muscle via the circulation. Second, many amino acids (e.g., isoleucine, alanine, leucine, valine) can be converted into metabolic intermediates (i.e., compounds that may directly participate in bioenergetics) in muscle cells and directly contribute as fuel in the bioenergetic pathways (12).

IN SUMMARY

- The body uses carbohydrate, fat, and protein nutrients consumed daily to provide the necessary energy to maintain cellular activities both at rest and during exercise. During exercise, the primary nutrients used for energy are fats and carbohydrates, with protein contributing a relatively small amount of the total energy used.
- Glucose is stored in animal cells as a polysaccharide called glycogen.
- Fatty acids are the primary form of fat used as an energy source in cells. Fatty acids are stored as triglycerides in muscle and fat cells.
- Proteins are composed of amino acids, and twenty different amino acids are required to form the various proteins contained in cells. The use of protein as an energy source requires that cellular proteins be broken down into amino acids.

HIGH-ENERGY PHOSPHATES

The immediate source of energy for muscular contraction is the high-energy phosphate compound **adenosine triphosphate (ATP)** (33). Although ATP is not the only energy-carrying molecule in the cell, it is the most important one, and without sufficient amounts of ATP most cells die quickly.

Figure 3.10 at top portion:

Adenosine diphosphate (ADP)

+

Inorganic phosphate (P$_i$)

↓

Adenosine triphosphate (ATP)

Figure 3.10 The structural formation of adenosine triphosphate (ATP).

The structure of ATP consists of three main parts: (1) an adenine portion, (2) a ribose portion, and (3) three linked phosphates (figure 3.10). The formation of ATP occurs by combining **adenosine diphosphate (ADP)** and **inorganic phosphate (P$_i$)** and requires a rather large amount of energy. Some of this energy is stored in the chemical bond joining ADP and P$_i$. Accordingly, this bond is called a high-energy bond. When the enzyme **ATPase** breaks this bond, energy is released, and this energy can be used to do work (e.g., muscular contraction):

$$\text{ATP} \xrightarrow{\text{ATPase}} \text{ADP} + \text{P}_i + \text{Energy}$$

ATP is often called the universal energy donor. It couples the energy released from the breakdown of foodstuffs into a usable form of energy required by all cells. For example, figure 3.11 presents a model depicting ATP as the universal energy donor in the cell. The cell uses exergonic reactions (breakdown of foodstuffs) to form ATP via endergonic reactions. This newly formed ATP can then be used to drive the energy-requiring processes in the cell. Therefore, energy-liberating reactions are linked to energy-requiring reactions like two meshed gears.

BIOENERGETICS

Muscle cells store limited amounts of ATP. Therefore, because muscular exercise requires a constant supply of ATP to provide the energy needed for contraction, metabolic pathways must exist in the cell with the capability to produce ATP rapidly. Indeed, muscle cells can produce ATP by any one or a combination of

Figure 3.11 A model of ATP as the universal energy carrier of the cell. Exergonic reactions are shown as blue gears with arrows going down (these reactions produce a decrease in free energy); endergonic reactions are shown as green gears with arrows going up (these reaction produced an increase in free energy).

three metabolic pathways: (1) formation of ATP by **phosphocreatine (PC)** breakdown, (2) formation of ATP via the degradation of glucose or glycogen (called glycolysis), and (3) oxidative formation of ATP. Formation of ATP via the PC pathway and glycolysis does not involve the use of O_2; these pathways are called **anaerobic** (without O_2) pathways. Oxidative formation of ATP by the use of O_2 is termed **aerobic** metabolism. A detailed discussion of the operation of the three metabolic pathways involved in the formation of ATP during exercise follows.

Anaerobic ATP Production

The simplest and, consequently, the most rapid method of producing ATP involves the donation of a phosphate group and its bond energy from PC to ADP to form ATP (33, 36, 37):

$$PC + ADP \xrightarrow{\text{Creatine kinase}} ATP + C$$

The reaction is catalyzed by the enzyme creatine kinase. As rapidly as ATP is broken down to ADP + P_i

at the onset of exercise, ATP is resynthesized via the PC reaction. However, muscle cells store only small amounts of PC, and thus the total amount of ATP that can be formed via this reaction is limited. The combination of stored ATP and PC is called the **ATP-PC system** or the "phosphagen system." It provides energy for muscular contraction at the onset of exercise and during short-term, high-intensity exercise (i.e., lasting fewer than 5 seconds). PC reformation requires ATP and occurs only during recovery from exercise (11).

The importance of the ATP-PC system in athletics can be appreciated by considering short-term, intense exercise such as sprinting 50 meters, high jumping, performing a rapid weight-lifting move, or a football player racing 10 yards downfield. All these activities require only a few seconds to complete and thus need a rapid supply of ATP. The ATP-PC system provides a simple one-enzyme reaction to produce ATP for these types of activities. The fact that depletion of PC is likely to limit short-term, high-intensity exercise has led to the suggestion that ingesting large amounts of creatine can improve exercise performance (see The Winning Edge 3.1).

THE WINNING EDGE 3.1

Exercise Physiology Applied to Sports

Does Creatine Supplementation Improve Exercise Performance?

The depletion of phosphocreatine (PC) may limit exercise performance during short-term, high-intensity exercise (e.g., 100- to 200-meter dash) because the depletion of PC results in a reduction in the rate of ATP production by the ATP-PC system. Studies have shown that ingestion of large amounts of creatine monohydrate (20 grams/day) over a 5-day period results in increased stores of muscle PC (2, 6, 14, 19, 26, 39). This creatine supplementation has been shown to improve performance in laboratory settings during short-duration (e.g., 30 seconds), high-intensity stationary cycling exercise (14, 19, 24, 26, 39). However, results on the influence of creatine supplementation on performance during short-duration running and swimming are not consistent (2, 14, 19, 26, 39). This may be due to the fact that creatine supplementation results in a weight gain due to water retention. Therefore,

this increase in body weight may impair performance in weight-bearing activities such as running.

Studies suggest that creatine supplementation in conjunction with resistance exercise training results in an enhanced physiologic adaptation to weight training (2, 5, 15, 23, 32, 39). Specifically, these studies indicate that creatine supplementation combined with resistance training promotes an increase in both dynamic muscular strength and fat-free mass. Nonetheless, whether creatine supplementation improves isokinetic or isometric muscular strength remains controversial (2).

Does oral creatine supplementation result in adverse physiological side effects and pose health risks? Unfortunately, a definitive answer to this question is not available. Although anecdotal reports indicate that creatine supplementation can be associated with negative side effects such as nausea, neurological dysfunction, minor gastrointestinal distress, and muscle cramping, these reports are not well documented

(2, 7, 14, 20, 39). At present, due to limited data, a firm conclusion about the long-term health risks of creatine supplementation cannot be reached. However, current evidence suggests that creatine supplementation for up to eight weeks does not appear to produce major health risks, but the safety of more prolonged creatine supplementation has not been established.

An important issue related to the use of creatine and other dietary supplements is the possibility of contamination within the product; that is, the supplement product may contain other chemical compounds in addition to creatine (27). Indeed, this is an important safety issue in the "over-the-counter supplement" industry because a large study has reported a high level of variability in the purity of over-the-counter products (27). For more information on creatine and exercise performance, see Bemben and Lamont (2005) and Hespel and Derave (2007) in the Suggested Readings.

A CLOSER LOOK 3.2

Lactic Acid or Lactate?

In many textbooks, the terms "lactic acid" and "lactate" are used interchangeably. This is often confusing to students who ask, "Are lactic acid and lactate the same molecule?" The answer is that lactic acid and lactate are related but are technically different molecules. Here's the explanation: The term *lactate* refers to the salt of lactic acid (figure 3.12) (4). You may recall from another science course that when acids dissociate and release hydrogen ions, the remaining molecule is called the *conjugate base* of the acid. It follows that lactate is the conjugate base of lactic acid. Because of the close relationship between lactic acid and lactate, many authors use these terms interchangeably (3). Remembering the relationship between lactic acid and lactate will reduce confusion when you read about these molecules in future chapters within this text.

FIGURE 3.12 The ionization of lactic acid forms the conjugate base called lactate. At normal body pH, lactic acid will rapidly dissociate to form lactate.

A second metabolic pathway capable of producing ATP rapidly without the involvement of O_2 is termed **glycolysis.** Glycolysis involves the breakdown of glucose or glycogen to form two molecules of pyruvate or **lactate** (figure 3.13). Simply stated, glycolysis is an anaerobic pathway used to transfer bond energy from glucose to rejoin P_i to ADP. This process involves a series of enzymatically catalyzed, coupled reactions. Glycolysis occurs in the sarcoplasm of the muscle cell and produces a net gain of two molecules of ATP and two molecules of pyruvate or lactate per glucose molecule (see A Closer Look 3.2).

Let's consider glycolysis in more detail. First, the reactions between glucose and pyruvate can be considered as two distinct phases: (1) an energy investment phase, and (2) an energy generation phase (figure 3.13). The first five reactions make up the "energy investment phase" where stored ATP must be used to form sugar phosphates. Although the end result of glycolysis is energy producing (exergonic), glycolysis must be "primed" by the addition of ATP at two points at the beginning of the pathway (figures 3.14 and 3.15). The purpose of the ATP priming is to add phosphate groups (called phosphorylation) to glucose and to fructose 6-phosphate. Note that if glycolysis begins with glycogen as the substrate, the addition of only one ATP is required. That is, glycogen does not require phosphorylation by ATP, but is phosphorylated by inorganic phosphate instead (figure 3.14). The last five reactions of glycolysis represent the "energy generation phase" of glycolysis. Figure 3.15 points out that two molecules of ATP are produced at each of two separate reactions near the

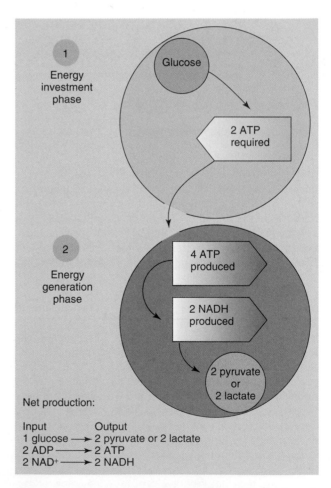

Net production:

Input	Output
1 glucose →	2 pyruvate or 2 lactate
2 ADP →	2 ATP
2 NAD+ →	2 NADH

Figure 3.13 Illustration of the two phases of glycolysis and the products of glycolysis. From *Biochemistry* by Mathews and van Holde. Copyright © 1990 by The Benjamin/Cummings Publishing Company. Reprinted by permission.

Figure 3.14 Illustration of the interaction between blood glucose and muscle glycogen for the provision of glucose for glycolysis. Regardless of the source of glucose for glycolysis, glucose must be phosphorylated to form glucose 6-phosphate as the first step in glycolysis. Note, however, that phosphorylation of glucose obtained from the blood requires 1 ATP, whereas the phosphorylation of glucose obtained from glycogen is achieved by using inorganic phosphate (P_i) located in the cell.

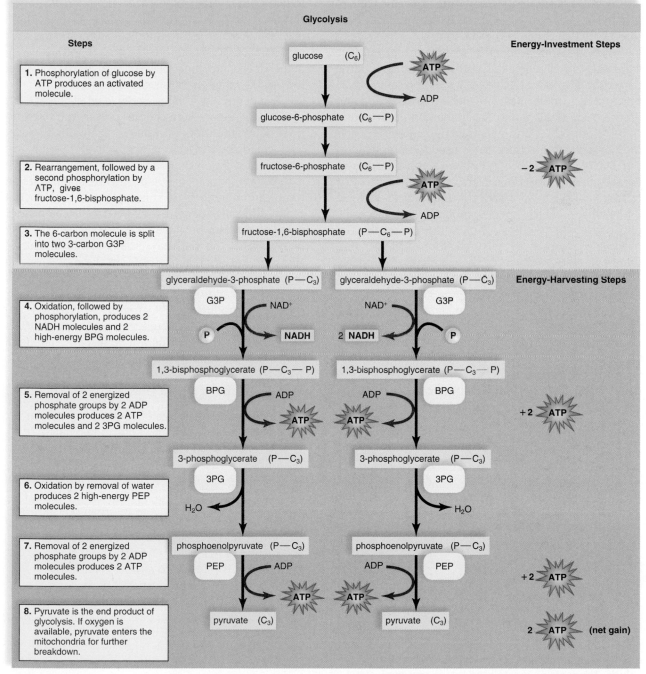

Figure 3.15 Summary of the anaerobic metabolism of glucose. Note that the end result of the anaerobic breakdown of one molecule of glucose is the production of two molecules of ATP and two molecules of pyruvate.

A CLOSER LOOK 3.3

NADH Is "Shuttled" into Mitochondria

NADH generated during glycolysis must be converted back to NAD$^+$ if glycolysis is to continue. As discussed in the text, the conversion of NADH to NAD$^+$ can occur by pyruvate accepting the hydrogens (forming lactate) or "shuttling" the hydrogens from NADH across the mitochondrial membrane. The "shuttling" of hydrogens across the mitochondrial membrane requires a specific transport system. Figure 4.9 (see chapter 4) illustrates this process. This transport system is located within the mitochondrial membrane and transfers NADH-released hydrogens from the cytosol into the mitochondria, where they can enter the electron transport chain.

end of the glycolytic pathway; thus, the net gain of glycolysis is two ATP if glucose is the substrate and three ATP if glycogen is the substrate.

Hydrogens are frequently removed from nutrient substrates in bioenergetic pathways and are transported by "carrier molecules." Two biologically important carrier molecules are nicotinamide adenine dinucleotide (NAD$^+$) and flavin adenine dinucleotide (FAD). Both NAD$^+$ and FAD transport hydrogens and their associated electrons to be used for later generation of ATP in the mitochondrion via aerobic processes. For the chemical reactions in glycolysis to proceed, two hydrogens must be removed from glyceraldehyde 3-phosphate, which then combines with inorganic phosphate (P$_i$) to form 1,3-diphosphoglycerate. The hydrogen acceptor in this reaction is NAD$^+$ (figure 3.15). Here, NAD$^+$ accepts one of the hydrogens, while the remaining hydrogen is free in solution. Upon accepting the hydrogen, NAD$^+$ is converted to its reduced form, NADH. Adequate amounts of NAD$^+$ must be available to accept the hydrogen atoms that must be removed from glyceraldehyde 3-phosphate if glycolysis is to continue (3, 31). How is NAD$^+$ reformed from NADH? There are two ways that the cell restores NAD$^+$ from NADH. First, if sufficient oxygen (O$_2$) is available, the hydrogens from NADH can be "shuttled" into the mitochondria of the cell and can contribute to the aerobic production of ATP (see A Closer Look 3.3). Second, if O$_2$ is not available to accept the hydrogens in the mitochondria, pyruvate can accept the hydrogens

to form lactate (figure 3.16). The enzyme that catalyzes this reaction is lactate dehydrogenase (LDH), with the end result being the formation of lactate and the reformation of NAD$^+$. Therefore, the reason for lactate formation is the "recycling" of NAD$^+$ (i.e., NADH converted to NAD$^+$) so that glycolysis can continue.

Again, glycolysis is the breakdown of glucose into pyruvate or lactate with the net production of two or three ATP, depending on whether the pathway began with glucose or glycogen, respectively. Figure 3.15 summarizes glycolysis in a simple flowchart. Glucose is a six-carbon molecule, and pyruvate and lactate are three-carbon molecules. This explains the production of two molecules of pyruvate or lactate from one molecule of glucose. Because O$_2$ is not directly involved in glycolysis, the pathway is considered anaerobic. However, in the presence of O$_2$ in the mitochondria, pyruvate can participate in the aerobic production of ATP. Thus, in addition to being an anaerobic pathway capable of producing ATP without O$_2$, glycolysis can be considered the first step in the aerobic degradation of carbohydrates. This will be discussed in detail in the next section, "Aerobic ATP Production."

IN SUMMARY

- The immediate source of energy for muscular contraction is the high-energy phosphate ATP. ATP is degraded via the enzyme ATPase as follows:

$$ATP \xrightarrow{ATPase} ADP + P_i + Energy$$

- Formation of ATP without the use of O$_2$ is termed *anaerobic metabolism*. In contrast, the production of ATP using O$_2$ as the final electron acceptor is referred to as *aerobic metabolism*.
- Muscle cells can produce ATP by any one or a combination of three metabolic pathways: (1) ATP-PC system, (2) glycolysis, and (3) oxidative formation of ATP.
- The ATP-PC system and glycolysis are two anaerobic metabolic pathways that are capable of producing ATP without O$_2$.

Figure 3.16 The addition of hydrogen atoms to pyruvate forms lactate and NAD$^+$, which can be used again in glycolysis. The reaction is catalyzed by the enzyme lactate dehydrogenase (LDH).

Hans Krebs and the Discovery of the "Krebs Cycle"

Hans Krebs (1900–1981) received the Nobel Prize for Physiology or Medicine in 1953 for his research on a series of important chemical reactions in cells that became known as the "Krebs cycle." Krebs was born in Germany and earned his MD degree from the University of Hamburg in 1925. After graduation from medical school, he moved to Berlin to study chemistry and became actively involved in biochemical research. The son of a Jewish physician, Hans Krebs was forced to leave Nazi Germany in 1933 for England. Upon arrival in England, Dr. Krebs continued his research at Cambridge University and later at the University of Sheffield and Oxford University.

During his distinguished research career, Hans Krebs made many important contributions to physiology and biochemistry. One of his first significant areas of research was how protein is metabolized in cells. An important outcome of this early work was the finding that the liver produces a nitrogenous waste product of protein metabolism called urea. Further work by Dr. Krebs and his colleague Kurt Henseleit (another German biochemist) led to the discovery of the series of reactions that produce urea (later known as the urea cycle).

Although Dr. Krebs's research on protein metabolism was important, he is best known for his discovery of the cellular reactions involving the substances formed from the breakdown of carbohydrates, fats, and proteins in the body. Specifically, in 1937, Dr. Krebs discovered the existence of a cycle of chemical reactions that combines the end product of carbohydrate breakdown (this product was later named acetyl-CoA) with oxaloacetic acid to form citric acid. Dr. Krebs's work showed that this cycle regenerates oxaloacetic acid through a series of intermediate compounds while liberating carbon dioxide and electrons. This cycle has been known by three different names, including the citric acid cycle and the tricarboxylic acid cycle. However, many biochemists (and this textbook) refer to this cycle as the Krebs cycle in recognition of Hans Krebs's contribution to this important discovery. The discovery of the Krebs cycle and how chemical foodstuffs are converted into usable energy was of vital importance to our basic understanding of cellular energy metabolism and paved the way for exercise physiologists to further investigate skeletal muscle bioenergetics during exercise.

Aerobic ATP Production

Aerobic production of ATP occurs inside the mitochondria and involves the interaction of two cooperating metabolic pathways: (1) the **Krebs cycle** and (2) the **electron transport chain.** The primary function of the Krebs cycle (also called the citric acid cycle) is to complete the oxidation (hydrogen removal) of carbohydrates, fats, or proteins using NAD^+ and FAD as hydrogen (energy) carriers. The importance of hydrogen removal is that hydrogens (by virtue of the electrons that they possess) contain the potential energy in the food molecules. This energy can be used in the electron transport chain to combine ADP + P_i to reform ATP. Oxygen does not participate in the reactions of the Krebs cycle but is the final hydrogen acceptor at the end of the electron transport chain (i.e., water is formed, $H_2 + O \rightarrow H_2O$). The process of aerobic production of ATP is termed oxidative phosphorylation. It is convenient to think of aerobic ATP production as a three-stage process (figure 3.17). Stage 1 is the generation of a key two-carbon molecule, acetyl-CoA. Stage 2 is the oxidation of acetyl-CoA in the Krebs cycle. Stage 3 is the process of **oxidative phosphorylation** (i.e., ATP formation) in the electron transport chain (i.e., respiratory chain). A detailed look at the Krebs cycle and electron transport chain follows.

Krebs Cycle The Krebs cycle is named after the biochemist Hans Krebs, whose pioneering research has increased our understanding of this rather complex pathway (see A Look Back—Important People in Science). Entry into the Krebs cycle requires preparation of a two-carbon molecule, acetyl-CoA. **Acetyl-CoA** can be formed from the breakdown of carbohydrates, fats, or proteins (figure 3.17). For the moment, let's focus on the formation of acetyl-CoA from pyruvate (pyruvate can be formed from both carbohydrates and proteins). Figure 3.18 depicts the cyclic nature of the reactions involved in the Krebs cycle. Note that pyruvate (three-carbon molecule) is broken down to form acetyl-CoA (two-carbon molecule), and the remaining carbon is given off as CO_2. Next, acetyl-CoA combines with oxaloacetate (four-carbon molecule) to form citrate (six carbons). What follows is a series of reactions to regenerate oxaloacetate and two molecules of CO_2, and the pathway begins all over again.

For every molecule of glucose entering glycolysis, two molecules of pyruvate are formed, and in the presence of O_2, they are converted to two molecules of acetyl-CoA. This means that each molecule of glucose results in two turns of the Krebs cycle. With this in mind, let's examine the Krebs cycle in more detail. The primary function of the Krebs cycle is to

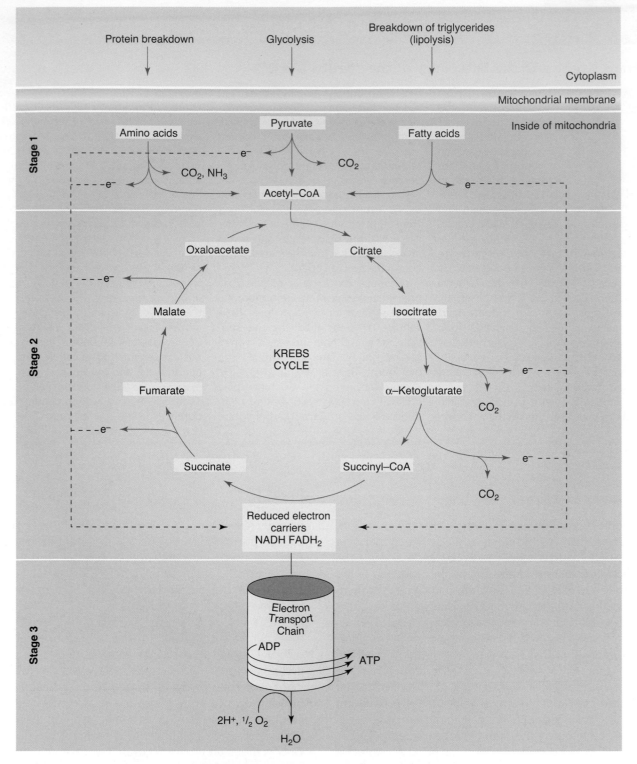

Figure 3.17 The three stages of oxidative phosphorylation. From Mathews and van Holde, B*iochemistry*, Diane Bowen, Ed. Copyright © 1990 Benjamin/Cummings Publishing Company, Menlo Park, CA. Reprinted by permission.

remove hydrogens and the energy associated with those hydrogens from various substrates involved in the cycle. Figure 3.18 illustrates that during each turn of the Krebs cycle, three molecules of NADH and one molecule of FADH are formed. For every pair of electrons passed through the electron transport chain from NADH to oxygen, enough energy is available to form 2.5 molecules of ATP (10). For every FADH molecule that is formed, enough energy is available to produce 1.5 molecules of ATP. Thus, in terms of ATP production, FADH is not as energy rich as NADH.

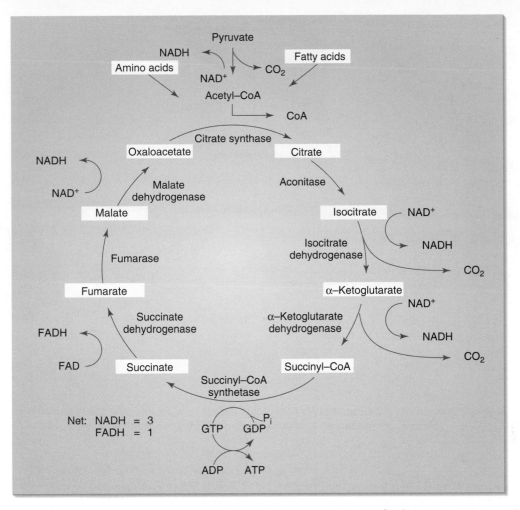

Figure 3.18 Compounds, enzymes, and reactions involved in the Krebs cycle. Note the formation of three molecules of NADH and one molecule of FADH per turn of the cycle.

In addition to the production of NADH and FADH, the Krebs cycle results in direct formation of an energy-rich compound, guanosine triphosphate (GTP) (figure 3.18). GTP is a high-energy compound that can transfer its terminal phosphate group to ADP to form ATP. The direct formation of GTP in the Krebs cycle is called substrate-level phosphorylation. It accounts for only a small amount of the total energy conversion in the Krebs cycle because most of the Krebs cycle energy yield (i.e., NADH and FADH) is taken to the electron transport chain to form ATP.

Up to this point we have focused on the role that carbohydrates play in producing acetyl-CoA to enter the Krebs cycle. How do fats and proteins undergo aerobic metabolism? The answer can be found in figure 3.19. Note that fats (triglycerides) are broken down to form fatty acids and glycerol. These fatty acids can then undergo a series of reactions to form acetyl-CoA (called beta oxidation; see A Closer Look 3.4 for details) and thus enter the Krebs cycle (8). Although glycerol can be converted into an intermediate of glycolysis in the liver, this does not occur to a great extent in human skeletal muscle. Therefore, glycerol is not an important direct muscle fuel source during exercise (13, 16).

As mentioned previously, protein is not considered a major fuel source during exercise, because it contributes only 2% to 15% of the fuel during exercise (9, 13, 25). Proteins can enter bioenergetic pathways in a variety of places. However, the first step is the breakdown of the protein into its amino acid subunits. What happens next depends on which amino acid is involved. For example, some amino acids can be converted to glucose or pyruvate, some to acetyl-CoA, and still others to Krebs-cycle intermediates. The role of proteins in bioenergetics is summarized in figure 3.19.

In summary, the Krebs cycle completes the oxidation of carbohydrates, fats, or proteins; produces CO_2; and supplies electrons to be passed through the electron transport chain to provide the energy for the aerobic production of ATP. Enzymes catalyzing Krebs-cycle reactions are located inside the mitochondria.

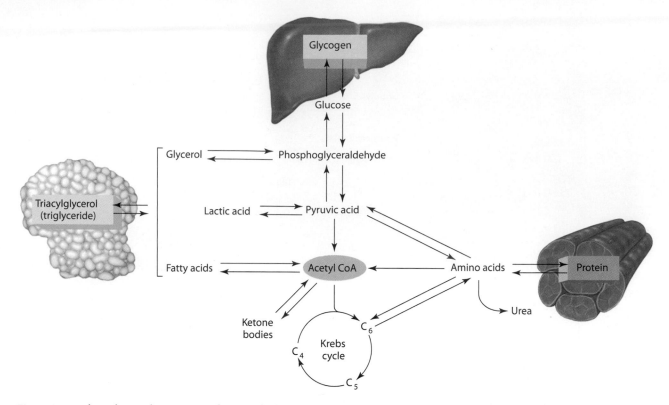

Figure 3.19 The relationships among the metabolism of proteins, carbohydrates, and fats. The overall interaction between the metabolic breakdown of these three foodstuffs is often referred to as the metabolic pool.

Electron Transport Chain The aerobic production of ATP (called oxidative phosphorylation) occurs in the mitochondria. The pathway responsible for this process is called the **electron transport chain** (also called the respiratory chain or cytochrome chain). Aerobic production of ATP is possible due to a mechanism that uses the potential energy available in reduced hydrogen carriers such as NADH and FADH to rephosphorylate ADP to ATP. The reduced hydrogen carriers do not directly react with oxygen. Instead, electrons removed from the hydrogen atoms are passed down a series of electron carriers known as cytochromes. During this passage of electrons down the cytochrome chain, enough energy is released to rephosphorylate ADP to form ATP at three sites (8) (figure 3.20). Interestingly, as electrons pass down the electron transport chain, highly reactive molecules called *free radicals* are formed. However, increased rates of electron flow through the electron transport chain do not increase in the rate of radical production in the mitochondrion (see Research Focus 3.1).

The hydrogen carriers that bring the electrons to the electron transport chain come from a variety of sources. Recall that two NADH are formed per glucose molecule that is degraded via glycolysis (figure 3.15). These NADH are outside the mitochondria, and their hydrogens must be transported across the mitochondrial membrane by special "shuttle" mechanisms. However, the bulk of the electrons that enter the electron transport chain come from those NADH and FADH molecules formed as a result of Krebs-cycle oxidation.

Figure 3.20 outlines the pathway for electrons entering the electron transport chain. Pairs of electrons from NADH or FADH are passed down a series of compounds that undergo oxidation and reduction, with enough energy being released to synthesize ATP at three places along the way. Notice that FADH enters the cytochrome pathway at a point just below the entry level for NADH (figure 3.20). This is important because the level of FADH entry bypasses one of the sites of ATP formation, and thus each molecule of FADH that enters the electron transport chain has enough energy to form only 1.5 ATP. In contrast, NADH entry into the electron transport chain results in the formation of 2.5 ATP (details will be mentioned later). At the end of the electron transport chain, oxygen accepts the electrons that are passed along and combines with hydrogen to form water. If O_2 is not available to accept those electrons, oxidative phosphorylation is not possible, and ATP formation in the cell must occur via anaerobic metabolism.

How does this ATP formation occur? The mechanism to explain the aerobic formation of ATP is known as the **chemiosmotic hypothesis.** As electrons are

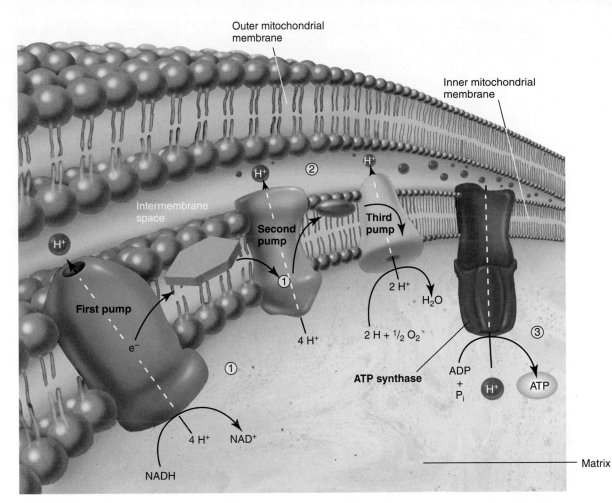

Figure 3.20 The steps leading to oxidative phosphorylation in the mitochondria. (1) Molecules within the electron transport chain function to pump H$^+$ from the mitochondrial matrix into the intermembrane space. (2) This results in an increased concentration of H$^+$ ions in the intermembrane space and therefore, a large H$^+$ gradient between the intermembrane space and the matrix of the mitochondria. (3) The movement of H$^+$ through the ATP synthase provides the energy required to produce ATP.

RESEARCH FOCUS 3.1

Free Radicals Are Formed in the Mitochondria

Although the passage of electrons down the electron transport chain performs an essential role in the process of aerobic ATP production, this pathway also produces free radicals (30) . Free radicals are molecules that have an unpaired electron in their outer orbital, which makes them highly reactive. That is, free radicals quickly react with other molecules in the cell, and this combi-

nation results in damage to the molecule combining with the radical.

Historically, it was believed that increased aerobic metabolism during exercise promotes increased production of free radicals in the mitochondria of the working muscles (30). However, new research indicates that this is not the case. Indeed, although exercise results in increased produc-

tion of free radicals in the active skeletal muscles, this increase in muscle free radical production is not due to oxidative phosphorylation in the mitochondrion (22). For additional information on the sources of free radical production during exercise, see Powers et al. (2008) in the Suggested Readings.

Beta Oxidation Is the Process of Converting Fatty Acids to Acetyl-CoA

Fats are stored in the body in the form of triglycerides within fat cells or in the muscle fiber itself. Release of fat from these storage depots occurs by the breakdown of triglycerides, which results in the liberation of fatty acids (see chapter 4). However, for fatty acids to be used as a fuel during aerobic metabolism, they must first be converted to acetyl-CoA. **Beta oxidation** is the process of oxidizing fatty acids to form acetyl-CoA. This occurs in the mitochondria and involves a series of enzymatically catalyzed steps, starting with an "activated fatty acid" and ending with the production of acetyl-CoA.

A simple illustration of this process is presented in figure 3.21. This process begins with the "activation" of the fatty acid; the activated fatty acid is then transported into the mitochondria, where the process of beta oxidation begins. In short, beta oxidation is a sequence of four reactions that "chops" fatty acids into two carbon fragments forming acetyl-CoA. Once formed, acetyl-CoA then becomes a fuel source for the Krebs cycle and leads to the production of ATP via the electron transport chain.

FIGURE 3.21 Illustration of beta oxidation. Beta oxidation occurs in the mitochondria and is the process of converting fatty acids into acetyl-CoA. The process begins after an activated fatty acid (i.e., fatty acyl-CoA) is transported into the mitochondria. This fatty acyl-CoA is broken into two carbon fragments, forming acetyl-CoA. This acetyl-CoA then enters the Krebs cycle and provides an energy source for the production of ATP within the electron transport chain.

transferred along the cytochrome chain, the energy released is used to "pump" hydrogens (protons; H^+) released from NADH and FADH from the inside of the mitochondria across the inner mitochondrial membrane (figure 3.20). This results in an accumulation of hydrogen ions within the space between the inner and outer mitochondrial membranes. The accumulation of H^+ is a source of potential energy that can be captured and used to recombine P_i with ADP to form ATP (17). For example, this collection of H^+ is similar to the potential energy of water at the top of a dam; when the water accumulates and runs over the top of

the dam, falling water becomes kinetic energy, which can be used to do work (17).

Three pumps move H^+ (i.e., protons) from mitochondrial matrix to the intermembrane space (figure 3.20). The first pump (using NADH) moves four H^+ into the intermembrane space for every two electrons that move along the electron transport chain. The second pump also transports four H^+ into the intermembrane space, while the third pump moves only two H^+ into the intermembrane space. As a result, there is a higher concentration of H^+ within the intermembrane space compared to that in the matrix; this gradient creates a strong drive for these H^+ to diffuse back into the matrix. However, because the inner mitochondrial membrane is not permeable to H^+, these ions can cross the membrane only through specialized H^+ channels (called *respiratory assemblies*). This idea is illustrated in figure 3.20. Notice that as H^+ cross the inner mitochondrial membrane through these channels, ATP is formed from the addition of phosphate to ADP (called *phosphorylation*). This occurs because the movement of H^+ across the inner mitochondrial membrane activates the enzyme ATP synthase, which is responsible for catalyzing the reaction:

$$ADP + P_i \rightarrow ATP$$

So, why is oxygen essential for the aerobic production of ATP? Remember that the purpose of the electron transport chain is to move electrons down a series of cytochromes to provide energy to drive ATP production in the mitochondria. This process, illustrated in figure 3.20, requires each element in the electron transport chain to undergo a series of oxidation-reduction reactions. If the last cytochrome (i.e., cytochrome a_3) remains in a reduced state, it would be unable to accept more electrons, and the electron transport chain would stop. However, when oxygen is present, the last cytochrome in the chain can be oxidized by oxygen. That is, oxygen, derived from the air we breathe, allows electron transport to continue by functioning as the final electron acceptor of the electron transport chain. This oxidizes cytochrome a3 and allows electron transport and oxidative phosphorylation to continue. At the last step in the electron transport chain, oxygen accepts two electrons that were passed along the electron transport chain from either NADH or FADH. This reduced oxygen molecule now binds with two protons (H^+) to form water (figure 3.20).

As mentioned earlier, NADH and FADH differ in the amount of ATP that can be formed from each of these molecules. Each NADH formed in the mitochondria donates two electrons to the electron transport system at the first proton pump (figure 3.20). These electrons are then passed to the second and third proton pumps until these electrons are finally passed along to oxygen. The first and second electron pumps transport four protons each, whereas the third electron pump transports two protons, for a total of ten. Because four protons are required to produce and transport one ATP from the mitochondria to the cytoplasm, the total ATP production from one NADH molecule is 2.5 ATP (10 protons/4 protons per ATP = 2.5 ATP). Note that ATP molecules do not exist in halves and that the decimal fraction of ATP indicates an average number of ATP molecules that are produced per NADH.

Compared to NADH, each FADH molecule produces less ATP because the electrons from FADH are donated later in the electron transport chain than those by NADH (figure 3.20). Therefore, the electrons from FADH activate only the second and third proton pumps. Because the first proton pump is bypassed, the electrons from FADH result in the pumping of six protons (four by the second pump and two by the third pump). Because four protons are required to produce and transport one ATP from the mitochondria to the cytoplasm, the total ATP production from one FAD molecule is 1.5 ATP (6 protons/4 protons per ATP = 1.5 ATP). See A Closer Look 3.5 for more details on the quantity of ATP produced in cells.

A CLOSER LOOK 3.5

A New Look at the ATP Balance Sheet

Historically, it was believed that aerobic metabolism of one molecule of glucose resulted in the production of thirty-eight ATP. However, more recent evidence indicates that this number overestimates the total ATP production and that only thirty-two molecules of ATP actually reach the cytoplasm . The explanation for this conclusion is that new evidence indicates that the energy provided by NADH and FADH is required not only for ATP production but also to transport ATP across the mitochondrial membrane. This added energy cost of ATP metabolism reduces the estimates of the total ATP yield from glucose. Specific details of this process follow.

For many years it was believed that for every three H^+ produced, one molecule of ATP was produced and could be used for cellular energy. Although it is true that approximately three H^+ must pass through the H^+ channels (i.e., respiratory assemblies) to produce one ATP, it is now known that another H^+ is required to move the ATP molecule across the mitochondrial membrane into the cytoplasm. The ATP and H^+ are transported into the cytoplasm in exchange for ADP and P_i, which are transported into the mitochondria to resynthesize ATP. Therefore, while the theoretical yield of ATP from glucose is thirty-eight molecules, the actual ATP yield, allowing for the energy cost of transport, is only thirty-two molecules of ATP per glucose. For details of how these numbers are obtained, see the section "Aerobic ATP Tally."

- Oxidative phosphorylation or aerobic ATP production occurs in the mitochondria as a result of a complex interaction between the Krebs cycle and the electron transport chain. The primary role of the Krebs cycle is to complete the oxidation of substrates and form NADH and FADH to enter the electron transport chain. The end result of the electron transport chain is the formation of ATP and water. Water is formed by oxygen-accepting electrons; hence, the reason we breathe oxygen is to use it as the final acceptor of electrons in aerobic metabolism.

AEROBIC ATP TALLY

It is now possible to compute the overall ATP production as a result of the aerobic breakdown of glucose or glycogen. Let's begin by counting the total energy yield of glycolysis. Recall that the net ATP production of glycolysis was two ATP per glucose molecule. Further, when O_2 is present in the mitochondria, two NADH produced by glycolysis can then be shuttled into the mitochondria with the energy used to synthesize an additional five ATP (table 3.2). Thus, glycolysis can produce two ATP directly via substrate-level

phosphorylation and an additional five ATP by the energy contained in the two molecules of NADH.

How many ATP are produced as a result of the oxidation-reduction activities of the Krebs cycle? Table 3.3 shows that two NADH are formed when pyruvate is converted to acetyl-CoA, which results in the formation of 5 ATP. Note that two GTP (similar to ATP) are produced via substrate-level phosphorylation. A total of six NADH and two FADH are produced in the Krebs cycle from one glucose molecule. Hence, the six NADH formed via the Krebs cycle results in the production of a total of 15 ATP (6 NADH × 2.5 ATP per NADH = 15 ATP), with three ATP being produced from the two FADH. Therefore, the total ATP yield for the aerobic degradation of glucose is thirty-two ATP. The aerobic ATP yield for glycogen breakdown is thirty-three ATP, because the net glycolytic production of ATP by glycogen is one ATP more than that of glucose.

EFFICIENCY OF OXIDATIVE PHOSPHORYLATION

How efficient is oxidative phosphorylation as a system of converting energy from foodstuffs into biologically usable energy? This can be calculated by computing the ratio of the energy contained in the

---

TABLE 3.2 Aerobic ATP Tally from the Breakdown of One Molecule of Glucose

Metabolic Process	High-Energy Products	ATP from Oxidative Phosphorylation	ATP Subtotal
Glycolysis	2 ATP	—	2 (total if anaerobic)
	2 NADH*	5	7 (if aerobic)
Pyruvate to acetyl-CoA	2 NADH	5	12
Krebs cycle	2 GTP	—	14
	6 NADH	15	29
	2 FADH**	3	32
			Grand total: 32 ATP

*2.5 ATP per NADH
**1.5 ATP per FADH

TABLE 3.3 Factors Known to Affect the Activity of Rate-Limiting Enzymes of Metabolic Pathways Involved in Bioenergetics

Pathway	Rate-Limiting Enzyme	Stimulators	Inhibitors
ATP-PC system	Creatine kinase	ADP	ATP
Glycolysis	Phosphofructokinase	AMP, ADP, P_i, pH↑	ATP, CP, citrate, pH↓
Krebs cycle	Isocitrate dehydrogenase	ADP, Ca^{++}, NAD^+	ATP, NADH
Electron transport chain	Cytochrome oxidase	ADP, P_i	ATP

ATP molecules produced via aerobic respiration divided by the total potential energy contained in the glucose molecule. For example, a mole (a mole is 1 gram molecular weight) of ATP, when broken down, has an energy yield of 7.3 kcal. The potential energy released from the oxidation of a mole of glucose is 686 kcal. Thus, an efficiency figure for aerobic respiration can be computed as follows (18):

$$\text{Efficiency of respiration} = \frac{32 \text{ moles ATP/mole glucose} \times 7.3 \text{ kcal/mole ATP}}{686 \text{ kcal/mole glucose}}$$

Therefore, the efficiency of aerobic respiration is approximately 34%, with the remaining 66% of the free energy of glucose oxidation being released as heat.

IN SUMMARY

- The aerobic metabolism of one molecule of glucose results in the production of 32 ATP molecules, whereas the aerobic ATP yield for glycogen breakdown is 33 ATP.
- The overall efficiency of aerobic respiration is approximately 34%, with the remaining 66% of the energy being released as heat.

CONTROL OF BIOENERGETICS

The biochemical pathways that result in the production of ATP are regulated by very precise control systems. Each of these pathways contains a number of reactions that are catalyzed by specific enzymes. In general, if ample substrate is available, an increase in the number of enzymes present results in an increased rate of chemical reactions. Therefore, the regulation of one or more enzymes in a biochemical pathway would provide a means of controlling the rate of that particular pathway. Indeed, metabolism is regulated by the control of enzymatic activity. Most metabolic pathways have one enzyme that is considered "rate limiting." This rate-limiting enzyme determines the speed of the particular metabolic pathway involved.

How does a rate-limiting enzyme control the speed of reactions? First, as a rule, rate-limiting enzymes are found early in a metabolic pathway. This position is important because products of the pathway might accumulate if the rate-limiting enzyme were located near the end of a pathway. Second, the activity of rate-limiting enzymes is regulated by modulators. Modulators are substances that increase or decrease enzyme activity. Enzymes that are regulated by modulators are called *allosteric enzymes*. In the control of energy metabolism, ATP is the classic example of an inhibitor, whereas ADP and P_i are examples of substances that stimulate enzymatic activity (31). The

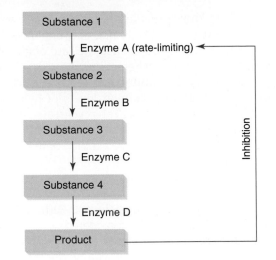

Figure 3.22 An example of a "rate-limiting" enzyme in a simple metabolic pathway. Here, a buildup of the product serves to inhibit the rate-limiting enzyme, which in turn slows down the reactions involved in the pathway.

fact that large amounts of cellular ATP would inhibit the metabolic production of ATP is logical because large amounts of ATP would indicate that ATP usage in the cell is low. An example of this type of negative feedback is illustrated in figure 3.22. In contrast, an increase in cell levels of ADP and P_i (low ATP) would indicate that ATP utilization is high. Therefore, it makes sense that ADP and P_i stimulate the production of ATP to meet the increased energy need.

Control of ATP-PC System

Phosphocreatine breakdown is regulated by creatine kinase activity. Creatine kinase is activated when sarcoplasmic concentrations of ADP increase and is inhibited by high levels of ATP. At the onset of exercise, ATP is split into ADP + P_i to provide energy for muscular contraction. This immediate increase in ADP concentrations stimulates creatine kinase to trigger the breakdown of PC to resynthesize ATP. If exercise is continued, glycolysis and finally aerobic metabolism begin to produce adequate ATP to meet the muscles' energy needs. The increase in ATP concentration, coupled with a reduction in ADP concentration, inhibits creatine kinase activity (table 3.3). Regulation of the ATP-PC system is an example of a "negative feedback" control system, which was introduced in chapter 2.

Control of Glycolysis

Although several factors control glycolysis, the most important rate-limiting enzyme in glycolysis is **phosphofructokinase (PFK)** (1). Note that PFK is located near the beginning of glycolysis (figure 3.15).

Table 3.3 lists known regulators of PFK. When exercise begins, ADP + P$_i$ levels rise and enhance PFK activity, which serves to increase the rate of glycolysis. In contrast, at rest, when cellular ATP levels are high, PFK activity is inhibited and glycolytic activity is slowed. Further, high cellular levels of hydrogen ions or citrate (produced via Krebs cycle) also inhibit PFK activity (35). Similar to the control of the ATP-PC system, regulation of PFK activity operates via negative feedback.

Another important regulatory enzyme in carbohydrate metabolism is phosphorylase, which is responsible for degrading glycogen to glucose. Although this enzyme is not technically considered a glycolytic enzyme, the reaction catalyzed by phosphorylase plays an important role in providing the glycolytic pathway with the necessary glucose at the origin of the pathway. With each muscle contraction, calcium (Ca^{++}) is released from the sarcoplasmic reticulum in muscle. This rise in sarcoplasmic Ca^{++} concentration indirectly activates phosphorylase, which immediately begins to break down glycogen to glucose for entry into glycolysis. Additionally, phosphorylase activity may be stimulated by high levels of the hormone epinephrine. Epinephrine is released at a faster rate during heavy exercise and results in the formation of the compound cyclic AMP (see chapter 5). It is cyclic AMP, not epinephrine, that directly activates phosphorylase. Thus, the influence of epinephrine on phosphorylase is indirect.

Control of Krebs Cycle and Electron Transport Chain

The Krebs cycle, like glycolysis, is subject to enzymatic regulation. Although several Krebs cycle enzymes are regulated, the rate-limiting enzyme is **isocitrate dehydrogenase.** Isocitrate dehydrogenase, like PFK, is inhibited by ATP and stimulated by increasing levels of ADP + P$_i$ (31). Further, growing evidence suggests that increased levels of calcium (Ca^{++}) in the mitochondria also stimulates isocitrate dehydrogenase activity (29). This is a logical signal to turn on energy metabolism in muscle cells, because an increase in free calcium in muscle is the signal to begin muscular contraction (see chapter 8).

The electron transport chain is also regulated by the amount of ATP and ADP + P$_i$ present (31). The rate-limiting enzyme in the electron transport chain is cytochrome oxidase. When exercise begins, ATP levels decline, ADP + P$_i$ levels increase, and cytochrome oxidase is stimulated to begin aerobic production of ATP. When exercise stops, cellular levels of ATP increase and ADP + P$_i$ concentrations decline, and thus the electron transport activity is reduced when normal levels of ATP, ADP, and P$_i$ are reached.

IN SUMMARY

- Metabolism is regulated by enzymatic activity. An enzyme that controls the rate of a metabolic pathway is termed the *rate-limiting enzyme.*
- The rate-limiting enzyme for glycolysis is phosphofructokinase, and the rate-limiting enzymes for the Krebs cycle and electron transport chain are isocitrate dehydrogenase and cytochrome oxidase, respectively.
- In general, cellular levels of ATP and ADP + P$_i$ regulate the rate of metabolic pathways involved in the production of ATP. High levels of ATP inhibit further ATP production, whereas low levels of ATP and high levels of ADP + P$_i$ stimulate ATP production. Evidence also exists that calcium may stimulate aerobic energy metabolism.

INTERACTION BETWEEN AEROBIC/ANAEROBIC ATP PRODUCTION

It is important to emphasize the interaction of anaerobic and aerobic metabolic pathways in the production of ATP during exercise. Although it is common to hear someone speak of aerobic versus anaerobic exercise, in reality the energy to perform most types of exercise comes from a combination of anaerobic and aerobic sources (11). This point is illustrated in The Winning Edge 3.2. Notice that the contribution of anaerobic ATP production is greater in short-term, high-intensity activities, whereas aerobic metabolism predominates in longer activities. For example, approximately 90% of the energy required to perform a 100-meter dash would come from anaerobic sources, with most of the energy coming via the ATP-PC system. Similarly, energy to run 400 meters (i.e., 55 seconds) would be largely anaerobic (70–75%). However, ATP and PC stores are limited, and thus glycolysis must supply much of the ATP during this type of event(11).

On the other end of the energy spectrum, events like the marathon (i.e., 26.2-mile race) rely on aerobic production of ATP for the bulk of the needed energy. Where does the energy come from in events of moderate length (i.e., 2 to 30 minutes)? The Winning Edge 3.2 provides an estimation of the percentage anaerobic/aerobic yield in events over a wide range of durations. Although these estimates are based on laboratory measurements of running or exercising on a cycle ergometer, they can be related

Exercise Physiology Applied to Sports

Contributions of Anaerobic/Aerobic Energy Production During Various Sporting Events

Because sports differ widely in both the intensity and the duration of physical effort, it is not surprising that the source of energy production differs widely among sporting events. Figure 3.23 provides an illustration of the anaerobic versus aerobic energy production during selected sports. Knowledge of the interaction between the anaerobic and aerobic energy production in exercise is useful to coaches and trainers in planning conditioning programs for athletes. See chapter 21 for more details.

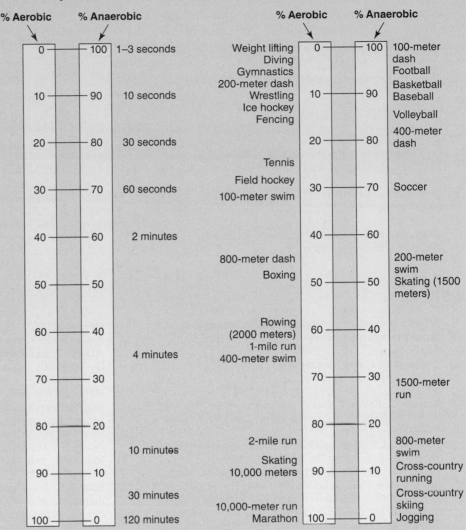

FIGURE 3.23 Contribution of anaerobic and aerobically produced ATP for use during sports.

to other athletic events that require intense effort by comparing the length of time spent in the activity. In review, the shorter the duration of all-out activity, the greater the contribution of anaerobic energy production; conversely, the longer the duration, the greater the contribution of aerobic energy production. A more detailed discussion of the metabolic responses to various types of exercise is presented in chapter 4.

IN SUMMARY

- Energy to perform exercise comes from an interaction of anaerobic and aerobic pathways.
- In general, the shorter the activity (high intensity), the greater the contribution of anaerobic energy production. In contrast, long-term activities (low to moderate intensity) utilize ATP produced from aerobic sources.

STUDY QUESTIONS

1. List and briefly discuss the function of the three major components of cell structure.
2. Briefly explain the concept of coupled reactions.
3. Define the following terms: (1) *bioenergetics*, (2) *endergonic reactions*, and (3) *exergonic reactions*.
4. Discuss the role of enzymes as catalysts. What is meant by the expression "energy of activation"?
5. Where does glycolysis, the Krebs cycle, and oxidative phosphorylation take place in the cell?
6. Define the terms *glycogen*, *glycogenolysis*, and *glycolysis*.

7. What are high-energy phosphates? Explain the statement that "ATP is the universal energy donor."
8. Define the terms *aerobic* and *anaerobic*.
9. Briefly discuss the function of glycolysis in bioenergetics. What role does NAD^+ play in glycolysis?
10. Discuss the operation of the Krebs cycle and the electron transport chain in the aerobic production of ATP. What is the function of NAD^+ and FAD in these pathways?
11. What is the efficiency of the aerobic degradation of glucose?
12. What is the role of oxygen in aerobic metabolism?
13. What are the rate-limiting enzymes for the following metabolic pathways? ATP-PC system? Glycolysis? Krebs cycle? Electron transport chain?
14. Briefly discuss the interaction of anaerobic versus aerobic ATP production during exercise.
15. Discuss the chemiosmotic theory of ATP production.
16. Briefly discuss the impact of changes in both temperature and pH on enzyme activity.
17. Discuss the relationship between lactic acid and lactate.

SUGGESTED READINGS

Bemben, M., and H. Lamont. 2005. Creatine supplementation and exercise performance. *Sports Medicine* 35:107–25.

Fox, S. 2009. *Human Physiology*. New York, NY: McGraw-Hill Companies.

Hespel P., and W. Derave. 2007. Ergogenic effects of creatine in sports and rehabilitation. *Sub-cellular Biochemistry* 46: 245–59.

Houston, M. 2006. *Biochemistry Primer for Exercise Science*. Champaign, IL: Human Kinetics.

Karp, G. 2009. *Cell and Molecular Biology: Concepts and Experiments*. Hoboken, NJ. Wiley Publishers.

Powers, S., and M. Jackson. 2008. Exercise-induced oxidative stress: Cellular mechanisms and impact on muscle force production. *Physiological Review* 88: 1243–76.

Widmaier, E., H. Raff, and K. Strang. 2008. *Vander's Human Physiology*. New York, NY. McGraw-Hill.

REFERENCES

1. **Alberts B, Johnson A, Lewis J, Raff M, Roberts K, and Walter P.** *Molecular Biology of the Cell*. New York: Garland Science, 2007.
2. **Bemben MG, and Lamont HS.** Creatine supplementation and exercise performance: recent findings. *Sports Medicine (Auckland, NZ)* 35: 107–125, 2005.
3. **Brooks G, Fahey T, and Baldwin K.** *Exercise Physiology: Human Bioenergetics and Its Applications*. New York: McGraw-Hill, 2005.
4. **Brooks GA.** Cell-cell and intracellular lactate shuttles. *The Journal of Physiology* 587: 5591–5600, 2009.
5. **Camic CL, Hendrix CR, Housh TJ, Zuniga JM, Mielke M, Johnson GO, Schmidt RJ, and Housh DJ.** The effects of polyethylene glycosylated creatine supplementation on muscular strength and power. *Journal of Strength and Conditioning Research/National Strength & Conditioning Association* 24: 3343–3351, 2010.
6. **Cribb PJ, Williams AD, Stathis CG, Carey MF, and Hayes A.** Effects of whey isolate, creatine, and resistance training on muscle hypertrophy. *Medicine and Science in Sports and Exercise* 39: 298–307, 2007.
7. **Dalbo VJ, Roberts MD, Stout JR, and Kerksick CM.** Putting to rest the myth of creatine supplementation leading to muscle cramps and dehydration. *British Journal of Sports Medicine* 42: 567–573, 2008.
8. **Devlin T.** *Textbook of Biochemistry with Clinical Correlations*. Hoboken: Wiley, 2010.
9. **Dolny DG, and Lemon PW.** Effect of ambient temperature on protein breakdown during prolonged exercise. *J Appl Physiol* 64: 550–555, 1988.
10. **Fox S.** *Human Physiology*. New York: McGraw-Hill, 2009.
11. **Gastin PB.** Energy system interaction and relative contribution during maximal exercise. *Sports Medicine (Auckland, NZ)* 31: 725–741, 2001.
12. **Gibala MJ.** Protein metabolism and endurance exercise. *Sports Medicine (Auckland, NZ)* 37: 337–340, 2007.
13. **Gollnick PD.** Metabolism of substrates: energy substrate metabolism during exercise and as modified by training. *Fed Proc* 44: 353–357, 1985.
14. **Greenhaff PL.** Creatine and its application as an ergogenic aid. *Int J Sport Nutr* 5 Suppl: S100–110, 1995.
15. **Hespel P, and Derave W.** Ergogenic effects of creatine in sports and rehabilitation. *Sub-cellular Biochemistry* 46: 245–259, 2007.
16. **Holloszy JO, and Coyle EF.** Adaptations of skeletal muscle to endurance exercise and their metabolic consequences. *J Appl Physiol* 56: 831–838, 1984.
17. **Houston M.** *Biochemistry Primer for Exercise Science*. Champaign: Human Kinetics, 2006.
18. **Jequier E, and Flatt J.** Recent advances in human bioenergetics. *News in Physiological Sciences* 1: 112–114, 1986.
19. **Juhn MS, and Tarnopolsky M.** Oral creatine supplementation and athletic performance: a critical review. *Clin J Sport Med* 8: 286–297, 1998.
20. **Juhn MS, and Tarnopolsky M.** Potential side effects of oral creatine supplementation: a critical review. *Clin J Sport Med* 8: 298–304, 1998.
21. **Karp G.** *Cell and Molecular Biology: Concepts and Experiments*. Hoboken, NJ: Wiley, 2009.
22. **Kavazis AN, Talbert EE, Smuder AJ, Hudson MB, Nelson WB, and Powers SK.** Mechanical ventilation induces diaphragmatic mitochondrial dysfunction and increased oxidant production. *Free Radical Biology & Medicine* 46: 842–850, 2009.
23. **Kerksick CM, Wilborn CD, Campbell WI, Harvey TM, Marcello BM, Roberts MD, Parker AG, Byars AG, Greenwood LD, Almada AL, Kreider RB, and Greenwood M.** The effects of creatine monohydrate supplementation with and without D-pinitol on resistance training adaptations. *Journal of Strength and Conditioning Research/National Strength & Conditioning Association* 23: 2673–2682, 2009.
24. **Law YL, Ong WS, GillianYap TL, Lim SC, and Von Chia E.** Effects of two and five days of creatine loading on muscular strength and anaerobic power in trained athletes. *Journal of Strength and Conditioning Research/National Strength & Conditioning Association* 23: 906–914, 2009.

25. **Lemon PW, and Mullin JP.** Effect of initial muscle glycogen levels on protein catabolism during exercise. *J Appl Physiol* 48: 624–629, 1980.

26. **Maughan RJ.** Creatine supplementation and exercise performance. *Int J Sport Nutr* 5: 94–101, 1995.

27. **Maughan RJ, King DS, and Lea T.** Dietary supplements. *J Sports Sci* 22: 95–113, 2004.

28. **McArdle W, Katch F, and Katch V.** *Exercise Physiology: Energy, Nutrition, and Human Performance.* Baltimore: Lippincott Williams & Wilkins, 2006.

29. **McCormack J, and Denton R.** Signal transduction by intramitochondrial calcium in mammalian energy metabolism. *News in Physiological Sciences* 9: 71–76, 1994.

30. **Powers SK, and Jackson MJ.** Exercise-induced oxidative stress: cellular mechanisms and impact on muscle force production. *Physiological Reviews* 88: 1243–1276, 2008.

31. **Pratt CW, and Cornely, K.** *Essential Biochemistry.* Hoboken: Wiley, 2011.

32. **Rawson ES, and Volek JS.** Effects of creatine supplementation and resistance training on muscle strength and weightlifting performance. *Journal of Strength and Conditioning Research/National Strength & Conditioning Association* 17: 822–831, 2003.

33. **Reed S.** *Essential Physiological Biochemistry: An Organ-Based Approach.* Hoboken: Wiley, 2010.

34. **Robergs RA, Ghiasvand F, and Parker D.** Biochemistry of exercise-induced metabolic acidosis. *American Journal of Physiology* 287: R502–516, 2004.

35. **Spriet LL.** Phosphofructokinase activity and acidosis during short-term tetanic contractions. *Can J Physiol Pharmacol* 69: 298–304, 1991.

36. **Tymoczko J, Berg J, and Stryer L.** *Biochemistry: A Short Course.* New York: W. H. Freeman, 2009.

37. **Voet D, and Voet JG.** *Biochemistry.* Hoboken: Wiley, 2010.

38. **West J.** *Best and Taylor's Physiological Basis of Medical Practice.* Baltimore: Lippincott Williams & Wilkins, 2001.

39. **Williams MH, and Branch JD.** Creatine supplementation and exercise performance: an update. *J Am Coll Nutr* 17: 216–234, 1998.

4

Exercise Metabolism

■ Objectives

By studying this chapter, you should be able to do the following:

1. Discuss the relationship between exercise intensity/duration and the bioenergetic pathways that are most responsible for the production of ATP during various types of exercise.

2. Describe, graphically, the change in oxygen uptake during the transition from rest to steady state exercise, and then recovery from exercise. Identify the oxygen deficit, oxygen requirement, and oxygen debt (excess post-exercise oxygen uptake).

3. Describe, graphically, the changes in oxygen uptake and blood lactate during an incremental (graded) exercise test. Identify the lactate threshold and maximal oxygen uptake ($\dot{V}O_2$ max).

4. Discuss several possible explanations for the sudden rise in blood-lactate concentration during incremental exercise.

5. List the factors that regulate fuel selection during exercise.

6. Describe the changes in the respiratory exchange ratio (R) with increasing intensities of exercise and during prolonged exercise of moderate intensity.

7. Describe the types of carbohydrates and fats used during increasing intensities of exercise and during prolonged exercise of moderate intensity.

8. Describe the lactate shuttle, with examples of how it is used during exercise.

■ Key Terms

anaerobic threshold
Cori cycle
excess post-exercise oxygen
   consumption (EPOC)
free fatty acid (FFA)
gluconeogenesis
graded (or incremental)
   exercise test
lactate threshold
lipase
lipolysis
maximal oxygen uptake
   ($\dot{V}O_2$ max)
oxygen debt
oxygen deficit
respiratory exchange ratio (R)

Exercise poses a serious challenge to the bioenergetic pathways in the working muscle. For example, during heavy exercise the body's total energy expenditure may increase fifteen to twenty-five times above expenditure at rest. Most of this increase in energy production is used to provide ATP for contracting skeletal muscles, which may increase their energy utilization 200 times over utilization at rest (1). Clearly, skeletal muscles have a great capacity to produce and use large quantities of ATP during exercise. This chapter describes: (1) the metabolic responses at the beginning of exercise and during recovery from exercise; (2) the metabolic responses to high-intensity, incremental, and prolonged exercise; (3) the selection of fuels used to produce ATP; and (4) how exercise metabolism is regulated.

We begin with an overview of the energy requirements of the body at rest, followed by a discussion of which bioenergetic pathways are activated at the onset of exercise.

ENERGY REQUIREMENTS AT REST

Recall that homeostasis is defined as a steady and unchanging internal environment (see chapter 2). During resting conditions, the healthy human body is in homeostasis, and therefore the body's energy requirement is also constant. At rest, almost 100% of the energy (i.e., ATP) required to sustain bodily functions is produced by aerobic metabolism. It follows that resting blood lactate levels are also steady and low (e.g., 1.0 millimole per liter).

Because the measurement of oxygen (O_2) consumption (oxygen consumed by the body) is an index of aerobic ATP production, measurement of O_2 consumption during rest provides an estimate of the body's "baseline" energy requirement. At rest, the total energy requirement of an individual is relatively low. For example, a 70-kilogram young adult would consume approximately 0.25 liter of oxygen each minute; this translates to a relative O_2 consumption of 3.5 ml of O_2 per kilogram (body weight) per minute. As mentioned earlier, muscular exercise can greatly increase the body's need for energy. Let's begin our discussion of exercise metabolism by considering which bioenergetic pathways are active during the transition from rest to exercise.

REST-TO-EXERCISE TRANSITIONS

Assume you are standing alongside a treadmill with its belt moving at 7 mph, and you jump onto the belt and start running. Within one step, you go from zero mph to 7 mph, and in that one step your muscles increase their rate of ATP production from that

(a)

(b)

(c)

Figure 4.1 The time course of speed (*a*), rate of ATP use (*b*), and oxygen uptake ($\dot{V}O_2$) (*c*) in the transition from rest to submaximal exercise.

required for standing to that required for running at 7 mph (see Figure 4.1a and b). If ATP production did not increase instantaneously, you would have fallen off the back of the treadmill! What metabolic changes must occur in skeletal muscle at the beginning of exercise to provide the necessary energy to continue movement? Similar to measurement of O_2 consumption during rest, measurement of O_2 consumption during exercise can provide information about aerobic metabolism during exercise. For example, in the transition from rest to light or moderate exercise, O_2 consumption increases rapidly and reaches a steady state within 1 to 4 minutes (11, 21, 89) (figure 4.1c).

The fact that O_2 consumption does not increase instantaneously to a steady-state value means that anaerobic energy sources contribute to the overall production of ATP at the beginning of exercise. Indeed, much evidence suggests that at the onset of exercise the ATP-PC system is the first active bioenergetic pathway, followed by glycolysis and, finally, aerobic energy production (3, 16, 37, 66, 94). This is shown in figure 4.2a, in which the PC concentration in muscle falls dramatically during a three-minute bout of exercise. Figure 4.2b shows that the production of ATP from PC was highest in the first minute of exercise and fell off after that, due in part to the systematic reduction in the PC store. Figure 4.2c shows that glycolysis was already contributing ATP during the first minute of exercise and increased during the second minute (9). The effectiveness of these two anaerobic systems in the first minutes of exercise is such that ATP levels in muscle are virtually unchanged, even though ATP is being used at a much higher rate (107). However, as the steady state O_2 consumption is reached, the body's ATP requirement is met via aerobic metabolism. The major point to be emphasized concerning the bioenergetics of rest-to-work transitions is that several energy systems are involved. In other words, the energy needed for exercise is not provided by simply turning on a single bioenergetic pathway, but rather by a mixture of several metabolic systems operating with considerable overlap.

The term **oxygen deficit** applies to the lag in oxygen uptake at the beginning of exercise. Specifically, the oxygen deficit is defined as the difference between oxygen uptake in the first few minutes of exercise and an equal time period after steady state has been obtained (81, 87). This is represented as the shaded area in the left portion of figure 4.1c. What causes this lag in oxygen uptake at the onset of exercise? Is it due to inadequate oxygen delivery to the muscle, or is it a failure of oxidative phosphorylation to increase immediately when exercise begins (74)? Dr. Bruce Gladden answers those questions in Ask the Expert 4.1.

Trained subjects reach the steady state $\dot{V}O_2$ faster than untrained subjects, resulting in a smaller oxygen deficit (58, 89). What is the explanation for this difference? It seems likely that the trained subjects have a better-developed aerobic bioenergetic capacity, resulting from either cardiovascular or muscular adaptations induced by endurance training (31, 58, 87, 89). Practically speaking, this means that aerobic ATP production is active earlier at the beginning of exercise and results in less production of lactate and H^+ in the trained individual when compared to the untrained individual. Chapter 13 provides a detailed analysis of this adaptation to training.

Figure 4.2   Figure 2a shows the rapid change of phosphocreatine (PC) concentration in muscle during a 3-minute bout of exercise. Figures 2b and 2c show the rate of ATP production during this 3-minute bout from PC and glycolysis, respectively.

IN SUMMARY

- In the transition from rest to light or moderate exercise, oxygen uptake increases rapidly, generally reaching a steady state within 1 to 4 minutes.
- The term oxygen deficit applies to the lag in oxygen uptake at the beginning of exercise.
- The failure of oxygen uptake to increase instantly at the beginning of exercise means that anaerobic pathways contribute to the overall production of ATP early in exercise. After a steady state is reached, the body's ATP requirement is met via aerobic metabolism.

ASK THE EXPERT 4.1

Oxygen Uptake Kinetics at the Onset of Constant Work-Rate Exercise: Questions and Answers with Dr. Bruce Gladden

Bruce Gladden, Ph.D., a professor in the Department of Kinesiology at Auburn University, is an internationally known expert in muscle metabolism during exercise. Dr. Gladden's research has addressed important questions relative to those factors that regulate oxygen consumption in skeletal muscle during exercise. Examples of Dr. Gladden's work can be found in prestigious international physiology journals. In this feature, Dr. Gladden answers questions about the time course of oxygen consumption at the onset of submaximal exercise.

QUESTION: What is so important about the oxygen consumption response at the onset of submaximal, constant work-rate exercise?

ANSWER: First, it is critical to realize that O_2 consumption is a direct indicator of the energy supplied by oxidative phosphorylation (i.e., the oxidative or aerobic energy system). The fact that there is a "lag" or delay before oxygen consumption rises to a steady-state level tells us that aerobic metabolism (i.e., oxidative phosphorylation in the mitochondria) is not fully activated at the onset of exercise. The importance of this response is that it can provide information about the control or regulation of oxidative phosphorylation. Further, this delayed response tells us that the anaerobic energy systems must also be activated to supply the needed energy at the beginning of exercise; i.e., there is an oxygen deficit.

QUESTION: Why does oxidative phosphorylation not achieve full activation instantaneously at the onset of exercise?

ANSWER: Historically, two alternative hypotheses have been offered. First, it has been suggested that there is an inadequate oxygen supply to the contracting muscles at exercise onset. What this means is that in at least some mitochondria, at least some of the time, there may not be molecules of oxygen available to accept electrons at the end of the electron transport chains. Clearly, if this is correct, the oxidative phosphorylation rate and therefore the whole body oxygen consumption would be restricted. The second hypothesis holds that there is a delay because the stimuli for oxidative phosphorylation require some time to reach their final levels and to have their full effects for a given exercise intensity. As discussed in chapter 3, the electron transport chain is stimulated by ADP and P_i (e.g., table 3.3). At the onset of exercise, the concentrations of ADP and P_i are barely above resting levels because the ATP concentration is being maintained by PC and accelerated glycolysis. However, the concen-

trations of ADP and P_i will continue to rise as PC is broken down, gradually providing additional stimulation to "turn on" oxidative phosphorylation until this aerobic pathway is providing essentially 100% of the energy requirement of the exercise. The key point is that these regulators of oxidative phosphorylation rate do not instantaneously rise from resting concentrations to the steady-state concentration levels. This has sometimes been referred to as the "inertia of metabolism."

QUESTION: Which of the two hypotheses is correct?

ANSWER: This is a difficult question because the two hypotheses are not mutually exclusive. My research with numerous colleagues (especially Drs. Bruno Grassi, Mike Hogan, and Harry Rossiter) provides support for the second hypothesis (i.e., "slowness" in the stimuli required to fully activate oxidative phosphorylation). Nevertheless, oxygen supply limitation can also play a role, a role that likely becomes more important at higher exercise intensities. None of the possible regulators or controllers of oxidative phosphorylation should be considered separately. All of them interact with each other to provide the overall stimulus to oxidative phosphorylation under any given exercise condition.

RECOVERY FROM EXERCISE: METABOLIC RESPONSES

If a subject is running on the treadmill at a speed that can be maintained comfortably for 20 or 30 minutes, and then jumps off to the side, the metabolic rate ($\dot{V}O_2$) does not fall instantaneously from the steady state value measured during the exercise to the resting $\dot{V}O_2$ value associated with standing by the treadmill. The metabolic rate remains elevated for several minutes immediately following exercise. This is shown in figure 4.3a, with a steady-state $\dot{V}O_2$ being achieved by minute 3 of exercise, and the oxygen

uptake returning to resting levels by 5 minutes after exercise. In contrast, Figure 4.3b shows the subject doing non-steady state exercise that can be maintained for only 6 minutes before exhaustion occurs. In this case, the subject could not meet the oxygen requirement for the task as shown by the much larger oxygen deficit, and the subject's $\dot{V}O_2$ is still not back to the resting level by 14 minutes after exercise. Clearly, the magnitude and duration of this elevated post-exercise metabolic rate are influenced by the intensity of the exercise (5, 48, 87). The reason(s) for this observation will be discussed shortly.

Historically, the term **oxygen debt** has been applied to the elevated oxygen uptake (above resting

(a)

(b)

Figure 4.3 Oxygen deficit and the excess post-exercise O_2 consumption (EPOC) during moderate exercise (*a*) and during heavy, exhausting exercise (*b*).

levels) following exercise. The prominent British physiologist A. V. Hill (59) first used the term O_2 debt and reasoned that the excess oxygen consumed (above rest) following exercise was repayment for the O_2 deficit incurred at the onset of exercise (see A Look Back—Important People in Science). Evidence collected in the 1920s and 1930s by Hill and other researchers in Europe and the United States suggested that the oxygen debt could be divided into two portions: the rapid portion immediately following exercise (i.e., approximately 2 to

3 minutes post-exercise) and the slow portion, which persisted for greater than 30 minutes after exercise. The rapid portion is represented by the steep decline in oxygen uptake following exercise, and the slow portion is represented by the slow decline in O_2 across time following exercise (figure 4.3a or b). The rationale for the two divisions of the O_2 debt was based on the belief that the rapid portion of the O_2 debt represented the oxygen that was required to resynthesize stored ATP and PC and replace tissue stores of O_2 (~20% of the O_2 debt),

A.V. Hill Was a Pioneer in Exercise Physiology

Archibald Vivian (A. V.) Hill (1886–1977) received the Nobel Prize for Physiology or Medicine in 1922 for his research on heat production in skeletal muscle. This work precisely described the magnitude of heat production in isolated skeletal muscle during both contraction and relaxation. Professor Hill was born in Bristol, England, and his family had little money to support his education. Nonetheless, he was both motivated and resourceful as he earned scholarships to support his studies in mathematics and natural sciences (chemistry, physics, and physiology) at Trinity College, Cambridge.

After graduation, Hill was encouraged to focus on physiology by one of his teachers, Dr. Walter Fletcher. Hill initiated his physiology research career at Cambridge in 1909 and began to investigate the nature of muscular contraction using frog muscle as a model. Hill later held faculty positions at Manchester University (1920–1923) and at University College, London (1923–1951).

In addition to his Nobel Prize winning research on heat production in skeletal muscle, A. V. Hill made many other contributions to our understanding of exercise physiology. For example, he was the first physiologist to demonstrate that contracting skeletal muscle can produce energy anaerobi-cally. This work was important because the general view at the time was that all energy for muscular performance was derived from aerobic metabolism. A. V. Hill also introduced the concept of the oxygen debt (i.e., oxygen consumption following exercise), and he was the first scientist to clearly describe the concept of maximal oxygen consumption in exercising humans. Other important scientific contributions of Hill include his discovery of heat production in nerves and the force-velocity equation in skeletal muscle.

For more information on A. V. Hill and his scientific contributions to exercise physiology, see the paper by Bassett in the Suggested Readings.

---

while the slow portion of the debt was due to the oxidative conversion of lactate to glucose in the liver (~80% of the O_2 debt).

Contradicting previous beliefs, recent evidence has shown that only about 20% of the oxygen debt is used to convert the lactate produced during exercise to glucose (the process of glucose synthesis from non-carbohydrate sources is called **gluconeogenesis**) (13, 16). Therefore, the notion that the "slow" portion of the O_2 debt is due entirely to oxidative conversion of lactate to glucose does not appear to be accurate. Several investigators have argued that the term *oxygen debt* be eliminated from the literature, because the elevated oxygen consumption following exercise does not appear to be entirely due to the "borrowing" of oxygen from the body's oxygen stores (13, 14, 16, 41). In recent years, several replacement terms have been suggested. One such term is **EPOC,** which stands for "**excess post-exercise oxygen consumption**" (14, 41).

If the EPOC is not exclusively used to convert lactate to glucose, why does oxygen consumption remain elevated post-exercise? Several possibilities exist. First, at least part of the O_2 consumed immediately following exercise is used to restore PC in muscle and O_2 stores in blood and tissues (11, 41).

Restoration of both PC and oxygen stores in muscle is completed within two to three minutes of recovery (54). This is consistent with the classic view of the rapid portion of the oxygen debt. Further, heart rate and breathing remain elevated above resting levels for several minutes following exercise; therefore, both of these activities require additional O_2 above resting levels. Other factors that may result in the EPOC are an elevated body temperature and specific circulating hormones. Increases in body temperature result in an increased metabolic rate (called the Q_{10} effect) (18, 52, 91). Further, it has been argued that high levels of epinephrine or norepinephrine result in increased oxygen consumption after exercise (43). However, both of these hormones are rapidly removed from the blood following exercise and therefore may not exist long enough to have a significant impact on the EPOC.

Earlier it was mentioned that the EPOC was greater following high-intensity exercise when compared to the EPOC following light-to-moderate work. This difference in EPOC is due to differences in the amount of body heat gained, the total PC depleted, the higher lactate levels, and the elevated blood levels of epinephrine and norepinephrine (48). First, assuming similar ambient conditions (i.e., temperature/relative humidity) and equal exercise time, high-intensity exercise will result in greater body heat gain than that gained by light exercise. Second, depletion of PC is dependent on exercise intensity. Because high-intensity exercise would utilize more PC, additional oxygen would be required during recovery for resynthesis. Third, even though only a small percentage of the lactate is converted to glucose, the elevated lactate levels would result in a greater level of gluconeogenesis, and its associated energy cost. Finally, intense exercise results in greater blood concentrations of lactate, epinephrine, and norepinephrine when compared to light work. All these factors may contribute to the EPOC being greater following intense exercise than following light

Removal of Lactate Following Exercise

What happens to the lactate that is formed during exercise? Classical theory proposed that the majority of the post-exercise lactate was converted into glucose in the liver and resulted in an elevated post-exercise oxygen uptake (i.e., O_2 debt). However, recent evidence suggests that this is not the case and that lactate is mainly oxidized after exercise (13, 16). That is, lactate is converted to pyruvate and used as a substrate by the heart and skeletal muscle. It is estimated that approximately 70% of the lactate produced during exercise is oxidized, while 20% is converted to glucose and the remaining 10% is converted to amino acids.

Figure 4.4 demonstrates the time course of lactate removal from the blood following strenuous exercise. Note that lactate removal is more rapid if continuous light exercise is performed as compared to a resting recovery. The explanation for these findings is linked to the fact that light exercise enhances oxidation of lactate by the working muscle (32, 42, 57). It is estimated that the optimum intensity of recovery exercise to promote blood lactate removal is around 30% to 40% of $\dot{V}O_2$ max (32). Higher exercise intensi-

ties would likely result in an increased muscle production of lactate and therefore hinder removal.

A recent study set the intensity of the active recovery at a percentage of the lactate threshold (LT), rather than a percentage of $\dot{V}O_2$ max. They found that when subjects did their active recovery at intensities just below the LT (the point at which lactate accumulation occurs) blood lactate was removed faster than at lower intensities (e.g., 40% to 60% of the LT) (83).

Due to the increase in muscle oxidative capacity observed with endurance

FIGURE 4.4 Blood lactate removal following strenuous exercise. Note that lactate can be removed more rapidly from the blood during recovery if the subject engages in continuous light exercise.

training, some authors have speculated that trained subjects might have a greater capacity to remove lactate during recovery from intense exercise (6, 8). Unfortunately, human studies examining the effects of training on the rate of blood lactate decline (following heavy exercise) have yielded conflicting results. However, two well-designed investigations have reported no differences in blood lactate disappearance between trained and untrained subjects during resting recovery from a maximal exercise bout (6, 38).

exercise. Figure 4.5 contains a summary of factors thought to contribute to the excess post-exercise oxygen consumption. Further, see A Closer Look 4.1 for more details on removal of lactate following exercise.

IN SUMMARY

- The oxygen debt (also called excess post-exercise oxygen consumption [EPOC]) is the O_2 consumption above rest following exercise.
- Several factors contribute to the EPOC. First, some of the O_2 consumed early in the recovery period is used to resynthesize stored PC in the muscle and replace O_2 stores in both muscle and blood. Other factors that contribute to the "slow" portion of the EPOC include an elevated body temperature, O_2 required to convert lactate to glucose (gluconeogenesis), and elevated blood levels of epinephrine and norepinephrine.

METABOLIC RESPONSES TO EXERCISE: INFLUENCE OF DURATION AND INTENSITY

The point was made in chapter 3 that short-term, high-intensity exercise lasting less than 10 seconds utilizes primarily anaerobic metabolic pathways to produce ATP. In contrast, an event like the marathon makes primary use of aerobic ATP production to provide the needed ATP for work. However, events lasting longer than 10 to 20 seconds and less than 10 minutes generally produce the needed ATP for muscular contraction via a combination of both anaerobic and aerobic pathways. In fact, most sports use a combination of anaerobic and aerobic pathways to produce the ATP needed for muscular contraction. The next three sections consider which bioenergetic pathways are involved in energy production in specific types of exercise.

Factors Contributing to Excess Post-Exercise Oxygen Consumption

Figure 4.5 A summary of factors that might contribute to excess post-exercise oxygen consumption (EPOC). See text for details.

Short-Term, Intense Exercise

The energy to perform short-term exercise of high intensity comes primarily from anaerobic metabolic pathways. Whether the ATP production is dominated by the ATP-PC system or glycolysis depends primarily on the length of the activity (1, 3, 66, 72). For example, the energy to run a 50-meter dash or to complete a single play in a football game comes principally from the ATP-PC system. In contrast, the energy to complete the 400-meter dash (i.e., 55 seconds) comes from a combination of the ATP-PC system, glycolysis, and aerobic metabolism, with glycolysis producing most of the ATP. In general, the ATP-PC system can supply almost all the needed ATP for work for events lasting 1 to 5 seconds; intense exercise lasting longer than 5 seconds begins to utilize the ATP-producing capability of glycolysis. It should be emphasized that the transition from the ATP-PC system to an increased dependence upon glycolysis during exercise is not an abrupt change but rather a gradual shift from one pathway to another.

Events lasting longer than 45 seconds use a combination of all three energy systems (i.e., ATP-PC, glycolysis, and aerobic systems). This point was emphasized in figure 3.23 in chapter 3. In general, intense exercise lasting approximately 60 seconds utilizes 70%/30% (anaerobic/aerobic) energy production, whereas events lasting 2 to 3 minutes utilize anaerobic and aerobic bioenergetic pathways almost equally to supply the needed ATP (see figure 3.23). Clearly, the contribution of aerobic energy production to the total energy requirement increases with the duration of exercise.

IN SUMMARY

- During high-intensity, short-term exercise (i.e., 2 to 20 seconds), the muscle's ATP production is dominated by the ATP-PC system.
- Intense exercise lasting more than 20 seconds relies more on anaerobic glycolysis to produce much of the needed ATP.
- Finally, high-intensity events lasting longer than 45 seconds use a combination of the ATP-PC system, glycolysis, and the aerobic system to produce the needed ATP for muscular contraction, with a 50%/50% (anaerobic/aerobic) contribution needed for exercise lasting between 2 and 3 minutes.

Prolonged Exercise

The energy to perform long-term exercise (i.e., more than 10 minutes) comes primarily from aerobic metabolism. A steady-state oxygen uptake can generally be maintained during submaximal, moderate-intensity exercise. However, two exceptions to this rule exist. First, prolonged exercise in a hot/humid environment results in a "drift" upward of oxygen uptake; therefore, a steady state is not maintained in this type of exercise, even though the work rate is constant (91) (see figure 4.6a). Second, continuous exercise at a high relative work rate (i.e., >75% $\dot{V}O_2$ max) results in a slow rise in oxygen uptake across time (52) (figure 4.6b). In each of these two types of exercise, the drift upward in $\dot{V}O_2$ is due principally to the effects of increasing body temperature and to rising blood levels of the hormones epinephrine and norepinephrine (18, 41, 43, 52, 70). Both of these variables tend to increase the metabolic rate, resulting in increased oxygen uptake across time. Use of a drug that blocks the receptors that epinephrine and norepinephrine bind to (to block their effects) results in an elimination of the drift in $\dot{V}O_2$, confirming the link between the two (70). In contrast, even though an 8-week endurance training program was shown to reduce the drift in $\dot{V}O_2$ during heavy exercise, it was not linked to a lower body temperature (20). Clearly, additional research is needed to explain the causes of this drift in $\dot{V}O_2$ in heavy exercise.

IN SUMMARY

- The energy to perform prolonged exercise (i.e., more than 10 minutes) comes primarily from aerobic metabolism.
- A steady-state oxygen uptake can generally be maintained during prolonged, moderate-intensity exercise. However, exercise in a hot/humid environment or exercise at a high relative work rate results in an upward "drift" in oxygen consumption over time; therefore, a steady state is not obtained in these types of exercise.

(a)

(b)

Figure 4.6 Comparison of oxygen uptake ($\dot{V}O_2$) across time during prolonged exercise in a hot and humid environment (*a*) and during prolonged exercise at a high relative work rate (>75% $\dot{V}O_2$ max) (*b*). Note that in both conditions there is a steady "drift" upward in $\dot{V}O_2$. See text for details.

Incremental Exercise

The maximal capacity to transport and utilize oxygen during exercise (**maximal oxygen uptake, or $\dot{V}O_2$ max**) is considered by many exercise scientists to be the most valid measurement of cardiovascular fitness. Indeed, **incremental exercise tests** (also called **graded exercise tests**) are often employed by physicians to examine patients for possible heart disease and by exercise scientists to determine a subject's cardiovascular fitness. These tests are usually conducted on a treadmill or a cycle ergometer. However, an arm crank ergometer can be employed for testing paraplegics or athletes whose sport involves arm work (e.g., swimmers). The test generally begins with the subject performing a brief warm-up, followed by an increase in the work rate every 1 to 3 minutes until the subject cannot maintain the desired power output. This increase in work rate can be achieved on the treadmill by increasing either the speed of the treadmill or the incline. On the cycle or arm ergometer, the increase in power output is obtained by increasing the resistance against the flywheel.

Figure 4.7 illustrates the change in oxygen uptake during a typical incremental exercise test on a cycle

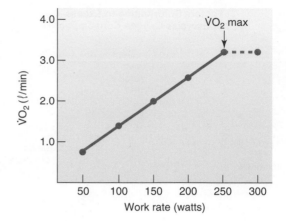

Figure 4.7 Changes in oxygen uptake ($\dot{V}O_2$) during an incremental exercise test. The observed plateau in $\dot{V}O_2$ represents $\dot{V}O_2$ max.

ergometer. Oxygen uptake increases as a linear function of the work rate until $\dot{V}O_2$ max is reached. When $\dot{V}O_2$ max is reached, an increase in power output does not result in an increase in oxygen uptake; thus, $\dot{V}O_2$ max represents a "physiological ceiling" for the ability of the oxygen transport system to deliver O_2 to contracting muscles. In the classic presentation of this test, the $\dot{V}O_2$ levels off or exhibits a "plateau" when the subject completes one stage further in the test; figure 4.7 shows this as a dashed line. The reason for using a dashed line is that many subjects do not demonstrate this plateau at the end of an incremental test; they simply cannot do one more stage beyond the one at which $\dot{V}O_2$ max was achieved. However, there are ways to demonstrate that the highest value reached is $\dot{V}O_2$ max (30, 64, 65, 96) (see chapter 17 for details). The physiological factors that influence $\dot{V}O_2$ max include the following: (1) the maximum ability of the cardiorespiratory system to deliver oxygen to the contracting muscle; and (2) the muscle's ability to take up the oxygen and produce ATP aerobically. Both genetics and exercise training are known to influence $\dot{V}O_2$ max; this will be discussed in chapter 13.

Lactate Threshold It is generally believed that most of the ATP production used to provide energy for muscular contraction during the early stages of an incremental exercise test comes from aerobic sources (78, 88, 99). However, as the exercise intensity increases, blood levels of lactate begin to rise in an exponential fashion (figure 4.8). This appears in untrained subjects around 50% to 60% of $\dot{V}O_2$ max, whereas it occurs at higher work rates in trained subjects (i.e., 65%–80% $\dot{V}O_2$ max) (46). Early on, a common term used to describe the point of a systematic rise in blood lactate during incremental exercise was the **anaerobic threshold** (15, 29, 36, 60, 69, 90, 110, 112, 116), because of the obvious link between anaerobic metabolism and the appearance of lactate.

Figure 4.8 Changes in blood lactate concentration during incremental exercise. The sudden rise in lactate is known as the lactate threshold.

Figure 4.9 Failure of the mitochondrial "hydrogen shuttle" system to keep pace with the rate of glycolytic production of NADH + H$^+$ results in the conversion of pyruvate to lactate.

However, because of arguments over terminology (see below), a more neutral term, the **lactate threshold,** has been widely adopted (28, 32, 104).

Another commonly used term that is related to the systematic rise in the blood lactate concentration is the *onset of blood lactate accumulation* (abbreviated as OBLA). This term, OBLA, differs from the lactate threshold in one important way. Rather than describing the blood lactate inflection point, the OBLA is defined as the exercise intensity (or oxygen consumption) at which a specific blood lactate concentration is reached (e.g., 4 millimoles per liter) (14, 55, 104). To avoid confusion, we will refer to the sudden rise in blood lactate levels during incremental exercise as the lactate threshold.

Some investigators believed that this sudden rise in the blood lactate concentration during incremental exercise represented a point of increasing reliance on anaerobic metabolism (i.e., glycolysis) (27, 108–112). Consequently, the term anaerobic threshold was adopted. The basic argument against the term *anaerobic threshold* centers around the question of whether the rise in blood lactate during incremental exercise is due to a lack of oxygen (hypoxia) in the working muscle or occurs for other reasons. Historically, rising blood lactate levels have been considered an indication of increased anaerobic metabolism within the contracting muscle because of low levels of O_2 in the individual muscle cells (110, 112). However, whether the end product of glycolysis is pyruvate or lactate depends on a variety of factors. First, if the rate of glycolysis is rapid, NADH production may exceed the transport capacity of the shuttle mechanisms that move hydrogens from the sarcoplasm into the mitochondria (101, 103, 115). Indeed, blood levels of epinephrine and norepinephrine begin to rise at 50% to 65% of $\dot{V}O_2$ max during incremental exercise and have been shown to stimulate the glycolytic rate; this increase in glycolysis increases the rate of NADH

production (103). Failure of the shuttle system to keep up with the rate of NADH production by glycolysis would result in pyruvate accepting some "unshuttled" hydrogens, and the formation of lactate could occur independent of whether the muscle cell had sufficient oxygen for aerobic ATP production (figure 4.9).

A second explanation for the formation of lactate in exercising muscle is related to the enzyme that catalyzes the conversion of pyruvate to lactate. The enzyme responsible for this reaction is lactate dehydrogenase (LDH), and it exists in several forms (different forms of the same enzyme are called isozymes). Recall that the reaction is as follows:

$$\begin{array}{ccc} CH_3 & LDH & CH_3 \\ | & & | \\ C = O + NADH + H^+ \leftrightarrow H - C - OH + NAD \\ | & & | \\ COO^- & & COO^- \\ \text{Pyruvate} & & \text{Lactate} \end{array}$$

This reaction is reversible in that lactate can be converted back to pyruvate under the appropriate conditions. Human skeletal muscle can be classified into three fiber types (see chapter 8). One of these is a "slow" fiber (sometimes called slow-twitch), whereas the remaining two are called "fast" fibers (sometimes called fast-twitch). As the names imply, fast fibers are recruited during intense, rapid exercise, whereas slow fibers are used primarily during low-intensity activity. The LDH isozyme found in fast fibers has a greater affinity for attaching to pyruvate, promoting the formation of lactate (62, 99). In contrast, slow fibers contain an LDH form that promotes the conversion of lactate to pyruvate. Therefore, lactate formation might occur in fast fibers during exercise simply because of the type of LDH present. Thus, lactate production would again be independent of oxygen availability in the muscle cell. Early in an incremental exercise test it is likely that slow fibers are the first called into action. However, as the exercise intensity increases, the amount of muscular force produced must be

Exercise Physiology Applied to Sports

Does Lactate Cause Muscle Soreness?

A belief among some athletes and coaches is that lactate production during exercise is a primary cause of delayed-onset muscle soreness (i.e., soreness occurring 24 to 48 hours after exercise). Nonetheless, physiological evidence indicates that lactate is not a primary cause of this type of muscle soreness. Several lines of "physiological reasoning" can be used to support this position. First, although lactate production occurs in active skeletal muscle during high-intensity exercise, lactate removal from the muscle and blood is rapid following an exercise session. In fact, blood levels of lactate return to resting levels within 60 minutes after exercise (see A Closer Look 4.1). Therefore, it seems unlikely that lactate production during a single exercise bout would result in muscle soreness 1 or 2 days later.

A second argument against lactate causing delayed-onset muscle soreness is that if lactate production caused muscle soreness, power athletes would experience soreness after each workout. Clearly, this is not the case. Indeed, well-conditioned power athletes (e.g., track sprinters) rarely experience muscle soreness after a routine training session.

If lactate is not the cause of delayed-onset muscle soreness, what is the cause? Growing evidence indicates that this type of muscle soreness originates from microscopic injury to muscle fibers. This kind of injury results in a slow cascade of biochemical events leading to inflammation and edema within the injured muscles. Because these events are slow to develop, the resulting pain generally doesn't appear until 24 to 48 hours after exercise. Details of the events leading to delayed-onset muscle soreness are discussed in chapter 21.

---

increased. This increased muscular force is supplied by recruiting more and more fast fibers. Therefore, the involvement of more fast fibers may result in increased lactate production and thus may be responsible for the lactate threshold.

A final explanation for the lactate threshold may be related to the rate of removal of lactate from the blood during incremental exercise. When a researcher removes a blood sample from an exercising subject, the concentration of lactate in that sample is the difference between the amount of lactate entry into the blood and the rate of lactate removal from the blood. At any given time during exercise, some muscles are producing lactate and releasing it into the blood, and some tissues (e.g., liver, skeletal muscles, heart, etc.) are removing lactate. Therefore, the concentration of lactate in the blood at any given time can be expressed mathematically in the following way:

$$\text{Blood lactate concentration} = \text{Lactate entry into the blood} - \text{Blood lactate removal}$$

Thus, a rise in the blood lactate concentration can occur due to either an increase in lactate production or a decrease in lactate removal. Recent evidence suggests that the rise in blood lactate levels in animals during incremental exercise may be the result of both an increase in lactate production and a decrease in the rate of lactate removal (16, 35). See chapter 13 for a discussion of how endurance training affects lactate production. Also, see The Winning Edge 4.1.

To summarize, controversy exists over both the terminology and the mechanism to explain the sudden rise in blood lactate concentration during incremental exercise. It is possible that any one or a combination of the explanations (including lack of O_2) might explain the lactate threshold. Figure 4.10 contains a summary of possible mechanisms to explain the lactate threshold. The search for definitive evidence to explain the mechanism(s) altering the blood lactate concentration during incremental exercise will continue for years to come.

Practical Use of the Lactate Threshold Regardless of the physiological mechanism to explain the

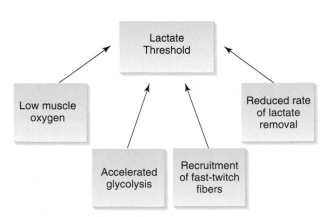

Figure 4.10 Possible mechanisms to explain the lactate threshold during incremental exercise. See text for details.

lactate threshold, it has important implications for predicting sports performance and perhaps in planning training programs for endurance athletes. For example, several studies have demonstrated that the lactate threshold used in combination with other physiological measurements (e.g., $\dot{V}O_2$ max), is a useful predictor of success in distance running (39, 79). Further, the lactate threshold might serve as a guideline for coaches and athletes in planning the level of exercise intensity needed to optimize training results (e.g., choose a training heart rate based on the LT). This is discussed in more detail in chapters 16 and 21.

IN SUMMARY

- Oxygen uptake increases in a linear fashion during incremental exercise until $\dot{V}O_2$ max is reached.
- The point at which there is a sudden increase in the blood lactate concentration during an incremental (graded) exercise test is termed the *lactate threshold*.
- Controversy exists over the mechanism to explain the sudden rise in blood lactate concentration during incremental exercise. It is possible that any one or a combination of the following factors might provide an explanation for the lactate threshold: (1) low muscle oxygen, (2) accelerated glycolysis due to epinephrine and norepinephrine, (3) recruitment of fast muscle fibers, and (4) a reduced rate of lactate removal.
- The lactate threshold has practical uses, such as predicting endurance performance and as a marker of training intensity.

ESTIMATION OF FUEL UTILIZATION DURING EXERCISE

A noninvasive technique that is commonly used to estimate the percent contribution of carbohydrate or fat to energy metabolism during exercise is the ratio of carbon dioxide output ($\dot{V}CO_2$) to the volume of oxygen consumed ($\dot{V}O_2$) (40, 114). This $\dot{V}CO_2/\dot{V}O_2$ ratio is called the **respiratory exchange ratio (R).** During steady-state conditions, the $\dot{V}CO_2/\dot{V}O_2$ ratio is often termed the respiratory quotient (RQ), as it is thought to reflect CO_2 production and O_2 consumption by the mitochondria of the active muscles. For simplicity, we will refer to the $\dot{V}CO_2/\dot{V}O_2$ ratio as the respiratory exchange ratio (R). How can the R be used to estimate whether fat or carbohydrate is being used as a fuel? The answer is related to the fact that fat and carbohydrate differ in the amount of O_2 used and CO_2

produced during oxidation. When using R as a predictor of fuel utilization during exercise, the role that protein contributes to ATP production during exercise is ignored. This is reasonable because protein generally plays a small role as a substrate during physical activity. Therefore, the R during exercise is often termed a "nonprotein R."

Let's consider the R for fat first. When fat is oxidized, O_2 combines with carbon to form CO_2 and joins with hydrogen to form water. The chemical relationship is as follows:

Fat (palmitic acid) $C_{16}H_{32}O_2$
Oxidation: $C_{16}H_{32}O_2 + 23\,O_2 \rightarrow 16\,CO_2 + 16\,H_2O$
Therefore, the $R = \dot{V}CO_2 \div \dot{V}O_2 = 16\,CO_2 \div 23\,O_2$
$\qquad = 0.70$

For R to be used as an estimate of substrate utilization during exercise, the subject must have reached a steady state. This is important because only during steady-state exercise are the $\dot{V}CO_2$ and $\dot{V}O_2$ reflective of O_2 uptake and CO_2 production in the tissues. For example, if a person is hyperventilating (i.e., breathing too much for a particular metabolic rate), excessive CO_2 loss from the body's CO_2 stores (see chapter 10) could bias the ratio of $\dot{V}CO_2$ to $\dot{V}O_2$ and invalidate the use of R to estimate which fuel is being consumed.

Carbohydrate oxidation also results in a predictable ratio of the volume of oxygen consumed to the amount of CO_2 produced. The oxidation of carbohydrate results in a R of 1.0:

Glucose $= C_6H_{12}O_6$
Oxidation: $C_6H_{12}O_6 + 6\,O_2 \rightarrow 6\,CO_2 + 6\,H_2O$
$R = \dot{V}CO_2 \div \dot{V}CO_2 = 6\,CO_2 \div 6\,O_2 = 1.0$

Fat oxidation requires more O_2 than carbohydrate oxidation because carbohydrate contains more O_2 than fat (104). The caloric equivalent of one liter of oxygen is approximately 4.70 kcal when fat alone is used, and approximately 5.0 kcal when carbohydrates alone are used. Consequently, you obtain about 6% more energy (ATP) per liter of oxygen when using carbohydrate, compared to fat, as the sole fuel for exercise.

It is unlikely that either fat or carbohydrate would be the only substrate used during most types of submaximal exercise. Therefore, the exercise R would likely be somewhere between 1.0 and 0.70. Table 4.1 lists a range of R values and the percentage of fat or carbohydrate metabolism they represent. Note that a nonprotein R of 0.85 represents a condition wherein fat and carbohydrate contribute equally as energy substrates. Further, notice that the higher the R, the greater the role of carbohydrate as an energy source, and the lower the R, the greater the contribution of fat. Table 4.1 shows how the caloric equivalent of oxygen changes with the mixture of fuel used (71).

TABLE 4.1	Percentage of Fat and Carbohydrate Metabolized as Determined by a Nonprotein Respiratory Exchange Ratio (R) and the Caloric Equivalent for Oxygen ($kcal \cdot L^{-1} O_2$)		
R	% Fat	% Carbohydrate	$kcal \cdot L^{-1} O_2$
0.70	100	0	4.69
0.75	83	17	4.74
0.80	67	33	4.80
0.85	50	50	4.86
0.90	33	67	4.92
0.95	17	83	4.99
1.00	0	100	5.05

Note: Values are from Knoebel (71).

IN SUMMARY

- The respiratory exchange ratio (R) is the ratio of carbon dioxide produced to the oxygen consumed ($\dot{V}CO_2/\dot{V}O_2$).
- For R to be used as an estimate of substrate utilization during exercise, the subject must have reached a steady state. This is important because only during steady-state exercise are the $\dot{V}CO_2$ and $\dot{V}O_2$ reflective of metabolic exchange of gases in tissues.
- The caloric equivalent for oxygen is 4.7 kcal/L when fat alone is used and 5.0 kcal/L when carbohydrate alone is used, about a 6% difference.

FACTORS GOVERNING FUEL SELECTION

Proteins contribute less than 2% of the substrate used during exercise of less than 1 hour's duration. However, the role of proteins as a fuel source may increase slightly during prolonged exercise (i.e., 3 to 5 hours' duration). During this type of exercise, the total contribution of protein to the fuel supply may reach 5% to 10% during the final minutes of work (10, 14, 63, 75, 76, 93, 113). Therefore, proteins play only a minor role as a substrate during exercise, with fat and carbohydrate serving as the major sources of energy during activity in the healthy individual consuming a balanced diet. Whether fat or carbohydrate is the primary substrate during work is determined by several factors, including diet, the intensity and duration of exercise, and whether the subject is endurance trained. For example, high-fat and low-carbohydrate diets promote a high rate of fat metabolism. In regard to exercise intensity, low-intensity exercise relies primarily on fat as fuel, whereas carbohydrate is the primary energy source during high-intensity exercise. Fuel selection is also influenced by the duration of exercise. During low-intensity, prolonged exercise, there is a progressive increase in the amount of fat oxidized by the working muscles. Endurance-trained subjects use more fat and less carbohydrate than less-fit subjects during prolonged exercise at the same intensity. In the next two sections we discuss in detail the influence of exercise intensity and duration on fuel selection. The role of endurance training is discussed in detail in chapter 13, and diet and performance is covered in chapter 23.

Exercise Intensity and Fuel Selection

Again, fats are a primary fuel source for muscle during low-intensity exercise (i.e., 30% $\dot{V}O_2$ max), whereas carbohydrate is the dominant substrate during high-intensity exercise (i.e., 70% $\dot{V}O_2$ max) (19, 23, 84, 98). The influence of exercise intensity on muscle fuel selection is illustrated in figure 4.11. Note that as the exercise intensity increases, there is a progressive increase in carbohydrate metabolism and a decrease in fat metabolism. Also notice that as the exercise intensity increases, there is an exercise intensity at which the energy derived from carbohydrate exceeds that of fat; this work rate has been labeled the *crossover point* (19). That is, as the exercise intensity increases above the crossover point, a progressive shift occurs from fat to carbohydrate metabolism.

What causes this shift from fat to carbohydrate metabolism as the exercise intensity increases? Two primary factors are involved: (1) recruitment of fast fibers and (2) increasing blood levels of epinephrine. As the exercise intensity increases, more and more fast muscle fibers are recruited (45). These fibers have an abundance of glycolytic enzymes but few

Figure 4.11 Illustration of the "crossover" concept. Note that as the exercise intensity increases, there is a progressive increase in the contribution of carbohydrate as a fuel source.

McArdle's Syndrome: A Genetic Error in Muscle Glycogen Metabolism

McArdle's syndrome is a genetic disease in which the person is born with a gene mutation and cannot synthesize the enzyme phosphorylase. This metabolic disorder prevents the individual from breaking down muscle glycogen as a fuel source during exercise. This inability to use glycogen during exercise also prevents the muscle from producing lactate, as indicated by the observation that blood lactate levels do not increase in McArdle's patients during high-intensity exercise. It should be no surprise then that during submaximal exercise McArdle's patients use more fat as a fuel compared to control subjects (86). However, despite rising levels of fatty acids in the blood of McArdle's patients, they are not able to oxidize more fat. This indicates that carbohydrate availability limits fat oxidation even during steady state exercise in these patients. See the section "Interaction of Fat/Carbohydrate Metabolism" below for more on this.

An unfortunate side effect of this genetic disorder is that McArdle's patients often complain of exercise intolerance and muscle pain during exertion. This clinical observation provides a practical illustration of the importance of muscle glycogen as an energy source during exercise. McArdle's syndrome is but one of many genetic disorders of metabolism. See van Adel and Tarnopolsky's review on these metabolic myopathies in Suggested Readings.

---

mitochondrial and lipolytic enzymes (enzymes responsible for fat breakdown). In short, this means that fast fibers are better equipped to metabolize carbohydrates than fats. Therefore, the increased recruitment of fast fibers results in greater carbohydrate metabolism and less fat metabolism (19).

A second factor that regulates carbohydrate metabolism during exercise is epinephrine. As exercise intensity increases, there is a progressive rise in blood levels of epinephrine. High levels of epinephrine increase phosphorylase activity, which causes an increase in muscle glycogen breakdown; this results in an increased rate of glycolysis and lactate production (19). Interestingly, there are some individuals who lack phosphorylase and cannot produce lactate (see Clinical Applications 4.1). This increased production of lactate inhibits fat metabolism by reducing the availability of fat as a substrate (106). The lack of fat as a substrate for working muscles under these conditions dictates that carbohydrate will be the primary fuel (see chapter 5 for more details on how this occurs).

Many individuals use exercise as a means of keeping body weight and body fat in check, and you are probably familiar with pieces of exercise equipment having a selection for a "fat burning" workout. In such a workout the emphasis is on low intensity and long duration. But is that really the best way to burn fat? See A Closer Look 4.2 for the answer.

Exercise Duration and Fuel Selection

During prolonged (i.e., greater than 30 minutes), moderate-intensity (40% to 59% $\dot{V}O_2$max) exercise, there is a gradual shift from carbohydrate metabolism toward an increasing reliance on fat as a substrate (4, 44, 61, 73, 84, 92). Figure 4.13 demonstrates this point.

What factors control the rate of fat metabolism during prolonged exercise? Fat metabolism is regulated by those variables that control the rate of fat breakdown (a process called lipolysis). Triglycerides are broken down into **free fatty acids (FFAs)** and glycerol by enzymes called **lipases.** These lipases are generally inactive until stimulated by the hormones epinephrine, norepinephrine, and glucagon (61). For example, during low-intensity, prolonged exercise, blood levels of epinephrine rise, which increases lipase activity and thus promotes lipolysis. This increase in lipolysis results in an increase in blood and muscle levels of FFA and promotes fat metabolism. In general, **lipolysis** is a slow process, and an increase in fat metabolism occurs only after several minutes of exercise. This point is illustrated in figure 4.13 by the slow increase in fat metabolism across time during prolonged submaximal exercise.

The mobilization of FFA into the blood is inhibited by the hormone insulin and high blood levels of lactate. Insulin inhibits lipolysis by direct inhibition of lipase activity. Normally, blood insulin levels decline during prolonged exercise (see chapter 5). However, if a high-carbohydrate meal or drink is consumed 30 to 60 minutes prior to exercise, blood glucose levels rise and more insulin is released from the pancreas. This elevation in blood insulin results in diminished lipolysis and a reduction in fat metabolism, leading to a greater use of carbohydrate as a fuel.

Interaction of Fat/Carbohydrate Metabolism

During short-term exercise it is unlikely that muscle stores of glycogen or blood glucose levels would be depleted. However, during prolonged exercise (e.g., greater than 2 hours) muscle and liver stores of

Exercise and Fat Metabolism: Is Low-Intensity Exercise Best for Burning Fat?

What intensity of exercise is optimal for burning fat? It is often assumed that the intensity of exercise must be kept very low to burn fat as a fuel. It is true that at low exercise intensities a high percentage of the total energy expenditure during exercise is derived from fat. It follows that as the exercise intensity increases, the percentage of fat used as fuel decreases (figure 4.11). However, a key point to consider is that the total rate of fat oxidation during exercise is typically greatest at higher exercise intensities that are below the lactate threshold. An appreciation of this point can be gained from figures 4.11 and 4.13. For example, during exercise at 20% of $\dot{V}O_2$ max, it is estimated that about 60% of the total energy expended would come from fat (figure 4.11). By comparison, during exercise at 50% of $\dot{V}O_2$ max, about 40% of the total energy expended would be obtained from fat (figure 4.11). Nonetheless, because the total rate of energy expenditure is 2.5 times greater at 50% $\dot{V}O_2$ max compared to 20% $\dot{V}O_2$ max, the absolute amount of fat metabolized is 33% higher during exercise at 50% $\dot{V}O_2$ max (figure 4.12). Therefore, expressing energy derived from fat as a percentage without consideration of the total energy expenditure is often misleading.

FIGURE 4.12 Illustration of the rate of fat metabolism during exercise at varying intensities in an untrained subject.* Note that when comparing exercise at 20, 50, 80, and 100% of $\dot{V}O_2$ max, the greatest absolute amount of fat was metabolized at 50% of $\dot{V}O_2$ max. Therefore, when designing an exercise program to reduce body fat stores, it is important to consider both the total rate of energy expenditure and the percentage of energy that is derived from fat metabolism. It is important to appreciate that this illustration is not intended to represent the "ideal" exercise intensity for all subjects to optimize fat metabolism. It is simply intended to make the point that there is an optimal exercise intensity to use fat as a fuel source and that this intensity depends upon both the percentage of energy derived from fat and the total rate of energy expenditure.

*The data presented in this example are based upon measurements obtained from an untrained male subject (body weight 89 kilograms; $\dot{V}O_2$ max 4.0 liters/min; lactate threshold 60% of $\dot{V}O_2$ max).

Figure 4.13 Shift from carbohydrate metabolism toward fat metabolism during prolonged exercise.

glycogen can reach very low levels (14, 24, 45, 50, 56). This is important because depletion of muscle and blood carbohydrate stores results in muscular fatigue (50). Why do low muscle glycogen levels produce fatigue? Recent evidence suggests the following answer. Depletion of available carbohydrate reduces the rate of glycolysis, and therefore the concentration of pyruvate in the muscle is also reduced (50). This lowers the rate of aerobic production of ATP by reducing the number of Krebs-cycle compounds (intermediates). In human muscle with adequate glycogen stores, submaximal exercise (i.e., 70% $\dot{V}O_2$ max) results in a ninefold increase (above resting values) in the number of Krebs-cycle intermediates (97). This elevated pool of Krebs-cycle intermediates is required for the Krebs cycle to "speed up" in an effort to meet the high ATP demands during exercise. Pyruvate (produced via glycolysis) is important in providing this increase in Krebs-cycle intermediates. For example, pyruvate is a precursor of several Krebs-cycle intermediates (e.g., oxaloacetate, malate). When the rate of glycolysis is reduced due to the unavailability of glucose or glycogen, pyruvate levels in the sarcoplasm decline, and the levels of Krebs-cycle intermediates decrease as well.

Exercise Physiology Applied to Sports

Carbohydrate Feeding via Sports Drinks Improves Endurance Performance

The depletion of muscle and blood carbohydrate stores can contribute to muscular fatigue during prolonged exercise. Therefore, can the ingestion of carbohydrates during prolonged exercise improve endurance performance? The clear answer to this question is yes! Studies investigating the effects of carbohydrate feeding through "sports drinks" have convincingly shown that carbohydrate feedings during submaximal (i.e., 70% $\dot{V}O_2$ max), long-duration (e.g., 90 minutes) exercise can improve endurance performance (26, 80). How much carbohydrate is required to improve performance? In general, carbohydrate feedings of 30 to 60 grams per hour are required to enhance performance.

Current questions include whether the addition of protein to these sport drinks will provide additional benefits to performance. You will see more on this in chapter 23, in addition to the role of carbohydrate loading in the days prior to the performance of endurance races (e.g., a marathon).

This decline in Krebs-cycle intermediates slows the rate of Krebs-cycle activity, with the end result being a reduction in the rate of aerobic ATP production. This reduced rate of muscle ATP production limits muscular performance and may result in fatigue.

It is important to appreciate that a reduction in Krebs-cycle intermediates (due to glycogen depletion) results in a diminished rate of ATP production from fat metabolism, because fat can be metabolized only via Krebs-cycle oxidation. Hence, when carbohydrate stores are depleted in the body, the rate at which fat is metabolized is also reduced (97). Therefore, "fats burn in the flame of carbohydrates" (103). The role that depletion of body carbohydrate stores may play in limiting performance during prolonged exercise is introduced in The Winning Edge 4.2 and is further discussed in both chapters 19 and 23.

Body Fuel Sources

In this section we outline the storage sites in the body for carbohydrates, fats, and proteins. Further, we define the role that each of these fuel storage sites plays in providing energy during exercise. Finally, we discuss the use of lactate as a fuel source during work.

Sources of Carbohydrate During Exercise Carbohydrate is stored as glycogen in both the muscle and the liver (see table 4.2). Muscle glycogen stores provide a direct source of carbohydrate for muscle energy metabolism, whereas liver glycogen stores serve as a means of replacing blood glucose. For example, when blood glucose levels decline during prolonged exercise, liver glycogenolysis is stimulated and glucose is released into the blood. This glucose

TABLE 4.2 Principal Storage Sites of Carbohydrate and Fat in the Body of a Healthy, Nonobese (20% Body Fat), 70-kg Male Subject

Note that dietary intake of carbohydrate influences the amount of glycogen stored in both the liver and muscle. Mass units for storage are grams (g) and kilograms (kg). Energy units are kilocalories (kcal) and kilojoules (kJ). Data are from references 29, 31, and 62.

| Storage Site | CARBOHYDRATE (CHO) | | |
	Mixed Diet	High-CHO Diet	Low-CHO Diet
Liver glycogen	60 g (240 kcal or 1,005 kJ)	90 g (360 kcal or 1,507 kJ)	<30 g (120 kcal or 502 kJ)
Glucose in blood and extracellular fluid	10 g (40 kcal or 167 kJ)	10 g (40 kcal or 167 kJ)	10 g (40 kcal or 167 kJ)
Muscle glycogen	350 g (1,400 kcal or 5,860 kJ)	600 g (2,400 kcal or 10,046 kJ)	300 g (1,200 kcal or 5,023 kJ)

| Storage Site | FAT |
	Mixed Diet
Adipocytes	14 kg (107,800 kcal or 451,251 kJ)
Muscle	0.5 kg (3,850 kcal or 16,116 kJ)

Figure 4.15   Percentage of energy derived from the four major sources of fuel during submaximal exercise (i.e., 65%–75% $\dot{V}O_2$ max). Data are from trained endurance athletes.

Figure 4.14   Influence of exercise intensity on muscle fuel source. Data are from highly trained endurance athletes.

can then be transported to the contracting muscle and used as fuel.

Carbohydrate used as a substrate during exercise comes from both glycogen stores in muscle and from blood glucose (22, 25, 45, 67, 102). The relative contribution of muscle glycogen and blood glucose to energy metabolism during exercise varies as a function of the exercise intensity and duration. Blood glucose plays the greater role during low-intensity exercise, whereas muscle glycogen is the primary source of carbohydrate during high-intensity exercise (see figure 4.14). As mentioned earlier, the increased glycogen usage during high-intensity exercise can be explained by the increased rate of glycogenolysis that occurs due to recruitment of fast-twitch fibers and elevated blood epinephrine levels.

During the first hour of submaximal prolonged exercise, much of the carbohydrate metabolized by muscle comes from muscle glycogen. However, as muscle glycogen levels decline across time, blood glucose becomes an increasingly important source of fuel (see figure 4.15).

Sources of Fat During Exercise   When an individual consumes more energy (i.e., food) than he or she expends, this additional energy is stored in the form of fat. A gain of 3500 kcal of energy results in the storage of 1 pound of fat. Most fat is stored in the form of triglycerides in adipocytes (fat cells), but some is stored in muscle cells as well (see table 4.2). As mentioned

earlier, the major factor that determines the role of fat as a substrate during exercise is its availability to the muscle cell. To be metabolized, triglycerides must be degraded to FFA (three molecules) and glycerol (one molecule). When triglycerides are split, FFA can be converted into acetyl-CoA and enter the Krebs cycle.

Which fat stores are used as a fuel source varies as a function of the exercise intensity and duration. For example, plasma FFAs (i.e., FFA from adipocytes) are the primary source of fat during low-intensity exercise. At higher work rates, metabolism of muscle triglycerides increases (see figure 4.14). At exercise intensities between 65% and 85% $\dot{V}O_2$ max, the contribution of fat as a muscle fuel source is approximately equal between plasma FFA and muscle triglycerides (23, 53, 95).

The contribution of plasma FFA and muscle triglycerides to exercise metabolism during prolonged exercise is summarized in figure 4.15. Note that at the beginning of exercise, the contribution of plasma FFA and muscle triglycerides is equal. However, as the duration of exercise increases, there is a progressive rise in the role of plasma FFA as a fuel source.

Sources of Protein During Exercise   To be used as a fuel source, proteins must first be degraded into amino acids. Amino acids can be supplied to muscle from the blood or from the amino acid pool in the fiber itself. Again, the role that protein plays as a substrate during exercise is small and is principally dependent on the availability of branch-chained amino acids and the amino acid alanine (7, 49). Skeletal muscle can directly metabolize branched-chain amino acids (e.g., valine, leucine, isoleucine) to produce ATP (47, 63). Further, in the liver, alanine can be converted to glucose and returned via the blood to skeletal muscle to be utilized as a substrate.

Any factor that increases the amino acid pool (amount of available amino acids) in the liver or in

The Cori Cycle: Lactate as a Fuel Source

During exercise, some of the lactate that is produced by skeletal muscles is transported to the liver via the blood (51, 105). Upon entry into the liver, lactate can be converted to glucose via gluconeogenesis. This "new" glucose can be released into the blood and transported back to skeletal muscles to be used as an energy source during exercise. The cycle of lactate-to-glucose between the muscle and liver is called the **Cori cycle** and is illustrated in figure 4.16.

Glucose

Glucose

Glucose

Pyruvate

Glucose-6-phosphate

Bloodstream

Pyruvate

Lactate

Lactate

Lactate

FIGURE 4.16 The Cori cycle. During intense exercise, lactate is formed in muscle fibers. The lactate formed in muscle can then be transported via the blood to the liver and converted to glucose by gluconeogenesis.

skeletal muscle can theoretically enhance protein metabolism (63, 77). One such factor is prolonged exercise (i.e., more than 2 hours). Numerous investigators have demonstrated that enzymes capable of degrading muscle proteins (proteases) are activated during long-term exercise (2, 33, 34, 85). The mechanism responsible for activation of these proteases during prolonged exercise appears to be exercise-induced increases in calcium levels within muscle fibers during exercise (2, 82). Indeed, several families of proteases are activated by increases in cellular levels of calcium (2, 82). Regardless of the mechanism responsible for protease activation during exercise, the practical aspect of this finding is that during the course of prolonged exercise, proteases become activated and amino acids are liberated from their parent proteins. This rise in the amino acid pool results in an increase in the use of amino acids as fuel during exercise (84).

Lactate as a Fuel Source During Exercise For many years, lactate was considered to be a waste product of glycolysis with limited metabolic use. However, new evidence has shown that lactate is not necessarily a waste product but can play a beneficial role during exercise by serving as both a substrate for the liver to synthesize glucose (see A Closer Look 4.3) and as a direct fuel source for skeletal muscle and the heart (12, 16, 53). That is, in slow skeletal muscle fibers and the heart, lactate removed from the blood can be converted to pyruvate, which can then be transformed to acetyl-CoA. This acetyl-CoA can then enter the Krebs cycle and contribute to oxidative metabolism. The concept that lactate can be produced

ASK THE EXPERT 4.2

The Lactate Shuttle: An Important Concept in Muscle Metabolism During Exercise: Questions and Answers with Dr. George Brooks

Dr. George Brooks is a professor in the Department of Integrative Physiology at the University of California-Berkeley. Professor Brooks is an internationally recognized exercise physiologist, and he has published more than 200 scientific papers on a variety of topics related to exercise metabolism. Dr. Brooks first coined the term "lactate shuttle" in 1985, and his laboratory performed much of the original research that defines the role that lactate plays as a fuel source during exercise. Dr. Brooks received the American College of Sports Medicine's Honor Award, the highest award offered by that organization, for his major contributions to our understanding of exercise metabolism. Here, Dr. Brooks answers questions related to the production and fate of lactate produced in skeletal muscle during exercise.

QUESTION: The concept of the lactate shuttle originated from your work over 20 years ago, and your research group has continued to provide new information about this important topic. Given that the concept of the lactate shuttle continues to evolve, what is your contemporary definition of the "lactate shuttle"?

ANSWER: In the broadest sense, the lactate shuttle is defined as the formation of lactate in one cell compartment and use in another compartment. That is, the compartments may be in the cell that pro-duced the lactate or in an adjacent cell or far removed cells in the body. Originally we believed that the main functions of the lactate shuttle were to provide oxidizable fuel and a gluconeogenic precursor. Now, we also recognize that lactate is a signaling molecule and may serve other functions in the body.

QUESTION: Which body tissues receive the most benefit from circulating lactate during prolonged exercise?

ANSWER: This is a difficult question to answer. Nonetheless, most lactate formed during exercise is used as a fuel in slow (Type I) skeletal muscle fibers and heart. Further, liver uptake of lactate from the blood is important because the use of lactate to form glucose (i.e., gluconeogenesis) in the liver is a basic and important physiological process, for without it hypoglycemia could occur in prolonged exercise.

QUESTION: In addition to your original concept of the cell-to-cell lactate shuttle, your group has recently discovered the existence of an "intracellular lactate shuttle." Can you please provide a brief description of the intracellular lactate shuttle?

ANSWER: The original Cell-Cell lactate shuttle was based on the concept of fiber type heterogeneity. The origi-nal idea was that recruitment of fast (Type II) fibers would result in lactate production, thus providing fuel for adjacent slow (Type I) muscle fibers and the heart. However, it became apparent that the lactate shuttle operated all the time, even at rest when Type II muscle fibers were not actively contracting. So, we recognized the presence of another component of the lactate shuttle, an intracellular component. In the most simple terms, the intracellular lactate shuttle refers to the concept that lactate can be produced within the cytoplasm of a muscle fiber and then taken up by mitochondria in the same fiber for use as a fuel source.

QUESTION: Is lactate shuttling always beneficial?

ANSWER: So far as we can tell, in normal physiology the answer appears to be "yes." However, we have recently shown that lactate transporters exist in cancer cells, including mitochondria of cancer cells (68). One way to think of cancer cells is that their runaway cell proliferation is fueled by lactate shuttle mechanisms. In fact, recognizing that fact, one group (100) has shown that poisoning lactate transport proteins is one way to kill cancer cells. Hence, today we and others are trying to figure out ways to disrupt lactate shuttling in tumors.

---

in one tissue and then transported to another to be used as an energy source has been termed the *lactate shuttle* (12, 13, 15–17). See Ask the Expert 4.2 for more details on the lactate shuttle.

IN SUMMARY

- The regulation of fuel selection during exercise is under complex control and is dependent upon several factors, including diet and the intensity and duration of exercise.

- In general, carbohydrates are used as the major fuel source during high-intensity exercise.
- During prolonged exercise, there is a gradual shift from carbohydrate metabolism toward fat metabolism.
- Proteins contribute less than 2% of the fuel used during exercise of less than one hour's duration. During prolonged exercise (i.e., 3 to 5 hours' duration), the total contribution of protein to the fuel supply may reach 5% to 10% during the final minutes of prolonged work.

STUDY QUESTIONS

1. Identify the predominant energy systems used to produce ATP during the following types of exercise:
   a. short-term, intense exercise (i.e., less than 10 seconds' duration)
   b. 400-meter dash
   c. 20-kilometer race (i.e., 12.4 miles)
2. Graph the change in oxygen uptake during the transition from rest to steady-state, submaximal exercise. Label the oxygen deficit. Where does the ATP come from during the transition period from rest to steady state?
3. Graph the change in oxygen uptake during recovery from exercise. Label the excess post-exercise oxygen consumption (EPOC) (i.e., oxygen debt).
4. How does modern theory of EPOC differ from the classical oxygen debt theory proposed by A. V. Hill?
5. Graph the change in oxygen uptake and blood lactate concentration during incremental exercise. Label the point on the graph that might be considered the lactate threshold or lactate inflection point, and $\dot{V}O_2$ max.
6. Discuss several possible reasons why blood lactate begins to rise rapidly during incremental exercise.
7. Briefly explain how the respiratory exchange ratio is used to estimate which substrate is being utilized during exercise. What is meant by the term nonprotein R?
8. List the factors that play a role in the regulation of carbohydrate metabolism during exercise.
9. Discuss the influence of exercise intensity on muscle fuel selection.
10. How does the duration of exercise influence muscle fuel selection?
11. List those variables that regulate fat metabolism during exercise.
12. What is the "lactate shuttle" and how is it demonstrated during exercise?

SUGGESTED READINGS

Bassett, D. R. 2002. Scientific contributions of A. V. Hill: Exercise physiology pioneer. *Journal of Applied Physiology* 93:1567–82.

Brooks, G., T. Fahey, and K. Baldwin. 2005. *Exercise Physiology: Human Bioenergetics and Its Applications*, 4th ed. New York: McGraw-Hill Companies.

Fox, S. 2011. *Human Physiology*. New York: McGraw-Hill Companies.

Gladden, L. B. 2004. Lactate metabolism: A new paradigm for the third millennium. *Journal of Physiology* 558:5–30.

Mooren, F., and K. Volker, eds. 2011. *Molecular and Cellular Exercise Physiology*. Champaign, IL: Human Kinetics.

Svedahl, K., and B. MacIntosh. 2003. Anaerobic threshold: The concept and methods of measurement. *Canadian Journal of Applied Physiology* 28:299–323.

Van Adel, B. A. and M. A. Tarnopolsky. 2009. Metabolic myopathies: Update 2009. *J Clin Neuromusc Dis.*10:97–121.

Widmaier, E., H. Raff, and K. Strang. 2006. *Vander's Human Physiology*, 10th ed. New York: McGraw-Hill Companies.

REFERENCES

1. **Armstrong R.** Biochemistry: energy liberation and use. In: *Sports Medicine and Physiology*, edited by Strauss R. Philadelphia: W. B. Saunders, 1979.
2. **Arthur GD, Booker TS, and Belcastro AN.** Exercise promotes a subcellular redistribution of calcium-stimulated protease activity in striated muscle. *Can J Physiol Pharmacol* 77: 42–47, 1999.
3. **Åstrand P.** *Textbook of Work Physiology*. Champaign: Human Kinetics, 2003.
4. **Ball-Burnett M, Green HJ, and Houston ME.** Energy metabolism in human slow and fast twitch fibres during prolonged cycle exercise. *J Physiol* 437: 257–267, 1991.
5. **Barnard RJ, and Foss ML.** Oxygen debt: effect of beta-adrenergic blockade on the lactacid and alactacid components. *J Appl Physiol* 27: 813–816, 1969.
6. **Bassett DR, Jr., Merrill PW, Nagle FJ, Agre JC, and Sampedro R.** Rate of decline in blood lactate after cycling exercise in endurance-trained and -untrained subjects. *J Appl Physiol* 70: 1816–1820, 1991.
7. **Bates P.** Exercise and protein turnover in the rat. *Journal of Physiology* (London) 303: 41P, 1980.
8. **Belcastro AN, and Bonen A.** Lactic acid removal rates during controlled and uncontrolled recovery exercise. *J Appl Physiol* 39: 932–936, 1975.
9. **Bendahan D, Mattei JP, Ghattas B, Confort-Gouny S, LeGuern ME, and Cozzone PJ.** Citrulline/malate promotes aerobic energy production in human exercising muscle. *Br J Sports Med* 36: 282–289, 2002.
10. **Berg A, and Keul J.** Serum alanine during long-lasting exercise. *International Journal of Sports Medicine* 1: 199–202, 1980.
11. **Boutellier U, Giezendanner D, Cerretelli P, and di Prampero PE.** After effects of chronic hypoxia on $\dot{V}O_2$ kinetics and on O_2 deficit and debt. *Eur J Appl Physiol Occup Physiol* 53: 87–91, 1984.
12. **Brooks G.** Lactate production under fully aerobic conditions: the lactate shuttle during rest and exercise. *Federation Proceedings* 45: 2924–2929, 1986.
13. **Brooks G.** Lactate: glycolytic end product and oxidative substrate during sustained exercise in mammals— the lactate shuttle. In: *Circulation, Respiration, and Metabolism*, edited by Berlin GR. Springer-Verlag, 1985.
14. **Brooks G, Fahey T, and Baldwin K.** *Exercise Physiology: Human Bioenergetics and Its Applications*. New York: McGraw-Hill, 2005.
15. **Brooks GA.** Anaerobic threshold: review of the concept and directions for future research. *Med Sci Sports Exerc* 17: 22–34, 1985.

16. **Brooks GA.** The lactate shuttle during exercise and recovery. *Med Sci Sports Exerc* 18: 360–368, 1986.

17. **Brooks GA, Dubouchaud H, Brown M, Sicurello JP, and Butz CE.** Role of mitochondrial lactate dehydrogenase and lactate oxidation in the intracellular lactate shuttle. *Proc Natl Acad Sci USA* 96: 1129–1134, 1999.

18. **Brooks GA, Hittelman KJ, Faulkner JA, and Beyer RE.** Temperature, skeletal muscle mitochondrial functions, and oxygen debt. *Am J Physiol* 220: 1053–1059, 1971.

19. **Brooks GA, and Mercier J.** Balance of carbohydrate and lipid utilization during exercise: the "crossover" concept. *J Appl Physiol* 76: 2253–2261, 1994.

20. **Casaburi R, Storer TW, Ben-Dov I, and Wasserman K.** Effect of endurance training on possible determinants of $\dot{V}O_2$ during heavy exercise. *J Appl Physiol* 62: 199–207, 1987.

21. **Cerretelli P, Shindell D, Pendergast DP, Di Prampero PE, and Rennie DW.** Oxygen uptake transients at the onset and offset of arm and leg work. *Respir Physiol* 30: 81–97, 1977.

22. **Coggin A.** Plasma glucose metabolism during exercise in humans. *Sports Medicine* 11: 102–124, 1991.

23. **Coyle EF.** Substrate utilization during exercise in active people. *Am J Clin Nutr* 61: 968S–979S, 1995.

24. **Coyle EF, Coggan AR, Hemmert MK, and Ivy JL.** Muscle glycogen utilization during prolonged strenuous exercise when fed carbohydrate. *J Appl Physiol* 61: 165–172, 1986.

25. **Coyle EF, Hamilton MT, Alonso JG, Montain SJ, and Ivy JL.** Carbohydrate metabolism during intense exercise when hyperglycemic. *J Appl Physiol* 70: 834–840, 1991.

26. **Coyle EF, and Montain SJ.** Carbohydrate and fluid ingestion during exercise: are there trade-offs? *Med Sci Sports Exerc* 24: 671–678, 1992.

27. **Davis JA.** Anaerobic threshold: review of the concept and directions for future research. *Med Sci Sports Exerc* 17: 6–21, 1985.

28. **Davis JA, Rozenek R, DeCicco DM, Carizzi MT, and Pham PH.** Comparison of three methods for detection of the lactate threshold. *Clin Physiol Funct Imaging* 27: 381–384, 2007.

29. **Davis JA, Vodak P, Wilmore JH, Vodak J, and Kurtz P.** Anaerobic threshold and maximal aerobic power for three modes of exercise. *J Appl Physiol* 41: 544–550, 1976.

30. **Day JR, Rossiter HB, Coats EM, Skasick A, and Whipp BJ.** The maximally attainable $\dot{V}O_2$ during exercise in humans: the peak vs. maximal issue. *J Appl Physiol* 95: 1910–1907, 2003.

31. **Dodd S, Powers S, O'Malley N, Brooks E, and Sommers H.** Effects of beta-adrenergic blockade on ventilation and gas exchange during incremental exercise. *Aviat Space Environ Med* 59: 718–722, 1988.

32. **Dodd S, Powers SK, Callender T, and Brooks E.** Blood lactate disappearance at various intensities of recovery exercise. *J Appl Physiol* 57: 1462–1465, 1984.

33. **Dohm GL, Beecher GR, Warren RQ, and Williams RT.** Influence of exercise on free amino acid concentrations in rat tissues. *J Appl Physiol* 50: 41–44, 1981.

34. **Dohm GL, Puente FR, Smith CP, and Edge A.** Changes in tissue protein levels as a result of endurance exercise. *Life Sci* 23: 845–849, 1978.

35. **Donovan CM, and Brooks GA.** Endurance training affects lactate clearance, not lactate production. *Am J Physiol* 244: E83–92, 1983.

36. **England P.** The effect of acute thermal dehydration on blood lactate accumulation during incremental exercise. *Journal of Sports Sciences* 2: 105–111, 1985.

37. **Essen B, and Kaijser L.** Regulation of glycolysis in intermittent exercise in man. *J Physiol* 281: 499–511, 1978.

38. **Evans BW, and Cureton KJ.** Effect of physical conditioning on blood lactate disappearance after supramaximal exercise. *Br J Sports Med* 17: 40–45, 1983.

39. **Farrell PA, Wilmore JH, Coyle EF, Billing JE, and Costill DL.** Plasma lactate accumulation and distance running performance. *Med Sci Sports* 11: 338–344, 1979.

40. **Fox S.** *Human Physiology.* New York: McGraw-Hill, 2011.

41. **Gaesser GA, and Brooks GA.** Metabolic bases of excess post-exercise oxygen consumption: a review. *Med Sci Sports Exerc* 16: 29–43, 1984.

42. **Gladden LB.** Net lactate uptake during progressive steady-level contractions in canine skeletal muscle. *J Appl Physiol* 71: 514–520, 1991.

43. **Gladden LB, Stainsby WN, and MacIntosh BR.** Norepinephrine increases canine skeletal muscle $\dot{V}O_2$ during recovery. *Med Sci Sports Exerc* 14: 471–476, 1982.

44. **Gollnick P, and Saltin B.** Fuel for muscular exercise: role of fat. In: *Exercise, Nutrition, and Energy Metabolism*, edited by Horton E, and Terjung R. New York: Macmillan, 1988.

45. **Gollnick PD.** Metabolism of substrates: energy substrate metabolism during exercise and as modified by training. *Fed Proc* 44: 353–357, 1985.

46. **Gollnick PD, Bayly WM, and Hodgson DR.** Exercise intensity, training, diet, and lactate concentration in muscle and blood. *Med Sci Sports Exerc* 18: 334–340, 1986.

47. **Goodman M.** Amino acid and protein metabolism. In: *Exercise, Nutrition, and Energy Metabolism*, edited by Horton E, and Terjung R. New York: Macmillan, 1988.

48. **Gore CJ, and Withers RT.** Effect of exercise intensity and duration on postexercise metabolism. *J Appl Physiol* 68: 2362–2368, 1990.

49. **Graham T.** Skeletal muscle amino acid metabolism and ammonia production during exercise. In: *Exercise Metabolism.* Champaign: Human Kinetics, 1995.

50. **Green H.** How important is endogenous muscle glycogen to fatigue during prolonged exercise? *Canadian Journal of Physiology and Pharmacology* 69: 1991.

51. **Green H, Halestrap A, Mockett C, O'Toole D, Grant S, and Ouyang J.** Increases in muscle MCT are associated with reductions in muscle lactate after a single exercise session in humans. *Am J Physiol Endocrinol Metab* 282: E154–160, 2002.

52. **Hagberg JM, Mullin JP, and Nagle FJ.** Oxygen consumption during constant-load exercise. *J Appl Physiol* 45: 381–384, 1978.

53. **Hargreaves M.** Skeletal muscle carbohydrate metabolism during exercise. In: *Exercise Metabolism.* Champaign: Human Kinetics, 1995.

54. **Harris RC, Edwards RH, Hultman E, Nordesjo LO, Nylind B, and Sahlin K.** The time course of phosphorylcreatine resynthesis during recovery of the quadriceps muscle in man. *Pflugers Arch* 367: 137–142, 1976.

55. **Heck H, Mader A, Hess G, Mucke S, Muller R, and Hollmann W.** Justification of the 4-mmol/l lactate threshold. *Int J Sports Med* 6: 117–130, 1985.

56. **Helge JW, Rehrer NJ, Pilegaard H, Manning P, Lucas SJ, Gerrard DF, and Cotter JD.** Increased fat oxidation and regulation of metabolic genes with ultraendurance exercise. *Acta Physiol (Oxf)* 191: 77–86, 2007.

57. **Hermansen L, and Stensvold I.** Production and removal of lactate during exercise in man. *Acta Physiol Scand* 86: 191–201, 1972.

58. **Hickson RC, Bomze HA, and Hollozy JO.** Faster adjustment of O_2 uptake to the energy requirement of exercise in the trained state. *J Appl Physiol* 44: 877–881, 1978.

59. **Hill A.** The oxidative removal of lactic acid. *Journal of Physiology* (London) 48: x–xi, 1914.

60. **Hollmann W.** Historical remarks on the development of the aerobic-anaerobic threshold up to 1966. *Int J Sports Med* 6: 109–116, 1985.

61. **Holloszy J.** Utilization of fatty acids during exercise. In: *Biochemistry of Exercise VII*, edited by Taylor A. Champaign: Human Kinetics, 1990, p. 319–328.

62. **Holloszy JO.** Muscle metabolism during exercise. *Arch Phys Med Rehabil* 63: 231–234, 1982.

63. **Hood DA, and Terjung RL.** Amino acid metabolism during exercise and following endurance training. *Sports Med* 9: 23–35, 1990.

64. **Howley ET.** $\dot{V}O_2$ max and the plateau—needed or not? *Med Sci Sports Exer* 39: 101–102, 2007.

65. **Howley ET, Bassett DR, and Welch HG.** Criteria for maximal oxygen uptake: review and commentary. *Med Sci Sports Exer* 27: 1292–1301, 1995.

66. **Hultman E.** Energy metabolism in human muscle. *J Physiol* 231: 56P, 1973.

67. **Hultman E, and Sjoholm H.** Substrate availability. In: *Biochemistry of Exercise*, edited by Knuttgen H, Vogel J, and Poortmans J. Champaign: Human Kinetics, 1983.

68. **Hussien R, and Brooks GA.** Mitochondrial and plasma membrane lactate transporter and lactate dehydrogenase isoform expression in breast cancer cell lines. *Physiological Genomics* doi:10.1152: PG-00177-02010, 2010.

69. **Jones NL, and Ehrsam RE.** The anaerobic threshold. *Exerc Sport Sci Rev* 10: 49–83, 1982.

70. **Kalis JK, Freund BJ, Joyner MJ, Jilka SM, Nittolo J, and Wilmore JH.** Effect of β-blockade on the drift in O_2 consumption during prolonged exercise. *J Appl Physiol* 64: 753–758, 1988.

71. **Knoebel KL.** Energy metabolism. In: *Physiology*, edited by Selkurt E. Boston: Little Brown & Co., 1984, p. 635–650.

72. **Knuttgen HG, and Saltin B.** Muscle metabolites and oxygen uptake in short-term submaximal exercise in man. *J Appl Physiol* 32: 690–694, 1972.

73. **Ladu MJ, Kapsas H, and Palmer WK.** Regulation of lipoprotein lipase in muscle and adipose tissue during exercise. *J Appl Physiol* 71: 404–409, 1991.

74. **Lai N, Gladden LB, Carlier PG, and Cabrera ME.** Models of muscle contraction and energetics. *Drug Discovery Today: Disease Models, Kinetic Models* 5: 273–288, 2009.

75. **Lemon PW, and Mullin JP.** Effect of initial muscle glycogen levels on protein catabolism during exercise. *J Appl Physiol* 48: 624–629, 1980.

76. **Lemon PW, and Nagle FJ.** Effects of exercise on protein and amino acid metabolism. *Med Sci Sports Exerc* 13: 141–149, 1981.

77. **MacLean DA, Spriet LL, Hultman E, and Graham TE.** Plasma and muscle amino acid and ammonia responses during prolonged exercise in humans. *J Appl Physiol* 70: 2095–2103, 1991.

78. **Mader A, and Heck H.** A theory of the metabolic origin of "anaerobic threshold." *Int J Sports Med* 7 Suppl 1: 45–65, 1986.

79. **Marti B, Abelin T, and Howald H.** A modified fixed blood lactate threshold for estimating running speed for joggers in 16-km races. *Scandinavian Journal of Sports Sciences* 9: 41–45, 1987.

80. **Maughan R.** Carbohydrate-electrolyte solutions during prolonged exercise. Perspectives in exercise science and sports medicine. In: *Ergogenics: Enhancements of Performance in Exercise and Sport*, edited by Lamb D, and Williams MH. New York: McGraw-Hill, 1991.

81. **Medbo JI, Mohn AC, Tabata I, Bahr R, Vaage O, and Sejersted OM.** Anaerobic capacity determined by maximal accumulated O_2 deficit. *J Appl Physiol* 64: 50–60, 1988.

82. **Menconi MJ, Wei W, Yang H, Wray CJ, and Hasselgren PO.** Treatment of cultured myotubes with the calcium ionophore A23187 increases proteasome activity via a CaMK II-caspase-calpain-dependent mechanism. *Surgery* 136: 135–142, 2004.

83. **Menzies P, Menzies C, McIntyre L, Paterson P, Wilson J, and Kemi OJ.** Blood lactate clearance during active recovery after an intense running bout depends on the intensity of the active recovery. *J Sport Sciences* 28: 975–982, 2010.

84. **Mooren F, and Volker K.** *Molecular and Cellular Exercise Physiology*. Champaign: Human Kinetics, 2011.

85. **Ordway GA, Neufer PD, Chin ER, and DeMartino GN.** Chronic contractile activity upregulates the proteasome system in rabbit skeletal muscle. *J Appl Physiol* 88: 1134–1141, 2000.

86. **Ørngreen MC, Jeppesen TD, Andersen ST, Taivassalo T, Hauerslev S, Preisler N, Haller RG, van Hall G, and Vissing J.** Fat metabolism during exercise in patients with McArdle disease. *Neurology* 72: 718–724, 2009.

87. **Powers S.** Oxygen deficit-debt relationships in ponies during submaximal treadmill exercise. *Respiratory Physiology* 70: 251–263, 1987.

88. **Powers SK, Byrd RJ, Tulley R, and Callender T.** Effects of caffeine ingestion on metabolism and performance during graded exercise. *Eur J Appl Physiol Occup Physiol* 50: 301–307, 1983.

89. **Powers SK, Dodd S, and Beadle RE.** Oxygen uptake kinetics in trained athletes differing in $\dot{V}O_2$ max. *Eur J Appl Physiol Occup Physiol* 54: 306–308, 1985.

90. **Powers SK, Dodd S, and Garner R.** Precision of ventilatory and gas exchange alterations as a predictor of the anaerobic threshold. *Eur J Appl Physiol Occup Physiol* 52: 173–177, 1984.

91. **Powers SK, Howley ET, and Cox R.** Ventilatory and metabolic reactions to heat stress during prolonged exercise. *J Sports Med Phys Fitness* 22: 32–36, 1982.

92. **Powers SK, Riley W, and Howley ET.** Comparison of fat metabolism between trained men and women during prolonged aerobic work. *Res Q Exerc Sport* 51: 427–431, 1980.

93. **Refsum HE, Gjessing LR, and Stromme SB.** Changes in plasma amino acid distribution and urine amino acids excretion during prolonged heavy exercise. *Scand J Clin Lab Invest* 39: 407–413, 1979.

94. **Riley WW, Jr., Powers SK, and Welch HG.** The effect of two levels of muscular work on urinary creatinine excretion. *Res Q Exerc Sport* 52: 339–347, 1981.

95. **Romijn JA, Coyle EF, Sidossis LS, Gastaldelli A, Horowitz JF, Endert E, and Wolfe RR.** Regulation of endogenous fat and carbohydrate metabolism in relation to exercise intensity and duration. *Am J Physiol* 265: E380–391, 1993.

96. **Rossiter HB, Kowalchuk JM, and Whipp BJ.** A test to establish maximum O_2 uptake despite no plateau in the O_2 uptake response to ramp incremental exercise. *J Appl Physiol* 100: 2006.

97. **Sahlin K, Katz A, and Broberg S.** Tricarboxylic acid cycle intermediates in human muscle during prolonged exercise. *Am J Physiol* 259: C834–841, 1990.

98. **Saltin B, and Gollnick P.** Fuel for muscular exercise: Role of carbohydrate. In: *Exercise, Nutrition, and Energy Metabolism*, edited by Horton E, and Terjung R. New York: Macmillan, 1988, p. 45–71.

99. **Skinner JS, and McLellan TH.** The transition from aerobic to anaerobic metabolism. *Res Q Exerc Sport* 51: 234–248, 1980.

100. **Sonveaux P, Végran F, Schroeder T, Wergin MC, Verrax J, Rabbani ZN, De Saedeleer CJ, Kennedy KM, Diepart C, Jordan BF, Kelley MJ, Gallez B, Wahl ML, Feron O, and Dewhirst MW.** Targeting lactate-fueled respiration selectively kills hypoxic tumor cells in mice. *Journal of Clinical Investigation* 118: 3930–3942, 2008.

101. **Stainsby WN.** Biochemical and physiological bases for lactate production. *Med Sci Sports Exerc* 18: 341–343, 1986.

102. **Stanley WC, and Connett RJ.** Regulation of muscle carbohydrate metabolism during exercise. *Faseb J* 5: 2155–2159, 1991.

103. **Stryer L.** *Biochemistry*. New York: W. H. Freeman, 2002.

104. **Svedahl K, and MacIntosh BR.** Anaerobic threshold: the concept and methods of measurement. *Can J Appl Physiol* 28: 299–323, 2003.

105. **Tonouchi M, Hatta H, and Bonen A.** Muscle contraction increases lactate transport while reducing sarcolemmal MCT4, but not MCT1. *Am J Physiol Endocrinol Metab* 282: E1062–1069, 2002.

106. **Turcotte L.** Lipid metabolism during exercise. In: *Exercise Metabolism*. Champaign: Human Kinetics, 1995, p. 99–130.

107. **van Hall G.** Lactate kinetics in human tissues at rest and during exercise. *Acta Physiol* 199: 499–508, 2010.

108. **Wasserman K.** Anaerobiosis, lactate, and gas exchange during exercise: the issues. *Federation Proceedings* 45: 2904–2909, 1986.

109. **Wasserman K, Beaver WL, and Whipp BJ.** Mechanisms and patterns of blood lactate increase during exercise in man. *Med Sci Sports Exerc* 18: 344–352, 1986.

110. **Wasserman K, and McIlroy MB.** Detecting the threshold of anaerobic metabolism in cardiac patients during exercise. *Am J Cardiol* 14: 844–852, 1964.

111. **Wasserman K, Whipp BJ, and Davis JA.** Respiratory physiology of exercise: metabolism, gas exchange, and ventilatory control. *Int Rev Physiol* 23: 149–211, 1981.

112. **Wasserman K, Whipp BJ, Koyl SN, and Beaver WL.** Anaerobic threshold and respiratory gas exchange during exercise. *J Appl Physiol* 35: 236–243, 1973.

113. **White TP, and Brooks GA.** [U-14C]glucose, -alanine, and -leucine oxidation in rats at rest and two intensities of running. *Am J Physiol* 240: E155–165, 1981.

114. **Widmaier E, Raff H, and Strang K.** *Vander's Human Physiology*. New York: McGraw-Hill, 2006.

115. **Wilson DF, Erecinska M, Drown C, and Silver IA.** Effect of oxygen tension on cellular energetics. *Am J Physiol* 233: C135–140, 1977.

116. **Yoshida T.** Effect of dietary modifications on the anaerobic threshold. *Sports Medicine* 3: 4–9, 1986.

5

Cell Signaling and the Hormonal Responses to Exercise

■ Objectives

By studying this chapter, you should be able to do the following:

1. Describe the concept of hormone-receptor interaction.
2. Identify the four factors influencing the concentration of a hormone in the blood.
3. Describe the mechanism by which steroid hormones act on cells.
4. Describe the "second messenger" hypothesis of hormone action.
5. Describe the role of the hypothalamus-releasing factors in the control of hormone secretion from the anterior pituitary gland.
6. Describe the relationship of the hypothalamus to the secretion of hormones from the posterior pituitary gland.
7. Identify the site of release, stimulus for release, and the predominant action of the following hormones: epinephrine, norepinephrine, glucagon, insulin, cortisol, aldosterone, thyroxine, growth hormone, estrogen, and testosterone.
8. Discuss the use of testosterone (an anabolic steroid) and growth hormone on muscle growth and their potential side effects.
9. Contrast the role of plasma catecholamines with intracellular factors in the mobilization of muscle glycogen during exercise.
10. Briefly discuss the following four mechanisms by which blood glucose homeostasis is maintained: mobilizing glucose from liver glycogen stores; mobilizing plasma free fatty acids from adipose tissue; synthesizing glucose from amino acids and glycerol in the liver; and blocking glucose entry into cells.
11. Graphically describe the changes in the following hormones during graded and prolonged exercise, and discuss how those changes influence the four mechanisms used to maintain the blood glucose concentration: insulin, glucagon, cortisol, growth hormone, epinephrine, and norepinephrine.
12. Describe the effect of changing hormone and substrate levels in the blood on the mobilization of free fatty acids from adipose tissue.

■ Outline

■ Key Terms

acromegaly
adenylate cyclase
adiponectin
adrenal cortex
adrenocorticotrophic hormone (ACTH)
aldosterone
alpha receptors
anabolic steroid
androgenic steroid
androgens
angiotensin I and II
anterior pituitary
antidiuretic hormone (ADH)
beta receptors
calcitonin
calmodulin
catecholamines
cortisol
cyclic AMP
diabetes mellitus

diacylglycerol
endocrine gland
endorphin
epinephrine (E)
estrogens
follicle-stimulating hormone (FSH)
G protein
glucagon
glucocorticoids
growth hormone (GH)
hormone
hypothalamic somatostatin
hypothalamus
inositol triphosphate
insulin
insulin-like growth factors (IGFs)
leptin
luteinizing hormone (LH)
melanocyte-stimulating hormone (MSH)
mineralocorticoids

neuroendocrinology
norepinephrine (NE)
pancreas
phosphodiesterase
phospholipase C
pituitary gland
posterior pituitary gland
prolactin
protein kinase C
releasing hormone
renin
second messenger
sex steroids
somatostatin
steroids
testosterone
thyroid gland
thyroid-stimulating hormone (TSH)
thyroxine (T_4)
triiodothyronine (T_3)

As presented in chapter 4, the fuels for muscular exercise include muscle glycogen and fat, plasma glucose and free fatty acids, and to a lesser extent, amino acids. These fuels must be provided at an optimal rate for activities as diverse as the 400-meter run and the 26-mile, 385-yard marathon, or performance will suffer. What controls the mixture of fuel used by the muscles? What stimulates the adipose tissue to release more FFA? How is the liver made aware of the need to replace the glucose that is being removed from the blood by exercising muscles? If glucose is not replaced, a hypoglycemic (low blood glucose) condition will occur. Hypoglycemia is a topic of crucial importance in discussing exercise as a challenge to homeostasis. Blood glucose is the primary fuel for the central nervous system (CNS), and without optimal CNS function during exercise, the chance of fatigue and the risk of serious injury increase. Although blood glucose was used as an example, it should be noted that sodium, calcium, potassium, and water concentrations, as well as blood pressure and pH, are also maintained within narrow limits during exercise. It should be no surprise then that there are a variety of automatic control systems maintaining these variables within these limits.

Chapter 2 presented an overview of automatic control systems that maintain homeostasis. In that context, you also were introduced to cell signaling—the fact that a wide variety of signals, some acting locally and others reaching all tissues, are needed for our adaption to a single bout of exercise, or to repeated bouts of exercise (training) that lead to changes in muscle structure and function. Although this chapter focuses primarily on one category of cell signaling, endocrine signals—the other types of

signals (i.e., autocrine, paracrine, and synaptic) are crucial—not only muscular adaptations, but also the health-related benefits, such as reduced risks of type 2 diabetes and coronary heart disease. This chapter provides additional information on cell signaling, with an emphasis on **neuroendocrinology,** a branch of physiology dedicated to the systematic study of control systems. The first part of the chapter presents a brief introduction to each hormone, indicates the factors controlling its secretion, and discusses its role in homeostasis. Following that, we discuss how **hormones** control the delivery of carbohydrates and fats during exercise.

NEUROENDOCRINOLOGY

Two of the major homeostatic systems involved in the control and regulation of various functions (cardiovascular, renal, metabolic, etc.) are the nervous and endocrine systems. Both are structured to sense information, organize an appropriate response, and then deliver the message to the proper organ or tissue. Often the two systems work together to maintain homeostasis; the term neuroendocrine response is reflective of that interdependence. The two systems differ in the way the message is delivered: The endocrine system releases hormones (endocrine signals) into the blood to circulate to tissues, whereas nerves use neurotransmitters (synaptic signals) to relay messages from one nerve to the other, or from a nerve to a tissue.

Endocrine glands release hormones (chemical messengers) directly into the blood, which carries the hormone to a tissue to exert an effect. It is the binding of the hormone to a specific protein receptor that allows the hormone to exert its effect. In that way, the hormone can circulate to all tissues while affecting only a few—those with the specific receptor.

Hormones can be divided into several classes based on chemical makeup: amino acid derivatives, peptides/protein, and **steroids.** The chemical structure influences the way in which the hormone is transported in the blood and the manner in which it exerts its effect on the tissue. For example, while steroid hormones' lipid-like structure requires that they be transported bound to plasma protein (to "dissolve" in the plasma), that same lipid-like structure allows them to diffuse through cell membranes to exert their effects. This is discussed in detail in a later section, "Stimulation of DNA in the Nucleus." Hormones exist in very small quantities in the blood and are measured in microgram (10^{-6} g), nanogram (10^{-9}g), and picogram (10^{-12} g) amounts. It wasn't until the 1950s that analytical techniques were improved to the point of allowing measurement of these low plasma concentrations (83).

Blood Hormone Concentration

The effect a hormone exerts on a tissue is directly related to the concentration of the hormone in the plasma and the number of active receptors to which it can bind. The hormone concentration in the plasma is dependent upon the following factors:

- the rate of secretion of the hormone from the endocrine gland,
- the rate of metabolism or excretion of the hormone,
- the quantity of transport protein (for some hormones), and
- changes in the plasma volume.

Control of Hormone Secretion   The rate at which a hormone is secreted from an endocrine gland is dependent on the magnitude of the input and whether it is stimulatory or inhibitory in nature. The input in every case is a chemical one, be it an ion (e.g., Ca^{++}) or a substrate (e.g., glucose) in the plasma, a neurotransmitter, such as acetylcholine or norepinephrine, or another hormone. Most endocrine glands are under the direct influence of more than one type of input, which may either reinforce or interfere with each other's effect. An example of this interaction is found in the control of **insulin** release from the pancreas. Figure 5.1 shows that the **pancreas,** which produces insulin, responds to changes in plasma glucose and amino acids, norepinephrine released from sympathetic neurons as well as circulating epinephrine, parasympathetic neurons, which release acetylcholine, and a variety of hormones. Elevations of plasma glucose and amino acids increase

Figure 5.1   The secretion of a hormone can be modified by a number of factors, some exerting a positive influence and others, a negative influence. From A. J. Vander et al., *Human Physiology: The Mechanisms of Body Function*, 4th ed. Copyright © 1985 McGraw-Hill, Inc., New York. Reprinted by permission.

insulin secretion (+), whereas an increase in sympathetic nervous system activity (epinephrine and norepinephrine) decreases (−) insulin secretion. This magnitude of inhibitory versus excitatory input determines whether there will be an increase or a decrease in the secretion of insulin.

Metabolism and Excretion of Hormones   The concentration of a hormone in the plasma is also influenced by the rate at which it is metabolized (inactivated) and/or excreted. Inactivation can take place at or near the receptor or in the liver, the major site for hormone metabolism. In addition, the kidneys can metabolize a variety of hormones, or excrete them in their free (active) form. In fact, the rate of excretion of a hormone in the urine has been used as an indicator of its rate of secretion during exercise (8, 34, 64, 65). Because blood flow to the kidneys and liver decreases during exercise, the rate at which hormones are inactivated or excreted decreases. This results in an elevation of the plasma level of the hormone over and above that due to higher rates of secretion.

Transport Protein   The concentration of some hormones is influenced by the quantity of transport protein in the plasma. Steroid hormones and thyroxine are transported bound to plasma proteins. For a hormone to exert its effect on a cell, it must be "free" to interact with the receptor and not "bound" to the transport protein. The amount of free hormone is dependent on the quantity of transport protein and the capacity and affinity of the protein to bind the hormone molecules. *Capacity* refers to the maximal quantity of hormone that can be bound to the transport protein, and *affinity* refers to the tendency of the transport protein to bind to the hormone. An increase in the quantity, capacity, or affinity of transport protein would reduce the amount of free hormone and its effect on tissue (43, 76). For example, high levels of estrogen during pregnancy increase the quantity of thyroxine's transport protein, causing a reduction in free thyroxine. The **thyroid gland** produces more thyroxine to counteract this effect.

Plasma Volume Changes in plasma volume will change the hormone concentration independent of changes in the rate of secretion or inactivation of the hormone. During exercise, plasma volume decreases due to the movement of water out of the cardiovascular system. This causes a small increase in the concentration of hormones in the plasma. By measuring changes in plasma volume, it is possible to "correct" the concentration of the hormone to obtain a more accurate assessment of endocrine gland activity (76).

IN SUMMARY

- Endocrine glands release hormones directly into the blood to alter the activity of tissues possessing receptors to which the hormone can bind.
- The free plasma hormone concentration determines the magnitude of the effect at the tissue level.
- The free hormone concentration can be changed by altering the rate of secretion or inactivation of the hormone, the quantity of transport protein, and the plasma volume.

Hormone-Receptor Interaction

Hormones are carried by the circulation to all tissues, but they affect only certain tissues. Tissues responsive to specific hormones have specific protein receptors capable of binding those hormones. These protein receptors should not be viewed as static fixtures associated with cells, but like any cellular structures, they are subject to change. The number of receptors varies from 500 to 100,000 per cell, depending on the receptor. Receptor number may decrease when exposed to a chronically elevated level of a hormone (down-regulation), resulting in a diminished response for the same hormone concentration. The opposite case, chronic exposure to a low concentration of a hormone, may lead to an increase in receptor number (up-regulation), with the tissue becoming very responsive to the available hormone. Because there are a finite number of receptors on or in a cell, a situation can arise in which the concentration of a hormone is so high that all receptors are bound to the hormone; this is called saturation. Any additional increase in the plasma hormone concentration will have no additional effect (37). Further, because the receptors are specific to a hormone, any chemical similar in "shape" will compete for the limited receptor sites. A major way in which endocrine function is studied is to use chemicals (drugs) to block receptors and observe the consequences. For example, patients with heart disease may receive a drug that blocks the receptors to which epinephrine (adrenaline) binds; this prevents the heart rate from getting too high during exercise. After the hormone binds to a receptor, cellular activity is altered by a variety of mechanisms.

Mechanisms of Hormone Action Mechanisms by which hormones modify cellular activity include:

- alteration of membrane transport mechanisms,
- altering activity of DNA in the nucleus to initiate or suppress the synthesis of a specific protein, and
- activation of special proteins in the cells by "second messengers."

Membrane Transport After binding to a receptor on a membrane, the major effect of some hormones is to activate carrier molecules in or near the membrane to increase the movement of substrates or ions from outside to inside the cell. For example, insulin binds to receptors on the surface of the cell and mobilizes glucose transporters located in the membrane of the cell. The transporters link up with glucose on the outside of the cell membrane where the concentration of glucose is high, and the glucose transporter diffuses to the inside of the membrane to release glucose for use in the cell (72). If an individual does not have adequate insulin, as exists in uncontrolled diabetes, glucose accumulates in the plasma because the glucose transporters in the membrane are not activated.

Altering Activity of DNA in the Nucleus Due to their lipid-like nature, steroid hormones diffuse easily through cell membranes, where they become bound to a protein receptor in the cytoplasm of the cell. Figure 5.2 shows that the steroid-receptor complex enters the nucleus and binds to a specific protein linked to DNA, which contains the instruction codes for protein synthesis. This activates (or, in a few cases, suppresses) genes that lead to the synthesis of a specific messenger RNA (mRNA) that carries the codes from the nucleus to the cytoplasm where the specific protein is synthesized. Although thyroid hormones are not steroid hormones, they act in a similar manner. These processes—the activation of DNA and the synthesis of specific protein—take time to turn on (making the hormones involved "slow-acting" hormones), but their effects are longer lasting than those generated by "second messengers" (48).

Second Messengers Many hormones, because of their size or highly charged structure, cannot easily cross cell membranes. These hormones exert their effects by binding to a receptor on the membrane

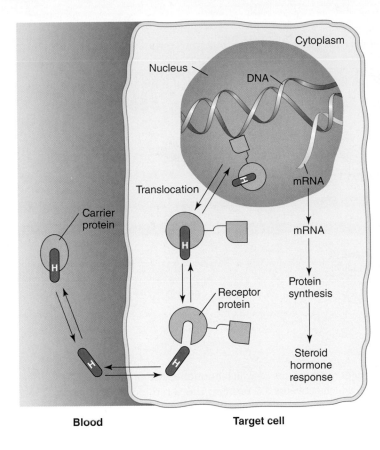

Figure 5.2 The mechanism by which steroid hormones act on target cells. A steroid hormone, represented by the letter H, is transported in plasma bound to a carrier protein. The steroid hormone diffuses through the plasma membrane, binds to a cytoplasmic protein receptor, and is transported to the nucleus where it binds to DNA. This stimulates mRNA synthesis that, in turn, leads to protein synthesis and brings about a change in cellular activity.

surface and activating a **G protein** located in the membrane of the cell. The G protein is the link between the hormone-receptor interaction on the surface of the membrane and the subsequent events inside the cell. The G protein may open an ion channel to allow Ca^{++} to enter the cell, or it may activate an enzyme in the membrane. If the G protein activates **adenylate**

cyclase, then **cyclic AMP** (cyclic 3′,5′-adenosine mono-phosphate) is formed from ATP (see figure 5.3). In turn, the cyclic AMP concentration increases in the cell and activates proteins, which directly alter cellular activity. For example, this mechanism is used to break down glycogen to glucose (by activating phosphorylase) and break down triglyceride molecules to free

Figure 5.3 The cyclic AMP "second messenger" mechanism by which hormones act on target cells. A hormone binds to a receptor on the plasma membrane, which activates a G protein. The G protein activates adenylate cyclase, which causes ATP to be converted to cyclic AMP. The cyclic AMP activates enzymes that bring about cellular responses.

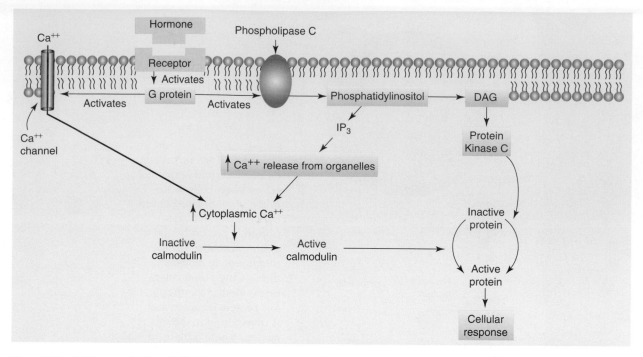

Figure 5.4 Calcium and phospholipase C second messenger mechanisms by which hormones act on target cells. A hormone binds to a receptor on the plasma membrane, which activates a G protein. The G protein may activate a calcium channel to allow calcium to enter the cell, activate calmodulin, and bring about cellular change. The G protein may also activate phospholipase C, which causes phosphotidylinositol to be broken down into inositol triphosphate (IP_3) and diacylglycerol (DAG). The IP3 causes release of calcium from intracellular organelles and activates calmodulin, and the DAG activates protein kinase C to bring about additional cellular responses.

fatty acids (by activating hormone sensitive lipase [HSL]). The cyclic AMP is inactivated by **phosphodiesterase,** an enzyme that converts cyclic AMP to 5'AMP. Factors that interfere with phosphodiesterase activity, such as caffeine, would increase the effect of the hormone by allowing cyclic AMP to exert its effect for a longer period of time. For example, caffeine may exert this effect on adipose tissue, causing free fatty acids to be mobilized at a faster rate (see chapter 25).

If the G protein activates a Ca^{++} ion channel, Ca^{++} enters the cell and binds to and activates a protein called calmodulin. The activated calmodulin influences cellular activity in much the same way as cyclic AMP does (see figure 5.4). Last, a G protein may activate a membrane-bound enzyme **phospholipase C.** When this occurs, a phospholipid in the membrane, phosphatidylinositol, is hydrolyzed into two intracellular molecules, **inositol triphosphate,** which causes Ca^{++} release from intracellular stores, and **diacylglycerol.** The diacylglycerol activates **protein kinase C** that, in turn, activates proteins in the cell (see figure 5.4). Cyclic AMP, Ca^{++}, inositol triphosphate, and diacylglycerol are viewed as **second messengers** in the events following the hormone's binding to a receptor on the cell membrane. These second messengers should not be viewed as being independent of one another, because changes in one can affect the action of the others (134).

Tyrosine Kinase In contrast to the above, insulin does not use these second messenger mechanisms to bring about its effects on the cell. Insulin binds to a tyrosine kinase receptor's alpha (α) subunits, which reside outside the cell (see figure 5.5). This binding causes the beta (β) subunits (located inside the cell) to phosphorylate themselves. The activated tyrosine kinase receptor phosphorylates signaling proteins that lead to the movement of glucose transporters (GLUT4) to the membrane so glucose can enter the cell; it also activates the enzyme glycogen synthase to form glycogen from the glucose molecules brought into the cell (105).

IN SUMMARY

- The hormone-receptor interaction triggers events at the cell, and changing the concentration of the hormone, the number of receptors on the cell, or the affinity of the receptor for the hormone will all influence the magnitude of the effect.
- Hormones bring about their effects by modifying membrane transport, activating/suppressing genes to alter protein synthesis, and activating second messengers (cyclic AMP, Ca^{++}, inositol triphosphate, and diacylglycerol).

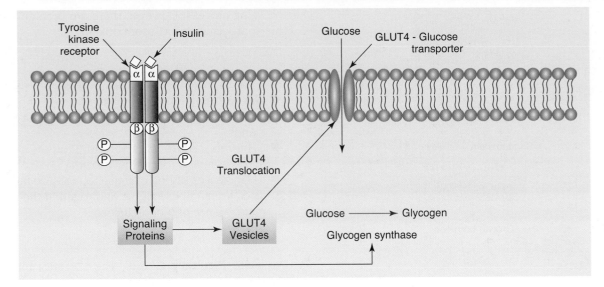

Figure 5.5 Insulin receptor. Insulin binds to the tyrosine kinase receptor's alpha (α) subunits, which reside outside the cell. This binding causes the beta (β) subunits (located inside the cell) to phosphorylate themselves and activate signaling proteins. The signaling proteins (l) cause GLUT4 (glucose transporters) to be mobilized from the cytoplasm to the plasma membrane to allow glucose to enter the cell, and (2) activates glycogen synthase to synthesize glycogen from glucose.

HORMONES: REGULATION AND ACTION

This section presents the major **endocrine glands,** their hormones and how they are regulated, the effects the hormones have on tissues, and how some of the hormones respond to exercise. This information is essential to discuss the role of the neuroendocrine system in the mobilization of fuel for exercise.

Hypothalamus and the Pituitary Gland

The **pituitary gland** is located at the base of the brain, attached to the hypothalamus. The gland has two lobes—the anterior lobe (adenohypophysis), which is a true endocrine gland, and the posterior lobe (neurohypophysis), which is neural tissue extending from the hypothalamus. Both lobes are under the direct control of the hypothalamus. In the case of the **anterior pituitary,** hormone release is controlled principally by chemicals (**releasing hormones** or factors) that originate in neurons located in the hypothalamus. These releasing hormones stimulate or inhibit the release of specific hormones from the anterior pituitary. The **posterior pituitary gland** receives its hormones from special neurons originating in the hypothalamus. The hormones move down the axon to blood vessels in the posterior hypothalamus where they are discharged into the general circulation (77).

Anterior Pituitary Gland The anterior pituitary hormones include **adrenocorticotrophic hormone (ACTH), follicle-stimulating hormone (FSH), luteinizing hormone (LH), melanocyte-stimulating hormone (MSH), thyroid-stimulating hormone (TSH), growth hormone (GH),** and **prolactin.** While prolactin directly stimulates the breast to produce milk, the majority of the hormones secreted from the anterior pituitary control the release of other hormones. TSH controls the rate of thyroid hormone formation and secretion from the thyroid gland; ACTH stimulates the production and secretion of **cortisol** in the adrenal cortex; LH stimulates the production of testosterone in the testes and estrogen in the ovaries; and GH stimulates the release of **insulin-like growth factors (IGFs)** from the liver and other tissues. However, IGFs can be produced by a variety of other means. In fact, the IGF-1 produced in muscle due to muscle contraction is associated with muscle hypertrophy (52, 80). However, as we will see, growth hormone exerts important effects on protein, fat, and carbohydrate metabolism (77).

Growth Hormone Growth hormone (GH) is secreted from the anterior pituitary gland and exerts profound effects on the growth of all tissues through the action of IGFs. Growth hormone secretion is controlled by releasing hormones secreted from the **hypothalamus.** Growth hormone-releasing hormone (GHRH) stimulates GH release from the anterior pituitary, whereas another factor, **hypothalamic somatostatin,** inhibits it. The GH and IGF levels in blood

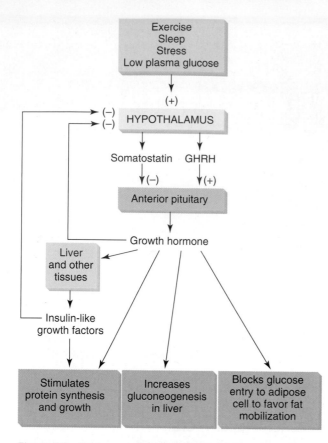

Figure 5.6 Summary of the positive and negative input to the hypothalamus, influencing growth hormone secretion. From A. J. Vander et al., *Human Physiology: The Mechanisms of Body Function*, 4th ed. Copyright © 1985 McGraw-Hill, Inc., New York. Reprinted by permission.

exert a negative feedback effect on the continued secretion of GH. As shown in figure 5.6, additional input to the hypothalamus that can influence the secretion of GH includes exercise, stress (broadly defined), a low plasma-glucose concentration, and sleep (133). However, exercise is the most potent stimulus (139). GH and IGFs stimulate tissue uptake of amino acids, the synthesis of new protein, and long-bone growth. In addition, GH spares plasma glucose by:

- opposing the action of insulin to reduce the use of plasma glucose,
- increasing the synthesis of new glucose in the liver (gluconeogenesis), and
- increasing the mobilization of fatty acids from adipose tissue.

Given these characteristics, it should be no surprise that GH increases with exercise to help maintain the plasma glucose concentration (this will be covered in detail in a later section, "Permissive and Slow-Acting Hormones"). Growth hormone, because of its role in protein synthesis, is being used by some athletes to enhance muscle mass and by the elderly to slow down

the aging process. However, there are problems with this approach (see A Closer Look 5.1).

IN SUMMARY

- The hypothalamus controls the activity of both the anterior pituitary and posterior pituitary glands.
- GH is released from the anterior pituitary gland and is essential for normal growth.
- GH increases during exercise to mobilize fatty acids from adipose tissue and to aid in the maintenance of blood glucose.

Posterior Pituitary Gland   The posterior pituitary gland provides a storage site for two hormones, oxytocin and antidiuretic hormone (ADH, also called vasopressin), which are produced in the hypothalamus to which the posterior pituitary is attached. Oxytocin is a powerful stimulator of smooth muscle, especially at the time of childbirth, and is also involved in the milk "let down" response needed for the release of milk from the breast.

Antidiuretic Hormone Antidiuretic hormone **(ADH)** does what its name implies: It reduces water loss from the body. ADH favors the reabsorption of water from the kidney tubules back into the capillaries to maintain body fluid. Two major stimuli cause an increased secretion of ADH:

- high plasma osmolality (a low water concentration) that can be caused by excessive sweating without water replacement, and
- a low plasma volume, which can be due either to the loss of blood or to inadequate fluid replacement.

There are osmoreceptors in the hypothalamus that sense the water concentration in the interstitial fluid. When the plasma has a high concentration of particles (low water concentration), the osmoreceptors shrink, and a neural reflex to the hypothalamus stimulates ADH release, which causes a reduction in water loss at the kidney. If the osmolality of the plasma is normal, but the volume of plasma is low, stretch receptors in the left atrium initiate a reflex leading to ADH release to attempt to maintain body fluid. During exercise, plasma volume decreases and osmolality increases, and for exercise intensities in excess of 60% of $\dot{V}O_2$ max, ADH secretion is increased, as shown in figure 5.7 (22). This favors the conservation of water to maintain plasma volume (136). Recently, it has been hypothesized that non-osmotic signals associated with exercise may override the usual controls and lead to excessive water retention and dilution of

A CLOSER LOOK 5.1

Growth Hormone and Performance

An excess of growth hormone (GH) during childhood is tied to gigantism, whereas an inadequate secretion causes dwarfism. The latter condition requires the administration of GH (along with other growth-promoting hormones) during the growing years if the child is to regain his or her normal position on the growth chart. In addition, in GH-deficient adults, therapeutic doses of GH cause increases in fat oxidation, $\dot{V}O_2$ max and strength, and improves body composition (139). GH was originally obtained by extracting it from the pituitary glands of cadavers—an expensive and time-consuming proposition. Due to the success of genetic engineering, recombinant human GH (rhGH) is now available.

If an excess of GH occurs during adulthood, a condition called **acromegaly** occurs. The additional GH during adulthood does not affect growth in height because the epiphyseal growth plates at the ends of the long bones have closed. Unfortunately, the excess GH causes permanent deformities, as seen in a thickening of the bones in the face, hands, and feet. Until recently, the usual cause of acromegaly was a tumor in the anterior pituitary gland that resulted in excess secretion of GH. This is no longer the case. In a drive to take advantage of the anabolic effects of GH, young adults with normal GH levels are injecting the now readily available human GH, along with other hormones (see A Closer Look 5.3). Does GH work on these individuals? Based on three recent reviews there appears to be consensus on the following (61, 84, 139):

- Normal adults show an increase in lean body mass, but this is due more to an increase in water retention than an increase in cell mass.
- There are minimal gains in lean body mass, muscle mass, and strength in men when GH is used with resistance training, compared to the use of resistance training alone.
- There are a variety of adverse events when GH is used, and these events are dose dependent. Adverse events include suppression of the GH/IGF axis, water retention and edema, joint and muscle aches, and an increased risk of injection-related diseases (e.g., HIV/AIDS).

In addition, a recent systematic review of the research on the safety and efficacy of GH on healthy older adults (mean age, 69 years) found many more adverse effects than benefits and recommended that GH not be used as an antiaging therapy (85).

Concern over the use of GH is so great that some have recommended that it be reclassified as a "controlled substance" to reduce its availability. One of the central problems in controlling the abuse of GH is the difficulty of distinguishing rhGH from what is produced naturally. New immunoassay techniques are making such detection and differentiation possible, but the effect of exercise on natural GH, coupled with its short half-life, complicates the problem of detection (119). However, Rennie (109) makes an interesting counterpoint to this concern about detection: Because no evidence exists that GH is a muscle-building hormone, does all the attention promote its abuse? This would be a good paper for the class to read to debate the merits of this view.

Figure 5.7 Percent change in the plasma antidiuretic hormone (ADH) concentration with increasing exercise intensity.

the body's sodium concentration, which may result in hyponatremia (low blood sodium). This has potentially deadly consequences (see chapter 23 for more on this) (56).

Thyroid Gland

The thyroid gland is stimulated by TSH to synthesize two iodine-containing hormones: **triiodothyronine (T_3)** and **thyroxine (T_4)**. T_3 contains three iodine atoms and T_4 contains four. TSH is also the primary stimulus for the release of T_3 and T_4 into the circulation, where they are bound to plasma proteins. Remember, it is the "free" hormone concentration (that which is not bound to plasma proteins) that is important in bringing about an effect on tissue. T_4 is released from the thyroid gland in much larger amounts compared to T_3. However, after release, most of the T_4 is converted to T_3, the more potent of the thyroid hormones.

Thyroid Hormones Thyroid hormones are central in establishing the overall metabolic rate (i.e., a hypothyroid [low T_3] individual would be characterized as being lethargic and hypokinetic). It is this effect of the hormone that has been linked to weight-control problems, but only a small percentage of obese individuals are hypothyroid. T_3 and T_4 act as permissive hormones in that they permit other hormones to exert their full effect. There is a relatively long latent period between the time T_3 and T_4 are elevated and the time when their effects are observed. The latent period is 6 to 12 hours for T_3 and 2 to 3 days for T_4. However, once initiated, their effects are long lasting (48). The control of T_3 and T_4 secretion is another example of the negative feedback mechanism introduced in chapter 2. At rest, as the plasma concentrations of T_3 and T_4 increase, they inhibit the release of TSH-releasing hormone from the hypothalamus as well as TSH itself. This self-regulating system ensures the necessary level of T_3 and T_4 for the maintenance of a normal metabolic rate. During exercise, the "free" hormone concentration increases due to changes in the binding characteristic of the transport protein, and the hormones are taken up at a faster rate by tissues. To counter the higher rate of removal of T_3 and T_4, TSH secretion increases and causes an increased secretion of these hormones from the thyroid gland (130). A recent study suggests that the exercise-induced increases in prolactin and cortisol (see later) also influence TSH release (51). Last, evidence suggests that resistance training has little effect on the pituitary (TSH)-thyroid (T_3, T_4) function (2).

IN SUMMARY

■ Thyroid hormones T_3 and T_4 are important for maintaining the metabolic rate and allowing other hormones to bring about their full effect.

Calcitonin The thyroid gland also secretes **calcitonin,** which is involved in a minor way in the regulation of plasma calcium (Ca^{++}), a crucial ion for normal muscle and nerve function. The secretion of this hormone is controlled by another negative feedback mechanism. As the plasma Ca^{++} concentration increases, calcitonin release is increased. Calcitonin blocks the release of Ca^{++} from bone and stimulates Ca^{++} excretion at the kidneys to lower the plasma Ca^{++} concentration. As the Ca^{++} concentration is decreased, the rate of calcitonin secretion is reduced. Current evidence indicates that calcitonin is not increased as a result of exercise, an appropriate response given its function (88).

Parathyroid Gland

Parathyroid hormone is the primary hormone involved in plasma Ca^{++} regulation. The parathyroid gland releases parathyroid hormone in response to a low plasma Ca^{++} concentration. The hormone stimulates bone to release Ca^{++} into the plasma and simultaneously increases the renal absorption of Ca^{++}; both raise the plasma Ca^{++} level. Parathyroid hormone also stimulates the kidney to convert a form of vitamin D (vitamin D_3) into a hormone that increases the absorption of Ca^{++} from the gastrointestinal tract. Parathyroid hormone increases during both intense and prolonged exercise (10, 88). The increase is related to a lower Ca^{++} concentration and the exercise-induced increases in plasma H^+ and catecholamine concentrations (88).

Adrenal Gland

The adrenal gland is really two different glands—the adrenal medulla, which secretes the **catecholamines, epinephrine (E),** and **norepinephrine (NE),** and the **adrenal cortex,** which secretes steroid hormones.

Adrenal Medulla The adrenal medulla is part of the sympathetic nervous system. Eighty percent of the gland's hormonal secretion is epinephrine, which affects receptors in the cardiovascular and respiratory systems, gastrointestinal (GI) tract, liver, other endocrine glands, muscle, and adipose tissue. E and NE are involved in the maintenance of blood pressure and the plasma glucose concentration. Their role in the cardiovascular system is discussed in chapter 9, and their involvement in the mobilization of substrate for exercise is discussed later in this chapter in the section "Fast-Acting Hormones." E and NE also respond to strong emotional stimuli, and they form the basis for Cannon's "fight or flight" hypothesis of how the body responds to challenges from the environment (14). Cannon's view was that the activation of the sympathetic nervous system prepared you either to confront a danger or to flee from it. Statements by sportscasters, such as "The adrenalin must really be pumping now," are a rough translation of this hypothesis. See A Look Back—Important People in Science for more on Dr. Walter B. Cannon.

E and NE bind to adrenergic (from adrenaline, the European name for epinephrine) receptors on target tissues. The **receptors** are divided into two major classes: **alpha (α)** and **beta (β),** with subgroups (α_1 and α_2; β_1, β_2, and β_3). E and NE bring about their effects via the second messenger mechanisms mentioned earlier. The response generated in the target tissue, both size and direction (inhibitory or excitatory), is dependent on the receptor type and whether E or NE is involved. This is an example of how important the receptors are in determining the cell's response to a hormone. Table 5.1 summarizes the effects of E and NE relative

Walter B. Cannon (1871–1945) and the Fight or Flight Response

Walter B. Cannon was born and raised in Wisconsin and attended Harvard College from 1892 to 1896. He then entered Harvard University to study medicine. During his first year, he worked in Dr. Henry Bowditch's lab and began to use the new technique of X-rays to study gastrointestinal motility. He completed his medical degree in 1900 and stayed on as an instructor in the Department of Physiology, of which Bowditch was chairman. Bowditch was a well-known physiologist who was one of the five founders of the American Physiological Society. Two years later, Dr. Cannon was promoted to assistant professor, and in 1906 he succeeded Dr. Bowditch as chairman of the department—a post he held until his retirement in 1942.

Dr. Cannon's research included work on gastrointestinal motility and the physiology of the emotions. He developed the concept of the emergency function of the sympathetic nervous system—the "fight or flight" response—the importance of epinephrine and norepinephrine in mobilizing the resources to the body to stay and fight, or to take flight in times of extreme stress. In addition to these important contributions, he also was responsible for the development of the concept of homeostasis—the idea that a dynamic constancy exists in the internal environment that is maintained by complex regulatory systems, of which the neuroendocrine system, described in this chapter, is a major part. Homeostasis is one of the most fundamental theories in biology, and a theme that we use through this textbook.

Dr. Cannon provided outstanding leadership, not only to the physiology department at Harvard, but to the broader field of physiology. He was the sixth president of the American Physiological Society (1914–16), and he spoke out strongly on a number of social and political issues, including fighting anti-vivisectionists, as did his mentor, Dr. Bowditch, before him. He published several important textbooks, including *Bodily Changes in Pain, Fear, and Rage* (1915), *The Wisdom of the Body* (1932), and *The Way of an Investigator* (1945), the latter being an autobiography that describes his personal experiences as a scientist. It provides keen insights for those interested in pursuing the life of a scientist. Dr. Cannon is regarded as the greatest American physiologist of the first half of the twentieth century.

For those interested in more detail about this man's life, see *Walter B. Cannon, The Life and Times of a Young Scientist* (1987) and *Walter B. Cannon, Science and Society* (2000), both published by Harvard University Press.

American Physiological Society (http:www.the-aps.org/about/pres/introwbc.htm)

to the type of adrenergic receptor involved (123). The different receptors cause changes in the cell's activity by increasing or decreasing the cyclic AMP or Ca^{++} concentrations. From this table it can be seen that if a cell experienced a loss of β_1 receptors and a gain in α_2 receptors, the same epinephrine concentration would bring about very different effects in the cell.

TABLE 5.1	**Adrenergic Receptor Subtypes: The Physiological Responses to Epinephrine and Norepinephrine**			
Receptor Type	Effect of E/NE	Membrane-Bound Enzyme	Intracellular Mediator	Effects on Various Tissues
β_1	E = NE	Adenylate cyclase	↑cyclic AMP	↑Heart rate ↑Glycogenolysis ↑Lipolysis
β_2	E >> > NE	Adenylate cyclase	↑cyclic AMP	↑Bronchodilation ↑Vasodilation
β_3	NE > E	Adenylate cyclase	↑cyclic AMP	↑Lipolysis
α_1	E ≥ NE	Phospholipase C	↑Ca^{++}	↑Phosphodiesterase ↑Vasoconstriction
α_2	E ≥ NE	Adenylate cyclase	↓cyclic AMP	Opposes action of β_1 and β_2 receptors ↓Insulin secretion

From J. Tepperman and H. M. Tepperman (129), Brunton, Lazo, and Parker (12), and Zouhal, et al. (149).

- The adrenal medulla secretes the catecholamines epinephrine (E) and norepinephrine (NE). E is the adrenal medulla's primary secretion (80%), and NE is primarily secreted from the adrenergic neurons of the sympathetic nervous system.
- Epinephrine and norepinephrine bind to α- and β-adrenergic receptors and bring about changes in cellular activity (e.g., increased heart rate, mobilization of fatty acids from adipose tissue) via second messengers.

Figure 5.8 Parallel increases in renin activity, angiotensin II, and aldosterone with increasing intensities of exercise. Data are expressed as the percent change from resting values.

Adrenal Cortex The adrenal cortex secretes a variety of steroid hormones having rather distinct physiological functions. The hormones can be grouped into three categories:

- **mineralocorticoids** (aldosterone), involved in the maintenance of the Na^+ and K^+ concentrations in plasma,
- **glucocorticoids** (cortisol), involved in plasma glucose regulation, and
- **sex steroids** (androgens and estrogens), which support prepubescent growth, with androgens being associated with post-pubescent sex drive in women.

The chemical precursor common to all of these steroid hormones is cholesterol; although the final active hormones possess minor structural differences, their physiological functions differ greatly.

Aldosterone Aldosterone (mineralocorticoid) is an important regulator of Na^+ reabsorption and K^+ secretion at the kidney. Aldosterone is directly involved in Na^+/H_2O balance and, consequently, plasma volume and blood pressure (see chapter 9). There are two levels of control over aldosterone secretion. The release of aldosterone from the adrenal cortex is controlled directly by the plasma K^+ concentration. An increase in K^+ concentration increases aldosterone secretion, which stimulates the kidney's active transport mechanism to secrete K^+ ions. This control system uses the negative feedback loop we have already seen. Aldosterone secretion is also controlled by another more complicated mechanism. A decrease in plasma volume, a fall in blood pressure at the kidney, or an increase in sympathetic nerve activity to the kidney stimulates special cells in the kidney to secrete an enzyme called **renin.** Renin enters the plasma and converts renin substrate (angiotensinogen) to **angiotensin I,** which is, in turn, converted to **angiotensin II** by angiotensin-converting enzyme (ACE) in the lungs. Angiotensin II is a powerful

vasoconstrictor, and individuals with hypertension may be prescribed an ACE inhibitor to lower blood pressure. Angiotensin II stimulates aldosterone release, which increases Na^+ reabsorption. The stimuli for aldosterone and ADH secretion are also the signals that stimulate thirst, a necessary ingredient to restore body fluid volume. During light exercise little or no change occurs in plasma renin activity or aldosterone (100). However, when a heat load is imposed during light exercise, both renin and aldosterone secretion are increased (38). When exercise intensity approaches 50% $\dot{V}O_2$ max (figure 5.8), renin, angiotensin, and aldosterone increase in parallel, showing the linkage within this homeostatic system (87, 130). Further, liver production of renin substrate increases to maintain the plasma concentration (93).

Cortisol The primary glucocorticoid secreted by the adrenal cortex is cortisol. By a variety of mechanisms, cortisol contributes to the maintenance of plasma glucose during long-term fasting and exercise. These mechanisms:

- promote the breakdown of tissue protein (by inhibiting protein synthesis) to form amino acids, which are then used by the liver to form new glucose (gluconeogenesis),
- stimulate the mobilization of free fatty acids from adipose tissue,
- stimulate liver enzymes involved in the metabolic pathway leading to glucose synthesis, and
- block the entry of glucose into tissues, forcing those tissues to use more fatty acids as fuel (48, 133).

A summary of cortisol's actions and its regulation is presented in figure 5.9. Cortisol secretion is controlled in the same manner as thyroxine. The

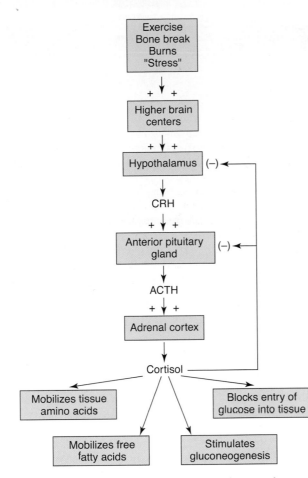

Figure 5.9 Control of cortisol secretion, showing the balance of positive and negative input to the hypothalamus, and cortisol's influence on metabolism.

hypothalamus secretes corticotrophic-releasing hormone (CRH), which causes the anterior pituitary gland to secrete more ACTH into the general circulation. ACTH binds to receptors on the adrenal cortex and increases cortisol secretion. As the cortisol level increases, CRH and ACTH are inhibited in another negative feedback system. However, the hypothalamus, like any brain center, receives neural input from other areas of the brain. This input can influence the secretion of hypothalamic-releasing hormones beyond the level seen in a negative feedback system. More than 70 years ago, Hans Selye observed that a wide variety of stressful events such as burns, bone breaks, and heavy exercise led to predictable increases in ACTH and cortisol; he called this response the General Adaptation Syndrome (GAS). A key point in this response was the release of ACTH and cortisol to aid in the adaptation. His GAS had three stages: (a) the alarm reaction, involving cortisol secretion, (b) the stage of resistance, where repairs are made, and (c) the stage of exhaustion, in which repairs are not adequate, and sickness or death results (121). The usefulness of the GAS is seen in times of "stress"

caused by tissue damage. Cortisol stimulates the breakdown of tissue protein to form amino acids, which can then be used at the site of the tissue damage for repair. While it is clear that muscle tissue is a primary source of amino acids, the functional overload of muscle with resistance or endurance training can prevent the muscle atrophy the glucocorticoids can cause (3, 57, 58). Throughout this section we summarize the role of hormones secreted from various endocrine glands. A Closer Look 5.2 provides a new addition to this list that will have profound implications in our understanding of obesity and its disease-related consequences.

IN SUMMARY

■ The adrenal cortex secretes aldosterone (mineralocorticoid), cortisol (glucocorticoid), and estrogens and androgens (sex steroids).
■ Aldosterone regulates Na^+ and K^+ balance. Aldosterone secretion increases with strenuous exercise, driven by the renin-angiotensin system.
■ Cortisol responds to a variety of stressors, including exercise, to ensure that fuel (glucose and free fatty acids) is available, and to make amino acids available for tissue repair.

Pancreas

The pancreas is both an exocrine and an endocrine gland. The exocrine secretions include digestive enzymes and bicarbonate, which are secreted into ducts leading to the small intestine. The hormones, released from groups of cells in the endocrine portion of the pancreas called the islets of Langerhans, include insulin, **glucagon,** and **somatostatin.**

Insulin   Insulin is secreted from beta (β) cells of the islets of Langerhans. Insulin is the most important hormone during the absorptive state, when nutrients are entering the blood from the small intestine. Insulin stimulates tissues to take up nutrient molecules such as glucose and amino acids and store them as glycogen, proteins, and fats. Insulin's best-known role is in the facilitated diffusion of glucose across cell membranes. A lack of insulin causes an accumulation of glucose in the plasma because the tissues cannot take it up. The plasma glucose concentration can become so high that reabsorption mechanisms in the kidney are overwhelmed and glucose is lost to the urine, taking large volumes of water with it. This condition is called **diabetes mellitus.**

As mentioned earlier in this chapter, insulin secretion is influenced by a variety of factors: plasma glucose concentration, plasma amino acid concentration, sympathetic and parasympathetic nerve

Adipose Tissue Is an Endocrine Organ

Many of you know that a connection exists between the obesity epidemic in this country and the dramatic increase in the number of people with type 2 diabetes and other chronic diseases (e.g., coronary artery disease, cancer). However, until recently, the direct link or cause between obesity and these diseases has remained a mystery. Fortunately, new evidence provides clues as to why too much adipose tissue has a negative impact on health.

Adipose tissue has been viewed, simply, as the principal storage site for fat, primarily triglycerides. When caloric intake exceeds expenditure, fat stores increase. Conversely, when caloric intake cannot meet energy demands, adipose tissue releases free fatty acids into the circulation to provide energy for the cells. Over the past 15 years this picture of adipose tissue as a passive energy supply depot changed markedly as it became clear that adipose tissue secretes a variety of very important hormones and is responsible for other factors that have a direct effect on metabolism and energy balance.

In the mid-1990s the hormone **leptin** was discovered. This hormone, secreted by adipose cells (adipocytes), influences appetite through a direct effect on the "feeding centers" in the hypothalamus. Two lines of evidence support this position. Mice that lack the gene to make leptin cannot regulate their appetite; they overeat and become

obese. Consistent with that, when leptin is injected into these mice, they reduce food intake, increase energy expenditure, and lose weight. In addition, leptin acts on peripheral tissues to enhance insulin sensitivity (allowing insulin to act) and promotes the oxidation of free fatty acids in muscle. **Adiponectin** is another hormone secreted by adipocytes. This hormone also increases insulin sensitivity and increases fatty acid oxidation in muscle (36, 46, 137).

As fat mass increases, leptin secretion also increases, but strangely, food intake is not restrained. Another molecule that blocks leptin's signal from reaching the hypothalamus is also produced, leading to what is known as leptin resistance. In contrast, adiponectin secretion decreases with an increase in fat mass, leading to a reduced sensitivity of tissues to insulin (insulin resistance) and the development of type 2 diabetes (a condition in which there is plenty of insulin, but the tissues are unresponsive to it).

In addition, as fat mass increases, adipocytes produce a variety of proinflammatory cytokines (e.g., tumor necrosis factor alpha [TNF-α]), and obesity is now recognized as contributing to a state of low-grade systemic inflammation (96, 116). See chapter 6 for more on inflammation. Adiponectin has the ability to suppress this systemic inflammation, but because its secretion is

reduced in obesity, it cannot carry out that role. These proinflammatory cytokines (also called adipokines or adipocytokines in adipose tissue) can lead to both insulin resistance and atherosclerosis (36, 46, 137).

Given the importance of adiponectin in insulin sensitivity, one might expect that exercise, which is known to improve insulin sensitivity (see chapter 17), would increase its concentration. Interestingly, neither an acute bout of exercise nor exercise training has any effect on the adiponectin concentration in blood. In contrast, the adiponectin level increases when there is a decrease in fat mass, whether it is brought about by exercise, diet, or a combined intervention. This suggests that the positive effects of exercise and weight loss on insulin sensitivity are independent and occur by different pathways. The same appears to be true for leptin; it is more responsive to changes in body weight than any exercise intervention (6, 9, 81, 127).

Clearly, adipose tissue is not a simple passive depot for energy storage, but is directly involved in appetite, energy expenditure, and the development of inflammation-related diseases, including cardiovascular disease and type 2 diabetes. It is clear that being physically active and maintaining a normal body weight are reasonable goals to minimize the risks of developing chronic diseases.

---

stimulation, and various hormones. The rate of secretion of insulin is dependent on the level of excitatory and inhibitory input to the beta cells of the pancreas (see figure 5.1). The blood glucose concentration is a major source of input that is part of a simple negative feedback loop; as the plasma glucose concentration increases (following a meal), the beta cells directly monitor this increase and secrete additional insulin to enhance tissue uptake of glucose. This increased uptake lowers the plasma glucose concentration, and insulin secretion is reduced (48, 83).

Glucagon Glucagon, secreted from the alpha (α) cells in the islets of Langerhans, exerts effects

opposite those of insulin. Glucagon secretion increases in response to a low plasma glucose concentration, which is monitored by the alpha cells. Glucagon stimulates both the mobilization of glucose from liver stores (glycogenolysis) and free fatty acids from adipose tissue (to spare blood glucose as a fuel). Last, along with cortisol, glucagon stimulates gluconeogenesis in the liver. Glucagon secretion is also influenced by factors other than the glucose concentration, notably the sympathetic nervous system (129). A complete description of the role of insulin and glucagon in the maintenance of blood glucose during exercise is presented later in this chapter in "Fast-Acting Hormones."

IN SUMMARY

- Insulin is secreted by the β cells of the islets of Langerhans in the pancreas and promotes the storage of glucose, amino acids, and fats.
- Glucagon is secreted by the α cells of the islets of Langerhans in the pancreas and promotes the mobilization of glucose and fatty acids.

Somatostatin Pancreatic somatostatin is secreted by the delta cells of the islets of Langerhans. Pancreatic somatostatin secretion is increased during the absorptive state, and it modifies the activity of the GI tract to control the rate of entry of nutrient molecules into the circulation. It may also be involved in the regulation of insulin secretion (129).

Testes and Ovaries

Testosterone and **estrogen** are the primary sex steroids secreted by the testes and ovaries, respectively. These hormones are not only important in establishing and maintaining reproductive function, they determine the secondary sex characteristics associated with masculinity and femininity.

Testosterone Testosterone is secreted by the interstitial cells of the testes and is controlled by interstitial cell stimulating hormone (ICSH—also known as LH), which is produced in the anterior pituitary. LH is, in turn, controlled by a releasing hormone secreted by the hypothalamus. Sperm production from the seminiferous tubules of the testes requires follicle-stimulating hormone (FSH) from the anterior pituitary and testosterone. Figure 5.10 shows testosterone secretion to be controlled by a negative feedback loop involving the anterior pituitary gland and the hypothalamus. Sperm production is controlled, in part, by another negative feedback loop involving the hormone inhibin (83, 133).

Testosterone is both an anabolic (tissue building) and androgenic (promoter of masculine characteristics) steroid because it stimulates protein synthesis and is responsible for the characteristic changes in boys at adolescence that lead to the high muscle-mass to fat-mass ratio. The plasma testosterone concentration is increased 10% to 37% during prolonged submaximal work (135), during exercise taken to maximum levels (25), and during endurance or strength training workouts (74). Some feel that these small changes are due to a reduction in plasma volume or to a decrease in the rate of inactivation and removal of testosterone (130). However, others have concluded on the basis of a parallel increase in the LH concentration that the increase in plasma testosterone is due to an increased rate of production (25).

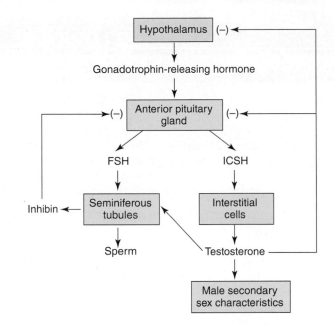

Figure 5.10 Control of testosterone secretion and sperm production by hypothalamus and anterior pituitary.

Although the testosterone response to exercise is small, and the concentration returns to resting values two hours after exercise (74), evidence exists that the resting plasma concentration is lower in both endurance-trained and resistance-trained males (5, 50). In one study, high-mileage (108 km · wk⁻¹) runners had lower levels of testosterone, sperm count, and sperm motility compared to moderate-mileage (54 km · wk⁻¹) runners (28). However, values were still in the normal range. Most readers probably recognize testosterone or one of its synthetic analogs as one of the most abused drugs in the drive to increase muscle mass and performance. Such use is not without its problems (see A Closer Look 5.3).

Estrogen and Progesterone Estrogen is a group of hormones that exerts similar physiological effects. These hormones include estradiol, estrone, and estriol. Estrogen stimulates breast development, female fat deposition, and other secondary sex characteristics (see figure 5.11). During the early part of the menstrual cycle called the follicular phase, LH stimulates the production of **androgens** in the follicle, which are subsequently converted to estrogens under the influence of FSH. Following ovulation, the luteal phase of the menstrual cycle begins, and both estrogens and progesterone are produced by the corpus luteum, a secretory structure occupying the space where the ovum was located (133). How does exercise affect these hormones, and vice versa? In one study (75), the plasma levels of LH, FSH, estradiol, and progesterone were measured at rest and at three different work rates during both the follicular and luteal phases of the menstrual cycle. The patterns of response of

Anabolic Steroids and Performance

Testosterone, as both an anabolic and an **androgenic steroid**, causes size changes as well as male secondary sexual characteristics, respectively. Due to these combined effects, scientists developed steroids to maximize the anabolic effects and minimize the androgenic effects. However, these effects can never be completely separated. These synthetic steroids were originally developed to promote tissue growth in patients who had experienced atrophy as a result of prolonged bed rest. Before long the thought occurred that these **anabolic steroids** might be helpful in developing muscle mass and strength in athletes.

Numerous studies were conducted to determine whether or not these steroids would bring about the desired changes, but a consensus was not achieved (4, 142, 143). The variation in results in published studies was related to the different tests used to measure body composition and strength, the study participants (novice or experienced), the length of the study, and training methods (146). In most of these studies the scientists used the recommended therapeutic dosage, as required by committees approving research with human subjects. Unfortunately, the "results" of many personal studies conducted in various gyms and weight-training facilities throughout the world disagreed with these scientific results. Why the disagreement in results between the controlled scientific studies and these latter "studies"? In the weight room it was not uncommon for a person look-

ing for greater "strength through chemistry" to take 10 to 100 times the recommended therapeutic dosage! In effect, it was difficult to compare the results of the controlled scientific studies with those done in the gym.

By the mid-1980s, the steroid problem had reached a level that prompted both professional and college sport teams to institute testing of athletes to control drug use. Olympic and Pan-American athletes were also tested to disqualify those who used the steroid. The problem escalated when athletes started to take pure testosterone rather than the anabolic steroid. Part of the reason for the switch was to reduce the chance of detection when drug testing was conducted, and part was related to the availability of testosterone. The following statements, taken from a recent position stand, provide a good summary of what we know about the use of these steroids, and what should be done to curb their abuse (61):

- Androgen use causes, in a concentration-dependent manner, increases in lean body mass, muscle mass, and strength in men.
- When androgens and resistance training are combined, greater gains are realized than with either intervention alone.
- The adverse effects in men include suppression of the hypothalamic-pituitary-gonadal axis, mood and behavior disorders, increased risk of cardiovascular disease, liver

dysfunction with oral androgens, insulin resistance, glucose intolerance, acne, and gynecomastia (breast development).
- The adverse effects in women are similar to that of men, but in addition, the androgens may have virilizing effects, such as enlargement of the clitoris, deepening of the voice, hirsutism, and change in body build. These changes may not be reversible when androgen use is stopped.

Recent studies using an online survey of those who use anabolic steroids provides some insights into the problem: the majority of users were noncompetitive body builders and nonathletes, used more than one anabolic steroid, and took them in megadose amounts, compared to what was recommended (98, 102). However, there is evidence that the prevalence of use among teenagers has decreased (61). Although the press highlights abuse by "winners" of the Tour de France (Floyd Landis) or Olympic Gold (Marion Jones), it is clear that the problem is much broader than realized by the general public. The same position stand mentioned above emphasizes the need for continued efforts to educate the athletes, coaches, parents, physicians, athletic trainers, and the general public about androgen use and abuse (61). For more information on a list of prohibited substances, go to the World Anti-Doping Agency's website: (www.wada-ama.org).

---

these hormones during graded exercise were very similar in the two phases of the menstrual cycle (75). Figure 5.12 shows only small changes in progesterone and estradiol with increasing intensities of work. Given that LH and FSH changed little or not at all during the luteal phase, the small increases in progesterone and estradiol were believed to be due to changes in plasma volume and to a decreased rate of removal rather than an increased rate of secretion (13, 130).

The effect of the phase of the menstrual cycle on exercise metabolism is not clear cut. This is due, in part, to variations in the research design, methods of measurement, and intensity of exercise used in the

studies. Based on a recent review, the following statements can be made (97):

- Anaerobic performances are not affected by menstrual cycle phase.
- The effect of menstrual cycle phase on time-trial endurance performances is mixed, and it has been suggested that the focus of future research be on ultra-endurance events.
- Glucose mobilization is lower during the luteal phase when exercise intensity is high enough to create an energy demand for carbohydrate. However, when exercise takes place soon after

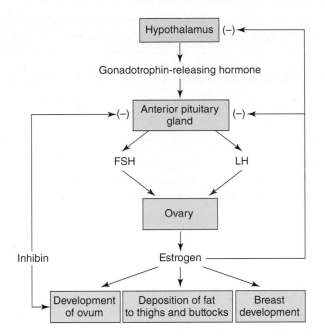

Figure 5.11 Role of estrogen in the development of female secondary sex characteristics and maturation of the ovum.

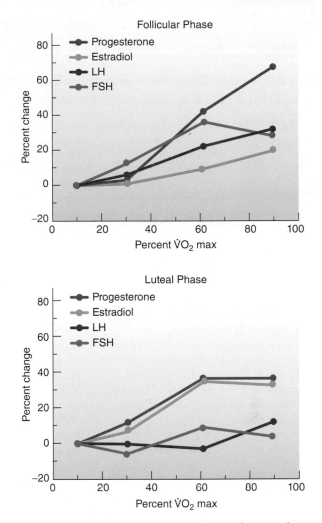

Figure 5.12 Percent change (from resting values) in the plasma FSH, LH, progesterone, and estradiol concentrations during graded exercise in the follicular and luteal phases of the menstrual cycle.

a meal or when glucose is provided during the exercise, the impact of menstrual cycle phase is reduced or eliminated.

■ Although animal studies show that estrogen increases lipolysis and plasma FFA, human studies do not support these findings.

■ There is an increase in protein catabolism at rest and during exercise in the luteal phase. This appears to be due to the effect of progesterone, since estrogen has the opposite effect.

In addition, there is general agreement that there are no menstrual cycle phase effects on $\dot{V}O_2$ max and the lactate, plasma volume, heart rate, and ventilation responses to exercise (144). Further, there does not appear to be an increased risk of heat illness during the luteal phase of the menstrual cycle, even though body temperature is higher (89).

There is an ongoing debate about whether estrogen influences indices of muscle damage, inflammation, and tissue repair. Animal studies provide consistent evidence that estrogen offers protective benefits; however, studies on humans fail to confirm these results (32). For those interested in having a ringside seat in this debate, read the Point: Counterpoint on this topic in which Tiidus and Enns debate Huber and Clarkson (131).

Because female athletes have a 4- to 6-fold greater risk of anterior cruciate injury compared to male athletes, there is interest as to whether the phase of the menstrual cycle might influence the risk. A review by Zazulak et al. (148) suggests that greater knee laxity occurs at 10–14 days into the cycle, compared to days 15–28, and the latter was greater than that measured during days 1–9. However, biomechanical analysis of the forces and the magnitude of knee flexion experienced when doing jumping tasks showed no differences between phases of the menstrual cycle or between genders (17).

Although the changes in estrogen and progesterone during an acute exercise bout are small, concern is being raised about the effect of chronic heavy exercise on the menstrual cycle of athletes. The two principal menstrual disorders are primary amenorrhea (absence of menstrual cycles in a girl who has not menstruated by 15 years of age) and secondary amenorrhea (onset of amenorrhea sometime after menarche). The incidence of menstrual disorders in athletes varies greatly but is higher in aesthetic, endurance, and weight-class sports, and at younger ages, higher training volumes, and lower body weights. Typically, the prevalence of amenorrhea in college-age women is about 2% to 5%. In contrast, in collegiate runners the incidence ranged from about 3% to 60% as training volume increased from <10 miles (16 km) to >68 miles (113 km) per week, and body weight decreased from >60 kg to <50 kg. In addition, the

Reproductive Disorders and Low Bone Mass in Female Athletes
Questions and Answers with Dr. Anne B. Loucks

Dr. Loucks is Professor of Biological Sciences at Ohio University. She is a productive researcher in the area of reproductive and skeletal disorders in female athletes, the author of numerous research articles and reviews on this topic, and is recognized internationally as an expert in the field. Dr. Loucks was involved in the development and revision of the American College of Sports Medicine's position stand on the Female Athlete Triad. Dr. Loucks's many accomplishments in research and scholarship were recognized by the American College of Sports Medicine in 2008 when she received that organization's prestigious Citation Award.

QUESTION: Are reproductive disorders in female athletes caused by low body fatness?

ANSWER: No. Very few studies find any difference in body composition between amenorrheic and eumenorrheic athletes. Secretion of gonadotropin-releasing hormone by the hypothamus is regulated, in part, by the availability of metabolic fuels. Further, hypothalamic reproductive disorders have been induced, prevented, and reversed by changing energy availability (i.e., dietary energy intake minus exercise energy expenditure), without any change in body composition. These disorders may be clinical (i.e., symptomatic: amenorrhea and oligomenorrhea) or subclinical (i.e., asymptomatic: luteal deficiency and anovulation). Most athletes acquire hypothalamic reproductive disorders by not eating enough each day to compensate for the energy they expend in exercise training that day, but no one should assume that a reproductive disorder is of hypothalamic origin. Because amenorrhea is a symptom of many diseases, a medical examination and endocrine measurements are needed to diagnose an athlete's reproductive disorder correctly so that she can receive appropriate care.

QUESTION: Is the low bone mass in some female athletes caused by amenorrhea?

ANSWER: Not entirely. Like other tissues, bone constantly turns over in a cycle of formation and resorption. Low estrogen levels in amenorrheic athletes do increase the rate of bone resorption, and bone mass does decline in proportion to the number of menstrual cycles missed. However, hormone replacement therapy and the restoration of normal menstrual cycles does not fully restore bone mass in women with hypothalamic amenorrhea. The reason is that low energy availability reduces the rate of bone formation by suppressing anabolic hormones such as thyroid hormone, insulin, and insulin-like growth factor-1. This hazard is especially acute during adolescence, when a faster rate of formation than resorption is needed for normal skeletal development.

QUESTION: What has research taught us about why female athletes do not eat enough?

ANSWER: Some athletes undereat obsessively as they express clinical mental illnesses classified as eating disorders. Other athletes undereat rationally as part of a temporary goal-oriented, but mismanaged, plan for optimizing body size and composition for success in their chosen sports. Many receive poor nutritional counseling and overdo it. Others undereat inadvertently, because prolonged exercise suppresses appetite—most extremely in those who eat the high-carbohydrate diet recommended for endurance sports. Athletes in endurance sports need to eat by discipline (i.e., specific amounts of particular foods at planned times) instead of by appetite. Young female athletes may also undereat for reasons unrelated to sport. Worldwide, regardless of BMI, about twice as many young women as men perceive themselves as overweight, so that 5-to-9 times as many young lean women as men are actively trying to lose weight.

QUESTION: What are the most important issues remaining to be solved?

ANSWER: We think we know how much athletes need to eat to compensate for their increased level of physical activity and thereby to prevent or reverse hypothalamic reproductive disorders, but we know very little about how to get them to do so. Therefore, we need applied research for developing practical procedures for monitoring and managing energy availability. We need to learn more about how the energy availability requirements of growing adolescents differ from those of full-grown adults. We also need to learn why some women appear to be more susceptible than others to the disruption of reproductive function by low energy availability. And finally, we need to learn more about the endocrine mechanisms mediating the influence of energy availability on reproductive and skeletal health.

---

incidence is much higher in younger (69%) than older (9%) runners (107). Special attention is now being directed at the issue of secondary amenorrhea because the chronically low estradiol levels can have a deleterious effect on bone mineral content. Osteoporosis, usually associated with the elderly (see chapter 17), is common in athletes with amenorrhea (59). Interested readers are referred to Redman and Loucks's review of the possible causes of exercise-induced menstrual cycle irregularities (107). What is most interesting is that exercise itself may not suppress reproductive function, but rather the impact of the energy cost of the exercise on energy availability. For some first-hand insights into this issue, see Ask the Expert 5.1.

Table 5.2 contains a summary of the information on each of the endocrine glands, their secretion(s), actions, controlling factors, the stimuli that elicit a response, and the effect of exercise on the hormonal response. This would be a good place to stop and review before proceeding to the discussion of the hor- monal control of muscle glycogen mobilization and the maintenance of the plasma glucose concentration during exercise. However, before we leave this section, we need to introduce you to a new member of the endocrine gland family—muscle itself (see A Closer Look 5.4).

TABLE 5.2	Summary of Endocrine Glands, Their Hormones, Their Action, Factors Controlling Their Secretion, Stimuli That Elicit a Response, and the Effect of Exercise				
Endocrine Gland	Hormone	Action	Controlling Factors	Stimuli	Exercise Effect
Anterior pituitary	Growth hormone (GH)	Increases growth, FFA mobilization, and gluconeo- genesis; decreases glucose uptake	Hypothalamic GH-releasing hormone; hypothalamic somatostatin	Exercise; "stress"; low blood glucose	↑
	Thyroid- stimulating hormone	Increases T_3 and T_4 production and secretion	Hypothalamic TSH-releasing hormone (TSH)	Low plasma T_3 and T4	↑
	Adrenocorti- cotrophic hormone (ACTH)	Increases cortisol synthesis secretion	Hypothalamic ACTH-releasing hormone	"Stress"; bone breaks; heavy exercise; burns, etc.	?
	Gonadotrophins: follicle stimulating hormone (FSH); luteinizing hormone (LH)	Female: estrogen and progesterone production and ovum development Male: testosterone production and sperm development	Hypothalamic gonadotrophic- releasing hormone Females: plasma estrogen and progesterone Males: plasma testosterone	Cyclic or intermittent firing of neurons in the hypothalamus	Small or no change
	Endorphins	Block pain by acting on opiate receptors in brain	ACTH-releasing hormone	"Stress"	↑ for exercise $\geq 70\%$ $\dot{V}O_2$ max
Posterior pituitary	Antidiuretic hormone (ADH) (vasopressin)	Decreases water loss at kidney; increases peripheral resistance	Hypothalamic neurons	Plasma volume; plasma osmolality	↑
Thyroid	Triiodothyronine (T_3); thyroxine (T_4)	Increases metabolic rate, mobilization of fuels, growth	TSH; plasma T_3 and T_4	Low T_3 and T_4	↑ "Free" T_3 and T_4
	Calcitonin	Decreases plasma calcium	Plasma calcium	Elevated plasma calcium	?
Parathyroid	Parathyroid hormone	Increases plasma calcium	Plasma calcium	Low plasma calcium	↑

TABLE 5.2 (Continued)

Endocrine Gland	Hormone	Action	Controlling Factors	Stimuli	Exercise Effect
Adrenal cortex	Cortisol	Increases gluconeogenesis, FFA mobilization and protein synthesis; decreases glucose utilization	ACTH	See ACTH, above	↑ Heavy exercise; ↓ light exercise
	Aldosterone	Increases potassium secretion and sodium reabsorption at kidney	Plasma potassium concentration and renin-angiotensin system	Low blood pressure and plasma volume; elevated plasma potassium and sympathetic activity to kidney	↑
Adrenal medulla	Epinephrine (80%); norepinephrine (20%)	Increases glycogenolysis, FFA mobilization, heart rate, stroke volume, and peripheral resistance	Output of baroreceptors; glucose receptor in hypothalamus; brain and spinal centers	Low blood pressure, and blood glucose; too much "stress"; emotion	↑
Pancreas	Insulin	Increases glucose amino acid, and FFA uptake into tissues	Plasma glucose and amino acid concentrations; autonomic nervous system	Elevated plasma glucose and amino acid concentrations; decreased epinephrine and norepinephrine	↓
	Glucagon	Increases glucose and FFA mobilization; gluconeogenesis	Plasma glucose and amino acid concentrations; autonomic nervous system	Low plasma glucose and amino acid concentrations; elevated epinephrine and norepinephrine	↑
Testes	Testosterone	Protein synthesis; secondary sex characteristics; sex drive; sperm Production	FSH and LH (ICSH)	Increased FSH and LH	Small ↑
Ovaries	Estrogen	Fat deposition; secondary sex characteristics; ovum development	FSH and LH	Increased FSH and LH	Small ↑

Muscle as an Endocrine Gland

Three of the major causes of death are cardiovascular disease, diabetes, and cancer. These diseases are linked to the presence of a low-grade chronic inflammation as shown by elevated blood levels of proinflammatory cytokines such as tumor necrosis factor alpha (TNF-α). What is important to know is that doing moderate-to-vigorous physical activity on a regular basis (e.g., 3 to 5 d/wk) is associated with positive health outcomes, including a reduction in the risk of type 2 diabetes, heart disease, and certain cancers. What is the connection between exercise and the reduced risk of these diseases? Until recently, little was known about the connection, but now it appears that it is muscle itself that brings about these favorable changes (11, 90, 101). Over the past 10 years it has become clear that muscle is an endocrine organ—that is—it

produces small signaling molecules called myokines (muscle cytokines) when it contracts. Some of these myokines act locally as autocrine agents to stimulate glucose uptake and increase fatty acid oxidation, and as paracrine agents to promote blood vessel growth in muscle. However, other myokines are released into the blood so that they can act as hormones and affect a variety of tissues and organs. For example, some myokines can increase liver production of glucose and stimulate triglyceride breakdown in adipose tissue to provide free fatty acids for fuel (11, 90, 101).

Interleukin 6 (IL-6) is the principal myokine produced by muscle during exercise. IL-6 can act as both a proinflammatory cytokine and an anti-inflammatory cytokine—that is—it can both promote inflammation and reduce it. IL-6 is the first myokine to

appear in the muscle and blood during exercise, and plasma IL-6 levels can be elevated 100-fold compared to resting conditions. It is important that other proinflammatory cytokines typically produced with an acute infection (e.g., TNF-α) do not normally increase with exercise, suggesting that the IL-6 released during exercise promotes an anti-inflammatory environment. Consistent with that, IL-6 has been shown to inhibit the production of TNF-α and stimulate the production of other anti-inflammatory cytokines (101).

In short, the anti-inflammatory environment provided by regular participation in exercise is linked to a reduction in chronic inflammation and a reduced risk of heart disease, type 2 diabetes, and certain cancers. We will see more about these myokines in later chapters.

IN SUMMARY

- Testosterone and estrogen establish and maintain reproductive function and determine secondary sex characteristics.
- Chronic exercise (training) can decrease testosterone levels in males and estrogen levels in females. The latter adaptation has potentially negative consequences related to osteoporosis.

HORMONAL CONTROL OF SUBSTRATE MOBILIZATION DURING EXERCISE

The type of substrate and the rate at which it is utilized during exercise depend to a large extent on the intensity and duration of the exercise. During strenuous exercise there is an obligatory demand for carbohydrate oxidation that must be met; fatty acid oxidation cannot substitute. In contrast, there is an increase in fat oxidation during prolonged, moderate exercise as carbohydrate fuels are depleted (62). Although diet and the training state of the person are important (see chapters 13, 21, and 23), the factors of intensity and duration of exercise ordinarily have prominence. Because of this, our discussion of the

hormonal control of substrate mobilization during exercise will be divided into two parts. The first will deal with the control of muscle glycogen utilization, and the second with the control of glucose mobilization from the liver and free fatty acids (FFA) from adipose tissue.

Muscle-Glycogen Utilization

At the onset of most types of exercise, and for the entire duration of very strenuous exercise, muscle glycogen is the primary carbohydrate fuel for muscular work (118). The intensity of exercise, which is inversely related to exercise duration, determines the rate at which muscle glycogen is used as a fuel. Figure 5.13 shows a series of lines describing the rates of glycogen breakdown for various exercise intensities expressed as a percent of $\dot{V}O_2$ max (118). The heavier the exercise, the faster glycogen is broken down. This process of glycogen breakdown (glycogenolysis) is initiated by second messengers, which activate protein kinases in the muscle cell (described in figure 5.3). Plasma epinephrine, a powerful stimulator of cyclic AMP formation when bound to β-adrenergic receptors on a cell, was believed to be primarily responsible for glycogenolysis. Figure 5.14 also shows a family of lines, the slopes of which describe how fast plasma E changes with increasing intensities of exercise (78).

Figure 5.13 Glycogen depletion in the quadriceps muscle during bicycle exercise of increasing exercise intensities.

Figure 5.14 Changes in the plasma epinephrine concentration during exercises of different intensities and durations.

Figure 5.15 Changes in muscle glycogen due to 2 minutes of work at 1200 kpm/min, before and after propranolol administration. Blocking the beta-adrenergic receptors had no effect on glycogen breakdown.

Clearly, the data presented in figures 5.13 and 5.14 are consistent with the view that a linkage exists between changes in plasma E during exercise and the increased rate of glycogen degradation. However, there is more to this story.

To test the hypothesis that glycogenolysis in muscle is controlled by circulating E during exercise, investigators had subjects take propranolol, a drug that blocks both β_1- and β_2-adrenergic receptors on the cell membrane. This procedure should block glycogenolysis because cyclic AMP formation would be affected. In the control experiment, subjects worked for 2 minutes at an intensity of exercise that caused the muscle glycogen to be depleted to half its initial value and the muscle lactate concentration to be elevated tenfold. Surprisingly, as shown in figure 5.15, when the subjects took the propranolol and repeated the test on another day, there was no difference in glycogen depletion or lactate formation (53). Other experiments have also shown that β-adrenergic blocking drugs have little effect on slowing the rate of glycogen breakdown during exercise (132). How can this be?

As mentioned in chapter 3, enzymatic reactions in a cell are under the control of both intracellular and extracellular factors. In the aforementioned example with propranolol, plasma E may not have been able to activate adenylate cyclase to form the cyclic AMP needed to activate the protein kinases to initiate glycogen breakdown. However, when a muscle cell is stimulated to contract, Ca^{++}, which is stored in the sarcoplasmic reticulum, floods the cell. Some Ca^{++} ions are used to initiate contractile events (see chapter 8), but other Ca^{++} ions bind to **calmodulin,** which, in turn, activates the protein kinases needed for glycogenolysis (see figure 5.4). In this case, the increased intracellular Ca^{++} (rather than cAMP) is the initial event stimulating muscle glycogen breakdown. Figure 5.16 summarizes these events. Experiments in which the increased secretion

Figure 5.16 The breakdown of muscle glycogen, glycogenolysis, can be initiated by either the Ca^{++}-calmodulin mechanism or the cyclic AMP mechanism. When a drug blocks the β-receptor, glycogenolysis can still occur.

of catecholamines was blocked during exercise confirmed the propranolol experiments, showing that an intact sympathoadrenal system was not necessary to initiate glycogenolysis in skeletal muscle (16).

Observations of glycogen-depletion patterns support this view. Individuals who do heavy exercise with one leg will cause elevations in plasma E, which circulates to all muscle cells. The muscle glycogen, however, is depleted only from the exercised leg (67), suggesting that intracellular factors (e.g., Ca^{++}) are more responsible for these events. Further, in experiments in which individuals engaged in intermittent, intense exercise interspersed with a rest period (interval work), the glycogen was depleted faster from fast-twitch fibers (31, 33, 44). The plasma E concentration should be the same outside both fast- and slow-twitch muscle fibers, but the glycogen was depleted at a faster rate from the fibers used in the activity. This is reasonable because a "resting" muscle fiber should not be using glycogen (or any other fuel) at a high rate. The rate of glycogenolysis would be expected to parallel the rate at which ATP is used by the muscle, and this has been shown to be the case, independent of E (108). This discussion does not mean that E cannot or does not cause glycogenolysis (18, 145). There is ample evidence to show that a surge of E will, in fact, cause this to occur (73, 123–125).

IN SUMMARY

- Glycogen breakdown to glucose in muscle is under the dual control of epinephrine-cyclic AMP and Ca^{++}-calmodulin. The latter's role is enhanced during exercise due to the increase in Ca^{++} from the sarcoplasmic reticulum. In this way the delivery of fuel (glucose) parallels the activation of contraction.

Blood Glucose Homeostasis During Exercise

As mentioned in the introduction, a focal point of hormonal control systems is the maintenance of the plasma glucose concentration during times of inadequate carbohydrate intake (fasting/starvation) and accelerated glucose removal from the circulation (exercise). In both cases, body energy stores are used to meet the challenge, and the hormonal response to these two different situations, exercise and starvation, is quite similar.

The plasma glucose concentration is maintained through four processes that:

- mobilize glucose from liver glycogen stores,
- mobilize plasma FFA from adipose tissue to spare plasma glucose,

- synthesize new glucose in the liver (gluconeogenesis) from amino acids, lactate, and glycerol, and
- block glucose entry into cells to force the substitution of FFA as a fuel.

The overall aim of these four processes is to provide fuel for work while maintaining the plasma glucose concentration. This is a major task when you consider that the liver may have only 80 grams of glucose before exercise begins, and the rate of blood glucose oxidation approaches 1 g/min in heavy exercise or in prolonged ($\geq$3 hours) moderate exercise (20, 24).

Although the hormones will be presented separately, keep in mind that each of the four processes is controlled by more than one hormone, and all four processes are involved in the adaptation to exercise. Some hormones act in a "permissive" way, or are "slow acting," while others are "fast-acting" controllers of substrate mobilization. For this reason, this discussion of the hormonal control of plasma glucose will be divided into two sections—one dealing with permissive and slow-acting hormones and the other dealing with fast-acting hormones.

Permissive and Slow-Acting Hormones Thyroxine, cortisol, and growth hormone are involved in the regulation of carbohydrate, fat, and protein metabolism. These hormones are discussed in this section because they either facilitate the actions of other hormones or respond to stimuli in a slow manner. Remember that to act in a permissive manner the hormone concentration doesn't have to change. However, as you will see, in certain stressful situations permissive hormones can achieve such elevated plasma concentrations that they act directly to influence carbohydrate and fat metabolism rather than to simply facilitate the actions of other hormones.

Thyroid Hormones The discussion of substrate mobilization during exercise must include the thyroid hormones T_3 and T_4, whose free concentrations do not change dramatically from resting to the exercising state. As mentioned earlier, T_3 and T_4 are important in establishing the overall metabolic rate and in allowing other hormones to exert their full effect (permissive hormone). They accomplish this latter function by influencing either the number of receptors on the surface of a cell (for other hormones to interact with) or the affinity of the receptor for the hormone. For example, without T_3, epinephrine has little effect on the mobilization of free fatty acids from adipose tissue. During exercise there is an increase in "free" T_3 due to changes in the binding characteristics of the transport protein (130). T_3 and T_4 are removed from the plasma by tissues during exercise at a greater rate than at rest. In turn, TSH secretion from the anterior

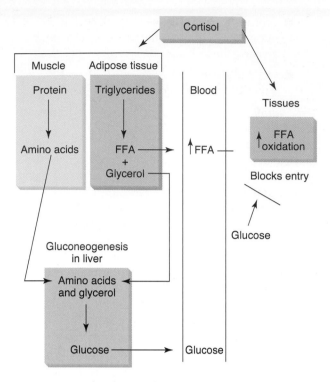

Figure 5.17 Role of cortisol in the maintenance of plasma glucose.

Figure 5.18 Percent change (from resting values) in the plasma cortisol concentration with increasing exercise intensity.

pituitary is increased to stimulate the secretion of T_3 and T_4 from the thyroid gland to maintain the plasma level (42). Low levels of T_3 and T_4 (hypothyroid state) would interfere with the ability of other hormones to mobilize fuel for exercise (100, 130).

Cortisol The primary glucocorticoid in humans is cortisol. As figure 5.17 shows, cortisol (48):

- stimulates FFA mobilization from adipose tissue,
- mobilizes tissue protein to yield amino acids for glucose synthesis in the liver (gluconeogenesis), and
- decreases the rate of glucose utilization by cells.

There are problems, however, when attempting to describe the cortisol response to exercise. Given the General Adaptation Syndrome (GAS) of Selye, events other than exercise can influence the cortisol response. Imagine how a naive subject might view a treadmill test on first exposure. The wires, noise, nose clip, mouthpiece, and blood sampling could all influence the level of arousal of the subject and result in a cortisol response that is not related to a need to mobilize additional substrate. Results supporting such a proposition were reported in the following study (106). Twelve subjects walked on a treadmill at five times their resting metabolic rate (5 METs) for 30 minutes, and blood samples were taken for cortisol analysis. Ten of the twelve subjects showed a decrease in cortisol due to the exercise, while the other two,

who were anxious, had an increase. Clearly, the perception of the subject can influence the cortisol response to mild exercise.

As exercise intensity increases, one might expect the cortisol secretion to increase. This is true, but only within certain limits. For example, Bonen (8) showed that the urinary excretion of cortisol was not changed by exercise at 76% $\dot{V}O_2$ max for 10 minutes, but was increased about twofold when the duration was extended to 30 minutes. Davies and Few (26) extended our understanding of the cortisol response to exercise when they studied subjects who completed several 1-hour exercise bouts. Each test was set at a constant intensity between 40% and 80% $\dot{V}O_2$ max. Exercise at 40% $\dot{V}O_2$ max resulted in a decrease in plasma cortisol over time, while the response was considerably elevated for exercise at 80% $\dot{V}O_2$ max. Figure 5.18 shows the plasma cortisol concentration measured at 60 minutes into each of the exercise tests plotted against % $\dot{V}O_2$ max. When the exercise intensity exceeded 60% $\dot{V}O_2$ max, the cortisol concentration increased; below that, the cortisol concentration decreased. What caused these changes? Using radioactive cortisol as a tracer, the researchers found that during light exercise cortisol was removed faster than the adrenal cortex secreted it, and during intense exercise the increase in plasma cortisol was due to a higher rate of secretion that could more than match the rate of removal, which had doubled.

What is interesting is that for low-intensity, long-duration exercise where the effects of cortisol would go a long way in maintaining the plasma glucose concentration, the concentration of cortisol does not change very much. Even if it did, the effects on metabolism would not be immediately noticeable. The direct effect of cortisol is mediated through the stimulation of DNA and the resulting mRNA formation, which leads to protein synthesis, a slow process. In essence, cortisol, like thyroxine, exerts a permissive effect on substrate mobilization during acute exercise, allowing other fast-acting hormones such as epinephrine and glucagon to deal with glucose and FFA mobilization. Support for this was provided in a study in which a drug was used to lower plasma cortisol before and during submaximal exercise; the overall metabolic response was not affected compared to a normal cortisol condition (29). Given that athletic competitions (triathlon, ultra marathon, most team sports) can result in tissue damage, the reason for changes in the plasma cortisol concentration might not be for the mobilization of fuel for exercising muscles. In these situations, cortisol's role in dealing with tissue repair might come to the forefront.

Growth Hormone   Growth hormone plays a major role in the synthesis of tissue protein, acting either directly or through the enhanced secretion of IGFs from the liver. However, GH can also influence fat and carbohydrate metabolism. Figure 5.19 shows that growth hormone supports the action of cortisol; it:

- decreases glucose uptake by tissue,
- increases FFA mobilization, and
- enhances gluconeogenesis in the liver.

The net effect is to preserve the plasma glucose concentration.

Describing the plasma GH response to exercise is as difficult as describing cortisol's response to exercise because GH can also be altered by a variety of physical, chemical, and psychological stresses (23, 47, 128). Given that, the earlier comments about cortisol should be kept in mind. Figure 5.20a shows plasma GH to increase with increasing intensities of exercise, achieving, at maximal work, values twenty-five times those at rest (128). Figure 5.20b shows the plasma GH concentration to increase over time during 60 minutes of exercise at 60% $\dot{V}O_2$ max (13). What is interesting, compared to other hormonal responses, is that the trained runners had a higher response compared to a group of nonrunners (see "Fast-Acting Hormones"). By

Figure 5.20   (a) Percent change (from resting values) in the plasma growth hormone concentration with increasing exercise intensity. (b) Percent change (from resting values) in the plasma growth hormone concentration during exercise at 60% $\dot{V}O_2$ max for runners and nonrunners (controls).

60 minutes, values for both groups were about five to six times those measured at rest. It must be added that the increased GH response at the same workload, shown by trained individuals, has not been universally observed. Some report lower responses following training (91, 126). In conclusion, GH, a hormone primarily concerned with protein synthesis, can achieve plasma concentrations during exercise that can exert a direct but "slow-acting" effect on carbohydrate and fat metabolism.

Figure 5.19   Role of plasma growth hormone in the maintenance of plasma glucose.

IN SUMMARY

- The hormones thyroxine, cortisol, and growth hormone act in a permissive manner to support the actions of other hormones during exercise.
- Growth hormone and cortisol also provide a "slow-acting" effect on carbohydrate and fat metabolism during exercise.

Liver   Adipose tissue   Tissues

Figure 5.21   Role of catecholamines in substrate mobilization.

Figure 5.22   Percent change (from resting values) in the plasma epinephrine and norepinephrine concentrations during exercise at ~60% $\dot{V}O_2$ max.

Fast-Acting Hormones   In contrast to the aforementioned "permissive" and slow-acting hormones, there are very fast-responding hormones whose actions quickly return the plasma glucose to normal. Again, although each will be presented separately, they behave collectively and in a predictable way during exercise to maintain the plasma glucose concentration (19).

Epinephrine and Norepinephrine   Epinephrine and norepinephrine have already been discussed relative to muscle glycogen mobilization. However, as figure 5.21 shows, they are also involved in the following (21, 113):

- the mobilization of glucose from the liver,
- the mobilization of FFA from adipose tissue, and
- interference with the uptake of glucose by tissues.

Although plasma NE can increase ten- to twentyfold during exercise and can achieve a plasma concentration that can exert a physiological effect (122), the primary means by which NE acts is when released from sympathetic neurons onto the surface of the tissue under consideration. The plasma level of NE is usually taken as an index of overall sympathetic nerve activity, but there is evidence that muscle sympathetic nerve activity during exercise may be a better indicator than that of plasma NE (120). Epinephrine, released from the adrenal medulla, is viewed as the primary catecholamine in the mobilization of glucose from the liver and FFA from adipose tissue (27, 39).

Figure 5.22 shows plasma E and NE to increase linearly with duration of exercise (66, 103, 149). These changes are related to cardiovascular adjustments to exercise—the increased heart rate and blood pressure—as well as to the mobilization of fuel. These responses favor the mobilization of glucose and FFA to maintain the plasma glucose concentration. While it is sometimes difficult to separate the effect of E from NE, E seems to be more responsive to changes in the plasma glucose concentration. A low plasma glucose concentration stimulates a receptor in the hypothalamus to increase E secretion while having

only a modest effect on plasma NE. In contrast, when the blood pressure is challenged, as during an increased heat load, the primary catecholamine involved is norepinephrine (103). Epinephrine binds to β-adrenergic receptors on the liver and stimulates the breakdown of liver glycogen to form glucose for release into the plasma. For example, when arm exercise is added to existing leg exercise, the adrenal medulla secretes a large amount of E. This causes the liver to release more glucose than muscles are using, and the blood glucose concentration actually increases (79). What happens if we block the effects of E and NE? If β-adrenergic receptors are blocked with propranolol (a β-adrenergic receptor blocking drug), the plasma glucose concentration is more difficult to maintain during exercise, especially if the subject has fasted (132). In addition, since the propranolol blocks β-adrenergic receptors on adipose tissue cells, fewer FFAs are released, and the muscles have to rely more on its limited glycogen supply for fuel (41).

Figure 5.23 shows that endurance training causes a very rapid decrease in the plasma E and NE responses to a fixed exercise bout. Within 3 weeks, the concentration of both catecholamines is greatly reduced (140). Paralleling this rapid decrease in E and NE with endurance exercise training is a reduction in glucose mobilization (92). In spite of this, the plasma glucose concentration is maintained because there is also a reduction in glucose uptake by muscle at the same fixed workload following endurance training (112, 141). Interestingly, during a very stressful event, a trained individual has a greater capacity to secrete E than an untrained individual does. In addition, when exercise is performed at the same relative workload (% $\dot{V}O_2$ max) after training (in contrast to the same fixed workload as in figure 5.23), the plasma NE concentration is higher. This suggests that physical training, which stimulates the sympathetic nervous system on a regular basis, increases its capacity to respond to extreme challenges (149).

Figure 5.23 Changes in plasma epinephrine and norepinephrine responses to a fixed workload over 7 weeks of endurance training.

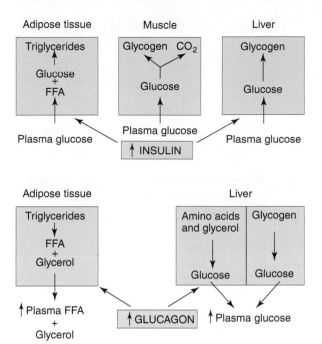

Figure 5.24 Effect of insulin and glucagon on glucose and fatty acid uptake and mobilization.

Insulin and Glucagon These two hormones will be discussed together because they respond to the same stimuli but exert opposite actions relative to the mobilization of liver glucose and adipose tissue FFA. In fact, the ratio of glucagon to insulin provides control over the mobilization of these fuels (19, 134). Further, they account for the vast majority of the glucose mobilized from the liver during moderate to vigorous exercise (21). Figure 5.24 shows insulin to be the primary hormone involved in the uptake and storage of glucose and FFA, and glucagon to cause the mobilization of those fuels from storage, as well as increase gluconeogenesis.

Given that insulin is directly involved in the uptake of glucose into tissue, and that glucose uptake by muscle can increase seven- to twentyfold during exercise (35), what should happen to the insulin concentration during exercise? Figure 5.25a shows that the insulin concentration decreases during exercise of increasing intensity (40, 54, 104); this, of course, is an appropriate response. If exercise were associated with an increase in insulin, the plasma glucose would be taken up into all tissues (including adipose tissue) at a faster rate, leading to an immediate hypoglycemia. The lower insulin concentration during exercise favors the mobilization of glucose from the liver and FFA from adipose tissue, both of which are necessary to maintain the plasma glucose concentration. Figure 5.25b shows that the plasma insulin concentration decreases during moderate-intensity, long-term exercise (49).

Figure 5.25 (a) Percent change (from resting values) in the plasma insulin concentration with increasing intensities of exercise. (b) Percent change (from resting values) in the plasma insulin concentration during prolonged exercise at 60% $\dot{V}O_2$ max showing the effect of endurance training on that response.

Figure 5.26 Percent change (from resting values) in the plasma glucagon concentration during prolonged exercise at 60% V̇O₂ max showing the effect of endurance training on that response.

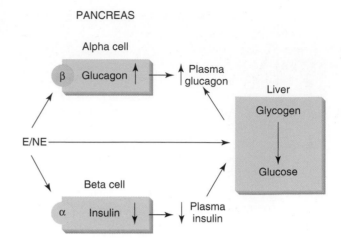

Figure 5.27 Effect of epinephrine and norepinephrine on insulin and glucagon secretion from the pancreas during exercise.

With plasma insulin decreasing with long-term exercise, it should be no surprise that the plasma glucagon concentration increases (49). This increase in plasma glucagon (shown in figure 5.26) favors the mobilization of FFA from adipose tissue and glucose from the liver, as well as an increase in gluconeogenesis. Overall, the reciprocal responses of insulin and glucagon favor the maintenance of the plasma glucose concentration at a time when the muscle is using plasma glucose at a high rate. Figure 5.26 also shows that following an endurance training program, the glucagon response to a fixed exercise task is diminished to the point that there is no increase during exercise. In effect, endurance training allows the plasma glucose concentration to be maintained with little or no change in insulin and glucagon. This is related in part to an increase in glucagon sensitivity in the liver (30, 82), a decrease in glucose uptake by muscle (112), and an increase in the muscle's use of fat as a fuel.

These findings raise several questions. If the plasma glucose concentration is relatively constant during exercise, and the plasma glucose concentration is a primary stimulus for insulin and glucagon secretion, what causes the insulin secretion to decrease and glucagon secretion to increase? The answer lies in the multiple levels of control over hormonal secretion mentioned earlier in the chapter (see figure 5.1). There is no question that changes in the plasma glucose concentration provide an important level of control over the secretion of glucagon and insulin (41). However, when the plasma glucose concentration is relatively constant, the sympathetic nervous system can modify the secretion of insulin and glucagon. Figure 5.27 shows that E and NE stimulate α-adrenergic receptors on the beta cells of the pancreas to decrease insulin secretion during exercise when the plasma glucose concentration is normal.

Figure 5.27 also shows that E and NE stimulate β-adrenergic receptors on the alpha cells of the pancreas to increase glucagon secretion when the plasma glucose concentration is normal (21). These effects have been confirmed through the use of adrenergic receptor blocking drugs. When phentolamine, an α-adrenergic receptor blocker, is given, insulin secretion increases with exercise. When propranolol, a β-adrenergic receptor blocker, is given, the glucagon concentration remains the same or decreases with exercise (86). Figure 5.28 summarizes the effect the sympathetic nervous system has on the mobilization of fuel for muscular work. Endurance training decreases the sympathetic nervous system response to a fixed exercise bout, resulting in less stimulation of

Figure 5.28 Effect of increased sympathetic nervous system activity on free fatty acid and glucose mobilization during submaximal exercise.

adrenergic receptors on the pancreas and less change in insulin and glucagon (see figures 5.25b and 5.26).

The observation that plasma insulin decreases with prolonged, submaximal exercise raises another question. How can exercising muscle take up glucose seven to twenty times faster than at rest if the insulin concentration is decreasing? Part of the answer lies in the large (ten- to twentyfold) increase in blood flow to muscle during exercise. Glucose delivery is the product of muscle blood flow and the blood glucose concentration. Therefore, during exercise, more glucose and insulin are delivered to muscle than at rest, and because the muscle is using glucose at a higher rate, a gradient for its facilitated diffusion is created (70, 112, 141). Another part of the answer relates to exercise-induced changes in the number of glucose transporters in the membrane. It has been known for some time that acute (a single bout) and chronic (training program) exercise increase a muscle's sensitivity to insulin so that less insulin is needed to have the same effect on glucose uptake into tissue (7, 55, 71). The effects of insulin and exercise on glucose transport are additive, suggesting that two separate pools of glucose transporters are activated or translocated in the membrane (45, 69, 71, 138). Interestingly, hypoxia brings about the same effect as exercise, but it is not an additive effect, suggesting that hypoxia and exercise recruit the same transporters (15). What is there about exercise that could cause these changes in glucose transporters?

Part of the answer lies in the high intramuscular Ca^{++} concentration that exists during exercise. The Ca^{++} appears to recruit inactive glucose transporters so that more glucose is transported for the same concentration of insulin (15, 63, 70). This improved glucose transport remains following exercise and facilitates the filling of muscle glycogen stores (see chapter 23). Repeated exercise bouts (training) reduce whole-body insulin resistance, making exercise an important part of therapy for the diabetic (70, 95, 147). Consistent with this, bed rest (94) and limb immobilization (111) increase insulin resistance. However, it is clear that glucose transporters in contracting muscle are regulated by more than changes in the calcium concentration. Factors such as protein kinase C, nitric oxide, AMP-activated protein kinase, and others play a role (110, 115, 117).

In summary, figures 5.29a and 5.29b show the changes in epinephrine, norepinephrine, growth hormone, cortisol, glucagon, and insulin to exercise of varying intensity and duration. The decrease in insulin and the increase in all the other hormones favor the mobilization of glucose from the liver, FFA from adipose tissue, and gluconeogenesis in the liver, while inhibiting the uptake of glucose. These combined actions maintain homeostasis relative to the plasma glucose concentration so that the central nervous system and the muscles can have the fuel they need.

IN SUMMARY

■ Plasma glucose is maintained during exercise by increasing liver glucose mobilization, using more plasma FFA, increasing gluconeogenesis, and decreasing glucose uptake by tissues. The decrease in plasma insulin and the increase in plasma E, NE, GH, glucagon, and cortisol during exercise control these mechanisms to maintain the glucose concentration.

■ Glucose is taken up seven to twenty times faster during exercise than at rest—even with the decrease in plasma insulin. The increases in intracellular Ca^{++} and other factors are associated with an increase in the number of glucose transporters that increase the membrane transport of glucose.

■ Training causes a reduction in E, NE, glucagon, and insulin responses to exercise.

Figure 5.29   (a) Summary of the hormonal responses to exercise of increasing intensity. (b) Summary of the hormonal responses to moderate exercise of long duration.

Hormone-Substrate Interaction

In the examples mentioned previously, insulin and glucagon responded as they did during exercise with a normal plasma glucose concentration due to the influence of the sympathetic nervous system. It must be mentioned that if there were a sudden change in the plasma glucose concentration during exercise, these hormones would respond to that change. For example, if the ingestion of glucose before exercise caused an elevation of plasma glucose, the plasma concentration of insulin would increase. This hormonal change would reduce FFA mobilization and force the muscle to use additional muscle glycogen (1).

During intense exercise, plasma glucagon, GH, cortisol, E, and NE are elevated and insulin is decreased. These hormonal changes favor the mobilization of FFA from adipose tissue that would spare carbohydrate and help maintain the plasma glucose concentration. If this is the case, why does plasma FFA use decrease with increasing intensities of exercise (114)? Part of the answer seems to be that there is an upper limit in the adipose cell's ability to deliver FFA to the circulation during exercise. For example, in trained subjects, the rate of release of FFA from adipose tissue was the highest at 25% $\dot{V}O_2$ max, and decreased at 65% and 85% $\dot{V}O_2$ max (114). Given that the hormone sensitive lipase (HSL) involved in triglyceride breakdown to FFA and glycerol is under stronger hormonal stimulation at the higher work rates, the FFA actually appears to be "trapped" in the adipose cell (60, 114). This may be due to a variety of factors, one of which is lactate. Figure 5.30a shows that as the blood lactate concentration increases, the plasma FFA concentration decreases (68). The elevated lactate has been linked to an increase in alpha glycerol phosphate, the activated form of glycerol needed to make triglycerides. In effect, as fast as the

FFA becomes available from the breakdown of triglycerides, the alpha glycerol phosphate recycles the FFA to generate a new triglyceride molecule (see figure 5.30b). In addition, the elevated H^+ concentration (associated with the high lactate level) can inhibit hormone sensitive lipase. The result is that the FFAs are not released from the adipose cell (99). Other explanations of the reduced availability of adipose tissue FFA during heavy exercise include a reduced blood supply to adipose tissue, resulting in less FFA to transport to muscle (39, 114), and an inadequate amount of albumin, the plasma protein needed to transport the FFA in the plasma (60). The result is that FFAs are not released from the adipose cell, the plasma FFA level falls, and the muscle must use more carbohydrate as a fuel. One of the effects of endurance training is to decrease the lactate concentration at any fixed work rate, which reduces this inhibition to FFA mobilization from adipose tissue. When this is combined with the training-induced increase in mitochondria, the trained person can use more fat as a fuel, spare the limited carbohydrate stores, and improve performance.

IN SUMMARY

■ The plasma FFA concentration decreases during heavy exercise even though the adipose cell is stimulated by a variety of hormones to increase triglyceride breakdown to FFA and glycerol. This may be due to (a) the higher H^+ concentration, which may inhibit hormone sensitive lipase, (b) the high levels of lactate during heavy exercise that promote the resynthesis of triglycerides, (c) an inadequate blood flow to adipose tissue, or (d) insufficient albumin needed to transport the FFA in the plasma.

(a)

(b)

Figure 5.30 (*a*) Changes in plasma free fatty acids due to increases in lactic acid. (*b*) Effect of lactate and H^+ on the mobilization of free fatty acids from the adipose cell.

STUDY QUESTIONS

1. Draw and label a diagram of a negative feedback mechanism for hormonal control using cortisol as an example.
2. List the factors that can influence the blood concentration of a hormone.
3. Discuss the use of testosterone and growth hormone as aids to increase muscle size and strength, and discuss the potential long-term consequences of such use.
4. List each endocrine gland, the hormone(s) secreted from that gland, and its (their) action(s).
5. Describe the two mechanisms by which muscle glycogen is broken down to glucose (glycogenolysis) for use in glycolysis. Which one is activated at the same time as muscle contraction?
6. Identify the four mechanisms involved in maintaining the blood glucose concentration.
7. Draw a summary graph of the changes in the following hormones with exercise of increasing intensity or duration: epinephrine, norepinephrine, cortisol, growth hormone, insulin, and glucagon.
8. What is the effect of training on the responses of epinephrine, norepinephrine, and glucagon to the same exercise task?
9. Briefly explain how glucose can be taken into the muscle at a high rate during exercise when plasma insulin is reduced. Include the role of glucose transporters.
10. Explain how free fatty acid mobilization from the adipose cell decreases during maximal work in spite of the cell being stimulated by all the hormones to break down triglycerides.
11. Discuss the effect of glucose ingestion on the mobilization of free fatty acids during exercise.

REFERENCES

1. **Ahlborg G, and Felig P.** Influence of glucose ingestion on fuel-hormone response during prolonged exercise. *Journal of Applied Physiology: Respiratory, Environmental and Exercise Physiology* 41: 683–688, 1976.
2. **Alen M, Pakarinen A, and Hakkinen K.** Effects of prolonged training on serum thyrotropin and thyroid hormones in elite strength athletes. *Journal of Sports Sciences* 11: 493–497, 1993.
3. **Almon RR, and Dubois DC.** Fiber-type discrimination in disuse and glucocorticoid-induced atrophy. *Medicine and Science in Sports and Exercise* 22: 304–311, 1990.
4. **American College of Sports Medicine.** *The Use of Anabolic-Androgenic Steroids in Sports*. In *Position Stands and Opinion Statements*. Indianapolis: The American College of Sports Medicine, 1984.
5. **Arce JC, De Souza MJ, Pescatello LS, and Luciano AA.** Subclinical alterations in hormone and semen profile in athletes. *Fertility and Sterility* 59: 398–404, 1993.
6. **Berggren JR, Hulver MW, and Houmard JA.** Fat as an endocrine organ: influence of exercise. *Journal of Applied Physiology: Respiratory, Environmental and Exercise Physiology* 99: 757–764, 2005.
7. **Berggren JR, Tanner CJ, Koves TR, Muoio DM, and Houmard JA.** Glucose uptake in muscle cell cultures from endurance-trained men. *Medicine and Science in Sports and Exercise* 37: 579–584, 2005.
8. **Bonen A.** Effects of exercise on excretion rates of urinary free cortisol. *Journal of Applied Physiology: Respiratory, Environmental and Exercise Physiology* 40: 155–158, 1976.
9. **Bouassida A, Chamari K, Zaouali M, Feki Y, Zbidi A, and Tabka Z.** Review on leptin and adiponectin responses and adaptations to acute and chronic exercise. *British Journal of Sports Medicine* 44: 620–630, 2010.
10. **Bouassida A, Latiri I, Bouassida S, Zalleg D, Zaouali M, Feki Y, Gharbi N, Zbidi A, and Tabka Z.** Parathyroid hormone and physcial exercise: a brief review. *J Sport Science and Medicine* 5: 367–374, 2006.
11. **Brandt C, and Pedersen BK.** The role of exercise-induced myokines in muscle homeostasis and the defense against chronic disease. *Journal of Biomedicine and Biotechnology* 2010: Article ID: 520258., 2010.
12. **Brunton L, Lazo JS, and Parker KL, editors.** *Goodman & Gilman's The Pharmacological Basis of Therapeutics*. New York: McGraw-Hill, 2005.
13. **Bunt JC, Boileau RA, Bahr JM, and Nelson RA.** Sex and training differences in human growth hormone levels during prolonged exercise. *Journal of Applied Physiology: Respiratory, Environmental and Exercise Physiology* 61: 1796–1801, 1986.
14. **Cannon W.** *Bodily Changes in Pain, Hunger, Fear and Rage*. Boston: Charles T. Branford Company, 1983.
15. **Cartee GD, Douen AG, Ramlal T, Klip A, and Holloszy JO.** Stimulation of glucose transport in skeletal muscle by hypoxia. *Journal of Applied Physiology: Respiratory, Environmental and Exercise Physiology* 70: 1593–1600, 1991.
16. **Cartier LJ, and Gollnick PD.** Sympathoadrenal system and activation of glycogenolysis during muscular activity. *Journal of Applied Physiology: Respiratory, Environmental and Exercise Physiology* 58: 1122–1127, 1985.
17. **Chaudhari AM, Lindenfeld TN, Andriacchi TP, Hewett TE, Riccobene J, Myer GD, and Noyes FR.** Knee and hip loading patterns at different phases in the menstrual cycle: implications for the gender difference in anterior cruciate ligament injury rates. *The American Journal of Sports Medicine* 35: 793–800, 2007.
18. **Christensen NJ, and Galbo H.** Sympathetic nervous activity during exercise. *Annual Review of Physiology* 45: 139–153, 1983.
19. **Coggan AR.** Plasma glucose metabolism during exercise in humans. *Sports Medicine* (Auckland, NZ) 11: 102–124, 1991.
20. **Coggan AR, and Coyle EF.** Carbohydrate ingestion during prolonged exercise: effects on metabolism and performance. *Exercise and Sport Sciences Reviews* 19: 1–40, 1991.
21. **Coker RH, and Kjaer M.** Glucoregulation during exercise: the role of the neuroendocrine system. *Sports Medicine* (Auckland, NZ) 35: 575–583, 2005.
22. **Convertino VA, Keil LC, and Greenleaf JE.** Plasma volume, renin, and vasopressin responses to graded exercise after training. *Journal of Applied Physiology: Respiratory, Environmental and Exercise Physiology* 54: 508–514, 1983.
23. **Copinschi G, Hartog M, Earll JM, and Havel RJ.** Effect of various blood sampling procedures on serum levels of immunoreactive human growth hormone. *Metabolism: Clinical and Experimental* 16: 402–409, 1967.

24. **Coyle EF.** Substrate utilization during exercise in active people. *The American Journal of Clinical Nutrition* 61: 968S–979S, 1995.
25. **Cumming DC, Brunsting LA, 3rd, Strich G, Ries AL, and Rebar RW.** Reproductive hormone increases in response to acute exercise in men. *Medicine and Science in Sports and Exercise* 18: 369–373, 1986.
26. **Davies CT, and Few JD.** Effects of exercise on adrenocortical function. *Journal of Applied Physiology: Respiratory, Environmental and Exercise Physiology* 35: 887–891, 1973.
27. **De Glisezinski I, Larrouy D, Bajzova M, Koppo K, Polak J, Berlan M, Bulow J, Langin D, Marques MA, Lafontan M, and Stich V.** Adrenaline but not noradrenaline is a determinant of exercise-induced lipid mobilization in human subcutaneous adipose tissue. *The Journal of Physiology* 13: 3393–3404, 2009.
28. **De Souza MJ, Arce JC, Pescatello LS, Scherzer HS, and Luciano AA.** Gonadal hormones and semen quality in male runners. A volume threshold effect of endurance training. *Int J Sports Med* 15: 383–391, 1994.
29. **Del Corral P, Howley ET, Hartsell M, Ashraf M, and Younger MS.** Metabolic effects of low cortisol during exercise in humans. *Journal of Applied Physiology: Respiratory, Environmental and Exercise Physiology* 84: 939–947, 1998.
30. **Drouin R, Lavoie C, Bourque J, Ducros F, Poisson D, and Chiasson JL.** Increased hepatic glucose production in response to glucagon in trained subjects. *The American Journal of Physiology* 274: E23–28, 1998.
31. **Edgerton VR.** *Glycogen depletion in specific types of human skeletal muscle fibers in intermittent and continuous exercise.* Verlag Basel: Birkhauser, 1975, p. 402–415.
32. **Enns DL, and Tiidus PM.** The influence of estrogen on skeletal muscle-sex matters. *Sports Medicine* 40: 41–58, 2010.
33. **Essen B.** Glycogen depletion of different fibre types in human skeletal muscle during intermittent and continuous exercise. *Acta Physiologica Scandinavica* 103: 446–455, 1978.
34. **Euler U.** *Sympatho-Adrenal Activity and Physical Exercise.* New York: Karger, Basal, 1969, p. 170–181.
35. **Felig P, and Wahren J.** Fuel homeostasis in exercise. *The New England Journal of Medicine* 293: 1078–1084, 1975.
36. **Fischer-Posovszky P, Wabitsch M, and Hochberg Z.** Endocrinology of adipose tissue—an update. *Hormone and Metabolic Research (Hormon- und Stoffwechselforschung = Hormones et metabolisme)* 39: 314–321, 2007.
37. **Fox SI.** *Human Physiology.* New York: McGraw-Hill, 2002.
38. **Francesconi RP, Sawka MN, and Pandolf KB.** Hypohydration and heat acclimation: plasma renin and aldosterone during exercise. *Journal of Applied Physiology: Respiratory, Environmental and Exercise Physiology* 55: 1790–1794, 1983.
39. **Frayn KN.** Fat as a fuel: emerging understanding of the adipose tissue-skeletal muscle axis. *Acta Physiologica Scandinavica* 199: 509–518, 2010.
40. **Galbo H, Holst JJ, and Christensen NJ.** Glucagon and plasma catecholamine responses to graded and prolonged exercise in man. *Journal of Applied Physiology: Respiratory, Environmental and Exercise Physiology* 38: 70–76, 1975.
41. **Galbo H, Holst JJ, Christensen NJ, and Hilsted J.** Glucagon and plasma catecholamines during beta-receptor blockade in exercising man. *Journal of Applied Physiology: Respiratory, Environmental and Exercise Physiology* 40: 855–863, 1976.
42. **Galbo H, Hummer L, Peterson IB, Christensen NJ, and Bie N.** Thyroid and testicular hormone responses to graded and prolonged exercise in man. *European Journal of Applied Physiology and Occupational Physiology* 36: 101–106, 1977.
43. **Ganong WF.** *Review of Medical Physiology.* Los Altos: Lange Medical Publications, 1979.
44. **Gollnick PD.** *Glycogen Depletion Patterns in Human Skeletal Muscle Fibers after Varying Types and Intensities of Exercise.* Verlag Basel: Birkhauser, 1975.
45. **Goodyear LJ, and Kahn BB.** Exercise, glucose transport, and insulin sensitivity. *Annual Review of Medicine* 49: 235–261, 1998.
46. **Greenberg AS, and Obin MS.** Obesity and the role of adipose tissue in inflammation and metabolism. *The American Journal of Clinical Nutrition* 83: 461S–465S, 2006.
47. **Greenwood FC, and Landon J.** Growth hormone secretion in response to stress in man. *Nature* 210: 540–541, 1966.
48. **Guyton AC.** *Textbook of Medical Physiology.* Philadelphia: W. B. Saunders, 1986.
49. **Gyntelberg F, Rennie MJ, Hickson RC, and Holloszy JO.** Effect of training on the response of plasma glucagon to exercise. *Journal of Applied Physiology: Respiratory, Environmental and Exercise Physiology* 43: 302–305, 1977.
50. **Hackney AC.** Endurance training and testosterone levels. *Sports Medicine (Auckland, NZ)* 8: 117–127, 1989.
51. **Hackney AC, and Dobridge JD.** Thyroid hormones and the relationship of cortisol and prolactin: influence of prolonged, exhaustive exercise. *Polish Journal of Endocrinology* 60: 252–257, 2009.
52. **Hameed M, Harridge SD, and Goldspink G.** Sarcopenia and hypertrophy: a role for insulin-like growth factor-1 in aged muscle? *Exercise and Sport Sciences Reviews* 30: 15–19, 2002.
53. **Harris RC, Bergström J, and Hultman E.** *The Effect of Propranolol on Glycogen Metabolism during Exercise.* New York: Plenum Press, 1971, p. 301–305.
54. **Hartley LH, Mason JW, Hogan RP, Jones LG, Kotchen TA, Mougey EH, Wherry FE, Pennington LL, and Ricketts PT.** Multiple hormonal responses to prolonged exercise in relation to physical training. *Journal of Applied Physiology: Respiratory, Environmental and Exercise Physiology* 33: 607–610, 1972.
55. **Heath GW, Gavin JR, 3rd, Hinderliter JM, Hagberg JM, Bloomfield SA, and Holloszy JO.** Effects of exercise and lack of exercise on glucose tolerance and insulin sensitivity. *Journal of Applied Physiology: Respiratory, Environmental and Exercise Physiology* 55: 512–517, 1983.
56. **Hew-Butler T.** Arginine vasopressin, fluid balance and exercise. *Sports Medicine* 40: 459–479, 2010.
57. **Hickson RC, Czerwinski SM, Falduto MT, and Young AP.** Glucocorticoid antagonism by exercise and androgenic-anabolic steroids. *Medicine and Science in Sports and Exercise* 22: 331–340, 1990.
58. **Hickson RC, and Marone JR.** Exercise and inhibition of glucocorticoid-induced muscle atrophy. *Exercise and Sport Sciences Reviews* 21: 135–167, 1993.
59. **Highet R.** Athletic amenorrhoea. An update on aetiology, complications and management. *Sports Medicine (Auckland, NZ)* 7: 82–108, 1989.
60. **Hodgetts V, Coppack S, Frayn K, and Hockaday T.** Factors controlling fat mobilization from human subcutaneous adipose tissue during exercise. *Journal of Applied Physiology* 71: 445–451, 1991.
61. **Hoffman JR, Kraemer WJ, Bhasin S, Storer T, Ratamess NA, Haff GG, Willoughby DS, and Rogol AD.** Position stand on androgen and human growth hormone use. *J Strength and Conditioning Research* 23 (Supplement 5): S1–59, 2009.

62. **Holloszy JO, Kohrt WM, and Hansen PA.** The regulation of carbohydrate and fat metabolism during and after exercise. *Front Biosci* 3: D1011–1027, 1998.

63. **Holloszy JO, and Narahara HT.** Enhanced permeability to sugar associated with muscle contraction. Studies of the role of Ca++. *The Journal of General Physiology* 50: 551–562, 1967.

64. **Howley ET.** The effect of different intensities of exercise on the excretion of epinephrine and norepinephrine. *Medicine and Science in Sports* 8: 219–222, 1976.

65. **Howley ET.** *The Excretion of Catecholamines as an Index of Exercise Stress.* Springfield: Charles C Thomas, 1980, p. 171–183.

66. **Howley ET, Cox RH, Welch HG, and Adams RP.** Effect of hyperoxia on metabolic and catecholamine responses to prolonged exercise. *Journal of Applied Physiology: Respiratory, Environmental and Exercise Physiology* 54: 59–63, 1983.

67. **Hultman E.** *Physiological Role of Muscle Glycogen in Man with Special Reference to Exercise.* New York: The American Heart Association, 1967, p. 1–114.

68. **Issekutz B, and Miller H.** Plasma free fatty acids during exercise and the effect of lactic acid. *Proceedings of the Society of Experimental Biology and Medicine* 110: 237–239, 1962.

69. **Ivy JL.** Role of exercise training in the prevention and treatment of insulin resistance and non-insulin-dependent diabetes mellitus. *Sports Medicine* (Auckland, NZ) 24: 321–336, 1997.

70. **Ivy JL.** The insulin-like effect of muscle contraction. *Exercise and Sport Sciences Reviews* 15: 29–51, 1987.

71. **Ivy JL, Young JC, McLane JA, Fell RD, and Holloszy JO.** Exercise training and glucose uptake by skeletal muscle in rats. *Journal of Applied Physiology: Respiratory, Environmental and Exercise Physiology* 55: 1393–1396, 1983.

72. **James DE.** The mammalian facilitative glucose transporter family. *News Physiol. Sci.* 10, 67–71, 1995.

73. **Jansson E, Hjemdahl P, and Kaijser L.** Epinephrine-induced changes in muscle carbohydrate metabolism during exercise in male subjects. *Journal of Applied Physiology: Respiratory, Environmental and Exercise Physiology* 60: 1466–1470, 1986.

74. **Jensen J, Oftebro H, Breigan B, Johnsson A, Ohlin K, Meen HD, Stromme SB, and Dahl HA.** Comparison of changes in testosterone concentrations after strength and endurance exercise in well trained men. *European Journal of Applied Physiology and Occupational Physiology* 63: 467–471, 1991.

75. **Jurkowski JE, Jones NL, Walker C, Younglai EV, and Sutton JR.** Ovarian hormonal responses to exercise. *Journal of Applied Physiology: Respiratory, Environmental and Exercise Physiology* 44: 109–114, 1978.

76. **Kargotich S, Goodman C, Keast D, Fry RW, Garcia-Webb P, Crawford PM, and Morton AR.** Influence of exercise-induced plasma volume changes on the interpretation of biochemical data following high-intensity exercise. *Clin J Sport Med* 7: 185–191, 1997.

77. **Keizer HA, and Rogol AD.** Physical exercise and menstrual cycle alterations. What are the mechanisms? *Sports Medicine* (Auckland, NZ) 10: 218–235, 1990.

78. **Kjaer M.** Epinephrine and some other hormonal responses to exercise in man: with special reference to physical training. *Int J Sports Med* 10: 2–15, 1989.

79. **Kjaer M, Kiens B, Hargreaves M, and Richter EA.** Influence of active muscle mass on glucose homeostasis during exercise in humans. *Journal of Applied Physiology: Respiratory, Environmental and Exercise Physiology* 71: 552–557, 1991.

80. **Kostek MC, Delmonico MJ, Reichel JB, Roth SM, Douglass L, Ferrell RE, and Hurley BF.** Muscle strength response to strength training is influenced by insulin-like growth factor 1 genotype in older adults. *Journal of Applied Physiology: Respiratory, Environmental and Exercise Physiology* 98: 2147–2154, 2005.

81. **Kraemer RR, and Castracane VD.** Exercise and humoral mediators of peripheral energy balance: ghrelin and adiponectin. *Exp Biol Med* 232: 184–194, 2007.

82. **Lavoie C.** Glucagon receptors: effect of exercise and fasting. *Canadian Journal of Applied Physiology* (*Revue canadienne de physiologie appliquee*) 30: 313–327, 2005.

83. **Laycock JF, and Wise PH.** *Essential Endocrinology.* New York: Oxford University Press, 1983.

84. **Liu H, Bravata DM, Olkin I, Friedlander AL, Liu V, Roberts B, Bendavid E, Saynina O, Salpeter SR, Garber AM, and Hoffman AR.** Systematic review: the effects of growth hormone on athletic performance. *Annals of Internal Medicine* 148: 2008.

85. **Liu H, Bravata DM, Olkin I, Nayak S, Roberts B, Garber AM, and Hoffman AR.** Systematic review: the safety and efficacy of growth hormone in the healthy elderly. *Annals of Internal Medicine* 146: 104–115, 2007.

86. **Luyckx AS, and Lefebvre PJ.** Mechanisms involved in the exercise-induced increase in glucagon secretion in rats. *Diabetes* 23: 81–93, 1974.

87. **Maher JT, Jones LG, Hartley LH, Williams GH, and Rose LI.** Aldosterone dynamics during graded exercise at sea level and high altitude. *Journal of Applied Physiology: Respiratory, Environmental and Exercise Physiology* 39: 18–22, 1975.

88. **Maïmoun L, and Sultan C.** Effect of physical activity on calcium homeostasis and calciotrophic hormones: a review. *Calcif Tissue Int* 85: 277–286, 2009.

89. **Marsh SA, and Jenkins DG.** Physiological responses to the menstrual cycle: implications for the development of heat illness in female athletes. *Sports Medicine* (Auckland, NZ) 32: 601–614, 2002.

90. **Mathur N, and Pedersen BK.** Exercise as a means to control low-grade systemic inflammation. *Mediators of Inflammation* 2008: 1–6, 2008.

91. **McMurray RG, and Hackney AC.** Interactions of metabolic hormones, adipose tissue and exercise. *Sports Medicine* (Auckland, NZ) 35: 393–412, 2005.

92. **Mendenhall LA, Swanson SC, Habash DL, and Coggan AR.** Ten days of exercise training reduces glucose production and utilization during moderate-intensity exercise. *The American Journal of Physiology* 266: E136–143, 1994.

93. **Metsarinne K.** Effect of exercise on plasma renin substrate. *Int J Sports Med* 9: 267–269, 1988.

94. **Mikines KJ, Richter EA, Dela F, and Galbo H.** Seven days of bed rest decrease insulin action on glucose uptake in leg and whole body. *Journal of Applied Physiology: Respiratory, Environmental and Exercise Physiology* 70: 1245–1254, 1991.

95. **Mikines KJ, Sonne B, Tronier B, and Galbo H.** Effects of acute exercise and detraining on insulin action in trained men. *Journal of Applied Physiology: Respiratory, Environmental and Exercise Physiology* 66: 704–711, 1989.

96. **Ogawa W, and Kasuga M.** Fat stress and liver resistance. *Science* 322: 1483–1484, 2008.

97. **Oosthuyse T, and Bosch AN.** The effect of the menstrual cycle on exercise metabolism. *Sports Medicine* 40: 207–227, 2010.

98. **Parkinson AB, and Evans NA.** Anabolic androgenic steroids: a survey of 500 users. *Medicine and Science in Sports and Exercise* 38: 644–651, 2006.

99. **Paul P.** FFA metabolism of normal dogs during steady-state exercise at different work loads. *Journal of Applied Physiology: Respiratory, Environmental and Exercise Physiology* 28: 127–132, 1970.
100. **Paul P.** *Uptake and Oxidation of Substrates in the Intact Animal during Exercise.* New York: Plenum Press, 1971, p. 225–248.
101. **Pedersen BK.** Edward F. Adolph Distinguished Lecture: Muscle as an endocrine organ: IL-6 and other myokines. *Journal of Applied Physiology: Respiratory, Environmental and Exercise Physiology* 107: 1006–1014, 2009.
102. **Perry PJ, Lund BC, Deninger MJ, Kutscher EC, and Schneider J.** Anabolic steroid use in weightlifters and bodybuilders: an internet survey of drug utilization. *Clin J Sport Med* 15: 326–330, 2005.
103. **Powers SK, Howley ET, and Cox R.** A differential catecholamine response during prolonged exercise and passive heating. *Medicine and Science in Sports and Exercise* 14: 435–439, 1982.
104. **Pruett ED.** Glucose and insulin during prolonged work stress in men living on different diets. *Journal of Applied Physiology: Respiratory, Environmental and Exercise Physiology* 28: 199–208, 1970.
105. **Raven PH, Johnson GB, Losos JB, Mason KA, and Singer SR.** *Biology.* New York: McGraw-Hill, 2008.
106. **Raymond LW, Sode J, and Tucci JR.** Adrenocortical response to non-exhaustive muscular exercise. *Acta Endocrinologica* 70: 73–80, 1972.
107. **Redman LM, and Loucks AB.** Menstrual disorders in athletes. *Sports Medicine (Auckland, NZ)* 35: 747–755, 2005.
108. **Ren JM, and Hultman E.** Regulation of glycogenolysis in human skeletal muscle. *Journal of Applied Physiology: Respiratory, Environmental and Exercise Physiology* 67: 2243–2248, 1989.
109. **Rennie MJ.** Claims for the anabolic effects of growth hormone: a case of the emperor's new clothes? *British Journal of Sports Medicine* 37: 100–105, 2003.
110. **Richter EA, Derave W, and Wojtaszewski JF.** Glucose, exercise and insulin: emerging concepts. *The Journal of Physiology* 535: 313–322, 2001.
111. **Richter EA, Kiens B, Mizuno M, and Strange S.** Insulin action in human thighs after one-legged immobilization. *Journal of Applied Physiology: Respiratory, Environmental and Exercise Physiology* 67: 19–23, 1989.
112. **Richter EA, Kristiansen S, Wojtaszewski J, Daugaard JR, Asp S, Hespel P, and Kiens B.** Training effects on muscle glucose transport during exercise. *Advances in Experimental Medicine and Biology* 441: 107–116, 1998.
113. **Rizza R, Haymond M, Cryer P, and Gerich J.** Differential effects of epinephrine on glucose production and disposal in man. *The American Journal of Physiology* 237: E356–362, 1979.
114. **Romijn JA, Coyle EF, Sidossis LS, Gastaldelli A, Horowitz JF, Endert E, and Wolfe RR.** Regulation of endogenous fat and carbohydrate metabolism in relation to exercise intensity and duration. *The American Journal of Physiology* 265: E380–391, 1993.
115. **Ryder JW, Chibalin AV, and Zierath JR.** Intracellular mechanisms underlying increases in glucose uptake in response to insulin or exercise in skeletal muscle. *Acta Physiologica Scandinavica* 171: 249–257, 2001.
116. **Sabio G, Das M, Mora A, Zhang Z, Jun JY, Ko HJ, Barrett T, Kim JK, and Davis RJ.** A stress signaling pathway in adipose tissue regulates hepatic insulin resistance. *Science* 322: 1539–1543, 2008.
117. **Sakamoto K, and Goodyear LJ.** Invited review: intracellular signaling in contracting skeletal muscle. *Journal of Applied Physiology: Respiratory, Environmental and Exercise Physiology* 93: 369–383, 2002.
118. **Saltin B, and Karlsson J.** *Muscle Glycogen Utilization during Work of Different Intensities.* New York: Plenum Press, 1971.
119. **Saugy M, Robinson N, Saudan C, Baume N, Avois L, and Mangin P.** Human growth hormone doping in sport. *British Journal of Sports Medicine* 40 Suppl 1: i35–39, 2006.
120. **Seals DR, Victor RG, and Mark AL.** Plasma norepinephrine and muscle sympathetic discharge during rhythmic exercise in humans. *Journal of Applied Physiology: Respiratory, Environmental and Exercise Physiology* 65: 940–944, 1988.
121. **Selye H.** *The Stress of Life.* New York: McGraw-Hill, 1976.
122. **Silverberg AB, Shah SD, Haymond MW, and Cryer PE.** Norepinephrine: hormone and neurotransmitter in man. *The American Journal of Physiology* 234: E252–256, 1978.
123. **Spriet LL, Ren JM, and Hultman E.** Epinephrine infusion enhances muscle glycogenolysis during prolonged electrical stimulation. *Journal of Applied Physiology: Respiratory, Environmental and Exercise Physiology* 64: 1439–1444, 1988.
124. **Stainsby WN, Sumners C, and Andrew GM.** Plasma catecholamines and their effect on blood lactate and muscle lactate output. *Journal of Applied Physiology: Respiratory, Environmental and Exercise Physiology* 57: 321–325, 1984.
125. **Stainsby WN, Sumners C, and Eitzman PD.** Effects of catecholamines on lactic acid output during progressive working contractions. *Journal of Applied Physiology: Respiratory, Environmental and Exercise Physiology* 59: 1809–1814, 1985.
126. **Stokes K.** Growth hormone responses to sub-maximal and sprint exercise. *Growth Horm IGF Res* 13: 225–238, 2003.
127. **Sun Y, Xun K, Wang C, Zhao H, Bi H, Chen X, and Wang Y.** Adiponectin, an unlocking adipocytokine. *Cardiovascular Therapeutics* 27: 59–75, 2009.
128. **Sutton J, and Lazarus L.** Growth hormone in exercise: comparison of physiological and pharmacological stimuli. *Journal of Applied Physiology: Respiratory, Environmental and Exercise Physiology* 41: 523–527, 1976.
129. **Tepperman J, and Tepperman HM.** *Metabolic and Endocrine Physiology.* Chicago: Year Book Medical Publishers, 1987.
130. **Terjung R.** *Endocrine Response to Exercise.* New York: Macmillan, 1979.
131. **Tiidus PM, Enns DL, Hubal MJ, and Clarkson PM.** Point:counterpoint: estrogen and sex do/do not influence post-exercise indexes of muscle damage, inflammation, and repair. *Journal of Applied Physiology: Respiratory, Environmental and Exercise Physiology* 106: 1010–1015, 2009.
132. **Van Baak MA.** β-adrenoceptor blockade and exercise: an update. *Sports Medicine* 5: 209–225, 1988.
133. **Vander AJ, Sherman JH, and Luciano DS.** *Human Physiology: The Mechanisms of Body Function.* New York: McGraw-Hill, 1985.
134. **Voet D, and Voet JG.** *Biochemistry.* New York: John Wiley & Sons, 1995.
135. **Vogel RB, Books CA, Ketchum C, Zauner CW, and Murray FT.** Increase of free and total testosterone during submaximal exercise in normal males. *Medicine and Science in Sports and Exercise* 17: 119–123, 1985.
136. **Wade CE.** Response, regulation, and actions of vasopressin during exercise: a review. *Medicine and Science in Sports and Exercise* 16: 506–511, 1984.

137. **Waki H, and Tontonoz P.** Endocrine functions of adipose tissue. *Annual Review of Pathology* 2: 31–56, 2007.

138. **Wallberg-Henriksson H, Constable SH, Young DA, and Holloszy JO.** Glucose transport into rat skeletal muscle: interaction between exercise and insulin. *Journal of Applied Physiology: Respiratory, Environmental and Exercise Physiology* 65: 909–913, 1988.

139. **Widdowson WM, Healy M-L, Sönksen PH, and Gibney J.** The physiology of growth hormone and sport. *Growth Hormone & IGF Research* 19: 308–319, 2009.

140. **Winder WW, Hagberg JM, Hickson RC, Ehsani AA, and McLane JA.** Time course of sympathoadrenal adaptation to endurance exercise training in man. *Journal of Applied Physiology: Respiratory, Environmental and Exercise Physiology* 45: 370–374, 1978.

141. **Wojtaszewski JF, and Richter EA.** Glucose utilization during exercise: influence of endurance training. *Acta Physiologica Scandinavica* 162: 351–358, 1998.

142. **Wright JE.** *Anabolic Steroids and Athletics.* New York: Macmillan, 1980.

143. **Wright JE.** *Anabolic Steroids and Sports.* New York: Sports Science Consultants, 1982.

144. **Xanne A, and Janse de Jonge X.** Effects of the menstrual cycle on exercise performance. *Sports Medicine* (Auckland, NZ) 33: 833–851, 2003.

145. **Yakovlev NN, and Viru AA.** Adrenergic regulation of adaptation to muscular activity. *Int J Sports Med* 6: 255–265, 1985.

146. **Yesalis CE, and Bahrke MS.** Anabolic-androgenic steroids. Current issues. *Sports Medicine* (Auckland, NZ) 19: 326–340, 1995.

147. **Young JC, Enslin J, and Kuca B.** Exercise intensity and glucose tolerance in trained and nontrained subjects. *Journal of Applied Physiology: Respiratory, Environmental and Exercise Physiology* 67: 39–43, 1989.

148. **Zazulak BT, Paterno M, Myer GD, Romani WA, and Hewett TE.** The effects of the menstrual cycle on anterior knee laxity: a systematic review. *Sports Medicine* (Auckland, NZ) 36: 847–862, 2006.

149. **Zouhal H, Jacob C, Delamarche P, and Gratas-Delamarche A.** Catecholamines and the effects of exercise, training, and gender. *Sports Medicine* 38: 401–423, 2008.

6

Exercise and the Immune System

The concept of homeostasis and the control systems that regulate the internal environment were introduced in chapter 2. The immune system is a critical homeostatic system that recognizes, attacks, and destroys foreign agents in the body. Obviously, this is important because the body is constantly under attack from foreign agents (e.g., bacteria, viruses, and fungi) that promote infection. By protecting the body against infection, the immune system plays an important role in maintaining homeostasis in the body.

Everyone has suffered from the unpleasant symptoms (i.e., runny nose and fever) of an upper respiratory tract infection (URTI). These URTIs are commonly referred to as colds and are caused by more than 200 different viruses (16). Currently, URTIs are the most common types of infections worldwide and the average adult suffers from two to five colds a year (10, 25). Although colds are not usually life threatening in healthy individuals, colds have many negative consequences because of increased health care costs and lost days from work, school, and exercise training (12). Because of the high occurrence of colds, these illnesses present a real concern to the health of athletes and the general population. Since exercise and other stresses (e.g., emotional stress, loss of sleep, etc.) are known to influence the immune system, it is important to understand the relationship between physical activity and the immune system. Therefore, this chapter is designed to introduce the primary components of the immune system and to discuss how exercise training impacts this important homeostatic system. We begin with a brief overview of how the immune system works to prevent infection.

OVERVIEW OF THE IMMUNE SYSTEM

The term **immunity** refers to all of the mechanisms used in the body to protect against foreign agents. The origin of this term is from the Latin term *immunitas* (meaning "freedom from")(4). Immunity results from a well-coordinated immune system that consists of both cellular and chemical components that provide overlapping protection against infectious agents. This overlapping of immune system components is designed to ensure that these redundant systems are efficient in protecting the body against infection from pathogens (disease-causing agents) such as bacteria, viruses, and fungi. The redundancy of the immune system is achieved by the teamwork of two arms of the immune system referred to as the innate and acquired immune system (also called the adaptive or specific immune system). A short introduction to these two immune systems follows.

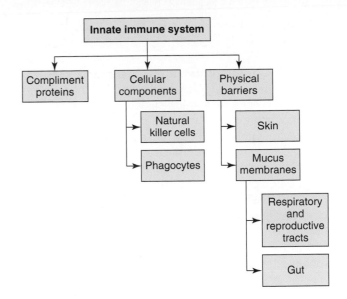

Figure 6.1 Major components of innate immunity. See text for complete details.

Innate Immune System

Humans and other animals are born with an innate, nonspecific, immune system that is made up of a diverse collection of both cellular and protein elements. This system provides both external and internal defenses against foreign invaders (figure 6.1). The external defense is the first line of innate defense and is composed of the physical barriers such as the skin and the mucus membranes (i.e., mucosa) that line our respiratory, digestive (gut), and genitourinary tracts. So, in order to cause trouble, bacteria and other foreign agents must cross these barriers. An invader that crosses the physical barrier of skin or mucosa is greeted by a second line of innate defense. This internal defense is composed of both specialized cells (e.g., phagocytes and natural killer cells) designed to destroy the invader, and a group of proteins called the complement system, which is located in the blood and tissues. The complement system is composed of more than twenty different proteins that work together to destroy foreign invaders; this system also signals other components of the immune system that the body has been attacked. Let's discuss each of these components of innate immunity in more detail.

Physical Barriers Again, the first line of defense against invaders is the physical barrier of the skin and the mucosa. Although we tend to think about the skin as being the primary barrier against foreign agents, the area covered by the skin is only about 2 square meters (28). In contrast, the area covered by the mucosa (i.e., respiratory, digestive, and genitourinary tracts) measures about 400 square meters (an area about the size of two tennis courts) (28). The key point here is that there is a larger perimeter that must be defended to keep unwanted foreign agents from entering the body.

Cellular Components (Phagocytes and Natural Killer Cells) Phagocytes and natural killer cells are specialized cells that are designed to attack and kill invading pathogens. Both cells are members of the leukocyte family of blood cells. Leukocytes (white blood cells) are a group of special cells designed to recognize and wipe out foreign invaders and form the second line of defense against foreign agents. A complete discussion of leukocytes and their function is beyond the scope of this chapter. Therefore, we will provide only a "big picture" overview of leukocytes and will focus our discussion on a few key leukocytes (phagocytes and natural killer cells) that play major roles in the innate immune system.

Where do leukocytes come from? All blood cells (red and white) are made in the blood marrow, where they are produced from common "self-renewing" stem cells. These cells are self-renewing because when stem cells divide into two daughter cells, one of the daughter cells remains a stem cell, whereas the second daughter cell becomes a mature blood cell. This strategy of renewal ensures that there will always be stem cells available to produce mature blood cells.

When stem cells divide, the maturing daughter cell must make a choice as to what type of blood it will become when it matures. These choices are not random but are highly regulated by complicated control systems. Figure 6.2 illustrates the process of stem cells forming a bi-potential stem cell that then can

form a variety of different leukocytes. Table 6.1 provides a brief description of the function of each of these leukocytes. In the next segments we discuss three important leukocytes that participate in innate immunity by protecting against both bacterial and viral infections.

Phagocytes are cells that engulf foreign agents in a process called phagocytosis. To remove unwanted bacteria, the body produces several different types of phagocytes which participate in the innate immune system. Two key phagocytes are macrophages and neutrophils. Together, these important phagocytes form an important line of defense against infection.

As illustrated in Figure 6.2, macrophages are derived from monocytes. **Macrophages** are located in tissues throughout the body and are often called "professional" phagocytes because they make their living destroying bacteria (28). When bacteria enter the body, macrophages recognize these invading cells and reach out to attach to the bacteria. This results in the bacteria being engulfed into a pouch (vesicle) which is moved inside the macrophage. When the bacterium is engulfed by the macrophage, the bacterium is killed by powerful chemicals and enzymes contained within the macrophage (4).

Macrophages can also contribute to innate immunity in two other important ways. First, when macrophages are destroying bacteria, they give off chemicals to increase the amount of blood flow to the infected site. This increased blood flow brings additional leukocytes to the area to take part in the battle of removing the invading microbes.

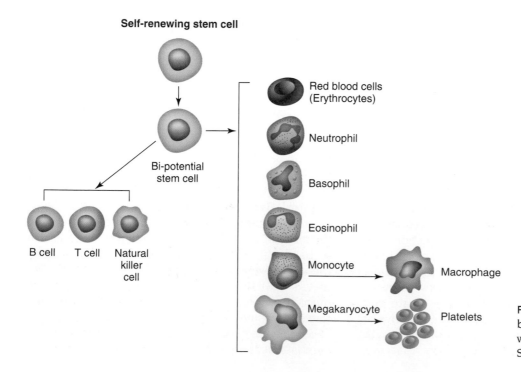

Figure 6.2 The formation of blood cells from stem cells within the bone marrow. See text for details.

TABLE 6.1 A Brief Overview of Leukocytes (White Blood Cells) and Their Function in Protecting Against Foreign Invaders

Leukocyte (White Blood Cell)	Site Produced	Innate or Acquired Immunity	Functions
Neutrophils	Bone marrow	Innate	1. Phagocytosis 2. Release chemicals involved in inflammation (vasodilators, chemotaxins, etc.)
Basophils	Bone marrow	Innate	Release chemicals (e.g., histamine) involved in inflammation
Eosinophils	Bone marrow	Innate	1. Destroy multicellular parasites 2. Involved in hypersensitivity reactions
Monocytes	Bone marrow	Innate	Precursors of macrophages—Macrophages are important phagocytes involved in innate immunity.
Megakaryocytes	Bone marrow	Not involved in immune function	Precursors of platelets—Platelets play an important role in blood clotting
B cell (also called B lymphocyte)	Bone marrow-activated in peripheral lymphoid organs	Acquired	1. Initiate antibody mediated reactions 2. Precursors of plasma cells—mature plasma cells secrete antibodies
T cell (also called T lymphocyte)	Bone marrow-activated in thymus	Acquired	Several different types of T cells exist collectively, these cells participate in cell-mediated responses of the acquired immune system
Natural killer cells	Bone marrow	Innate	1. Bind directly to virus-infected cells and cancer cells to kill them 2. Function as killer cells in antibody-dependent immune response

Further, during the battle with bacteria, macrophages also produce proteins called cytokines. **Cytokines** are cell signals that regulate the immune system by facilitating communication between cells within the immune system (4). For example, some cytokines alert immune cells that the battle is on and cause these cells to exit the blood to help fight the rapidly multiplying bacteria (28). In this case, cytokines serve as a chemoattractant. Chemoattractants are chemicals that recruit other immune system players to the battle site to assist in protecting the body from infection. Other cytokines promote fever, stimulate production of other components of the immune response, and promote inflammation (8).

Macrophages are not the only phagocytes involved in innate immunity. Indeed, neutrophils may be the most important phagocyte in innate immunity (28). **Neutrophils** are leukocytes that also participate as phagocytes during a bacterial invasion. Neutrophils have been called professional killers that are "on call" in the blood (28). After neutrophils have been summoned to the infected area, these important phagocytes exit the blood and become activated to begin destroying the foreign

invaders. Similar to macrophages, neutrophils also produce cytokines that can alert other immune cells. Further, activated neutrophils also release chemicals that promote increased blood flow to the infected area.

In addition to the professional phagocytes (i.e., macrophages and neutrophils), another key cellular component of the innate immune system is the **natural killer cell.** These cells are produced in the bone marrow from stem cells (figure 6.2) and are "on call" to fight an infection. Most natural killer cells are found in the blood, liver, or spleen and when called to fight an infection, these cells exit the blood and move to the battle ground to take part in the fight. When they reach the battle site (i.e., location of the bacteria), natural killer cells play two key roles in defending us against infections. First, natural killer cells can destroy virus-infected cells, bacteria, parasites, fungi, and cancer cells. Second, natural killer cells also give off cytokines that help with immune defense. So, natural killer cells are an important part of the innate immune system because they are versatile "killers" of foreign agents, including bacteria, viruses, cancer cells, and other unwanted invaders of the body.

A CLOSER LOOK 6.1

Inflammation Is a Normal Part of the Immune Response

The word *inflammation* comes from the Latin word *inflammare*, which means "to set on fire." **Inflammation** is a normal part of the biological response to harmful stimuli, such as bacteria entering the body. In short, the goal of inflammation is to restore homeostasis by helping the injured tissue return to its normal state. Inflammation can be classified as either acute or chronic. A brief explanation of the differences between acute and chronic inflammation follows.

Acute Inflammation   The following example illustrates an acute inflammatory response. At some time in your life you have probably experienced a small cut on your finger or hand. In this case, the break in your skin allows bacteria to enter through the wound and results in an acute (i.e., brief) and localized inflammatory response. The clinical signs of localized inflammation are redness, swelling, heat, and pain. This occurs because of a cascade of events triggered by the innate immune system. The redness, swelling, and heat around the injured tissue results from the increased blood flow to the damaged area. This increased blood flow is triggered by the release of chemicals from phagocytes that are summoned to the infected area. Indeed, both macrophages and neutrophils release chemicals (e.g., bradykinin) that promote vasodilation (i.e., widening of the diameter of blood vessels). This vasodilation increases blood flow and fluid collection (i.e., edema) around the injured tissue. The pain associated with this type of local inflammatory response comes from chemicals (e.g., kinins) that stimulate pain receptors in the inflamed area.

Chronic Inflammation   Typically, a small cut on your finger results in acute inflammation that is resolved within a few days when the immune system removes the invading bacteria, a scab forms, and the tissue returns to normal. However, chronic (i.e., unending) systemic inflammation occurs in situations of persistent infection (e.g., tuberculosis) or constant activation of the immune response as seen in diseases such as cancer, heart failure, rheumatoid arthritis, or chronic obstructive lung disease. Interestingly, both obesity and aging are also associated with chronic inflammation (1, 2). Regardless of the cause, chronic inflammation is associated with increased circulating cytokines and the so-called "acute phase proteins" such as c-reactive protein. This is significant because chronically elevated blood levels of both cytokines and c-reactive proteins are thought to contribute to the risk of many diseases, including heart disease and cancer (1).

It is also important to appreciate that chronic systemic inflammation is not "all or none" but can exist in differing levels that are often described as "high grade" or "low grade" inflammation. A severe "high grade" level of inflammation might occur in patients suffering from certain types of cancers or rheumatoid arthritis. In contrast, even in the absence of diagnosed diseases, low grade inflammation can exist in both older and obese individuals (2). The health significance of "low grade" systemic inflammation is a hot topic in medicine because low grade inflammation has been linked to increased risks of cancer, Alzheimer, diabetes, and heart disease (1, 2). However, whether chronic inflammation actually causes all of these diseases or merely accompanies them is currently unknown.

To summarize, phagocytes (macrophages and neutrophils) and natural killer cells are important cellular components of the innate immune system and form the second line of defense against infection. Collectively, these cells remove dangerous invading agents and protect the body against infection whenever the physical barriers of defense are compromised (e.g., skin wound). When these cellular components of the innate immune system are activated following an infection, a physiologic response known as inflammation occurs. The hallmark signs of inflammation are redness, swelling, heat, and pain. More details about inflammation can be found in A Closer Look 6.1.

Complement System   The **complement system** plays an important role in innate immunity and consists of numerous proteins that circulate in the blood in inactive forms. Like phagocytes and natural killer cells, the complement system is another component of the innate defense against infection. The more than 20 proteins that make up the complement system are produced primarily by the liver and are present in high concentrations in the blood and tissues (28). When the body is exposed to a foreign agent (e.g. bacterium), the complement system is activated to attack the invader. These activated complement proteins recognize the surface of the bacterium as a foreign agent and attach to the surface of the foreign cell. This triggers a rapid series of events resulting in the binding of more and more complement proteins on the surface of the bacteria. The addition of multiple complement proteins to the surface of the bacterium forms a "hole" (i.e., channel) in the surface of the bacterium. And once a bacterium has a hole in its membrane, the bacterium dies.

In addition to forming membrane attack complexes, the complement system also performs two other jobs in innate immunity. The second function is to "tag" the cell surface of invading bacteria so that other cellular components (e.g., phagocytes) of the innate immune system can recognize and kill the invader. The third and final role of complement proteins is to serve as chemoattractants. As mentioned earlier, a chemoattractant recruits other

Edward Jenner Was the Pioneer of the Smallpox Vaccine

Edward Jenner (1749–1823) was an English physician who played a major role in developing the smallpox vaccine. Because of this accomplishment, he is sometimes referred to as the "father of immunology." Here is the story behind Jenner's discovery of the smallpox vaccine.

One of the first clues that the immune system was adaptive came in 1796 when Jenner began vaccinating the English against smallpox. During the life of Jenner, smallpox was a huge health problem, and approximately 30 percent of the people infected with smallpox died. In fact, hundreds of thousands of people died from the disease and many others were horribly disfigured (28). Two observations led

Edward Jenner to develop a vaccination procedure against smallpox. First, Jenner observed that milkmaids often contracted a disease called cowpox, which caused them to develop lesions that were similar to the sores associated with smallpox. Second, Jenner also observed that the milkmaids that contracted cowpox almost never got smallpox, which, as it turns out, is a close relative of the cowpox virus (28). Based upon these observations, Jenner reasoned that exposure to a small amount of cowpox virus can promote immunity against smallpox.

To test this hypothesis, Jenner decided to perform a bold experiment. He collected pus from the sores of milkmaids infected with cowpox. He then injected this fluid into the arm of a young boy named James Phipps. This inoculation produced a fever but no

great illness resulted. A few weeks following this treatment, Jenner then injected Phipps with pus collected from sores of a patient infected with smallpox. This daring experiment was a huge success because, remarkably, the young boy did not contract smallpox. However, Phipps was still able to contract other childhood diseases (e.g., measles). This illustrates one of the hallmarks of the adaptive immune system. That is, the acquired immune system adapts to defend against specific invaders.

Obviously, Jenner's experiments on this young boy would not be performed today because of ethical concerns. Nonetheless, we can be thankful that Jenner's experiments were a success because it paved the way for future vaccines that have saved the lives of countless numbers of people around the world.

---

immune players to the battle site to assist in protecting the body from infection.

To summarize, the complement system performs several important jobs when the body is invaded by foreign agents. This system can destroy invaders by building a membrane attack complex that can punch a hole in the surface of the invading bacterium. Second, it can enhance the function of other cells (e.g., phagocyges) within the immune system by tagging the invading agent for destruction. Third, it can alert other cells in the immune system that the body is being attacked. Most important, all these functions of the complement system can act rapidly to protect the body during invasion.

Acquired Immune System

Over 95 percent of all animals get along fine with only the innate immune system to protect them (28). However, for humans and other vertebrates, Mother Nature developed another layer of protection against disease, the acquired immune system. This system of immunity adapts to protect us against almost any type of invader. The primary purpose of the acquired immune system is to protect us against viruses because the innate immune system cannot eliminate many viruses (28). The first evidence that the acquired immune system existed was provided by Dr. Edward Jenner in the 1790s (see A Look Back—Important People in Science).

The acquired immune system is composed of highly specialized cells and processes that prevent or eliminate invading pathogens. This adaptive immune response provides us with the ability to recognize and remember specific pathogens (i.e., to generate immunity) and to mount stronger attacks each time a repeating pathogen is encountered. Therefore, this system is sometimes called the *adaptive immune system* because it prepares itself for future pathogen challenges.

The major cells involved in the acquired immune system are B cells (also called B lymphocytes) and T cells (also called T lymphocytes). Both B and T cells are members of the leukocyte family of blood cells that have their origin from stem cells located within bone marrow (Fig. 6.2). A brief overview of how B and T cells function in acquired immunity follows.

B Cells These cells play a key role in specific immunity and combat both bacterial infections and viral infections by secreting antibodies into the blood. **B cells** function as antibody factories and can produce more than 100 million different types of antibodies that are required to protect us against a wide variety of invading antigens. Antibodies (also called immunoglobulins) are proteins manufactured by B cells to help fight against foreign substances called *antigens*. Antigens are any substance that stimulates the immune system to produce antibodies. For example, bacteria, viruses, or fungi are all antigens. Further, antigens can also be substances called allergens that promote an allergic response. Common allergens include pollen, animal dander, dust, and the contents of certain foods. When the body is confronted by these antigens, B cells respond by producing antibodies to protect against this invasion.

Although the body can produce more than 100 million different antibodies, there are five general classes of antibodies, and each has a different function. The five classes of antibodies are IgG, IgA, IgM, IgD, and IgE. The abbreviation Ig stands for immunoglobulin (i.e., antibody). A detailed discussion of the specific function of each of these classes of antibodies exceeds the goals of this chapter. However, an example of how two classes of antibodies function is useful in understanding the role of antibodies in protection against disease.

When B cells are activated by an invading antigen, IgM is one of the first antibodies produced. Producing this large antibody early during an infection is a good strategy because IgM antibodies can protect against invaders in two important ways. First, IgM antibodies can activate the complement cascade to assist in removing the unwanted invader. In fact, the term *complement* was coined by immunologists when they discovered that antibodies were much more effective in dealing with invaders if they are complemented by other proteins—the complement system (28). Second, IgM antibodies are good at neutralizing viruses by binding to them and preventing the virus from infecting cells. Hence, because of these combined properties, the IgM is the perfect "first" antibody to protect against viral or bacterial invasions (28).

IgG antibodies are another important class of antibodies. These antibodies circulate in the blood and other body fluids and defend against invading bacteria and viruses (31). The binding of IgG antibodies with bacterial or viral antigens activates other immune cells (e.g., macrophages, neutrophils, and natural killer cells) that destroy these invaders and protect us against disease.

T Cells   **T cells** are a family of immune cells produced in the bone marrow. T cells and B cells differ in several ways. First, while B cells mature in the bone marrow, T cells mature in a specialized immune organ called the thymus; this is why they are called T cells. Further, T cells do not produce antibodies but specialize in recognizing protein antigens in the body. There are three main types of T cells: (1) Killer T cells (also called cytotoxic T cells; (2) Helper T cells; and (3) Regulatory T cells. Killer T cells are a potent weapon against viruses because they can recognize and kill virus-infected cells (6). Helper T cells secrete cytokines that have a dramatic effect on other immune system cells. In this

way, helper T cells serve as the quarterback of the immune system by directing the action of other immune cells. Finally, as the name implies, the regulatory T cells are involved in regulation of immune function. Specifically, these cells play a role in inhibiting responses to both self-antigens (i.e., preventing the immune system from attacking normal body cells) and foreign antigens. In this way, regulatory T cells help to regulate self-tolerance and prevent autoimmune diseases (4).

IN SUMMARY

- The human immune system is a complex and redundant system designed to protect us against invading pathogens.
- A healthy immune system requires the teamwork of two layers of immune protection: (1) innate immune system and (2) acquired immune system.
- The innate system provides the first line of defense against foreign invaders and is composed of three major components: (1) Physical barriers such as the skin and the mucous membranes that line our respiratory, digestive, and genitourinary tracts; (2) specialized cells (e.g., phagocytes and natural killer cells) designed to destroy invaders, and (3) a group of proteins called the complement system, which are located throughout the body to protect against invaders.
- The acquired immune system adapts to protect against almost any type of invading pathogen. The primary purpose of the acquired immune system is to provide protection against viruses that the innate immune system cannot provide. B and T cells are the major cells involved in the acquired immune system. B cells produce antibodies, whereas T cells specialize in recognizing and removing antigens in the body.

EXERCISE AND THE IMMUNE SYSTEM

Compared to most areas of research in exercise physiology, exercise and the immune system is a relatively new topic of study. However, interest in the field of exercise immunology has grown rapidly during the past two decades. In the following sections we will discuss several important topics related to the effects of exercise on resistance to infection.

Exercise and Resistance to Infection

The concept that exercise can have both a positive and a negative effect on the risk of infection is almost two

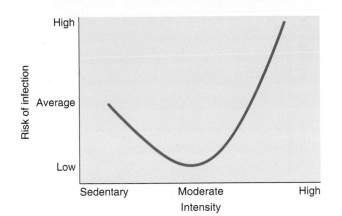

Figure 6.3 "J" shaped model of the relationship between varying amounts of exercise and the risk of URTI. This model suggests that moderate aerobic exercise reduces the risk of infection, whereas high intensity/long-duration exercise may increase the risk of infection (19).

decades old. This idea was introduced by Dr. David Nieman when he described the risk of an upper-respiratory tract infection (URTI) as a J-shaped curve that changed as a function of the intensity and amount of exercise being performed (figure 6.3). Note in figure 6.3 that people engaging in regular bouts of moderate exercise are at a lower risk of an URTI compared to sedentary individuals and people who engage in intense and/or long-duration exercise sessions. For example, marathon runners represent those at the high end of the exercise intensity and duration scale. Indeed, running a marathon increases the risk of an URTI in the days following the run (24). In the next two segments, we discuss the reasons why moderate- and high-intensity exercise have different effects on the risk of infection.

Moderate Aerobic Exercise Protects Against Infection Many studies support the concept that people who engage in regular bouts of moderate aerobic exercise catch fewer colds (i.e., URTIs) than both sedentary individuals and people who engage in high-intensity/long-duration exercise (22, 23). For example, both epidemiological and randomized studies consistently report that regular exercise results in an 18–67% reduction in the risk of URTI(9). Interestingly, this exercise-induced protection against infection can be achieved with many types of aerobic activity (e.g., walking, jogging, cycling, swimming, sports play, and aerobic dance). In general, it appears that 20–40 minutes of moderate intensity exercise (i.e., 40–60% of $\dot{V}O_2$ max) is adequate to promote a beneficial effect on the immune system. Importantly, this exercise-induced reduction in the risk of URTI occurs in both men and women of all ages (22).

The explanation as to why moderate intensity exercise protects against URTI remains a topic of debate. Nonetheless, there are several possible reasons to explain why exercise reduces the risk of infection. First, each bout of moderate aerobic exercise causes an increase in blood levels of natural killer cells, neutrophils, and antibodies (9). Therefore, an acute bout of exercise provides a positive boost to both the innate immune system (natural killer cells and neutrophils) and the acquired immune system (antibodies). Note that this exercise-induced boost in immune function is transient and that the immune system returns to pre-exercise levels within 3 hours. Nonetheless, it seems that each bout of exercise improves immune function against pathogens over a short time period, which results in a reduced risk of infection (22). Other factors might also contribute to the positive impact of routine exercise on the reduced risk of infection. For example, people who engage in regular exercise may also benefit from an improved psychological well-being (i.e., less emotional stress), good nutritional status, and a healthy lifestyle (e.g., adequate sleep). Each of these factors has been linked to a reduced risk of infection and therefore may also be a connection between regular exercise and lowered risk for URTI.

Although it is clear that aerobic exercise provides protection against colds, it remains unknown if resistance exercise training provides the same level of protection against infection. This is because few studies have systematically investigated the impact of resistance exercise on immune function. Nonetheless, based on the available evidence, it appears that an acute bout of resistance exercise results in a transient increase in natural killer cells (15). However, this immune boost is temporary because blood levels of primary immune cells return to normal within a short period following a resistance training session (5). To summarize, it seems possible that regular bouts of resistance exercise might protect against infection, but additional research is required to firmly establish that resistance exercise alone is effective in providing protection against URTIs.

High-Intensity/Long-Duration Aerobic Exercise Increases the Risk of Infection

The idea that athletes engaged in intense training are more susceptible to infections originated from anecdotal reports from coaches and athletes. For instance, the marathon runner Alberto Salazar reported that he caught 12 colds in 12 months while training for the 1984 Olympic marathon (17). Because Salazar was engaged in intense exercise training, many people reasoned that the high level of exercise training was responsible for his increased number of colds. However, anecdotal reports do not prove cause and effect, and scientific studies were required to determine if intense exercise training leads to an increased risk of infection. In general, many studies support the concept that athletes engaged in intensive endurance training suffer a higher incidence of URTI compared to sedentary individuals or people engaged in moderate exercise (figure 6.3) (9, 21, 24). For example, compared to the general population, evidence indicates that sore throats and flu-like symptoms are more common in athletes involved in intense training (11, 24). Indeed, the risk of developing an URTI is two- to sixfold higher in athletes following a marathon compared to the general public (24). This increased risk of illness is a concern for athletes because even minor infections can impair exercise performance and the ability to sustain intense exercise training (27). Further, prolonged viral infections are often associated with the development of persistent fatigue, which poses another threat to the athlete (7).

There are several reasons why high-intensity and long-duration exercise promotes an increased risk of infection (9). First, prolonged (>90 minutes) and intense exercise has a temporary depressive effect on the immune system. For example, after a marathon, the following major changes occur in immune function:

- Decreased blood levels of B cells, T cells, and natural killer cells
- Decreases in natural killer cell activity and T-cell function
- Decreases in nasal neutrophil phagocytosis
- Decreases in nasal and salivary IgA levels
- Increases in pro- and anti-inflammatory cytokines

Collectively, these changes result in a depression of the immune system's ability to defend against invading pathogens. It has been argued that this immune suppression following a marathon provides an "open window," during which viruses and bacteria can gain a foothold and increase the risk of infection (see figure 6.4).

The biological reason to explain why intense exercise promotes immune dysfunction is probably related to the immunosuppressive effects of stress hormones such as cortisol (8). You may recall from chapter 5 that prolonged strenuous exercise results in large increases in the circulating levels of cortisol. High cortisol levels has been reported to depress immune system function in several ways (8). For example, high levels of cortisol can inhibit the function of specific cytokines, suppress natural killer cell function, and depress both the production and function of T cells (20).

Although strenuous exercise can depress immune function, other factors may also contribute to the increased risk of infection in athletes engaged in intense training. For example, athletes engaged in intense training may also be exposed to other potential stressors, including a lack of sleep, mental stress, increased exposure to pathogens due to large crowds, air travel, and inadequate diet to support immune

Figure 6.4 The open window theory is a potential explanation for why high-intensity exercise increases the risk of infection. In brief, prolonged exercise (e.g., marathon-type exertion) leads to immune dysfunction that increases the likelihood for opportunistic upper respiratory tract infections (21).

health (see the Ask the Expert feature for more details on diet and immune health). Each of these factors has been reported to have a negative impact on immune function and therefore could contribute to the increased incidence of URTIs in athletes (9). Figure 6.5 summarizes the factors that may explain why athletes engaged in intense training are at a greater risk of infection.

Finally, do weeks of intense exercise training result in a chronic state of immune depression? The answer to this question is no, because following an acute bout of exercise, circulating leukocyte number and function return to pre-exercise levels within 3–24 hours (8). Further, comparisons of leukocyte number and other markers of immune function between athletes and nonathletes do not differ markedly (8). Therefore, in the resting state, immune function is not different between athletes and nonathletes.

Factors affecting susceptibility to infection in athletes

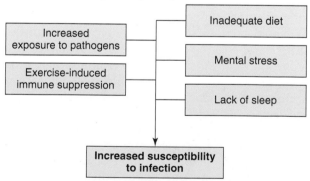

Figure 6.5 Several factors may explain why athletes engaged in intense training are at a greater risk of infection; these include increased exposure to pathogens, exercise-induced immune suppression, inadequate diet, mental stress, and lack of sleep.

Dr. David Nieman, a professor in the Department of Health, Leisure, and Exercise Science at Appalachian State University, is an internationally known expert on stress and human immune function. Specifically, Dr. Nieman's research has addressed numerous important questions related to the impact of both exercise and nutrition on the risk of infection in athletes. In this feature, Dr. Nieman answers questions about the impact of diet and nutritional supplements on immune function in athletes.

QUESTION: Nutritional deficiencies have been shown to impair immune function. What nutritional advice can you provide to athletes regarding the importance of adequate energy intake and the balance of macronutrient consumption during periods of intense training?

ANSWER: Low energy intake leading to rapid weight loss and muscle wasting has a profound, negative effect on immune function. However, when energy intake matches energy expenditure, a wide range in the macronutrient and micronutrient content of the diet is compatible with healthy immune function. Low energy intake is just one of several lifestyle factors that influence immune function, and others include heavy exertion, mental stress, sleep disruption, and poor hygienic practices. All of these factors together can seriously undermine immune function, increasing the risk for certain infections, including upper respiratory tract infection (URTI).

QUESTION: Some reports suggest that consumption of carbohydrate (30–60 g CHO/hour) during prolonged exercise can reduce the degree of exercise-induced immunosuppression. How strong is the experimental evidence to support this claim?

ANSWER: Multiple research teams have investigated this question since the mid-1990s. In general, ingesting 30 to 60 grams carbohydrate during each hour of running, cycling, or similar aerobic exercise keeps the blood glucose higher when compared to no-carbohydrate conditions, lowers blood levels of stress hormones such as cortisol and epinephrine, and as a result, takes the edge off post-exercise immune inflammatory responses. Nonetheless, consumption of carbohydrates during exercise does not protect against the transient decrease in immune function that is experienced by athletes after long exercise bouts.

QUESTION: Numerous advertisements claim that specific nutritional supplements can improve immune function and reduce the risk of infection. In your opinion, are there nutritional supplements that can provide the athlete with increased protection against the risk of URTI?

ANSWER: There is a growing realization that extra vitamins, minerals, and amino acids do not provide countermeasure immune benefits for healthy and well-fed athletes during heavy training. As a result, the focus has shifted to other types of nutritional components such as probiotics, bovine colostrum, β-glucan, flavonoids, and polyphenols such as quercetin, resveratrol, curcumin, and epigallicatechin-3-gallate (EGCG), N-3 polyunsaturated fatty acids (N-3 PUFAs or fish oil), herbal supplements, and unique plant extracts (e.g., green tea extract, black currant extract, tomato extract with lycopene, anthocyanin-rich extract from bilberry, polyphenol-rich pomegranate fruit extract). More well-designed studies with human subjects are needed before enthusiastic support is given to any of these supplements. Some exert impressive effects when cultured with specialized cells and in animal-based models, but then fail when studied under double-blinded, placebo-controlled conditions in human athletes.

IN SUMMARY

- Exercise can have both a positive and a negative effect on the risk of infection. The relationship between the intensity/amount of exercise and the risk of developing an URTI is described as a J-shaped curve (figure 6.3). This J-shaped curve illustrates that moderate intensity aerobic exercise decreases the risk of infection, whereas high-intensity/prolonged exercise increases the risk of infection.
- Regular aerobic exercise can reduce the risk of infection in several ways. In particular, an acute bout of moderate exercise increases blood levels of antibodies, natural killer cells, and neutrophils that provide a positive boost to the immune system.
- The fact that moderate aerobic exercise provides a transient boost to the immune system is another example of how regular exercise can enhance a control system in the body to preserve homeostasis. Indeed, by protecting the body against infection, the immune system plays an important role in maintaining homeostasis.
- High-intensity/long-duration exercise has been shown to have a temporary depressive effect on the immune system. This acute immune suppression following an intense exercise session provides an "open window" during which viruses and bacteria can grow, resulting in an infection.

EXERCISING IN ENVIRONMENTAL EXTREMES: INCREASED RISK FOR INFECTION?

Exercise in environmental extremes (e.g., heat, cold, and high altitude) can increase circulating stress hormones such as cortisol (30). Given that high levels of cortisol can depress immune function, does exercise in environmental extremes result in immune depression and increase the risk of infection? Let's review the evidence regarding the effects of exercise in hot, cold, and high-altitude environments on the immune system.

Exercising in a hot versus cool environment results in significant increases in body temperature and elevates circulating levels of stress hormones (30). In theory, this increase in circulating stress hormones could pose a threat to immune function. Nonetheless, laboratory studies indicate that exercise in a hot environment does not significantly impair the function of key cells involved in immune function (e.g., neutrophils and natural killer cells) (26, 30). Therefore, exercising in the heat does not pose a greater threat to immune function than exercise in a cool environment.

It is commonly believed that being exposed to cold weather increases the susceptibility to URTIs. Indeed, the use of the term "colds" may have come from the belief that cold exposure causes URTI (30). Several studies have investigated the impact of short- and long-term cold exposure with/without exercise on key elements of the immune system. Collectively, these investigations provide limited evidence to indicate that cold exposure increases your risk of infection. For example, both acute exposure and repeated bouts of cold exposure increase the number of circulating neutrophils, T- and B-cells, and natural killer cells in non-exercising subjects (13). Therefore, cold exposure alone does not have a negative impact on the immune system; indeed, cold exposure appears to have a positive effect on the immune system (30). Studies also demonstrate that exercise in a cold environment does not suppress immune function (30). Therefore, current evidence does not support the popular belief that short- or long-term cold exposure, with or without exercise, suppresses immune function and increases the risk of infection (30).

Endurance exercise performed at high altitudes (e.g., >6,000 feet above sea level) impairs performance and is associated with increased levels of stress hormones that could depress immune function. Nonetheless, laboratory studies indicate that acute exercise at simulated high altitude does not impair immune function. In fact, a single bout of exercise in a simulated high-altitude condition results in increased circulating levels of leukocytes (14). In contrast to these laboratory studies, field studies conducted in the mountains suggest that living and exercising at high altitude depresses immune function and increases the risk of URTI (3, 29). The increased risk of infection that occurs during prolonged exposure to high altitudes may arise from a combination of stresses, such as low arterial oxygen levels, high altitude-related sleep disorders, and acute mountain sickness. Regardless of the mechanisms involved, high-altitude exposure combined with exercise appears to impair the immune system and increase the risk of URTI (30).

IN SUMMARY

- Although exercise in the heat can increase circulating levels of stress hormones, exercising in a hot environment does not pose a greater threat to immune function compared to exercise in a cool environment.
- Research does not support the popular belief that short- or long-term cold exposure, with or without exercise, suppresses immune function and increases the risk of infection.
- Prolonged high altitude exposure (i.e., living in the mountains) combined with exercise can increase the risk of URTI.

SHOULD YOU EXERCISE WHEN YOU HAVE A COLD?

Anyone who exercises on a regular basis has been faced with the decision of whether to skip a workout or exercise during a cold. This is often a difficult decision because of the uncertainty as to whether a bout of exercise will worsen your illness or perhaps make you feel better. The next time that you are faced with a cold, here are some general guidelines to follow when you are making the decision as to whether you should exercise or take the day off. It is typically okay to exercise with a cold if your symptoms are above the neck (18). That is, if your cold symptoms are limited to a runny nose, nasal congestion, and a mild sore throat (18). Nonetheless, you should probably reduce the intensity of workout during a cold and avoid high-intensity/long-duration workouts. If your cold symptoms get worse with physical activity, stop exercise and rest. You can restart your workout routine gradually as you begin to feel better.

In contrast to the advice above, there are some situations when you should not exercise. For example, postpone your workout if your cold symptoms are below the neck (i.e., chest congestion, cough, or stomach pain). Further, don't exercise if you have a fever, general fatigue, or widespread muscle aches (18). You can resume training when the below-the-neck cold symptoms have passed and your fever is no longer present.

IN SUMMARY

■ It is reasonable to exercise during a cold if your symptoms are limited to a runny nose, nasal congestion, and a mild sore throat.

■ It is not wise to exercise if your cold symptoms are below the neck (i.e., chest congestion, cough, or stomach pain). Also, don't exercise if you have a fever, general fatigue, or widespread muscle aches.

STUDY QUESTIONS

1. Describe how the innate and acquired immune systems work as a unit to protect the body against infection.
2. Define the key components that make up the innate immune system (e.g., macrophages, neutrophils, natural killer cells, and complement system), and describe how these elements protect against infection.
3. List the primary components of the acquired immune system (e.g., B cells, antibodies, and T cells), and explain how they protect against infection.
4. Describe the differences between acute and chronic inflammation.
5. Outline the effects of moderate exercise training on the immune system and the risk of infection.
6. Explain how an acute bout of intense and prolonged (>90 minutes) exercise impacts immune function and the risk of infection.
7. Discuss the impact of exercise in hot, cold, and high-altitude environments on the immune system and the risk of infection.
8. Discuss the guidelines for deciding whether it is wise to exercise when you have a cold.

SUGGESTED READINGS

Coico RaS, G. 2009. *Immunology: A Short Course*. Hoboken, NJ: Wiley-Blackwell.

Gleeson M. 2006. *Immune Function in Sport and Exercise*. Philadelphia, PA: Elsevier.

Somppayrac L. 2008. *How the Immune System Works*. Malden, MA: Blackwell Publishing.

University of California, Berkeley. 2008, January. Is inflammation the root of all disease? *Wellness Newsletter*.

REFERENCES

1. **Ahmad A, Banerjee S, Wang Z, Kong D, Majumdar AP, and Sarkar FH.** Aging and inflammation: etiological culprits of cancer. *Current Aging Science* 2: 174–186, 2009.
2. **Balistreri CR, Caruso C, and Candore G.** The role of adipose tissue and adipokines in obesity-related inflammatory diseases. *Mediators of Inflammation* 2010: 802078, 2010.
3. **Chouker A, Demetz F, Martignoni A, Smith L, Setzer F, Bauer A, Holzl J, Peter K, Christ F, and Thiel M.** Strenuous physical exercise inhibits granulocyte activation induced by high altitude. *J Appl Physiol* 98: 640–647, 2005.
4. **Coico R, and Sunshine G.** *Immunology: A Short Course*. Hoboken: Wiley-Blackwell, 2009.
5. **Flynn MG, Fahlman M, Braun WA, Lambert CP, Bouillon LE, Brolinson PG, and Armstrong CW.** Effects of resistance training on selected indexes of immune function in elderly women. *J Appl Physiol* 86: 1905–1913, 1999.
6. **Fox S.** *Human Physiology*. Boston: McGraw-Hill, 2009.
7. **Friman G, and Ilback NG.** Acute infection: metabolic responses, effects on performance, interaction with exercise, and myocarditis. *International Journal of Sports Medicine* 19 Suppl 3: S172–182, 1998.
8. **Gleeson M.** *Immune Function in Sport and Exercise*. Philadelphia: Elsevier, 2006.
9. **Gleeson M.** Immune function in sport and exercise. *J Appl Physiol* 103: 693–699, 2007.
10. **Graham N.** The epidemiology of acute respiratory tract infections in children and adults: a global perspective. *Epidemiological Reviews* 12: 149–178, 1990.
11. **Heath GW, Ford ES, Craven TE, Macera CA, Jackson KL, and Pate RR.** Exercise and the incidence of upper respiratory tract infections. *Medicine and Science in Sports and Exercise* 23: 152–157, 1991.
12. **Heath GW, Macera CA, and Nieman DC.** Exercise and upper respiratory tract infections. Is there a relationship? *Sports Medicine* (Auckland, NZ) 14: 353–365, 1992.
13. **Jansky L, Pospisilova D, Honzova S, Ulicny B, Sramek P, Zeman V, and Kaminkova J.** Immune system of cold-exposed and cold-adapted humans. *European Journal of Applied Physiology and Occupational Physiology* 72: 445–450, 1996.
14. **Klokker M, Kjaer M, Secher NH, Hanel B, Worm L, Kappel M, and Pedersen BK.** Natural killer cell response to exercise in humans: effect of hypoxia and epidural anesthesia. *J Appl Physiol* 78: 709–716, 1995.
15. **Miles MP, Kraemer WJ, Grove DS, Leach SK, Dohi K, Bush JA, Marx JO, Nindl BC, Volek JS, and Mastro AM.** Effects of resistance training on resting immune parameters in women. *European Journal of Applied Physiology* 87: 506–508, 2002.
16. **Monto A.** Epidemiology of viral infections. *American Journal of Medicine* 112: 4S–12S, 2002.
17. **Nieman DC.** Can too much exercise increase the risk of sickness? *Sports Science Exchange* 11 (suppl): 69, 1998.
18. **Nieman DC.** Current perspective on exercise immunology. *Current Sports Medicine Reports* 2: 239–242, 2003.
19. **Nieman DC.** Exercise, upper respiratory tract infection, and the immune system. *Medicine and Science in Sports and Exercise* 26: 128–139, 1994.
20. **Nieman DC.** Immune response to heavy exertion. *J Appl Physiol* 82: 1385–1394, 1997.

21. **Nieman DC.** Marathon training and immune function. *Sports Medicine* (Auckland, NZ) 37: 412–415, 2007.

22. **Nieman DC, Henson DA, Austin MD, and Sha W.** Upper respiratory tract infection is reduced in physically fit and active adults. *British Journal of Sports Medicine* 2010.

23. **Nieman DC, Henson DA, Gusewitch G, Warren BJ, Dotson RC, Butterworth DE, and Nehlsen-Cannarella SL.** Physical activity and immune function in elderly women. *Medicine and Science in Sports and Exercise* 25: 823–831, 1993.

24. **Nieman DC, Johanssen LM, Lee JW, and Arabatzis K.** Infectious episodes in runners before and after the Los Angeles Marathon. *The Journal of Sports Medicine and Physical Fitness* 30: 316–328, 1990.

25. **NIH.** The common cold. http://wwwniaidnihgov/topics/commoncold, 2010.

26. **Peake J, Peiffer JJ, Abbiss CR, Nosaka K, Okutsu M, Laursen PB, and Suzuki K.** Body temperature and its effect on leukocyte mobilization, cytokines and markers of neutrophil activation during and after exercise. *European Journal of Applied Physiology* 102: 391–401, 2008.

27. **Roberts JA.** Viral illnesses and sports performance. *Sports Medicine* (Auckland, NZ) 3: 298–303, 1986.

28. **Somppayrac L.** *How the Immune System Works.* Malden: Blackwell Publishing, 2008.

29. **Tiollier E, Schmitt L, Burnat P, Fouillot JP, Robach P, Filaire E, Guezennec C, and Richalet JP.** Living high-training low altitude training: effects on mucosal immunity. *European Journal of Applied Physiology* 94: 298–304, 2005.

30. **Walsh NP, and Whitham M.** Exercising in environmental extremes: a greater threat to immune function? *Sports Medicine* (Auckland, NZ) 36: 941–976, 2006.

31. **Widmaier E, H. Raff, and K. Strang.** *Vander's Human Physiology.* Boston: McGraw-Hill, 2008.

7

The Nervous System: Structure and Control of Movement

The nervous system provides the body with a rapid means of internal communication that allows us to move about, talk, and coordinate the activity of billions of cells. Thus, neural activity is critically important in the body's ability to maintain homeostasis. The purpose of this chapter is to present an overview of the nervous system, with emphasis on neural control of voluntary movement. We will begin with a brief discussion of the general function of the nervous system.

GENERAL NERVOUS SYSTEM FUNCTIONS

The nervous system is the body's means of perceiving and responding to events in the internal and external environments. Receptors capable of sensing touch, pain, temperature changes, and chemical stimuli send information to the **central nervous system (CNS)** concerning changes in our environment. The CNS can respond to these stimuli in several ways. The response may be involuntary movement (e.g., rapid removal of a hand from a hot surface) or alteration in the rate of release of some hormone from the endocrine system (see chapter 5). In addition to integrating body activities and controlling voluntary movement, the nervous system is responsible for storing experiences (memory) and establishing patterns of response based on previous experiences (learning). The four major functions of the nervous system that will be discussed in this chapter are as follows (5):

1. Control of the internal environment (nervous system works with endocrine system)
2. Voluntary control of movement
3. Programming of spinal reflexes
4. Assimilation of experiences necessary for memory and learning

ORGANIZATION OF THE NERVOUS SYSTEM

Anatomically, the nervous system can be divided into two main parts: the CNS and the **peripheral nervous system (PNS).** The CNS is the portion of the nervous system contained in the skull (brain) and the spinal cord; the PNS consists of nerve cells (neurons) outside the CNS (see figure 7.1). Recall from your previous courses in physiology that the term *innervation* refers to the supply of nerves to a particular organ (e.g., skeletal muscle). In other words, the term innervation means that nerves are connected to a particular organ.

The PNS can be further subdivided into two sections: (1) the sensory portion and (2) the motor portion.

Figure 7.1 Overview of the anatomical divisions of the nervous system.

The sensory division is responsible for transmission of neuron impulses from sense organs (receptors) to the CNS. These sensory nerve fibers, which conduct information toward the CNS, are called **afferent fibers.** The motor portion of the PNS can be further subdivided into the somatic motor division (which innervates skeletal muscle) and autonomic motor division (which innervates involuntary effector organs like smooth muscle in the gut, cardiac muscle, and glands). Motor nerve fibers, which conduct impulses away from the CNS, are referred to as **efferent fibers.** The relationships between the CNS and the PNS are visualized in figure 7.2.

IN SUMMARY

- The nervous system is the body's means of perceiving and responding to events in the internal and external environments. Receptors capable of sensing touch, pain, temperature, and chemical stimuli send information to the CNS concerning changes in our environment. The CNS responds by either voluntary movement or a change in the rate of release of some hormone from the endocrine system, depending on which response is appropriate.
- The nervous system is divided into two major divisions: (1) the central nervous system and (2) the peripheral nervous system. The central nervous system includes the brain and the spinal cord, whereas the peripheral nervous system includes the nerves outside the central nervous system.

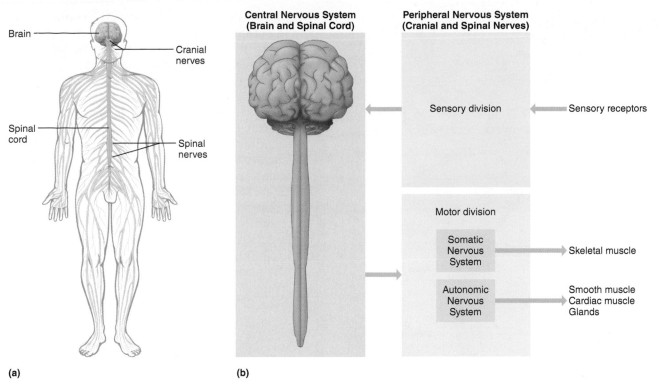

Brain

Cranial
nerves

Spinal
cord

Spinal
nerves

**Central Nervous System
(Brain and Spinal Cord)**

**Peripheral Nervous System
(Cranial and Spinal Nerves)**

Sensory division ← Sensory receptors

Motor division

Somatic
Nervous
System → Skeletal muscle

Autonomic
Nervous
System → Smooth muscle
Cardiac muscle
Glands

(a)   (b)

Figure 7.2 The relationship between the motor and sensory fibers of the peripheral nervous system (PNS) and the central nervous system (CNS).

Structure of the Neuron

The functional unit of the nervous system is the **neuron.** Anatomically, neurons are cells that can be divided into three regions: (1) **cell body,** (2) **dendrites,** and (3) **axon** (see figure 7.3). The center of operation for the neuron is the cell body, or soma, which contains the nucleus. Narrow, cytoplasmic attachments extend from the cell body and are called dendrites. **Dendrites** serve as a receptive area that can conduct electrical impulses toward the cell body. The **axon** (also called the nerve fiber) carries the electrical message away from the cell body toward another neuron or effector organ. Axons vary in length from a few millimeters to a meter (14). Each neuron has only one axon; however, the axon can divide into several collateral branches that terminate at other neurons, muscle cells, or glands (figure 7.3). Contact points between an axon of one neuron and the dendrite of another neuron are called **synapses** (see figure 7.4).

In large nerve fibers like those innervating skeletal muscle, the axons are covered with an insulating layer of cells called **Schwann cells.** The membranes of Schwann cells contain a large amount of a lipid-protein substance called myelin, which forms a discontinuous sheath that covers the outside of the axon. The gaps or spaces between the myelin segments along the axon are called nodes of Ranvier and play an important role in neural transmission. In general, the larger the diameter of the axon, the greater the speed

of neural transmission (14). Thus, those axons with large myelin sheaths conduct impulses more rapidly than small, nonmyelinated fibers. Damage or destruction of myelin along myelinated nerve fibers results in nervous system dysfunction. Indeed, damage to myelin is the basis for the neurological disease multiple sclerosis (see Clinical Applications 7.1 for more information about multiple sclerosis).

Electrical Activity in Neurons

Neurons are considered "excitable tissue" because of their specialized properties of irritability and conductivity. **Irritability** is the ability of the dendrites and neuron cell body to respond to a stimulus and convert it to a neural impulse. **Conductivity** refers to the transmission of the impulse along the axon. In simple terms, a nerve impulse is an electrical signal carried the length of the axon. This electrical signal is initiated by a stimulus that causes a change in the electrical charge of the neuron. Let's begin our discussion with a definition of the resting membrane potential.

Resting Membrane Potential At rest, all cells (including neurons) are negatively charged on the inside of the cell with respect to the charge that exists outside the cell. This negative charge is the result of an unequal distribution of charged ions (ions are elements with a positive or negative charge) across the cell membrane. Thus, a neuron is polarized, and this

Figure 7.3   The parts of a neuron.

electrical charge difference is called the **resting membrane potential.** The magnitude of the resting membrane potential varies from –5 to –100 mv depending upon the cell type. The resting membrane potential of neurons is generally in the range of –40 mv to –75 mv (58) (figure 7.5).

Let's discuss the resting membrane potential in more detail. Cellular proteins, phosphate groups, and other nucleotides are negatively charged (anions) and are fixed inside the cell because they cannot cross the cell membrane. Because these negatively charged molecules are unable to leave the cell, they attract positively charged ions (cations) from the extracellular fluid. This results in an accumulation of a net positive charge on the outside surface of the membrane and a net negative charge on the inside surface of the membrane.

The magnitude of the resting membrane potential is primarily determined by two factors: (1) the permeability of the plasma membrane to different ion

Figure 7.5   Illustration of the resting membrane potential in cells. Compared to the outside of the cell, more negatively charged (fixed) ions exist inside the cell; this results in a negative resting membrane potential. Also, notice that both sodium and potassium can diffuse across the plasma member with potassium diffusing from the inside of the cell to the extracellular fluid, whereas sodium diffuses into the cell from the extracellular fluid.

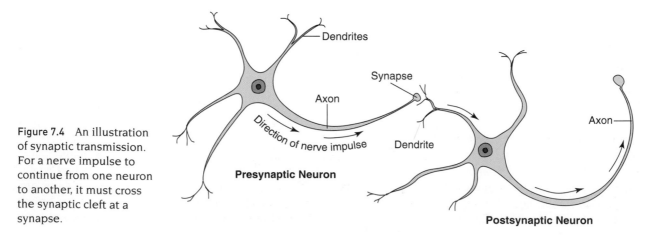

Figure 7.4   An illustration of synaptic transmission. For a nerve impulse to continue from one neuron to another, it must cross the synaptic cleft at a synapse.

CLINICAL APPLICATIONS 7.1

Multiple Sclerosis and Nervous System Function

Multiple sclerosis (MS) is a neurological disease that progressively destroys the myelin sheaths of axons in multiple areas of the central nervous system. Although the exact cause of MS is not known, the MS-mediated destruction of myelin has an inherited (i.e., genetic) component and is due to an immune system attack on myelin. Destruction of the myelin sheath prohibits the normal conduction of nerve impulses, resulting in a progressive loss of nervous system function. The pathology of MS is characterized by general fatigue, muscle weakness, poor motor control, loss of balance, and mental depression (62). Therefore, patients with MS often have difficulties in performing activities of daily living and suffer from a low quality of life.

Although there is no known cure for MS, growing evidence indicates that regular exercise, including both endurance and resistance exercise, can improve the functional capacity of patients suffering from this neurological disorder (60–63). For example, recent studies reveal that MS patients engaging in a regular exercise program exhibit increased muscular strength and endurance resulting in an improved quality of life (9, 60). Importantly, regular exercise may also reduce the mental depression associated with MS (60, 62). However, because of limited research, the amount and types of exercise that provide the optimum benefit for MS remains unknown (1).

---

species and (2) the difference in ion concentrations between the intracellular and extracellular fluids (64). Although numerous intracellular and extracellular ions exist, sodium, potassium, and chloride ions are present in the greatest concentrations and therefore play the most important role in generating the resting membrane potential (64). The concentrations of sodium, potassium, chloride, and calcium are illustrated in figure 7.6. Notice that the concentration of sodium is much greater on the outside of the cell, whereas the concentration of potassium is much greater on the inside of the cell. For comparative purposes, the intracellular and extracellular concentrations of calcium and chloride are also illustrated (figure 7.6).

The permeability of the neuron membrane to potassium, sodium, and other ions is regulated by proteins within the membrane that function as channels that can be opened or closed by "gates" within the channel. This concept is illustrated in figure 7.7. Notice that ions can move freely across the cell

Figure 7.6 Concentrations of ions across a typical cell membrane. Although the body contains many different ions, sodium, potassium, and chloride ions exist in the largest concentrations and therefore play the most important roles in determining the resting membrane potential in cells.

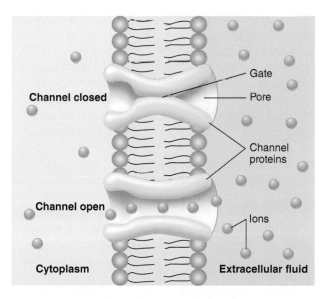

Figure 7.7 Illustration of channels that regulate ion passage across the plasma membrane. Ion channels are composed of proteins that span the entire membrane from the inside to the outer surface. Ion passage through the channels is regulated by the opening or closing of "gates" that serve as doors in the middle of the channel. For example, when channels are open (i.e., gate is open) ions are free to pass through the channel (lower portion of figure). In contrast, when the channel gate is closed, ions' movement through the channel is halted (upper portion of figure).

membrane when the channel is open, whereas closure of the channel gate prevents ion movement. Because the concentration of potassium (+ charge) is high inside the cell and the concentration of sodium (+ charge) is high outside the cell, a change in the membrane's permeability to either potassium or sodium would result in a movement of these charged ions down their concentration gradients. That is, sodium would enter the cell, and potassium would leave the cell. At rest, almost all the sodium channels are closed, whereas a few potassium channels are open. This means that there are more potassium ions leaving the cell than sodium ions "leaking" into the cell. This results in a net loss of positive charges from the inside of the membrane, thus making the resting membrane potential negative. In short, the negative membrane potential in a resting neuron is due primarily to the diffusion of potassium out of the cell, caused by (1) the higher permeability of the membrane for potassium than sodium and (2) the concentration gradient for potassium from inside to outside the cell.

As mentioned previously, a small number of ions are always moving across the cell membrane. If potassium ions continued to diffuse out of the cell and the sodium ions continued to diffuse into the cell, the concentration gradients for these ions would decrease. This would result in a loss of the negative membrane potential. What prevents this from happening? The cell membrane has a sodium/potassium pump that uses energy from ATP to maintain the intracellular/extracellular concentrations by pumping sodium out of the cell and potassium into the cell. Interestingly, this pump not only maintains the concentration gradients that are needed to maintain the resting membrane potential, but it also helps to generate the potential because it exchanges three sodium ions for every two potassium ions (5, 62) (figure 7.8).

Action Potential Research that explained how neurons transmit impulses from the periphery to the brain was completed in England more than 50 years ago. A neural message is generated when a stimulus of sufficient strength reaches the neuron membrane and opens sodium gates, which allows sodium ions to diffuse into the neuron, making the inside more and more positive (depolarizing the cell). When depolarization reaches a critical value called "threshold," the sodium gates open and an **action potential,** or nerve impulse, is formed (see figures 7.9 and 7.10b). After an action potential has been generated, a sequence of ionic exchanges occurs along the axon to propagate the nerve impulse. This ionic exchange along the neuron occurs in a sequential fashion at the nodes of Ranvier (figure 7.3).

Repolarization occurs immediately following depolarization, resulting in a return of the resting membrane potential with the nerve ready to be stimulated again (figures 7.9 and 7.10). How does repolarization occur? Depolarization, with a slight time delay, causes a brief increase in membrane permeability to potassium. As a result, potassium leaves the cell rapidly, making the inside of the membrane more negative (see figure 7.10c). Further, after the depolarization stimulus is removed, the sodium gates within the cell membrane close, and sodium entry into the cell is slowed (therefore, few positive charges are entering the cell). The combined result of these activities quickly restores the resting membrane potential to the original negative charge. To summarize, the events leading to neuron depolarization and repolarization are illustrated step-by-step in figure 7.10a–c. That is, the resting membrane potential is illustrated in figure 7.10a, whereas the events that lead to an action potential are highlighted in figure 7.10b. Finally, the ionic movements that lead to repolarization of the neuron are illustrated in figure 7.10c.

All-or-None Law The development of a nerve impulse is considered to be an "all-or-none" response and is referred to as the "all-or-none" law of action potentials. This means that if a nerve impulse is initiated, the impulse will travel the entire length of the axon without a decrease in voltage. In other words, the neural impulse is just as strong after traveling the length of the axon as it was at the initial point of stimulation.

A mechanical analogy of the all-or-none law is the firing of a gun (62). That is, the speed of the bullet leaving the gun does not depend upon how hard you pulled the trigger. Indeed, firing a gun is all or none; you cannot fire a gun halfway.

Neurotransmitters and Synaptic Transmission As mentioned previously, neurons communicate with other neurons at junctions called synapses. A **synapse** is a small gap (20–30 nanometers) between the synaptic endfoot of the presynaptic neuron and a dendrite of a postsynaptic neuron (see figure 7.11).

Communication between neurons occurs via a process called synaptic transmission. Synaptic transmission occurs when sufficient amounts of a specific neurotransmitter (a neurotransmitter is a chemical messenger that neurons use to communicate with each other) are released from synaptic vesicles contained in the presynaptic neuron (figure 7.11). The nerve impulse results in the synaptic vesicles releasing stored neurotransmitter into the synaptic cleft (space between presynaptic neuron and postsynaptic membrane; see figure 7.11). Neurotransmitters that cause the depolarization of membranes are termed excitatory transmitters. After release into the synaptic cleft, these neurotransmitters bind to "receptors" on the target membrane, which produces a series of

Figure 7.8 Exchange of sodium and potassium across the plasma membrane by the sodium/potassium pump. The sodium/potassium pump requires energy (ATP) and is therefore an active transport pump that moves three molecules of sodium out of the cell and returns two molecules of potassium into the cell. The sodium/potassium pump process is summarized by steps 1 through 6.

graded depolarizations in the dendrites and cell body (3, 4, 25, 30, 39, 53). These graded depolarizations are known as **excitatory postsynaptic potentials (EPSPs).** If sufficient amounts of the neurotransmitter are released, the postsynaptic neuron is depolarized to threshold and an action potential is generated.

EPSPs can bring the postsynaptic neuron to threshold in two ways: (1) temporal summation and (2) spatial summation. The summing of several EPSPs

from a single presynaptic neuron over a short time period is termed **temporal summation** ("temporal" refers to time). The number of EPSPs required to bring the postsynaptic neuron to threshold varies, but it is estimated that the addition of up to fifty EPSPs might be required to produce an action potential within some neurons. Nonetheless, one means by which an action potential can be generated is through rapid, repetitive excitation from a single excitatory presynaptic neuron.

Figure 7.9 An action potential is produced by an increase in sodium conductance into the neuron. As sodium enters the neuron, the charge becomes more and more positive, and an action potential is generated.

A second means of achieving an action potential at the postsynaptic membrane is to sum EPSPs from several different presynaptic inputs (i.e., several different axons), known as spatial summation. In **spatial summation,** concurrent EPSPs come into a postsynaptic neuron from numerous different excitatory inputs. As with temporal summation, up to fifty EPSPs arriving simultaneously on the postsynaptic membrane may be required to produce an action potential (5).

A common neurotransmitter, which also happens to be the transmitter at the nerve/muscle junction, is acetylcholine. Upon release into the synaptic cleft, acetylcholine binds to receptors on the postsynaptic membrane and opens "channels" that permit sodium to enter the nerve or muscle cell. As discussed above, when enough sodium enters the postsynaptic membrane of a neuron or muscle, depolarization results. To prevent chronic depolarization of the postsynaptic neuron, the neurotransmitter must be broken down into less-active molecules via enzymes located within

Figure 7.10 (*a*) At rest, the membrane is about −70 millivolts. (*b*) When the membrane reaches threshold, sodium channels open, some sodium ions diffuse inward, and the membrane is depolarized. (*c*) When the potassium channels open, potassium channels diffuse outward, and the membrane is repolarized.

Sending neuron

Nerve impulse

Axon

Endfeet

Neural
impulse

Dendrite

Receiving neuron

Neural impulse

Endfoot
(or terminal bouton)

Synaptic vesicle

Synaptic cleft

Neurotransmitter
molecule

Presynaptic membrane

Postsynaptic membrane

Figure 7.11 The basic structure of a chemical synapse. In this idealized drawing, the basic elements of the synapse can be seen: the terminal of the presynaptic axon containing synaptic vesicles, the synaptic cleft, and the postsynaptic membrane. From A. J. Vander et al., *Human Physiology: The Mechanisms of Body Function*, 8th edition. Copyright 2001 McGraw-Hill, Inc., New York. Reprinted by permission.

the synaptic cleft. In the case of acetylcholine, the degrading enzyme is called acetylcholinesterase. This enzyme breaks down acetylcholine into acetyl and choline and thus removes the stimulus for depolarization (14). Following breakdown of the neurotransmitter, the post synaptic membrane repolarizes and is prepared to receive additional neurotransmitters and generate a new action potential. Note that not all neurotransmitters are excitatory. In fact, some neurotransmitters have just the opposite effect of excitatory

transmitters (5). These inhibitory transmitters cause a hyperpolarization (increased negativity) of the postsynaptic membrane. This hyperpolarization of the membrane is called an **inhibitory postsynaptic potential,** or **IPSP.** The end result of an IPSP is that the neuron develops a more negative resting membrane potential, is pushed further from threshold, and thus resists depolarization. In general, whether a neuron reaches threshold or not is dependent on the ratio of the number of EPSPs to the number of IPSPs. For example, a neuron that is simultaneously bombarded by an equal number of EPSPs and IPSPs will not reach threshold and generate an action potential. On the other hand, if the EPSPs outnumber the IPSPs, the neuron is moved toward threshold and an action potential may be generated.

Acetylcholine is an interesting example of a neurotransmitter that can be both inhibitory and excitatory. While acetylcholine produces depolarization of skeletal muscle, it causes a hyperpolarization of the heart, slowing the heart rate. This occurs because the combination of acetylcholine with receptors in the heart causes the opening of membrane channels that allow potassium to diffuse out of the cell (21). Therefore, an outward diffusion of potassium produces a hyperpolarization of heart tissue, and the membrane potential is moved further away from the threshold valve.

IN SUMMARY

- Nerve cells are called neurons and are divided anatomically into three parts: (1) the cell body, (2) dendrites, and (3) the axon. Axons are generally covered by Schwann cells, with gaps between these cells called nodes of Ranvier.
- Neurons are specialized cells that respond to physical or chemical changes in their environment. At rest, neurons are negatively charged in the interior with respect to the electrical charge outside the cell. This difference in electrical charge is called the resting membrane potential.
- A neuron "fires" when a stimulus changes the permeability of the membrane, allowing sodium to enter at a high rate, which depolarizes the cell. When the depolarization reaches threshold, an action potential or nerve impulse is initiated. Repolarization occurs immediately following depolarization due to an increase in membrane permeability to potassium and a decreased permeability to sodium.
- Neurons communicate with other neurons at junctions called synapses. Synaptic transmission occurs when sufficient amounts of a specific neurotransmitter are released from the presynaptic neuron. Upon release, the neurotransmitter binds to a receptor on the post synaptic membrane.
- Neurotransmitters can be excitatory or inhibitory. An excitatory transmitter increases neuronal permeability to sodium and results in excitatory postsynaptic potentials (EPSPs). Inhibitory neurotransmitters cause the neuron to become more negative (hyperpolarized). This hyperpolarization of the membrane is called an inhibitory postsynaptic potential (IPSP).

SENSORY INFORMATION AND REFLEXES

The CNS receives a constant bombardment of messages from receptors throughout the body about changes in both the internal and external environment. These receptors are sense organs that change forms of energy in the "real world" into the energy of nerve impulses, which are conducted to the CNS by sensory neurons. A complete discussion of sense organs is beyond the scope of this chapter, so we will limit our discussion to those receptors responsible for position sense and muscle chemoreceptors (i.e., receptors that are sensitive to changes in the chemical environment of muscles). Receptors that provide the CNS with information about body position are called **proprioceptors,** or kinesthetic receptors, and include muscle spindles, Golgi tendon organs, and joint receptors.

Joint Proprioceptors

The term **kinesthesia** means conscious recognition of the position of body parts with respect to one another as well as recognition of limb-movement rates (32, 33, 42, 48, 49). These functions are accomplished by extensive sensory devices in and around joints. There are three principal types of joint proprioceptors: (1) free nerve endings, (2) Golgi-type receptors, and (3) Pacinian corpuscles. The most abundant of these are free nerve endings, which are sensitive to touch and pressure. These receptors are stimulated strongly at the beginning of movement; they adapt (i.e., become less sensitive to stimuli) slightly at first, but then transmit a steady signal until the movement is complete (7, 17, 29, 48). A second type of position receptor, Golgi-type receptors (not to be confused with Golgi tendon organs found in muscle tendons), are found in ligaments around joints. These receptors are not as abundant as free nerve endings, but they work in a similar manner. Pacinian corpuscles are found in the tissues around joints and adapt rapidly following the initiation of movement. This rapid adaptation presumably helps detect the rate of joint rotation (29). To summarize, the joint receptors work together to provide the body with a conscious means of recognition of the orientation of body parts as well as feedback about the rates of limb movement.

Muscle Proprioceptors

Skeletal muscle contains several types of sensory receptors. These include chemoreceptors, muscle spindles, and Golgi tendon organs (29, 34, 49). Chemoreceptors are specialized free nerve endings that send information to the central nervous system in

1. Muscle spindles detect stretch of the muscle.

2. Sensory neurons conduct action potentials to the spinal cord.

3. Sensory neurons synapse with alpha motor neurons.

4. Stimulation of the alpha motor neurons causes the muscle to contract and resist being stretched.

Figure 7.12 The structure of muscle spindles and their location in skeletal muscle.

response to changes in muscle pH, concentrations of extracellular potassium, and changes in O_2 and CO_2 tensions. Chemoreceptors may play a role in cardiopulmonary regulation during exercise and will be discussed in more detail in chapters 9 and 10.

For the nervous system to properly control skeletal muscle movements, it must receive continuous sensory feedback from the contracting muscle. This sensory feedback includes (1) information concerning the tension developed by a muscle and (2) an account of the muscle length. Golgi tendon organs (GTOs) provide the central nervous system with feedback concerning the tension developed by the muscle, whereas the muscle spindle provides sensory information concerning the relative muscle length (8, 34, 49). A discussion of each sensory organ follows.

Muscle Spindle As previously stated, the **muscle spindle** functions as a length detector. Muscle spindles are found in large numbers in most human locomotor muscles (24, 49). Muscles that require the finest degree of control, such as the muscles of the hands, have the highest density of spindles. In contrast, muscles that are responsible for gross movements (e.g., quadriceps) contain relatively few spindles.

The muscle spindle is composed of several thin muscle cells (called intrafusal fibers) that are surrounded by a connective tissue sheath. Like normal skeletal muscle fibers (called extrafusal fibers), muscle spindles insert into connective tissue within the muscle. Therefore, muscle spindles run parallel with muscle fibers (see figure 7.12).

Muscle spindles contain two types of sensory nerve endings. The primary endings respond to dynamic changes in muscle length. The second type of sensory ending is called the secondary ending, and it does not respond to rapid changes in muscle length, but provides the central nervous system with continuous information concerning static muscle length.

In addition to the sensory neurons, muscle spindles are innervated by gamma motor neurons, which stimulate the intrafusal fibers to contract simultaneously along with extrafusal fibers. Gamma motor neuron stimulation causes the central region of the intrafusal fibers to shorten, which serves to tighten the spindle. The need for contraction of the intrafusal fibers can be explained as follows: When skeletal muscles are shortened by motor neuron stimulation, muscle spindles are passively shortened along with the skeletal muscle fibers. If the intrafusal fibers did not compensate accordingly, this shortening would result in "slack" in the spindle and make them less sensitive. Therefore, their function as length detectors would be compromised.

Muscle spindles are responsible for the observation that rapid stretching of skeletal muscles results in a reflex contraction. This is called the stretch reflex

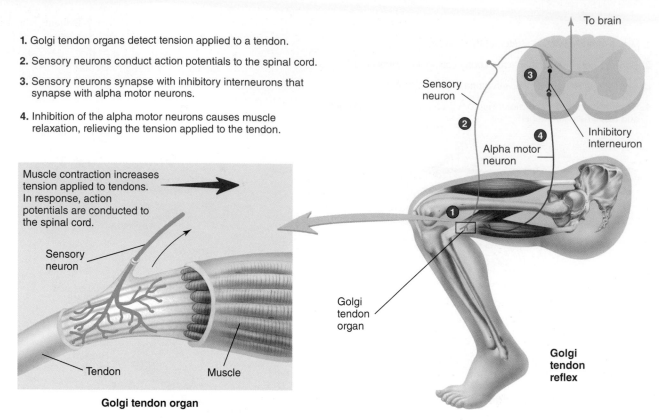

1. Golgi tendon organs detect tension applied to a tendon.

2. Sensory neurons conduct action potentials to the spinal cord.

3. Sensory neurons synapse with inhibitory interneurons that synapse with alpha motor neurons.

4. Inhibition of the alpha motor neurons causes muscle relaxation, relieving the tension applied to the tendon.

To brain

Sensory neuron

Inhibitory interneuron

Alpha motor neuron

Golgi tendon reflex

Muscle contraction increases tension applied to tendons. In response, action potentials are conducted to the spinal cord.

Sensory neuron

Golgi tendon organ

Tendon

Muscle

Golgi tendon organ

Figure 7.13 The Golgi tendon organ is located in series with muscle and serves as a "tension monitor" that acts as a protective device for muscle. See text for details.

or myotatic reflex; it is present in all muscles but is most dramatic in the extensor muscles of the limbs. The so-called knee-jerk reflex is often evaluated by the physician by tapping the patellar tendon with a rubber mallet. The blow by the mallet stretches the entire muscle and thus "excites" the primary nerve endings located in muscle spindles. The neural impulse from the muscle spindle synapses at the spinal cord level with a motor neuron, which then stimulates the extrafusal fibers of the extensor muscle, resulting in an isotonic contraction.

The function of the muscle spindle is to assist in the regulation of movement and to maintain posture. This is accomplished by the muscle spindle's ability to detect and cause the central nervous system (CNS) to respond to changes in the length of skeletal muscle fibers. The following practical example shows how the muscle spindle assists in the control of movement. Suppose a student is holding a single book in front of him or her with the arm extended. This type of load poses a tonic stretch on the muscle spindle, which sends information to the CNS concerning the final length of the extrafusal muscle fibers. If a second book is suddenly placed upon the first book, the muscles would be suddenly stretched (arm would drop) and a burst of impulses from the muscle spindle would alert the CNS about the change in muscle length due to the increased load. The ensuing reflex

would recruit additional motor units to raise the arm back to the original position. Generally, this type of reflex action results in an overcompensation. That is, more motor units are recruited than are needed to bring the arm back to the original position. However, immediately following the overcompensation movement, an additional adjustment rapidly occurs and the arm is quickly returned to the original position.

Golgi Tendon Organs The **Golgi tendon organs (GTOs)** continuously monitor the tension produced by muscle contraction. Golgi tendon organs are located within the tendon and thus are in series with the extrafusal fibers (figure 7.13). In essence, GTOs serve as "safety devices" that help prevent excessive force during muscle contraction. When activated, GTOs send information to the spinal cord via sensory neurons, which in turn excite inhibitory neurons (i.e., send IPSPs). This inhibitory reflex prevents motor neurons from firing, reduces muscle force production, and therefore protects the muscle against contraction-induced injury. This process is pictured in figure 7.13.

It seems possible that GTOs play an important role in the performance of strength activities. For instance, the amount of force that can be produced by a muscle group may be dependent on the ability of the individual to voluntarily oppose the inhibition of the GTO. It seems possible that the inhibitory influences of the GTO could be gradually reduced in response to strength training (20). This would allow an individual to produce a greater amount of muscle force and, in many cases, improve sport performance.

Finally, the GTO is also responsible for a reflex known as the inverse stretch reflex (also called inverse myotatic reflex). As the name implies, the inverse stretch reflex is the opposite of the stretch reflex and results in decreased muscle tension by GTO-mediated inhibition of motor neurons in the spinal cord supplying the muscle. Here's how the inverse stretch reflex works. A vigorous contraction of a muscle group activates the GTO. The GTO responds by sending a message to the spinal cord to inhibit motor neuron firing and reduce the amount of force generated by the muscle. Interestingly, passive stretching of a muscle also activates the GTO and results in relaxation of the stretched muscle.

Muscle Chemoreceptors

Skeletal muscles contain chemoreceptors that respond to chemical changes in the muscle (26–28, 35). Specifically, these receptors are a type of free nerve ending and are sensitive to changes in the chemical environment surrounding muscle; they send information to the CNS via slow conducting fibers classified as group III (myelinated) and group IV (unmyelinated) fibers. Scientific debate continues about the complete list of factors that stimulate muscle chemoreceptors. However, changes in the concentration of hydrogen ions, carbon dioxide, and/or potassium around muscle are known to be potent stimulators of these receptors. The physiological role of muscle chemoreceptors is to provide the CNS with information about the metabolic rate of muscular activity. This information may be important in the regulation of the cardiovascular and pulmonary responses to exercise (6, 28, 35) and is discussed in chapters 9 and 10.

Withdrawal Reflex

A reflex arc is the nerve pathway from the receptor to the CNS and from the CNS along a motor pathway back to the effector organ. Reflex contraction of skeletal muscles can occur in response to sensory input and is not dependent on the activation of higher brain centers. One purpose of a reflex is to provide a rapid means of removing a limb from a source of pain. Consider the case of a person touching a sharp object. The obvious reaction to this painful stimulus is to quickly remove the hand from the source of pain. This rapid removal is accomplished via reflex action. Again, the pathways for this neural reflex are as follows (21): (1) a sensory nerve (pain receptor) sends a nerve impulse to the spinal column; (2) interneurons

within the spinal cord are excited and in turn stimulate motor neurons; (3) the excited interneurons cause depolarization of specific motor neurons, which control the flexor muscles necessary to withdraw the limb from the point of injury. The antagonistic muscle group (e.g., extensors) is simultaneously inhibited via IPSPs. This simultaneous excitatory and inhibitory activity is known as **reciprocal inhibition** (see figure 7.14).

Another interesting feature of the withdrawal reflex is that the opposite limb is extended to support the body during the removal of the injured limb. This event is called the crossed-extensor reflex and is illustrated by the left portion of figure 7.14. Notice that the extensors are contracting as the flexors are inhibited.

IN SUMMARY

- Proprioceptors are position receptors located in joint capsules, ligaments, and muscles. The three most abundant joint and ligament receptors are free nerve endings, Golgi-type receptors, and Pacinian corpuscles. These receptors provide the body with a conscious means of recognizing the orientation of body parts as well as feedback about the rates of limb movement.
- Muscle chemoreceptors are sensitive to changes in the chemical environment surrounding muscle and send information back to the CNS about the metabolic rate of muscular activity.
- The muscle spindle functions as a length detector in muscle.
- Golgi tendon organs continuously monitor the tension developed during muscular contraction. In essence, Golgi tendon organs serve as safety devices that help prevent excessive force during muscle contractions.
- Reflexes provide the body with a rapid, unconscious means of reacting to some stimuli.

SOMATIC MOTOR FUNCTION AND MOTOR NEURONS

The term *somatic* refers to the outer (i.e., nonvisceral) regions of the body. The somatic motor portion of the peripheral nervous system is responsible for carrying neural messages from the spinal cord to skeletal muscle fibers. These neural messages are the signals for muscular contraction to occur. Muscular contraction will be discussed in detail in chapter 8.

The organization of the somatic motor nervous system is illustrated in figure 7.15. The somatic neuron

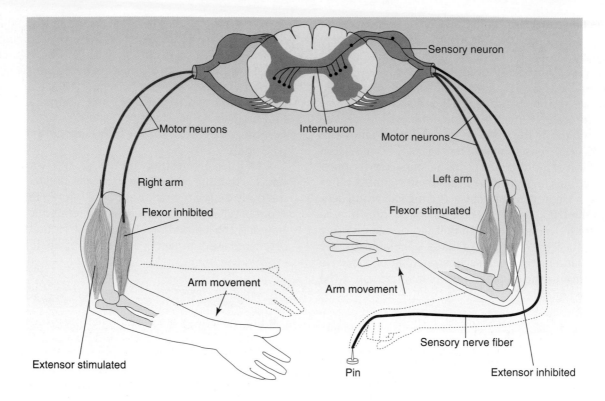

Figure 7.14 When the flexor muscle on one side of the body is stimulated to contract via a withdrawal reflex, the extensor on the opposite side also contracts.

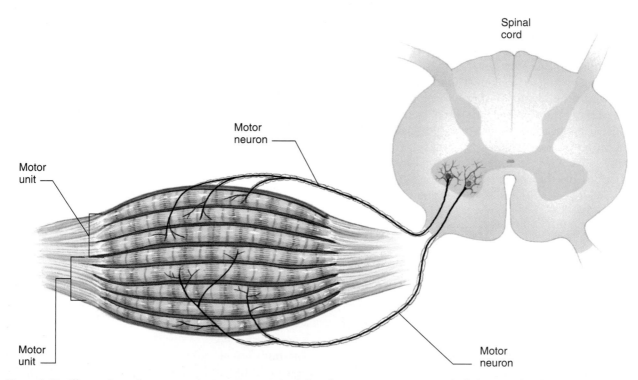

Figure 7.15 Illustration of a motor unit. A motor unit is defined as a motor neuron and all the muscle fibers it innervates.

that innervates skeletal muscle fibers is called a **motor neuron** (also called an alpha motor neuron). Note that the cell body of motor neurons is located within the spinal cord (figure 7.15). The axon of the

motor neuron leaves the spinal cord as a spinal nerve and extends to the muscle that it is responsible for innervating. After the axon reaches the muscle, the axon splits into collateral branches; each collateral

Motor Unit Recruitment and the Size Principle

As introduced in the text, motor unit recruitment is the progressive activation of more and more muscle fibers by the successive recruitment of additional motor units. Recall that a motor unit consists of one motor neuron and all of the muscle fibers that it is responsible for activating. All muscles in the body contain many motor units, and the fibers belonging to a motor unit are spread out across the entire muscle. When a single motor unit is activated, all the muscle fibers innervated by the motor neuron are stimulated to contract. The activation of a single motor unit results in a weak muscle contraction (i.e., limited force production). To increase muscle force production, more motor units must be recruited. This process of motor unit recruitment occurs in an orderly fashion beginning with the smallest motor neurons and eventually activating larger and larger motor neurons (37). This concept was developed by Elwood Henneman and is known as the size principle.

Henneman proposed that the mechanism responsible for the size principle was that the smaller motor neurons had a smaller surface area and would produce a larger EPSP, which would reach threshold sooner, resulting in an action potential. Further, he predicted that larger motor neurons (with a larger surface area) would produce smaller EPSPs; therefore, these motor neurons would be more difficult to depolarize and achieve an action potential. Taken together, the size principle predicts that motor unit recruitment will occur in order of their increasing size, with the smallest motor neurons firing first, followed by larger and larger motor neurons.

To better understand how the size principle works, let's discuss the three main types of motor units in the body:

1. Type S (slow)—These small motor neurons innervate the slow and high oxidative muscle fibers. These fibers are called type I muscle fibers; muscle fiber types are discussed in detail in chapter 8.

2. Type FR (fast, fatigue resistant)— These larger motor neurons innervate the "intermediate" muscle fibers (called type IIa fibers).

3. Type FF (fast, fatigable)—These are the largest motor neurons and innervate the "fast" muscle fibers (called type IIx fibers).

An incremental exercise test is a good example to illustrate how the size principle works during exercise. Recall from chapter 4 that an incremental exercise test consists of numerous stages lasting 1–3 minutes per stage. The test begins at a low work rate and with each progressive stage, the work rate increases until the subject cannot maintain the desired power output. So, during the first stage of a graded exercise test, only a low level of muscle force production is required; therefore, you would recruit only the slow, type S motor units. As the test progresses, you will need to produce more muscular force and therefore you will recruit more and more of the type S motor units and eventually progress to the type FR motor units. As the exercise test becomes more difficult, any further increase in muscle force production would come from recruiting the type FF motor units. The size principle and its role in muscle force production is mentioned again in chapter 8.

---

branch innervates a single muscle fiber. Each motor neuron and all the muscle fibers that it innervates is known as a **motor unit.**

When a single motor neuron is activated, all of the muscle fibers that it innervates are stimulated to contract. However, note that the number of muscle fibers that a motor neuron innervates is not constant and varies from muscle to muscle. The number of muscle fibers innervated by a single motor neuron is called the innervation ratio (i.e., number of muscle fibers/motor neuron). In muscle groups that require fine motor control, the innervation ratio is low. For example, the innervation ratio of the extraocular muscles (i.e., muscles that regulate eye movement) is 23/1. In contrast, innervation ratios of large muscles that are not involved in fine motor control (e.g., leg muscles) may range from 1,000/1 to 2,000/1.

One of the ways that the central nervous system can increase the force of muscle contraction is by increasing the number of motor units that are recruited. The term *motor unit recruitment* refers to the progressive activation of more and more motor neurons. Recruitment of additional motor units activates more muscle fibers, which increases the strength of a voluntary muscle contraction. In general, motor units are recruited in an orderly fashion as a function of their size. For example, when a muscle is initially activated to lift a light weight, the first motor units to fire are small in size; this results in a limited amount of force generation. However, when more force is required (i.e., lifting a heavy weight), there is a progressive increase in the recruitment of more large motor neurons to increase muscle force production. This orderly and sequential recruitment of larger motor units is called the **size principle** (37). For more details on the size principle see A Closer Look 7.1, and for information on the scientist that discovered this important principle of neurophysiology, see Important People in Science.

Elwood Henneman Discovered the Size Principle of Motor Neuron Recruitment

Elwood Henneman (1915–1995) was an American scientist who was interested in understanding how the nervous system controls the actions of skeletal muscles. Dr. Henneman completed his medical education at McGill University, and following his postdoctoral training at Johns Hopkins he became a faculty member at Harvard.

Although Dr. Henneman's research advanced our understanding of many aspects of the nervous system, one of his most important discoveries was that the susceptibility of a motor neuron to "fire" is a function of its size.

That is, the smallest motor neurons are the most easily excited, whereas large motor neurons are the least susceptible to excitation. This important discovery is referred to as the *size principle* (also called the *Henneman size principle*) and is discussed in A Closer Look 7.1.

Dr. Henneman's research interest in skeletal muscles developed from his lifelong pursuit of sports and physical activity. During his undergraduate studies, Henneman was a star on the Harvard tennis team. Dr. Henneman was also an excellent downhill skier, and he remained physically active throughout his life. In fact, his strong physique is credited with allowing him to survive a series of major operations,

including installation of an artificial aortic valve, coronary bypass surgery, and an aortic aneurysm (i.e., tear in the aorta). The latter operation was described as "colorful" because the aneurysm occurred when Dr. Henneman was delivering a lecture to Harvard medical students. He diagnosed the problem himself from behind the speakers' podium and ordered a student in the front row to call the hospital and alert the surgery department that Professor Henneman would be arriving to the emergency room with an aortic aneurysm. Although this was a close call, Dr. Henneman survived the surgery and remained active in science until his death.

IN SUMMARY

- The somatic motor portion of the peripheral nervous system is responsible for carrying neural messages from the spinal cord to skeletal muscle fibers.
- A motor neuron and all the muscle fibers that it innervates are known as a motor unit.
- The number of muscle fibers innervated by a single motor neuron is called the innervation ratio (i.e., number of muscle fibers/motor neuron).
- The size principle is defined as the progressive recruitment of motor units beginning with the smallest motor neurons and progressing to larger and larger motor neurons.

VESTIBULAR APPARATUS AND EQUILIBRIUM

Before we begin a discussion of how the brain controls motor functions, it is important to appreciate how the body maintains balance (i.e., equilibrium). The **vestibular apparatus,** an organ located in the inner ear, is responsible for maintaining general equilibrium. Although a detailed discussion of the anatomy of the vestibular apparatus will not be presented here, a brief discussion of the function of the vestibular apparatus is appropriate. The receptors contained within the vestibular apparatus are sensitive to any change in head

position or movement direction (5, 25, 47). Movement of the head excites these receptors, and nerve impulses are sent to the CNS regarding this change in position. Specifically, these receptors provide information about linear acceleration and angular acceleration. This mechanism allows us to have a sense of acceleration or deceleration when running or traveling by car. Further, a sense of angular acceleration helps us maintain balance when the head is turning or spinning (e.g., performing gymnastics or diving).

The neural pathways involved in the control of equilibrium are outlined in figure 7.16. Any head movement results in the stimulation of receptors in

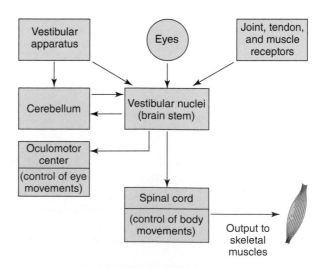

Figure 7.16 The role of the vestibular apparatus in the maintenance of equilibrium and balance.

the vestibular apparatus, which transmits neural information to the cerebellum and the vestibular nuclei located in the brain stem. Further, the vestibular nuclei relay a message to the oculomotor center (controls eye movement) and to neurons in the spinal cord that control movements of the head and limbs. Thus, the vestibular apparatus controls head and eye movement during physical activity, which serves to maintain balance and visually track the events of movement. In summary, the vestibular apparatus is sensitive to the position of the head in space and to sudden changes in the direction of body movement. Its primary function is to maintain equilibrium and preserve a constant plane of head position. Failure of the vestibular apparatus to function properly would prevent the accurate performance of any athletic task that requires head movement. Since most sporting events require at least some head movement, the importance of the vestibular apparatus is obvious.

IN SUMMARY

- The vestibular apparatus is responsible for maintaining general equilibrium and is located in the inner ear. Specifically, these receptors provide information about linear and angular acceleration.

MOTOR CONTROL FUNCTIONS OF THE BRAIN

The brain can be conveniently subdivided into three parts: the brain stem, cerebrum, and cerebellum. Figure 7.17 demonstrates the anatomical relationship of these components. Each of these structures makes important contributions to the regulation of movement. The next several paragraphs will outline the brain's role in regulating the performance of sports skills.

Brain Stem

The **brain stem** is located inside the base of the skull just above the spinal cord. It consists of a complicated series of nerve tracts and nuclei (clusters of neurons) and is responsible for many metabolic functions, cardiorespiratory control, and some highly complex reflexes. The major structures of the brain stem are the medulla, pons, and midbrain. In addition, there is a series of complex neurons scattered throughout the brain stem that is collectively called the reticular formation. The reticular formation receives and integrates information from all regions of the CNS and works with higher brain centers in controlling muscular activity (5).

Figure 7.17 The anatomical relationship among the cerebrum, the cerebellum, and the brain stem.

In general, the neuronal circuits in the brain stem are thought to be responsible for the control of eye movement and muscle tone, equilibrium, support of the body against gravity, and many special reflexes. One of the most important roles of the brain stem in control of locomotion is that of maintaining postural tone. That is, centers in the brain stem provide the nervous activity necessary to maintain normal upright posture and therefore support the body against gravity. It is clear that the maintenance of upright posture requires that the brain stem receive information from several sensory modalities (e.g., vestibular receptors, pressure receptors of the skin, vision). Damage to any portion of the brain stem results in impaired movement control(5, 13, 25).

Cerebrum

The **cerebrum** is the large dome of the brain that is divided into right and left cerebral hemispheres. The outermost layer of the cerebrum is called the cerebral cortex and is composed of tightly arranged neurons. Although the cortex is only about one-fourth of an inch thick, it contains over eight million neurons. The cortex performs three very important motor behavior functions (14): (1) the organization of complex movement, (2) the storage of learned experiences, and (3) the reception of sensory information. We will limit our discussion to the role of the cortex in the organization of movement. The portion of the cerebral cortex that is most concerned with voluntary movement is the motor cortex. Although the motor cortex plays a significant role in motor control, it appears that input to the motor cortex from subcortical structures (i.e., cerebellum, etc.) is absolutely essential for coordinated movement to occur (14, 23, 55). Thus, the **motor cortex** can be described as the final relay point upon which subcortical inputs are focused. After the motor cortex sums these inputs, the final movement plan is formulated and the motor commands are sent to the spinal cord. This "movement plan" can be modified by both subcortical and spinal centers, which supervise the fine details of the movement.

Cerebellum

The **cerebellum** lies behind the pons and medulla (figure 7.17). Although complete knowledge about cerebellar function is not currently available, much is known about the role of this structure in movement control. It is clear that the cerebellum plays an important role in coordinating and monitoring complex movement. This work is accomplished via connections leading from the cerebellum to the motor cortex, the brain stem, and the spinal cord. Evidence exists to suggest that the primary role of the cerebellum is to

aid in the control of movement in response to feedback from proprioceptors (29, 55). Further, the cerebellum may initiate fast, ballistic movements via its connection with the motor cortex (5). Damage to the cerebellum results in poor movement control and muscular tremor that is most severe during rapid movement. Head injuries due to sport-related injuries can lead to damage and dysfunction in both the cerebrum and/or cerebellum. For an overview of sport-related concussions, see Clinical Applications 7.2.

Role of the Brain in Exercise-Induced Fatigue

Everyone has experienced fatigue during an exercise training session. Indeed, prolonged or high intensity exercise results in fatigue, which limits human performance. In theory, exercise-induced fatigue can be due to central factors (e.g., higher brain centers and/or motor neurons) or peripheral factors (fatigue within skeletal muscle fibers). Let's discuss the possible role of the brain in exercise-induced fatigue in more detail.

In regard to fatigue within the exercising muscle fibers, it is clear that prolonged or intense contractions can disturb muscle homeostasis and impair the ability of muscle fibers to generate force (45, 46). However, it is also possible that exercise-induced fatigue could result from dysfunction of the central nervous system (i.e., central fatigue) resulting in a reduced motor output to the exercising skeletal muscles (43, 52, 56). This type of central fatigue could occur during prolonged endurance exercise due to the depletion of excitatory neurotransmitters in the motor cortex. This depletion of excitatory neurotransmitters would limit the activation of motor neurons and the muscle fibers that they innervate. In fact, some investigators have proposed that higher brain centers act as a "governor" to control exercise tolerance (40, 41). This "central governor" theory of fatigue proposes that exercise-induced fatigue is regulated by the action of a central (brain) control center that regulates exercise performance (40). It is proposed that this type of control system would limit muscle activation during exercise by reducing motor output from higher brain centers. A theorized advantage of the central governor theory of exercise fatigue is that this system would protect the body against catastrophic disturbances in homeostasis by promoting fatigue and the cessation of exercise before damage occurs.

So, is exercise-induced fatigue controlled solely by the brain, as predicted by the central governor theory? Unfortunately, the answer to this question remains unknown. Nonetheless, current evidence suggests that both central and peripheral factors can contribute to exercise-induced fatigue, and that the

Sport-Related Concussions

Although head injuries can occur in many activities, sports with the greatest risk of head injury include football, gymnastics, ice hockey, wrestling, and boxing. Other sporting activities that pose a significant risk for head injury include horse racing, motorcycle and automobile racing, martial arts, soccer, and rugby.

A forceful blow to the head during sports (e.g., a football collision) can result in a brain injury that is classified by the amount of damage to brain tissue. One of the most common brain injuries in sports is the concussion, and it is estimated that approximately 3.8 million sports-related concussions occur each year in the U.S. (22, 51). A concussion is defined as a complex brain injury resulting from a traumatic force to the head, neck, or body (36). Concussions differ in their degree of severity, but most concussions share several common features (see table 7.1). Note that a concussion does not always result in a loss of consciousness. Indeed, only 10% of athletes who suffer a sport-related concussion are rendered unconscious (2).

Interestingly, girls appear to have a higher rate of concussion than boys in the same sport (e.g., basketball) (11, 22). The reason for this difference is unknown, but some experts suggest that gender differences exist in the ability to withstand equivalent blows to the head and neck (11, 22). It is also possible that, compared to female athletes, some male athletes may be reluctant to report their head injuries to coaches or parents for fear of being removed from athletic competition (22). Therefore, the incidence of concussion in male athletes may be underestimated (22). If this is the case, the occurrence of concussions may not differ between girls and boys.

What health risks are associated with sustaining a concussion? In general, most concussions result in a short-lived impairment of brain function that typically resolves naturally within a few days (36). Nonetheless, there are some atypical outcomes of a concussion that present serious health risks. These major health risks associated with a concussion include (51): (1) permanent brain damage or death associated with delayed brain swelling; (2) second-impact syndrome; (3) same season repeat concussion; and (4) late-life consequences of repeated concussions. A brief discussion of these concussion-related risks follows.

The risk of permanent brain damage or death in most sports is low. For example, although American football is considered a high risk sport for head injury, it is estimated that only 1 out of every 20,500 football players develop a permanent brain injury each year (51). The second-impact syndrome occurs when an athlete who has sustained an initial concussion suffers a second head injury before the first injury has healed. This second-impact syndrome promotes brain vascular congestion, which can progress to cerebral swelling and death. Also, after sustaining a concussion, the brain is in a state of vulnerability for an extended period. Therefore, an additional risk of a sports-related concussion is the increased vulnerability to a second concussion within the same season (51). This concussion-related health risk is often called the *same-season repeat concussion*. A final health risk of suffering a concussion is the possibility that a brain injury early in life increases the risk of late-life degenerative brain disorders (e.g., Alzheimer's disease) (51). Indeed, one study suggests that retired professional American football players are at a higher risk for early onset of Alzheimer's disease than a nonathletic population (19). Therefore, although the typical concussion does not pose an acute life-threatening injury, several post-concussion health risks exist. For more details on sports-related concussions, see Halstead and Walter (2010) in the Suggested Readings.

TABLE 7.1	Signs and Symptoms of a Concussion		
Physical	**Cognitive**	**Emotional**	**Sleep**
Headache	Difficulty remembering	Irritability	Drowsiness
Nausea	Difficulty concentrating	Sadness	Sleeping more than usual
Vomiting	Feeling mentally "foggy"	Emotional	Sleeping less than usual
Visual problems	Answers questions slowly	Nervousness	Difficulty falling asleep

relative contribution of central or peripheral factors may depend upon the environmental conditions and the type of exercise (e.g., intensity and duration) performed to induce fatigue. Therefore, the "central governor" theory of exercise-induced fatigue remains a theory, and future research will be required to support or reject this concept (57). More will be said about muscle fatigue in chapter 8.

■ The brain can be subdivided into three parts: (1) the brain stem, (2) the cerebrum, and (3) the cerebellum.

■ The motor cortex controls motor activity with the aid of input from subcortical areas.

■ Prolonged endurance exercise can deplete excitatory neurotransmitters in higher brain centers (i.e., motor cortex) and reduce motor neuron activation. This type of exercise-induced fatigue (i.e., central fatigue) results from a reduced activation of motor neurons and the muscle fibers that they innervate.

MOTOR FUNCTIONS OF THE SPINAL CORD

One motor function of the spinal cord has already been discussed (withdrawal reflex). The precise role of spinal reflexes in the control of movement is still being debated. However, there is increasing evidence that normal motor function is influenced by spinal reflexes. In fact, some authors claim that reflexes play a major role in the control of voluntary movements. These investigators believe that the events that underlie volitional movement are built on a variety of spinal reflexes (5, 23, 59). Support for this idea comes from the demonstration that spinal reflex neurons are directly affected by descending neural traffic from the brain stem and cortical centers.

The spinal cord makes a major contribution to the control of movement by the preparation of spinal centers to perform the desired movement. The spinal mechanism by which a voluntary movement is translated into appropriate muscle action is termed *spinal tuning*. Spinal tuning appears to operate in the following way: Higher brain centers of the motor system are concerned with only the general parameters of movement. The specific details of the movement are refined at the spinal cord level via interaction of spinal cord neurons and higher brain centers. In other words, although the general pattern of the anticipated movement is controlled by higher motor centers, additional refinement of this movement may occur by a complex interaction of spinal cord neurons and higher centers (5). Thus, it appears that spinal centers play an important role in volitional movement.

■ Evidence exists that the spinal cord plays an important role in voluntary movement with groups of neurons controlling certain aspects of motor activity.

■ The spinal mechanism by which a voluntary movement is translated into appropriate muscle action is termed *spinal tuning*.

CONTROL OF MOTOR FUNCTIONS

Watching a highly skilled athlete perform a sports skill is exciting, but it really does not help us to appreciate the complex integration of the many parts of the nervous system required to perform this act. A pitcher throwing a baseball seems to the observer to be accomplishing a simple act, but in reality this movement consists of a complex interaction of higher brain centers with spinal reflexes performed together with precise timing. How the nervous system produces a coordinated movement has been one of the major unresolved mysteries facing neurophysiologists for many decades. Although progress has been made toward answering the basic question of "How do humans control voluntary movement?," much is still unknown about this process. Our purpose here will be to provide the reader with a simplistic overview of the brain and the control of movement.

Traditionally, it was believed that the motor cortex controlled voluntary movement with little input from subcortical areas. However, evidence suggests that this is not the case (23, 55). Although the motor cortex is the final executor of movement programs, it appears that the motor cortex does not give the initial signal to move, but rather is at the end of the chain of neurophysiological events involved in volitional movement (44). The first step in performing a voluntary movement occurs in subcortical and cortical motivational areas, which play a key role in consciousness. This conscious "prime drive" sends signals to the so-called association areas of the cortex (different from the motor cortex), which forms a "rough draft" of the planned movement from a stock of stored subroutines (12, 38). Information concerning the nature of the plan of movement is then sent to both the cerebellum and the basal nuclei (clusters of neurons located in the cerebral hemispheres) (see figure 7.18). These structures cooperate to convert the "rough draft" into precise temporal and spatial excitation programs (23). The cerebellum is possibly more important for making fast movements, whereas the basal nuclei are more responsible for slow or deliberate movements. From the cerebellum and basal nuclei, the precise program is sent through the thalamus to the motor cortex, which forwards the message down to spinal neurons for "spinal tuning" and finally to skeletal muscle (16, 18). Feedback to the CNS from muscle receptors and proprioceptors allows for modification of motor programs if necessary. The ability to change movement patterns allows the individual to correct "errors" in the original movement plan.

To summarize, the control of voluntary movement is complex and requires the cooperation of many areas of the brain as well as several subcortical areas.

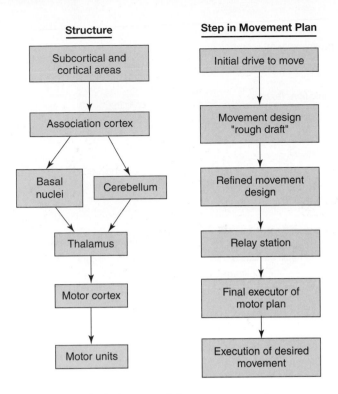

Structure	Step in Movement Plan
Subcortical and cortical areas	Initial drive to move
Association cortex	Movement design "rough draft"
Basal nuclei / Cerebellum	Refined movement design
Thalamus	Relay station
Motor cortex	Final executor of motor plan
Motor units	Execution of desired movement

Figure 7.18 Block diagram of the structures and processes leading to voluntary movement.

Recent evidence suggests that the motor cortex does not by itself formulate the signals required to initiate voluntary movement. Instead, the motor cortex receives input from a variety of cortical and subcortical structures. Feedback to the CNS from muscle and joint receptors allows for adjustments to improve the movement pattern. Much is still unknown about the details of the control of complex movement, and this topic provides an exciting frontier for future research.

IN SUMMARY

- Control of voluntary movement is complex and requires the cooperation of many areas of the brain as well as several subcortical areas.
- The first step in performing a voluntary movement occurs in subcortical and cortical motivational areas, which send signals to the association cortex, which forms a "rough draft" of the planned movement.
- The movement plan is then sent to both the cerebellum and the basal nuclei. These structures cooperate to convert the "rough draft" into precise temporal and spatial excitation programs.
- The cerebellum is important for making fast movements, whereas the basal nuclei are more responsible for slow or deliberate movements.

- From the cerebellum and basal nuclei, the precise program is sent through the thalamus to the motor cortex, which forwards the message down to spinal neurons for "spinal tuning" and finally to skeletal muscle.
- Feedback to the CNS from muscle receptors and proprioceptors allows for the modification of motor programs if necessary.

AUTONOMIC NERVOUS SYSTEM

The **autonomic nervous system** plays an important role in maintaining **homeostasis.** In contrast to somatic motor nerves, autonomic motor nerves innervate effector organs (e.g., smooth muscle, cardiac muscle), which are not usually under voluntary control. Autonomic motor nerves innervate cardiac muscle, glands, and smooth muscle found in airways, the gut, and blood vessels. In general, the autonomic nervous system operates below the conscious level, although some individuals apparently can learn to control some portions of this system. Although involuntary, it appears that the function of the autonomic nervous system is closely linked to emotion. For example, all of us have experienced an increase in heart rate following extreme excitement or fear. Further, the secretions from the digestive glands and sweat glands are affected by periods of excitement. It should not be surprising that participation in intense exercise results in an increase in autonomic activity.

The autonomic nervous system can be separated both functionally and anatomically into two divisions: (1) **sympathetic division** and (2) **parasympathetic division** (see figure 7.19). Most organs receive dual innervation by both the parasympathetic and sympathetic branches of the autonomic nervous system (62). In general, the sympathetic portion of the autonomic nervous system tends to activate an organ (e.g., increases heart rate), whereas parasympathetic impulses tend to inhibit it (e.g., slows heart rate). Therefore, the activity of a particular organ can be regulated according to the ratio of sympathetic/parasympathetic impulses to the tissue. In this way, the autonomic nervous system may regulate the activities of involuntary muscles (i.e., smooth muscle) and glands in accordance with the needs of the body (see chapter 5).

The sympathetic division of the autonomic nervous system has its cell bodies of the preganglionic neurons in the thoracic and lumbar regions of the spinal cord. These fibers leave the spinal cord and enter the sympathetic ganglia (figure 7.19). The neurotransmitter between the preganglionic neurons and postganglionic

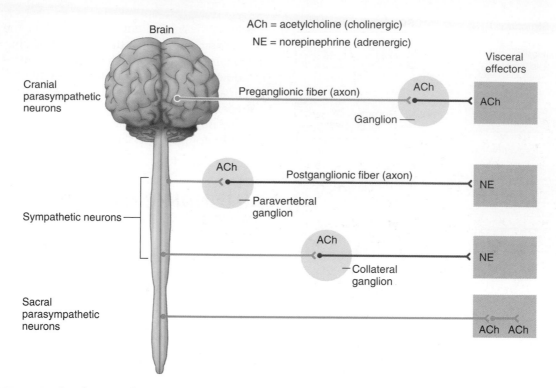

ACh = acetylcholine (cholinergic)
NE = norepinephrine (adrenergic)

Figure 7.19 A simple schematic demonstrating the neurotransmitters of the autonomic nervous system.

neurons is acetylcholine. Postganglionic sympathetic fibers leave these sympathetic ganglia and innervate a wide variety of tissues. The neurotransmitter released at the effector organ is primarily norepinephrine. Recall from chapter 5 that norepinephrine exerts its action on the effector organ by binding to either an alpha or a beta receptor on the membrane of the target organ (21). Following sympathetic stimulation, norepinephrine is removed in two ways: (1) reuptake into the postganglionic fiber; and/or (2) broken down into nonactive by-products (21).

The parasympathetic division of the autonomic nervous system has its cell bodies located within the brain stem and the sacral portion of the spinal cord. Parasympathetic fibers leave the brain stem and the spinal cord and converge on ganglia in a wide variety of anatomical areas. Acetylcholine is the neurotransmitter in both preganglionic and postganglionic fibers. After parasympathetic nerve stimulation, acetylcholine is released and rapidly degraded by the enzyme acetyl-cholinesterase.

At rest, the activities of the sympathetic and parasympathetic divisions of the autonomic nervous system are in balance. However, during a bout of exercise, the activity of the parasympathetic nervous system decreases and activation of the sympathetic nervous system increases. A major role of the sympathetic nervous system during exercise is to regulate blood flow to the working muscles (54). This is achieved by increasing cardiac output and a redistribution of blood flow toward the contracting muscles (discussed in chapter 9). At the cessation of exercise, sympathetic activity decreases and parasympathetic activity increases, allowing the body to return to a resting state (15).

IN SUMMARY

- The autonomic nervous system is responsible for maintaining the constancy of the body's internal environment.
- Anatomically and functionally, the autonomic nervous system can be divided into two divisions: (1) the sympathetic division and (2) the parasympathetic division.
- In general, the sympathetic portion (releasing norepinephrine) tends to excite an organ, whereas the parasympathetic portion (releasing acetylcholine) tends to inhibit the same organ.

EXERCISE ENHANCES BRAIN HEALTH

Although it is well known that regular exercise can benefit overall health, research now indicates that exercise can also improve brain (cognitive) function, particularly in later life. Maintaining brain health

Figure 7.20 Regular exercise targets many aspects of brain function and has broad positive benefits on overall brain health. Specifically, exercise promotes an increase in several brain growth factors that lead to improved brain health by improving cognition, neurogenesis, and vascular function.

throughout life is an important goal, and both mental stimulation (e.g., reading) and exercise are interventions that can contribute to good brain health. Therefore, daily exercise is a simple and inexpensive way to help maintain the health of the central nervous system.

How strong is the evidence that regular exercise improves brain function and protects against age-related deterioration? In short, the evidence is extremely strong. Specifically, numerous studies reveal that exercise targets many aspects of brain

function and has broad effects on overall brain health, learning, memory, and depression, particularly in older populations (8). Moreover, regular exercise can protect against several types of dementia (e.g., Alzheimer's disease) and certain types of brain injury (e.g., stroke) (8, 50). Therefore, exercise increases brain health, just as it improves body health, and thus represents an important lifestyle intervention to improve brain function and resistance to neurodegenerative diseases (10, 31).

How does exercise enhance brain health? Regular aerobic exercise promotes a cascade of brain growth factor signaling that (1) enhances learning and memory; (2) stimulates neurogenesis (i.e., formation of new neurons); (3) improves brain vascular function and blood flow; and (4) attenuates the mechanisms driving depression (7). In addition to these central mechanisms, exercise also reduces several peripheral risk factors for cognitive decline, including inflammation, hypertension, and insulin resistance (8). Figure 7.20 summarizes the exercise-induced cascade of events that lead to improved brain function and health.

IN SUMMARY

- Research indicates that exercise can improve brain (cognitive) function, particularly in older individuals.

STUDY QUESTIONS

1. Identify the location and functions of the central nervous system.
2. Draw a simple chart illustrating the organization of the nervous system.
3. Define *synapses*.
4. Define *membrane potential* and *action potential*.
5. Discuss an IPSP and an EPSP. How do they differ?
6. What are proprioceptors? Give some examples.
7. Describe the location and function of the vestibular apparatus.
8. What is meant by the term *spinal tuning*?
9. List the possible motor functions played by the brain stem, the motor cortex, and the cerebellum.
10. Describe the divisions and functions of the autonomic nervous system.
11. Define the terms *motor unit* and *innervation ratio*.
12. Briefly describe the positive benefits of exercise on brain function.
13. How does regular exercise maintain neuronal health?
14. Describe the withdrawal reflex.
15. Outline the functions of both muscle spindles and the Golgi tendon organ.
16. Describe the general anatomical design of a muscle spindle and discuss its physiological function.
17. Discuss the function of Golgi tendon organs in monitoring muscle tension.

SUGGESTED READINGS

Colcombe, S. J. et al. 2006. Aerobic exercise training increases brain volume in aging humans. *The Journals of Gerontology. Series A, Biological Sciences and Medical Sciences* 61:1166–70.

Cotman, C. W., N. Berchtold, and L. Christie. 2007. Exercise builds brain health: Key roles of growth factor cascades and inflammation. *Trends in Neuroscience* 30: 464–72.

Fox, S. 2009. *Human Physiology*. New York, NY: McGraw-Hill Companies.

Halstead, M. E., and Walter, K. D. 2010. American Academy of Pediatrics. Clinical report—sport-related concussion in children and adolescents. *Pediatrics* 126: 597–615.

Roatta, S., and Farina, D. 2010. Sympathetic actions on the skeletal muscle. *Exercise and Sports Science Review* 38: 31–35.

REFERENCES

1. **Asano M, Dawes DJ, Arafah A, Moriello C, and Mayo NE.** What does a structured review of the effectiveness of exercise interventions for persons with multiple sclerosis tell us about the challenges of designing trials? *Multiple Sclerosis* (Houndmills, Basingstoke, England) 15: 412–421, 2009.
2. **Bailes J.** Sports-related concussion: what we know in 2009—a neurosurgeon's perspective. *Journal of the International Neuropsychological Society* 15: 509–511, 2009.
3. **Barchas JD, Akil H, Elliott GR, Holman RB, and Watson SJ.** Behavioral neurochemistry: neuroregulators and behavioral states. *Science* 200: 964–973, 1978.
4. **Barde YA, Edgar D, and Thoenen H.** New neurotrophic factors. *Annu Rev Physiol* 45: 601–612, 1983.
5. **Brodal P.** *Central Nervous System.* New York: Oxford University Press, 2010.
6. **Busse MW, Maassen N, and Konrad H.** Relation between plasma K+ and ventilation during incremental exercise after glycogen depletion and repletion in man. *The Journal of Physiology* 443: 469–476, 1991.
7. **Clark FJ, and Burgess PR.** Slowly adapting receptors in cat knee joint: can they signal joint angle? *Journal of Neurophysiology* 38: 1448–1463, 1975.
8. **Cotman CW, Berchtold NC, and Christie LA.** Exercise builds brain health: key roles of growth factor cascades and inflammation. *Trends Neurosci* 30: 464–472, 2007.
9. **De Souza-Teixeira F, Costilla S, Ayan C, Garcia-Lopez D, Gonzalez-Gallego J, and de Paz JA.** Effects of resistance training in multiple sclerosis. *International Journal of Sports Medicine* 30: 245–250, 2009.
10. **Desai AK, Grossberg GT, and Chibnall JT.** Healthy brain aging: a road map. *Clinics in Geriatric Medicine* 26: 1–16, 2010.
11. **Dick RW.** Is there a gender difference in concussion incidence and outcomes? *British Journal of Sports Medicine* 43 Suppl 1: i46–50, 2009.
12. **Dietz V.** Human neuronal control of automatic functional movements: interaction between central programs and afferent input. *Physiological Reviews* 72: 33–69, 1992.
13. **Eccles JC.** *The Understanding of the Brain.* New York: McGraw-Hill, 1977.
14. **Fox S.** *Human Physiology.* New York: McGraw-Hill, 2009.
15. **Freeman JV, Dewey FE, Hadley DM, Myers J, and Froelicher VF.** Autonomic nervous system interaction with the cardiovascular system during exercise. *Prog Cardiovasc Dis* 48: 342–362, 2006.
16. **Fregni F, and Pascual-Leone A.** Hand motor recovery after stroke: tuning the orchestra to improve hand motor function. *Cogn Behav Neurol* 19: 21–33, 2006.
17. **Goodwin GM, McCloskey DI, and Matthews PB.** The contribution of muscle afferents to kinaesthesia shown by vibration induced illusions of movement and by the effects of paralysing joint afferents. *Brain* 95: 705–748, 1972.
18. **Grillner S.** Control of locomotion in bipeds, tetrapods, and fish. In: *Handbook of Physiology: The Nervous System Motor Control.* Washington, DC: American Physiological Society, 1981, p. 1179–1236.
19. **Guskiewicz KM, Marshall SW, Bailes J, McCrea M, Cantu RC, Randolph C, and Jordan BD.** Association between recurrent concussion and late-life cognitive impairment in retired professional football players. *Neurosurgery* 57: 719–726; discussion 719–726, 2005.
20. **Hakkinen K, Pakarinen A, Kyrolainen H, Cheng S, Kim DH, and Komi PV.** Neuromuscular adaptations and serum hormones in females during prolonged power training. *International Journal of Sports Medicine* 11: 91–98, 1990.
21. **Hall J.** *Guyton and Hall: Texbook of Medical Physiology.* Philadelphia: Saunders, 2011.
22. **Halstead ME, and Walter KD.** American Academy of Pediatrics. Clinical report—sport-related concussion in children and adolescents. *Pediatrics* 126: 597–615, 2010.
23. **Henatsch HD, and Langer HH.** Basic neurophysiology of motor skills in sport: a review. *International Journal of Sports Medicine* 6: 2–14, 1985.
24. **Hunt CC.** Mammalian muscle spindle: peripheral mechanisms. *Physiological Reviews* 70: 643–663, 1990.
25. **Kandel E, Schwartz J, and Jessell D.** *Principles of Neural Science.* Stamford: Appleton & Lange, 2000.
26. **Kaufman MP, Rybicki KJ, Waldrop TG, and Ordway GA.** Effect of ischemia on responses of group III and IV afferents to contraction. *J Appl Physiol* 57: 644–650, 1984.
27. **Kaufman MP, Waldrop TG, Rybicki KJ, Ordway GA, and Mitchell JH.** Effects of static and rhythmic twitch contractions on the discharge of group III and IV muscle afferents. *Cardiovasc Res* 18: 663–668, 1984.
28. **Kniffki K, Mense S, and Schmidt R.** Muscle receptors with fine afferent fibers which may evoke circulatory reflexes. *Circulation Research* 48 (Suppl.): 25–31, 1981.
29. **Konczak J, Corcos DM, Horak F, Poizner H, Shapiro M, Tuite P, Volkmann J, and Maschke M.** Proprioception and motor control in Parkinson's disease. *Journal of Motor Behavior* 41: 543–552, 2009.
30. **Krieger DT, and Martin JB.** Brain peptides (first of two parts). *N Engl J Med* 304: 876–885, 1981.
31. **Marks BL, Katz LM, and Smith JK.** Exercise and the aging mind: buffing the baby boomer's body and brain. *The Physician and Sportsmedicine* 37: 119–125, 2009.
32. **Matthews PB.** Muscle afferents and kinaesthesia. *Br Med Bull* 33: 137–142, 1977.
33. **McAuley E, Kramer AF, and Colcombe SJ.** Where does Sherrington's muscle sense originate? *Annual Review of Neuroscience* 5: 189–218, 1982.
34. **McCloskey D.** Sensing position and movements of the fingers. *News in Physiological Sciences* 2: 226–230, 1987.
35. **McCloskey DI, and Mitchell JH.** Reflex cardiovascular and respiratory responses originating in exercising muscle. *The Journal of Physiology* 224: 173–186, 1972.
36. **McCrory P, Meeuwisse W, Johnston K, Dvorak J, Aubry M, Molloy M, and Cantu R.** Consensus statement on concussion in sport—the Third International Conference on Concussion in Sport held in Zurich, November 2008. *The Physician and Sportsmedicine* 37: 141–159, 2009.
37. **Mendell LM.** The size principle: a rule describing the recruitment of motoneurons. *Journal of Neurophysiology* 93: 3024–3026, 2005.
38. **Morton SM, and Bastian AJ.** Cerebellar contributions to locomotor adaptations during splitbelt treadmill walking. *J Neurosci* 26: 9107–9116, 2006.
39. **Nicoll RA, Malenka RC, and Kauer JA.** Functional comparison of neurotransmitter receptor subtypes in mammalian central nervous system. *Physiological Reviews* 70: 513–565, 1990.

40. **Noakes TD.** The central governor model of exercise regulation applied to the marathon. *Sports Medicine (Auckland, NZ)* 37: 374–377, 2007.

41. **Noakes TD, St Clair Gibson A, and Lambert EV.** From catastrophe to complexity: a novel model of integrative central neural regulation of effort and fatigue during exercise in humans: summary and conclusions. *British Journal of Sports Medicine* 39: 120–124, 2005.

42. **O'Donovan MJ.** Developmental regulation of motor function: an uncharted sea. *Med Sci Sports Exerc* 17: 35–43, 1985.

43. **Ogoh S, and Ainslie PN.** Cerebral blood flow during exercise: mechanisms of regulation. *J Appl Physiol* 107: 1370–1380, 2009.

44. **Petersen TH, Rosenberg K, Petersen NC, and Nielsen JB.** Cortical involvement in anticipatory postural reactions in man. *Experimental Brain Research Experimentelle Hirnforschung* 193: 161–171, 2009.

45. **Place N, Bruton JD, and Westerblad H.** Mechanisms of fatigue induced by isometric contractions in exercising humans and in mouse isolated single muscle fibres. *Clinical and Experimental Pharmacology & Physiology* 36: 334–339, 2009.

46. **Powers SK, and Jackson MJ.** Exercise-induced oxidative stress: cellular mechanisms and impact on muscle force production. *Physiological Reviews* 88: 1243–1276, 2008.

47. **Pozzo T, Berthoz A, Lefort L, and Vitte E.** Head stabilization during various locomotor tasks in humans. II. Patients with bilateral peripheral vestibular deficits. *Experimental Brain Research Experimentelle Hirnforschung* 85: 208–217, 1991.

48. **Proske U.** Kinesthesia: the role of muscle receptors. *Muscle & Nerve* 34: 545–558, 2006.

49. **Proske U, and Gandevia SC.** The kinaesthetic senses. *The Journal of Physiology* 587: 4139–4146, 2009.

50. **Radak Z, Hart N, Sarga L, Koltai E, Atalay M, Ohno H, and Boldogh I.** Exercise plays a preventive role against Alzheimer's disease. *J Alzheimers Dis* 20: 777–783, 2010.

51. **Randolph C, and Kirkwood MW.** What are the real risks of sport-related concussion, and are they modifiable? *J Int Neuropsychol Soc* 15: 512–520, 2009.

52. **Rasmussen P, Nielsen J, Overgaard M, Krogh-Madsen R, Gjedde A, Secher NH, and Petersen NC.** Reduced muscle activation during exercise related to brain oxygenation and metabolism in humans. *The Journal of Physiology* 588: 1985–1995.

53. **Redman S.** Monosynaptic transmission in the spinal cord. *News in Physiological Sciences* 1: 171–174, 1986.

54. **Roatta S, and Farina D.** Sympathetic actions on the skeletal muscle. *Exerc Sport Sci Rev* 38: 31–35, 2010.

55. **Sage GH.** *Motor Learning and Control: A Neuropsychological Approach.* New York: McGraw-Hill, 1984.

56. **Saldanha A, Nordlund Ekblom MM, and Thorstensson A.** Central fatigue affects plantar flexor strength after prolonged running. *Scandinavian Journal of Medicine & Science in Sports* 18: 383–388, 2008.

57. **Shephard RJ.** Is it time to retire the "central governor"? *Sports Medicine (Auckland, NZ)* 39: 709–721, 2009.

58. **Shier D, Butler J, and Lewis R.** *Hole's Human Anatomy and Physiology.* New York: McGraw-Hill, 2007.

59. **Soechting J, and Flanders M.** Arm movements in three-dimensional space: computation, theory, and observation. In: *Exercise and Sport Science Reviews,* edited by Holloszy J. Baltimore: Lippincott Williams & Wilkins, 1991, p. 389–418.

60. **Stroud NM, and Minahan CL.** The impact of regular physical activity on fatigue, depression and quality of life in persons with multiple sclerosis. *Health and Quality of Life Outcomes* 7: 68, 2009.

61. **White LJ, and Castellano V.** Exercise and brain health—implications for multiple sclerosis: part 1—neuronal growth factors. *Sports Medicine (Auckland, NZ)* 38: 91–100, 2008.

62. **White LJ, and Dressendorfer RH.** Exercise and multiple sclerosis. *Sports Medicine (Auckland, NZ)* 34: 1077–1100, 2004.

63. **White LJ, McCoy SC, Castellano V, Gutierrez G, Stevens JE, Walter GA, and Vandenborne K.** Resistance training improves strength and functional capacity in persons with multiple sclerosis. *Multiple Sclerosis (Houndmills, Basingstoke, England)* 10: 668–674, 2004.

64. **Widmaier E, Raff H, and Strang K.** *Vander's Human Physiology.* New York: McGraw-Hill, 2006.

8

Skeletal Muscle: Structure and Function

The human body contains more than 600 skeletal muscles, which constitute 40% to 50% of the total body weight (61). Skeletal muscle performs three important functions: (1) force generation for locomotion and breathing, (2) force generation for postural support, and (3) heat production during periods of cold stress. The most obvious function of skeletal muscle is to enable an individual to move freely and breathe. New evidence also suggests that skeletal muscles are endocrine organs and play an important role in the regulation of a variety of organ systems in the body. This concept was introduced in chapter 5 and will be discussed again in chapter 13.

Skeletal muscles are attached to bones by tough connective tissue called tendons. One end of the muscle is attached to a bone that does not move (origin), and the opposite end is fixed to a bone (insertion) that is moved during muscular contraction. A variety of different movements are possible, depending on the type of joint and muscles involved.

Muscles that decrease joint angles are called **flexors,** and muscles that increase joint angles are called **extensors.**

Given the role of skeletal muscles in determining sports performance, a thorough understanding of muscle structure and function is important to the exercise scientist, physical educator, physical therapist, and coach. Therefore, this chapter will discuss the structure and function of skeletal muscle.

STRUCTURE OF SKELETAL MUSCLE

Skeletal muscle is composed of several kinds of tissue. These include muscle cells (also called muscle fibers) themselves, nerve tissue, blood, and various types of connective tissue. Figure 8.1 displays the relationship between muscle and the various connective tissues.

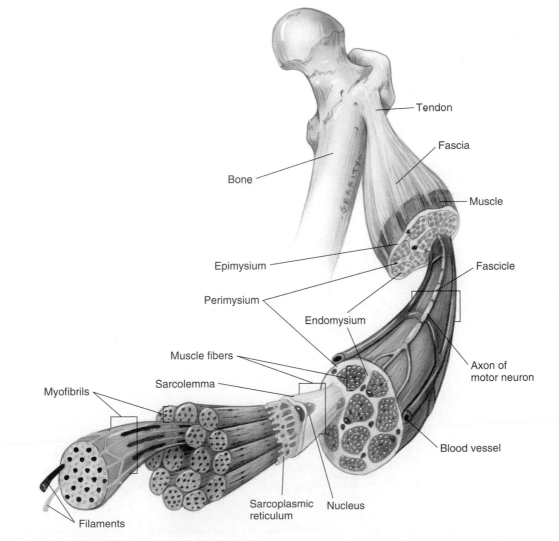

Figure 8.1   Connective tissue surrounding skeletal muscle.

Individual muscles are separated from each other and held in position by connective tissue called fascia. Three separate layers of connective tissue exist in skeletal muscle. The outermost layer that surrounds the entire muscle is called the **epimysium.** As we move inward from the epimysium, connective tissue called the **perimysium** surrounds individual bundles of muscle fibers. These individual bundles of muscle fibers are called a **fascicle.** Each muscle fiber within the fasciculus is surrounded by connective tissue called the **endomysium.** Just below the endomysium and surrounding each muscle fiber is another layer of protective tissue called the basement membrane.

Despite their unique shape, muscle fibers have many of the same organelles that are present in other cells. That is, they contain mitochondria, lysosomes, and so on. However, unlike most other cells in the body, muscle cells are multinucleated (i.e., have many nuclei). One of the most distinctive features of the microscopic appearance of skeletal muscles is their striated appearance (see figure 8.2). These stripes are produced by alternating light and dark bands that appear across the length of the fiber; these dark bands contain the primary muscle contractile proteins and will be discussed in detail later.

Each individual muscle fiber is a thin, elongated cylinder that generally extends the length of the muscle. The cell membrane surrounding the muscle fiber cell is called the **sarcolemma.** Located above the sarcolemma and below the basal lamina are a group of muscle precursor cells called satellite cells. **Satellite cells** are undifferentiated cells that play a key role in muscle growth and repair (81). If muscle fibers are destroyed (i.e., due to injury or disease), they cannot be replaced by cell division. However, satellite cells may also contribute to muscle growth during strength training by dividing and contributing nuclei to existing muscle fibers. Increasing the number of nuclei within muscle fibers enhances the fibers' ability to synthesize proteins and, therefore, assists in muscle growth (81).

The addition of nuclei to growing muscle fibers is a strategy used by the fiber to maintain a constant ratio of cell volume per nucleus. The volume of cytoplasm surrounding an individual nucleus is termed the myonuclear domain (1). The biological significance of the myonuclear domain is that a single nucleus can sustain the necessary gene expression (i.e., production of proteins) only for a limited area of cell volume. Therefore, to maintain a constant myonuclear domain, new nuclei (obtained from satellite

Figure 8.2   The microstructure of muscle. Note that a skeletal muscle fiber contains numerous myofibrils, each consisting of units called sarcomeres.

cells) are incorporated into skeletal muscle fibers during growth (47, 49, 79). It follows that to maintain a stable myonuclear domain, nuclei are lost from fibers during atrophy.

Beneath the sarcolemma lies the sarcoplasm (also called cytoplasm), which contains the cellular proteins, organelles, and myofibrils. **Myofibrils** are numerous threadlike structures that contain the contractile proteins (figure 8.2). In general, myofibrils are composed of two major types of protein filaments: (1) thick filaments composed of the protein **myosin** and (2) thin filaments composed primarily of the protein **actin.** The arrangement of these two protein filaments gives skeletal muscle its striated appearance (figure 8.2). Located on the actin molecule itself are two additional proteins, troponin and tropomyosin. These proteins make up only a small portion of the

muscle, but they play an important role in the regulation of the contractile process.

Myofibrils can be further subdivided into individual segments called **sarcomeres.** Sarcomeres are divided from each other by a thin sheet of structural proteins called a Z *line* or Z-*disk*. Myosin filaments are located primarily within the dark portion of the sarcomere, which is called the A *band*, while actin filaments occur principally in the light regions of the sarcomere called I *bands* (figure 8.2). In the center of the sarcomere is a portion of the myosin filament with no overlap of the actin. This is the H *zone*.

Within the sarcoplasm of muscle is a network of membranous channels that surrounds each myofibril and runs parallel with it. These channels are called the **sarcoplasmic reticulum** and are storage sites for calcium (figure 8.3). Remember from your

Sarcolemma

Triad of the reticulum:

Terminal cisternae

Transverse tubule

Sarcoplasmic reticulum

Mitochondria

Waldrop

Myofibrils

A band

I band

Z line

Nucleus

Figure 8.3 Within the sarcoplasm of muscle is a network of channels called the sarcoplasmic reticulum and the transverse tubules.

previous physiology course(s) that calcium release from the sarcoplasmic reticulum plays an important role in triggering muscular contraction. Another set of membranous channels called the **transverse tubules** extends from the sarcolemma into the muscle fiber and passes completely through the fiber. These transverse tubules pass between two enlarged portions of the sarcoplasmic reticulum called the **terminal cisternae.** All of these parts serve a function in muscular contraction and are discussed in further detail later in this chapter.

NEUROMUSCULAR JUNCTION

Each skeletal muscle cell is connected to a nerve fiber branch coming from a nerve cell. These nerve cells are called **motor neurons,** and they extend outward from the spinal cord. The motor neuron and all the muscle fibers it innervates are called a **motor unit.** Stimulation from motor neurons initiates the contraction process. The site where the motor neuron and muscle cell meet is called the **neuromuscular junction.** At this junction the sarcolemma forms a pocket that is called the motor end plate (see figure 8.4).

The end of the motor neuron does not physically make contact with the muscle fiber but is separated by a short gap called the synaptic cleft (also called the neuromuscular cleft). When a nerve impulse reaches the end of the motor nerve, the neurotransmitter acetylcholine is released and diffuses across the synaptic cleft to bind with receptor sites on the motor end plate. This causes an increase in the permeability of the sarcolemma to sodium, resulting in a depolarization called the **end-plate potential (EPP).** The EPP is always large enough to exceed threshold and is the signal to begin the contractile process.

IN SUMMARY

- The human body contains more than 600 voluntary skeletal muscles, which constitute 40% to 50% of the total body weight. Skeletal muscle performs three major functions: (1) force production for locomotion and breathing, (2) force production for postural support, and (3) heat production during cold stress.
- Individual muscle fibers are composed of hundreds of threadlike protein filaments called myofibrils. Myofibrils contain two major types of contractile protein: (1) actin (part of the thin filaments) and (2) myosin (major component of the thick filaments).
- The region of cytoplasm surrounding an individual nucleus is termed the myonuclear domain. The importance of the myonuclear domain is that a single nucleus is responsible for the gene expression for its surrounding cytoplasm.
- Motor neurons extend outward from the spinal cord and innervate individual muscle fibers. The site where the motor neuron and muscle cell meet is called the neuromuscular junction. Acetylcholine is the neurotransmitter that stimulates the muscle fiber to depolarize, which is the signal to start the contractile process.

Motor neuron fiber
Nerve fiber branches
Muscle fiber nucleus
Motor end plate
Myofibril of muscle fiber

Mitochondria
Synaptic vesicles
Synaptic cleft
Folded sarcolemma
Motor end plate

Figure 8.4 The connecting point between a motor neuron and a single muscle fiber is called the neuromuscular junction. The neurotransmitter acetylcholine is stored in synaptic vesicles at the end of the nerve fiber.

A LOOK BACK—IMPORTANT PEOPLE IN SCIENCE

Andrew F. Huxley Developed the "Sliding Filament Theory of Muscle Contraction"

Andrew Huxley (1917–) received the Nobel Prize for Physiology and Medicine in 1963 for his research on nerve transmission. Huxley was born in London, England, and was educated at the University of Cambridge. After graduation he accepted a research position at Cambridge and worked from 1941–1952 on nerve conduction. In 1952, he changed his research focus and began to study the mechanisms responsible for muscular contraction.

During his distinguished research career, Huxley made many important contributions to physiology. One of his first significant areas of research was the process of how neural transmission occurs. Working with Alan Hodgkin, the pair hypothesized that neural transmission (i.e., development of an action potential) occurs due to ions passing through ion channels on cell membranes. This hypothesis was confirmed years later, and Dr. Huxley and Dr. Hodgkin shared the Nobel Prize in 1963 for this work.

Although he won the Nobel Prize for his research on neural transmission, Professor Huxley is probably best known for his work on how skeletal muscles contract. Dr. Huxley and his research colleagues developed the "sliding filament theory of muscle contraction," and many investigators have since confirmed the basic principles of this original theory. Professor Huxley remains a faculty member in the Department of Physiology at University College (London).

MUSCULAR CONTRACTION

Muscular contraction is a complex process involving a number of cellular proteins and energy production systems. The final result is a sliding of actin over myosin, which causes the muscle to shorten and therefore develop tension. Although complete details of muscular contraction at the molecular level continue to be debated, the basic process of muscular contraction is well defined. The process of muscular contraction is best explained by the **sliding filament model** of contraction, which is now often called the **swinging lever-arm model** of muscle contraction (31, 40, 69). For a historical overview of the sliding filament theory of muscle contraction, see A Look Back—Important People in Science.

Overview of the Sliding Filament/ Swinging Lever-Arm Model

The general process of muscular contraction is illustrated in figure 8.5. Muscle fibers contract by a shortening of their myofibrils due to actin sliding over the myosin. This results in a reduction in the distance from Z line to Z line. Understanding the details of how muscular contraction occurs requires an appreciation of the microscopic structure of the myofibril. Note that the "heads" of the myosin cross-bridges are oriented toward the actin molecule (see figure 8.6). The actin and myosin filaments slide across each other during muscular contraction due to the action of the numerous cross-bridges extending out as "arms" from

myosin and attaching to actin. The binding of the myosin cross-bridge to actin results in an orientation of cross-bridges so that they can pull the actin from each side toward the center. This "pulling" of actin over the myosin molecule results in muscle shortening and the generation of force.

The term excitation-contraction coupling refers to the sequence of events in which a nerve impulse (action potential) reaches the muscle membrane and leads to muscle shortening by cross-bridge activity. This process will be discussed step-by-step next. Let's begin with a discussion of the energy source for contraction.

Energy for Contraction

The energy for muscular contraction comes from the breakdown of ATP by the enzyme myosin ATPase (21, 32, 36, 37, 41, 43). This enzyme is located on the "head" of the myosin cross-bridge. Recall that the bioenergetic pathways responsible for the synthesis of ATP were discussed earlier, in chapter 3; they are summarized in figure 8.7. The breakdown of ATP to ADP and inorganic phosphate (Pi) and the release of energy serves to energize the myosin cross-bridges, which in turn pull the actin molecules over myosin and thus shorten the muscle (25, 37, 50, 58, 59, 75).

Note that a single contraction cycle or "power stroke" of all the cross-bridges in a muscle would shorten the muscle by only 1% of its resting length (88). Because some muscles can shorten up to 60% of their resting length, it is clear that the contraction cycle must be repeated over and over again (59).

Figure 8.5 When a skeletal muscle contracts, (*a*) individual sarcomeres shorten as thick (myosin) and thin (actin) filaments slide past one another. (*b*) Photograph taken with electron microscope that illustrates a sarcomere shortening during muscle contraction (magnification is 23,000×).

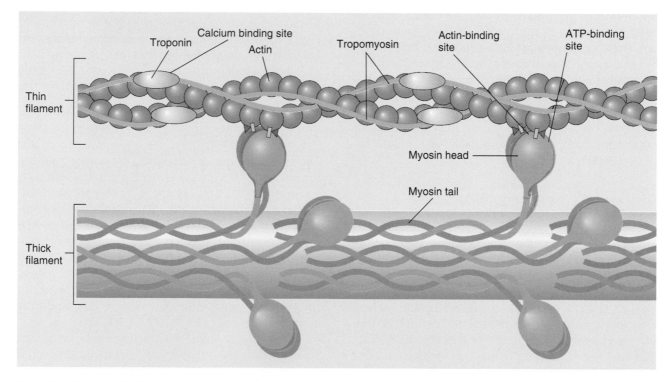

Figure 8.6 Proposed relationships among troponin, tropomyosin, myosin cross-bridges, and calcium. Note that when Ca^{++} binds to troponin, tropomyosin is removed from the active sites on actin, and cross-bridge attachment can occur.

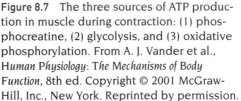

Figure 8.7 The three sources of ATP production in muscle during contraction: (1) phosphocreatine, (2) glycolysis, and (3) oxidative phosphorylation. From A. J. Vander et al., *Human Physiology: The Mechanisms of Body Function*, 8th ed. Copyright © 2001 McGraw-Hill, Inc., New York. Reprinted by permission.

Regulation of Excitation-Contraction Coupling

Relaxed muscles are easily stretched, which demonstrates that at rest, actin and myosin are not firmly attached and therefore are unbound. What regulates the interaction of actin and myosin and thus regulates muscle contraction? The first step in the process of muscular contraction begins with a nerve impulse arriving at the neuromuscular junction. The action potential from the motor neuron causes the release of acetylcholine into the synaptic cleft of the neuromuscular junction; acetylcholine binds to receptors on the motor end plate, producing an end-plate potential that leads to depolarization of the muscle cell (59). This depolarization (i.e., excitation) is conducted down the transverse tubules deep into the muscle fiber. When the action potential reaches the sarcoplasmic reticulum, calcium is released and diffuses into the muscle to bind to a protein called troponin. This is the "trigger" step in the control of muscular contraction because the regulation of contraction is a function of two regulatory proteins, **troponin** and **tropomyosin,** which are located on the actin molecule. Troponin and tropomyosin regulate muscular contraction by controlling the interaction of actin and myosin.

To understand how troponin and tropomyosin control muscular contraction, one needs to appreciate the anatomical relationship between actin, troponin, and tropomyosin (see figure 8.6). Notice that the actin filament is formed from many protein subunits arranged in a double row and twisted. Tropomyosin

is a thin molecule that lies in a groove between the double rows of actin. Attached directly to the tropomyosin is the protein troponin. This arrangement allows troponin and tropomyosin to work together to regulate the attachment of the actin and myosin cross-bridges. In a relaxed muscle, tropomyosin blocks the active sites on the actin molecule where the myosin cross-bridges must attach to produce a contraction. The trigger for contraction to occur is linked to the release of stored calcium (Ca^{++}) from a region of the sarcoplasmic reticulum termed the **lateral sac,** or sometimes called the *terminal cisternae* (51, 72). In a resting (relaxed) muscle the concentration of Ca^{++} in the sarcoplasm is very low. However, when a nerve impulse arrives at the neuromuscular junction, it travels down the transverse tubules to the sarcoplasmic reticulum and causes the release of Ca^{++}. Much of this Ca^{++} binds to troponin (see figure 8.6), which causes a position change in tropomyosin such that the active sites on the actin are uncovered. This permits the binding of a "cocked or energized" myosin cross-bridge on the actin molecule. The cross-bridge binding initiates the release of energy stored within the myosin molecule; this produces an angular movement of each cross-bridge, resulting in muscle shortening. Attachment of "fresh" ATP to the myosin cross-bridges breaks the myosin cross-bridge bound to actin. The enzyme ATPase again hydrolyzes (i.e., breaks down) the ATP attached to the myosin cross-bridge and provides the energy necessary for cocking (i.e., energizing) the myosin cross-bridge for reattachment to another active site on an actin molecule. This contraction cycle can be repeated as long

A CLOSER LOOK 8.1

Step-by-Step Summary of Excitation-Contraction Coupling

Excitation

The process of excitation is illustrated in steps 1 and 2 in figure 8.8 and involves two processes:

1. The generation of an action potential in a motor neuron causes the release of acetylcholine into the synaptic cleft of the neuromuscular junction.

2. Acetylcholine binds with receptors on the motor end-plate, producing an end-plate potential, which leads to a depolarization that is conducted down the transverse tubules deep into the muscle fiber. This depolarization results in calcium being released from the sarcoplasmic reticulum.

Contraction

The steps involved in muscular contraction are illustrated in figure 8.9 and are listed in sequential order here (30, 37, 58, 75):

1. In the resting state, the myosin cross-bridges are not connected to actin (no force generation; step 1, figure 8.9).

2. When the depolarization (i.e., neural stimulation) reaches the sarcoplasmic reticulum, Ca^{++} is released into the sarcoplasm. The Ca^{++} then binds to troponin, which causes a shift in the position of tropomyosin to uncover the "active sites" on the actin. The breakdown of ATP (hydrolysis) (step 2, figure 8.9) results in an "energized" or "cocked" myosin cross-bridge (step 3, figure 8.9), which then forms a strong bond at the active site on actin (step 4, figure 8.9).

3. Inorganic phosphate is now released from the myosin cross-bridge and the energized cross-bridge pulls the actin molecule (step 5, figure 8.9).

4. Cross-bridge movement is completed by the release of ADP from the myosin cross-bridge. Note, at this point within the contraction cycle, the myosin cross-bridge remains bound with actin (step 6, figure 8.9).

5. Attachment of ATP to the myosin cross-bridge allows the myosin cross-bridge to break the strong binding state and form a weak binding state. In this weak binding state, ATP is broken down to $ADP + P_i +$ energy, and the released energy is used to "energize" and cock the myosin cross-bridge (step 1, figure 8.9). This contraction cycle can be repeated as long as Ca^{++} and ATP are present (i.e., step 1 moves to step 2 and the cycle continues).

The contraction cycle is broken when action potentials stop and the sarcoplasmic reticulum actively removes Ca^{++} from the sarcoplasm (figure 8.8, steps 5–6).

---

as free Ca^{++} is available to bind to troponin and ATP can be hydrolyzed to provide the energy. Failure of the muscle to maintain homeostasis (e.g., due to inadequate Ca^{++} levels, high levels of hydrogen ion, etc.) results in impaired cross-bridge movement, and fatigue occurs. The causes of exercise-induced muscle fatigue will be introduced in a forthcoming segment.

The signal to stop contraction is the absence of the nerve impulse at the neuromuscular junction. When this occurs, an energy-requiring Ca^{++} pump located within the sarcoplasmic reticulum begins to move Ca^{++} back into the sarcoplasmic reticulum. This removal of Ca^{++} from troponin causes tropomyosin to move back to cover the binding sites on the actin molecule, and cross-bridge interaction ceases. Figure 8.8 illustrates the basic steps involved in muscle contraction and relaxation.

A Closer Look 8.1 contains a step-by-step summary of the events that occur during excitation and muscular contraction. For a detailed discussion of molecular events involved in skeletal muscle contraction, see references (10, 25, 28, 30, 31, 37–39, 58, 59, 75). Time spent learning the microstructure of muscle and the events that lead to contraction will pay dividends later, as this material is important to a thorough understanding of exercise physiology.

IN SUMMARY

- The process of muscular contraction can be best explained by the sliding filament/swinging cross-bridge model, which proposes that muscle shortening occurs due to movement of the actin filament over the myosin filament.
- The steps leading to muscular contraction are (see figure 8.9 for a detailed, step-by-step illustration):
  a. The nerve impulse travels down the transverse tubules and reaches the sarcoplasmic reticulum, and Ca^{++} is released.
  b. Ca^{++} binds to the protein troponin.
  c. Ca^{++} binding to troponin causes a position change in tropomyosin away from the "active sites" on the actin molecule and binding between actin and myosin.
  d. Muscular contraction occurs by multiple cycles of cross-bridge activity. Shortening will continue as long as energy is available and Ca^{++} is free to bind to troponin. When neural activity ceases at the neuromuscular junction, Ca^{++} is removed from the sarcoplasm and actively pumped into the sarcoplasmic reticulum by the Ca^{++} pump. This results in tropomyosin moving to cover the active site on actin, and the muscle relaxes.

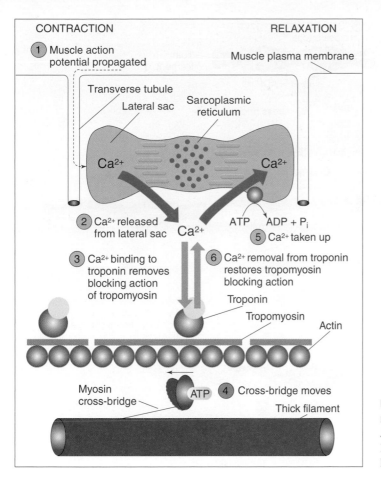

CONTRACTION

① Muscle action
potential propagated

RELAXATION

Muscle plasma membrane

Transverse tubule

Lateral sac   Sarcoplasmic reticulum

Ca^{2+} Ca^{2+}

② Ca^{2+} released
from lateral sac Ca^{2+}

ATP   ADP + P_i

⑤ Ca^{2+} taken up

③ Ca^{2+} binding to
troponin removes
blocking action
of tropomyosin

⑥ Ca^{2+} removal from troponin
restores tropomyosin
blocking action

Troponin

Tropomyosin

Actin

Myosin
cross-bridge   ATP

④ Cross-bridge moves

Thick filament

Figure 8.8 Illustration of the steps involved in muscle excitation, contraction, and relaxation. From A. J. Vander et al., *Human Physiology: The Mechanisms of Body Function*, 8th ed. Copyright © 2001 McGraw-Hill, Inc., New York. Reprinted by permission.

EXERCISE AND MUSCLE FATIGUE

High-intensity exercise or prolonged, submaximal exercise results in a decline in the muscle's ability to generate power. This decrease in muscle power output is called fatigue. Specifically, muscle fatigue is defined as a reduction in muscle power output that can result from a decrease in both muscle force generation and shortening velocity. The onset of muscle fatigue during exercise is illustrated in figure 8.10. Note that muscle fatigue differs from injury to the muscle because muscle fatigue is reversible by a few hours of rest, whereas recovery from muscle damage may take days to weeks to fully recover (30).

The causes of exercise-induced muscle fatigue are complex and not fully understood. Depending upon the type of exercise and the environmental conditions, fatigue may result in disturbances in the central nervous system and/or peripheral factors within skeletal muscle (2). The concept of "central nervous system fatigue" was introduced in chapter 7,

and we will focus on peripheral (i.e., skeletal muscle) fatigue here.

Although the exact causes of muscle fatigue remain controversial, it is established that an individual's state of fitness, nutritional status, fiber type composition, and the intensity and duration of exercise all effect the fatigue process (30). Further, regardless of the cause of muscle fatigue, the end result is a decline in muscle force generation due to impaired force production at the cross-bridge level. An overview of the potential contributors to exercise-induced muscle fatigue follows.

The causes of muscle fatigue are complex and vary depending upon the type of exercise performed. For example, muscle fatigue resulting from high-intensity exercise lasting approximately 60 seconds (e.g., sprinting 400 meters) may be due to several factors, including an accumulation of lactate, hydrogen ions, ADP, inorganic phosphate, and free radicals within the active muscle fibers (30). Collectively, the accumulation of these metabolites disrupts muscle homeostasis and diminishes the number of cross bridges bound to actin, resulting in diminished force production (30, 76, 78).

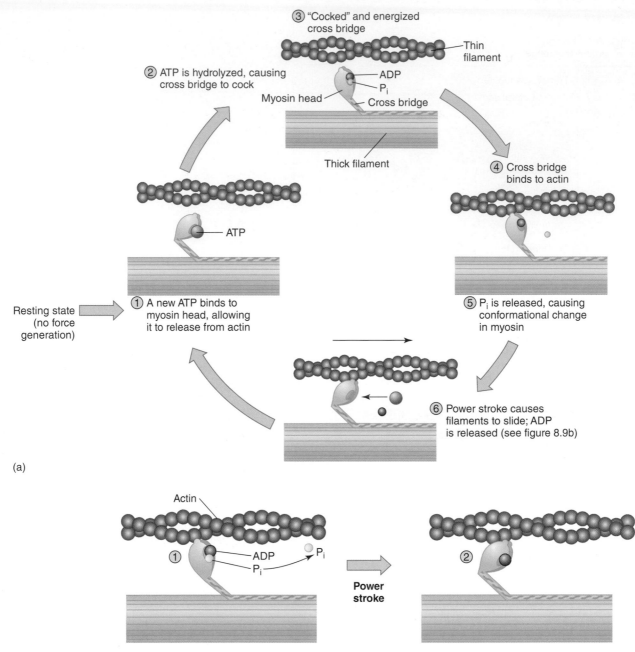

Figure 8.9 (*a*) Step-by-step illustration of the cross-bridge cycle that causes sliding of the filaments and muscle contraction. The hydrolysis (breakdown) of ATP is required for the activation of the cross-bridge, and the binding of new ATP is required for the cross-bridge release from actin at the end of the cycle. See text for more details. (*b*) Illustration of the cross-bridge stroke. The myosin head has been activated by the splitting of ATP into ADP and P_i which remain bound to the cross-bridge. At this point, the myosin head has formed a bond with actin, forming a cross-bridge between the thick and thin filaments. After the inorganic phosphate (P_i) leaves the cross-bridge, the myosin head moves, producing the power stroke that moves the actin filament.

Muscular fatigue that occurs in the later stages of an endurance event lasting 2 to 4 hours (i.e., marathon running) may also involve an accumulation of free radicals in the muscle, but other factors such as disturbances in muscle/extracellular electrolyte homeostasis and depletion of muscle glycogen may also contribute to this type of muscle fatigue (30, 78). Muscle fatigue and the limiting factors to exercise performance are discussed in more detail in chapter 19.

Onset of fatigue

Contraction time

Figure 8.10 Muscular fatigue is characterized by a reduced ability to generate force.

IN SUMMARY

- Muscle fatigue is defined as a reduction in muscle power output that results from decreased muscle force generation and shortening velocity.
- The causes of exercise-induced muscle fatigue are complex and vary depending upon the type of exercise performed.

EXERCISE-ASSOCIATED MUSCLE CRAMPS

Almost everyone has experienced muscle cramps during or following a prolonged or intense exercise session. Muscle cramps can be painful and result from spasmodic, involuntary skeletal muscle contractions. Although numerous theories have been proposed to explain the cause of cramps, the exact cause of exercise-induced muscle cramps remains an open debate. Currently, there are two primary theories to explain exercise-induced muscle cramping: (1) electrolyte depletion and dehydration theory and (2) altered neuromuscular control theory.

The electrolyte depletion and dehydration theory predicts that exercise-induced muscle cramps occur due to electrolyte imbalances in the blood and extracellular fluid (8, 9). Supporters of this theory argue that exercise-induced loss of body water and sodium via sweating results in electrolyte imbalances that trigger muscle contractions by causing motor nerve terminals to spontaneously discharge. To date, most of the support for the electrolyte/dehydration theory comes from anecdotal clinical observations (66). Further, several recent scientific studies do not support this theory (66). Nonetheless, before this theory can be completely rejected, additional studies are required.

The altered neuromuscular control theory contends that exercise-associated muscle cramps occur due to abnormal activity of both the muscle spindle and Golgi tendon organ. In short, this theory proposes that exercise-induced muscle fatigue results in increased muscle spindle activity and decreased Golgi tendon activity (67). This abnormal function of these two muscle-sense organs results in increased firing of the motor neurons located in the spinal cord, which results in involuntary muscle contractions (i.e., cramps). Evidence to support this theory is growing, and abnormal reflex activity is likely a key factor that promotes exercise-related muscle cramps. For example, evidence to support this theory comes from the observation that passive stretching of the cramping muscle can relieve the cramp. It appears that passive stretching relieves muscle cramps by invoking the inverse stretch reflex. Recall from chapter 7 that the inverse stretch reflex occurs by activation of the Golgi tendon organ. That is, stretching of a muscle activates the Golgi tendon organ, which inhibits motor neurons in the spinal cord, resulting in muscle relaxation. Therefore, the fact that stretching the cramping muscle often relieves cramping provides evidence to support the concept that impaired neuromuscular control is present in exercise-induced muscle cramping.

In summary, the exact cause of muscle cramps associated with exercise remains a debated topic. However, growing evidence indicates that exercise-associated muscle cramps are due to abnormal spinal reflex activity, which is linked with muscle fatigue. Nonetheless, it seems possible that following prolonged exercise in a hot environment, electrolyte imbalances can also be a contributory factor to muscle cramps under this type of exercise condition.

IN SUMMARY

- Muscle cramps are spasmodic and involuntary skeletal muscle contractions.
- The exact cause of exercise-induced muscle cramps remains unclear. Nonetheless, mounting research indicates that many cases of exercise-associated muscle cramps occur due to abnormal spinal reflex activity that occurs as a by-product of muscle fatigue.

FIBER TYPES

Human skeletal muscle can be divided into major classes based on the histochemical or biochemical characteristics of the individual fibers. How fibers are "typed" is discussed in A Closer Look 8.2. Specifically, muscle fibers are classified into two general categories: (1) slow, type I fibers (also called slow twitch fibers); and (2) fast, type II fibers (also called fast-twitch fibers) (16, 18, 26, 27, 46). Only one type of slow (type I) muscle fiber exists in human muscle, whereas two subcategories of fast, type II fibers exist: (a) type IIa fibers and (b) type IIx fibers. Though some muscles are composed of predominantly fast or slow

How Are Skeletal Muscle Fibers Typed?

The relative percentage of fast or slow fibers contained in a particular muscle can be estimated by removing a small piece of muscle (via a procedure called a biopsy) and performing histochemical analysis of the individual muscle cells. A common method uses a histochemical procedure that divides muscle fibers into three categories based on the specific "isoform" of myosin found in the fiber. This technique uses selective antibodies that recognize and "tag" each of the different myosin proteins (e.g., type I, type IIa, and type IIx) found in human muscle fibers. Specifically, this method involves the binding of a high affinity antibody to each unique myosin protein. This technique can then identify different muscle fibers due to color differences across the varying muscle fiber types. Figure 8.11 is an example of a muscle cross-section after immunohistochemical staining for a skeletal muscle membrane pro-

FIGURE 8.11 Immunohistochemical staining of a cross-sectional area of a skeletal muscle. The red staining is dystrophin protein, which is located within the membrane that surrounds a skeletal muscle fiber. The blue cells are type I fibers, whereas the green cells are type IIa fibers. The cells that appear black are type IIx muscle fibers.

tein (dystrophin), as well as immunohistochemical staining for type I, IIa, and IIx skeletal muscle fibers (10, 45, 41, 56).

One of the inherent problems with fiber typing in humans is that a muscle biopsy is usually performed on only one muscle group. Therefore, a single sample from one muscle is not representative of the entire body. A further complication is that a small sample of fibers taken from a single area of the muscle may not be truly representative of the total fiber population of the muscle biopsied (3, 71). Therefore, it is difficult to make a definitive statement concerning the whole body percentage of muscle fiber types based on the staining of a single muscle biopsy.

---

fibers, most muscles in the body contain a mixture of both slow and fast fiber types. The percentage of the respective fiber types contained in skeletal muscles can be influenced by genetics, blood levels of hormones, and the exercise habits of the individual. From a practical standpoint, the fiber composition of skeletal muscles plays an important role in performance in both power and endurance events (11, 70). A brief overview of how muscle fibers are identified in the laboratory is presented in A Closer Look 8.2.

Overview of Biochemical and Contractile Characteristics of Skeletal Muscle

Before discussing the specific characteristics of specific muscle fiber types, let's discuss the general biochemical and contractile properties of skeletal muscle that are important to muscle function.

Biochemical Properties of Muscle The three primary biochemical characteristics of muscle that are important to muscle function are (1) the oxidative capacity, (2) the type of myosin isoform, and (3) the

abundance of contractile protein within the fiber. The oxidative capacity of a muscle fiber is determined by the number of mitochondria, the number of capillaries surrounding the fiber, and the amount of myoglobin within the fiber. A large number of mitochondria provides a greater capacity to produce ATP aerobically. A high number of capillaries surrounding a muscle fiber ensures that the fiber will receive adequate oxygen during periods of contractile activity. Myoglobin is similar to hemoglobin in the blood in that it binds O_2, and it also acts as a "shuttle" mechanism for O_2 between the cell membrane and the mitochondria. Therefore, a high myoglobin concentration improves the delivery of oxygen from the capillary to the mitochondria where it will be used. Collectively, the significance of these biochemical characteristics is that a muscle fiber with a high concentration of myoglobin, along with a high number of mitochondria and capillaries, will have a high aerobic capacity and therefore will be fatigue resistant during prolonged bouts of submaximal exercise.

The second important biochemical characteristic of muscle fiber is that the different myosin isoforms differ in their myosin ATPase activity. Many isoforms of ATPase exist, and the various isoforms differ in their activities (i.e., speed that they break down ATP). Muscle fibers that contain ATPase isoforms with high ATPase activity will degrade ATP rapidly; this results in a high speed of muscle shortening. Conversely, muscle fibers with low ATPase activities shorten at slow speeds.

Finally, the third important biochemical characteristic of muscle fibers that influences contractile properties is the abundance of contractile proteins (i.e., actin and myosin) in the muscle fiber. Indeed, fibers that contain large amounts of actin and myosin generate more force than fibers with low levels of these key contractile proteins. The details about fiber type differences in the levels of actin and myosin will be discussed in more detail later.

Contractile Properties of Skeletal Muscle In comparing the contractile properties of muscle fiber types, four performance characteristics are important: (1) maximal force production, (2) speed of contraction, (3) maximal power output, and (4) muscle fiber efficiency. Let's discuss each of these characteristics briefly.

First, maximal force production of a muscle fiber is compared by expressing how much force the fiber produces per unit of fiber cross-sectional area. This property of a skeletal muscle fiber is called the fiber specific tension or specific force production. In other words, specific tension is the force production divided by the size of the fiber (e.g., specific force = force/fiber cross-sectional area).

A second key contractile property of muscle fibers is the speed of contraction. The contraction speed of muscle fibers is compared by measuring the maximal shortening velocity (called Vmax) of individual fibers. Vmax represents the highest speed at which a fiber can shorten. Because muscle fibers shorten by cross-bridge movement (called cross-bridge cycling), Vmax is determined by the rate of cross-bridge cycling. The key biochemical factor that regulates fiber Vmax is the myosin ATPase activity. Therefore, fibers with high myosin ATPase activities (e.g., fast fibers) possess a high Vmax, whereas fibers with low myosin ATPase activities possess a low Vmax (e.g., slow fibers).

A third important contractile property of a muscle fiber is the maximal power output. The power of a muscle fiber is determined by both the force generation and the shortening velocity. Specifically, the maximal power output of a muscle fiber is defined as the product of force generation multiplied by the shortening velocity (i.e., power = force × shortening velocity). Therefore, muscle fibers with a high force generating capacity and a fast shortening velocity can produce a high power output. In contrast, muscle fibers that possess slow shortening velocities and/or a low force generating capacity are not capable of producing power outputs.

Finally, the efficiency of contraction is the fourth important contractile property of a skeletal muscle fiber. The efficiency of a muscle fiber is a measure of the muscle fiber's economy. That is, an efficient fiber would require less energy to perform a certain amount of work compared to a less-efficient fiber. In practice, this measurement is made by dividing the amount of energy used (i.e., ATP used) by the amount of force produced. In the next segment, we discuss how individual fiber types differ across these four key contractile properties.

Characteristics of Individual Fiber Types

Three major muscle fiber types exist in human skeletal muscle (two subtypes of fast fibers—identified as type IIx and IIa; and a slow fiber—identified as type I). Let's begin our discussion of muscle fiber types by examining the biochemical and contractile properties of both slow and fast fibers.

Slow (Type I) Fibers Only one type of slow fiber exists in humans—type I. **Type I fibers** (also called slow-oxidative or **slow-twitch fibers**) contain large numbers of oxidative enzymes (i.e., high mitochondrial volume) and are surrounded by more capillaries than fast, type II fibers. In addition, type I fibers contain higher concentrations of myoglobin than fast fibers. The high concentration of myoglobin, the large number of capillaries, and the high mitochondrial enzyme activities provide type I fibers with a large capacity for aerobic metabolism and a high resistance to fatigue.

In regard to contractile properties (shortening velocity and force generation), type I fibers possess a slower maximal shortening velocity (Vmax) compared to fast fibers (figure 8.12) (19, 57). The mechanism to explain this fact was presented earlier (i.e., type I fibers possess a lower myosin ATPase activity compared to fast fibers).

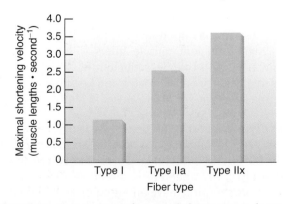

Figure 8.12 Comparison of maximal shortening velocities between fiber types. Data are from reference 20.

(a) Specific force

(b) Maximal power

Figure 8.13 Comparison of (a) maximal specific force production and (b) maximal power output between muscle fiber types. Data are from Capepari et al. (19).

Further, type I fibers produce a lower specific tension than fast fibers do (figure 8.13) (19). The explanation for this observation is that type I fibers contain less actin and myosin per cross-sectional area than fast type II fibers do. This is important because the amount of force generated by a muscle fiber is directly related to the number of myosin cross-bridges bound to actin (i.e., the force generating state) at any given time. Simply stated, the more cross-bridges generating force, the greater the force production. Therefore, fast fibers exert more force than slow fibers because they contain more myosin cross-bridges per cross-sectional area of fiber than do slow fibers.

Finally, type I fibers are more efficient than fast fibers (23). This is important because at any given work rate, highly efficient muscle fibers will require less energy (i.e., ATP) than less efficient fibers. The difference in efficiency between slow and fast fibers is likely due to a lower rate of ATP turnover in slow fibers (23).

Fast (Type IIa and IIx) Fibers Two subtypes of fast fibers exist in humans: (1) type IIx and (2) type IIa. **Type IIx fibers** (sometimes called **fast-twitch fibers** or fast-glycolytic fibers) have a relatively small number of mitochondria, have a limited capacity for aerobic metabolism, and have less resistant to fatigue than slow fibers (33, 55). However, these fibers are rich in glycolytic enzymes, which provide them with a large anaerobic capacity (54).

The fastest skeletal muscle fiber in many small animals (e.g., rats) is the type IIb fiber. For several years it was believed that the fastest fiber in human skeletal muscle was also a "type IIb" fiber. However, it is now established that the fastest muscle fiber in humans is the type IIx fiber. The story behind this change in scientific thinking follows: In the late 1980s, German and Italian scientists independently discovered a new fast muscle fiber, named type IIx, in rodent skeletal muscle (6, 64). Since the discovery of this type IIx fiber in rodents, it has been determined that this type of myosin is similar in structure to that contained in the fastest muscle fiber in humans (63, 65). Therefore, throughout this textbook we will refer to type IIx fibers as the fastest skeletal muscle fiber type in humans (24).

The specific tension of type IIx fibers is similar to type IIa fibers but is greater than type I fibers (figure 8.13) (19). Further, the myosin ATPase activity in type IIx fibers is higher than other fiber types, resulting in the highest Vmax of all fiber types (figure 8.12). It follows that type IIx fibers generate the highest power output of all muscle fiber types (figure 8.13) (19).

Type IIx fibers are less efficient than all other fiber types. This low efficiency is due to the high myosin ATPase activity, which results in a greater energy expenditure per unit of work performed (23).

The second type of fast fiber is the **type IIa fiber** (also called **intermediate fibers** or fast-oxidative glycolytic fibers). These fibers contain biochemical and fatigue characteristics that are between type IIx and type I fibers. Therefore, conceptually, type IIa fibers can be viewed as a mixture of both type I and type IIx fiber characteristics. The comparisons of contractile properties between type IIa and IIx fibers are illustrated in figures 8.12 and 8.13.

Finally, it is important to appreciate that regular exercise training can modify both the biochemical and contractile properties of human muscle fibers and can result in the conversion of fast fibers into slow fibers. A detailed discussion of exercise-induced changes in skeletal muscle fibers will be presented in chapter 13 (5, 12, 35, 56).

IN SUMMARY

- Human skeletal muscle fiber types can be divided into three general classes of fibers based on their biochemical and contractile properties. Two categories of fast fibers exist, type IIx and type IIa. One type of slow fiber exists, type I fibers.
- The biochemical and contractile properties characteristic of all muscle fiber types are summarized in table 8.1.

TABLE 8.1	Characteristics of Human Skeletal Muscle Fiber Types		
	FAST FIBERS		**SLOW FIBERS**
Characteristic	Type IIx	Type IIa	Type I
Number of mitochondria	Low	High/moderate	High
Resistance to fatigue	Low	High/moderate	High
Predominant energy system	Anaerobic	Combination	Aerobic
ATPase activity	Highest	High	Low
Vmax (speed of shortening)	Highest	High	Low
Efficiency	Low	Moderate	High
Specific tension	High	High	Moderate

■ Although classifying skeletal muscle fibers into three general groups is a convenient system to study the properties of muscle fibers, it is important to appreciate that human skeletal muscle fibers exhibit a wide range of contractile and biochemical properties. That is, the biochemical and contractile properties of type IIx, type IIa, and type I fibers represent a continuum instead of three neat packages.

Fiber Types and Performance

Numerous studies have reported several interesting facts concerning the percentages of fast and slow muscle fibers found in humans. First, there are no apparent sex or age differences in fiber distribution (54). Second, the average sedentary man or woman possesses approximately 50% slow fibers. Third, highly successful power athletes (e.g., sprinters, etc.) typically possess a large percentage of fast fibers, whereas endurance athletes generally have a high percentage of slow fibers (22, 26, 73). Table 8.2 presents some examples of the percentage of slow and fast fibers found in successful athletes.

It is clear from table 8.2 that considerable variation in the percentage of various fiber types exists even among successful athletes competing in the same event or sport. Indeed, although the percentage of type I (slow) muscle fibers is highly correlated with an individual's $\dot{V}O_2$ max, the percentage of type I fibers can explain only 40% of the variation in $\dot{V}O_2$ max between individuals (68). Furthermore, two equally successful 10,000-meter runners have been shown to differ in the percentage of slow fibers that each possesses. For example, runner A might be found to possess 70% slow fibers, whereas runner B possesses 85% slow fibers. This observation demonstrates that an individual's muscle fiber composition is not the only variable that determines success in athletic events (22). In fact, success in athletic performance is due to a complex interaction of psychological, biochemical, neurological, cardiopulmonary, and biomechanical factors (14, 15, 48, 80).

IN SUMMARY

■ Successful power athletes (e.g., sprinters) generally possess a large percentage of fast muscle fibers and therefore a low percentage of slow, type I fibers.
■ In contrast to power athletes, endurance athletes (e.g., marathoners) typically possess a high percentage of slow muscle fibers and a low percentage of fast fibers.
■ Although muscle fiber types are known to play a role in sport performance, considerable variation exists among successful athletes competing in the same sport.

MUSCLE ACTIONS

The process of skeletal muscle force generation has historically been referred to as a "muscle contraction." However, to describe both lengthening and shortening actions of a muscle as a contraction can be confusing. Therefore, the term **muscle action** has been proposed to describe the process of muscle force development. This term is now commonly used to describe different types of muscular contractions.

Several types of muscle actions exist. For example, it is possible for skeletal muscle to generate force

TABLE 8.2	Typical Muscle Fiber Composition in Elite Athletes	
Sport	% Slow Fibers (Type I)	% Fast Fibers (Types IIx and IIa)
Distance runners	70–80	20–30
Track sprinters	25–30	70–75
Nonathletes	47–53	47–53

Data from references 20 and 82.

(a)

(b)

Figure 8.14 (*a*) Isometric actions occur when a muscle exerts force but does not shorten. (*b*) Concentric actions occur when a muscle contracts and shortens.

without a large amount of muscle shortening. This might occur when an individual attempts to perform a "curl" with a dumbbell weight that he or she cannot move (see figure 8.14a). What happens here is that muscle tension increases, but the dumbbell does not move, and therefore neither does the body part that applies the force. This kind of muscle force development is called an **isometric action** and is referred to as a static exercise. Isometric actions are common in the postural muscles of the body, which act to maintain a static body position during periods of standing or sitting.

In contrast to isometric muscle actions, most types of exercise or sports activities require muscle actions that result in the movement of body parts. Exercise that involves movement of body parts is called **dynamic** exercise (formally called isotonic exercise). Two types of muscle actions can occur during dynamic exercise: (1) concentric and (2) eccentric. A muscle action that results in muscular shortening with movement of a body part is called a **concentric action** (figure 8.14b). An **eccentric action** occurs when a muscle is activated and force is produced, but the muscle lengthens. Table 8.3 summarizes the classifications of exercise and muscle action types.

Note that eccentric muscle actions can result in high stress within the sarcomere. This eccentric action

Type of Exercise	Muscle Action	Muscle Length Change
Dynamic	Concentric	Decreases
	Eccentric	Increases
Static	Isometric	No change

TABLE 8.3 Summary of the Classifications of Exercise and Muscle Action Types

induced stress on the muscle is often associated with muscle fiber injury, resulting in a loss of muscle force generating capacity and muscle soreness due to inflammation and swelling of the muscle fiber. More details about exercise-induced muscle injury and soreness are presented in chapter 21.

SPEED OF MUSCLE ACTION AND RELAXATION

If a muscle is given a single stimulus, such as a brief electrical shock applied to the nerve innervating it, the muscle responds with a simple **twitch.** The movement of the muscle can be recorded on a special recording device, and the time periods for contraction and relaxation can be studied. Figure 8.15 illustrates the time course of a simple twitch in an isolated frog muscle. Notice that the twitch can be divided into three phases. First, immediately after the stimulus, there is a brief latent period (lasting a few milliseconds) prior to the beginning of muscle shortening. The second phase of the twitch is the contraction phase, which lasts approximately 40 milliseconds. Finally,

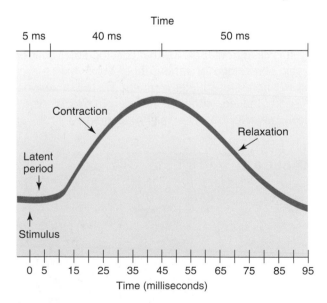

Figure 8.15 A recording of a simple twitch. Note the three time periods (latent period, contraction, and relaxation) following the stimulus.

the muscle returns to its original length during the relaxation period, which lasts about 50 milliseconds and thus is the longest of the three phases.

The timing of the phases in a simple twitch varies among muscle fiber types. The variability in speed of contraction arises from differences in the responses of the individual fiber types that make up muscles. Individual muscle fibers behave much like individual neurons in that they exhibit all-or-none responses to stimulation. To contract, an individual muscle fiber must receive an appropriate amount of stimulation. However, fast fibers contract in a shorter time period when stimulated than do slow fibers. The explanation for this observation is as follows: The speed of shortening is greater in fast fibers than in slow fibers because the sarcoplasmic reticulum in fast fibers releases Ca^{++} at a faster rate, and fast fibers possess a higher ATPase activity compared to the slow fiber types (19, 26, 29, 62). The higher ATPase activity results in a more rapid splitting of ATP and a quicker release of the energy required for contraction.

FORCE REGULATION IN MUSCLE

As stated earlier, the amount of force generated in a single muscle fiber is related to the number of myosin cross-bridges making contact with actin. However, the amount of force exerted during muscular contraction in a group of muscles is complex and dependent on three primary factors. (1) number and types of motor units recruited, (2) the initial length of the muscle, and (3) the nature of the neural stimulation of the motor units (4, 18, 20, 29). A discussion of each of these factors follows.

First, variations in the strength of contraction within an entire muscle depend on both the type and the number of muscle fibers that are stimulated to contract (i.e., recruited). Recall from chapter 7 that motor units are recruited according to the size principle, and if only a few motor units are recruited, the force is small. It follows that if more motor units are stimulated, the force increases. Figure 8.16 illustrates this point. Note that as the stimulus is increased, the force of contraction is increased due to the recruitment of additional motor units. Also, recall that fast fibers exert a greater specific force than do slow fibers. Therefore, the types of motor units recruited also influence force production.

A second factor that determines the force exerted by a muscle is the initial length of the muscle at the time of contraction. There exists an "ideal" length of the muscle fiber. The explanation for the existence of an ideal length is related to the overlap between actin and myosin. For instance, when the resting length is longer than optimal, the overlap between actin and myosin is limited and few cross-bridges can attach.

Figure 8.16 The relationship between increasing stimulus strength and the force of contraction. Weak stimuli do not activate many motor units and do not produce great force. In contrast, increasing the stimulus strength recruits more and more motor units and thus produces more force.

This concept is illustrated in figure 8.17. Note that when the muscle is stretched to the point where there is no overlap of actin and myosin, cross-bridges cannot attach and thus tension cannot be developed. At the other extreme, when the muscle is shortened to about 60% of its resting length, the Z lines are very close to the thick myosin filaments; thus, only limited additional shortening can occur.

A final factor that can affect the amount of force a muscle exerts upon contraction is the nature of the neural stimulation. Simple muscle twitches studied under experimental conditions reveal some interesting, fundamental properties about how muscles function. However, normal body movements involve sustained contractions that are not simple twitches. The sustained contractions involved in normal body movements can be closely replicated in the laboratory if a series of stimulations are applied to the muscle. The recording pictured in figure 8.18 represents what occurs when successive stimuli are applied to the muscle. The first few contractions represent simple twitches. Note that as the frequency of stimulations is increased, the muscle does not have time to relax between stimuli, and the force appears to be additive. This response is called **summation** (addition of successive twitches). If the frequency of stimuli is increased further, individual contractions are blended in a single, sustained contraction called **tetanus.** A tetanic contraction will continue until the stimuli are stopped or the muscle fatigues.

In addition to the previous discussion of the physiological factors that impact muscle force production, both aging and disease can also impact muscle's ability to generate force. Indeed, it is well established that aging results in a loss of muscle mass which reduces muscle force production. Also, several common diseases, such as diabetes and cancer, can also impair muscle function. Finally, specific

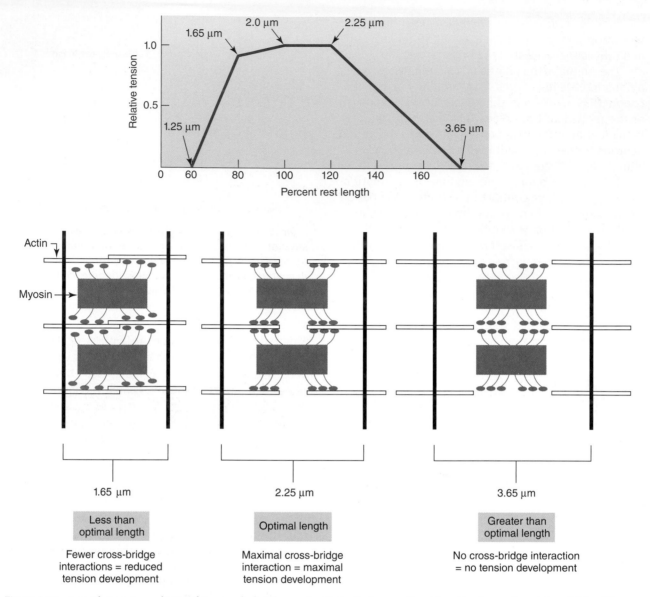

Figure 8.17 Length-tension relationships in skeletal muscle. Note that an optimal length of muscle exists, which will produce maximal force when stimulated. Lengths that are above or below this optimal length result in a reduced amount of force when stimulated.

Figure 8.18 Recording showing the change from simple twitches to summation, and finally tetanus. Peaks to the left represent simple twitches, while increasing the frequency of the stimulus results in summation of the twitches, and finally tetanus.

muscle diseases (e.g., muscular dystrophy) can also have a negative impact on muscle force production (see Clinical Applications 8.1 for more details).

Muscular contractions that occur during normal body movements are tetanic contractions. These sustained contractions result from a series of rapidly repeated neural impulses conducted by the motor neurons that innervate those motor units involved in the movement. It is important to appreciate that in the body, neural impulses to various motor units do not arrive at the same time as they do in the laboratory-induced tetanic contraction. Instead, various motor units are stimulated to contract at different times. Thus, some motor units are contracting while some are relaxing. This type of tetanic contraction results in a smooth contraction and aids in sustaining a coordinated muscle contraction.

Both Diseases and Aging Can Negatively Impact Muscle Function

Many common diseases and old age can have a negative influence on the ability of skeletal muscle to exert force. Let's discuss the impact of old age and several widespread diseases on muscle function.

Aging and Muscle Loss Aging is associated with a loss of muscle mass (called sarcopenia) (77). The age-related decline in muscle mass begins around age 25 and occurs across the lifetime. However, the rate of age-related muscle loss occurs in two distinct phases. The first is a "slow" phase of muscle loss, in which 10% of muscle mass is lost from age 25 to 50 years. Thereafter, there is a rapid loss in muscle mass. In fact, from age 50 to 80 years, an additional 40% of muscle mass is lost. Thus, by age 80, one-half of the total skeletal muscle mass is lost. Also, aging results in a loss of fast fibers (particularly type IIx) and an increase in slow fibers (52). From a clinical perspective, severe age-related sarcopenia can have negative health consequences because it increases the risk of falls in the elderly and reduces the ability to perform activities of daily living, which results

in a loss of independence (52). Researchers are actively studying the mechanisms to explain age-related sarcopenia in hopes of the discovery of therapeutic treatments. It is important to note that regular bouts of resistance exercise remains one of the most useful and practical means to delay age-related muscle loss.

Diabetes The incidence of type II diabetes is rapidly increasing worldwide. Unfortunately, uncontrolled diabetes is associated with a progressive loss of muscle mass. Therefore, uncontrolled diabetes combined with aging has the potential to accelerate age-related loss of skeletal muscle mass (17). Notably, both aerobic and resistance exercise training have been shown to be protective against diabetes-induced muscle loss.

Cancer Up to 50% of cancer patients suffer from a rapid loss of skeletal muscle mass (74). This type of disease-related muscle loss is called cachexia (7). Cancer-mediated loss of skeletal muscle results in patient weakness and may account for up to 20% of deaths in cancer patients (34). Because of the clinical significance of cachexia,

investigators are developing methods to counteract cancer-induced cachexia. Some of the most promising therapies include regular exercise combined with nutritional interventions (44).

Muscular Dystrophy Muscular dystrophy refers to a group of hereditary muscle diseases that weaken skeletal muscles. Collectively, these diseases are characterized by defects in muscle proteins that result in a progressive muscle weakness and a loss of muscle fibers. Although more than 100 different types of muscular dystrophy exist, Duchene muscular dystrophy is the most common childhood form of this disease. The prognosis for people with muscular dystrophy varies with the type of muscular dystrophy. Some forms of muscular dystrophy can be mild and progress slowly over a normal life span. In contrast, other forms of this disorder produce severe muscle weakness along with the loss of the ability to walk and breathe without assistance. Although scientists continue to study muscular dystrophy, there are currently few clinical options to successfully treat the most severe forms of this disease.

FORCE-VELOCITY/POWER-VELOCITY RELATIONSHIPS

In most physical activities, muscular force is applied through a range of movement. For instance, an athlete performing the shot put applies force against the shot over a specified range of movement prior to release. How far the shot travels is a function of both the speed of the shot upon release and the angle of release. Because success in many athletic events is dependent on speed, it is important to appreciate some of the basic concepts underlying the relationship between muscular force and the speed of movement. The relationship between speed of movement and muscular force is shown in figure 8.19.

Two important points emerge from an examination of figure 8.19:

1. At any absolute force exerted by the muscle, the velocity or speed of movement is greater in

muscles that contain a high percentage of fast fibers when compared to muscles that possess predominantly slow fibers.

2. The maximum velocity of muscle shortening is greatest at the lowest force (i.e., resistance against the muscle). In short, the greatest speed of movement is generated at the lowest workloads (11, 42). This principle holds true for both slow and fast fibers.

What is the physiological explanation for the force-velocity curve? The answer lies in the analysis of the cross-bridge connections between actin and myosin. Recall that the amount of force generated by a muscle is determined by the number of cross-bridges attached between actin and myosin. Also, note that the cross-bridge connections between actin and myosin require a certain amount of time to make this connection. Therefore, during rapid muscle shortening (i.e., high velocity movement), the actin-myosin filaments move past each other at a fast rate. This rapid

Figure 8.19 Muscle force-velocity relationships. Note that at any given speed of movement, muscle groups with a high percentage of fast fibers exert more *force* than those with muscle groups that contain primarily slow fibers.

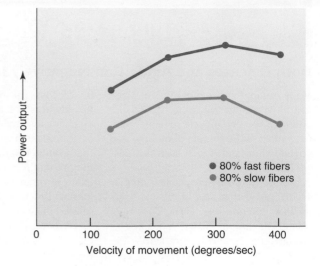

Figure 8.20 Muscle power-velocity relationships. In general, the power produced by a muscle group increases as a function of velocity of movement. At any given speed of movement, muscles that contain a large percentage of fast fibers produce more *power* than those muscles that contain primarily slow fibers.

shortening restricts the number of cross-bridges that can make a connection and therefore limits muscle force production. Conversely, as muscle shortening velocity decreases, more cross-bridges have time to connect, and muscle force production increases.

The data contained in figure 8.19 also demonstrate that fast fibers are capable of producing greater muscular force at a faster speed than slow fibers. The biochemical mechanism to explain this observation is related to the fact that fast fibers possess higher ATPase activity than do slow fibers (26, 29). Therefore, ATP is broken down more rapidly in fast fibers when compared to slow fibers. Further, calcium release from the sarcoplasmic reticulum is faster following neural stimulation in fast fibers than in slow fibers (29, 60).

The relationship between force and movement speed has practical importance for the physical therapist, athlete, or physical educator. The message is simply that athletes who possess a high percentage of fast fibers would seem to have an advantage in power-type athletic events. This may explain why successful sprinters and weight lifters typically possess a relatively high percentage of fast fibers.

As might be expected, the fiber-type make-up of a muscle influences the power-velocity curve (see figure 8.20). The peak power that can be generated by muscle is greater in muscle that contains a high percentage of fast fibers than in muscle that is largely composed of slow fibers. As with the force-velocity curve, two important points should be retained from the examination of the power-velocity curve:

1. At any given velocity of movement, the peak power generated is greater in muscle that contains a high percentage of fast fibers than in muscle with a high percentage of slow fibers. This difference is due to the aforementioned biochemical differences between fast and slow

fibers. Again, athletes who possess a high percentage of fast fibers can generate more power than athletes with predominantly slow fibers.

2. The peak power generated by any muscle increases with increasing velocities of movement up to a movement speed of 200 to 300 degrees/second. The reason for the plateau of power output with increasing movement speed is that muscular force decreases with increasing speed of movement (see figure 8.19). Therefore, with any given muscle group there is an optimum speed of movement that will elicit the greatest power output.

IN SUMMARY

- The amount of force generated during muscular contraction is dependent on the following factors: (1) types and number of motor units recruited, (2) the initial muscle length, and (3) the nature of the motor units' neural stimulation.
- The addition of muscle twitches is termed *summation*. When the frequency of neural stimulation to a motor unit is increased, individual contractions are fused in a sustained contraction called *tetanus*.
- The peak force generated by muscle decreases as the speed of movement increases. However, in general, the amount of power generated by a muscle group increases as a function of movement velocity.

STUDY QUESTIONS

1. List the principal functions of skeletal muscles.
2. List the principal proteins contained in skeletal muscle.
3. Outline the contractile process. Use a step-by-step format illustrating the entire process, beginning with the nerve impulse reaching the neuromuscular junction.
4. Outline the mechanical and biochemical properties of human skeletal muscle fiber types.
5. Discuss those factors thought to be responsible for regulating force during muscular contractions.
6. Define the term *summation*.
7. Graph a simple muscle twitch and a contraction that results in tetanus.
8. Discuss the relationship between force and speed of movement during a muscular contraction.

SUGGESTED READINGS

Cairns, S., A. Knicker, M. Thompson, and G. Sjogaard. 2005. Evaluation of models used to study neuromuscular fatigue. *Exercise and Sport Science Reviews* 33:9–16.

Fox, S. 2010. *Human Physiology*. New York: McGraw-Hill Companies.

Harridge, S. D. R. 2007. Plasticity of human skeletal muscle: Gene expression to in vivo function. *Experimental Physiology* 92(5):783–97.

Leiber, R. 2010. *Skeletal Muscle Structure, Function, and Plasticity: The Physiological Basis of Rehabilitation*. New York: Lippincott Williams & Wilkins.

MacIntosh, B., P. Gardiner, and A. McComas. 2005. *Skeletal Muscle-Form and Function*. Champaign, IL: Human Kinetics Publishers.

Segerstrom A. B. et al. 2011. Relation between cycling exercise capacity, fiber-type composition, and lower extremity muscle strength and muscle endurance. *J Strength Cond Res* 25: 16–22.

Widmaier, E., H. Raff, and K. Strang. 2010. *Vander's Human Physiology* (10th ed.). New York: McGraw-Hill Companies.

REFERENCES

1. **Allen DL, Roy RR, and Edgerton VR.** Myonuclear domains in muscle adaptation and disease. *Muscle Nerve* 22: 1350–1360, 1999.
2. **Ament W, and Verkerke GJ.** Exercise and fatigue. *Sports Med* 39: 389–422, 2009.
3. **Armstrong R.** Differential inter- and intramuscular responses to exercise: considerations in use of the biopsy technique. In: *Biochemistry of Exercise*, edited by Knuttgen H, Vogel J, and Poortmans J. Champaign: Human Kinetics, 1983.
4. **Armstrong R, and Laughlin H.** Muscle function during locomotion in mammals. In: *Circulation, Respiration, and Metabolism*, edited by Giles R. New York: Springer-Verlag, 1985, p. 56–63.
5. **Baldwin KM, Klinkerfuss GH, Terjung RL, Mole PA, and Holloszy JO.** Respiratory capacity of white, red, and intermediate muscle: adaptative response to exercise. *Am J Physiol* 222: 373–378, 1972.
6. **Bar A, and Pette D.** Three fast myosin heavy chains in adult rat skeletal muscle. *FEBS Lett* 235: 153–155, 1988.
7. **Bennani-Baiti N, and Walsh D.** What is cancer anorexia-cachexia syndrome? A historical perspective. *The Journal of the Royal College of Physicians of Edinburgh* 39: 257–262, 2009.
8. **Bergeron MF.** Exertional heat cramps: recovery and return to play. *J Sport Rehabil* 16: 190–196, 2007.
9. **Bergeron MF.** Heat cramps: fluid and electrolyte challenges during tennis in the heat. *J Sci Med Sport* 6: 19–27, 2003.
10. **Billeter R, and Hoppeler H.** Muscular basis of strength. In: *Strength and Power in Sport*, edited by Komi P. Oxford: Blackwell scientific Publishing, 1992.
11. **Bobbert MF, Ettema GC, and Huijing PA.** The force-length relationship of a muscle-tendon complex: experimental results and model calculations. *Eur J Appl Physiol Occup Physiol* 61: 323–329, 1990.
12. **Booth FW, and Thomason DB.** Molecular and cellular adaptation of muscle in response to exercise: perspectives of various models. *Physiol Rev* 71: 541–585, 1991.
13. **Bottinelli R, Canepari M, Reggiani C, and Stienen GJ.** Myofibrillar ATPase activity during isometric contraction and isomyosin composition in rat single skinned muscle fibres. *J Physiol* 481 (Pt 3): 663–675, 1994.
14. **Brooks G, Fahey T, White T, and Baldwin KM.** *Exercise Physiology: Human Bioenergetics and Its Applications.* New York: McGraw-Hill, 1985.
15. **Brooks G, Fahey T, White T, and Baldwin KM.** *Fundamentals of Human Performance.* New York: Macmillan, 1987.
16. **Buchthal F, and Schmalbruch H.** Contraction times and fibre types in intact human muscle. *Acta Physiol Scand* 79: 435–452, 1970.
17. **Buford TW, Anton SD, Judge AR, Marzetti E, Wohlgemuth SE, Carter CS, Leeuwenburgh C, Pahor M, and Manini TM.** Models of accelerated sarcopenia: critical pieces for solving the puzzle of age-related muscle atrophy. *Ageing Research Reviews* 9: 369–383, 2010.
18. **Burke R.** The control of muscle force: motor unit recruitment and firing pattern. In: *Human Muscle Power*, edited by Jones N, McCartney N, and McComas A. Champaign: Human Kinetics, 1986.
19. **Canepari M, Pellegrino MA, D'Antona G, and Bottinelli R.** Single muscle fiber properties in aging and disuse. *Scand J Med Sci Sports* 20: 10–19, 2010.
20. **Carlson F, and Wilkie D.** *Muscle Physiology.* Englewood Cliffs: Prentice-Hall, 1974.
21. **Conley KE.** Cellular energetics during exercise. *Adv Vet Sci Comp Med* 38A: 1–39, 1994.
22. **Costill DL, Fink WJ, and Pollock ML.** Muscle fiber composition and enzyme activities of elite distance runners. *Med Sci Sports* 8: 96–100, 1976.
23. **Coyle EF, Sidossis LS, Horowitz JF, and Beltz JD.** Cycling efficiency is related to the percentage of type I muscle fibers. *Med Sci Sports Exerc* 24: 782–788, 1992.
24. **D'Antona G, Lanfranconi F, Pellegrino MA, Brocca L, Adami R, Rossi R, Moro G, Miotti D, Canepari M, and Bottinelli R.** Skeletal muscle hypertrophy and structure and function of skeletal muscle fibres in male body builders. *J Physiol* 570: 611–627, 2006.

25. **Ebashi S.** Excitation-contraction coupling and the mechanism of muscle contraction. *Annu Rev Physiol* 53: 1–16, 1991.

26. **Edgerton V.** Morphological basis of skeletal muscle power output. In: *Human Muscle Power*, edited by Jones N, McCartney N, and McComas A. Champaign: Human Kinetics, 1986, p. 43–58.

27. **Edgerton V.** Muscle fiber activation and recruitment. In: *Biochemistry of Exercise*, edited by Knuttgen H, Vogel J, and Poortmans J. Champaign: Human Kinetics, 1983.

28. **Edman K.** Contractile performance of skeletal muscle fibers. In: *Strength and Power in Sport*, edited by Komi P. Oxford: Blackwell scientific Publishing, 1992, p. 96–114.

29. **Faulker J, Claflin D, and McCully K.** Power output of fast and slow fibers from human skeletal muscles. In: *Human Muscle Power*, edited by Jones N, McCartney N, and McComas A. Champaign: Human Kinetics, 1986.

30. **Fitts RH.** The cross-bridge cycle and skeletal muscle fatigue. *J Appl Physiol* 104: 551–558, 2008.

31. **Geeves MA, and Holmes KC.** The molecular mechanism of muscle contraction. *Adv Protein Chem* 71: 161–193, 2005.

32. **Gollnick PD, and Saltin B.** Significance of skeletal muscle oxidative enzyme enhancement with endurance training. *Clin Physiol* 2: 1–12, 1982.

33. **Green H.** Muscle power: fiber type recruitment, metabolism, and fatigue. In: *Human Muscle Power*, edited by Jones N, McCartney N, and McComas A. Champaign: Human Kinetics, 1986.

34. **Gullett N, Rossi P, Kucuk O, and Johnstone PA.** Cancer-induced cachexia: a guide for the oncologist. *Journal of the Society for Integrative Oncology* 7: 155–169, 2009.

35. **Gunning P, and Hardeman E.** Multiple mechanisms regulate muscle fiber diversity. *Faseb J* 5: 3064–3070, 1991.

36. **Holloszy JO.** Muscle metabolism during exercise. *Arch Phys Med Rehabil* 63: 231–234, 1982.

37. **Holmes KC.** The swinging lever-arm hypothesis of muscle contraction. *Curr Biol* 7: R112–118, 1997.

38. **Holmes KC, and Geeves MA.** The structural basis of muscle contraction. *Philosophical Transactions of the Royal Society of London* 355: 419–431, 2000.

39. **Holmes KC, Schroder RR, Sweeney HL, and Houdusse A.** The structure of the rigor complex and its implications for the power stroke. *Philosophical Transactions of the Royal Society of London* 359: 1819–1828, 2004.

40. **Huxley HE.** Past, present and future experiments on muscle. *Philosophical Transactions of the Royal Society of London* 355: 539–543, 2000.

41. **Kodama T.** Thermodynamic analysis of muscle ATPase mechanisms. *Physiol Rev* 65: 467–551, 1985.

42. **Kojima T.** Force-velocity relationship of human elbow flexors in voluntary isotonic contraction under heavy loads. *Int J Sports Med* 12: 208–213, 1991.

43. **Lieber RL.** *Skeletal Muscle Structure, Function, and Plasticity.* Philadelphia: Lippincott Williams and Wilkins, 2010.

44. **Lowe SS.** Physical activity and palliative cancer care. *Recent Results in Cancer Research (Fortschritte der Krebsforschung)* 186: 349–365, 2011.

45. **Lowey S.** Cardiac and skeletal muscle myosin polymorphism. *Med Sci Sports Exerc* 18: 284–291, 1986.

46. **MacIntosh B, Gardiner P, and McComas A.** *Skeletal Muscle—Form and Function.* Champaign: Human Kinetics, 2005.

47. **Mantilla CB, Sill RV, Aravamudan B, Zhan WZ, and Sieck GC.** Developmental effects on myonuclear domain size of rat diaphragm fibers. *J Appl Physiol* 104: 787–794, 2008.

48. **McArdle W, Katch F, and Katch V.** *Exercise Physiology: Energy, Nutrition, and Human Performance.* Baltimore: Lippincott Williams & Wilkins, 2001.

49. **McClung JM, Kavazis AN, DeRuisseau KC, Falk DJ, Deering MA, Lee Y, Sugiura T, and Powers SK.** Caspase-3 regulation of diaphragm myonuclear domain during mechanical ventilation-induced atrophy. *Am J Respir Crit Care Med* 175: 150–159, 2007.

50. **Metzger J.** Mechanism of chemomechanical coupling in skeletal muscle during work. In: *Energy Metabolism in Exercise and Sport*, edited by Lamb D, and Gisolfi C. New York: McGraw-Hill, 1992, p. 1–43.

51. **Moss RL, Diffee GM, and Greaser ML.** Contractile properties of skeletal muscle fibers in relation to myofibrillar protein isoforms. *Rev Physiol Biochem Pharmacol* 126: 1–63, 1995.

52. **Narici MV, and Maffulli N.** Sarcopenia: characteristics, mechanisms and functional significance. *British Medical Bulletin* 95: 139–159, 2010.

53. **Noakes TD, and St Clair Gibson A.** Logical limitations to the "catastrophe" models of fatigue during exercise in humans. *Br J Sports Med* 38: 648–649, 2004.

54. **Pette D.** *Plasticity of Muscle.* New York: Walter de Gruyter, 1980.

55. **Pette D, and Spamer C.** Metabolic properties of muscle fibers. *Fed Proc* 45: 2910–2914, 1986.

56. **Pette D, and Staron RS.** Cellular and molecular diversities of mammalian skeletal muscle fibers. *Rev Physiol Biochem Pharmacol* 116: 1–76, 1990.

57. **Powers SK, Criswell D, Herb RA, Demirel H, and Dodd S.** Age-related increases in diaphragmatic maximal shortening velocity. *J Appl Physiol* 80: 445–451, 1996.

58. **Rayment I, Holden HM, Whittaker M, Yohn CB, Lorenz M, Holmes KC, and Milligan RA.** Structure of the actin-myosin complex and its implications for muscle contraction. *Science* 261: 58–65, 1993.

59. **Ruegg J.** *Calcium in Muscle Activation.* Berlin: Springer-Verlag, 1992.

60. **Ruegg JC.** Excitation-contraction coupling in fast- and slow-twitch muscle fibers. *Int J Sports Med* 8: 360–364, 1987.

61. **Saladin K.** *Anatomy and Physiology.* Boston: McGraw-Hill, 2010.

62. **Saltin B, and Gollnick PD.** Skeletal muscle adaptability: significance for metabolism and performance. In: *Handbook of Physiology*, edited by Peachy L, Adrian R, and Geiger S. Bethesda: American Physiological Society, 1983.

63. **Sant'Ana Pereira J, Ennion S, Moorman A, Goldspink G, and Sargeant A.** The predominant fast myHC's in human skeletal muscle corresponds to the rat IIa and IIx and not IIb (A26). In: *Annual Meeting of Society for Neuroscience*, 1994.

64. **Schiaffino S, Gorza L, Sartore S, Saggin L, Ausoni S, Vianello M, Gundersen K, and Lomo T.** Three myosin heavy chain isoforms in type 2 skeletal muscle fibres. *J Muscle Res Cell Motil* 10: 197–205, 1989.

65. **Schiaffino S, and Reggiani C.** Myosin isoforms in mammalian skeletal muscle. *J Appl Physiol* 77: 493–501, 1994.

66. **Schwellnus MP.** Cause of exercise associated muscle cramps (EAMC)—altered neuromuscular control, dehydration or electrolyte depletion? *Br J Sports Med* 43: 401–408, 2009.

67. **Schwellnus MP, Derman EW, and Noakes TD.** Aetiology of skeletal muscle "cramps" during exercise: a novel hypothesis. *J Sports Sci* 15: 277–285, 1997.

68. **Segerstrom AB, Holmback AM, Hansson O, Elgzyri T, Eriksson KF, Ringsberg K, Groop L, Wollmer P, and Thorsson O.** Relation between cycling exercise capacity, fiber-type composition, and lower extremity muscle strength and muscle endurance. J *Strength Cond Res* 25: 16–22, 2011.

69. **Sellers JR.** Fifty years of contractility research post sliding filament hypothesis. J *Muscle Res Cell Motil* 25: 475–482, 2004.

70. **Simoneau JA, Lortie G, Boulay MR, Marcotte M, Thibault MC, and Bouchard C.** Inheritance of human skeletal muscle and anaerobic capacity adaptation to high-intensity intermittent training. *Int J Sports Med* 7: 167–171, 1986.

71. **Snow D, and Harris R.** Thoroughbreds and greyhounds: biochemical adaptations in creatures of nature and man. In: *Circulation, Respiration, and Metabolism*, edited by Giles R. New York: Springer-Verlag, 1985, p. 227–239.

72. **Tate CA, Hyek MF, and Taffet GE.** The role of calcium in the energetics of contracting skeletal muscle. *Sports Med* 12: 208–217, 1991.

73. **Tesch PA, Thorsson A, and Kaiser P.** Muscle capillary supply and fiber type characteristics in weight and power lifters. J *Appl Physiol* 56: 35–38, 1984.

74. **Tisdale MJ.** Mechanisms of cancer cachexia. *Physiol Rev* 89: 381–410, 2009.

75. **Vale RD.** Getting a grip on myosin. *Cell* 78: 733–737, 1994.

76. **Vandenboom R.** The myofibrillar complex and fatigue: a review. *Can J Appl Physiol* 29: 330–356, 2004.

77. **Vinciguerra M, Musaro A, and Rosenthal N.** Regulation of muscle atrophy in aging and disease. *Adv Exp Med Biol* 694: 211–233, 2010.

78. **Westerblad H, and Allen DG.** Cellular mechanisms of skeletal muscle fatigue. *Adv Exp Med Biol* 538: 563–570; discussion 571, 2003.

79. **White RB, Bierinx AS, Gnocchi VF, and Zammit PS.** Dynamics of muscle fibre growth during postnatal mouse development. BMC *Developmental Biology* 10: 21, 2010.

80. **Wilmore J, and Costill DL.** *Training for Sport and Activity: The Physiological Basis of the Conditioning Process.* Champaign: Human Kinetics, 1993.

81. **Wozniak AC, Kong J, Bock E, Pilipowicz O, and Anderson JE.** Signaling satellite-cell activation in skeletal muscle: markers, models, stretch, and potential alternate pathways. *Muscle Nerve* 31: 283–300, 2005.

9

Circulatory Responses to Exercise

■ Objectives

By studying this chapter, you should be able to do the following:

1. Give an overview of the design and function of the circulatory system.
2. Describe the cardiac cycle and the associated electrical activity recorded via the electro-cardiogram.
3. Discuss the pattern of redistribution of blood flow during exercise.
4. Outline the circulatory responses to various types of exercise.
5. Identify the factors that regulate local blood flow during exercise.
6. List and discuss those factors responsible for regulation of stroke volume during exercise.
7. Discuss the regulation of cardiac output during exercise.

■ Outline

■ Key Terms

arteries
arterioles
atrioventricular node (AV node)
autoregulation
capillaries
cardiac accelerator nerves
cardiac output
cardiovascular control center
central command
diastole
diastolic blood pressure
double product
electrocardiogram (ECG)
heart rate variability
intercalated discs
mixed venous blood
myocardium
pulmonary circuit
sinoatrial node (SA node)
stroke volume
systole
systolic blood pressure
vagus nerve
veins
venules

William Harvey Developed the First Complete Theory of the Circulatory System

William Harvey (1578–1657) was born in Flokestone, England, in 1578. He was educated at both King's College and the University of Cambridge. He later studied medicine at the University of Padua in Italy. After completion of his medical studies in 1602, he returned to England and quickly became a fellow of the Royal College of Physicians and later served as the personal physician of King James I in 1618.

Dr. Harvey was fascinated by anatomical studies, and King James I encouraged him to pursue research to improve the practice of medicine. As a researcher, William Harvey made many important discoveries about how the cardiovascular system operates. First, by observing the action of the heart in small animals, Harvey proved that the heart expels blood during each contraction. Further, he also discovered that valves exist in veins and correctly identified them as restricting the flow of blood in one direction. Dr. Harvey's work on the circulatory system was summarized in a book published in 1628 titled *An Anatomical Study of the Motion of the Heart and of the Blood in Animals*. This text explained Harvey's theories on how the heart propelled blood through a circular course throughout the body and was the first published record to accurately describe how the circulatory system works in humans and other animals.

One of the major challenges to homeostasis posed by exercise is the increased muscular demand for oxygen; during heavy exercise the demand may be fifteen to twenty-five times greater than at rest. The primary purpose of the cardiorespiratory system is to deliver adequate amounts of oxygen and remove wastes from body tissues. Further, the circulatory system also transports nutrients and aids in temperature regulation. It is important to remember that the respiratory system and the circulatory system function together as a "coupled unit"; the respiratory system adds oxygen and removes carbon dioxide from the blood, while the circulatory system is responsible for the delivery of oxygenated blood and nutrients to tissues in accordance with their needs. In simple terms, the "cardiopulmonary system" works as a unit to maintain oxygen and carbon dioxide homeostasis in body tissues. A British physician, William Harvey, proposed the first complete theory about how the cardiovascular system works in humans (see A Look Back—Important People in Science).

To meet the increased oxygen demands of muscle during exercise, two major adjustments of blood flow must be made: (1) an increased **cardiac output** (i.e., increased amount of blood pumped per minute by the heart) and (2) a redistribution of blood flow from inactive organs to the active skeletal muscles. However, while the needs of the muscles are being met, other tissues, such as the brain, cannot be denied blood flow. This is accomplished by maintaining blood pressure, the driving force behind blood flow. A thorough understanding of the cardiovascular responses to exercise is important for the student of exercise physiology. Therefore, this chapter describes the design and function of the circulatory system and how it responds during exercise.

ORGANIZATION OF THE CIRCULATORY SYSTEM

The human circulatory system is a closed loop that circulates blood to all body tissues. Circulation of blood requires the action of a muscular pump, the heart, that creates the "pressure head" needed to move blood through the system. Blood travels away from the heart in **arteries** and returns to the heart by way of **veins.** The system is considered "closed" because arteries and veins are continuous with each other through smaller vessels. Arteries branch extensively to form a "tree" of smaller vessels. As the vessels become microscopic they form **arterioles,** which eventually develop into "beds" of much smaller vessels called **capillaries.** Capillaries are the smallest and most numerous of blood vessels; all exchanges of oxygen, carbon dioxide, and nutrients between tissues and the circulatory system occur across capillary beds. Blood passes from capillary beds to small venous vessels called **venules.** As venules move back toward the heart, they increase in size and become veins. Major veins empty directly into the heart. The mixture of venous blood from both the upper and lower body that accumulates in the right side of the heart is termed **mixed venous blood.** Mixed venous blood therefore represents an average of venous blood from the entire body.

Structure of the Heart

The heart is divided into four chambers and is often considered to be two pumps in one. The right atrium and right ventricle form the right pump, and the left atrium and left ventricle combine to make the left

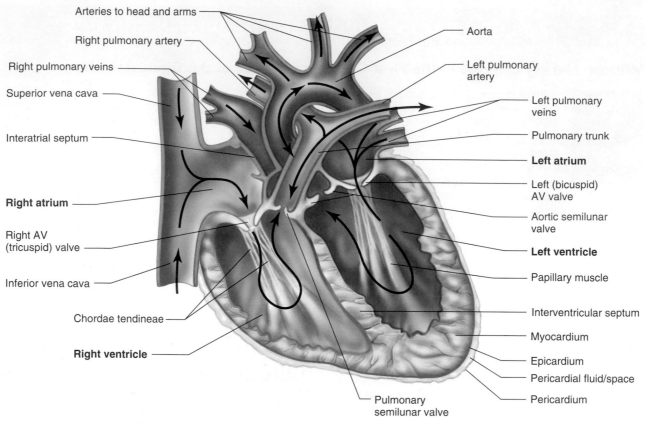

Labels (left side, top to bottom):
Arteries to head and arms
Right pulmonary artery
Right pulmonary veins
Superior vena cava
Interatrial septum
Right atrium
Right AV (tricuspid) valve
Inferior vena cava
Chordae tendineae
Right ventricle

Labels (right side, top to bottom):
Aorta
Left pulmonary artery
Left pulmonary veins
Pulmonary trunk
Left atrium
Left (bicuspid) AV valve
Aortic semilunar valve
Left ventricle
Papillary muscle
Interventricular septum
Myocardium
Epicardium
Pericardial fluid/space
Pericardium

Label (bottom):
Pulmonary semilunar valve

Figure 9.1 Anterior view of the heart.

pump (see figure 9.1). The right side of the heart is separated from the left side by a muscular wall called the interventricular septum. This septum prevents the mixing of blood from the two sides of the heart.

Blood movement within the heart is from the atria to the ventricles, and from the ventricles blood is pumped into the arteries. To prevent backward movement of blood, the heart contains four one-way valves. The right and left atrioventricular valves connect the atria with the right and left ventricles, respectively (figure 9.1). These valves are also known as the tricuspid valve (right atrioventricular valve) and the bicuspid valve (left atrioventricular valve). Backflow from the arteries into the ventricles is prevented by the pulmonary semilunar valve (right ventricle) and the aortic semilunar valve (left ventricle).

Pulmonary and Systemic Circuits

As mentioned previously, the heart can be considered as two pumps in one. The right side of the heart pumps blood that is partially depleted of its oxygen content and contains an elevated carbon dioxide content as a result of gas exchange in the various tissues of the body. This blood is delivered from the right heart into the lungs through the **pulmonary circuit.** At the lungs, oxygen is loaded into the blood and

carbon dioxide is released. This "oxygenated" blood then travels to the left side of the heart and is pumped to the various tissues of the body via the systemic circuit (figure 9.2).

IN SUMMARY

- The purposes of the cardiovascular system are the following: (1) the transport of O_2 to tissues and removal of wastes, (2) the transport of nutrients to tissues, and (3) the regulation of body temperature.
- The heart is two pumps in one. The right side of the heart pumps blood through the pulmonary circulation, and the left side of the heart delivers blood to the systemic circulation.

HEART: MYOCARDIUM AND CARDIAC CYCLE

To better appreciate how the circulatory system adjusts to the stress of exercise, it is important to understand elementary details of heart muscle structure as well as the electrical and mechanical activities of the heart.

O₂

CO₂

Pulmonary circuit

O₂-poor,
CO₂-rich
blood

O₂-rich,
CO₂-poor
blood

Systemic circuit

CO₂

O₂

Figure 9.2 Illustration of the systemic and pulmonary circulations. As depicted by the color change from blue to red, blood becomes fully oxygenated as it flows through the lungs and then loses some oxygen (color changes from red to blue) as it flows through the other organs and tissues.

Myocardium

The wall of the heart is composed of three layers: (1) an outer layer called the epicardium, (2) a muscular middle layer, the myocardium, and (3) an inner layer

known as the endocardium (see figure 9.3). It is the **myocardium,** or heart muscle, that is responsible for contracting and forcing blood out of the heart. The myocardium receives its blood supply via the right and left coronary arteries, which branch off the aorta and encircle the heart. The coronary veins run alongside the arteries and drain all coronary blood into a larger vein called the coronary sinus, which deposits blood into the right atrium.

Maintaining a constant blood supply to the heart via the coronary arteries is critical because, even at rest, the heart has a high demand for oxygen and nutrients. When coronary blood flow is disrupted (i.e., blockage of a coronary blood vessel) for more than several minutes, permanent damage to the heart occurs. This type of injury results in the death of cardiac muscle cells and is commonly called a heart attack, or myocardial infarction (see chapter 17). The number of heart cells that die from this insult determines the severity of a heart attack. That is, a "mild" heart attack may damage only a small portion of the heart, whereas a "major" heart attack may destroy a large number of heart cells (fibers). A major heart attack greatly diminishes the heart's pumping capacity; therefore, minimizing the amount of injury to the heart during a heart attack is important. Importantly, strong evidence indicates that exercise training can provide cardiac protection during a heart attack (see Clinical Applications 9.1).

Heart muscle differs from skeletal muscle in several ways. First, cardiac muscle fibers are shorter than skeletal muscle fibers and are connected in a tight series. Further, cardiac fibers are typically branched, whereas skeletal muscle fibers are elongated and do not branch. Also, cardiac muscle contraction is involuntary, whereas skeletal muscle contractions are under voluntary control.

Another difference between cardiac fibers and skeletal muscle fibers is that, unlike skeletal muscle fibers, heart muscle fibers are all interconnected via **intercalated discs.** These intercellular connections permit the transmission of electrical impulses from one fiber to another. Intercalated discs are nothing more than leaky membranes that allow ions to cross from one fiber to another. Therefore, when one heart fiber is depolarized to contract, all connecting heart fibers also become excited and contract as a unit. This arrangement is called a functional syncytium. Heart muscle cells in the atria are separated from ventricular muscle cells by a layer of connective tissue that does not permit the transmission of electrical impulses. Hence, the atria contract separately from the ventricles.

One more difference between heart and skeletal muscle fibers is that human heart fibers cannot be divided into different fiber types. The ventricular myocardium is considered to be a homogenous

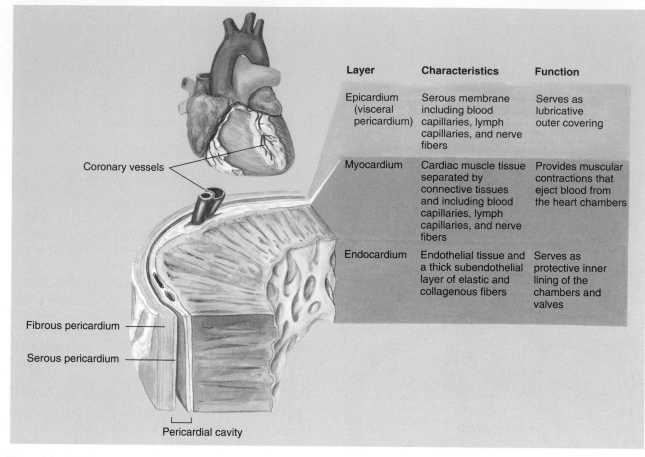

Layer	Characteristics	Function
Epicardium (visceral pericardium)	Serous membrane including blood capillaries, lymph capillaries, and nerve fibers	Serves as lubricative outer covering
Myocardium	Cardiac muscle tissue separated by connective tissues and including blood capillaries, lymph capillaries, and nerve fibers	Provides muscular contractions that eject blood from the heart chambers
Endocardium	Endothelial tissue and a thick subendothelial layer of elastic and collagenous fibers	Serves as protective inner lining of the chambers and valves

Coronary vessels

Fibrous pericardium

Serous pericardium

Pericardial cavity

Figure 9.3 The heart wall is composed of three distinct layers: (1) epicardium, (2) myocardium, and (3) endocardium.

muscle containing one primary fiber type that has similarities to the type I, slow fibers found in skeletal muscle. In this regard, heart muscle fibers are highly aerobic and contain large numbers of mitochondria. Note, however, that cardiac muscle fibers contain many more mitochondria than type I, slow skeletal muscle fibers. This fact highlights the importance of continuous aerobic metabolism in the heart.

Although heart muscle and skeletal muscle differ in many ways, they are also similar in several ways. For example, both heart and skeletal muscle fibers are striated and contain the same contractile proteins: actin and myosin. Further, both heart and skeletal muscle fibers require calcium to activate the myofilaments (17), and both fibers contract via the sliding filament model of contraction (see chapter 8). In addition, like skeletal muscle, heart muscle can alter its force of contraction as a function of the degree of overlap of actin-myosin filaments due to changes in fiber length. Table 9.1 contains a point-by-point comparison of the structural/functional similarities and differences between cardiac and skeletal muscle fibers.

Cardiac Cycle

The cardiac cycle refers to the repeating pattern of contraction and relaxation of the heart. The contraction phase is called **systole** and the relaxation period is called **diastole.** Generally, when these terms are used alone, they refer to contraction and relaxation of the ventricles. However, note that the atria also contract and relax; therefore, there is an atrial systole and diastole. Atrial contraction occurs during ventricular diastole, and atrial relaxation occurs during ventricular systole. The heart thus has a two-step pumping action. The right and left atria contract together, which empties atrial blood into the ventricles. Approximately 0.1 second after the atrial contraction, the ventricles contract and deliver blood into both the systemic and pulmonary circuits.

At rest, contraction of the ventricles during systole ejects about two-thirds of the blood in the ventricles, leaving about one-third in the ventricles. The ventricles then fill with blood during the next diastole. A healthy twenty-one-year-old female might have an average resting heart rate of 75 beats per minute. This means that the total cardiac cycle lasts 0.8 second,

CLINICAL APPLICATIONS 9.1

Exercise Training Protects the Heart

It is now well established that regular exercise training is cardioprotective. Indeed, many epidemiological studies have provided evidence that regular exercise can reduce the incidence of heart attacks and that the survival rate of heart attack victims is greater in active people than in sedentary ones. Recent experiments provide direct evidence that regular endurance exercise training reduces the amount of cardiac damage that occurs during a heart attack (26, 28, 29). The protective effect of exercise is illustrated in figure 9.4. Notice that exercise training can reduce the magnitude of cardiac injury during a heart attack by approximately 60%. This is significant because the number of cardiac cells that are destroyed during a heart attack determines the patient's chances of a full, functional recovery.

Animal experiments indicate that exercise-induced protection against myocardial injury during a heart attack can be achieved quickly (29). For example, it appears that as few as 3–5 consecutive days of aerobic exercise (~60 minutes/day) can provide significant cardiac protection against heart attack-mediated damage to the heart muscle (29).

How does exercise training alter the heart and provide cardioprotection during a heart attack? A definitive answer to this question is not available. Nonetheless, evidence suggests that the exercise-training induced improvement in the heart's ability to resist permanent injury during a heart attack is linked to improvements in the heart's antioxidant capacity (i.e., the ability to remove free radicals) (26, 28, 29). Furthermore, recent evidence suggests that alterations in cardiac mitochondria also play a role in exercise-induced cardioprotection (18). For more details see Powers et al. (2008) in the Suggested Readings.

FIGURE 9.4 Regular endurance exercise protects the heart against cell death during a heart attack. Note that during a myocardial infarction (i.e., heart attack), exercise trained individuals suffer significantly less cardiac injury compared to untrained individuals. Data are from reference 88.

TABLE 9.1	A Comparison of the Structural and Functional Differences/Similarities Between Heart Muscle and Skeletal Muscle	
Structural Comparison	**Heart Muscle**	**Skeletal Muscle**
Contractile proteins: actin and myosin	Present	Present
Shape of muscle fibers	Shorter than skeletal muscle fibers and branching	Elongated—no branching
Nuclei	Single	Multiple
Z discs	Present	Present
Striated	Yes	Yes
Cellular junctions	Yes—intercalated discs	No junctional complexes
Connective tissue	Endomysium	Epimysium, perimysium, and endomysium
Functional Comparison		
Energy production	Aerobic (primarily)	Aerobic and anaerobic
Calcium source (for contraction)	Sarcoplasmic reticulum and extracellular calcium	Sarcoplasmic reticulum
Neural control	Involuntary	Voluntary
Regeneration potential	None—no satellite cells present	Some possibilities via satellite cells

Figure 9.5 Increases in heart rate during exercise are achieved primarily through a decrease in the time spent in diastole; however, at high heart rates, the length of time spent in systole also decreases.

with 0.5 second spent in diastole and the remaining 0.3 second dedicated to systole (17) (see figure 9.5). If the heart rate increases from 75 beats per minute to 180 beats per minute (e.g., heavy exercise), there is a reduction in the time spent in both systole and diastole (11). This point is illustrated in figure 9.5. Note that a rising heart rate results in a greater time reduction in diastole, whereas systole is less affected.

Pressure Changes During the Cardiac Cycle During the cardiac cycle, the pressure within the heart chambers rises and falls. When the atria are relaxed, blood flows into them from the venous circulation. As these chambers fill, the pressure inside gradually increases. Approximately 70% of the blood entering the atria during diastole flows directly into the ventricles through the atrioventricular valves before the atria contract. Upon atrial contraction, atrial pressure rises and forces most of the remaining 30% of the atrial blood into the ventricles.

Pressure in the ventricles is low while they are filling, but when the atria contract, the ventricular pressure increases slightly. Then as the ventricles contract, the pressure rises sharply, which closes the atrioventricular valves and prevents backflow into the atria. As soon as ventricular pressure exceeds the pressure of the pulmonary artery and the aorta, the pulmonary and aortic valves open and blood is forced into both pulmonary and systemic circulations. Figure 9.6 illustrates the changes in ventricular pressure as a function of time during the resting cardiac cycle. Note the occurrence of two heart sounds that are produced by the closing of the atrioventricular valves (first heart sound) and the closing of the aortic and pulmonary valves (second heart sound).

Arterial Blood Pressure

Blood exerts pressure throughout the vascular system, but is greatest within the arteries, where it is generally measured and used as an indication of health. Blood pressure is the force exerted by blood against the arterial walls and is determined by how much blood is pumped and the resistance to blood flow.

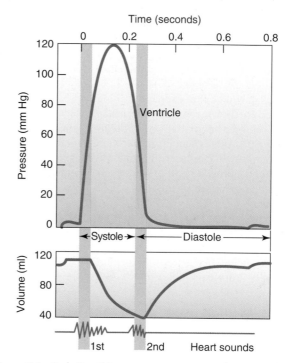

Figure 9.6 Relationship among pressure, volume, and heart sounds during the cardiac cycle. Notice the change in ventricular pressure and volume during the transition from systole to diastole.

Arterial blood pressure can be estimated by the use of a sphygmomanometer (see A Closer Look 9.1). The normal blood pressure of an adult male is 120/80, while that of adult females tends to be lower (110/70). The larger number in the expression of blood pressure is the systolic pressure expressed in millimeters of mercury (mm Hg). The lower number in the blood pressure ratio is the diastolic pressure, again expressed in mm Hg. **Systolic blood pressure** is the pressure generated as blood is ejected from the heart during ventricular systole. During ventricular relaxation (diastole), the arterial blood pressure decreases and represents **diastolic blood pressure.** The difference between systolic and diastolic blood pressure is called the pulse pressure.

The average pressure during a cardiac cycle is called *mean arterial pressure.* Mean arterial blood pressure

A CLOSER LOOK 9.1

Measurement of Arterial Blood Pressure

Arterial blood pressure is not usually measured directly but is estimated using an instrument called a sphygmomanometer (see figure 9.7). This device consists of an inflatable arm cuff connected to a column of mercury. The cuff can be inflated by a bulb pump, with the pressure in the cuff measured by the rising column of mercury. For example, a pressure of 100 mm of mercury (mm Hg) would be enough force to raise the column of mercury upward a distance of 100 mm.

Blood pressure is measured in the following way: The rubber cuff is placed around the upper arm so it surrounds the brachial artery. Air is pumped into the cuff so that the pressure around the arm exceeds arterial pressure. Because the pressure applied around the arm is greater than arterial pressure, the brachial artery is squeezed shut and blood flow is stopped. If a stethoscope is placed over the brachial artery (just below the cuff), no sounds are heard, since there is no blood flow. However, if the air control valve is slowly opened to release air, the pressure in the cuff begins to decline, and soon the pressure around the arm reaches a point that is equal to or just slightly below arterial pressure. At this point blood begins to spurt through the artery and a sharp sound (known as Korotkoff sounds) can be heard through the stethoscope. The pressure (i.e., height of mercury column) at which the first tapping sound is heard represents systolic blood pressure.

As the cuff pressure continues to decline, a series of increasingly louder sounds can be heard. When the pressure in the cuff is equal to or slightly below diastolic blood pressure, the sounds heard through the stethoscope cease. Therefore, resting diastolic blood pressure represents the height of the mercury column when the sounds disappear.

1. No sound is heard because there is no blood flow when the cuff pressure is high enough to keep the brachial artery closed.

2. **Systolic pressure** is the pressure at which a Korotkoff sound is first heard. When cuff pressure decreases and is no longer able to keep the brachial artery closed during systole, blood is pushed through the partially opened brachial artery to produce turbulent blood flow and a sound. The brachial artery remains closed during diastole.

3. As cuff pressure continues to decrease, the brachial artery opens even more during systole. At first, the artery is closed during diastole, but, as cuff pressure continues to decrease, the brachial artery partially opens during diastole. Turbulent blood flow during systole produces Korotkoff sounds, although the pitch of the sounds changes as the artery becomes more open.

4. **Diastolic pressure** is the pressure at which the sound disappears. Eventually, cuff pressure decreases below the pressure in the brachial artery and it remains open during systole and diastole. Nonturbulent flow is reestablished and no sounds are heard.

FIGURE 9.7   A sphygmomanometer is used to measure arterial blood pressure.

is important because it determines the rate of blood flow through the systemic circuit.

Determination of mean arterial pressure is not easy. It is not a simple average of systolic and diastolic pressure, because diastole generally lasts longer than systole. However, mean arterial pressure can be estimated at rest in the following way:

Mean arterial pressure = DBP + .33 (pulse pressure)

Here, DBP is the diastolic blood pressure, and the pulse pressure is the difference between systolic and diastolic pressures. Let's consider a sample calculation of mean arterial pressure at rest.

For example, suppose an individual has a blood pressure of 120/80 mm Hg. The mean arterial pressure would be:

**Mean arterial pressure = 80 mm Hg
+ .33(120 − 80)
= 80 mm Hg + 13
= 93 mm Hg**

Note that this equation cannot be used to compute mean arterial blood pressure during exercise because it is based on the timing of the cardiac cycle at rest. That is, arterial blood pressure rises during systole and falls during diastole across the cardiac cycle. Therefore, to accurately estimate the average arterial blood pressure at any time, systolic and diastolic blood pressure must be measured and the amount of time spent in both systole and diastole must be known. Recall that the time spent in systole and diastole differs between rest and exercise. For example, the formula estimates that the time spent in systole occupies 33% of the total cardiac cycle at rest. However, during maximal exercise, systole may account for 66% of the total cardiac cycle time. Therefore, any formula designed to estimate mean arterial blood pressure must be adjusted to reflect the time spent in systole and diastole.

High blood pressure (called hypertension) is classified as blood pressures above 140/90 mm HG. Unfortunately, approximately 31% of all adults (>18 years old) in the United States have hypertension (13). Hypertension is generally classified into one of two categories: (1) primary, or essential hypertension, and (2) secondary hypertension. The cause of primary hypertension is multifactorial; that is, there are several factors whose combined effects produce hypertension. This type of hypertension constitutes 95% of all reported cases of hypertension in the United States. Secondary hypertension is a result of some known disease process, and thus the hypertension is "secondary" to another disease.

Hypertension can lead to a variety of health problems. For example, hypertension increases the workload on the left ventricle, resulting in an adaptive increase in the muscle mass of the left heart (called left ventricular hypertrophy). In the early phases of hypertension-induced left ventricular hypertrophy, the increase in cardiac mass helps to maintain the heart's pumping ability. However, with time, this left ventricular hypertrophy changes the organization and function of cardiac muscle fibers, resulting in diminished pumping capacity of the heart, which can lead to heart failure. Further, the presence of hypertension is a major risk factor for developing arteriosclerosis and heart attacks. Finally, hypertension also increases the risk of kidney damage and the rupture of a cerebral blood vessel resulting in localized brain injury (i.e., a stroke).

Factors That Influence Arterial Blood Pressure

Mean arterial blood pressure is determined by two factors: (1) cardiac output and (2) total vascular resistance. Cardiac output is the amount of blood pumped from the heart, and total vascular resistance is the sum of resistance to blood flow provided by all systemic blood vessels. Mathematically, mean arterial blood pressure is defined as the product of cardiac output times total vascular resistance, as given in the following equation:

Mean arterial blood pressure = (cardiac output × total vascular resistance)

Therefore, an increase in either cardiac output or vascular resistance results in an increase in mean arterial blood pressure. In the body, mean arterial blood pressure depends on a variety of physiological factors, including cardiac output, blood volume, resistance to flow, and blood viscosity. These relationships are summarized in figure 9.8. An increase in any of these variables results in an increase in arterial blood pressure. Conversely, a decrease in any of these variables causes a decrease in blood pressure.

How is blood pressure regulated? Acute (short-term) regulation of blood pressure is achieved by the sympathetic nervous system, whereas long-term regulation of blood pressure is primarily a function of the kidneys (4). The kidneys regulate blood pressure by controlling blood volume.

Pressure receptors (called baroreceptors) in the carotid artery and the aorta are sensitive to changes in arterial blood pressure. An increase in arterial pressure triggers these receptors to send impulses to the **cardiovascular control center,** which responds by decreasing sympathetic activity. A reduction in sympathetic activity may lower cardiac output and/or reduce vascular resistance, which in turn lowers blood pressure. Conversely, a decrease in blood pressure results in a reduction of baroreceptor activity to

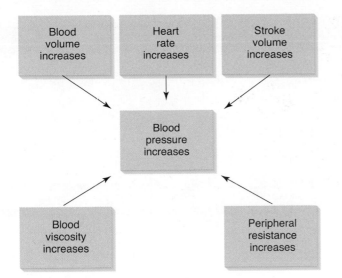

Figure 9.8 Some factors that influence arterial blood pressure.

Electrical Activity of the Heart

Many myocardial cells have the unique potential for spontaneous electrical activity (i.e., each has an intrinsic rhythm). However, in the normal heart, spontaneous electrical activity is limited to a special region located in the right atrium. This region, called the **sinoatrial node (SA node),** serves as the pacemaker for the heart (see figure 9.9). Spontaneous electrical activity in the SA node occurs due to a decay of the resting membrane potential via inward diffusion of sodium during diastole. When the SA node reaches the depolarization threshold and "fires," the wave of depolarization spreads over the atria, resulting in atrial contraction. The wave of atrial depolarization cannot directly cross into the ventricles but must be transported by way of specialized conductive tissue. This specialized conductive tissue radiates from a small mass of muscle tissue called the **atrioventricular node (AV node).** This node, located in the floor of the right atrium, connects the atria with the ventricles by a pair of conductive pathways called the *right and left bundle branches* (figure 9.9). Note that atrial-mediated depolarization of the AV node is delayed by approximately 0.10 second. This time delay is important because it allows atrial contraction to empty atrial blood into the ventricles prior to ventricular depolarization and contraction. Upon reaching the ventricles,

the brain. This causes the cardiovascular control center to respond by increasing sympathetic outflow, which raises blood pressure back to normal. For a complete discussion of blood-pressure regulation, see Courneya (2010) or Fox (2010) in the Suggested Readings.

1. Action potentials originate in the sinoatrial (SA) node (the pacemaker) and travel across the wall of the atrium (*arrows*) from the SA node to the atrioventricular (AV) node.

2. Action potentials pass through the AV node and along the atrioventricular (AV) bundle, which extends from the AV node, through the fibrous skeleton, into the interventricular septum.

3. The AV bundle divides into right and left bundle branches, and action potentials descend to the apex of each ventricle along the bundle branches.

4. Action potentials are carried by the Purkinje fibers from the bundle branches to the ventricular walls.

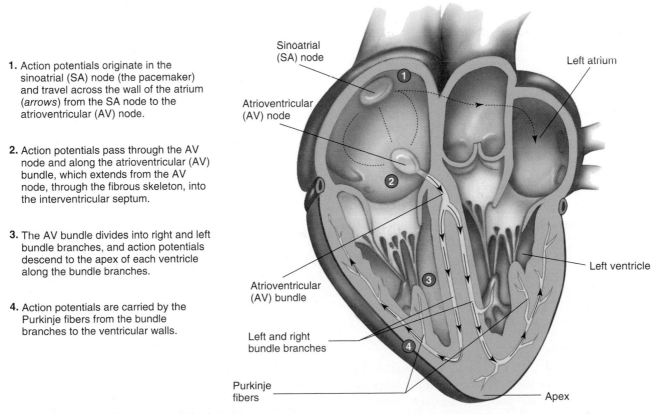

Figure 9.9 Conduction system of the heart.

A CLOSER LOOK 9.2

Diagnostic Use of the ECG During Exercise

Cardiologists are physicians who specialize in diseases of the heart and vascular system. One of the diagnostic procedures commonly used to evaluate cardiac function is to make ECG measurements during an incremental exercise test (commonly called a stress test). This allows the physician to observe changes in blood pressure as well as changes in the patient's ECG during periods of exercise-induced stress.

The most common cause of heart disease is the collection of fatty plaque (called atherosclerosis) inside coronary vessels. This collection of plaque reduces blood flow to the myocardium. The adequacy of blood flow to the heart is relative—it depends on the metabolic demand placed on the heart. An obstruction to a coronary artery, for example, may allow suffi-

cient blood flow at rest, but may be inadequate during exercise due to increased metabolic demand placed on the heart. Therefore, a graded exercise test may serve as a "stress test" to evaluate cardiac function.

An example of an abnormal exercise ECG is illustrated in figure 9.10. Myocardial ischemia (reduced blood

FIGURE 9.10
Depression of the S-T segment of the electrocardiogram as a result of myocardial ischemia.

flow) may be detected by changes in the S-T segment of the ECG. Notice the depressed S-T segment in the picture on the right when compared to the normal ECG on the left. This S-T segment depression suggests to the physician that ischemic heart disease may be present and that additional diagnostic procedures may be warranted.

these conductive pathways branch into smaller fibers called Purkinje fibers. The Purkinje fibers then spread the wave of depolarization throughout the ventricles.

A recording of the electrical changes that occur in the myocardium during the cardiac cycle is called an **electrocardiogram (ECG).** Analysis of ECG waveforms allows the physician to evaluate the heart's ability to conduct impulses and therefore determine if electrical problems exist. Further, analysis of the ECG during exercise is often used in the diagnosis of coronary artery disease (see A Closer Look 9.2). Figure 9.11 illustrates a normal ECG pattern. Notice that the ECG pattern contains several different deflections, or waves, during each cardiac cycle. Each of these distinct waveforms is identified by different letters. The first deflection on the ECG is called the P wave and represents the depolarization of the atria. The second wave, the QRS complex, represents the depolarization of the ventricles and occurs approximately 0.10 second following the P wave. The final deflection, the T wave, is the result of ventricular repolarization. Notice that atrial repolarization is usually not visible on the ECG because it occurs at the same time as the QRS complex (figure 9.12). That is, atrial repolarization is "hidden" by the QRS complex.

Finally, figure 9.13 illustrates the relationship between changes in the intraventricular pressure and the ECG. Note that the QRS complex (i.e., depolarization of the ventricles) occurs at the beginning of

systole, whereas the T wave (i.e., repolarization of the ventricles) occurs at the beginning of diastole. Also, notice that the rise in intraventricular pressure at the beginning of systole results in the first heart sound, due to closure of the atrioventricular valves (AV valves), and that the fall in intraventricular pressure at the end of systole results in the second heart sound, due to the closure of the aortic and pulmonary semilunar valves.

IN SUMMARY

- The contraction phase of the cardiac cycle is called *systole* and the relaxation period is called *diastole*.
- The pacemaker of the heart is the SA node.
- The average blood pressure during a cardiac cycle is called *mean arterial blood pressure*.
- Blood pressure can be increased by one or all of the following factors:
  a. increase in blood volume,
  b. increase in heart rate,
  c. increased blood viscosity,
  d. increase in stroke volume, and/or
  e. increased peripheral resistance.
- A recording of the electrical activity of the heart during the cardiac cycle is called the *electrocardiogram (ECG)*.

Figure 9.11 The normal electrocardiogram during rest.

CARDIAC OUTPUT

Cardiac output ($\dot{Q}$) is the product of the heart rate (HR) and the **stroke volume** (SV) (amount of blood pumped per heartbeat):

$$\dot{Q} = HR \times SV$$

Thus, cardiac output can be increased due to a rise in either heart rate or stroke volume. During exercise in the upright position (e.g., running, cycling, etc.), the increase in cardiac output is due to an increase in both heart rate and stroke volume. Table 9.2 presents typical values at rest and during maximal exercise for heart rate, stroke volume, and cardiac output in both untrained and highly trained endurance athletes. The gender differences in stroke volume and cardiac output are due mainly to differences in body sizes between men and women (2) (see table 9.2).

Regulation of Heart Rate

During exercise, the quantity of blood pumped by the heart must change in accordance with the elevated skeletal muscle oxygen demand. Because the SA node controls heart rate, changes in heart rate often involve factors that influence the SA node. The two most prominent factors that influence heart rate are the parasympathetic and sympathetic nervous systems (25).

The parasympathetic fibers that supply the heart arise from neurons in the cardiovascular control center in the medulla oblongata and make up a portion of the **vagus nerve** (4). Upon reaching the heart, these fibers make contact with both the SA node and the AV node (see figure 9.14). When stimulated, these nerve endings release acetylcholine, which causes a decrease in the activity of both the SA and AV nodes due to hyperpolarization (i.e., moving the resting membrane potential further from threshold). The end result is a reduction of heart rate. Therefore, the parasympathetic nervous system acts as a braking system to slow down heart rate.

Even at rest, the vagus nerves carry impulses to the SA and AV nodes (25). This is often referred to as parasympathetic tone. As a consequence, changes in parasympathetic activity can cause heart rate to increase or decrease. For instance, a decrease in parasympathetic tone to the heart can elevate heart rate, whereas an increase in parasympathetic activity causes a slowing of heart rate.

Key

■ Wave of depolarization

■ Wave of repolarization

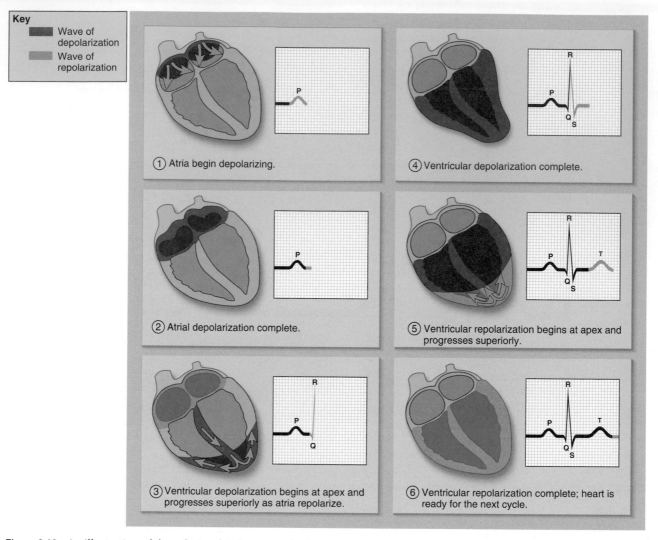

① Atria begin depolarizing.

② Atrial depolarization complete.

③ Ventricular depolarization begins at apex and progresses superiorly as atria repolarize.

④ Ventricular depolarization complete.

⑤ Ventricular repolarization begins at apex and progresses superiorly.

⑥ Ventricular repolarization complete; heart is ready for the next cycle.

Figure 9.12 An illustration of the relationship between the heart's electrical events and the recording of the ECG. Panels 1–2 illustrate atrial depolarization and the formation of the P wave. Panels 3–4 illustrate ventricular depolarization and formation of the QRS complex. Finally, panels 5–6 illustrate repolarization of the ventricles and formation of the T wave.

Figure 9.13 The relationship between changes in the intraventricular pressure and the ECG. Notice that the QRS complex (i.e., depolarization of the ventricles) occurs at the beginning of systole and the rise in ventricular pressure. Further, note that the T wave (repolarization of the ventricles) occurs at the same time that the ventricles relax at the beginning of diastole.

TABLE 9.2	Typical Resting and Maximal Exercise Values for Stroke Volume (SV), Heart Rate (HR), and Cardiac Output ($\dot{Q}$) for College-Age Untrained Subjects and Trained Endurance Athletes (Body Weights: Male = 70 kg; Female = 50 kg)					
Subject	HR (beats/min)		SV (ml/beat)		$\dot{Q}$ (l/min)	
Rest						
Untrained male	72	×	70	=	5.00	
Untrained female	75	×	60	=	4.50	
Trained male	50	×	100	=	5.00	
Trained female	55	×	80	=	4.40	
Max Exercise						
Untrained male	200	×	110	=	22.0	
Untrained female	200	×	90	=	18.0	
Trained male	190	×	180	=	34.2	
Trained female	190	×	125	=	23.8	

Note that values are rounded off. Data from references 3, 22, and 68.

Studies have shown that the initial increase in heart rate during exercise, up to approximately 100 beats per minute, is due to a withdrawal of parasympathetic tone (34). At higher work rates, stimulation of the SA and AV nodes by the sympathetic nervous system is responsible for increases in heart rate (34). Sympathetic fibers reach the heart by means of the **cardiac accelerator nerves,** which innervate both the SA node and the ventricles (figure 9.14). Endings of these fibers release norepinephrine upon stimulation, which act on

Figure 9.14 The activities of the SA and AV nodes can be altered by both the sympathetic and parasympathetic nervous systems.

Chapter Nine Circulatory Responses to Exercise

CLINICAL APPLICATIONS 9.2

Beta-Blockade and Exercise Heart Rate

Beta-adrenergic blocking medications (beta-blockers) are commonly prescribed for patients with coronary artery disease and/or hypertension. Although there are many different classes of these drugs, all these medications compete with epinephrine and norepinephrine for beta-adrenergic receptors in the heart. The end result is that beta-blockers reduce heart rate and the vigor of myocardial contraction, thus reducing the oxygen requirement of the heart.

In clinical exercise physiology, it is important to appreciate that all beta-blocking drugs will decrease resting heart rate as well as exercise heart rate.

Indeed, individuals on beta-blocking medications will exhibit lower exercise heart rates during both submaximal and maximal exercise. This is an important fact that should be considered when prescribing exercise and interpreting the exercise test results of individuals using beta-blocking medications.

---

beta receptors in the heart and cause an increase in both heart rate and the force of myocardial contraction. (See Clinical Applications 9.2.)

At rest, a normal balance between parasympathetic tone and sympathetic activity to the heart is maintained by the cardiovascular control center in the medulla oblongata. The cardiovascular control center receives impulses from various parts of the circulatory system relative to changes in important parameters (e.g., blood pressure, blood oxygen tension), and it relays motor impulses to the heart in response to a changing cardiovascular need. For example, an increase in resting blood pressure above normal stimulates pressure receptors in the carotid arteries and the arch of the aorta, which in turn send impulses to the cardiovascular control center (figure 9.14). In response, the cardiovascular control center increases parasympathetic activity to the heart to slow the heart rate and reduce cardiac output. This reduction in cardiac output causes blood pressure to decline back toward normal.

Another regulatory reflex involves pressure receptors located in the right atrium. In this case, an increase in right atrial pressure signals the cardiovascular control center that an increase in venous return has occurred; hence, to prevent a backup of blood in the systemic venous system, an increase in cardiac output must result. The cardiovascular control center responds by sending sympathetic accelerator nerve impulses to the heart, which increase heart rate and cardiac output. The end result is that the increase in cardiac output lowers right atrial pressure back to normal, and venous blood pressure is reduced.

Finally, a change in body temperature can influence heart rate. An increase in body temperature above normal results in an increase in heart rate, whereas lowering of body temperature below normal causes a reduction in heart rate (34). For example, exercise in a hot environment results in increased body temperatures and higher heart rates than if the same exercise was performed in a cool environment. This topic is discussed in more detail in chapter 12.

Heart Rate Variability

As discussed previously, heart rate is regulated by the autonomic nervous system (i.e., balance between the parasympathetic and sympathetic nervous systems). The term **heart rate variability** (HRV) refers to the variation in the time between heartbeats (19). In practice, the time interval (expressed in milliseconds) between two heartbeats can be measured as the R-R time interval using an ECG tracing, as illustrated in figure 9.11. The HRV is then calculated as the standard deviation of the R-R time interval during a selected time period. A wide variation in HRV is considered to be a good index of a "healthy" balance between the sympathetic and parasympathetic nervous systems, whereas low HRV indicates an imbalance exists in autonomic regulation.

The physiological significance of HRV is that the time variation between heartbeats reflect autonomic balance and is an excellent noninvasive screening tool for many diseases. For example, low HRV has been shown to predict future cardiovascular events, such as sudden cardiac death. Further, low HRV is an independent risk factor for the development of cardiovascular disease, including heart failure, myocardial infarction, and hypertension (20). Epidemiological studies have also established that low HRV is an excellent predictor of increased cardiovascular morbidity and mortality in patients with existing cardiovascular disease.

What is the physiological cause of low HRV variability? Again, the autonomic nervous system regulates many cardiovascular parameters including both heart rate and HRV. Recall that heart rate can be elevated by increasing sympathetic activity or decreased by increasing parasympathetic (vagal) activity. The balance between the effects of the sympathetic and parasympathetic systems, the two opposite-acting branches of the autonomic nervous system, is referred to as the *sympathovagal balance* and is reflected in the beat-to-beat changes of the cardiac cycle (19).

Numerous factors can influence the sympathovagal balance and thus impact HRV. For example, with advancing age or some disease states, there is a decrease in parasympathetic tone at rest (19) or an increase in sympathetic nervous system outflow (8). This results in a disturbance in sympathovagal balance and a decrease in HRV. Some specific examples of diseases that promote a decrease in HRV are as follows: HRV is decreased in patients suffering from depression, hypertension, and heart disease, and in individuals following a myocardial infarction (19). Importantly, research indicates that physical inactivity promotes a decrease in HRV, whereas regular bouts of aerobic exercise results in increased HRV (19). Therefore, investigation of the types of exercise and specific training programs that have positive influences on HRV has become an important area of research.

Regulation of Stroke Volume

Stroke volume, at rest or during exercise, is regulated by three variables: (1) the end-diastolic volume (EDV), which is the volume of blood in the ventricles at the end of diastole; (2) the average aortic blood pressure; and (3) the strength of ventricular contraction.

EDV is often referred to as "preload," and it influences stroke volume in the following way. Two physiologists, Frank and Starling, demonstrated that the strength of ventricular contraction increased with an enlargement of EDV (i.e., stretch of the ventricles). This relationship has become known as the Frank-Starling law of the heart. The increase in EDV results in a lengthening of cardiac fibers, which improves the force of contraction in a manner similar to that seen in skeletal muscle (discussed in chapter 8). The mechanism to explain the influence of fiber length on cardiac contractility is that an increase in the length of cardiac fibers increases the number of myosin cross-bridge interactions with actin, resulting in increased force production. A rise in cardiac contractility results in an increase in the amount of blood pumped per beat; the relationship between EDV volume and stroke volume is illustrated in figure 9.15.

The principal variable that influences EDV is the rate of venous return to the heart. An increase in venous return results in a rise in EDV and therefore an increase in stroke volume. Increased venous return and the resulting increase in EDV play a key role in the increase in stroke volume observed during upright exercise.

What factors regulate venous return during exercise? There are three principal mechanisms: (1) constriction of the veins (venoconstriction), (2) pumping action of contracting skeletal muscle (called the

Figure 9.15 An illustration of the relationship between ventricular end-diastolic volume and stroke volume. Notice the increase in stroke volume when venous return increases above the normal resting level.

muscle pump), and (3) pumping action of the respiratory system (respiratory pump).

1. Venoconstriction. Venoconstriction increases venous return by reducing the volume capacity of the veins to store blood. The end result of a reduced volume capacity in veins is to move blood back toward the heart. Venoconstriction occurs via a reflex sympathetic constriction of smooth muscle in veins draining skeletal muscle, which is controlled by the cardiovascular control center (4).

2. Muscle pump. The muscle pump is a result of the mechanical action of rhythmic skeletal muscle contractions. Therefore, when muscles contract during exercise, they compress veins and push blood back toward the heart. Between contractions, blood refills the veins and the process is repeated. Blood is prevented from flowing away from the heart between contractions by one-way valves located in large veins (figure 9.16). During sustained muscular contractions (isometric exercise), the muscle pump cannot operate, and venous return to the heart is reduced.

3. Respiratory pump. The rhythmic pattern of breathing also provides a mechanical pump by which venous return is promoted. The respiratory pump works in the following way. During inspiration, the pressure within the thorax (chest) decreases and abdominal pressure increases. This creates a flow of venous blood from the abdominal region into the thorax and therefore promotes venous return. Although quiet breathing (rest) aids in venous return, the role of the respiratory pump is enhanced during exercise due to the greater respiratory rate and depth. Indeed, recent evidence indicates that the respiratory pump is the predominant factor that promotes venous return to the heart during upright exercise (22).

A second variable that affects stroke volume is the aortic pressure (mean arterial pressure). In order

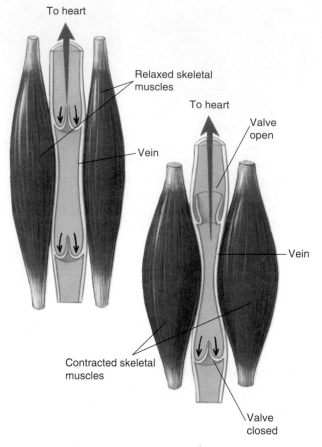

Figure 9.16 The action of the one-way venous valves. Contraction of skeletal muscles helps to pump blood toward the heart, but is prevented from pushing blood away from the heart by closure of the venous valves.

Figure 9.17 Effects of sympathetic stimulation of the heart on stroke volume. Note that sympathetic stimulation results in an increase in stroke volume at any given diastolic volume; that is, sympathetic stimulation increases ventricular contractility via an increased level of intracellular calcium resulting in a higher myosin cross-bridge interaction with actin.

to eject blood, the pressure generated by the left ventricle must exceed the pressure in the aorta. Therefore, aortic pressure or mean arterial pressure (called afterload) represents a barrier to the ejection of blood from the ventricles. Stroke volume is thus inversely proportional to the afterload; that is, an increase in aortic pressure produces a decrease in stroke volume. However, it is noteworthy that afterload is minimized during exercise due to arteriole dilation. This arteriole dilation in the working muscles reduces afterload and makes it easier for the heart to pump a large volume of blood.

The final factor that influences stroke volume is the effect of circulating catecholamines (i.e., epinephrine and norepinephrine) and direct sympathetic stimulation of the heart by cardiac accelerator nerves. Both of these mechanisms increase cardiac contractility by increasing the amount of calcium available to the myocardial cell (34). In particular, epinephrine and norepinephrine both increase in entry of extracellular calcium into the cardiac muscle fiber. The relationship between sympathetic stimulation of the

heart and stroke volume is illustrated in figure 9.17. Notice that compared to control conditions (i.e., limited sympathetic stimulation), increased sympathetic stimulation of the heart increases stroke volume at any level of EDV.

To summarize, stroke volume is regulated by three factors: EDV, cardiac contractility, and cardiac afterload. During upright exercise, the exercise-induced increases in stroke volume occur due to both increases in EDV and increased cardiac contractility due to circulating catecholamines and/or sympathetic stimulation. In contrast, an increase in cardiac afterload results in a decrease in stroke volume.

IN SUMMARY

- Cardiac output is the product of heart rate and stroke volume ($\dot{Q} = HR \times SV$). Figure 9.18 summarizes those variables that influence cardiac output during exercise.
- The pacemaker of the heart is the SA node. SA node activity is modified by the parasympathetic nervous system (slows HR) and the sympathetic nervous system (increases HR).
- Heart rate increases at the beginning of exercise due to a withdrawal of parasympathetic tone. At higher work rates, the increase in heart rate is achieved via an increased sympathetic outflow to the SA nodes.
- Stroke volume is regulated via (1) end-diastolic volume, (2) afterload (i.e., aortic blood pressure), and (3) the strength of ventricular contraction.
- Venous return increases during exercise due to (1) venoconstriction, (2) the muscle pump, and (3) the respiratory pump.

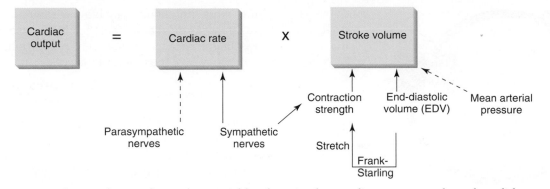

Figure 9.18 Factors that regulate cardiac output. Variables that stimulate cardiac output are shown by solid arrows, and factors that reduce cardiac output are shown by dotted arrows.

HEMODYNAMICS

One of the most important features of the circulatory system is that the system is a continuous "closed loop." Blood flow through the circulatory system results from pressure differences between the two ends of the system. To understand the physical regulation of blood flow to tissues, it is necessary to appreciate the interrelationships between pressure, flow, and resistance. The study of these factors and the physical principles of blood flow is called *hemodynamics.*

Physical Characteristics of Blood

Blood is composed of two principal components, plasma and cells. Plasma is the "watery" portion of blood that contains numerous ions, proteins, and hormones. The cells that make up blood are red blood cells (RBCs), platelets, and white blood cells. Red blood cells contain hemoglobin used for the transport of oxygen (see chapter 10). Platelets play an important role in blood clotting, and white blood cells are important in preventing infection (chapter 6).

The percentage of the blood that is composed of cells is called the hematocrit. That is, if 42% of the blood is cells and the remainder is plasma, the hematocrit is 42% (see figure 9.19). On a percentage basis, RBCs constitute the largest fraction of cells found in blood. Therefore, the hematocrit is principally influenced by increases or decreases in RBC numbers. The average hematocrit of a normal college-age male is 42%, and the hematocrit of a normal college-age female averages approximately 38%. These values vary among individuals and are dependent on a number of variables.

Blood is several times more viscous than water, and this viscosity increases the difficulty with which blood flows through the circulatory system. One of

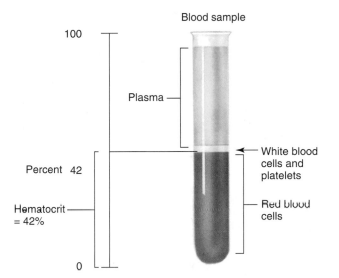

Figure 9.19 Blood cells become packed at the bottom of the test tube when blood is centrifuged; this leaves the plasma at the top of the tube. The percentage of whole blood that is composed of blood cells is termed the hematocrit.

the major contributors to viscosity is the concentration of RBCs found in the blood. Therefore, during periods of anemia (decreased RBCs), the viscosity of blood is lowered. Conversely, an increase in hematocrit results in an elevation in blood viscosity. The potential influence of changing blood viscosity on performance is discussed in chapter 25.

Relationships Among Pressure, Resistance, and Flow

As mentioned earlier, blood flow through the vascular system is dependent upon the difference in pressure at the two ends of the system. For example, if the pressures at the two ends of the vessel are equal, no flow will occur. In contrast, if the pressure is higher at one end of the vessel than the other, blood will flow

Figure 9.20 The flow of blood through the systemic circuit is dependent on the pressure difference (ΔP) between the aorta and the right atrium. In this illustration, the mean pressure in the aorta is 100 mm Hg, while the pressure in the right atrium is 0 mm Hg. Therefore, the "driving" pressure across the circuit is 100 mm Hg (100 − 0 = 100).

from the region of higher pressure to the region of lower pressure. The rate of flow is proportional to the pressure difference ($P_1 - P_2$) between the two ends of the tube. Figure 9.20 illustrates the "pressure head" driving blood flow in the systemic circulatory system under resting conditions. Here, the mean arterial pressure is 100 mm Hg (i.e., this is the pressure of blood in the aorta), while the pressure at the opposite end of the circuit (i.e., pressure in the right atrium) is 0 mm Hg. Therefore, the driving pressure across the circulatory system is 100 mm Hg (100 − 0 = 100).

It should be pointed out that the flow rate of blood through the vascular system is proportional to the pressure difference across the system, but it is inversely proportional to the resistance. Inverse proportionality is expressed mathematically by the placement of this variable in the denominator of a fraction, because a fraction decreases when the denominator increases. Therefore, the relationship between blood flow, pressure, and resistance is given by the equation

$$\text{Blood flow} = \frac{\Delta\ \text{Pressure}}{\text{Resistance}}$$

where Δ pressure means the difference in pressure between the two ends of the circulatory system. Notice that blood flow can be increased by either an increase in blood pressure or a decrease in resistance. A fivefold increase in blood flow could be generated by increasing pressure by a factor of five; however, this large increase in blood pressure would be hazardous to health. Fortunately, increases in blood flow during exercise are achieved primarily by a decrease in resistance with a small rise in blood pressure.

What factors contribute to the resistance of blood flow? Resistance to flow is directly proportional to the length of the vessel and the viscosity of blood. However,

the most important variable determining vascular resistance is the diameter of the blood vessel, because vascular resistance is inversely proportional to the fourth power of the radius of the vessel:

$$\text{Resistance} = \frac{\text{Length} \times \text{viscosity}}{\text{Radius}^4}$$

In other words, an increase in either vessel length or blood viscosity results in a proportional increase in resistance. However, reducing the radius of a blood vessel by one-half would increase resistance sixteen-fold (i.e., $2^4 = 16$)!

Sources of Vascular Resistance

Under most circumstances, the viscosity of blood and the length of the blood vessels are not manipulated in normal physiology. Therefore, the primary factor regulating blood flow through organs must be the radius of the blood vessel. Because the effect of changes in radius on changes in flow rate are magnified by a power of four, blood can be diverted from one organ system to another by varying degrees of vasoconstriction and vasodilation. This principle is used during heavy exercise to divert blood toward contracting skeletal muscle and away from less-active tissue. This concept is discussed in detail in the next section, "Changes in Oxygen Delivery to Muscle During Exercise."

The greatest vascular resistance in blood flow occurs in arterioles. This point is illustrated in figure 9.21. Note the large drop in arterial pressure that occurs across the arterioles; approximately 70% to 80% of the decline in mean arterial pressure occurs across the arterioles.

IN SUMMARY

- Blood is composed of two principal components: plasma and cells.
- Blood flow through the vascular system is directly proportional to the pressure at the two ends of the system and inversely proportional to resistance:

$$\text{Blood flow} = \frac{\Delta\ \text{Pressure}}{\text{Resistance}}$$

- The most important factor determining resistance to blood flow is the radius of the blood vessel. The relationship between vessel radius, vessel length, blood viscosity, and flow is

$$\text{Resistance} = \frac{\text{Length} \times \text{viscosity}}{\text{Radius}^4}$$

- The greatest vascular resistance to blood flow is offered in the arterioles.

Figure 9.21 Pressure changes across the systemic circulation. Notice the large pressure drop across the arterioles.

CHANGES IN OXYGEN DELIVERY TO MUSCLE DURING EXERCISE

During intense exercise, the metabolic need for oxygen in skeletal muscle increases many times over the resting value. To meet this rise in oxygen demand, blood flow to the contracting muscle must increase. As mentioned earlier, increased oxygen delivery to exercising skeletal muscle is accomplished via two mechanisms: (1) an increased cardiac output and (2) a redistribution of blood flow from inactive organs to the working skeletal muscle.

Changes in Cardiac Output During Exercise

Cardiac output increases during exercise in direct proportion to the metabolic rate required to perform the exercise task. This is shown in figure 9.22. Note that the relationship between cardiac output and percent maximal oxygen uptake is essentially linear. The increase in cardiac output during exercise in the upright position is achieved by an increase in both stroke volume and heart rate. However, in untrained or moderately trained subjects, stroke volume does not increase beyond a workload of 40% to 60% of $\dot{V}O_2$ max (figure 9.22). Therefore, at work rates greater than 40% to 60% $\dot{V}O_2$ max, the rise in cardiac output in these individuals is achieved by increases in heart rate alone. The examples presented in figure 9.22 for maximal heart rate, stroke volume, and cardiac output are typical values for

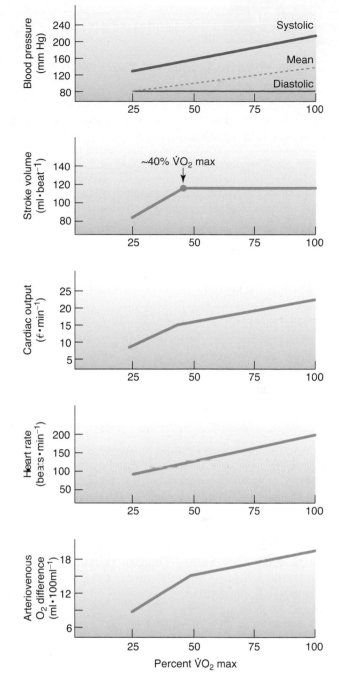

Figure 9.22 Changes in blood pressure, stroke volume, cardiac output, heart rate, and the arterial–mixed venous oxygen difference as a function of relative work rates. See text for details.

a 70-kg, active (but not highly trained) college-age male. See table 9.2 for examples of maximal stroke volume and cardiac output for trained men and women.

Note that although most experts agree that stroke volume reaches a plateau between 40–60% of $\dot{V}O_2$ max in untrained and moderately trained individuals, evidence exists that stroke volume does not plateau in highly trained athletes during running exercise. This point is discussed in more detail in Research Focus 9.1.

www.mhhe.com/powers8e

Chapter Nine   Circulatory Responses to Exercise   **207**

Stroke Volume Does Not Plateau in Endurance Athletes

It is widely accepted that during incremental exercise, stroke volume in active or untrained subjects reaches a plateau at a submaximal work rate (i.e., approximately 40–60% $\dot{V}O_2$ max) (figure 9.22). The physiological explanation for this plateau in stroke volume is that at high heart rates, the time available for ventricular filling is decreased.

Therefore, diastole and end-diastolic volume decrease. However, new evidence suggests that during incremental work rates, the stroke volume of endurance athletes (e.g., highly trained distance runners) does not plateau but continues to increase to $\dot{V}O_2$ max (14, 44). What is the explanation for this observation? It appears that compared

to untrained subjects, endurance athletes have improved ventricular filling during heavy exercise due to increased venous return. This increase in end-diastolic volume results in an increased force of ventricular contraction (Frank-Starling law) and an increase in stroke volume.

Maximal cardiac output tends to decrease in a linear fashion in both men and women after thirty years of age (12, 16). This is primarily due to a decrease in maximal heart rate with age (12). For example, because cardiac output equals heart rate times stroke volume, any decrease in heart rate would result in a decrease in cardiac output. The decrease in maximal heart rate with age in adults can be estimated by the following formula:

$$\text{Max HR} = 220 - \text{age (years)}$$

According to this formula, a twenty-year-old subject might have a maximal heart rate of 200 beats per minute ($220 - 20 = 200$), whereas a fifty-year-old would have a maximal heart rate of 170 beats per minute ($220 - 50 = 170$). However, this is only an estimate, and values can be 20 beats $\times$ min^{-1} higher or lower.

The above formula for adults is not a good predictor of maximal heart rate in children. In children (ages 7–17), the following formula can be used to predict maximal heart rate (21):

$$\text{Max HR} = 208 - .7 \times \text{age (years)}$$

According to this formula for children, a twelve-year-old child would have a maximal heart rate of 200 beats ($208 - 8 = 200$). Similar to the formula used to predict maximal heart rates in adults, the formula for children provides only an estimate of maximal heart rates, and wide variability in maximal heart rates can exist between different children (21).

Changes in Arterial-Mixed Venous O_2 Content During Exercise

Note in figure 9.22 the change in the arterial-mixed venous oxygen difference (a $-$ $\bar{v}O_2$ diff) that occurs during exercise. The a $-$ $\bar{v}O_2$ difference represents the amount of O_2 that is taken up from 100 ml of blood by the tissues during one trip around the systemic circuit. An increase in the a $-$ $\bar{v}O_2$ difference during exercise is due to an increase in the amount of O_2 taken up

and used for the oxidative production of ATP by skeletal muscle. The relationship between cardiac output ($\dot{Q}$), a $-$ $\bar{v}$ O_2 diff, and oxygen uptake is given by the Fick equation:

$$\dot{V}O_2 = \dot{Q} \times (a - \bar{v}\, O_2\ \text{diff})$$

Simply stated, the Fick equation says that $\dot{V}O_2$ is equal to the product of cardiac output and the a $-$ $\bar{v}$ O_2 diff. This means that an increase in either cardiac output or a $-$ $\bar{v}$ O_2 diff would elevate $\dot{V}O_2$.

Redistribution of Blood Flow During Exercise

To meet the increased oxygen demand of the skeletal muscles during exercise, it is necessary to increase muscle blood flow while reducing blood flow to less-active organs such as the liver, kidneys, and GI tract. Figure 9.23 points out that the change in blood flow to muscle and the splanchnic (pertaining to the viscera) circulation is dictated by the exercise intensity (metabolic rate). That is, the increase in muscle blood flow during exercise and the decrease in splanchnic blood flow change as a linear function of % $\dot{V}O_2$ max (34).

Figure 9.24 illustrates the change in blood flow to various organ systems between resting conditions and during maximal exercise. Several important points need to be stressed. First, at rest, approximately 15% to 20% of total cardiac output is directed toward skeletal muscle (2, 34). However, during maximal exercise, 80% to 85% of total cardiac output goes to contracting skeletal muscle (34). This is necessary to meet the huge increase in muscle oxygen requirements during intense exercise. Second, notice that during heavy exercise, the percentage of total cardiac output that goes to the brain is reduced compared to that during rest. However, the absolute blood flow that reaches the brain is slightly increased above resting values; this is due to the elevated cardiac output during exercise (6, 45). Further, although the percentage of total cardiac output that reaches the myocardium is the

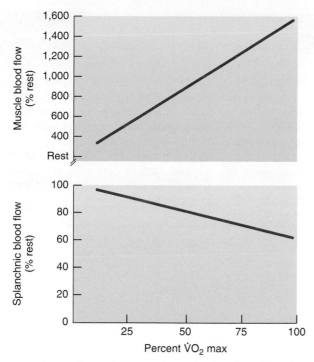

Figure 9.23 Changes in muscle and splanchnic blood flow as a function of exercise intensity. Notice the large increase in muscle blood flow as the work rate increases. Data from L. Rowell, *Human Circulation: Regulation During Physical Stress.* 1986: Oxford University Press, New York, NY.

same during maximal exercise as it is at rest, the total coronary blood flow is increased due to the increase in cardiac output during heavy exercise. Also, note that skin blood flow increases during both light and moderate exercise but decreases during maximal exercise (6). Finally, compared to rest, blood flow to abdominal organs is also decreased during maximal exercise (figure 9.24). This reduction in abdominal blood flow during heavy exercise is an important means of shifting blood flow away from "less-active" tissues and toward the working skeletal muscles.

Regulation of Local Blood Flow During Exercise

What regulates blood flow to various organs during exercise? Muscle as well as other body tissues have the unique ability to regulate their own blood flow in direct proportion to their metabolic needs. Blood flow to skeletal muscle during exercise is regulated in the following way. First, the arterioles in skeletal muscle have a high vascular resistance at rest. This is due to adrenergic sympathetic stimulation, which causes arteriole smooth muscle to contract (vasoconstriction) (41). This produces a relatively low blood flow to muscle at rest (4–5 ml per minute per 100 grams of muscle), but because muscles have a large mass, this accounts for 20% to 25% of total blood flow from the heart.

At the beginning of exercise, the initial skeletal muscle vasodilation that occurs is due to an intrinsic metabolic control (41). This type of blood flow regulation is termed **autoregulation,** and it is thought to be the most important factor in regulating blood flow to muscle during exercise. The increased metabolic rate of skeletal muscle during exercise causes local changes such as decreases in oxygen tension, increases in CO_2 tension, nitric oxide, potassium and adenosine concentrations, and a decrease in pH (increase in acidity) (see Research Focus 9.2). These local changes work together to cause vasodilation of arterioles feeding the contracting skeletal muscle (41). Vasodilation reduces the vascular resistance and therefore increases blood flow. As a result of these changes, blood delivery to contracting skeletal muscle during heavy exercise may rise fifteen to twenty times above that during rest (41). Further, arteriole vasodilation is combined with "recruitment" of the capillaries in skeletal muscle. At rest, only 50% to 80% of the capillaries in skeletal muscle are open at any one time; however, during intense exercise, almost all of the capillaries in contracting muscle may be open (34).

The level of vasodilation that occurs in arterioles and small arteries leading to skeletal muscle is regulated by the metabolic need of the muscle. That is, the intensity of exercise and the number of motor units recruited determine the overall need for blood flow to the muscle. For example, during low-intensity exercise, a relatively small number of motor units will be recruited into action, resulting in a relatively small demand for blood flow to these active muscle fibers. In contrast, high-intensity exercise would result in the recruitment of a large number of motor units and, therefore, result in increased production of local vasodilatory factors. Specifically, increased muscle contractile activity is associated with the production of numerous factors that promote blood vessel vasodilation; these include increases in the release of potassium from the muscle, CO_2 production, adenosine, and lactate/hydrogen ions (37). Moreover, an increase in the production and release of nitric oxide from endothelial cells of blood vessels also promotes vasodilation during exercise (see Research Focus 9.2). Collectively, these changes result in increased vasodilation of arterioles/small arteries and promote increased blood flow to the contracting muscle in order to match the metabolic demand.

While the vascular resistance in skeletal muscle decreases during exercise, vascular resistance to flow in the visceral organs and other inactivity tissue increases. This occurs due to an increased sympathetic output to these organs, which is regulated by the cardiovascular control center. As a result of the increase in visceral vasoconstriction during exercise (i.e., resistance increases), blood flow to the viscera can decrease to only 20% to 30% of resting values (34).

Nitric Oxide Is an Important Vasodilator

Research in the early 1990s led to the discovery of an important vasodilator called *nitric oxide*. Nitric oxide is produced in the endothelium of arterioles. After production, nitric oxide promotes smooth muscle relaxation in the arteriole, which results in vasodilation and therefore causes an increase in blood flow. Current evidence suggests that nitric oxide works in conjunction with other local factors in autoregulation of blood flow (41).

How important is nitric oxide in the autoregulation of muscle blood flow during exercise? It is generally agreed that production of nitric oxide is a requirement for the optimal regulation of muscle blood flow during exercise (41). Nonetheless, it appears that nitric oxide is one of several factors involved in regulation of muscle blood flow during exercise (37).

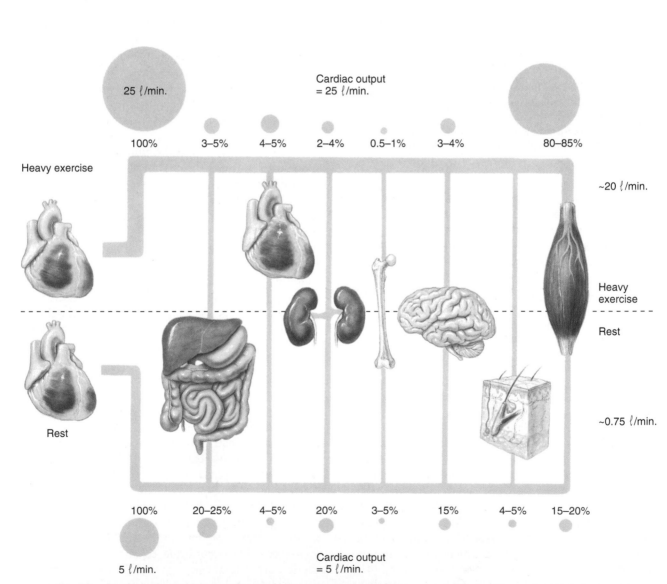

Figure 9.24 Distribution of cardiac output during rest and maximal exercise. At rest, the cardiac output is 5 ℓ/min. (bottom of figure); during maximum exercise, the cardiac output increased five-fold to 25 ℓ/min. Note the large increases in blood flow to the skeletal muscle and the reduction in flow to the liver/GI tract. From P. Åstrand and K. Rodahl, *Textbook of Work Physiology*, 3d ed. Copyright © 1986 McGraw-Hill, Inc., New York. Reprinted by permission of the authors.

IN SUMMARY

- Oxygen delivery to exercising skeletal muscle increases due to (1) an increased cardiac output and (2) a redistribution of blood flow from inactive organs to the contracting skeletal muscles.
- Cardiac output increases as a linear function of oxygen uptake during exercise. During exercise in the upright position, stroke volume reaches a plateau at approximately 40–60% of $\dot{V}O_2$ max; therefore, at work rates above 40–60% $\dot{V}O_2$ max, the rise in cardiac output is due to increases in heart rate alone.
- During exercise, blood flow to contracting muscle is increased, and blood flow to less-active tissues is reduced.
- Regulation of muscle blood flow during exercise is primarily regulated by local factors (called autoregulation). Autoregulation refers to intrinsic control of blood flow by change in local metabolites (e.g., oxygen tension, pH, potassium, adenosine, and nitric oxide) around arterioles.

CIRCULATORY RESPONSES TO EXERCISE

The changes in heart rate and blood pressure that occur during exercise reflect the type and intensity of exercise performed, the duration of exercise, and the environmental conditions under which the work was performed. For example, heart rate and blood pressure are higher during arm work when compared to leg work at a given oxygen uptake. Further, exercise in a hot/humid condition results in higher heart rates when compared to the same exercise in a cool environment. The next several sections discuss the cardiovascular responses to exercise during a variety of exercise conditions.

Emotional Influence

Submaximal exercise in an emotionally charged atmosphere results in higher heart rates and blood pressures when compared to the same work in a psychologically "neutral" environment. This emotional elevation in heart rate and blood pressure response to exercise is mediated by an increase in sympathetic nervous system activity. If the exercise is maximal (e.g., 400-meter dash), high emotion elevates the pre-exercise heart rate and blood pressure but does not generally alter the peak heart rate or blood pressure observed during the exercise itself.

Transition from Rest to Exercise

At the beginning of exercise there is a rapid increase in heart rate, stroke volume, and cardiac output. It has been demonstrated that heart rate and cardiac output begin to increase within the first second after muscular contraction begins (see figure 9.25). If the work rate is constant and below the lactate threshold, a steady-state plateau in heart rate, stroke volume, and cardiac output is reached within 2 to 3 minutes. This response is similar to that observed in oxygen uptake at the beginning of exercise (see chapter 4).

Recovery from Exercise

Recovery from short-term, low-intensity exercise is generally rapid. This is illustrated in figure 9.25. Notice that heart rate, stroke volume, and cardiac output all decrease rapidly back toward resting levels following this type of exercise. Recovery speed varies from individual to individual, with well-conditioned subjects demonstrating better recuperative powers than untrained subjects. In regard to recovery heart rates, the slopes of heart-rate decay following exercise are generally the same for

Figure 9.25 Changes in cardiac output, stroke volume, and heart rate during the transition from rest to submaximal constant intensity exercise and during recovery. See text for discussion. Data from L. Rowell, 1974, "Human Cardiovascular Adjustments to Exercise and Thermal Stress," American Physiological Society, Bethesda, MD: *Physiological Reviews*, 54:75–159; and L. Rowell, H*uman Circulation: Regulation During Physical Stress*. 1986: Oxford University Press, New York, NY.

trained and untrained subjects. However, trained subjects recover faster following exercise because they don't achieve as high a heart rate as untrained subjects during a particular exercise.

Recovery from long-term exercise is much slower than the response depicted in figure 9.25. This is particularly true when the exercise is performed in hot/humid conditions, because an elevated body temperature delays the fall in heart rate during recovery from exercise (36).

Incremental Exercise

The cardiovascular responses to dynamic incremental exercise are illustrated in figure 9.22. Heart rate and cardiac output increase in direct proportion to oxygen uptake. Further, blood flow to muscle increases as a function of oxygen uptake (see figure 9.23). This ensures that as the need to synthesize ATP to supply the energy for muscular contraction increases, the supply of O_2 reaching the muscle also increases. However, both cardiac output and heart rate reach a plateau at approximately 100% $\dot{V}O_2$ max (see figure 9.22). This point represents a maximal ceiling for oxygen transport to exercising skeletal muscles, and it is thought to occur simultaneously with the attainment of maximal oxygen uptake.

The increase in cardiac output during incremental exercise is achieved via a decrease in vascular resistance to flow and an increase in mean arterial blood pressure. The elevation in mean arterial blood pressure during exercise is due to an increase in systolic pressure, because diastolic pressure remains fairly constant during incremental work (see figure 9.22).

As mentioned earlier, the increase in heart rate and systolic blood pressure that occurs during exercise results in an increased workload on the heart. The increased metabolic demand placed on the heart during exercise can be estimated by examining the double product. The **double product** (also known as

rate-pressure product) is computed by multiplying heart rate times systolic blood pressure:

**Double product =
heart rate × systolic blood pressure**

Table 9.3 contains an illustration of changes in the double product during an incremental exercise test. The take-home message in table 9.3 is simply that increases in exercise intensity result in an elevation in both heart rate and systolic blood pressure; each of these factors increases the workload placed on the heart.

Careful examination of table 9.3 reveals that the double product during exercise at $\dot{V}O_2$ max is five times greater than the double product at rest. This implies that maximal exercise increases the workload on the heart by 500% over rest.

The practical application of the double product is that this measure can be used as a guideline to prescribe exercise for patients with coronary artery blockage. For example, suppose a patient develops chest pain (called angina pectoris) at a certain intensity of exercise due to myocardial ischemia at a double product of 30,000. Because chest pain appears at a double product of 30,000, the cardiologist or exercise physiologist would recommend that this patient perform types of exercise that result in a double product of 30,000. This would reduce the risk of the patient developing chest pain due to a high metabolic demand on the heart.

Arm Versus Leg Exercise

As mentioned earlier, at any given level of oxygen consumption, both heart rate and blood pressure are higher during arm work when compared to leg work (1, 24, 33) (see figure 9.26). The explanation for the higher heart rate seems to be linked to a greater sympathetic outflow to the heart during arm work when compared to leg exercise (2). Additionally, isometric exercise

TABLE 9.3 Changes in the Double Product (i.e., Heart Rate × Systolic Blood Pressure) During an Incremental Exercise Test in a Healthy 21-Year-Old Female Subject

Note that the double product is a dimensionless term that reflects the relative changes in the workload placed on the heart during exercise and other forms of stress.

Condition	Heart Rate (beats · min⁻¹)	Systolic Blood Pressure (mm Hg)	Double Product
Rest	75	110	8,250
Exercise			
25% $\dot{V}O_2$ max	100	130	13,000
50% $\dot{V}O_2$ max	140	160	22,400
75% $\dot{V}O_2$ max	170	180	30,600
100% $\dot{V}O_2$ max	200	210	42,000

Figure 9.26 Comparison of mean arterial blood pressure and heart rate during submaximal rhythmic arm and leg exercise.

Figure 9.27 Changes in cardiac output, stroke volume, and heart rate during prolonged exercise at a constant intensity. Notice that cardiac output is maintained by an increase in heart rate to offset the fall in stroke volume that occurs during this type of work.

also increases the heart rate above the expected value based on relative oxygen consumption (1).

The relatively large increase in blood pressure for arm work is due to a vasoconstriction in the inactive muscle groups (2). For example, the larger the muscle group (e.g., legs) involved in performing the exercise, the more resistance vessels (arterioles) that are dilated. Therefore, this lower peripheral resistance is reflected in lower blood pressure (because cardiac output × resistance = pressure).

Intermittent Exercise

If exercise is discontinuous (e.g., interval training), the extent of the recovery of heart rate and blood pressure between bouts depends on the level of subject fitness, environmental conditions (temperature, humidity), and the duration and intensity of the exercise. With a relatively light effort in a cool environment, there is generally complete recovery between exercise bouts within several minutes. However, if the exercise is intense or the work is performed in a hot/humid environment, there is a cumulative increase in heart rate between efforts, and thus recovery is not complete (38). The practical consequence of performing repeated bouts of light exercise is that many repetitions can be performed. In contrast, the nature of high-intensity exercise dictates that a limited number of efforts can be tolerated.

Prolonged Exercise

Figure 9.27 illustrates the change in heart rate, stroke volume, and cardiac output that occurs during prolonged exercise at a constant work rate. Note that cardiac output is maintained at a constant level throughout the duration of the exercise. However, as the duration of exercise increases, stroke volume declines while heart rate increases (6). Figure 9.27 demonstrates that the ability to maintain a constant cardiac output in the face of declining stroke volume is due to the increase in heart rate being equal in magnitude to the decline in stroke volume.

The increase in heart rate and decrease in stroke volume observed during prolonged exercise is often referred to as *cardiovascular drift* and is due to the influence of rising body temperature on dehydration and a reduction in plasma volume (5, 30, 34). A reduction in plasma volume acts to reduce venous return to the heart and therefore reduce stroke volume. If prolonged exercise is performed in a hot/humid environment, the increase in heart rate and decrease in stroke volume is exaggerated even more than depicted in figure 9.27 (27, 32). In fact, it is not surprising to find near-maximal heart rates during submaximal exercise in the heat. For example, it has been demonstrated that during a 2.5-hour marathon race at a work rate of 70% to 75% $\dot{V}O_2$ max, maximal heart rates may be maintained during the last hour of the race (10).

Does prolonged exercise at high heart rates pose a risk for cardiac injury? The answer to this question is almost always "no" for healthy individuals. However, sudden cardiac deaths have occurred in individuals of all ages during exercise. See Clinical Applications 9.3 for more details on sudden death during exercise.

Sudden Cardiac Death During Exercise

Sudden death is defined as an unexpected, natural, and nonviolent death occurring within the first six hours following the beginning of symptoms. Note that not all sudden deaths are due to cardiac events. In fact, in the United States, only 30% of sudden deaths in people between 14 and 21 years of age are cardiac in origin (40). How many of these cases of sudden death occur during exercise? Each year, fewer than 20 cases of sudden cardiac death during exercise are reported in the United States. Therefore, given that millions of people are actively engaged in sports and regular exercise in the United States, the likelihood that a healthy person will die from sudden cardiac death is extremely small. Across the world it is estimated that sudden cardiac death occurs in one out of 200,000 youth athletes (9). Again, the risk of sudden cardiac death in young athletes is limited.

The causes of sudden cardiac death are diverse and vary as a function of age. For example, in children and adolescents, most sudden cardiac deaths occur due to lethal cardiac arrhythmias (abnormal heart rhythm). These arrhythmias can arise from genetic anomalies in coronary arteries, cardiomyopathy (wasting of cardiac muscle due to disease), and/or myocarditis (inflammation of the heart) (3, 9, 40). In adults, coronary heart disease and cardiomyopathy are the most common causes of sudden cardiac death (40). Similar to sudden deaths in children, sudden cardiac deaths in adults are also generally associated with lethal cardiac arrhythmias.

Can a medical exam identify people at risk for sudden cardiac death during exercise? Yes. The combination of a medical history and a complete medical exam by a qualified physician can usually identify individuals with undetected heart disease or genetic defects that would place them at risk for sudden death during exercise.

IN SUMMARY

- The changes in heart rate and blood pressure that occur during exercise are a function of the type and intensity of exercise performed, the duration of exercise, and the environmental conditions.
- The increased metabolic demand placed on the heart during exercise can be estimated by examining the double product.
- At the same level of oxygen consumption, heart rate and blood pressure are greater during arm exercise than during leg exercise.
- The increase in heart rate that occurs during prolonged exercise is called cardiovascular drift.

REGULATION OF CARDIOVASCULAR ADJUSTMENTS TO EXERCISE

The cardiovascular adjustments at the beginning of exercise are rapid. Within one second after the commencement of muscular contraction there is a withdrawal of vagal outflow to the heart, which is followed by an increase in sympathetic stimulation of the heart (34). At the same time, there is a vasodilation of arterioles in active skeletal muscles and a reflex increase in the resistance of vessels in less-active areas. The end result is an increase in cardiac output to ensure that blood flow to muscle matches the metabolic needs (see figure 9.28). What is the signal to "turn on" the cardiovascular system at the onset of exercise? This question has puzzled physiologists for many years (15). At present, a complete answer is not available. However, recent advances in understanding cardiovascular control have led to the development of the *central command theory* (42).

The term **central command** refers to a motor signal developed within the brain (42). The central command theory of cardiovascular control argues that the initial cardiovascular changes at the beginning of dynamic

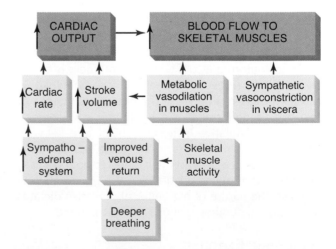

Figure 9.28 A summary of cardiovascular responses to exercise.

exercise (e.g., cycle ergometer exercise) are due to centrally generated cardiovascular motor signals, which set the general pattern of the cardiovascular response. However, it is believed that cardiovascular activity can be and is modified by heart mechanoreceptors, muscle chemoreceptors, muscle mechanoreceptors, and pressure-sensitive receptors (baroreceptors) located within the carotid arteries and the aortic arch (31, 42). Muscle chemoreceptors are sensitive to increases in muscle metabolites (e.g., potassium, lactic acid, etc.) and send messages to higher brain centers to "fine-tune" the cardiovascular responses to exercise (42). This type of peripheral feedback to the cardiovascular control center (medulla oblongata) has been termed the *exercise pressor reflex* (7, 23).

Muscle mechanoreceptors (e.g., muscle spindles, Golgi tendon organs) are sensitive to the force and speed of muscular movement. These receptors, like muscle chemoreceptors, send information to higher brain centers to aid in modification of the cardiovascular responses to a given exercise task (34, 35, 39, 43).

Finally, baroreceptors, which are sensitive to changes in arterial blood pressure, may also send afferent information back to the cardiovascular control center to add precision to the cardiovascular activity during exercise. These pressure receptors are important because they regulate arterial blood pressure around an elevated systemic pressure during exercise (34).

In review, the central command theory proposes that the initial signal to the cardiovascular system at the beginning of exercise comes from higher brain centers. However, fine-tuning of the cardiovascular response to a given exercise test is accomplished via a series of feedback loops from muscle chemoreceptors, muscle mechanoreceptors, and arterial baroreceptors (see figure 9.29). The fact that there appears to be some overlap among these three feedback systems during submaximal exercise suggests that redundancy in cardiovascular control exists (34). This is not surprising considering the importance of matching blood flow to the metabolic needs of exercising

Figure 9.29 A summary of cardiovascular control during exercise. See text for discussion.

skeletal muscle. Whether one or many of these feedback loops becomes more important during heavy exercise is not currently known and poses an interesting question for future research.

IN SUMMARY

- The central command theory of cardiovascular control during exercise proposes that the initial signal to "drive" the cardiovascular system at the beginning of exercise comes from higher brain centers.
- Although central command is the primary drive to increase heart rate during exercise, the cardiovascular response to exercise is fine-tuned by feedback from muscle chemoreceptors, muscle mechanoreceptors, and arterial baroreceptors to the cardiovascular control center.

STUDY QUESTIONS

1. What are the major purposes of the cardiovascular system?
2. Briefly, outline the design of the heart. Why is the heart often called "two pumps in one"?
3. Outline the cardiac cycle and the associated electrical activity recorded via the electrocardiogram.
4. Graph the heart rate, stroke volume, and cardiac output response to incremental exercise.
5. What factors regulate heart rate during exercise? Stroke volume?
6. How does exercise influence venous return?
7. What factors determine local blood flow during exercise?
8. Graph the changes that occur in heart rate, stroke volume, and cardiac output during prolonged exercise. What happens to these variables if the exercise is performed in a hot/humid environment?
9. Compare heart rate and blood pressure responses to arm and leg work at the same oxygen uptake. What factors might explain the observed differences?
10. Explain the central command theory of cardiovascular regulation during exercise.

SUGGESTED READINGS

Borjesson, M., and A. Pelliccia. 2009. Incidence and aetiology of sudden cardiac death in young athletes: An international perspective. *British Journal of Sports Medicine* 43: 644–48.

Courneya, C,, and M. Parker. 2010. *Cardiovascular Physiology: A Clinical Approach*. Philadelphia: Wolters Kluwer.

Coyle, E., and J. Gonzalez-Alonso. 2001. Cardiovascular drift during prolonged exercise: New perspectives. *Exercise and Sport Sciences Reviews* 29: 88–92.

Crandall, C., and J. Gonzalez-Alonso. 2010. Cardiovascular function in the heat-stressed human. *Acta Physiol (Oxf)* 199: 407–23.

Fox, S. 2010. *Human Physiology*. New York: McGraw-Hill Companies.

Powers, S. K., J. C. Quindry, and A. N. Kavazis. 2008. Exercise induced cardioprotection against myocardial ischemia reperfusion injury. *Free Radical Biology and Medicine* 44: 193–201.

Sarelius, I., and U. Pohl. 2010. Control of muscle blood flow during exercise: Local factors and integrative mechanisms. *Acta Physiol (Oxf)* 199: 349–65.

Williamson, J. W., P. J. Fadel, and J. H. Mitchell. 2006. New insights into central cardiovascular control during exercise in humans: A central command update. *Exp Physiol* 91: 51–58.

REFERENCES

1. **Asmussen E.** Similarities and dissimilarities between static and dynamic exercise. *Circulation Research* 48: 3–10, 1981.
2. **Åstrand P.** *Textbook of Work Physiology*. Champaign: Human Kinetics, 2003.
3. **Borjesson M, and Pelliccia A.** Incidence and aetiology of sudden cardiac death in young athletes: an international perspective. *British Journal of Sports Medicine* 43: 644–648, 2009.
4. **Courneya C, and Parker M.** *Cardiovascular Physiology: A Clinical Approach*. Philadelphia: Wolters Kluwer, 2010.
5. **Coyle EF, and Gonzalez-Alonso J.** Cardiovascular drift during prolonged exercise: new perspectives. *Exerc Sport Sci Rev* 29: 88–92, 2001.
6. **Crandall C, and Gonzalez-Alonso J.** Cardiovascular function in the heat-stressed human. *Acta Physiol (Oxf)* 199: 407–423, 2010.
7. **Duncan G, Johnson RH, and Lambie DG.** Role of sensory nerves in the cardiovascular and respiratory changes with isometric forearm exercise in man. *Clin Sci (Lond)* 60: 145–155, 1981.
8. **Feldman D, Elton TS, Menachemi DM, and Wexler RK.** Heart rate control with adrenergic blockade: clinical outcomes in cardiovascular medicine. *Vasc Health Risk Manag* 6: 387–397, 2010.
9. **Ferreira M.** Sudden cardiac death athletes: a systematic review. *Sports Medicine, Rehabilitation, Therapy, and Technology* 2: 1–6, 2010.
10. **Fox EL, and Costill DL.** Estimated cardiorespiratory response during marathon running. *Arch Environ Health* 24: 316–324, 1972.
11. **Fox S.** *Human Physiology*. New York: McGraw-Hill, 2010.
12. **Gerstenblith G, Renlund DG, and Lakatta EG.** Cardiovascular response to exercise in younger and older men. *Fed Proc* 46: 1834–1839, 1987.
13. **Gillespie C Kuklina EV, Briss PA, Blair NA, and Hong Y.** Vital signs: prevalence, treatment, and control of hypertension—United States, 1999–2002 and 2005–2008. *Morbidity and Mortality Weekly Report* 60: 103–108, 2011.
14. **Gledhill N, Cox D, and Jamnik R.** Endurance athletes' stroke volume does not plateau: major advantage is diastolic function. *Med Sci Sports Exerc* 26: 1116–1121, 1994.
15. **Gorman M, and Sparks H.** The unanswered question. *News in Physiological Sciences* 6: 191–193, 1991.
16. **Hagberg JM.** Effect of training on the decline of $\dot{V}O_2$ max with aging. *Fed Proc* 46: 1830–1833, 1987.
17. **Katz A.** *Physiology of the Heart*. Philadelphia: Wolters Kluwer Lippincott Williams and Wilkins, 2010.
18. **Kavazis AN, McClung JM, Hood DA, and Powers SK.** Exercise induces a cardiac mitochondrial phenotype that resists apoptotic stimuli. *Am J Physiol Heart Circ Physiol* 294: H928–935, 2008.
19. **Levy WC, Cerqueira MD, Harp GD, Johannessen KA, Abrass IB, Schwartz RS, and Stratton JR.** Effect of endurance exercise training on heart rate variability at rest in healthy young and older men. *Am J Cardiol* 82: 1236–1241, 1998.
20. **Liew R, and Chiam PT.** Risk stratification for sudden cardiac death after acute myocardial infarction. *Ann Acad Med Singapore* 39: 237–246, 2010.
21. **Mahon AD, Marjerrison AD, Lee JD, Woodruff ME, and Hanna LE.** Evaluating the prediction of maximal heart rate in children and adolescents. *Res Q Exerc Sport* 81: 466–471, 2010.
22. **Miller JD, Pegelow DF, Jacques AJ, and Dempsey JA.** Skeletal muscle pump versus respiratory muscle pump: modulation of venous return from the locomotor limb in humans. *J Physiol* 563: 925–943, 2005.
23. **Mitchell JH.** J. B. Wolffe memorial lecture. Neural control of the circulation during exercise. *Med Sci Sports Exerc* 22: 141–154, 1990.
24. **Mitchell JH, Payne FC, Saltin B, and Schibye B.** The role of muscle mass in the cardiovascular response to static contractions. *J Physiol* 309: 45–54, 1980.
25. **Mohrman D, and Heller L.** *Cardiovascular Physiology*. New York: McGraw Hill Lange, 2010.
26. **Powers SK, Demirel HA, Vincent HK, Coombes JS, Naito H, Hamilton KL, Shanely RA, and Jessup J.** Exercise training improves myocardial tolerance to in vivo ischemia-reperfusion in the rat. *Am J Physiol* 275: R1468–1477, 1998.
27. **Powers SK, Howley ET, and Cox R.** A differential catecholamine response during prolonged exercise and passive heating. *Med Sci Sports Exerc* 14: 435–439, 1982.
28. **Powers SK, Locke M, and Demirel HA.** Exercise, heat shock proteins, and myocardial protection from I-R injury. *Med Sci Sports Exerc* 33: 386–392, 2001.
29. **Powers SK, Quindry JC, and Kavazis AN.** Exercise-induced cardioprotection against myocardial ischemia-reperfusion injury. *Free Radic Biol Med* 44: 193–201, 2008.
30. **Raven P, and Stevens G.** Cardiovascular function during prolonged exercise. In: *Perspectives in Exercise Science and Sports Medicine: Prolonged Exercise*, edited by Lamb D, and Murray R. Indianapolis: Benchmark Press, 1988, p. 43–71.
31. **Raven PB, Fadel PJ, and Ogoh S.** Arterial baroreflex resetting during exercise: a current perspective. *Exp Physiol* 91: 37–49, 2006.

32. **Ridge B, and Pyke F.** Physiological responses to combinations of exercise and sauna. *Australian Journal of Science and Medicine in Sport* 18: 25–28, 1986.

33. **Rosiello RA, Mahler DA, and Ward JL.** Cardiovascular responses to rowing. *Med Sci Sports Exerc* 19: 239–245, 1987.

34. **Rowell LB**. *Human Circulation Regulation During Physical Stress*. New York: Oxford University Press, 1986.

35. **Rowell LB**. What signals govern the cardiovascular responses to exercise? *Med Sci Sports Exerc* 12: 307–315, 1980.

36. **Rubin SA**. Core temperature regulation of heart rate during exercise in humans. *J Appl Physiol* 62: 1997–2002, 1987.

37. **Sarelius I, and Pohl U.** Control of muscle blood flow during exercise: local factors and integrative mechanisms. *Acta Physiol (Oxf)* 199: 349–365, 2010.

38. **Sawka MN, Knowlton RG, and Critz JB**. Thermal and circulatory responses to repeated bouts of prolonged running. *Med Sci Sports* 11: 177–180, 1979.

39. **Tibes U.** Reflex inputs to the cardiovascular and respiratory centers from dynamically working canine muscles. Some evidence for involvement of group III or IV nerve fibers. *Circ Res* 41: 332–341, 1977.

40. **Virmani R, Burke AP, and Farb A.** Sudden cardiac death. *Cardiovasc Pathol* 10: 211–218, 2001.

41. **Whyte J, Laughlin, MH**. The effects of acute and chronic exercise on the vasculature. *Acta Physiologica* 199: 441–450, 2010.

42. **Williamson JW, Fadel PJ, and Mitchell JH**. New insights into central cardiovascular control during exercise in humans: a central command update. *Exp Physiol* 91: 51–58, 2006.

43. **Wyss CR, Ardell JL, Scher AM, and Rowell LB**. Cardiovascular responses to graded reductions in hindlimb perfusion in exercising dogs. *Am J Physiol* 245: H481–486, 1983.

44. **Zhou B, Conlee RK, Jensen R, Fellingham GW, George JD, and Fisher AG**. Stroke volume does not plateau during graded exercise in elite male distance runners. *Med Sci Sports Exerc* 33: 1849–1854, 2001.

45. **Zobl E.** Effect of exercise on the cerebral circulation and metabolism. *Journal of Applied Physiology* 20: 1289–1293, 1965.

Respiration During Exercise

■ Objectives

By studying this chapter, you should be able to do the following:

1. Explain the primary function of the pulmonary system.
2. Outline the major anatomical components of the respiratory system.
3. List the major muscles involved in inspiration and expiration at rest and during exercise.
4. Discuss the importance of matching blood flow to alveolar ventilation in the lung.
5. Explain how gases are transported across the blood-gas interface in the lung.
6. Discuss the major transportation modes of O_2 and CO_2 in the blood.
7. Discuss the effects of increasing temperature, decreasing pH, and increasing levels of 2–3 DPG on the oxygen-hemoglobin dissociation curve.
8. Describe the ventilatory response to constant load, steady-state exercise. What happens to ventilation if exercise is prolonged and performed in a high-temperature/humid environment?
9. Describe the ventilatory response to incremental exercise. What factors are thought to contribute to the alinear rise in ventilation at work rates above 50% to 70% of $\dot{V}O_2$ max?
10. Identify the location and function of chemoreceptors and mechanoreceptors that are thought to play a role in the regulation of breathing.
11. Discuss the neural-humoral theory of respiratory control during exercise.

■ Outline

alveolar ventilation ($\dot{V}_A$)
alveoli
anatomical dead space
aortic bodies
Bohr effect
bulk flow
carotid bodies
cellular respiration
deoxyhemoglobin

diaphragm
diffusion
hemoglobin
myoglobin
oxyhemoglobin
partial pressure
pleura
pulmonary respiration
residual volume (RV)

respiration
spirometry
tidal volume
total lung capacity (TLC)
ventilation
ventilatory threshold (Tvent)
vital capacity (VC)

The word **respiration** can have two definitions in physiology. These definitions can be divided into two separate but related subdivisions: (1) **pulmonary respiration** and (2) **cellular respiration.** Pulmonary respiration refers to ventilation (breathing) and the exchange of gases (O_2 and CO_2) in the lungs. Cellular respiration relates to O_2 utilization and CO_2 production by the tissues (see chapter 3). This chapter is concerned with pulmonary respiration, and the term respiration is used in the text as a synonym for pulmonary respiration. Because the pulmonary system plays a key role in maintaining blood-gas homeostasis (i.e., O_2 and CO_2 tensions) during exercise, an understanding of lung function during work is important for the student of exercise physiology. Therefore, this chapter will discuss the design and function of the respiratory system during exercise.

FUNCTION OF THE LUNG

The primary purpose of the respiratory system is to provide a means of gas exchange between the external environment and the body. That is, the respiratory system provides the individual with a means of replacing O_2 and removing CO_2 from the blood. The exchange of O_2 and CO_2 between the lung and blood occurs as a result of two processes: (1) ventilation and (2) diffusion. The term **ventilation** refers to the mechanical process of moving air into and out of the lungs. **Diffusion** is the random movement of molecules from an area of high concentration to an area of lower concentration. Because O_2 tension in the lungs is greater than in the blood, O_2 moves from the lungs into the blood. Similarly, the tension of CO_2 in the blood is greater than the tension of CO_2 in the lungs, and thus CO_2 moves from the blood into the lungs and is expired. Diffusion in the respiratory system occurs rapidly because there is a large surface area within the lungs and a very short diffusion distance between blood and gas in the lungs. The fact that the O_2 and CO_2 tension in the blood leaving the lungs is almost in complete equilibrium with the O_2 and CO_2 tension found within the lungs is testimony to the high efficiency of normal lung function.

The respiratory system also plays an important role in the regulation of the acid-base balance during heavy exercise. This important topic is introduced in this chapter and discussed in more detail in chapter 11.

IN SUMMARY

- The primary function of the pulmonary system is to provide a means of gas exchange between the environment and the body.
- The respiratory system also plays an important role in the regulation of the acid-base balance during exercise.

STRUCTURE OF THE RESPIRATORY SYSTEM

The human respiratory system is composed of a group of passages that filter air and transport it into the lungs, where gas exchange occurs within microscopic air sacs called **alveoli.** The major components of the respiratory system are pictured in figure 10.1. The organs of the respiratory system include the nose, nasal cavity, pharynx, larynx, trachea, bronchial tree, and the lungs themselves. The anatomical position of the lungs relative to the major muscle of inspiration, the diaphragm, is pictured in figure 10.2. Note that both the right and the left lungs are enclosed by a set of membranes called **pleura.** The visceral pleura adheres to the outer surface of the lung, whereas the parietal pleura lines the thoracic walls and the diaphragm. These two pleura are separated by a thin layer of fluid that acts as a lubricant, allowing a gliding action of one pleura on the other. The pressure in the pleural cavity (intrapleural pressure) is less than atmospheric and becomes even lower during inspiration, causing air to inflate the lungs. The fact that intrapleural pressure is less than atmospheric is important, because it prevents the collapse of the fragile air sacs within the lungs. More will be said about this later.

The air passages of the respiratory system are divided into two functional zones: (1) the conducting

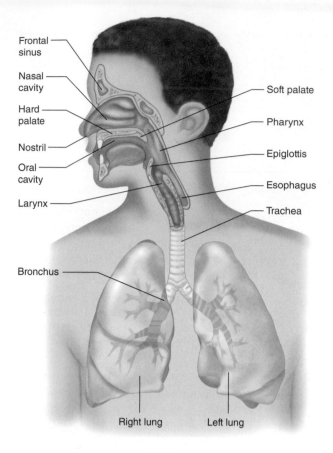

Figure 10.1 Major organs of the respiratory system.

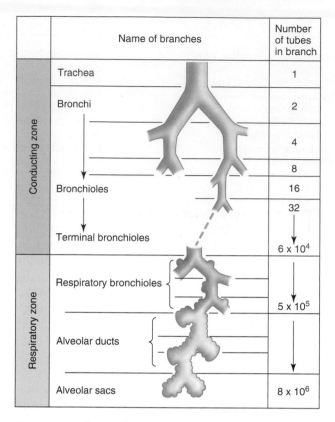

Figure 10.3 The conducting zones and respiratory zones of the pulmonary system.

	Name of branches		Number of tubes in branch
Conducting zone	Trachea		1
	Bronchi		2
			4
			8
	Bronchioles		16
			32
	Terminal bronchioles		6×10^4
Respiratory zone	Respiratory bronchioles		5×10^5
	Alveolar ducts		
	Alveolar sacs		8×10^6

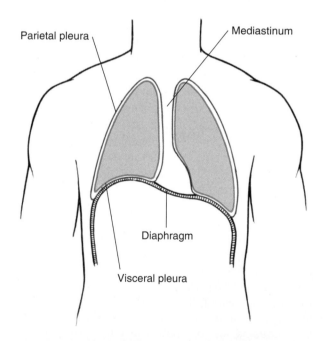

Figure 10.2 Position of the lungs, diaphragm, and pleura.

The region of the lung where gas exchange occurs is labeled the respiratory zone and includes the respiratory bronchioles and alveolar sacs. Respiratory bronchioles are included in this region because they contain small clusters of alveoli.

Conducting Zone

Air enters the trachea from the pharynx (throat), which receives air from both the nasal and oral cavities. At rest, healthy humans breathe through the nose. However, during moderate to heavy exercise, the mouth becomes the major passageway for air (33). For gas to enter or leave the trachea, it must pass through a valve-like opening called the *epiglottis*, which is located between the vocal cords.

The trachea branches into two primary bronchi (right and left) that enter each lung. The bronchial tree then branches several more times before forming bronchioles (bronchioles are small branches of the bronchial tree). The bronchioles then branch several times before they become the alveolar ducts leading to the alveolar sacs and respiratory zone of the lung (see figure 10.4).

The conducting zone of the respiratory system not only serves as a passageway for air, but also functions to filter and humidify the air as it moves toward

zone and (2) the respiratory zone (see figure 10.3). The conducting zone includes all those anatomical structures (e.g., trachea, bronchial tree, bronchioles) that air passes through to reach the respiratory zone.

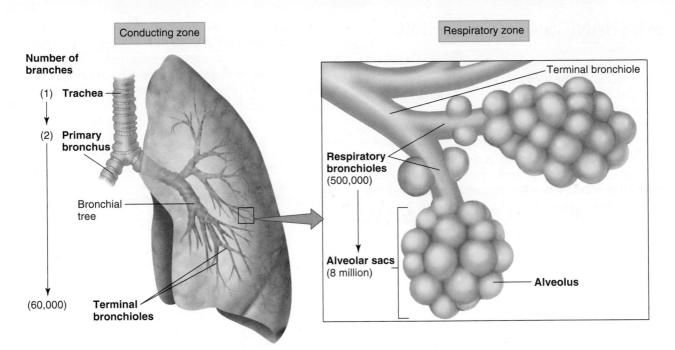

Respiratory zone

Number of
branches

(1) Trachea

(2) Primary
bronchus

Bronchial
tree

(60,000)

Terminal
bronchioles

Terminal bronchiole

Respiratory
bronchioles
(500,000)

Alveolar sacs
(8 million)

Alveolus

Figure 10.4 The bronchial tree consists of the passageways that connect the trachea and the alveoli.

the respiratory zone of the lung. Regardless of the temperature or humidity of the environment, the air that reaches the lung is warmed and is saturated with water vapor (67, 69). This warming and humidification of air prevents the delicate lung tissue from desiccation (drying out) during exercise when breathing is increased (67, 98).

Respiratory Zone

Gas exchange in the lungs occurs across about 300 million tiny alveoli. The enormous number of these structures provides the lung with a large surface area for diffusion. It is estimated that the total surface area available for diffusion in the human lung is 60 to 80 square meters (i.e., size of a tennis court). The rate of diffusion is further assisted by the fact that each alveolus is only one cell layer thick, so that the total blood-gas barrier is only two cell layers thick (alveolar cell and capillary cell) (see figure 10.5).

Although the alveoli provide the ideal structure for gas exchange, the fragility of these tiny "bubbles" presents some problems for the lung. For example, because of the surface tension (pressure exerted due to the properties of water) of the liquid lining the alveoli, relatively large forces develop, which tend to collapse alveoli. Fortunately, some of the alveolar cells (called type II, see figure 10.5) synthesize and release a material called *surfactant*, which lowers the surface tension of the alveoli and thus prevents their collapse (60).

IN SUMMARY

- Anatomically, the pulmonary system consists of a group of passages that filter air and transport it into the lungs where gas exchange occurs within tiny air sacs called *alveoli*.

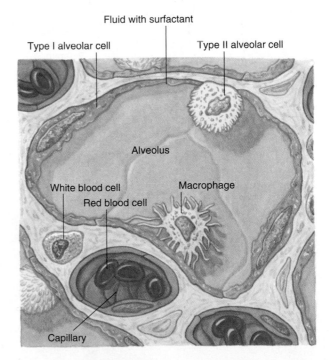

Fluid with surfactant

Type I alveolar cell

Type II alveolar cell

Alveolus

White blood cell

Macrophage

Red blood cell

Capillary

Figure 10.5 Relationship between type II alveolar cells and the alveolus.

MECHANICS OF BREATHING

As previously mentioned, movement of air from the environment to the lungs is called pulmonary ventilation and occurs via a process known as **bulk flow.** Bulk flow refers to the movement of molecules along a passageway due to a pressure difference between the two ends of the passageway. Thus, inspiration occurs due to the pressure in the lungs (intrapulmonary) being reduced below atmospheric pressure. Conversely, expiration occurs when the pressure within the lungs exceeds atmospheric pressure. The means by which this pressure change within the lungs is achieved is discussed within the next several paragraphs.

Inspiration

Any muscle capable of increasing the volume of the chest is considered to be an inspiratory muscle. The **diaphragm** is the most important muscle of inspiration and is the only skeletal muscle considered essential for life (32, 33, 66, 67, 89, 91, 93). This thin, dome-shaped muscle inserts into the lower ribs and is innervated by the phrenic nerves. When the diaphragm contracts, it forces the abdominal contents downward and forward. Further, the ribs are lifted outward. The outcome of these two actions is to reduce intrapleural pressure, which in turn causes the lungs to expand.

This expansion of the lungs results in a reduction in intrapulmonary pressure below atmospheric, which allows airflow into the lungs (figure 10.6).

During normal, quiet breathing the diaphragm performs most of the work of inspiration. However, during exercise, accessory muscles of inspiration are called into action to assist in breathing (71, 73, 97). These include the external intercostal muscles, pectoralis minor, the scalene muscles, and the sternocleidomastoids (see figure 10.7). Collectively, these muscles assist the diaphragm in increasing the volume of the thorax, which aids in inspiration (see A Closer Look 10.1).

Expiration

Expiration is passive during normal, quiet breathing. That is, no muscular effort is necessary for expiration to occur at rest. This is true because the lungs and chest walls are elastic and tend to return to their equilibrium position after expanding during inspiration (101). During exercise, expiration becomes active. The most important muscles involved in expiration are those found in the abdominal wall, which include the rectus abdominus and the internal oblique (67). When these muscles contract, the diaphragm is pushed upward and the ribs are pulled downward and inward. This results in an increase in intrapulmonary pressure and expiration occurs.

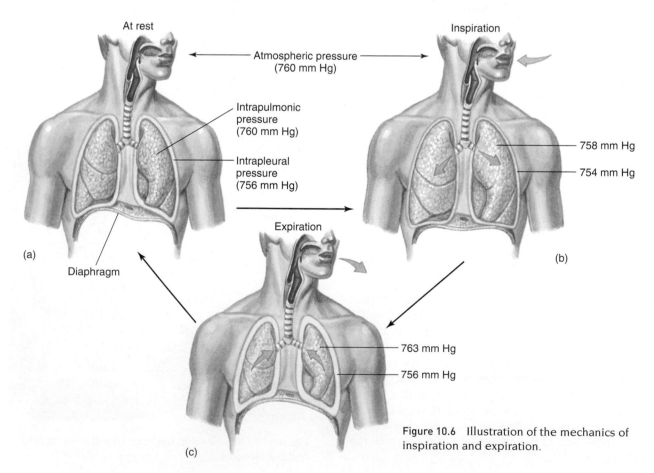

Figure 10.6 Illustration of the mechanics of inspiration and expiration.

Figure 10.7   The muscles of respiration. The principal muscles of inspiration are shown on the left side of the trunk; the principal muscles of expiration are shown on the right side.

A CLOSER LOOK 10.1

Respiratory Muscles and Exercise

Respiratory muscles are skeletal muscles that are functionally similar to locomotor muscles. Their primary task is to act upon the chest wall to move gas in and out of the lungs to maintain arterial blood gas and pH homeostasis. The importance of normal respiratory muscle function can be appreciated by considering that respiratory muscle failure due to disease or spinal cord injury would result in the inability to ventilate the lungs and maintain blood gas and pH levels within an acceptable range.

Muscular exercise results in an increase in pulmonary ventilation, and therefore an increased workload is placed on respiratory muscles. Historically, it was believed that respiratory muscles do not fatigue during exercise. However, growing evidence indicates that both prolonged exercise (e.g., 120 minutes) and high-intensity exercise (80–100% $\dot{V}O_2$ max) can promote respiratory muscle fatigue (110). The impact of respiratory muscle fatigue on exercise performance is discussed later in this chapter.

Do respiratory muscles adapt to regular exercise training in a similar manner to locomotor skeletal muscles? The answer to this question is yes! Regular endurance exercise training increases respiratory muscle oxidative capacity and improves respiratory muscle endurance (81, 82, 94, 106, 107). Further, new evidence reveals that exercise training also increases the oxidative capacity of upper airway muscles (108). This is important because these muscles play a key role in maintaining open airways to reduce the work of breathing during exercise. The effects of exercise training on skeletal muscles is discussed in detail in chapter 13. For more information on respiratory muscle adaptation to exercise, see Powers and Shanely (2004) in the Suggested Readings.

Exercise-Induced Asthma

Asthma is a disease that promotes a reversible narrowing of the airways. An asthma "attack" can be caused by both contraction of smooth muscle around the airways (called a bronchospasm) and a collection of mucus within the airway. This reduction in airway diameter results in an increased work of breathing, and individuals suffering from asthma generally report being short of breath (called dyspnea).

Although there are many potential causes of asthma (24, 72) some asthmatic patients develop a bronchospasm during or immediately after exercise. This type of asthma is called "exercise-induced asthma." When an individual experiences an asthma attack during exercise, breathing becomes labored and a wheezing sound is often heard during expiration. If the asthmatic attack is severe, it becomes impossible for the individual to exercise at even low intensities because of the dyspnea associated with the increased work of breathing. Asthma is an excellent example of how even a small decrease in airway diameter can result in a large increase in breathing resistance. See chapter 17 for more details on exercise and asthma.

Airway Resistance

At any rate of airflow into the lungs, the pressure difference that must be developed depends on the resistance of the airways. Airflow through the airways of the respiratory system can be mathematically defined by the following relationships:

$$\text{Airflow} = \frac{P_1 - P_2}{\text{Resistance}}$$

where $P_1 - P_2$ is the pressure difference at the two ends of the airway, and resistance is the resistance to flow offered by the airway. Airflow is increased anytime there is an increase in the pressure gradient across the pulmonary system, or if there is a decrease in airway resistance. This same relationship for blood flow was discussed in chapter 9.

What factors contribute to airway resistance? By far the most important variable contributing to airway resistance is the diameter of the airway. Airways that are reduced in size due to disease (chronic obstructive pulmonary disease, asthma, etc.) offer more resistance to flow than healthy, open airways. When the radius of an airway is reduced, the resistance to flow is increased markedly. Therefore, one can easily understand the effect of obstructive lung diseases (e.g., exercise-induced asthma) on increasing the work of breathing, especially during exercise when pulmonary ventilation is ten to twenty times greater than at rest (see Clinical Applications 10.1 and 10.2).

- The major muscle of inspiration is the diaphragm.

- Air enters the pulmonary system due to intra-pulmonary pressure being reduced below atmospheric pressure (bulk flow).
- At rest, expiration is passive. However, during exercise, expiration becomes active, using muscles located in the abdominal wall (e.g., rectus abdominus and internal oblique).
- The primary factor that contributes to airflow resistance in the pulmonary system is the diameter of the airway.

PULMONARY VENTILATION

Before beginning a discussion of ventilation, it is helpful to define some commonly used pulmonary physiology symbols:

1. V is used to denote volume.
2. $\dot{V}$ means volume per unit of time (generally one minute).
3. The subscripts $_{T, D, A, I, E}$ are used to denote tidal ($_T$), dead space ($_D$), alveolar ($_A$), inspired ($_I$), and expired ($_E$), respectively.

Pulmonary ventilation refers to the movement of gas into and out of the lungs. The amount of gas ventilated per minute is the product of the frequency of breathing (f) and the amount of gas moved per breath (**tidal volume**):

$$\dot{V} = V_T \times f$$

In a 70-kg man, the $\dot{V}$ at rest is generally around 7.5 liters/minute, with a tidal volume of 0.5 liter and a

Exercise and Chronic Obstructive Pulmonary Disease

Chronic obstructive pulmonary disease (COPD) is clinically identified by a decreased expiratory airflow resulting from increased airway resistance. Although COPD and asthma both result in blockage of the airways, these diseases differ in one key feature. Asthma is a reversible narrowing of the airways; that is, asthma can come and go. In contrast, COPD is a constant narrowing of the airways. Although COPD patients can experience some variation in airway blockage, these individuals always experience some level of airway obstruction.

Note that COPD is often the result of a combination of two separate lung diseases: (1) chronic bronchitis and (2) emphysema. Each of these individual diseases results in increased airway obstruction. Chronic bronchitis is a lung disorder that results in a constant production of mucus within airways, resulting in airway blockage. Emphysema causes a decreased elastic support of the airways, resulting in airway collapse and increased airway resistance. Two of the greatest risk factors in developing COPD are tobacco smoking and a family history of emphysema (116).

Because COPD patients have a constant narrowing of the airways, this airway resistance places an increased workload on respiratory muscles to move gas in and out of the lung. Recognition of this increased work of breathing leads to the sensation of being short of breath (dyspnea). Because the magnitude of dyspnea is closely linked to the amount of work performed by respiratory muscles, dyspnea in COPD patients is greatly increased during exercise. In patients with severe COPD, dyspnea may become so debilitating that the patient has difficulty in performing routine activities of daily living (e.g., walking to the bathroom, showering, etc.). See West (2007) in the Suggested Readings for more details on COPD and exercise.

---

frequency of 15. During maximal exercise, ventilation may reach 120 to 175 liters per minute, with a frequency of 40 to 50 breaths per minute and a tidal volume of approximately 3 to 3.5 liters.

It is important to understand that not all of the air that passes the lips reaches the alveolar gas compartment, where gas exchange occurs. Part of each breath remains in conducting airways (trachea, bronchi, etc.) and thus does not participate in gas exchange. This "unused" ventilation is called dead-space ventilation (V_D), and the space it occupies is known as **anatomical dead space.** The volume of inspired gas that reaches the respiratory zone is referred to as **alveolar ventilation ($\dot{V}_A$).** Thus, total minute ventilation can be subdivided into dead space ventilation and alveolar ventilation:

$$\dot{V} = \dot{V}_A + \dot{V}_D$$

Note that pulmonary ventilation is not equally distributed throughout the lung. The basal (bottom) region of the lung receives more ventilation than the apex (top region), particularly during quiet breathing (67). This changes to some degree during exercise, with the apical (top) regions of the lung receiving an increased percentage of the total ventilation (56).

IN SUMMARY

- Pulmonary ventilation refers to the amount of gas moved into and out of the lungs.
- The amount of gas moved per minute is the product of tidal volume times breathing frequency.

PULMONARY VOLUMES AND CAPACITIES

Pulmonary volumes can be measured via a technique known as **spirometry.** Using this procedure, the subject breathes into a device that is capable of measuring inspired and expired gas volumes. Modern spirometers use computer technology to measure pulmonary volumes and the rate of expired airflow (see figure 10.8). Figure 10.9 is a spirogram showing

Figure 10.8 Photograph of a computerized spirometer used to measure lung volumes. Courtesy of Sensormedics Corp.

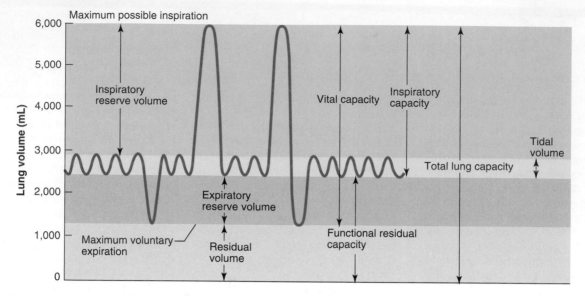

Figure 10.9   A spirogram showing lung volumes and capacities at rest.

the measurement of tidal volumes during quiet breathing and the various lung volumes and capacities that are defined in table 10.1. Several of these terms require special mention. First, **vital capacity (VC)** is defined as the maximum amount of gas that can be expired after a maximum inspiration. Second, the **residual volume (RV)** is the volume of gas remaining in the lungs after a maximum expiration. Finally, **total lung capacity (TLC)** is defined as

the amount of gas in the lungs after a maximum inspiration; it is the sum of the two lung volumes (VC + RV) just mentioned. Note that exercise training does not impact any of these lung volumes or capacities. More will be said about this later.

Clinically, spirometry is useful in diagnosing lung diseases such as chronic obstructive lung disease (COPD). For example, because of increased airway resistance, COPD patients will have a diminished

Measurement	Typical Value	Definition
TABLE 10.1	**Respiratory Volumes and Capacities for a 70-Kg Young Adult Male**	
Respiratory Volumes		
Tidal volume (TV)	500 mL	Amount of air inhaled or exhaled in one breath during quiet breathing
Inspiratory reserve volume (IRV)	3,000 mL	Amount of air in excess of tidal volume that can be inhaled with maximum effort
Expiratory reserve volume (ERV)	1,200 mL	Amount of air in excess of tidal volume that can be exhaled with maximum effort
Residual volume (RV)	1,300 mL	Amount of air remaining in the lungs after maximum expiration; that is, the amount of air that can never be voluntarily exhaled
Respiratory Capacities		
Vital capacity (VC)	4,700 mL	Amount of air that can be forcefully exhaled following a maximum inspiration VC = (ERV + TV + IRV)
Inspiratory capacity (IC)	3,500 mL	Maximum amount of air that can be inhaled following a normal expiration (IC = TV + IRV)
Functional residual capacity (FRC)	2,500 mL	Amount of air remaining in the lungs following a normal expiration (FRC = RV + ERV)
Total lung capacity (TLC)	6,000 mL	Maximum amount of air in the lungs at the end of a maximum inspiration (TLC = RV + VC)

vital capacity and a reduced rate of expired airflow during a maximal expiratory effort. An illustration of how spirometry can detect airway obstruction in patients follows. One of the easiest spirometric tests to detect airway blockage is the measurement of forced expiratory volume and vital capacity (VC). The forced expiratory volume (called FEV1) is the volume of gas expired in 1 second by a forced (maximal effort) expiration from a full inspiration. Vital capacity is the total amount of gas that can be expired during a maximal expiration following a full inspiration. A simple way to make these measures is illustrated in figure 10.8. The patient is comfortably seated in front of the spirometer and breathes through a rubber mouthpiece connected to the spirometer. The patient breathes in maximally and then maximally exhales. The spirometer records the expired volume of gas against time during the expiratory effort.

Figure 10.10 compares the measurements of FEV1 and VC in both a normal, healthy individual and a patient with COPD. Notice, in the normal individual, the vital capacity is 5.0 liters and the FEV1 was 4.0 liters. Therefore, the FEV in this healthy individual is 80% of the VC (i.e., 4.0/5.0 × 100 = 80%). Indeed, the normal ratio of FEV1 to VC in healthy individuals is 80% or higher.

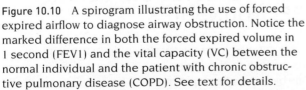

Figure 10.10   A spirogram illustrating the use of forced expired airflow to diagnose airway obstruction. Notice the marked difference in both the forced expired volume in 1 second (FEV1) and the vital capacity (VC) between the normal individual and the patient with chronic obstructive pulmonary disease (COPD). See text for details.

Now let's analyze the measurement of FEV1 and VC in the patient with COPD. Note that the rate at which air was expired in the COPD patient is much slower than in the healthy subject, so that only 1.0 liter of air is expired in the first second. Moreover, the vital capacity in the COPD patient is only 3.0 liters. Therefore, in this patient, the ratio of forced expired volume to vital capacity (1.0/3.0 × 100) is 33%. This value is much lower than the normal values for a normal individual (i.e., 80%) and is typical of a COPD patient with severe airway obstruction. For more information on the impact of COPD on exercise tolerance, see Clinical Applications 10.2.

IN SUMMARY

- Pulmonary volumes can be measured using spirometry.
- Vital capacity is the maximum amount of gas that can be expired after a maximal inspiration.
- Residual volume is the amount of gas left in the lungs after a maximal expiration.

DIFFUSION OF GASES

Prior to discussing diffusion of gases across the alveolar membrane into the blood, let's review the concept of **partial pressure.** According to Dalton's law, the total pressure of a gas mixture is equal to the sum of the pressures that each gas would exert independently. Thus, the pressure that each gas exerts independently can be calculated by multiplying the fractional composition of the gas by the absolute pressure (barometric pressure). Let's consider an example calculating the partial pressure of oxygen in air at sea level. The barometric pressure at sea level is 760 mm Hg (recall that barometric pressure is the force exerted by the weight of the gas contained within the atmosphere). The composition of air is generally considered to be as follows:

Gas	Percentage	Fraction
Oxygen	20.93	.2093
Nitrogen	79.04	.7904
Carbon dioxide	0.03	.0003
Total	100.0	

Therefore, the partial pressure of oxygen (PO_2) at sea level can be computed as:

$$PO_2 = 760 \times .2093$$
$$PO_2 = 159 \text{ mm Hg}$$

In a similar manner, the partial pressure of nitrogen can be calculated to be:

$$PN_2 = 760 \times .7904$$
$$PN_2 = 600.7 \text{ mm Hg}$$

Because O_2, CO_2, and N_2 make up almost 100% of the atmosphere, the total barometric pressure (P) can be computed as:

$$P \text{ (dry atmosphere)} = PO_2 + PN_2 + PCO_2$$

Diffusion of a gas across tissues is described by Fick's law of diffusion, which states that the rate of gas transfer (V gas) is proportional to the tissue area, the diffusion coefficient of the gas, and the difference in the partial pressure of the gas on the two sides of the tissue, and is inversely proportional to the thickness:

$$V \text{ gas} = \frac{A}{T} \times D \times (P_1 - P_2)$$

where A is the area, T is the thickness of the tissue, D is the diffusion coefficient of the gas, and $P_1 - P_2$ is the difference in the partial pressure between the two sides of the tissue. In simple terms, the rate of diffusion for any single gas is greater when the surface area for diffusion is large and the "driving pressure" between the two sides of the tissue is high. In contrast, an increase in tissue thickness impedes diffusion. The lung is well designed for the diffusion of gases across the alveolar membrane into and out of the blood. First, the total surface area available for diffusion is large. Second, the alveolar membrane is extremely thin. The fact that the lung is an ideal organ for gas exchange is important; during maximal exercise, the rate of O_2 uptake and CO_2 output may increase twenty to thirty times above resting condition.

The amount of O_2 or CO_2 dissolved in blood obeys Henry's law and is dependent on the temperature of blood, the partial pressure of the gas, and the solubility of the gas. Because the temperature of the blood does not change a great deal during exercise (i.e., 1–3° C), and the solubility of the gas remains constant, the major factor that determines the amount of dissolved gas is the partial pressure.

Figure 10.11 illustrates gas exchange via diffusion across the alveolar-capillary membranes and at the tissue level. Note that the PCO_2 and PO_2 of blood entering the lung are approximately 46 and 40 mm Hg, respectively. In contrast, the PCO_2 and PO_2 in alveolar gas are around 40 and 105 mm Hg, respectively. As a consequence of the difference in partial pressure across the blood-gas interface, CO_2 leaves the blood and diffuses into the alveolus, and O_2 diffuses from the alveolus into the blood. Blood leaving the lung has a PO_2 of approximately 95 mm Hg and a PCO_2 of 40 mm Hg.

IN SUMMARY

- Gas moves across the blood-gas interface in the lung due to simple diffusion.
- The rate of diffusion is described by Fick's law and diffusion is greater when the surface area is large and the driving pressure is high.

BLOOD FLOW TO THE LUNG

The pulmonary circulation begins at the pulmonary artery, which receives venous blood from the right ventricle (recall that this is mixed venous blood). Mixed venous blood is then circulated through the pulmonary capillaries where gas exchange occurs, and this oxygenated blood is returned to the left atrium via the pulmonary vein to be circulated throughout the body (see figure 10.12).

Recall that the rates of blood flow in the pulmonary and systemic circulation are equal. In the adult, the left and right ventricles of the heart have an output of approximately 5 liters/minute. However, the pressures in the pulmonary circulation are relatively low when compared to those in the systemic circulation (see chapter 9). This low-pressure system is due to low vascular resistance in the pulmonary circulation (67, 118). An interesting feature of pulmonary circulation is that during exercise, the resistance in the pulmonary vascular system falls due to the distension of vessels and the recruitment of previously unused capillaries. This decrease in pulmonary vascular resistance results in increased lung blood flow during exercise with relatively small increases in pulmonary arterial pressure.

When we are standing, considerable inequality of blood flow exists within the human lung due to gravity. For example, in the upright position, blood flow decreases almost linearly from bottom to top, reaching very low values at the top (apex) of the lung (see figure 10.13). This distribution may be altered during exercise and with a change in posture. During light exercise, blood flow to the apex of the lung is increased (19). This will improve gas exchange and will be discussed in the next section. When individuals lie on their backs (supine), blood flow becomes uniform within the lung. In contrast, measurements of blood flow in humans who are suspended upside down show that blood flow to the apex of the lung greatly exceeds that found in the base.

IN SUMMARY

- The pulmonary circulation is a low-pressure system with a rate of blood flow equal to that in the systemic circuit.
- In a standing position, most of the blood flow to the lung is distributed to the base of the lung due to gravitational force.

VENTILATION-PERFUSION RELATIONSHIPS

Thus far we have discussed pulmonary ventilation, blood flow to the lungs, and diffusion of gases across the blood-gas barrier in the lung. It seems reasonable to

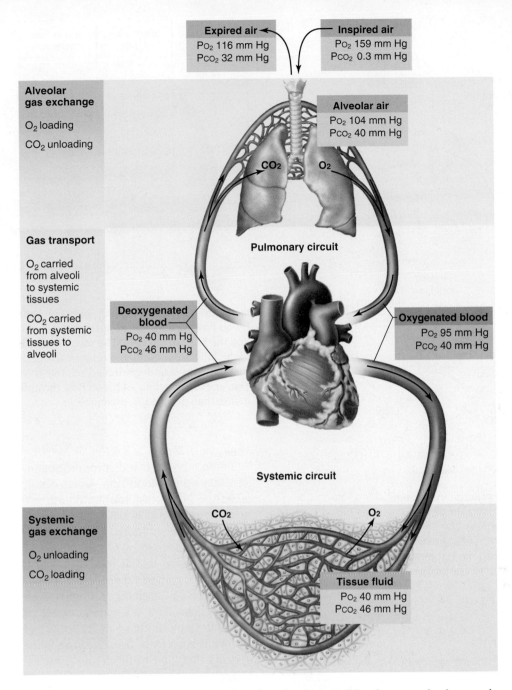

Expired air
Po_2 116 mm Hg
Pco_2 32 mm Hg

Inspired air
Po_2 159 mm Hg
Pco_2 0.3 mm Hg

Alveolar gas exchange

O_2 loading

CO_2 unloading

Alveolar air
Po_2 104 mm Hg
Pco_2 40 mm Hg

CO_2 O_2

Pulmonary circuit

Gas transport

O_2 carried from alveoli to systemic tissues

CO_2 carried from systemic tissues to alveoli

Deoxygenated blood
Po_2 40 mm Hg
Pco_2 46 mm Hg

Oxygenated blood
Po_2 95 mm Hg
Pco_2 40 mm Hg

Systemic circuit

Systemic gas exchange

O_2 unloading

CO_2 loading

CO_2 O_2

Tissue fluid
Po_2 40 mm Hg
Pco_2 46 mm Hg

Figure 10.11 Partial pressures of oxygen (PO_2) and carbon dioxide (PCO_2) in blood as a result of gas exchange in the lung and gas exchange between capillaries and tissues. Note that the alveolar PO_2 of 104 is a result of mixing atmospheric air (i.e., 159 mm Hg at sea level) with existing alveolar gas along with water vapor.

assume that if all these processes were adequate, normal gas exchange would occur in the lung. However, normal gas exchange requires a matching of ventilation to blood flow (perfusion, Q). In other words, an alveolus can be well ventilated, but if blood flow to the alveolus does not adequately match ventilation, normal gas exchange does not occur. Indeed, mismatching of ventilation and perfusion is responsible for most of the problems of gas exchange that occur due to lung diseases.

The ideal ventilation-to-perfusion ratio (V/Q) is 1.0 or slightly greater. That is, there is a one-to-one matching of ventilation to blood flow, which results in optimum gas exchange. Unfortunately, the V/Q ratio is generally not equal to 1.0 throughout the lung, but varies depending on the section of the lung being considered (32, 40, 57, 67, 117). This concept is illustrated in figure 10.14, where the V/Q ratio at the apex and the base of the lung is calculated for resting conditions.

Let's discuss the V/Q ratio in the apex of the lung first. Here, the ventilation (at rest) in the upper region of the lung is estimated to be 0.24 liter/minute, whereas the blood flow is considered to be 0.07 liter/minute.

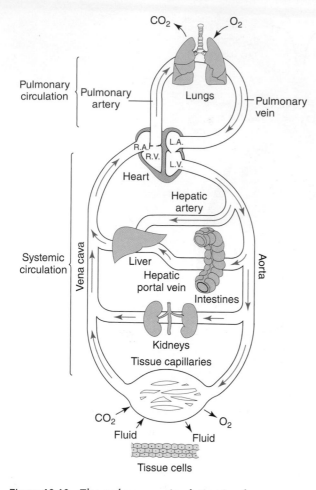

Figure 10.12 The pulmonary circulation is a low-pressure system that pumps mixed venous blood through the pulmonary capillaries for gas exchange. After the completion of gas exchange, this oxygenated blood is returned to the left heart chambers to be circulated throughout the body.

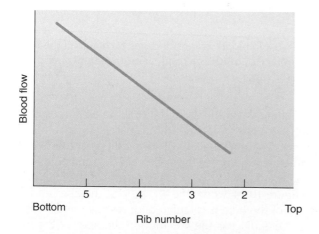

Figure 10.13 Regional blood flow within the lung. Note that there is a linear decrease in blood flow from the lower regions of the lung toward the upper regions.

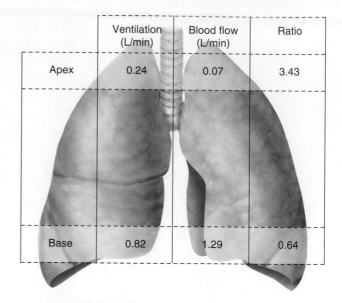

	Ventilation (L/min)	Blood flow (L/min)	Ratio
Apex	0.24	0.07	3.43
Base	0.82	1.29	0.64

Figure 10.14 The relationship between ventilation and blood flow (ventilation/perfusion ratios) at the top (apex) and the base of the lung. The ratios indicate that the base of the lung is overperfused relative to ventilation and that the apex is underperfused relative to ventilation. This uneven matching of blood flow to ventilation results in less than perfect gas exchange.

Thus, the V/Q ratio is 3.4 (i.e., 0.24/0.07 = 3.4). A large V/Q ratio represents a disproportionately high ventilation relative to blood flow, which results in poor gas exchange. In contrast, the ventilation at the base of the lung (figure 10.14) is 0.82 liter/minute, with a blood flow of 1.29 liters/minute (V/Q ratio = 0.82/1.29 = 0.64). A V/Q ratio less than 1.0 represents a greater blood flow than ventilation to the region in question. Although V/Q ratios less than 1.0 are not indicative of ideal conditions for gas exchange, in most cases V/Q ratios greater than 0.50 are adequate to meet the gas exchange demands at rest (117).

What effect does exercise have on the V/Q ratio? It appears that light-to-moderate exercise improves the V/Q relationship, whereas heavy exercise may result in a small V/Q inequality, and thus a minor impairment in gas exchange (56). Whether the increase in V/Q inequality is due to low ventilation or low perfusion is not clear. The possible effects of this V/Q mismatch on blood gases will be discussed later in the chapter.

IN SUMMARY

- Efficient gas exchange between the blood and the lung requires proper matching of blood flow to ventilation (called ventilation-perfusion relationships).
- The ideal ratio of ventilation to perfusion is 1.0 or slightly greater, because this ratio implies a perfect matching of blood flow to ventilation.

O₂ AND CO₂ TRANSPORT IN BLOOD

Although some O_2 and CO_2 are transported as dissolved gases in the blood, the major portion of O_2 and CO_2 transported via blood is done by O_2 combining with hemoglobin and CO_2 being transformed into bicarbonate (HCO_3^-). A complete discussion of how O_2 and CO_2 are transported in blood follows.

Hemoglobin and O₂ Transport

Approximately 99% of the O_2 transported in the blood is chemically bound to **hemoglobin,** which is a protein contained in the red blood cells (erythrocytes). Each molecule of hemoglobin can transport four O_2 molecules. The binding of O_2 to hemoglobin forms **oxyhemoglobin;** hemoglobin that is not bound to O_2 is referred to as **deoxyhemoglobin.**

The amount of O_2 that can be transported per unit volume of blood is dependent on the concentration of hemoglobin. Normal hemoglobin concentration for a healthy male and female is approximately 150 grams and 130 grams, respectively, per liter of blood. When completely saturated with O_2, each gram of hemoglobin can transport 1.34 ml of O_2 (67). Therefore, if hemoglobin is 100% saturated with O_2, the healthy male and female can transport approximately 200 ml and 174 ml of O_2, respectively, per liter of blood at sea level.

Oxyhemoglobin Dissociation Curve

The combination of O_2 with hemoglobin in the lung (alveolar capillaries) is called loading, and the release of O_2 from hemoglobin at the tissues is called unloading. Thus, loading and unloading are reversible reactions:

$$\textbf{Deoxyhemoglobin} + \textbf{O}_2 \longleftrightarrow \textbf{Oxyhemoglobin}$$

The factors that determine the direction of this reaction are (1) the PO_2 of the blood and (2) the affinity or bond strength between hemoglobin and O_2. A high PO_2 drives the reaction to the right (i.e., loading), whereas low PO_2 and a reduced affinity of hemoglobin for O_2 moves the reaction to the left (i.e., unloading). For example, a high PO_2 in the lungs results in an increase in arterial PO_2 and the formation of oxyhemoglobin (i.e., reaction moves right). In contrast, a low PO_2 in the tissue results in a decrease of PO_2 in the systemic capillaries and thus unloads O_2 to be used by the tissues (reaction moves left).

The effect of PO_2 on the combination of O_2 with hemoglobin is illustrated by the oxyhemoglobin dissociation curve (figure 10.15). This sigmoidal (S-shaped) curve has several interesting features. First, the percent hemoglobin saturated with O_2 (% HbO_2) increases sharply up to an arterial PO_2 of 40 mm Hg. At PO_2 values above 40 mm Hg, the increase in % HbO_2 rises slowly to a plateau around 90 to 100 mm Hg, at which the % HbO_2 is approximately 97%. At rest, the body's O_2 requirements are relatively low, and only about 25% of the O_2 transported in the blood is unloaded to the tissues. In contrast, during intense exercise, the mixed venous PO_2 can reach a value of 18 to 20 mm Hg, and the tissues can extract up to 90% of the O_2 carried by hemoglobin.

The shape of the oxyhemoglobin dissociation curve is well designed to meet human O_2 transport needs. The relatively flat portion of the curve (above a PO_2 of approximately 90 mm Hg) allows arterial PO_2 to oscillate from 90 to 100 mm Hg without a large drop in % HbO_2. This is important because there is a decline in arterial PO_2 with aging and upon ascent to high altitude. At the other end of the curve (steep portion, 0–40 mm Hg), small changes in PO_2 result in a release of large amounts of O_2 from hemoglobin. This is critical during exercise when tissue O_2 consumption is high.

Figure 10.15 The relationship between the partial pressure of O_2 in blood and the relative saturation of hemoglobin with O_2 is pictured here in the oxygen-hemoglobin dissociation curve. Notice the relatively steep portion of the curve up to PO_2 values of 40 mm Hg, after which there is a gradual rise to reach a plateau.

Effect of pH on O₂–Hb Dissociation Curve In addition to the effect of blood PO_2 on O_2 binding to hemoglobin, a change in acidity, temperature, or red blood cell (RBC) levels of 2,3-diphosphoglyceric acid (2–3 DPG) can affect the loading/unloading reaction. First, let's consider the effect of changing blood acid-base status on hemoglobin's affinity for O_2. The strength of the bond between O_2 and hemoglobin is weakened by a decrease in blood pH (increased acidity), which results in increased unloading of O_2 to the tissues. This is represented by a "right" shift in the oxyhemoglobin curve and is called the **Bohr effect** (see figure 10.16). A right shift in the oxyhemoglobin dissociation curve might be expected during heavy exercise due to the rise in blood hydrogen ion levels observed in this type of work. The mechanism to explain the Bohr effect is the fact that hydrogen ions (i.e., protons) bind to hemoglobin, which reduces its O_2 transport capacity. Therefore, when there is a higher-than-normal concentration of hydrogen ions in the blood (i.e., acidosis), there is a reduction in hemoglobin affinity for O_2. This facilitates the unloading of O_2 to the tissues during exercise, because the acidity level is higher in muscles.

Temperature Effect on O₂–Hb Dissociation Curve Another factor that affects hemoglobin affinity for O_2 is temperature. At a constant pH, the affinity of hemoglobin for O_2 is inversely related to blood temperature. That is, a decrease in temperature results in a left shift in the oxyhemoglobin curve, whereas an increase in temperature causes a right shift of the curve. This means that an increase in blood temperature weakens the bond between O_2 and hemoglobin, which assists in the unloading of O_2 to working muscle. Conversely, a decrease in blood temperature results in a stronger bond between O_2 and hemoglobin, which hinders O_2 release. The effect of increasing blood temperature on the oxyhemoglobin dissociation curve is presented in figure 10.17. During exercise, increased heat production in the contracting muscle would promote a right shift in the oxyhemoglobin dissociation curve and facilitate unloading of O_2 to the tissue.

2–3 DPG and the O₂–Hb Dissociation Curve A final factor that potentially can affect the shape of the oxyhemoglobin dissociation curve is the concentration of 2–3 DPG in red blood cells (RBCs). Red blood cells are unique in that they do not contain a nucleus or mitochondria. Therefore, they must rely on anaerobic glycolysis to meet the cell's energy needs. A by-product of RBC glycolysis is the compound 2–3 DPG, which can combine with hemoglobin and reduce hemoglobin's affinity for O_2 (i.e., right shift in oxyhemoglobin dissociation curve).

Red blood cell concentrations of 2–3 DPG are known to increase during exposure to altitude and in

Figure 10.16 The effect of changing blood pH on the shape of the oxygen-hemoglobin dissociation curve. A decrease in pH results in a rightward shift of the curve (Bohr effect), while an increase in pH results in a leftward shift of the curve.

Figure 10.17 The effect of changing blood temperature on the shape of the oxygen-hemoglobin dissociation curve. An increase in temperature results in a rightward shift in the curve, while a decrease in blood temperature results in a leftward shift in the curve.

anemia (low blood hemoglobin) (67). However, blood 2–3 DPG levels do not increase significantly during exercise at sea level (70, 99). Therefore, although an increase in blood 2–3 DPG can alter Hb-O_2 affinity, it appears that exercise at sea level does not increase 2–3 DPG in the red blood cell. Therefore, the right shift in the oxyhemoglobin curve during heavy exercise is not due to changes in 2–3 DPG but to the degree of acidosis and blood temperature elevation.

O_2 Transport in Muscle

Myoglobin is an oxygen-binding protein found in skeletal muscle fibers and cardiac muscle (not in blood) and acts as a "shuttle" to move O_2 from the muscle cell membrane to the mitochondria. Myoglobin is found in large quantities in slow-twitch fibers (i.e., high aerobic capacity), in smaller amounts in intermediate fibers, and in only limited amounts in fast-twitch fibers. Myoglobin is similar in structure to hemoglobin, but is about one-fourth the weight. The difference in structure between myoglobin and hemoglobin results in a difference in O_2 affinity between the two molecules. This point is illustrated in figure 10.18. Myoglobin has a greater affinity for O_2 than hemoglobin, and therefore the myoglobin-O_2 dissociation curve is much steeper than that of hemoglobin for PO_2 values below 20 mm Hg. The practical implication of the shape of the myoglobin-O_2 dissociation curve is that myoglobin discharges its O_2 at very low PO_2 values. This is important because the PO_2 in the mitochondria of contracting skeletal muscle may be as low as 1 to 2 mm Hg.

Myoglobin O_2 stores may serve as an "O_2 reserve" during transition periods from rest to exercise. At the beginning of exercise, there is a time lag between the onset of muscular contraction and an increased O_2 delivery to the muscle. Therefore, O_2 bound to myoglobin prior to the initiation of exercise serves to buffer the O_2 needs of the muscle until the cardio-pulmonary system can meet the new O_2 requirement. At the conclusion of exercise, myoglobin O_2 stores must be replenished, and this O_2 consumption above rest contributes to the O_2 debt (see chapter 4).

CO_2 Transport in Blood

Carbon dioxide is transported in the blood in three forms: (1) dissolved CO_2 (about 10% of blood CO_2 is transported this way), (2) CO_2 bound to hemoglobin (called carbaminohemoglobin; about 20% of blood CO_2 is transported via this form), and (3) bicarbonate (70% of CO_2 found in blood is transported as bicarbonate: HCO_3^-). The three forms of CO_2 transport in the blood are illustrated in figure 10.19.

Because most of the CO_2 that is transported in blood is transported as bicarbonate, this mechanism deserves special attention. Carbon dioxide can be converted to bicarbonate (within RBCs) in the following way:

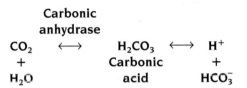

A high PCO_2 causes CO_2 to combine with water to form carbonic acid. This reaction is catalyzed by the enzyme carbonic anhydrase, which is found in RBCs. After formation, carbonic acid dissociates into a hydrogen ion and a bicarbonate ion. The hydrogen ion then binds to hemoglobin, and the bicarbonate

Figure 10.18 Comparison of the dissociation curve for myoglobin and hemoglobin. The steep myoglobin dissociation demonstrates a higher affinity for O_2 than hemoglobin.

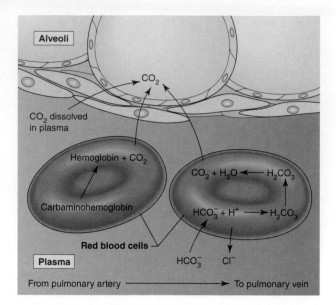

Figure 10.19 Carbon dioxide is released from the tissues and moves into the blood. Carbon dioxide is transported in three forms in the blood: (1) dissolved CO_2, (2) CO_2 combined with hemoglobin (carboxyhemoglobin), and (3) bicarbonate (HCO_3^-). Notice that as HCO_3^- moves out of the red blood cell, chloride (Cl^-) moves into the red blood cell (chloride shift) to maintain electrochemical balance in the cell.

Figure 10.20 Carbon dioxide is released from the blood into the pulmonary capillaries. At the time of CO_2 release in the lung, there is a "reverse chloride shift" and carbonic acid dissociates into CO_2 and H_2O.

ion diffuses out of the RBC into the plasma (figure 10.19). Because bicarbonate carries a negative charge (anion), the removal of a negatively charged molecule from a cell without replacement would result in an electrochemical imbalance across the cell membrane. This problem is avoided by the replacement of bicarbonate by chloride (Cl^-), which diffuses from the plasma into the RBC. This exchange of anions occurs in the RBC as blood moves through the tissue capillaries and is called the chloride shift (figure 10.19).

When blood reaches the pulmonary capillaries, the PCO_2 of the blood is greater than that of the alveolus, and thus CO_2 diffuses out of the blood across the blood-gas interface. At the lung, the binding of O_2 to Hb results in a release of the hydrogen ions bound to hemoglobin and promotes the formation of carbonic acid:

$$H^+ + HCO_3^- \longrightarrow H_2CO_3$$

Under conditions of low PCO_2 that exist at the alveolus, carbonic acid then dissociates into CO_2 and H_2O:

$$H_2CO_3 \longrightarrow CO_2 + H_2O$$

The release of CO_2 from the blood into the alveoli (figure 10.20) is removed from the body in the expired gas.

IN SUMMARY

- More than 99% of the O_2 transported in blood is chemically bonded with hemoglobin. The effect of the partial pressure of O_2 on the combination of O_2 with hemoglobin is illustrated by the S-shaped O_2-hemoglobin dissociation curve.
- An increase in body temperature and a reduction in blood pH results in a right shift in the O_2-hemoglobin dissociation curve and a reduced affinity of hemoglobin for O_2.
- Carbon dioxide is transported in blood in three forms: (1) dissolved CO_2 (10% is transported in this way), (2) CO_2 bound to hemoglobin (called carbaminohemoglobin; about 20% of blood CO_2 is transported via this form), and (3) bicarbonate (70% of CO_2 found in blood is transported as bicarbonate [HCO_3^-]).

VENTILATION AND ACID-BASE BALANCE

Pulmonary ventilation can play an important role in removing H^+ from the blood by the HCO_3^- reaction discussed previously (102). For example, an increase in CO_2 in blood or body fluids results in an increase in hydrogen ion accumulation and thus a decrease in pH. In contrast, removal of CO_2 from blood or body fluids may decrease hydrogen ion concentration and thus increase pH. Recall that the CO_2-carbonic anhydrase reaction occurs as follows:

$$\text{Lung} \longleftarrow$$
$$CO_2 + H_2O \longleftrightarrow H_2CO_3 \longleftrightarrow H^+ + HCO_3^-$$
$$\text{Muscle} \longrightarrow$$

Therefore, an increase in pulmonary ventilation causes exhalation of additional CO_2 and results in a reduction of blood PCO_2 and a lowering of hydrogen ion concentration. On the other side, a reduction in pulmonary ventilation would result in a buildup of CO_2 and an increase in hydrogen ion concentration (pH would decrease). The role of the pulmonary system in acid-base balance is discussed in detail in chapter 11.

IN SUMMARY

- An increase in pulmonary ventilation causes exhalation of additional CO_2, which results in a reduction of blood PCO_2 and a lowering of hydrogen ion concentration (i.e., pH increases).

VENTILATORY AND BLOOD-GAS RESPONSES TO EXERCISE

Before discussing ventilatory control during exercise, we should examine the ventilatory response to several types of exercise.

Rest-to-Work Transitions

The change in pulmonary ventilation observed in the transition from rest to constant-load submaximal exercise (i.e., below the lactate threshold) is pictured in figure 10.21. Note that expired ventilation ($\dot{V}_E$) increases abruptly at the beginning of exercise, followed by a slower rise toward a steady-state value (8, 21, 22, 38, 53, 80, 87, 120).

Figure 10.21 also points out that arterial tensions of PCO_2 and PO_2 are relatively unchanged during this type of exercise (35, 37, 113). However, note that arterial PO_2 decreases and arterial PCO_2 tends to increase slightly in the transition from rest to steady-state exercise (37). This observation suggests that the increase in alveolar ventilation at the beginning of exercise is not as rapid as the increase in metabolism.

Prolonged Exercise in a Hot Environment

Figure 10.22 illustrates the change in pulmonary ventilation during prolonged, constant-load, submaximal exercise (below the lactate threshold) in two different

Figure 10.21 The changes in ventilation and partial pressures of O_2 and CO_2 in the transition from rest to steady-state submaximal exercise.

environmental conditions. The neutral environment represents exercise in a cool, low-relative-humidity environment (19°C, 45% relative humidity). The second condition represented in figure 10.22 is a hot/high-humidity environment, which hampers heat loss from the body. The major point to appreciate from figure 10.22 is that ventilation tends to "drift" upward during prolonged work. The mechanism to explain this increase in $\dot{V}_E$ during work in the heat is an increase in blood temperature, which directly affects the respiratory control center (88).

Another interesting point to gain from figure 10.22 is that although ventilation is greater during exercise in a hot/humid environment when compared to work

Figure 10.22 Changes in ventilation and blood gas tensions during prolonged, submaximal exercise in a hot/humid environment.

Chapter Ten   Respiration During Exercise   **235**

in a cool environment, there is little difference in arterial PCO_2 between the two types of exercise. This finding suggests that the increase in ventilation seen during work in the heat is due to an increase in breathing frequency and dead-space ventilation (32).

Incremental Exercise

The ventilatory response for an elite male distance runner and an untrained college student during an incremental exercise test is illustrated in figure 10.23. In both subjects, ventilation increases as a linear function of oxygen uptake up to 50% to 75% of O_2 max, where ventilation begins to rise exponentially (114). This $\dot{V}_E$ "inflection point" has been called the **ventilatory threshold (Tvent)** (7, 55, 77, 78).

An interesting point that emerges from figure 10.23 is the startling difference between the highly trained elite athlete and the untrained subject in arterial PO_2

during heavy exercise. The untrained subject is able to maintain arterial PO_2 within 10 to 12 mm Hg of the normal resting value, whereas the highly trained distance runner shows a decrease of 30 to 40 mm Hg at near-maximal work (30, 32, 33). This drop in arterial PO_2, often observed in the healthy, trained athlete, is similar to that observed in exercising patients who have severe lung disease. However, not all healthy, elite endurance athletes develop low-arterial PO_2 values (low PO_2 is called *hypoxemia*) during heavy exercise. It appears that only about 40% to 50% of highly trained, male endurance athletes ($\dot{V}O_2$ max 4.5 l/min or 68 ml · kg · min^{-1}) show this marked hypoxemia (85, 93). In addition, the degree of hypoxemia observed in these athletes during heavy work varies considerably among individuals (30, 86, 93, 111). The reason for the subject differences is unclear.

A growing body of evidence also indicates that female endurance athletes also develop exercise-

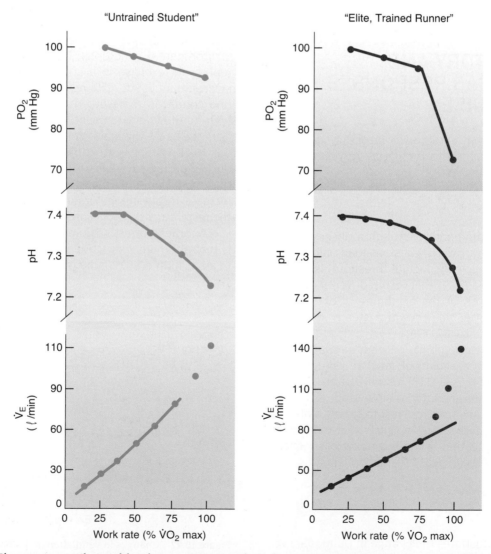

Figure 10.23 Changes in ventilation, blood-gas tensions, and pH during incremental exercise in a highly trained male distance runner and an untrained male college student.

induced hypoxemia (54, 58, 59, 61). In fact, it has been argued that the incidence of exercise-induced hypoxemia in highly trained and elite female athletes may be greater than males (54, 59, 61). Additional research is required to confirm or deny this prediction. Perhaps the most important question concerning exercise-induced hypoxemia in healthy athletes is, What factor(s) accounts for this failure of the pulmonary system? Unfortunately, a complete answer to this question is not available. Nonetheless, it appears that both ventilation-perfusion mismatch and diffusion limitations are likely contributors to exercise-induced hypoxemia in elite athletes (73, 93, 119). Diffusion limitations during intense exercise in elite athletes could occur due to a reduced amount of time that the red blood cells spend in the pulmonary capillary (31, 32, 34). This short red blood cell transit time in the pulmonary capillaries is due to the high cardiac outputs achieved by these athletes during high-intensity exercise and may be less than the time required for gas equilibrium to be achieved between the lung and blood (30, 96, 121).

IN SUMMARY

- At the onset of constant-load submaximal exercise, ventilation increases rapidly, followed by a slower rise toward a steady-state value. Arterial PO_2 and PCO_2 are maintained relatively constant during this type of exercise.
- During prolonged exercise in a hot/humid environment, ventilation "drifts" upward due to the influence of rising body temperature on the respiratory control center.
- Incremental exercise results in a linear increase in $\dot{V}_E$ up to approximately 50% to 70% of O_2 max; at higher work rates, ventilation begins to rise exponentially. This ventilatory inflection point has been called the *ventilatory threshold*.

CONTROL OF VENTILATION

Obviously, precise regulation of pulmonary gas exchange during rest and exercise is important in maintaining homeostasis by providing normal arterial O_2 content and maintenance of the acid-base balance within the body. Although the control of breathing has been actively studied by physiologists for many years, many unanswered questions remain. Let's begin our discussion of ventilatory control during exercise with a review of ventilatory regulation at rest.

Ventilatory Regulation at Rest

As mentioned earlier, inspiration and expiration are produced by the contraction and relaxation of the diaphragm during quiet breathing, and by accessory muscles during exercise. Contraction and relaxation of these respiratory muscles are directly controlled by somatic motor neurons in the spinal cord. Motor neuron activity, in turn, is directly controlled by the respiratory control center in the medulla oblongata.

Respiratory Control Center

Our understanding of the neural mechanisms that control breathing in humans remains incomplete. This is because the control of breathing cannot be investigated directly in humans for both ethical and technical reasons. Therefore, our current knowledge of the neural mechanisms that regulate breathing comes from animal experiments. These studies provide key insight into how mammals generate a respiratory rhythm. The leading hypothesis to explain the initiation of breathing is called the "group pacemaker hypothesis." This hypothesis proposes that the genesis of breathing comes from the firing of several clusters of neurons within the brain stem that serve as pacemakers. Specifically, the stimulus for inspiration comes from four distinct respiratory rhythm centers located within both the medulla oblongata and the pons regions of the brain stem (47). The rhythm generating centers in the medulla are named the preBötzinger Complex (preBötC) and the retrotrapezoid nucleus (RTN) (figure 10.24). The rhythm generating centers in the pons are composed of two clusters of neurons called the *pneumotaxic center* and the *caudal pons* (figure 10.24). The normal rhythm of breathing occurs due to an interaction between pacemaker neurons in each of these regions (7). At rest, the breathing rhythm appears to be dominated by pacemaker neurons in the preBötC with assistance from the other regulatory regions. During exercise the preBötC interacts with the other respiratory rhythm centers to regulate breathing to match the metabolic demand (100). The interaction between these respiratory pacemakers to control breathing involves both positive and negative feedback to achieve tight regulation. Finally, the concept of a group pacemaker suggests that the regulation of breathing is under redundant control. Additional research is required to fully describe how these different respiratory control centers work together to produce the precise level of respiratory control that exists in humans.

Input to the Respiratory Control Center Several types of receptors are capable of modifying the actions of neurons contained in the respiratory control center. In general, input to the respiratory control center can be classified into two types: (1) neural and (2) humoral (blood-borne). Neural input refers to afferent or efferent input to the respiratory control center from neurons that are excited by means other than blood-borne

Figure 10.24   Locations of the brain stem respiratory control centers.

Midbrain

Pons

Brain stem
respiratory — ┌ Pneumotaxic center
centers ├ Caudal pons
└ Retrotrapezoid nucleus

PreBötzinger complex

Medulla oblongata

stimuli. Humoral input to the respiratory control center refers to the influence of some blood-borne stimuli reaching a specialized chemoreceptor. This receptor reacts to the strength of the stimuli and sends the appropriate message to the medulla. A brief overview of each of these receptors will be presented prior to a discussion of ventilatory control during exercise.

Humoral Chemoreceptors   Chemoreceptors are specialized neurons that are capable of responding to changes in the internal environment. Traditionally, respiratory chemoreceptors are classified according to their location as being either *central chemoreceptors* or *peripheral chemoreceptors*.

Central Chemoreceptors   The central chemoreceptors are located in the medulla (anatomically separate from the respiratory center) and are affected by changes in PCO_2 and H^+ of the cerebrospinal fluid (CSF). An increase in either PCO_2 or H^+ of the CSF results in the central chemoreceptors sending afferent input into the respiratory center to increase ventilation (35).

Peripheral Chemoreceptors   The primary peripheral chemoreceptors are located in the aortic arch and at the bifurcation of the common carotid artery. The receptors located in the aorta are called **aortic bodies**, and those found in the carotid artery are **carotid bodies** (figure 10.25). These peripheral chemoreceptors respond to increases in arterial H^+ concentrations and PCO_2 (1, 4, 10, 49, 109, 116, 122). Additionally, the carotid bodies are sensitive to increases in blood potassium levels and decreases in arterial PO_2 (17, 49, 75). When comparing these two sets of peripheral chemoreceptors, it appears that the carotid bodies are more important (5, 11, 16, 35, 49, 50–52, 67, 103, 105, 113, 115).

Effect of Blood PCO_2, PO_2, and Potassium on Ventilation

How do the central and peripheral chemoreceptors respond to changes in chemical stimuli? The effects of increases in arterial PCO_2 on minute ventilation is shown in figure 10.26. Note that $\dot{V}_E$ increases as a linear function of arterial PCO_2. In general, a 1 mm Hg rise in PCO_2 results in a 2 liter/minute increase in $\dot{V}_E$ (35). The increase in $\dot{V}_E$ that results from a rise in arterial PCO_2 is likely due to CO_2 stimulation of both the carotid bodies and the central chemoreceptors (35, 76).

In healthy individuals breathing at sea level, changes in arterial PO_2 have little effect on the control

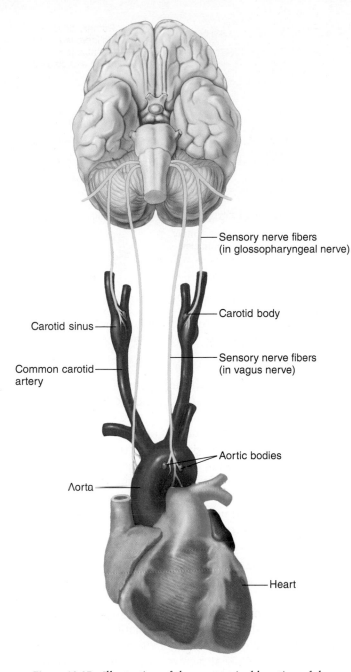

Figure 10.25 Illustration of the anatomical location of the peripheral chemoreceptors (i.e., aortic bodies and carotid bodies). The aortic chemoreceptors respond to arterial changes in arterial H^+ ion concentration (i.e., pH) and PCO_2. The carotid bodies also respond to arterial changes in arterial pH, PCO_2, and also changes in PO_2.

Labels on figure:
- Sensory nerve fibers (in glossopharyngeal nerve)
- Carotid sinus
- Carotid body
- Common carotid artery
- Sensory nerve fibers (in vagus nerve)
- Aortic bodies
- Aorta
- Heart

Figure 10.26 Changes in ventilation as a function of increasing arterial PCO_2. Notice that ventilation increases as a linear function of increasing PCO_2.

Figure 10.27 Changes in ventilation as a function of decreasing arterial PO_2. Note the existence of a "hypoxic threshold" for ventilation as arterial PO_2 declines.

of ventilation (67). However, exposure to an environment with a barometric pressure much lower than that at sea level (i.e., high altitude) can alter arterial PO_2 and stimulate the carotid bodies, which in turn signal the respiratory center to increase ventilation (49). The relationship between arterial PO_2 and $\dot{V}_E$ is illustrated in figure 10.27. The point on the $PO_2/\dot{V}_E$ curve where $\dot{V}_E$ begins to rise rapidly is often referred

to as the hypoxic threshold (*hypoxic* means low PO_2) (2). This hypoxic threshold usually occurs around an arterial PO_2 of 60 to 75 mm Hg. The chemoreceptors responsible for the increase in $\dot{V}_E$ following exposure to low PO_2 are the carotid bodies, because the aortic and central chemoreceptors in humans do not respond to changes in PO_2 (35, 67).

Increases in blood levels of potassium can also stimulate the carotid bodies and promote an increase in ventilation (17, 75). Because blood potassium levels rise during exercise due to a net potassium efflux from the contracting muscle, some investigators have suggested that potassium may play a role in regulating ventilation during exercise (17, 75). More will be said about this later.

Neural Input to the Respiratory Control Center

Evidence indicates that neural input to the respiratory control center can come from both efferent and afferent pathways. For example, impulses from the motor cortex (i.e., central command) can both control skeletal muscle and drive ventilation in proportion to the amount of work being performed (42, 43). In short, neural impulses originating in the motor cortex may pass through the medulla and "spill over," causing an increase in $\dot{V}_E$ that reflects the number of muscle motor units being recruited.

Afferent input to the respiratory control center during exercise may come from one of several peripheral receptors, such as the muscle spindles, Golgi tendon organs, or joint pressure receptors (25, 65, 104). In addition, it is possible that special chemoreceptors located in muscle may respond to changes in potassium and H^+ concentrations and send afferent information to the respiratory control center. This type of input to the medulla is considered afferent neural information because the stimuli are not humorally mediated. Finally, evidence suggests that the right ventricle of the heart contains mechanoreceptors that send afferent information back to the respiratory control center relative to increases in cardiac output (e.g., during exercise) (115). These mechanoreceptors might play important roles in providing afferent input to the respiratory control center at the onset of exercise.

Ventilatory Control During Submaximal Exercise

In the previous sections, we have discussed several possible sources of input to the respiratory control center. Let's now discuss how the body regulates breathing during exercise (9, 15, 18, 25–27, 41, 43, 46, 65, 79, 95, 113, 122). Current evidence suggests that the "primary" drive to increase ventilation during exercise is due to neural input from higher brain centers (central command) to the respiratory control center (29). However, the fact that arterial PCO_2 is tightly regulated during most types of submaximal exercise suggests that humoral chemoreceptors and afferent neural feedback from working muscles act to fine-tune breathing to match the metabolic rate and thus maintain a rather constant arterial PCO_2 (13, 14, 49, 74, 113). Therefore, ventilation during exercise is regulated by several overlapping factors that provide redundancy to the control system.

During prolonged exercise in a hot environment, ventilation can be influenced by factors other than those discussed previously. For example, the drift upward in $\dot{V}_E$ seen in figure 10.22 may be due to a direct influence of rising blood temperature on the respiratory control center, and rising blood catecholamines (epinephrine and norepinephrine) stimulating the carotid bodies to increase $\dot{V}_E$ (88).

To summarize, the increase in ventilation during submaximal exercise is due to an interaction of both neural and chemoreceptor input to the respiratory control center. Efferent neural mechanisms from higher brain centers (central command) provide the

*Act to fine-tune ventilation during exercise

Figure 10.28 A summary of respiratory control during submaximal exercise. See text for details.

primary drive to breathe during exercise, with humoral chemoreceptors and neural feedback from working muscles providing a means of precisely matching ventilation with the amount of CO_2 produced via metabolism. This redundancy in control mechanisms is not surprising when one considers the important role that respiration plays in sustaining life and maintaining a steady-state during exercise (48, 50). A summary of respiratory control during submaximal exercise appears in figure 10.28.

Ventilatory Control During Heavy Exercise

Controversy exists concerning the mechanism to explain the alinear rise in ventilation (ventilatory threshold) that occurs during an incremental exercise test. However, several factors may contribute to this rise. First, examination of figure 10.23 suggests that the alinear rise in $\dot{V}_E$ and the decrease in pH often occur simultaneously. Because rising hydrogen ion levels in blood have been shown to stimulate the carotid bodies and increase $\dot{V}_E$, it has been proposed that the rise in blood lactate, which occurs during incremental exercise, is the stimulus causing the alinear rise in $\dot{V}_E$ (i.e., ventilatory threshold). Based on this belief, it is common for researchers to estimate the lactate threshold noninvasively by measurement of the ventilatory threshold (6, 18, 112, 114). Nonetheless, this technique is not perfect; the ventilatory threshold and the lactate threshold do not always occur at the same work rate (44, 78).

What additional factors, other than rising blood lactate, might cause the alinear rise in $\dot{V}_E$ observed

A CLOSER LOOK 10.2

Training Reduces the Ventilatory Response to Exercise

Although exercise training does not alter the structure of the lung, endurance training does promote a decrease in ventilation during submaximal exercise at moderate-to-high-intensity work rates. For example, when comparisons are made at a fixed submaximal work rate, a training program can reduce exercise ventilation by 20% to 30% below pretraining levels (20, 23) (see figure 10.29).

What is the mechanism to explain this training-induced reduction in exercise ventilation? A definitive answer is not known. However, this training effect is likely due to changes in the aerobic capacity of the locomotor skeletal muscles. These training-induced changes result in less production of H+ ions and probably less afferent feedback from the working muscles to stimulate breathing (20).

FIGURE 10.29 Illustration of the effects of endurance training on ventilation during exercise.

during incremental exercise? The close relationship between blood potassium levels and ventilation during heavy exercise has led several investigators to speculate that potassium is an important factor in controlling ventilation during heavy exercise (17, 68, 75). Certainly, other secondary factors, such as rising body temperature and blood catecholamines, might also play a contributory role to the increasing $\dot{V}_E$ during heavy exercise. Further, it is likely that neural input to the respiratory control center influences the ventilatory pattern during incremental exercise. For example, as exercise intensity increases, motor unit recruitment may occur in a nonlinear fashion, and the associated efferent and afferent neural signals to the respiratory control center may promote the alinear rise in $\dot{V}_E$ seen at the ventilatory threshold (78).

To review, it is logical that the rise in blood hydrogen ions observed at the lactate threshold can stimulate ventilation and thus may be a key mechanism to explain the ventilatory threshold. However, secondary factors such as an increase in blood potassium levels, rising body temperature, elevated blood catecholamines, and possible neural influences might also contribute to ventilatory control during heavy exercise (see A Closer Look 10.2).

Although many investigators, including Jerome Dempsey, H. V. Forster, Brian Whipp, and Karl Wasserman, have all contributed to our understanding of the control of breathing during exercise, we highlight the career of Karl Wasserman (see Important People in Science).

IN SUMMARY

- Current evidence suggests that the normal rhythm of breathing is generated by the interaction between four separate respiratory rhythm centers located in the medulla oblongata and the pons. At rest, the breathing rhythm is dominated by pacemaker neurons in the preBötzinger Complex.
- During exercise the preBötzinger Complex interacts with the retrotrapezoid nucleus along with two additional regulatory centers in the pons to regulate breathing. The coupling of these respiratory control centers to regulate breathing involves both positive and negative feedback to achieve tight control.

A LOOK BACK—IMPORTANT PEOPLE IN SCIENCE

Karlman Wasserman—A Research Pioneer in Exercise and the Pulmonary System

Karl Wasserman was born in Brooklyn, New York, and completed both his PhD and MD degrees at Tulane University. Dr. Wasserman began his post-doctoral research career at Stanford University, working with the well-known pulmonary physiologist, Dr. Julius Comroe. Dr. Wasserman was later recruited to UCLA where he served as Division Chief in Pulmonary Medicine at Harbor-UCLA Medical Center for more than 30 years.

During his long and productive research career, Professor Wasserman and colleagues made major contributions to our understanding of exercise metabolism and how the lung functions during exercise. For example, Wasserman performed important studies that carefully described the exercise-induced changes in pulmonary ventilation and arterial blood gases. Further, Dr. Wasserman performed many of the early investigations of the lactate threshold (a.k.a., anaerobic threshold). He also published key studies on the efficiency of muscular exercise.

Another important accomplishment of the Wasserman research group was the development of a computerized system to measure pulmonary gas exchange on a breath-by-breath basis. This vital research tool is now commercially available and is widely used by exercise physiologists to measure breath-by-breath changes in gas exchange during exercise. This computerized system (often called a *metabolic cart*) allows the researcher or clinician to measure the size of each breath during exercise. Further, this system can measure the amount of oxygen consumed in the body during a short time period. One advantage of this breath-by-breath system is that it allows investigators to measure rapid changes (i.e., seconds) in breathing and whole body metabolism during exercise. Using this advanced system, Dr. Wasserman and colleagues performed many studies regarding the rapid changes in oxygen consumption at the beginning of exercise.

Dr. Wasserman's research also added greatly to our understanding of how breathing is controlled during exercise. Although Professor Wasserman has retired from UCLA, he remains active in exercise-related research projects and collaborates with scientists around the world. Clearly, Dr. Karl Wasserman was both a pioneer and a trailblazer in research involving exercise and the cardiopulmonary system.

IN SUMMARY *continued*

- Input into the respiratory control center to increase ventilation can come from both neural and chemoreceptor sources. Neural input may come from higher brain centers, or it may arise from receptors in the exercising muscle. Humoral chemoreceptor input may arise from both central chemoreceptors and peripheral chemoreceptors. The central chemoreceptors are sensitive to increases in PCO_2 and decreases in pH. The peripheral chemoreceptors (carotid bodies are the most important) are sensitive to increases in PCO_2 and decreases in PO_2 or pH. The primary drive to increase ventilation during exercise comes from higher brain centers (central command). Also, humoral chemoreceptors and neural feedback from working muscles act to fine-tune ventilation.

DO THE LUNGS ADAPT TO EXERCISE TRAINING?

It is well known that the muscular-skeletal system and the cardiovascular system are actively engaged during muscular exercise and that both organ systems undergo adaptive changes in response to regular endurance exercise. In contrast, it has been demonstrated that the lungs in physically trained individuals are not significantly different from the lungs in a sedentary individual (36, 62). More specifically, endurance exercise training (months to years) has no measurable effect on lung structure and resting pulmonary function that will improve pulmonary gas exchange during exercise (36, 62).

If both the cardiovascular system and skeletal muscles adapt to exercise training, why is the adaptability of pulmonary structures substantially less than these other links in the oxygen transport system? One answer to this question is that the structural capacity of the normal lung is "overbuilt" and exceeds the demand for oxygen and carbon dioxide transport in young adults during exercise (36). Therefore, in most individuals, adaptation of the lung to exercise training is not required for the lung to adequately perform the job of maintaining blood-gas homeostasis during exercise. However, one exception to this rule is the highly trained and elite endurance athlete. In these athletes, the inability of the lung to increase its gas exchange capabilities in response to exercise training results in a failure of the pulmonary system to match the high requirement for oxygen transfer across the blood-gas barrier during maximal exercise. This failure results in a reduction in the arterial oxygen content (i.e., hypoxemia). The impact of exercise-induced hypoxemia in elite athletes on exercise performance is discussed in the next section.

DOES THE PULMONARY SYSTEM LIMIT MAXIMAL EXERCISE PERFORMANCE?

Although some controversy exists (12), the pulmonary system is not generally considered to be the limiting factor during prolonged submaximal exercise (19, 28, 32, 39, 45). Although respiratory muscle failure can occur during certain disease states (e.g., obstructive lung disease), respiratory muscle fatigue is not thought to limit exercise in healthy humans exercising at low-to-moderate intensity at sea level (28, 39). Indeed, the major muscle of inspiration, the diaphragm, is a highly oxidative muscle that resists fatigue (83, 89, 90). The best evidence that the lungs and respiratory muscles are performing well during prolonged submaximal exercise (e.g., 75% $\dot{V}O_2$ max) is the observation that arterial oxygen content does not decrease during this type of work (84).

Historically, it has not been believed that the pulmonary system limits performance during high-intensity exercise at sea level (39, 45, 64). However, several studies question this idea. Indeed, new evidence suggests that the pulmonary system may limit exercise performance during high-intensity exercise (e.g., 95–100% $\dot{V}O_2$ max) in trained and untrained healthy subjects. For example, unloading the respiratory muscles (e.g., breathing a low-density helium/oxygen gas) during heavy exercise (90% $\dot{V}O_2$ max) improves exercise performance (63). This observation indicates that respiratory muscle fatigue may play a role in limiting human performance at extremely high work rates.

New evidence confirms that respiratory muscle fatigue occurs during high-intensity exercise (e.g., 10 minutes of exercise at 80–85% $\dot{V}O_2$ max) (3). For details on the impact of the respiratory system on exercise performance, see Ask the Expert 10.1. The

ASK THE EXPERT 10.1

The Pulmonary System and Exercise Performance
Questions and Answers with Dr. Jerome Dempsey

Jerome Dempsey, Ph.D., *a professor in the Department of Population Health Sciences at the University of Wisconsin–Madison, is an internationally known researcher in the field of pulmonary physiology. A significant portion of Dr. Dempsey's research has focused on respiratory gas exchange during exercise and the regulation of pulmonary gas exchange during intense exercise. Without question, Dr. Dempsey's research team has performed many of the "classic" studies that explore the mechanisms responsible for exercise-induced hypoxemia in elite athletes and the effects of exercise on respiratory muscle function. Here, Dr. Dempsey answers questions related to the role that the pulmonary system plays in exercise performance.*

QUESTION: Some investigators argue that "specific" training of the respiratory muscles can improve both submaximal and maximal exercise performance. How strong is the evidence to support these claims?

ANSWER: Early research on respiratory muscle training claimed large and unrealistic effects on exercise performance, but these studies did not include placebo controls. When exercise performance is a major outcome variable under consideration, it must be recognized that this has a large volitional component. Therefore it is essential that the placebo effect be included in the experimental design; i.e., the athletes in both the experimental or control groups must have an "expectation" that their performance will improve as a result of the "treatment." More recently, well-designed studies of respiratory muscle training have shown a small but significant 2–3% improvement in time-trial performance (> placebo group) as a result of several weeks of respiratory muscle training, using resistive inspiratory loading. So, if properly done, I believe respiratory muscle training does indeed have a significant, although small, positive influence on endurance performance.

QUESTION: What are the potential mechanism(s) to explain why respiratory muscle training improves exercise performance?

ANSWER: In the absence of direct evidence on this question, we can offer the following possibilities. During heavy-intensity endurance exercise, as the respiratory muscles fatigue (see below) this initiates a metaboreflex from the fatiguing muscles, which increases efferent sympathetic vasoconstrictor activity, which in turn causes a redistribution of blood flow—i.e., reduced blood flow to the limb locomotor muscles and (presumably) increased blood flow to the respiratory muscles. If respiratory muscle training delays the onset of respiratory muscle fatigue during endurance exercise, this will allow less vasoconstriction and therefore greater blood flow and O_2 transport to the limbs, thereby allowing a given intensity of exercise to be sustained longer. We need to add here that highly fit endurance athletes who have not undergone specific respiratory muscle training but who undergo high levels of daily whole body training also show better conditioned and less fatigable respiratory muscles.

(continued)

QUESTION: Does whole body endurance exercise promote respiratory muscle fatigue?

ANSWER: Yes, fatigue of both inspiratory and abdominal expiratory muscles has been demonstrated to result from heavy intensity endurance exercise in humans of widely varying fitness levels. The method used to quantify this fatigue requires specific electric or magnetic supermaximal stimulation of the motor nerves innervating the diaphragm or expiratory muscles and measurement of a significant reduction in force output of these muscles from pre- to post-exercise, with this fatigue lasting more than 30 to 60 minutes following the exercise. The exercise must be in excess of 80% to 85% of $\dot{V}O_2$ max and be sustained for at least several (>10–15) minutes to the point of volitional exhaustion. It is also known that exercise-induced respiratory muscle fatigue is caused both by the amount of sustained work exerted by the diaphragm (both force production and a high velocity of shortening) and also because of the limited amount of blood flow available; i.e., the available total cardiac output must be shared by both the respiratory and limb muscles during heavy exercise.

QUESTION: What are the physiologic effects of respiratory muscle fatigue?

ANSWER: These effects are revealed by the use of a special mechanical ventilator that is capable of unloading the respiratory muscles and substantially reducing the work of breathing during heavy exercise and thereby preventing diaphragm fatigue. Relief of a substantial amount of this high sustained level of respiratory muscle work reduces the rate of development of limb muscle fatigue during whole body exercise and significantly improves endurance exercise performance. Preventing respiratory muscle fatigue does *not* result in an improvement in ventilation or pulmonary gas exchange, apparently because there is sufficient reserve in the accessory respiratory muscles and even in the primary inspiratory and expiratory muscles to provide sufficient alveolar ventilation in healthy subjects. Rather, the major effect of preventing exercise-induced respiratory muscle fatigue is more likely the prevention of the respiratory muscle metaboreflex effects on increasing sympathetically mediated vasoconstriction and an improved vasodilation and blood flow to limb locomotor muscles (see above). Please note that these effects of reducing respiratory muscle work on alleviating the development of limb muscle fatigue and increasing exercise performance are present in normal healthy subjects exercising at sea level. These cardiovascular effects of exercise-induced respiratory muscle work are greatly enhanced under conditions of increased ventilation during exercise, such as occurs in healthy subjects in the hypoxia of high altitude and to an even greater extent in patients with chronic heart failure exercising at relatively mild levels at sea level.

---

pulmonary system may also limit performance during high-intensity exercise in the elite endurance athlete who exhibits exercise-induced hypoxemia. Recall that in approximately 40% to 50% of elite endurance athletes, arterial PO_2 declines during heavy exercise to a level that negatively affects their ability to transport oxygen to the working muscles (92, 96, 121) (figure 10.23). In these athletes, the pulmonary system cannot keep pace with the need for respiratory gas exchange at workloads near $\dot{V}O_2$ max (30–32, 85, 92, 93). This failure in pulmonary gas exchange may limit exercise performance in these subjects (92).

STUDY QUESTIONS

1. What is the primary function of the pulmonary system? What secondary functions does it serve?
2. List and discuss the major anatomical components of the respiratory system.
3. What muscle groups are involved in ventilation during rest? During exercise?
4. What is the functional significance of the ventilation-perfusion ratio? How would a high V/Q ratio affect gas exchange in the lung?
5. Discuss those factors that influence the rate of diffusion across the blood-gas interface in the lung.
6. Graph the relationship between hemoglobin-O_2 saturation and the partial pressure of O_2 in the blood. What is the functional significance of the shape of the O_2-hemoglobin dissociation curve? What factors affect the shape of the curve?

IN SUMMARY

- The pulmonary system does not limit exercise performance in healthy young subjects during prolonged submaximal exercise (e.g., work rates 90% $\dot{V}O_2$ max).
- In contrast to submaximal exercise, new evidence indicates that the respiratory system (i.e., respiratory muscle fatigue) may be a limiting factor in exercise performance at work rates >90% $\dot{V}O_2$ max. Further, incomplete pulmonary gas exchange may occur in some elite endurance athletes and limit exercise performance at high exercise intensities.

7. Discuss the modes of transportation for CO_2 in the blood.
8. Graph the ventilatory response in the transition from rest to constant-load submaximal exercise. What happens to ventilation if the exercise is prolonged and performed in a hot/humid environment? Why?
9. Graph the ventilatory response to incremental exercise. Label the ventilatory threshold. What factor(s) might explain the ventilatory threshold?
10. List and identify the functions of the chemoreceptors that contribute to the control of breathing.
11. What neural afferents might also contribute to the regulation of ventilation during exercise?
12. Discuss the control of ventilation during exercise.

SUGGESTED READINGS

Anderson, S., and P. Kippelen. 2005. Exercise-induced bronchoconstriction: Pathogenesis. *Current Allergy and Asthma Reports* 5:116–22.

Fox, S. 2010. *Human Physiology*. New York: McGraw-Hill Companies.

Levitzky, M. 2007. *Pulmonary Physiology*. New York: McGraw-Hill.

Powers, S., and R. Shanely. 2002. Exercise-induced changes in diaphragmatic bioenergetic and antioxidant capacity. *Exercise and Sport Science Reviews* 30:69–74.

West, J. 2007. *Pulmonary Pathophysiology*. Philadelphia: Lippincott Williams & Wilkins.

Widmaier, E., H. Raff, and K. Strang. 2010. *Vander's Human Physiology*. New York: McGraw-Hill Companies.

REFERENCES

1. **Allen CJ, and Jones NL.** Rate of change of alveolar carbon dioxide and the control of ventilation during exercise. J Physiol 355: 1–9, 1984.

2. **Asmussen E.** Control of ventilation in exercise. In: *Exercise and Sport Science Reviews*, edited by Terjung R. Philadelphia: Franklin Press, 1983.

3. **Babcock MA, Pegelow DF, Harms CA, and Dempsey JA.** Effects of respiratory muscle unloading on exercise-induced diaphragm fatigue. J Appl Physiol 93: 201–206, 2002.

4. **Band DM, Wolff CB, Ward J, Cochrane GM, and Prior J.** Respiratory oscillations in arterial carbon dioxide tension as a control signal in exercise. Nature 283: 84–85, 1980.

5. **Banzett RB, Coleridge HM, and Coleridge JC.** I. Pulmonary-CO_2 ventilatory reflex in dogs: effective range of CO_2 and results of vagal cooling. Respir Physiol 34: 121–134, 1978.

6. **Beaver WL, Wasserman K, and Whipp BJ.** A new method for detecting anaerobic threshold by gas exchange. J Appl Physiol 60: 2020–2027, 1986.

7. **Bellissimo N, Thomas SG, Goode RC, and Anderson GH.** Effect of short duration physical activity and ventilation threshold on subjective appetite and short-term energy intake in boys. Appetite 49: 644–651, 2007.

8. **Bennett FM, and Fordyce WE.** Characteristics of the ventilatory exercise stimulus. Respir Physiol 59: 55–63, 1985.

9. **Bennett FM, Tallman RD, Jr., and Grodins FS.** Role of VCO_2 in control of breathing of awake exercising dogs. J Appl Physiol 56: 1335–1339, 1984.

10. **Bisgard GE, Forster HV, Mesina J, and Sarazin RG.** Role of the carotid body in hyperpnea of moderate exercise in goats. J Appl Physiol 52: 1216–1222, 1982.

11. **Boon JK, Kuhlmann WD, and Fedde MR.** Control of respiration in the chicken: effects of venous CO_2 loading. Respir Physiol 39: 169–181, 1980.

12. **Boutellier U, and Piwko P.** The respiratory system as an exercise limiting factor in normal sedentary subjects. Eur J Appl Physiol Occup Physiol 64: 145–152, 1992.

13. **Brice AG, Forster HV, Pan LG, Funahashi A, Hoffman MD, Murphy CL, and Lowry TF.** Is the hyperpnea of muscular contractions critically dependent on spinal afferents? J Appl Physiol 64: 226–233, 1988.

14. **Brice AG, Forster HV, Pan LG, Funahashi A, Lowry TF, Murphy CL, and Hoffman MD.** Ventilatory and $PaCO_2$ responses to voluntary and electrically induced leg exercise. J Appl Physiol 64: 218–225, 1988.

15. **Brown DR, Forster HV, Pan LG, Brice AG, Murphy CL, Lowry TF, Gutting SM, Funahashi A, Hoffman M, and Powers S.** Ventilatory response of spinal cord-lesioned subjects to electrically induced exercise. J Appl Physiol 68: 2312–2321, 1990.

16. **Brown HV, Wasserman K, and Whipp BJ.** Effect of beta-adrenergic blockade during exercise on ventilation and gas exchange. J Appl Physiol 41: 886–892, 1976.

17. **Busse MW, Maassen N, and Konrad H.** Relation between plasma K+ and ventilation during incremental exercise after glycogen depletion and repletion in man. J Physiol 443: 469–476, 1991.

18. **Caiozzo VJ, Davis JA, Ellis JF, Azus JL, Vandagriff R, Prietto CA, and McMaster WC.** A comparison of gas exchange indices used to detect the anaerobic threshold. J Appl Physiol 53: 1184–1189, 1982.

19. **Capen RL, Hanson WL, Latham LP, Dawson CA, and Wagner WW, Jr.** Distribution of pulmonary capillary transit times in recruited networks. J Appl Physiol 69: 473–478, 1990.

20. **Casaburi R, Storer TW, and Wasserman K.** Mediation of reduced ventilatory response to exercise after endurance training. J Appl Physiol 63: 1533–1538, 1987.

21. **Casaburi R, Whipp BJ, Wasserman K, Beaver WL, and Koyal SN.** Ventilatory and gas exchange dynamics in response to sinusoidal work. J Appl Physiol 42: 300–301, 1977.

22. **Casaburi R, Whipp BJ, Wasserman K, and Stremel RW.** Ventilatory control characteristics of the exercise hyperpnea as discerned from dynamic forcing techniques. Chest 73: 280–283, 1978.

23. **Clanton TL, Dixon GF, Drake J, and Gadek JE.** Effects of swim training on lung volumes and inspiratory muscle conditioning. J Appl Physiol 62: 39–46, 1987.

24. **Coleridge H, and Coleridge J.** Airway axon reflexes—where now? News in Physiological Sciences 10: 91–96, 1995.

25. **Davidson AC, Auyeung V, Luff R, Holland M, Hodgkiss A, and Weinman J.** Prolonged benefit in post-polio syndrome from comprehensive rehabilitation: a pilot study. Disabil Rehabil 31: 309–317, 2009.

26. **Dejours P.** Control of respiration in muscular exercise. In: *Handbook of Physiology*, edited by Fenn W. Washington: American Physiological Society, 1964.

27. **Dempsey J.** Integration of motor, circulatory, respiratory, and metabolic control. In: *Handbook of Physiology: Exercise Section 12*, edited by Rawl L, and Sheppard J. New York: Oxford University Press, 1996.

28. **Dempsey J, Aaron E, and Martin B.** Pulmonary function during prolonged exercise. In: *Perspectives in Exercise and Sports Medicine: Prolonged Exercise*, edited by Lamb D, and Murray R. Indianapolis: Benchmark Press, 1988, p. 75–119.

29. **Dempsey J, Forster H, and Ainsworth D.** Regulation of hyperpnea, hyperventilation, and respiratory muscle recruitment during exercise. In: *Regulation of Breathing*, edited by Pack A, and Dempsey J. New York: Marcel Dekker, 1994, p. 1065–1034.

30. **Dempsey J, Hanson P, Pegelow D, Claremont A, and Rankin J.** Limitations to exercise capacity and endurance: pulmonary system. Can J Appl Sport Sci 7: 4–13, 1982.

31. **Dempsey J, Powers S, and Gledhill N.** Cardiovascular and pulmonary adaptation to physical activity. In: *Exercise, Fitness, and Health: A Consensus of Current Knowledge*, edited by Bouchard C. Champaign: Human Kinetics, 1990, p. 205–216.

32. **Dempsey JA.** J. B. Wolffe memorial lecture. Is the lung built for exercise? *Med Sci Sports Exerc* 18: 143–155, 1986.

33. **Dempsey JA, and Fregosi RF.** Adaptability of the pulmonary system to changing metabolic requirements. *Am J Cardiol* 55: 59D–67D, 1985.

34. **Dempsey JA, McKenzie DC, Haverkamp HC, and Eldridge MW.** Update in the understanding of respiratory limitations to exercise performance in fit, active adults. *Chest* 134: 613–622, 2008.

35. **Dempsey JA, Mitchell GS, and Smith CA.** Exercise and chemoreception. *Am Rev Respir Dis* 129: S31–34, 1984.

36. **Dempsey JA, Sheel AW, Haverkamp HC, Babcock MA, and Harms CA.** [The John Sutton Lecture: CSEP, 2002]. Pulmonary system limitations to exercise in health. *Can J Appl Physiol* 28 Suppl: S2–24, 2003.

37. **Dempsey JA, Vidruk EH, and Mitchell GS.** Pulmonary control systems in exercise: update. *Fed Proc* 44: 2260–2270, 1985.

38. **Dodd S, Powers S, O'Malley N, Brooks E, and Sommers H.** Effects of beta-adrenergic blockade on ventilation and gas exchange during the rest to work transition. *Aviat Space Environ Med* 59: 255–258, 1988.

39. **Dodd SL, Powers SK, Thompson D, Landry G, and Lawler J.** Exercise performance following intense, short-term ventilatory work. *Int J Sports Med* 10: 48–52, 1989.

40. **Domino KB, Eisenstein BL, Cheney FW, and Hlastala MP.** Pulmonary blood flow and ventilation-perfusion heterogeneity. *J Appl Physiol* 71: 252–258, 1991.

41. **Duffin J.** Neural drives to breathing during exercise. *Can J Appl Physiol* 19: 289–304, 1994.

42. **Eldridge FL, Millhorn DE, Kiley JP, and Waldrop TG.** Stimulation by central command of locomotion, respiration and circulation during exercise. *Respir Physiol* 59: 313–337, 1985.

43. **Eldridge FL, Millhorn DE, and Waldrop TG.** Exercise hyperpnea and locomotion: parallel activation from the hypothalamus. *Science* 211: 844–846, 1981.

44. **England P.** The effect of acute thermal dehydration on blood lactate accumulation during incremental exercise. *Journal of Sports Sciences* 2: 105–111, 1985.

45. **Fairbarn MS, Coutts KC, Pardy RL, and McKenzie DC.** Improved respiratory muscle endurance of highly trained cyclists and the effects on maximal exercise performance. *Int J Sports Med* 12: 66–70, 1991.

46. **Favier R, Desplanches D, Frutoso J, Grandmontagne M, and Flandrois R.** Ventilatory and circulatory transients during exercise: new arguments for a neuro-humoral theory. *J Appl Physiol* 54: 647–653, 1983.

47. **Feldman JL, and Del Negro CA.** Looking for inspiration: new perspectives on respiratory rhythm. *Nat Rev Neurosci* 7: 232–242, 2006.

48. **Forster H, and Pan L.** Exercise hyperpnea: characteristics and control. In: *The Lung: Scientific Foundations*, edited by Crystal R, and West J. New York: Raven Press, 1991, p. 1553–1564.

49. **Forster HV, and Smith CA.** Contributions of central and peripheral chemoreceptors to the ventilatory response to $CO_2/H+$. *J Appl Physiol* 108: 989–994, 2010.

50. **Green JF, Schertel ER, Coleridge HM, and Coleridge JC.** Effect of pulmonary arterial PCO_2 on slowly adapting pulmonary stretch receptors. *J Appl Physiol* 60: 2048–2055, 1986.

51. **Green JF, and Schmidt ND.** Mechanism of hyperpnea induced by changes in pulmonary blood flow. *J Appl Physiol* 56: 1418–1422, 1984.

52. **Green JF, and Sheldon MI.** Ventilatory changes associated with changes in pulmonary blood flow in dogs. *J Appl Physiol* 54: 997–1002, 1983.

53. **Grucza R, Miyamoto Y, and Nakazono Y.** Kinetics of cardiorespiratory response to dynamic and rhythmic-static exercise in men. *Eur J Appl Physiol Occup Physiol* 61: 230–236, 1990.

54. **Guenette JA, and Sheel AW.** Exercise-induced arterial hypoxaemia in active young women. *Appl Physiol Nutr Metab* 32: 1263–1273, 2007.

55. **Hagberg JM, Coyle EF, Carroll JE, Miller JM, Martin WH, and Brooke MH.** Exercise hyperventilation in patients with McArdle's disease. *J Appl Physiol* 52: 991–994, 1982.

56. **Hammond MD, Gale GE, Kapitan KS, Ries A, and Wagner PD.** Pulmonary gas exchange in humans during exercise at sea level. *J Appl Physiol* 60: 1590–1598, 1986.

57. **Hansen JE, Ulubay G, Chow BF, Sun XG, and Wasserman K.** Mixed-expired and end-tidal CO_2 distinguish between ventilation and perfusion defects during exercise testing in patients with lung and heart diseases. *Chest* 132: 977–983, 2007.

58. **Harms CA, McClaran SR, Nickele GA, Pegelow DF, Nelson WB, and Dempsey JA.** Effect of exercise-induced arterial O_2 desaturation on $\dot{V}O_2$max in women. *Med Sci Sports Exerc* 32: 1101–1108, 2000.

59. **Harms CA, McClaran SR, Nickele GA, Pegelow DF, Nelson WB, and Dempsey JA.** Exercise-induced arterial hypoxaemia in healthy young women. *J Physiol* 507 (Pt 2): 619–628, 1998.

60. **Hawgood S, and Shiffer K.** Structures and properties of the surfactant-associated proteins. *Annu Rev Physiol* 53: 375–394, 1991.

61. **Hopkins SR, Barker RC, Brutsaert TD, Gavin TP, Entin P, Olfert IM, Veisel S, and Wagner PD.** Pulmonary gas exchange during exercise in women: effects of exercise type and work increment. *J Appl Physiol* 89: 721–730, 2000.

62. **Hopkins SR, and Harms CA.** Gender and pulmonary gas exchange during exercise. *Exerc Sport Sci Rev* 32: 50–56, 2004.

63. **Johnson BD, Aaron EA, Babcock MA, and Dempsey JA.** Respiratory muscle fatigue during exercise: implications for performance. *Med Sci Sports Exerc* 28: 1129–1137, 1996.

64. **Johnson BD, and Dempsey JA.** Demand vs. capacity in the aging pulmonary system. *Exerc Sport Sci Rev* 19: 171–210, 1991.

65. **Kao F.** An experimental study of the pathways involved in exercise hyperpnea employing cross-circulation techniques. In: *The Regulation of Human Respiration*, edited by Cunningham D. Oxford: Blackwell, 1963.

66. **Kavazis AN, DeRuisseau KC, McClung JM, Whidden MA, Falk DJ, Smuder AJ, Sugiura T, and Powers SK.** Diaphragmatic proteasome function is maintained in the ageing Fisher 344 rat. *Exp Physiol* 92: 895–901, 2007.

67. **Levitzky M.** *Pulmonary Physiology.* New York: McGraw-Hill 2007.

68. **Lindinger MI, and Sjogaard G.** Potassium regulation during exercise and recovery. *Sports Med* 11: 382–401, 1991.

69. **Lumb AB.** *Nunn's Applied Respiratory Physiology.* Oxford: Butterworth-Heinemann, 2010.

70. **Mairbaurl H, Schobersberger W, Hasibeder W, Schwaberger G, Gaesser G, and Tanaka KR.** Regulation of red cell 2,3-DPG and $Hb-O_2$-affinity during acute exercise. *Eur J Appl Physiol Occup Physiol* 55: 174–180, 1986.

71. **McParland C, Mink J, and Gallagher CG.** Respiratory adaptations to dead space loading during maximal incremental exercise. *J Appl Physiol* 70: 55–62, 1991.

72. **Moreira A, Delgado L, and Carlsen KH.** Exercise-induced asthma: why is it so frequent in Olympic athletes? *Expert Rev Respir Med* 5: 1–3, 2011.

73. **Nielsen H.** Arterial desaturation during exercise in man: implications for O_2 uptake and work capacity. *Scandinavian Journal of Medicine in Science and Sports* 13: 339–358, 2003.

74. **Pan LG, Forster HV, Wurster RD, Brice AG, and Lowry TF.** Effect of multiple denervations on the exercise hyperpnea in awake ponies. *J Appl Physiol* 79: 302–311, 1995.

75. **Paterson DJ.** Potassium and ventilation in exercise. *J Appl Physiol* 72: 811–820, 1992.

76. **Paulev PE, Mussell MJ, Miyamoto Y, Nakazono Y, and Sugawara T.** Modeling of alveolar carbon dioxide oscillations with or without exercise. *Jpn J Physiol* 40: 893–905, 1990.

77. **Powers S.** Ventilatory threshold, running economy, and distance running performance. *Research Quarterly for Exercise and Sport* 54: 179–182, 1983.

78. **Powers S, and Beadle R.** Onset of hyperventilation during incremental exercise: a brief review. *Research Quarterly for Exercise and Sport* 56: 352–360, 1985.

79. **Powers SK, and Beadle RE.** Control of ventilation during submaximal exercise: a brief review. *J Sports Sci* 3: 51–65, 1985.

80. **Powers SK, Beadle RE, Thompson D, and Lawler J.** Ventilatory and blood gas dynamics at onset and offset of exercise in the pony. *J Appl Physiol* 62: 141–148, 1987.

81. **Powers SK, Coombes J, and Demirel H.** Exercise training-induced changes in respiratory muscles. *Sports Med* 24: 120–131, 1997.

82. **Powers SK, and Criswell D.** Adaptive strategies of respiratory muscles in response to endurance exercise. *Med Sci Sports Exerc* 28. 1115–1122, 1996.

83. **Powers SK, Criswell D, Lawler J, Martin D, Ji LL, Herb RA, and Dudley G.** Regional training-induced alterations in diaphragmatic oxidative and antioxidant enzymes. *Respir Physiol* 95: 227–237, 1994.

84. **Powers SK, Dodd S, Criswell DD, Lawler J, Martin D, and Grinton S.** Evidence for an alveolar-arterial PO_2 gradient threshold during incremental exercise. *Int J Sports Med* 12: 313–318, 1991.

85. **Powers SK, Dodd S, Lawler J, Landry G, Kirtley M, McKnight T, and Grinton S.** Incidence of exercise-induced hypoxemia in elite endurance athletes at sea level. *Eur J Appl Physiol Occup Physiol* 58: 298–302, 1988.

86. **Powers SK, Dodd S, Woodyard J, Beadle RE, and Church G.** Haemoglobin saturation during incremental arm and leg exercise. *Br J Sports Med* 18: 212–216, 1984.

87. **Powers SK, Dodd S, Woodyard J, and Mangum M.** Caffeine alters ventilatory and gas exchange kinetics during exercise. *Med Sci Sports Exerc* 18: 101–106, 1986.

88. **Powers SK, Howley ET, and Cox R.** Ventilatory and metabolic reactions to heat stress during prolonged exercise. *J Sports Med Phys Fitness* 22: 32–36, 1982.

89. **Powers SK, Lawler J, Criswell D, Dodd S, Grinton S, Bagby G, and Silverman H.** Endurance-training-induced cellular adaptations in respiratory muscles. *J Appl Physiol* 68: 2114–2118, 1990.

90. **Powers SK, Lawler J, Criswell D, Lieu FK, and Martin D.** Aging and respiratory muscle metabolic plasticity: effects of endurance training. *J Appl Physiol* 72: 1068–1073, 1992.

91. **Powers SK, Lawler J, Criswell D, Silverman H, Forster HV, Grinton S, and Harkins D.** Regional metabolic differences in the rat diaphragm. *J Appl Physiol* 69: 648–650, 1990.

92. **Powers SK, Lawler J, Dempsey JA, Dodd S, and Landry G.** Effects of incomplete pulmonary gas exchange on $\dot{V}O_2$ max. *J Appl Physiol* 66: 2491–2495, 1989.

93. **Powers SK, Martin D, Cicale M, Collop N, Huang D, and Criswell D.** Exercise-induced hypoxemia in athletes: role of inadequate hyperventilation. *Eur J Appl Physiol Occup Physiol* 65: 37–42, 1992.

94. **Powers SK, and Shanely RA.** Exercise-induced changes in diaphragmatic bioenergetic and antioxidant capacity. *Exerc Sport Sci Rev* 30: 69–74, 2002.

95. **Powers SK, Stewart MK, and Landry G.** Ventilatory and gas exchange dynamics in response to head-down tilt with and without venous occlusion. *Aviat Space Environ Med* 59: 239–245, 1988.

96. **Powers SK, and Williams J.** Exercise-induced hypoxemia in highly trained athletes. *Sports Med* 4: 46–53, 1987.

97. **Ramonatxo M, Mercier J, Cohendy R, and Prefaut C.** Effect of resistive loads on pattern of respiratory muscle recruitment during exercise. *J Appl Physiol* 71: 1941–1948, 1991.

98. **Reynolds HY.** Immunologic system in the respiratory tract. *Physiol Rev* 71: 1117–1133, 1991.

99. **Spodaryk K, and Zoladz JA.** The 2,3-DPG levels of human red blood cells during an incremental exercise test: relationship to the blood acid-base balance. *Physiol Res* 47: 17–22, 1998.

100. **St John WM, and Paton JF.** Role of pontile mechanisms in the neurogenesis of eupnea. *Respir Physiol Neurobiol* 143: 321–332, 2004.

101. **Stamenovic D.** Micromechanical foundations of pulmonary elasticity *Physiol Rev* 70: 1117–1134, 1990.

102. **Stringer W, Casaburi R, and Wasserman K.** Acid-base regulation during exercise and recovery in humans. *J Appl Physiol* 72: 954–961, 1992.

103. **Suzuki S, Suzuki J, and Okubo T.** Expiratory muscle fatigue in normal subjects. *J Appl Physiol* 70: 2632–2639, 1991.

104. **Tibes U.** Reflex inputs to the cardiovascular and respiratory centers from dynamically working canine muscles. Some evidence for involvement of group III or IV nerve fibers. *Circ Res* 41: 332–341, 1977.

105. **Trenchard D, Russell NJ, and Raybould HE.** Non-myelinated vagal lung receptors and their reflex effects on respiration in rabbits. *Respir Physiol* 55: 63–79, 1984.

106. **Vincent HK, Powers SK, Demirel HA, Coombes JS, and Naito H.** Exercise training protects against contraction-induced lipid peroxidation in the diaphragm. *Eur J Appl Physiol Occup Physiol* 79: 268–273, 1999.

107. **Vincent HK, Powers SK, Stewart DJ, Demirel HA, Shanely RA, and Naito H.** Short-term exercise training improves diaphragm antioxidant capacity and endurance. *Eur J Appl Physiol* 81: 67–74, 2000.

108. **Vincent HK, Shanely RA, Stewart DJ, Demirel HA, Hamilton KL, Ray AD, Michlin C, Farkas GA, and Powers SK.** Adaptation of upper airway muscles to chronic endurance exercise. *Am J Respir Crit Care Med* 166: 287–293, 2002.

109. **Virkki A, Polo O, Gyllenberg M, and Aittokallio T.** Can carotid body perfusion act as a respiratory controller? *J Theor Biol* 249: 737–748, 2007.

110. **Walker DJ, Walterspacher S, Schlager D, Ertl T, Roecker K, Windisch W, and Kabitz HJ.** Characteristics of diaphragmatic fatigue during exhaustive exercise until task failure. *Respir Physiol Neurobiol* 176: 14–20, 2011.

111. **Warren GL, Cureton KJ, Middendorf WF, Ray CA, and Warren JA.** Red blood cell pulmonary capillary transit time during exercise in athletes. *Med Sci Sports Exerc* 23: 1353–1361, 1991.

112. **Wasserman K.** The anaerobic threshold measurement to evaluate exercise performance. *Am Rev Respir Dis* 129: S35–40, 1984.

113. **Wasserman K.** CO_2 flow to the lungs and ventilatory control. In: *Muscular Exercise and the Lung*, edited by Dempsey J, and Reed C. Madison: University of Wisconsin Press, 1977.

114. **Wasserman K, Whipp BJ, Koyl SN, and Beaver WL.** Anaerobic threshold and respiratory gas exchange during exercise. *J Appl Physiol* 35: 236–243, 1973.

115. **Weissman ML, Jones PW, Oren A, Lamarra N, Whipp BJ, and Wasserman K.** Cardiac output increase and gas exchange at start of exercise. *J Appl Physiol* 52: 236–244, 1982.

116. **West J.** *Pulmonary Pathophysiology*. Philadelphia: Lippincott Williams & Wilkins, 2007.

117. **West J, and Wagner P.** Ventilation-perfusion relationships. In: *The Lung: Scientific Foundations*, edited by Crystal R, and West J. New York: Raven Press, 1991, p. 1289–1305.

118. **West JB.** *Respiratory Physiology: The Essentials*. Philadelphia: Wolters Kluwer/Lippincott Williams & Wilkins, 2008.

119. **Wetter TJ, Xiang Z, Sonetti DA, Haverkamp HC, Rice AJ, Abbasi AA, Meyer KC, and Dempsey JA.** Role of lung inflammatory mediators as a cause of exercise-induced arterial hypoxemia in young athletes. *J Appl Physiol* 93: 116–126, 2002.

120. **Whipp BJ, and Ward SA.** Physiological determinants of pulmonary gas exchange kinetics during exercise. *Med Sci Sports Exerc* 22: 62–71, 1990.

121. **Williams JH, Powers SK, and Stuart MK.** Hemoglobin desaturation in highly trained athletes during heavy exercise. *Med Sci Sports Exerc* 18: 168–173, 1986.

122. **Yamamoto WS, and Edwards MW, Jr.** Homeostasis of carbon dioxide during intravenous infusion of carbon dioxide. *J Appl Physiol* 15: 807–818, 1960.

11

Acid-Base Balance During Exercise

■ Objectives

By studying this chapter, you should be able to do the following:

1. Define the terms *acid*, *base*, and *pH*.
2. Discuss the importance of acid-base regulation to exercise performance.
3. List the principal intracellular and extracellular buffers.
4. Explain the role of respiration in the regulation of acid-base status during exercise.
5. Outline acid-base regulation during exercise.
6. Discuss the principal ways that hydrogen ions are produced during exercise.

■ Outline

■ Key Terms

acid
acidosis
alkalosis
base
buffer
hydrogen ion
ion
pH
respiratory compensation
strong acids
strong bases

Recall that an **ion** is any atom that is missing electrons or has gained electrons. Further, note that a hydrogen atom contains a single proton in its nucleus orbited by a single electron. A **hydrogen ion** is formed by the loss of the electron; molecules that release hydrogen ions are called *acids*. Substances that readily combine with hydrogen ions are termed *bases*. In physiology, the concentration of hydrogen ions is expressed in pH units. The pH of body fluids must be regulated (i.e., normal arterial blood pH = 7.40 ± .02) in order to maintain homeostasis. This regulation of the pH of body fluids is important because changes in hydrogen ion concentrations can alter the rates of enzyme-controlled metabolic reactions and modify numerous other normal body functions. Therefore, acid-base balance is primarily concerned with the regulation of hydrogen ion concentrations. Heavy exercise can present a serious challenge to hydrogen ion control systems due to hydrogen ion production, and hydrogen ions may limit performance in some types of intense activities (7, 14, 16, 20, 40). Therefore, given the potential detrimental influence of hydrogen ion accumulation on exercise performance, it is important to have an understanding of acid-base regulation.

ACIDS, BASES, AND pH

In biological systems, one of the simplest but most important ions is the hydrogen ion. The concentration of hydrogen ions influences the rates of chemical reactions, the shape and function of enzymes as well as other cellular proteins, and the integrity of the cell itself (10, 46).

An **acid** is defined as a molecule that releases hydrogen ions and thus can raise the hydrogen ion concentration of a solution above that of pure water. In contrast, a **base** is a molecule that is capable of combining with hydrogen ions and therefore lowers the hydrogen ion concentration of the solution.

Acids that give up hydrogen ions (ionize) more completely are called **strong acids.** For example, sulfuric acid is produced by the metabolism of sulfur-containing amino acids (e.g., cysteine) and is a strong acid. At normal body pH, sulfuric acid liberates almost all of its hydrogen ions and therefore elevates the hydrogen ion concentration of the body.

Bases that ionize more completely are defined as **strong bases.** The bicarbonate ion HCO_3^- is an example of a biologically important strong base. Bicarbonate ions are found in relatively large concentrations in blood and are capable of combining with hydrogen ions to form a weak acid called carbonic acid. The role of HCO_3^- in the regulation of acid-base balance during exercise will be discussed later in the chapter.

As stated earlier, the concentration of hydrogen ions is expressed in pH units on a scale that runs from 0 to 14. Solutions that contain pH values below 7 are acidic, whereas pH values above 7 are judged to be basic. The **pH** of a solution is defined as the negative logarithm of the hydrogen ion concentration (H⁺). Recall that a logarithm is the exponent that indicates the power to which one number must be raised to obtain another number. For instance, the logarithm of 100 to the base 10 is 2. Thus, the definition of pH can be written mathematically as:

$$pH = -\log_{10} [H^+]$$

As an example, if the [H⁺] = 40 nM (0.000000040 M), then the pH would be 7.40. A solution is considered neutral (in terms of acid-base status) if the concentration of H⁺ and hydroxyl ions (OH⁻) are equal. This is the case for pure water, in which the concentrations for both H⁺ and OH⁻ are 0.00000010 M. Thus, the pH of pure water is:

$$\textbf{pH (pure water)} = -\log_{10} [H^+]$$
$$= 7.0$$

Figure 11.1 shows the continuum of the pH scale. Note that as the hydrogen ion concentration increases, pH declines and the acidity of the blood increases, resulting in a condition termed **acidosis.** Conversely, as the hydrogen ion concentration decreases, pH increases and the solution becomes more basic (alkalotic). This condition is termed **alkalosis.** Conditions leading to acidosis or alkalosis are summarized in figure 11.2.

The normal arterial pH is 7.4, and in healthy people, this value varies less than 0.05 pH unit (42). Failure to maintain acid-base homeostasis in the body can have lethal consequences. Indeed, even small changes in blood pH can have negative effects on the function of organ systems. For example, both increases and decreases in arterial pH can promote abnormal electrical activity in the heart, resulting in rhythm disturbances (12, 42). Numerous disease states can result in acid-base disturbances in the body and are introduced in Clinical Applications 11.1.

Figure 11.1 The pH scale. If the pH of arterial blood drops below the normal value of 7.4, the resulting condition is termed acidosis. In contrast, if the pH increases above 7.4, blood alkalosis occurs.

CLINICAL APPLICATIONS 11.1

Conditions and Diseases That Promote Metabolic Acidosis or Alkalosis

As mentioned previously, failure to maintain acid-base homeostasis in the body can have serious consequences and can lead to dysfunction of essential organs. Indeed, even relatively small changes in arterial pH (i.e., 0.1–0.2 pH units) can have significant negative impact on organ function (12).

Metabolic acidosis occurs due to a gain in the amount of acid in the body. A number of conditions or disease states can promote metabolic acidosis. For example, long-term starvation (i.e.,

several days) can result in metabolic acidosis due to the production of keto-acids in the body as a by-product of fat metabolism. In extreme circumstances, the type of metabolic acidosis can result in death.

Diabetes is a common metabolic disease that promotes metabolic acidosis. Uncontrolled diabetes can result in a form of metabolic acidosis called diabetic ketoacidosis. Similar to starvation-induced acidosis, this form of acidosis is also due to the

overproduction of ketoacids due to high levels of fat metabolism. World-wide, numerous deaths occur each year from this form of acidosis (12, 42).

Metabolic alkalosis results from a loss of acids from the body. Conditions leading to metabolic alkalosis include severe vomiting and diseases such as kidney disorders that result in a loss of acids (12, 42). In both of these circumstances, the loss of acids results in an overabundance of bases in the body, leading to metabolic alkalosis.

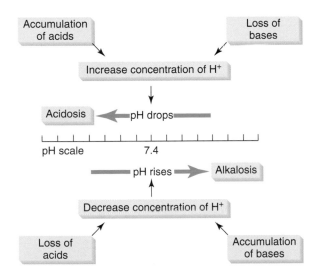

Figure 11.2   Acidosis results from an accumulation of acids or a loss of bases. Alkalosis results from a loss of acids or an accumulation of bases.

IN SUMMARY

- Acids are defined as molecules that can liberate hydrogen ions, which increases the hydrogen ion concentration of an aqueous solution.
- Bases are molecules that are capable of combining with hydrogen ions.
- The concentration of hydrogen ions in a solution is quantified by pH units. The pH of a solution is defined as the negative logarithm of the hydrogen ion concentration:

$$pH = -\log_{10} [H^+]$$

HYDROGEN ION PRODUCTION DURING EXERCISE

Much debate exists regarding the primary sites of hydrogen ion production during exercise (3, 28). Nonetheless, it is clear that high intensity exercise results in a marked decrease in muscle pH. Current evidence indicates that the exercise-induced decrease in muscle pH is due to multiple factors. Three important contributors to exercise-induced muscle acidosis are outlined below (11, 25).

1. Production of carbon dioxide and carbonic acid. Carbon dioxide, an end product in the oxidation of carbohydrates, fats, and proteins, can be regarded as an acid by virtue of its ability to react with water to form carbonic acid (H_2CO_3), which in turn dissociates to form H^+ and HCO_3^-:

$$CO_2 + H_2O \longleftrightarrow H^+ + HCO_3^-$$

Because CO_2 is a gas and can be eliminated by the lungs, it is often referred to as a *volatile acid*. During the course of a day, the body produces large amounts of CO_2 due to normal metabolism. During exercise, metabolic production of CO_2 increases and therefore adds an additional "volatile acid" load on the body.

2. Production of lactic acid and lactate. Several investigators argue that production of lactic acid in the muscle during heavy exercise is a key factor that causes the decrease in muscle pH (3).

www.mhhe.com/powers8e
Chapter Eleven   Acid-Base Balance During Exercise   **251**

Sport and Exercise-Induced Disturbances in Muscle Acid-Base Balance

What types of sports or exercise promote acid-base disturbances in skeletal muscle? In general, any sport or exercise activity requiring high-intensity muscular contractions that persist for 45 seconds or longer can produce significant amounts of hydrogen ions, resulting in a decrease in muscle and blood pH. Table 11.1 provides a list of popular sports and the risk of developing muscle acid-base disturbances in each sport. Note that the risk of acid-base disturbances is classified as being high, moderate, or low. For sports classified in the low-to-moderate risk category (e.g., soccer), the risk of muscle acid-base disturbance is often connected to effort of the competitor. That is, an aggressive athlete that is constantly playing at 100% effort is more likely to develop an acid-base imbalance compared to the athlete that plays at "half speed" during the game. Also, note that track and field races like the 5,000 and 10,000 meter runs are listed as moderate and low to-moderate risks for acid-base disturbances, respectively. In these types of track races, athletes may produce limited amounts of hydrogen ions during most of the race, but a sustained sprint to the finish during the last lap of these events could result in production of relatively large amounts of hydrogen ions and, therefore, result in acid-base disturbances in the muscle and blood.

Because acid-base disturbances can contribute to muscle fatigue and limit exercise performance, it is not surprising that some exercise scientists have investigated the possibility that increasing the buffering capacity of the blood results in improved exercise performance. One approach to this problem is to ingest large quantities of a buffer prior to exercise. A detailed discussion of this topic can be found in The Winning Edge 11.1.

However, the importance of lactic acid in exercise-induced acidosis has been questioned because it appears that lactate and not lactic acid is the primary product of glycolysis (36). Nonetheless, some lactic acid does exist in muscle and it appears likely that exercise-induced production of lactate may also contribute to exercise-induced muscle acidosis because the lactate ion is associated with a decrease in pH within the muscle cell (3, 28).

3. ATP breakdown. The breakdown of ATP for energy during muscle contraction results in the release of H^+ ions (36). For example, the breakdown of ATP results in the following reaction:

$$ATP + H_2O \longrightarrow ADP + HPO_4 + H^+$$

Therefore, the breakdown of ATP alone during exercise can be an important source of H^+ ions in contracting muscles.

In summary, scientific debate exists about the primary causes of exercise-induced acidosis. Nonetheless, it is clear that contracting muscles can produce H^+ from several sites; therefore, the cause of exercise-induced acidosis is likely due to the production of H^+'s from several different sources. A summary of three major metabolic processes that serve as primary sources of hydrogen ions in working skeletal muscle are illustrated in figure 11.3. Further, although high-intensity exercise of sufficient duration (i.e., >45 seconds) can significantly decrease muscle pH, not all sports or exercise activities produce large amounts of hydrogen ions. A detailed discussion of which sports or exercise activities pose the greatest risk of acid-base disturbances is contained in A Closer Look 11.1.

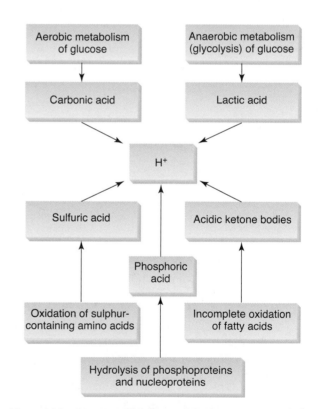

Figure 11.3 Sources of hydrogen ions in contracting skeletal muscles.

TABLE 11.1	Risk of Developing an Acid-Base Disturbance in Popular Sports
Sport	Risk of Acid-Base Disturbance
Baseball	Low
Basketball	Low-to-moderate
Boxing	Low-to-moderate
Cross-country skiing	Low
Football (American)	Low
100-meter sprint	Low
100-meter swim	High
400-meter run	High
800-meter run	High
1,500-meter run	Moderate-to-high
5,000-meter run	Moderate
10,000-meter run	Low-to-moderate
Marathon run	Low
Soccer	Low-to-moderate
Weight lifting (low repetitions)	Low
Volleyball	Low

IN SUMMARY

- High intensity exercise results in a marked decrease to both muscle and blood pH.
- This exercise-induced decrease in muscle pH is due to multiple factors, including (1) increased production of carbon dioxide; (2) increased production of both lactic acid and lactate; and (3) the release of H^+ ions during the breakdown of ATP.
- Only moderate-to-high intensity exercise or sports present a threat to acid-base disturbances during exercise (see table 11.1).

IMPORTANCE OF ACID-BASE REGULATION DURING EXERCISE

As discussed earlier, heavy exercise results in the production of large amounts of hydrogen ions. These hydrogen ions can exert a powerful effect on other molecules due to their small size and positive charge. Hydrogen ions exert their influence by attaching to molecules and thus altering their original size and shape (8, 14, 16, 33, 41). This change in size and shape may alter the normal function of the molecule (enzyme) and therefore influence metabolism in an important way.

An increase in the intramuscular hydrogen ion concentration can impair exercise performance in at least two ways. First, an increase in the hydrogen ion

concentration reduces the muscle cell's ability to produce ATP by inhibiting key enzymes involved in both anaerobic and aerobic production of ATP (8, 14, 19). Second, hydrogen ions compete with calcium ions for binding sites on troponin, thereby hindering the contractile process (8, 14, 45). This is discussed again in chapter 19.

IN SUMMARY

- Hydrogen ions can attach to molecules and alter their original size and function.
- Failure to maintain acid-base homeostasis during exercise can impair performance by inhibiting metabolic pathways responsible for the production of ATP or by interfering with the contractile process in the working muscle.

ACID-BASE BUFFER SYSTEMS

From the preceding discussion, it is clear that a rapid accumulation of hydrogen ions during heavy exercise can negatively influence muscular performance. Therefore, it is important that the body have control systems capable of regulating acid-base status to prevent drastic decreases or increases in pH. How does the body regulate pH? One of the most important means of regulating hydrogen ion concentrations in body fluids is by the aid of buffers. A **buffer** resists pH change by removing hydrogen ions when the hydrogen ion concentration increases, and releasing hydrogen ions when the hydrogen ion concentration falls.

Buffers often consist of a weak acid and its associated base (called a *conjugate base*). The ability of individual buffers to resist pH change is dependent upon two factors. First, individual buffers differ in their intrinsic physiochemical ability to act as buffers. Simply stated, some buffers are better than others. A second factor influencing buffering capacity is the concentration of the buffer present (22, 39). The greater the concentration of a particular buffer, the more effective the buffer can be in preventing pH change.

Intracellular Buffers

The first line of defense in protecting against pH change during exercise is in the cell itself. The most common intracellular buffers are proteins and phosphate groups (25, 39). Many intracellular proteins contain ionizable groups that are weak acids capable of accepting hydrogen ions. Intracellular phosphocreatine (see chapter 3) has been shown to be a useful

Exercise Physiology Applied to Sports

Ingestion of Sodium Buffers and Human Performance

Because exercise-induced disturbances in muscle acid-base balance have been linked to muscle fatigue and impaired sports performance, several studies have explored the possibility that ingestion of a sodium buffer can improve athletic performance. Although not all investigators have reported an improvement in human performance with the ingestion of sodium buffers (2), many studies have found that performance during high-intensity exercise is improved when athletes ingest a sodium buffer prior to exercise (6, 7, 26, 34, 37, 40). Two buffers that have been studied extensively are sodium bicarbonate and sodium citrate. In general, results from several studies suggest that boosting the blood-buffering capacity by ingestion of these buffers increases time to exhaustion during high-intensity exercise (e.g., 80–120% $\dot{V}O_2$ max). It seems likely that if ingestion of a buffer improves physical performance, it does so by increasing the extracellular buffering capacity, which in turn increases the transport of lactate and hydrogen ions out of the muscle fibers (38). This would reduce the interference of hydrogen ions on bioenergetic ATP production and/or the contractile process itself.

In deciding to use sodium bicarbonate or sodium citrate prior to a sporting event, an athlete should understand the risks associated with this decision. Ingestion of sodium bicarbonate in the doses required to improve blood-buffering capacity can cause gastrointestinal problems, including diarrhea and vomiting (7, 37). In contrast, the ingestion of sodium citrate has been reported to improve exercise performance without the same gastrointestinal side effects associated with sodium bicarbonate (24, 30, 31). Further, recent evidence suggests that supplementation with other potential buffers (e.g., beta-alanine) may also play a beneficial role in protecting against exercise-induced acidosis (39). Regardless of the type of buffer ingested, extremely large doses of any buffer could result in severe alkalosis and have serious health consequences. A final consideration in the use of any ergogenic aid is the legality of the drug. In regard to the use of acid-base buffers, numerous sports regulatory agencies have banned the use of sodium buffers during competition.

Buffer System	Constituents	Actions
Bicarbonate system	Sodium bicarbonate ($NaHCO_3$)	Converts strong acid into weak acid
	Carbonic acid (H_2CO_3)	Converts strong base into weak base
Phosphate system	Sodium phosphate ($Na_2HPO_4^-$)	Converts strong acid into weak acid
Protein system	COO^- group of a molecule	Accepts hydrogens in the presence of excess acid
	NH_3 group of a molecule	Accepts hydrogens in the presence of excess acid

TABLE 11.2 Chemical Acid-Base Buffer Systems

buffer at the onset of exercise (1, 22). Further, weak phosphoric acids are found in relatively large concentrations in cells and also serve as an intracellular buffer system. In addition, bicarbonate in muscle has been demonstrated to be a useful buffer during exercise (4, 16). A summary of the chemical action of intracellular buffer systems is presented in table 11.2.

Extracellular Buffers

The blood contains three principal buffer systems (4, 12, 16, 25): (1) proteins, (2) hemoglobin, and (3) bicarbonate. Blood proteins act as buffers in the extracellular compartment. Like intracellular proteins, these blood proteins contain ionizable groups that are weak acids and therefore act as buffers. However, because blood proteins are found in small quantities, their usefulness as buffers during heavy exercise is limited.

In contrast, hemoglobin is a particularly important protein buffer and is a major blood buffer during resting conditions. In fact, hemoglobin has approximately six times the buffering capacity of plasma proteins due to its high concentration (12, 25). Also contributing to the effectiveness of hemoglobin as a buffer is the fact that deoxygenated hemoglobin is a better buffer than oxygenated hemoglobin. As a result, after hemoglobin becomes deoxygenated in the capillaries, it is better able to bind hydrogen ions formed when CO_2 enters the blood from the tissues. Thus, hemoglobin helps to minimize pH changes caused by loading of CO_2 into the blood (12).

The bicarbonate buffer system is probably the most important buffer system in the body (4, 25). This fact has been exploited by some investigators who have demonstrated that an increase in blood bicarbonate concentration (ingestion of bicarbonate) results in an improvement in performance in some types of exercise (4, 7, 20, 26) (see The Winning Edge 11.1).

Peter Stewart Challenged Acid-Base Research by Proposing the Concept of "Strong Ion Difference"

Peter Stewart (1921–1993) was born and raised in Winnipeg, Canada. After completing his B.S. degree, he earned both his master's and Ph.D. degrees from the University of Minnesota. During a long and productive research career, Dr. Stewart served on the faculty of the University of Illinois, Emory University, and Brown University.

In the 1970s, Dr. Stewart developed a strong interest in acid-base regulation and started to mathematically analyze the variables involved in controlling the pH of body fluids. In 1981, he challenged the traditional concepts of acid-base control by publishing his book titled How to Understand Acid-Base Balance—A Quantitative Acid-Base Primer for Biology and Medicine. This book quickly stirred debate among researchers in acid-base balance. A brief synopsis of this controversy follows. Historically, it has been believed that the balance between the levels of hydrogen ions and bicarbonate ions determines the pH of body fluids. Dr. Stewart challenged this concept and argued that hydrogen ions and bicarbonate ions are not the independent variables that control acid-base. Instead, he suggested that these variables are dependent variables that are regulated by other factors, including the strong ion difference,* carbon dioxide levels, and the amount of weak and nonvolatile acids in body fluids. So, does this mean that calculating pH using the Henderson-Hasselbalch equation is of no value? The short answer to this question is no. However, Dr. Stewart's work demonstrates that the factors that regulate acid-base balance in the body are far more complex than originally believed.

Although many physiologists have accepted the science supporting Dr. Stewart's proposal of how acid-base balance is maintained, criticism of his concept of strong ion difference remains. A key criticism of the strong ion balance concept of acid-base control is the complexity of the chemistry and mathematics behind this model. Moreover, in practice, it is often difficult to measure all the variables required to calculate pH using Dr. Stewart's strong ion difference method. Therefore, in the foreseeable future, the traditional approach to acid-base balance seems certain to prevail.

*In Dr. Stewart's terminology, the strong ion difference is defined as the contrast between the number of strong cations (e.g., sodium, potassium, calcium, etc.) and strong anions (e.g., chloride, lactate, etc.) in body fluids (21). You can visit acid-base.org for Stewart's original text. A new edition of Stewart's Textbook of Clinical Acid Base Medicine was recently published and is listed in the suggested readings list (Kellum et al. 2009) (21).

The bicarbonate buffer system involves the weak acid H_2CO_3, which undergoes the following dissociation reaction:

$$CO_2 + H_2O \longleftrightarrow H_2CO_3^- \longleftrightarrow H^+ + HCO_3^-$$

The ability of bicarbonate-carbonic acid (H_2CO_3) to act as a buffer system is described mathematically by a relationship known as the Henderson-Hasselbalch equation:

$$pH = pKa + \log_{10}\left(\frac{HCO_3^-}{H_2CO_3}\right)$$

where pKa is the dissociation constant for H_2CO_3 and has a constant value of 6.1. In short, the Henderson-Hasselbalch equation states that the pH of a weak acid solution is determined by the ratio of the concentration of base (i.e., bicarbonate) in solution to the concentration of acid (i.e., carbonic acid). The normal pH of arterial blood is 7.4, and the ratio of bicarbonate to carbonic acid is 20 to 1. Let's consider an example using the Henderson-Hasselbalch equation to calculate arterial blood pH. Normally the concentration of blood bicarbonate is 24 mEq/l and the concentration of carbonic acid is 1.2 m Eq/l. Therefore, the blood pH can be calculated as follows:

$$pH = pKa + \log_{10}\left(\frac{24}{1.2}\right)$$

$$= 6.1 + \log_{10} 20$$
$$= 6.1 + 1.3$$
$$pH = 7.4$$

Although the traditional view of acid-base chemistry has considered the levels of bicarbonate and hydrogen ions as two primary determinants of pH, new ideas were advanced in the early 1980s that exposed the complexity of regulating pH balance in the body. These new concepts were launched by Peter Stewart and are introduced in A Look Back—Important People in Science.

IN SUMMARY

- The body maintains acid-base homeostasis by buffer-control systems. A buffer resists pH change by removing hydrogen ions when the pH declines and by releasing hydrogen ions when the pH increases.
- The principal intracellular buffers are proteins, phosphate groups, and bicarbonate.
- Primary extracellular buffers are bicarbonate, hemoglobin, and blood proteins.

RESPIRATORY INFLUENCE ON ACID-BASE BALANCE

The fact that the respiratory system contributes to acid-base balance during exercise was introduced in chapter 10. However, more details about how the respiratory system contributes to the control of pH will be presented here. Recall that CO_2 is considered a volatile acid because it can be readily changed from CO_2 to carbonic acid. Also, remember that it is the partial pressure of CO_2 in the blood that determines the concentration of carbonic acid. For example, according to Henry's law, the concentration of a gas in solution is directly proportional to its partial pressure. That is, as the partial pressure increases, the concentration of the gas in solution increases, and vice versa.

Because CO_2 is a gas, it can be eliminated by the lungs. Therefore, the respiratory system is an important regulator of blood carbonic acid and pH. To better understand the role of the lungs in acid-base balance, let's reexamine the carbonic acid dissociation equation:

$$CO_2 + H_2O \longleftrightarrow H_2CO_3 \longleftrightarrow H^+ + HCO_3^-$$

This relationship demonstrates that when the amount of CO_2 in the blood increases, the amount of H_2CO_3 increases, which lowers pH by elevating the acid concentration of the blood (i.e., the reaction moves to the right). In contrast, when the CO_2 content of the blood is lowered (i.e., CO_2 is "blown off" by the lungs), the pH of the blood increases because less acid is present (reaction moves to the left). Therefore, the respiratory system provides the body with a rapid means of regulating blood pH by controlling the amount of CO_2 present in the blood (17).

IN SUMMARY

- Respiratory control of acid-base balance involves the regulation of blood PCO_2.
- An increase in blood PCO_2 lowers pH, whereas a decrease in blood PCO_2 increases pH.

REGULATION OF ACID-BASE BALANCE VIA THE KIDNEYS

Because the kidneys do not play an important part in acid-base regulation during short-term exercise, only a brief overview of the kidney's role in acid-base balance will be presented here. The principal means by which the kidneys regulate hydrogen ion concentration is by increasing or decreasing the bicarbonate concentration (9–11, 23). When the hydrogen ion concentration increases in body fluids, the kidney responds by a reduction in the rate of bicarbonate excretion. This results in an increase in the blood bicarbonate concentration and therefore assists in buffering the increase in hydrogen ions. Conversely, when the pH of body fluids rises (hydrogen ion concentration decreases), the kidneys increase the rate of bicarbonate excretion. Therefore, by changing the amount of buffer present in body fluids, the kidneys aid in the regulation of the hydrogen ion concentration. The kidney mechanism involved in regulating the bicarbonate concentration is located in a portion of the kidney called the tubule, and acts through a series of complicated reactions and active transport across the tubular wall.

Why is the kidney not an important regulator of acid-base balance during exercise? The answer lies in the amount of time required for the kidney to respond to an acid-base disturbance. It takes several hours for the kidneys to react effectively in response to an increase in blood hydrogen ions (10, 46). Therefore, the kidneys respond too slowly to be of major benefit in the regulation of hydrogen ion concentration during exercise.

IN SUMMARY

- Although the kidneys play an important role in the long-term regulation of acid-base balance, the kidneys are not significant in the regulation of acid-base balance during exercise.

REGULATION OF ACID-BASE BALANCE DURING EXERCISE

During the final stages of an incremental exercise test or during near-maximal exercise of short duration, there is a decrease in both muscle and blood pH primarily due to the increase in the production of hydrogen ions by the muscle (13, 15, 29). This point is illustrated in figure 11.4, where the changes in blood and muscle pH during an incremental exercise test are graphed as a function of % $\dot{V}O_2$ max. Note that muscle and blood pH follow similar trends during this type of exercise, but that muscle pH is always 0.4 to 0.6 pH unit lower than blood pH (27, 32). This is because muscle hydrogen ion concentration is higher

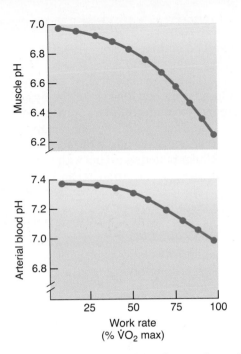

Figure 11.4 Changes in arterial blood pH and muscle pH during incremental exercise. Notice that arterial and muscle pH begin to fall together at work rates above 50% V̇O₂ max.

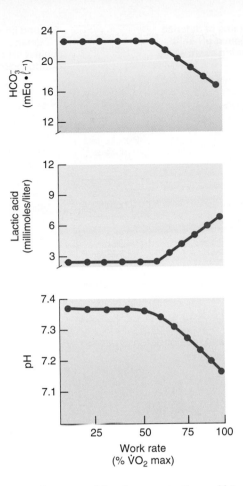

Figure 11.5 Changes in blood concentrations of bicarbonate and pH as a function of work rate.

than that of blood, and muscle buffering capacity is lower than that of blood.

The amount of hydrogen ions produced during exercise is dependent on (1) the exercise intensity, (2) the amount of muscle mass involved, and (3) the duration of the work (5, 13, 15). Exercise involving high-intensity leg work (e.g., running) may reduce arterial pH from 7.4 to a value of 7.0 within a few minutes (13, 18, 27, 35, 43). Further, repeated bouts of this type of exercise may cause blood pH to decline even further to a value of 6.8 (13). This blood pH value is the lowest ever recorded and would present a life-threatening situation if it were not corrected within a few minutes.

How does the body regulate acid-base balance during exercise? Because working muscles are the primary source of hydrogen ions during exercise, it is logical that the first line of defense against a rise in acid production resides in the individual muscle fibers. It is estimated that intracellular proteins contribute as much as 60% of the cell's buffering capacity, with an additional 20% to 30% of the total buffering capacity coming from muscle bicarbonate (25). The final 10% to 20% of muscle buffering capacity comes from intracellular phosphate groups.

Because the muscle's buffering capacity is limited, extracellular fluid (principally the blood) must possess a means of buffering hydrogen ions as well. The principal extracellular buffer and probably the most important buffer in the body is blood bicarbonate (25, 39). Hemoglobin and blood proteins assist in this buffer process but play only a minor role in blood buffering of hydrogen ions during exercise (25). Figure 11.5 illustrates the role of blood bicarbonate as a buffer during incremental exercise (44). Note that at approximately 50% to 60% of V̇O₂ max, blood pH begins to decline due to the rise in hydrogen ions in the blood. This increase in blood hydrogen ion concentration stimulates the carotid bodies, which then signal the respiratory control center to increase alveolar ventilation (i.e., ventilatory threshold; see chapter 10). An increase in alveolar ventilation results in the reduction of blood PCO₂ and therefore acts to reduce the acid load produced by exercise (17). The overall process of respiratory assistance in buffering lactic acid during exercise is referred to as **respiratory compensation** for metabolic acidosis.

First line of defense against pH shift during exercise

Second line of defense against pH shift during exercise

Cellular buffer systems
- Cell proteins
- Phosphate buffers
- Bicarbonate buffers

Blood buffer system
- Bicarbonate buffers — Respiratory compensation
- Blood proteins
- Hemoglobin

Figure 11.6 Lines of defense against pH change during intense exercise.

IN SUMMARY

- Figure 11.6 outlines the process of buffering exercise-induced acidosis.
- The first line of defense against exercise-produced hydrogen ions is the chemical buffer systems of the intracellular compartment and the blood. These buffer systems act rapidly to convert strong acids into weak acids.
- Intracellular buffering occurs with the aid of cellular proteins, bicarbonate, and phosphate groups. Blood buffering of hydrogen ions occurs through bicarbonate, hemoglobin, and blood proteins, with bicarbonate playing the most important role.
- Another line of defense against pH shift during exercise is respiratory compensation for metabolic acidosis.

STUDY QUESTIONS

1. Define the terms *acid, base, buffer, acidosis, alkalosis,* and *pH*.
2. Graph the pH scale. Label the pH values that represent normal arterial and intracellular pH.
3. List and briefly discuss the major sources of hydrogen ions produced in the muscle during exercise.
4. Why is the maintenance of acid-base homeostasis important to physical performance?
5. What are the principal intracellular and extracellular buffers?
6. Discuss respiratory compensation for metabolic acidosis. What would happen to blood pH if an individual began to hyperventilate at rest? Why?
7. Briefly, outline how the body resists pH change during exercise. Include in your outline both the cellular and blood buffer systems.

SUGGESTED READINGS

Fox, S. 2008. *Human Physiology*. New York: McGraw-Hill Companies.

Jones, N. L. (2008). An obsession with CO_2. *Appl Physiol Nutr Metab* 33:641–50.

Kellum, J., and P. Elbers (eds.). (2009). *Stewart's textbook of acid-base*. acid-base.org.

McNaughton, L. R., J. Siegler, and A. Midgley. (2008). Ergogenic effects of sodium bicarbonate. *Curr Sports Med Rep* 7: 230–36.

Widmaier, E., H. Raff, and K. Strang. 2006. *Vander's Human Physiology*, 10th ed. New York: McGraw-Hill Companies.

REFERENCES

1. **Adams GR, Foley JM, and Meyer RA.** Muscle buffer capacity estimated from pH changes during rest-to-work transitions. J *Appl Physiol* 69: 968–972, 1990.
2. **Aschenbach W, Ocel J, Craft L, Ward C, Spangenburg E, and Williams J.** Effect of oral sodium loading on high-intensity arm ergometry in college wrestlers. *Med Sci Sports Exerc* 32: 669–675, 2000.
3. **Boning D, and Maassen N.** Point: lactic acid is the only physicochemical contributor to the acidosis of exercise. J *Appl Physiol* 105: 358–359, 2008.
4. **Broch-Lips M, Overgaard K, Praetorius HA, and Nielsen OB.** Effects of extracellular $HCO_3(-)$ on fatigue, pHi, and K+ efflux in rat skeletal muscles. J *Appl Physiol* 103: 494–503, 2007.
5. **Cerretelli P, and Samaja M.** Acid-base balance at exercise in normoxia and in chronic hypoxia. Revisiting the "lactate paradox." *Eur J Appl Physiol* 90: 431–448, 2003.
6. **Coombes J, and McNaughton L.** The effects of bicarbonate ingestion on leg strength and power during isokinetic knee flexion and extension. *Journal of Strength and Conditioning Research* 7: 241–249, 1993.
7. **Costill DL, Verstappen F, Kuipers H, Janssen E, and Fink W.** Acid-base balance during repeated bouts of exercise: influence of HCO_3. *Int J Sports Med* 5: 228–231, 1984.
8. **Edwards R.** Biochemical bases of fatigue in exercise performance: catastrophe theory of muscular fatigue. In: *Biochemistry of Exercise*. Champaign: Human Kinetics, 1983.

9. **Fox E, Foss M, and Keteyian S.** *Fox's Physiological Basis for Exercise and Sport.* New York: McGraw-Hill, 1998.

10. **Fox S.** *Human Physiology.* New York: McGraw-Hill, 2010.

11. **Guyton A, and Hall J.** *Textbook of Medical Physiology.* Philadelphia: W. B. Saunders, 2005.

12. **Halperin M, Goldstein M, and Kamel K.** *Fluid, Electrolyte, and Acid-Base Physiology.* Philadelphia: Saunders, 2010.

13. **Hultman E, and Sahlin K.** Acid-base balance during exercise. In: *Exercise and Sport Science Reviews*, edited by Hutton R, and Miller D. Philadelphia: Franklin Institute Press, 1980, p. 41–128.

14. **Hultman E, and Sjoholm J.** Biochemical causes of fatigue. In: *Human Muscle Power*, edited by Jones N, McCartney N, and McComas A. Champaign: Human Kinetics, 1986.

15. **Itoh H, and Ohkuwa T.** Ammonia and lactate in the blood after short-term sprint exercise. *Eur J Appl Physiol Occup Physiol* 62: 22–25, 1991.

16. **Jones NL.** Hydrogen ion balance during exercise. *Clin Sci (Lond)* 59: 85–91, 1980.

17. **Jones NL.** An obsession with CO_2. *Appl Physiol Nutr Metab* 33: 641–650, 2008.

18. **Jones NL, Sutton JR, Taylor R, and Toews CJ.** Effect of pH on cardiorespiratory and metabolic responses to exercise. *J Appl Physiol* 43: 959–964, 1977.

19. **Karlsson J.** Localized muscular fatigue: role of metabolism and substrate depletion. In: *Exercise and Sport Science Reviews*, edited by Hutton R, and Miller D. Philadelphia: Franklin Institute Press, 1979, p. 1–42.

20. **Katz A, Costill DL, King DS, Hargreaves M, and Fink WJ.** Maximal exercise tolerance after induced alkalosis. *Int J Sports Med* 5: 107–110, 1984.

21. **Kellum J, and Elbers P** editors. *Stewart's textbook of acid-base.* acid-base.org, 2009.

22. **Kemp GJ, Tonon C, Malucelli E, Testa C, Liava A, Manners D, Trevisi E, Martinuzzi A, Barbiroli B, and Lodi R.** Cytosolic pH buffering during exercise and recovery in skeletal muscle of patients with McArdle's disease. *Eur J Appl Physiol* 105: 687–694, 2009.

23. **Kiil F.** Mechanisms of transjunctional transport of NaCl and water in proximal tubules of mammalian kidneys. *Acta Physiol Scand* 175: 55–70, 2002.

24. **Kowalchuk JM, Maltais SA, Yamaji K, and Hughson RL.** The effect of citrate loading on exercise performance, acid-base balance and metabolism. *Eur J Appl Physiol Occup Physiol* 58: 858–864, 1989.

25. **Laiken N, and Fanestil D.** Acid-base balance and regulation of hydrogen ion excretion. In: *Physiological Basis of Medical Practice*, edited by West J. Baltimore: Lippincott Williams & Wilkins, 1985.

26. **Linderman J, and Fahey TD.** Sodium bicarbonate ingestion and exercise performance. An update. *Sports Med* 11: 71–77, 1991.

27. **Linderman J, Fahey TD, Lauten G, Brooker AS, Bird D, Dolinar B, Musselman J, Lewis S, and Kirk L.** A comparison of blood gases and acid-base measurements in arterial, arterialized venous, and venous blood during short-term maximal exercise. *Eur J Appl Physiol Occup Physiol* 61: 294–301, 1990.

28. **Lindinger MI, and Heigenhauser GJ.** Counterpoint: lactic acid is not the only physicochemical contributor to the acidosis of exercise. *J Appl Physiol* 105: 359–361; discussion 361–362, 2008.

29. **Marsh GD, Paterson DH, Thompson RT, and Driedger AA.** Coincident thresholds in intracellular phosphorylation potential and pH during progressive exercise. *J Appl Physiol* 71: 1076–1081, 1991.

30. **McNaughton LR.** Sodium citrate and anaerobic performance: implications of dosage. *Eur J Appl Physiol Occup Physiol* 61: 392–397, 1990.

31. **McNaughton LR, Siegler J, and Midgley A.** Ergogenic effects of sodium bicarbonate. *Curr Sports Med Rep* 7: 230–236, 2008.

32. **Meyer RA, Adams GR, Fisher MJ, Dillon PF, Krisanda JM, Brown TR, and Kushmerick MJ.** Effect of decreased pH on force and phosphocreatine in mammalian skeletal muscle. *Can J Physiol Pharmacol* 69: 305–310, 1991.

33. **Nattie EE.** The alphastat hypothesis in respiratory control and acid-base balance. *J Appl Physiol* 69: 1201–1207, 1990.

34. **Nielsen HB, Hein L, Svendsen LB, Secher NH, and Quistorff B.** Bicarbonate attenuates intracellular acidosis. *Acta Anaesthesiol Scand* 46: 579–584, 2002.

35. **Robergs RA, Costill DL, Fink WJ, Williams C, Pascoe DD, Chwalbinska-Moneta J, and Davis JA.** Effects of warm-up on blood gases, lactate and acid-base status during sprint swimming. *Int J Sports Med* 11: 273–278, 1990.

36. **Robergs RA, Ghiasvand F, and Parker D.** Biochemistry of exercise-induced metabolic acidosis. *Am J Physiol Regul Integr Comp Physiol* 287: R502–516, 2004.

37. **Robertson RJ, Falkel JE, Drash AL, Swank AM, Metz KF, Spungen SA, and LeBoeuf JR.** Effect of induced alkalosis on physical work capacity during arm and leg exercise. *Ergonomics* 30: 19–31, 1987.

38. **Roth DA, and Brooks GA.** Lactate transport is mediated by a membrane-bound carrier in rat skeletal muscle sarcolemmal vesicles. *Arch Biochem Biophys* 279: 377–385, 1990.

39. **Sale C, Saunders B, and Harris RC.** Effect of beta-alanine supplementation on muscle carnosine concentrations and exercise performance. *Amino Acids* 39: 321–333, 2010.

40. **Siegler JC, and Gleadall-Siddall DO.** Sodium bicarbonate ingestion and repeated swim sprint performance. *J Strength Cond Res* 24: 3105–3111, 2010.

41. **Spriet LL.** Phosphofructokinase activity and acidosis during short-term tetanic contractions. *Can J Physiol Pharmacol* 69: 298–304, 1991.

42. **Stein J.** *Internal Medicine.* St. Louis: Mosby Year-Book, 2002.

43. **Street D, Bangsbo J, and Juel C.** Interstitial pH in human skeletal muscle during and after dynamic graded exercise. *J Physiol* 537: 993–998, 2001.

44. **Stringer W, Casaburi R, and Wasserman K.** Acid-base regulation during exercise and recovery in humans. *J Appl Physiol* 72: 954–961, 1992.

45. **Vollestad NK, and Sejersted OM.** Biochemical correlates of fatigue. A brief review. *Eur J Appl Physiol Occup Physiol* 57: 336–347, 1988.

46. **Widmaier E, Raff H, and Strang K.** *Vander's Human Physiology.* New York: McGraw-Hill, 2010.

Temperature Regulation

Body core temperature regulation is critical because cellular structures and metabolic pathways are affected by temperature. For example, enzymes that regulate metabolic pathways are greatly influenced by temperature changes. Indeed, an increase in body temperature above 45° C (normal core temperature is approximately 37° C) can destroy the normal protein structure of enzymes, resulting in death. Further, a decrease in body temperature below 34° C causes a slowed metabolism and abnormal cardiac function (arrhythmias), which can lead to death. Hence, people and many animals live their entire lives only a few degrees from their thermal death point. Therefore, it is clear that body temperature must be carefully regulated.

Animals that maintain a rather constant body core temperature are called **homeotherms.** The maintenance of a constant body temperature requires that heat loss must match the rate of heat production. To accomplish thermal regulation, the body is well equipped with both nervous and hormonal mechanisms that regulate metabolic rate as well as the amount of heat loss in response to body temperature changes. The temperature-maintenance strategy of homeotherms uses a "furnace" rather than a "refrigerator" to maintain body temperature at a constant level. That is, the body temperature is set near the high end of the survival range and is held constant by continuous metabolic heat production coupled with a small but continual heat loss. The rationale for this strategy seems to be that temperature regulation by heat conservation and generation is very efficient, whereas our cooling capacity is much more limited (5, 20).

Because contracting skeletal muscles produce large amounts of heat, long-term exercise in a hot/humid environment presents a serious challenge to temperature homeostasis. In fact, many exercise physiologists believe that overheating is the only serious threat to health that exercise presents to a healthy individual. This chapter discusses the principles of temperature regulation during exercise. The cardiovascular and pulmonary responses to exercise in a hot environment have already been discussed in chapters 9 and 10, respectively, and the influence of temperature on performance is discussed in chapter 24.

OVERVIEW OF HEAT BALANCE DURING EXERCISE

D. B. Dill and colleagues performed many of the first studies of heat stress in humans at the Harvard Fatigue Laboratory. This early research provided the scientific foundation for our current understanding of thermal stress and temperature regulation during exercise. See A Look Back—Important People in Science for a historical overview of the work of D. B. Dill.

Figure 12.1 During steady-state conditions, temperature homeostasis is maintained by an equal rate of body heat gain and heat loss.

The goal of temperature regulation is to maintain a constant core temperature and thus prevent overheating or overcooling. If the core temperature is to remain constant, the amount of heat lost must match the amount of heat gained (see figure 12.1). Consistent with that, if heat loss is less than heat production, there is a net gain in body heat and therefore body temperature rises; if heat loss exceeds heat production, there is a net loss in body heat and body temperature decreases.

During exercise, body temperature is regulated by making adjustments in the amount of heat that is lost. One of the important functions of the circulatory system is to transport heat. Blood is very effective in this function because it has a high capacity to store heat. When the body is attempting to lose heat, blood flow is increased to the skin as a means of promoting heat loss to the environment. In contrast, when the goal of temperature regulation is to prevent heat loss, blood is directed away from the skin and toward the interior of the body to prevent additional heat loss.

It is important to point out that within the body, temperature varies a great deal. That is, there is a gradient between core temperature (i.e., deep central areas, including the heart, lungs, abdominal organs) and the "shell" (skin) temperature. In extreme circumstances (i.e., exposure to very cold temperatures), the core temperature may be 20° C higher than the shell (33). However, such large core-to-shell gradients are rare, and the ideal difference between core and shell temperatures is approximately 4° C (3, 57). Even within the core, temperature varies from one organ to another. Because large differences in temperature exist between one body part and another, it is important to be specific as to where body temperature is being measured. Therefore, when discussing body temperature, it is important to be specific as to where the temperature measurements were obtained (i.e., skin temperature or core temperature) (3).

D. B. (Bruce) Dill Was a Pioneer in Environmental and Heat Stress Research

After earning his Ph.D. from Stanford University in 1925, **D. B. (Bruce) Dill** went to Harvard University to work with the renowned physiologist L. J. Henderson. Professor Henderson remains well-known today for his contributions to acid-base chemistry, including the Henderson-Hasselbalch equation introduced in chapter 11.

In 1927, Dr. Dill became one of the founding members of the Harvard Fatigue Laboratory. This important research laboratory was charged with investigating factors that influenced human fatigue, including the impact of extreme environments (i.e., heat, cold, and high altitude), exercise, nutrition, acid-base balance, and aging. During the 20-year existence of the Harvard Fatigue Laboratory, the work completed by Dr. Dill and his colleagues greatly advanced our understanding of both environmental and exercise physiology.

After the closure of the Harvard Fatigue Laboratory, Dr. Dill became the scientific director of the Medical Division of the Army Chemical Center, where he directed research until 1961. Dr. Dill's research at this Army research center produced many important outcomes, including research that led to better methods of cardiopulmonary resuscitation. These same procedures are still used today and have saved many lives around the world.

Following his mandatory retirement from the Army research center at age 70, Dr. Dill joined the faculty at Indiana University for a five-year research appointment. He then moved to Boulder City, Nevada, to become a research professor at the Desert Research Institute, University of Nevada–Las Vegas. At the Desert Research Institute, Dill continued his work on the physiological impact of heat stress, and he remained active in environmental stress research until his death at age 95. He presented his last lecture at a scientific conference at the age of 93. The topic discussed was the change in D. B. Dill's $\dot{V}O_2$ max during the past 60 years! In fact, at age 93, Bruce Dill was the oldest person to perform a $\dot{V}O_2$ max test. During Dr. Dill's long and productive scientific career, he coauthored numerous books and more than 300 research reports. Many of these studies laid the foundation for our current understanding of the impact of heat stress on human physiology and performance.

IN SUMMARY

- Homeotherms are animals that maintain a rather constant body core temperature. To maintain a constant core temperature, heat loss must match heat gain.
- Temperature varies markedly within the body. In general, there is a thermal gradient from deep body temperature (core temperature) to the shell (skin) temperature.

TEMPERATURE MEASUREMENT DURING EXERCISE

Measurements of deep-body temperatures can be accomplished with many different devices, including mercury thermometers, devices known as thermocouples or thermistors, and/or ingestible core temperature pills (9). In the laboratory setting, a common site of core temperature measurement is the rectum. Although rectal temperature is not the same as the temperature in the brain where temperature is regulated, it can be used to estimate changes in deep-body temperature during exercise. In addition, temperature measurements near the eardrum (called tympanic temperature) have been found to be a good estimate of the actual brain temperature. Another alternative is to measure the temperature of the esophagus as an indication of core temperature. Like rectal temperature, esophageal temperature is not identical to brain temperature, but it offers a measure of deep-body temperature.

Although the measurements of rectal, tympanic, and esophageal temperature can easily be performed in the laboratory setting, each of these techniques has limitations in a field setting. Indeed, it would be difficult to apply these temperature measurement techniques in athletes during an American football or soccer practice session. Nonetheless, the recent development of ingestible temperature sensor telemetry systems has made onfield core temperature measurement possible and allowed the investigation of core temperature changes in athletes during practice sessions (4, 41). These ingestible temperature sensors use low-power radio frequency transmissions to communicate with a temperature monitor. These probes have been shown to be both valid and reliable in measuring core temperature in football players during practice (4). Further, numerous other commercially available devices exist for the measurement of body temperature in the field setting and the validity of these products has been established (9).

Skin temperature can be measured by placing temperature sensors (thermistors) on the skin at various locations. The mean skin temperature can be calculated by assigning certain factors to each individual skin measurement in proportion to the fraction of the body's total surface area that each measurement represents. For example, mean skin temperature (Ts_s) can be estimated by the following formula (27):

$$T_s = (T_{forehead} + T_{chest} + T_{forearm} + T_{thigh} + T_{calf} +$$

$$T_{abdomen} + T_{back}) \div 7$$

where $T_{forehead}$, T_{chest}, $T_{forearm}$, T_{thigh}, T_{calf}, $T_{abdomen}$, and T_{back} represent skin temperatures measured on the forehead, chest, forearm, thigh, calf, abdomen, and back, respectively.

IN SUMMARY

- Measurements of deep-body temperatures can be accomplished via mercury thermometers, or devices known as *thermocouples* or *thermistors*. Common sites of measurement include the rectum, the ear (tympanic temperature), and the esophagus.
- Skin temperature can be measured by placing temperature sensors (thermistors) on the skin at various locations.

OVERVIEW OF HEAT PRODUCTION/HEAT LOSS

As previously stated, the goal of temperature regulation is to maintain a constant core temperature. This regulation is achieved by controlling the rate of heat production and heat loss. When out of balance, the body either gains or loses heat. The temperature control center is an area in the brain called the hypothalamus. The hypothalamus works like a thermostat by initiating an increase in heat production when body temperature falls and an increase in the rate of heat loss when body temperature rises. Temperature regulation is controlled by both physical and chemical processes. Let's begin our discussion of temperature regulation by introducing those factors that govern heat production and heat loss.

Heat Production

The body produces internal heat due to normal metabolic processes. At rest or during sleep, metabolic heat production is small; however, during intense exercise, heat production is large. Heat production in the body can be classified as (1) voluntary (exercise) or (2) involuntary (shivering or biochemical heat production caused by the secretion of hormones such as thyroxine and catecholamines) (see figure 12.2).

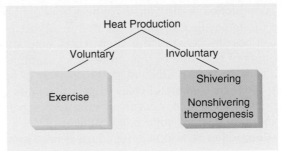

Figure 12.2 The body produces heat due to normal metabolic processes. Heat production can be classified as being either voluntary or involuntary.

Because the body is, at most, 20% to 30% efficient, 70% to 80% of the energy expended during exercise appears as heat. During heavy exercise, this can result in a large heat load. Indeed, work in a hot/humid environment serves as a serious test of the body's ability to lose heat.

Involuntary heat production by shivering is the primary means of increasing heat production during exposure to cold. Maximal shivering can increase the body's heat production by approximately five times the resting value (1, 5). In addition, release of thyroxine from the thyroid gland can also increase metabolic rate. Thyroxine acts by increasing the metabolic rate of all cells in the body (16). Finally, an increase in blood levels of catecholamines (epinephrine and norepinephrine) can cause an increase in the rate of cellular metabolism (16). The increase in heat production due to the combined influences of thyroxine and catecholamines is called nonshivering thermogenesis.

Heat Loss

Heat loss from the body may occur by four processes: (1) radiation, (2) conduction, (3) convection, and/or (4) evaporation. The first three of these heat-loss mechanisms require a temperature gradient to exist between the skin and the environment. **Radiation** is heat loss in the form of infrared rays. This involves the transfer of heat from the surface of one object to the surface of another, with no physical contact being involved (i.e., sun transferring heat to the earth via radiation). At rest in a comfortable environment (e.g., room temperature = 21° C), 60% of the heat loss occurs via radiation. This is possible because skin temperature is greater than the temperature of surrounding objects (walls, floor, etc.), and a net loss of body heat occurs due to the thermal gradient. Note that on a hot, sunny day when surface temperatures are greater than skin temperature, the body can also gain heat via radiation. Therefore, it is important to remember that radiation is heat transfer by infrared rays and can result in either heat loss or heat gain depending on the environmental conditions.

Conduction is the transfer of heat from the body into the molecules of cooler objects in contact with its surface. In general, the body loses only small amounts of heat due to this process. An example of heat loss due to conduction is the transfer of heat from the body to a metal chair while a person is sitting on it. The heat loss occurs as long as the chair is cooler than the body surface in contact with it.

Convection is a form of conductive heat loss in which heat is transmitted to either air or water molecules in contact with the body. In convective heat loss, air or water molecules are warmed and move away from the source of the heat and are replaced by cooler molecules. An example of forced convection is a fan moving large quantities of air past the skin; this would increase the number of air molecules coming in contact with the skin and thus promote heat loss. Practically speaking, the amount of heat loss due to convection is dependent on the magnitude of the airflow over the skin. Therefore, under the same wind conditions, cycling at high speeds would improve convective cooling when compared to cycling at slow speeds. Swimming in cool water (water temperature less than skin temperature) also results in convective heat loss. In fact, water's effectiveness in cooling is about 25 times greater than that of air at the same temperature.

The final means of heat loss is evaporation. Evaporation accounts for approximately 25% of the heat loss at rest, but under most environmental conditions it is the most important means of heat loss during exercise (44). In **evaporation,** heat is transferred from the body to water on the surface of the skin. When this water gains sufficient heat (energy), it is converted to a gas (water vapor), taking the heat away from the body. Evaporation occurs due to a vapor pressure gradient between the skin and the air. Vapor pressure is the pressure exerted by water molecules that have been converted to gas (water vapor). Evaporative cooling during exercise occurs in the following way. When body temperature rises above normal, the nervous system stimulates sweat glands to secrete sweat onto the surface of the skin. As sweat evaporates, heat is lost to the environment, which in turn lowers skin temperature.

Evaporation of sweat from the skin is dependent on three factors: (1) the temperature and relative humidity, (2) the convective currents around the body, and (3) the amount of skin surface exposed to the environment (3, 43). At high environmental temperatures, relative humidity is the most important factor influencing the rate of evaporative heat loss. High relative humidity reduces the rate of evaporation. In fact, when the relative humidity is near 100%, evaporation is limited. Therefore, cooling by way of evaporation is most effective under conditions of low humidity.

Why does high relative humidity reduce the rate of evaporation? The answer is linked to the fact that high relative humidity (RH) reduces the vapor pressure

TABLE 12.1	The Relationship Between Temperature and Relative Humidity (RH) on Vapor Pressure
50% RH Temperature °C	Vapor Pressure (mm Hg)
0	2.3
10	4.6
20	8.8
30	15.9
75% RH Temperature °C	Vapor Pressure (mm Hg)
0	3.4
10	6.9
20	13.2
30	23.9
100% RH Temperature °C	Vapor Pressure (mm Hg)
0	4.6
10	9.2
20	17.6
30	31.9

gradient between the skin and the environment. On a hot/humid day (e.g., RH = 80–90%), the vapor pressure in the air is close to the vapor pressure on moist skin. Therefore, the rate of evaporation is greatly reduced. High sweat rates during exercise in a hot/high humidity environment result in useless water loss. That is, sweating per se does not cool the skin; it is evaporation that cools the skin.

Let's explore in more detail those factors that regulate the rate of evaporation. The major point to keep in mind is that evaporation occurs due to a vapor pressure gradient. That is, for evaporative cooling to occur during exercise, the vapor pressure on the skin must be greater than the vapor pressure in the air. Vapor pressure is influenced by both temperature and relative humidity. This relationship is illustrated in table 12.1. Notice that at any given temperature, a rise in relative humidity results in increased vapor pressure. Practically speaking, this means that less evaporative cooling occurs during exercise on a hot/humid day when compared to a cool/low humidity day. For example, an athlete running on a hot/humid day (e.g., air temperature = 30° C; RH = 100%) might have a mean skin temperature in the range of 33°–34° C. The vapor pressure on the skin would be approximately 35 mm Hg and the air vapor pressure would be around 32 mm Hg (table 12.1). This small vapor pressure gradient between the skin and air (3 mm Hg) would permit only limited evaporation, and therefore little

A CLOSER LOOK 12.1

Calculation of Heat Loss via Evaporation

Knowledge that evaporation of 1,000 ml of sweat results in 580 kcal of heat loss makes it possible to calculate the sweat and evaporation rate necessary to maintain a specified body temperature during exercise. Consider the following example: John is working on a cycle ergometer at a $\dot{V}O_2$ of 2.0 liters · min⁻¹ (energy expenditure of 10.0 kcal · min⁻¹). If John exercises for 20 minutes at this metabolic rate and is 20% efficient, how much

evaporation would be necessary to prevent an increase in core temperature?[1] The total heat produced can be calculated as:

Total energy expenditure
= 20 min × 10 kcal/min
= 200 kcal

Total heat produced
= 200 kcal × .80[1]
= 160 kcal

The total evaporation necessary to prevent any heat gain would be computed as:

$$\frac{160 \text{ kcal}}{580 \text{ kcal/liter}} = .276 \text{ liter}^2$$
(evaporation necessary to prevent heat gain)

[1]If efficiency is 20%, then 80%, or .80, of the total energy expenditure must be released as heat.
[2]Assumes no other heat-loss mechanism is active.

cooling would occur. In contrast, the same athlete running on a cool/low humidity day (e.g., air temperature = 10° C; RH = 50%) might have a mean skin temperature of 30° C. The vapor pressure gradient between the skin and air under these conditions would be approximately 28 mm Hg (32 − 4 = 28) (table 12.1). This relatively large skin-to-air vapor pressure gradient would permit a relatively large evaporative rate, and therefore body cooling would occur under these conditions.

How much heat can be lost via evaporation during exercise? Heat loss due to evaporation can be calculated in the following manner. The body loses

0.58 kcal of heat for each ml of water that evaporates (68). Therefore, evaporation of 1 liter of sweat would result in a heat loss of 580 kcal (1,000 ml × 0.58 kcal/ml = 580 kcal). See A Closer Look 12.1 for additional examples of body heat loss calculations.

In summary, heat loss during exercise (other than swimming) in a cool/moderate environment occurs primarily due to evaporation. In fact, when exercise is performed in a hot environment (where air temperature is greater than skin temperature), evaporation is the only means of losing body heat. The means by which the body gains and loses heat during exercise are summarized in figure 12.3.

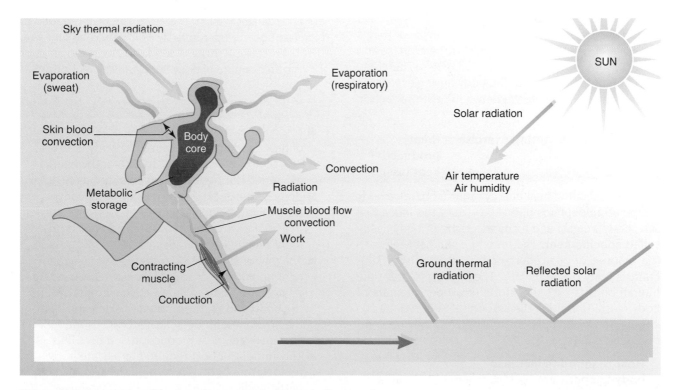

Figure 12.3 A summary of heat exchange mechanisms during exercise.

A CLOSER LOOK 12.2

Calculation of Body Temperature Increase During Exercise

Knowledge of the specific heat of the human body, along with information regarding how much heat is produced and lost from the body during exercise, permits the calculation of how much body temperature will increase during an exercise session. To better understand how to perform these calculations, let's consider the following example of an athlete performing an endurance training workout. For example, a well-trained distance runner performs a training session on an outdoor track. The weather on this day is relatively hot (30° C) and humid (60% relative humidity). The runner weighs 60 kg and performs a 40-minute workout at a $\dot{V}O_2$ of 3.0 liters $\cdot$ min^{-1} (i.e., energy expenditure of 15 kcal per minute). If this runner is 20% efficient and can lose only 60% of the heat produced during exercise, how much her or his body temperature increase during this exercise session?

The total heat storage and body temperature increase during exercise can be calculated in the following steps:

1. **Total energy expenditure**
   = 40 min × 15 kcal/min
   = 600 kcal

2. **Total heat produced**
   = 600 kcal × 0.80[1]
   = 480 kcal

3. **Total heat stored during exercise**
   = 480 kcal × 0.40[2]
   = 192 kcal

4. **Amount of heat storage required to increase body temperature by 1° C**
   = 0.83 kcal/kg × 60 kg[3]
   = 49.8 kcal

The increase in body temperature resulting from this exercise session can now be calculated as follows:

5. **Increase in body temperature (°C) during exercise = Total heat stored during exercise (specific heat × body mass)**
   = 192 kcal/49.8 kcal/°C
   = 3.86° C

In the current example, this exercise bout would result in an increase in body temperature by 3.86° C—that is, 192 kcal/(0.83 kcal/kg × 60 kg). Therefore, if the athlete began the training session with a body temperature of 37° C, the post-exercise body temperature would increase to 40.86° C (i.e., 37° C + 3.86° C).

[1]If the efficiency is 20%, then 80%, or 0.80, of the total energy expenditure must be released as heat.
[2]If the athlete can lose only 60% of the heat produced during exercise, the remaining 40%, or 0.40, of the heat produced must be stored as heat energy.
[3]The amount of heat required to increase body temperature by 1° C = (specific heat × body mass).

Heat Storage in the Body During Exercise

Now that we have discussed both heat production and heat loss, let's talk about heat storage in the body during exercise. As mentioned earlier, any heat that is produced by the working muscles during exercise and is not lost must be stored in body tissues. Therefore, the amount of heat gain in the body during exercise is computed as the difference between heat production and heat loss:

Body heat gain during exercise = (heat produced − heat loss)

The amount of heat energy required to raise body temperature depends upon the size of the individual (i.e., body weight) and a characteristic of body tissue called **specific heat.** The term specific heat refers to the amount of heat energy required to raise 1 kilogram of body tissue by 1° C. The specific heat for the human body is 0.83 kilocalorie (kcal) per kilogram of body mass. Therefore, the amount of heat required to elevate the body temperature by 1° C can be computed as follows:

Heat required to increase body temperature by 1° C = (specific heat × body mass)

For example, using the preceding equation, the amount of heat required to increase body temperature by 1° C in a 70-kg individual can be computed by multiplying the specific heat of the body (0.83 kcal/kg) by the individual's body weight (70 kg). Therefore, the heat required to increase body temperature by 1° C would be 58.1 kcal (i.e., 0.83 kcal/kg × 70 kg = 58.1 kcal). See A Closer Look 12.2 for an example of body heat gain calculations.

IN SUMMARY

- Muscular exercise can result in large amounts of heat production. Because the body is at most 20% to 30% efficient, 70% to 80% of the energy expended during exercise is released as heat.
- Body heat can be lost by evaporation, convection, conduction, and radiation. During exercise in a cool environment, evaporation is the primary avenue for heat loss.
- The rate of evaporation from the skin is dependent upon three factors: (1) temperature and relative humidity, (2) convective currents around the body, and (3) the amount of skin exposed to the environment. Body heat storage is the difference between heat production and heat loss.
- The amount of heat required to elevate body temperature by 1° C is termed the specific heat of the body.

BODY'S THERMOSTAT— HYPOTHALAMUS

Again, the body's temperature regulatory center is located in the hypothalamus. The **anterior hypothalamus** is primarily responsible for dealing with increases in body heat, whereas the **posterior hypothalamus** is responsible for reacting to a decrease in body temperature. In general, the hypothalamus operates much like a thermostat in your home—that is, it attempts to maintain a relatively constant core temperature around some "set point." The set-point temperature in humans is approximately 37° C.

The input to the temperature-regulating centers in the hypothalamus comes from receptors in both the skin and the core. Changes in environmental temperature are first detected by thermal receptors (both heat and cold) located in the skin. These skin temperature receptors transmit nerve impulses to the hypothalamus, which then initiates the appropriate response in an effort to maintain the body's set-point temperature. Further, heat-/cold-sensitive neurons are located in both the spinal cord and the hypothalamus itself, sensing changes in the core temperature.

An increase in core temperature above the set point results in the hypothalamus initiating a series of physiological actions aimed at increasing the amount of heat loss. First, the hypothalamus stimulates the sweat glands, which results in an increase in evaporative heat loss (25, 29). In addition, the vasomotor control center withdraws the normal vasoconstrictor tone to the skin, promoting increased skin blood flow and therefore allowing increased heat loss. Figure 12.4 illustrates the physiological responses associated with an increase in core temperature. When core temperature returns to normal, the stimulus to promote both sweating and vasodilation is removed. This is an example of a control system using negative feedback (see chapter 2).

Physiological Responses to Cold

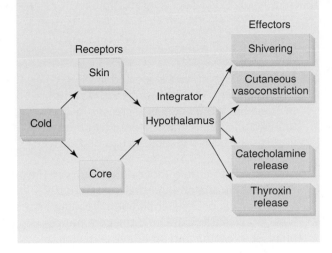

Figure 12.5 An illustration of the physiological responses to cold stress.

When cold receptors are stimulated in the skin or the hypothalamus, the thermoregulatory control center sets forth a plan of action to minimize heat loss and increase heat production. First, the vasomotor center directs peripheral blood vessels to vasoconstrict, which reduces heat loss (5, 23). Second, if core temperature drops significantly, involuntary shivering begins (5, 65). Additional responses include stimulation of the pilomotor center, which promotes piloerection (goosebumps). This piloerection reflex is an effective means of increasing the insulation space over the skin in fur-bearing animals, but is not an effective means of preventing heat loss in humans. Further, the hypothalamus indirectly increases thyroxine production and release, which increases cellular heat production (5). Finally, the posterior hypothalamus initiates the release of norepinephrine, which increases the rate of cellular metabolism (nonshivering thermogenesis). The physiological responses to a decrease in core temperature are summarized in figure 12.5.

Shift in the Hypothalamic Thermostat Set Point Due to Fever

A fever is an increase in body temperature above the normal range, and it may be caused by numerous bacterial/viral infections or brain disorders. During a fever, select proteins and other toxins secreted by bacteria can cause the set point of the hypothalamic thermostat to rise above the normal level. Substances that cause this effect are called pyrogens. When the set point of the hypothalamic thermostat is raised to a higher level than normal, all the mechanisms for raising body temperature are called into play (16). Within a few hours after the thermostat has been set

Physiological response to a "Heat Load"

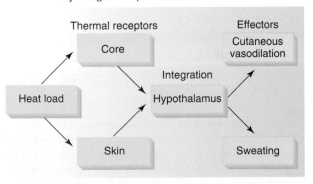

Figure 12.4 A summary illustration of the physiological responses to an increase in "heat load."

to a higher level, the body core temperature reaches this new level due to heat conservation.

Figure 12.6   Changes in metabolic energy production, evaporative heat loss, convective heat loss, and radiative heat loss during 25 minutes of submaximal exercise in a cool environment.

IN SUMMARY

- The body's thermostat is located in the hypothalamus. The anterior hypothalamus is responsible for reacting to increases in core temperature, while the posterior hypothalamus governs the body's responses to a decrease in temperature.
- An increase in core temperature results in the anterior hypothalamus initiating a series of physiological actions aimed at increasing heat loss. These actions include the commencement of sweating and an increase in skin blood flow.
- Cold exposure results in the posterior hypothalamus promoting physiological changes that increase body heat production (shivering) and reduce heat loss (cutaneous vasoconstriction).

THERMAL EVENTS DURING EXERCISE

Now that an overview of how the hypothalamus responds to different thermal challenges has been presented, let's discuss the thermal events that occur during submaximal constant-load exercise in a cool/moderate environment (i.e., low humidity and room temperature). Heat production increases during exercise due to muscular contraction and is directly proportional to the exercise intensity. The venous blood draining the exercising muscle distributes the excess heat throughout the body core. As core temperature increases, thermal sensors in the hypothalamus sense the increase in blood temperature, and the thermal integration center in the hypothalamus compares this increase in temperature with the set-point temperature and finds a difference between the two (18, 43, 46, 66). The response is to direct the nervous system to commence sweating and to increase blood flow to the skin (6, 45). These acts serve to increase body heat loss and minimize the increase in body temperature. At this point, the internal temperature reaches a new, elevated steady-state level (see figure 12.6). Note that this new steady-state core temperature does not represent a change in the set-point temperature, as occurs in fever (18, 43, 46, 70). Instead, the thermal regulatory center attempts to return the core temperature back to resting levels, but is incapable of doing so in the face of the sustained heat production associated with exercise.

Figure 12.6 also illustrates the roles of evaporation, convection, and radiation in heat loss during constant-load exercise in a moderate environment. Notice the constant but small role of convection and radiation in heat loss during this type of exercise. This is due to a constant temperature gradient between the skin and the room. In contrast, evaporation plays the most important role in heat loss during exercise in this type of environment (43, 46, 48).

During constant-load exercise, the core temperature increase is directly related to the exercise intensity and is independent of ambient temperature over a wide range of conditions (i.e., 8°–29° C with low relative humidity) (47). This point is illustrated in figure 12.7. Notice the linear rise in core temperature as the metabolic rate increases. The fact that it is the exercise intensity and not the environmental temperature that determines the rise in core temperature during

Figure 12.7   The relationship between metabolic rate and rectal temperature during constant load arm (●) and leg (●) exercise. From M. Nelson, 1938, "Die Regulation der Korpertemperatur bei Muskelarbeit" in *Scandinavica Archives Physiology*, 79:193. Copyright © 1938 Blackwell Scientific Publications, Ltd., Oxford, England. Reprinted by permission.

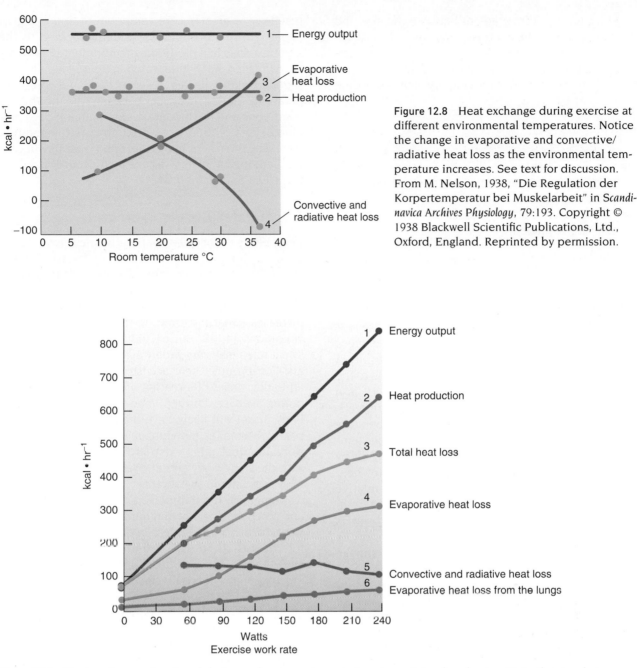

Figure 12.8 Heat exchange during exercise at different environmental temperatures. Notice the change in evaporative and convective/radiative heat loss as the environmental temperature increases. See text for discussion. From M. Nelson, 1938, "Die Regulation der Korpertemperatur bei Muskelarbeit" in *Scandinavica Archives Physiology*, 79:193. Copyright © 1938 Blackwell Scientific Publications, Ltd., Oxford, England. Reprinted by permission.

Figure 12.9 Heat exchange at rest and during cycle ergometer exercise at a variety of work rates. Note the steady increase in evaporative heat loss as a function of an increase in power output. In contrast, an increase in metabolic rate has essentially no influence on the rate of convective and radiative heat loss. From M. Nelson, 1938, "Die Regulation der Korpertemperatur bei Muskelarbeit" in *Scandinavica Archives Physiology*, 79:193. Copyright © 1938 Blackwell Scientific Publications, Ltd., Oxford, England. Reprinted by permission.

exercise suggests that the method of heat loss during continuous exercise is modified according to ambient conditions (31, 47). This concept is presented in figure 12.8, which shows heat loss mechanisms during constant-intensity exercise. Note that as the ambient temperature increases, the rate of convective and radiative heat loss decreases due to a decrease in the skin-to-room temperature gradient. This decrease in convective and radiative heat loss is matched by an increase in evaporative heat loss, and core temperature remains the same (see figure 12.8).

The relationship between exercise intensity and body heat production is illustrated in figure 12.9. Notice the linear increase in energy output (expenditure), heat production, and total heat loss as a function of exercise work rate. Further, note that convective and radiative heat loss are not increased as a function of exercise work rate. This is due to a relatively constant temperature gradient between the skin and the environment. In contrast, there is a consistent rise in evaporative heat loss with increments in exercise intensity. This observation reemphasizes the point that evaporation is the primary means of losing heat during exercise.

IN SUMMARY

- During constant intensity exercise, the increase in body temperature is directly related to the exercise intensity.
- Body heat production increases in proportion to exercise intensity.

HEAT INDEX—A MEASURE OF HOW HOT IT FEELS

The Heat Index (HI) is typically expressed in degrees Fahrenheit (F) (or Centigrade) and is a measure of how hot it feels when relative humidity is added to the actual air temperature. In other words, the HI is a measure of the body's perception of how hot it feels. The HI is calculated by combining the air temperature and relative humidity to compute an apparent temperature. As discussed previously, heat loss by evaporation is the most important means of heat loss during exercise (44). However, when the relative humidity is high (i.e., high water vapor saturation in the atmosphere), the evaporation rate of sweat is retarded. This means that heat is removed from the body at a lower rate, resulting in body heat storage and an increase in body temperature. Therefore, high humidity increases an individual's perception of how hot the environment feels. For example, if the air temperature is 82° F and the relative humidity is 80%, the calculated HI is 89° F. In this illustration, the environment feels like 89° F rather than the actual air temperature of 82° F. Figure 12.10 provides the HI over a range of relative humidity (%) values and temperatures.

EXERCISE IN A HOT ENVIRONMENT

Continuous exercise in a hot/humid environment poses a particularly stressful challenge to the maintenance of normal body temperature and fluid homeostasis. High heat and humidity reduce the body's ability to lose heat by radiation/convection and evaporation, respectively. This inability to lose heat during exercise in a hot/humid environment

results in a greater core temperature and a higher sweat rate (more fluid loss) when compared to the same exercise in a moderate environment (53–55, 57, 58, 63). This point is illustrated in figure 12.11. Notice the marked differences in sweat rates and core temperatures during exercise between the hot/humid conditions and the moderate environment. The combined effect of fluid loss and high core temperature increases the risk of **hyperthermia** (large rise in core temperature) and heat injury (see Clinical Applications 12.1 and chapter 24).

Sweat Rates During Exercise

In an effort to increase evaporative heat loss during exercise, humans rely on their ability to increase sweat production via eccrine sweat glands (i.e., sweat glands under sympathetic cholinergic control) (30). In this regard, exercise in a hot environment greatly increases sweat rates during training or competitive conditions (4, 19, 30, 61, 62). Note, however, that sweat rates may vary widely across different individuals. For example, heat-accustomed individuals have an earlier onset of sweating and a higher sweat rate during exercise. Further, large individuals (i.e., large body mass) will likely have higher sweat rates compared to smaller individuals. Finally, genetic variations in sweat rates exist such that two individuals with the same body size and level of heat adaptation may also differ in sweat rates.

American football players, wearing full uniforms and practicing in a hot and humid environment, experience some of the largest sweat rates ever recorded for athletes. Although several reasons exist for high sweat loss in these athletes, two major contributors are that many football players possess large body masses and that football uniforms retard heat loss (1, 24). For example, the average sweat loss in football players ranges from 4 to 5 liters per hour during a practice session in a hot and humid environment (19). Further, during preseason practice sessions where football athletes are practicing twice a day, the daily sweat loss ranged from 9 to 12 liters of water. Failure to replace this loss of fluid on a daily basis would result in progressive dehydration and increase the risk of heat injury (4, 61, 62). For more information on the importance of fluid replacement during exercise, see The Winning Edge 12.1.

Exercise Performance is Impaired in a Hot Environment

Performance during prolonged, submaximal exercise (e.g., a marathon or long triathlon) is impaired in a hot/humid environment (39). Further, athletic performance during intermittent, high-intensity exercise

Temperature °F (°C)	Relative Humidity (%)												
	40	45	50	55	60	65	70	75	80	85	90	95	100
110 (47)	136 (58)												
108 (43)	130 (54)	137 (58)											
106 (41)	124 (51)	130 (54)	137 (58)										
104 (40)	119 (48)	124 (51)	131 (55)	137 (58)									
102 (39)	114 (46)	119 (48)	124 (51)	130 (54)	137 (58)								
100 (38)	109 (43)	114 (46)	118 (48)	124 (51)	129 (54)	136 (58)							
98 (37)	105 (41)	109 (43)	113 (45)	117 (47)	123 (51)	128 (53)	134 (57)						
96 (36)	101 (38)	104 (40)	108 (42)	112 (44)	116 (47)	121 (49)	126 (52)	132 (56)					
94 (34)	97 (36)	100 (38)	103 (39)	106 (41)	110 (43)	114 (46)	119 (48)	124 (51)	129 (54)	135 (57)			
92 (33)	94 (34)	96 (36)	99 (37)	101 (38)	105 (41)	108 (42)	112 (44)	116 (47)	121 (49)	126 (52)	131 (55)		
90 (32)	91 (33)	93 (34)	95 (35)	97 (36)	100 (38)	103 (39)	106 (41)	109 (43)	113 (45)	117 (47)	122 (50)	127 (53)	132 (56)
88 (31)	88 (31)	89 (32)	91 (33)	93 (34)	95 (35)	98 (37)	100 (38)	103 (39)	106 (41)	110 (43)	113 (45)	117 (47)	121 (49)
86 (30)	85 (29)	87 (31)	88 (31)	89 (32)	91 (33)	93 (34)	95 (35)	97 (36)	100 (38)	102 (39)	105 (41)	108 (42)	112 (44)
84 (29)	83 (28)	84 (29)	85 (29)	86 (30)	88 (31)	89 (32)	90 (32)	92 (33)	94 (34)	96 (36)	98 (37)	100 (38)	103 (39)
82 (28)	81 (27)	82 (28)	83 (28)	84 (29)	84 (29)	85 (29)	86 (30)	88 (31)	89 (32)	90 (32)	91 (33)	93 (34)	95 (35)
80 (27)	80 (27)	80 (27)	81 (27)	81 (27)	82 (28)	82 (28)	83 (28)	84 (29)	84 (29)	85 (29)	86 (30)	86 (30)	87 (31)

Category	Heat Index
Extreme Danger	130°F or higher (54°C or higher)
Danger	105–129°F (41–54°C)
Extreme Caution	90–105°F (32–41°C)
Caution	80–90°F (27–32°C)

Figure 12.10 The relationship of relative humidity (%) and temperature and the Heat Index. Data obtained from National Weather Service–Tulsa.

Exercise-Related Heat Injuries Can Be Prevented

Heat injury during exercise can occur when the level of body heat production is high and environmental conditions (e.g., high ambient temperature and humidity) impede heat loss from the body. The primary cause of heat injury is hyperthermia (high body temperature). Increases in body temperature of 2° C to 3° C generally do not have ill effects (3, 7). Nonetheless, increases in body temperature above 40° C to 41° C can be associated with a variety of heat-related problems. Note that heat-related problems during exercise are not "all or none," but form a heat-injury continuum that can extend from a relatively minor problem (i.e., heat syncope) to a life-threatening, major medical emergency (i.e., heat stroke). The general symptoms of heat stress include nausea, headache, dizziness, reduced sweat rate, and the general inability to think rationally.

Each year in the United States, several heat-related problems in American football are reported. Nonetheless, heat-related illness during exercise can be prevented. To prevent overheating during exercise, the following guidelines are useful:

- Exercise during the coolest part of the day.
- Minimize both the intensity and duration of exercise on hot/humid days.
- Expose a maximal surface area of skin for evaporation (i.e., removal of clothing) during exercise.
- When removal of clothing during exercise is not possible (e.g., American football), provide frequent rest/cooldown breaks along with intermittent clothing shed (e.g., removal of helmet and upper clothing).
- To avoid dehydration during exercise, workouts should permit frequent water breaks (coupled with rest/cool-down).
- Rest/cool-down breaks during exercise should remove the athlete from radiant heat gain due to direct sunlight (e.g., sitting under a tent) and offer exposure to circulating, cool air (e.g., fans).
- Measure body weight at the beginning and end of a training (or practice) session to determine the amount of fluid replacement required to restore body water balance before the next training session.

When an athlete develops symptoms of heat injury, the obvious treatment is to stop exercising and immediately begin cooling the body (e.g., cold water immersion). Cold fluids with electrolytes should also be provided for rehydration. See chapter 24 for more details on the signs and symptoms of heat injury.

Figure 12.11 Differences in core temperature and sweat rate during 45 minutes of submaximal exercise in a hot/humid environment versus a cool environment

(e.g., Rugby, Soccer, 15-min time trial on cycle) is also compromised on a hot day (15, 26, 60). While the exact mechanism(s) responsible for this decreased exercise performance continue to be debated, prolonged exercise in a hot/humid environment can impede exercise performance in several ways; these include alterations in muscle metabolism, cardiovascular function/fluid balance, and central nervous system function. A brief discussion of each of these factors follows.

Several changes in muscle metabolism occur during exercise that can have a negative impact on exercise performance. First, during exercise in the heat, the rate of muscle glycogen degradation is increased with a parallel rise in both carbohydrate metabolism and lactate accumulation (21). This is important because muscle glycogen depletion and low blood glucose levels (i.e., hypoglycemia) are associated with muscle fatigue during prolonged exercise (21). Moreover, exercise-induced increases in muscle lactate levels and the associated decrease in muscle pH are also linked to muscle fatigue. Therefore, a collective depletion of muscle glycogen stores and high muscle lactate levels could contribute to muscle fatigue during prolonged exercise in the heat.

Prevention of Dehydration During Exercise

Athletic performance can be impaired by sweat-induced loss of body water (i.e., dehydration). Indeed, dehydration resulting in loss of 1% to 2% of body weight is sufficient to impair exercise performance (8, 39). Dehydration of greater than 3% of body weight further impairs physiological function and increases the risk of heat injury (8, 38). Therefore, prevention of dehydration during exercise is important to both maximize athletic performance and prevent heat injuries. Dehydration can be avoided by adherence to the following guidelines:

- Athletes should be well hydrated prior to beginning a workout or competition. This can be achieved by drinking 400 to 800 ml of fluid within three hours prior to exercise (37, 39).
- Athletes should consume 150 to 300 ml of fluid every 15 to 20 minutes during exercise (39). The actual volume of fluid ingested during each drinking period should be adjusted to environmental conditions (i.e., rate of sweat loss) and individual tolerances for drinking during exercise.
- To ensure rehydration following exercise, athletes should monitor fluid losses during exercise by recording body weight prior to the workout and then weighing immediately after the work-out session. To ensure proper rehydration following exercise, the individual should consume fluids equal to approximately 150% of the weight loss. For example, if an athlete loses 1 kg of body weight during a training session, he/she should consume 1.5 liters of fluid to achieve complete rehydration (39).
- Monitoring the color of urine between workouts is a practical way to judge hydration levels in athletes. For example, in a well-hydrated individual, urine is typically clear or the color of lemonade. In contrast, in dehydrated individuals, urine appears as a dark-yellow fluid.

Which is the optimal rehydration fluid—water or a well-formulated sports drink? The National Athletic Trainers Association has concluded that well-designed sports drinks are superior to water for rehydration following exercise (8). The rationale for this recommendation is that these beverages increase voluntary intake by athletes and allow for more effective rehydration. For more details on fluid replacement during and following exercise, please see Maughan (2010) in the Suggested Readings.

Another metabolic explanation for heat-induced muscular fatigue is that free radical production is increased in skeletal muscles during exercise in the heat (72). Recall that free radicals are molecules with an unpaired electron in their outer orbital (56). This is significant because molecules with unpaired electrons are highly reactive. That is, free radicals bind quickly with other molecules, and this combination results in damage to the molecule combining with the radical. Therefore, accelerated production of free radicals during exercise in the heat could contribute to muscle fatigue because of damage to muscle contractile proteins (56).

An additional contributor to impaired exercise performance in a hot/humid environment is that heat stress can result in cardiovascular strain and reduced muscle blood flow. Note, however, that reduced muscle blood flow does not contribute to poor exercise tolerance during light or moderate exercise because muscle blood flow is well maintained under these exercise conditions when dehydration does not occur (12). In contrast, during high intensity (i.e., near $\dot{V}O_2$ max) exercise performed in a hot/humid environment, there is a progressive decline in muscle blood flow. This reduction in muscle blood flow during exercise in the heat is due to a competition for blood between the working muscles and the skin. That is, as body temperature rises during exercise in a hot environment, blood flow moves away from the contracting muscle toward the skin to assist in cooling the body. Therefore, during high intensity exercise, reduced muscle blood flow can contribute to impaired exercise performance in the heat. In contrast, reduced muscle blood flow cannot explain the heat-induced reduction in exercise performance during light to moderate intensity work.

Further, both hyperthermia and dehydration can directly diminish exercise performance due to central nervous system impairment. Specifically, hyperthermia can act upon the central nervous system to reduce the mental drive for motor performance (21, 38, 40). Indeed, many studies have demonstrated that prolonged exercise in the heat can retard exercise performance due to changes in the central nervous system. For more details on this topic, see Hargreaves (2008) and Maughan et al. (2007) in the Suggested Readings.

In summary, exercise in the heat accelerates muscle fatigue and impairs exercise performance. It seems likely that heat-induced fatigue is not due to a single factor but probably results from a combination of metabolic events (10). Key factors that could

Exercise Performance in a Hot Environment
Questions and Answers with Dr. Michael Sawka

Michael Sawka, Ph.D., *is Director of the Thermal and Mountain Medicine Division at the United States Army Research Institute of Environmental Medicine. Dr. Sawka is an internationally recognized expert in both exercise physiology and environmental stress. Indeed, Dr. Sawka has authored more than 200 highly regarded research studies related to both exercise and environmental physiology. In particular, Dr. Sawka and his team have performed many studies investigating the impact of a hot environment on exercise performance. In this box feature, Dr. Sawka addresses three important questions related to exercise performance in the heat.*

QUESTION: Your work has established that environmental heat stress has a negative impact on aerobic exercise performance. However, how does heat stress impact performance in team sports, such as soccer or American football?

ANSWER: The performance of a team is dependent upon the individual athletes. If the individual athlete's performance is impaired, then it is likely the team's performance will also be suboptimal. In addition, team sports are greatly dependent upon cohesion and decision making, and there is evidence that heat stress and dehydration can degrade cognitive function, which will impact decision making and team cohesion.

QUESTION: Your group has extensively studied the mechanism(s) to explain why environmental heat stress impairs aerobic exercise performance. What are the primary explanations as to why a hot environment impairs aerobic performance?

ANSWER: Heat stress impairs aerobic exercise performance because of two primary reasons: (1) cardiovascular strain needed to support high skin blood flow; and (2) dehydration, which reduces plasma volume and thus increases cardiovascular strain. The high skin blood flow and plasma loss both act to reduce venous pressure and thus reduce cardiac filling. Despite a compensatory increase in heart rate and contractility, stroke volume will usually decline and thus make it difficult to maintain blood pressure and to sustain adequate blood flow to skeletal muscle and the brain. The net effect is that heat stress degrades maximal aerobic power and that any submaximal work rate is performed at a greater relative work rate (i.e., percent of maximal aerobic power), which also increases perception of effort. In addition, heat stress alters skeletal muscle metabolism (increased glycogen use and lactate accumulation) and may modify central nervous system function, which can contribute to impaired exercise performance.

QUESTION: Strong evidence indicates that heat acclimation improves exercise tolerance in hot environments. However, are there other strategies (e.g., precooling or hyperhydration) that athletes can utilize to improve aerobic performance in a hot environment?

ANSWER: By far the most effective strategies to sustain performance during heat stress are to achieve heat acclimation and maintain adequate hydration. There is some evidence that precooling and hyperhydration can help, but in my opinion their benefits are marginal and if improperly used might be counterproductive. Hyperhydration can slightly delay developing dehydration and slightly increase blood volume, thus helping to support the cardiovascular system. Nonetheless, any benefits are marginal and, depending upon the methods employed, could increase the likelihood of hyponatremia (i.e., low blood sodium levels), discomfort from increased urine output or headache. Precooling allows body temperature (skin and core) to be lower at the beginning of exercise, but the small benefits demonstrated in laboratory studies may be lost in real-life competition when athletes are exposed to the hot environment for a significant period before initiating competition. In addition, overcooling the skeletal muscles might initially impair muscle performance.

---

contribute to heat-related muscle fatigue are alterations in muscle metabolism, impaired cardiovascular function/fluid balance, and central nervous system dysfunction resulting in impaired neuromuscular function. Several strategies can be used by athletes to improve their exercise tolerance in a hot environment. For example, athletes can optimize exercise performance in the heat by becoming heat acclimated and consuming fluid before and during exercise. The process of physiological adaptation to heat (heat acclimation) will improve exercise tolerance and will be discussed later in this chapter.

Guidelines for the consumption of water before and during athletic performance are presented in The Winning Edge 12.1 and are also discussed in chapter 23. For more details on exercise performance in the heat, see Ask the Expert 12.1.

Gender and Age Differences in Thermoregulation

It the 1960s it was believed that, compared to men, women were less tolerant of exercise in a hot environment. However, these early studies did not match men and women at the same level of heat acclimation and similar body compositions (i.e., equal percent body fat). More recent studies have matched men and women for these characteristics, and the gender differences in heat tolerance are small (49).

Does aging impair one's ability to thermoregulate and exercise in the heat? This issue remains controversial, but growing evidence suggests that age per se does not limit one's ability to thermoregulate during exercise (14, 28, 30, 52). For example, well-controlled studies have concluded that exercise-conditioned old and young men show little difference in thermoregulation during exercise (52, 64). Further, a recent review of the literature on this subject has concluded that heat tolerance does not appear to be compromised by age in healthy and physically active older subjects (28, 30). Based upon the collective evidence, it appears that deconditioning (i.e., decline in $\dot{V}O_2$ max) and a lack of heat acclimatization in older subjects may explain why some of the earlier studies reported a decrease in thermotolerance with age.

Heat Acclimation

Regular exercise in a hot environment results in a series of physiological adjustments designed to minimize disturbances in homeostasis due to heat stress. The reversible physiological adaptation to changes in environmental conditions (e.g., heat stress) is called **acclimation.** A similar term, **acclimatization** also refers to adaptation to a new climatic condition (e.g.,

changes in temperature or altitude). Although these terms are often used interchangeably, the term *acclimation* is most appropriately used to refer to rapid (days to a few weeks) adaptation to environmental change, whereas *acclimatization* is most appropriately applied when environmental adaptation occurs over a long time period (many weeks to several months). In our discussion of improved heat tolerance, we will use the term acclimation to denote an improved tolerance to heat stress during a relatively short period (several days).

Individuals of all ages are capable of acclimating to a hot environment (28, 64). The end result of heat acclimation is a lower heart rate and core temperature during submaximal exercise (14). Although partial heat acclimation can occur by training in a cool environment, it is essential that athletes exercise in a hot environment to obtain maximal heat acclimation (2). Because an elevation in core temperature is the primary stimulus to promote heat acclimation, it is recommended that the athlete perform strenuous interval training or continuous exercise at an intensity exceeding 50% of the athlete's $\dot{V}O_2$ max in order to promote higher core temperatures (50) (see Research Focus 12.1).

The primary adaptations that occur during heat acclimation are an increased plasma volume, earlier onset of sweating, higher sweat rate, reduced salt loss in sweat, a reduced skin blood flow, and increased synthesis of heat shock proteins. It is interesting that heat adaptation occurs rapidly, with almost complete acclimation being achieved by 7–14 days after the first

RESEARCH FOCUS 12.1

Can Exercise Training in Cool Conditions Promote Heat Acclimation?

Athletes who train in cool environments often travel to warmer climates to compete. Without adequate heat acclimation, these athletes will be at a disadvantage compared to athletes who have developed a high level of heat adaptation by training in a hot/humid environment. Therefore, a key question is, "Can training in heavy clothing in a cool environment promote heat acclimation?" The answer to this question is yes, but the magnitude of the heat acclimation that is obtained by this method is generally less than the maximal level of acclimation that can be achieved by daily training in a hot/humid environment

(2, 13). Nonetheless, "artificial" heat training in heavy clothing in cool conditions appears to be better than attempting no heat acclimation measures (13).

On a related topic, most of us have witnessed individuals exercising in a rubber suit. These exercise suits are typically made of a rubberized vinyl that covers the entire body and prevents evaporative heat loss from the skin. While exercise in these suits will promote increased body temperature and therefore will contribute to heat acclimation, prolonged exercise in a rubber suit is a high-risk endeavor that could lead to high body temperatures

and heat injury. Therefore, wearing a rubber suit during exercise is not recommended because of the risk of hyperthermia associated with the prevention of evaporative heat loss. Also, note that while exercise in a rubber suit will encourage body water loss, exercise in a rubber suit does not necessarily result in the loss of body fat because to lose body fat, you must create an energy (i.e., caloric) deficit. Indeed, while a sweat-induced loss of body water does reduce your body weight, as soon as you replace these fluids by drinking, your body weight will return to normal. See chapter 18 for details on loss of body fat.

Figure 12.12 The number of days required to reach maximal heat acclimation during consecutive days of heat exposure. Note that heat maximal heat acclimation is achieved between 7–14 days following the initial heat exposure.

exposure (6, 51, 70) (figure 12.12). A brief discussion of each of these physiological adaptations follows.

Heat acclimation results in a 10% to 12% increase in plasma volume (17, 67). This increased plasma volume maintains central blood volume, stroke volume, and sweating capacity, and allows the body to store more heat with a smaller temperature gain.

A key aspect of heat acclimation is an earlier onset of sweating and an increase in the sweat rate. An earlier onset of sweating simply means that sweating begins rapidly after the commencement of exercise; this translates into less heat storage at the beginning of exercise and a lower core temperature. In addition, heat acclimation can increase the sweating capacity almost threefold above the rate achievable prior to heat adaptation (59, 71). Therefore, much more evaporative cooling is possible, which is a major advantage in minimizing heat storage during prolonged work.

Moreover, sweat losses of sodium and chloride are lower following heat acclimation, due to an increased secretion of aldosterone (11). While this adaptation results in a reduction of electrolyte loss and aids in reducing electrolyte disturbances during exercise in the heat, it does not minimize the need to replace water loss, which is higher than normal (see chapters 23 and 24).

Moreover, research indicates that an important part of heat acclimation includes the cellular production of heat shock proteins in skeletal muscle fibers and all other cells of the body. Heat shock proteins are members of a large family of proteins called "stress proteins," which were introduced in chapter 2. As the name implies, these stress proteins are synthesized in response to stress (e.g., heat) and are designed to prevent cellular damage due to heat or other stresses. Details of how heat shock proteins protect cells against heat stress are found in Research Focus 12.2.

In summary, regular bouts of exercise in a hot environment results in the rapid development of heat acclimation that reaches maximal adaptation within 7–14 days. This adaptation results in a reduced heart rate during submaximal exercise in the heat, decreased body core temperature, decreased psychological rating of perceived exertion, and improved exercise performance in a hot environment (34). The days required to reach maximal heat acclimation for these various physiological measures are summarized in figure 12.12, and an illustration of the impact of heat acclimation on heart rate and core temperature during exercise in the heat is illustrated in figure 12.13.

Loss of Acclimation

The rate of decay of heat acclimation is rapid, with reductions in heat tolerance occurring within a few days of inactivity (i.e., no heat exposure) (32). In this

---

RESEARCH FOCUS 12.2

Heat Acclimation and Heat Shock Proteins

Repeated bouts of prolonged exercise in a warm or hot environment result in many physiological adaptations that minimize disturbances in homeostasis due to heat stress. Collectively, these adaptations improve exercise tolerance in hot environments and reduce the risk of heat injury. Evidence indicates that an important part of this adaptive process is the synthesis of heat shock proteins in numerous tissues, including skeletal muscle and the heart (42). Heat shock proteins represent a family of "stress" proteins that are synthesized in response to cellular stress (i.e., heat, acidosis, tissue injury, etc.). Although heat shock proteins perform a variety of cellular functions, it is clear that these proteins protect cells from thermal injury by stabilizing and refolding damaged proteins. Indeed, heat shock proteins play an important role in the development of thermotolerance and protect body cells from the heat loads associated with prolonged exercise (42).

Figure 12.13 Illustration of the impact of heat acclimation on heart rate and core temperature during constant load submaximal (50% V̇O₂ max) exercise in a hot environment.

regard, studies have shown that heat tolerance can decline significantly within seven days of no heat exposure, and complete loss of heat tolerance can occur following twenty-eight days of no heat exposure (2). Therefore, repeated exposure to heat is required to maintain heat acclimation (69).

IN SUMMARY

- During prolonged exercise in a moderate environment, core temperature will increase gradually above the normal resting value and will reach a plateau at approximately 30 to 45 minutes.
- During exercise in a hot/humid environment, core temperature does not reach a plateau, but will continue to rise. Long-term exercise in this type of environment increases the risk of heat injury.
- Heat acclimation results in (1) an increase in plasma volume, (2) an earlier onset of sweating during exercise, (3) a higher sweat rate, (4) a reduction in the amount of electrolytes lost in sweat, (5) a reduction in skin blood flow, and (6) increased levels of heat shock protein in tissues.

EXERCISE IN A COLD ENVIRONMENT

Exercise in a cold environment enhances an athlete's ability to lose heat and therefore greatly reduces the chance of heat injury. In general, the combination of metabolic heat production and warm clothing prevents the development of **hypothermia** (large decrease in core temperature) during short-term work on a cold day. However, exercise in the cold for extended periods of time (e.g., a long triathlon), or swimming in cold water, may overpower the body's ability to prevent heat loss, and hypothermia may result. In such cases, heat production during exercise is not able to keep pace with heat loss. This is particularly true during swimming in extremely cold water (e.g., <15° C). Severe hypothermia may result in a loss of judgment, which increases the risk of further cold injury.

Individuals with a high percentage of body fat have an advantage over lean individuals when it comes to cold tolerance (23, 49). Large amounts of subcutaneous fat provide an increased layer of insulation from the cold. This additional insulation reduces the rate of heat loss and therefore improves cold tolerance. For this reason, women generally tolerate mild cold exposure better than men (49).

Participation in sports activities in the cold may present several other types of problems for the athlete. For example, hands exposed to cold weather become numb due to the reduction in the rate of neural transmission and reduced blood flow due to vasoconstriction. This results in a loss of dexterity and affects such skills as throwing and catching. In addition, exposed flesh is susceptible to frostbite, which may present a serious medical condition. Further details of the effects of a cold environment on performance are presented in chapter 24.

Cold Acclimation

Three major physiological adaptations occur when humans are chronically exposed to cold temperatures (35, 36). First, cold adaptation results in a reduction in the mean skin temperature at which shivering begins. That is, people who are cold acclimated begin shivering at a lower skin temperature when compared to unacclimated individuals. The explanation for this finding is that cold-acclimatized people maintain heat production with less shivering by increasing nonshivering thermogenesis. This is achieved by an increase in the release of norepinephrine, which results in an increase in metabolic heat production (7, 22).

A second physiological adjustment that occurs due to cold acclimation is that cold-adjusted individuals can maintain a higher mean hand-and-foot temperature during cold exposure when compared to unacclimated persons. Cold acclimation apparently results in improved intermittent peripheral vasodilation to increase blood flow (and heat flow) to both the hands and feet (35, 36).

The third and final physiological adaptation to cold is the improved ability to sleep in cold environments. Unacclimated people who try to sleep in cold environments will often shiver so much that sleep is impossible. In contrast, cold-acclimatized individuals can sleep comfortably in cold environments due to their elevated level of nonshivering thermogenesis. The exact time course of complete cold acclimation is not clear. However, subjects placed in a cold chamber begin to show signs of cold acclimation after one week (50).

IN SUMMARY

- Exercise in a cold environment enhances an athlete's ability to lose heat and therefore greatly reduces the chance of heat injury.
- Cold acclimation results in three physiological adaptations: (1) improved ability to sleep in cold environments, (2) increased nonshivering thermogenesis, and (3) a higher intermittent blood flow to the hands and feet. The overall goal of these adaptations is to increase heat production and maintain core temperature, which will make the individual more comfortable during cold exposure.

STUDY QUESTIONS

1. Define the following terms: (1) *homeotherm*, (2) *hyperthermia*, and (3) *hypothermia*.
2. Why does a significant increase in core temperature represent a threat to life?
3. Explain the comment that the term *body temperature* is a misnomer.
4. How is body temperature measured during exercise?
5. Briefly discuss the role of the hypothalamus in temperature regulation. How do the anterior hypothalamus and posterior hypothalamus differ in function?
6. List and define the four mechanisms of heat loss. Which of these avenues plays the most important part during exercise in a hot/dry environment?
7. Discuss the two general categories of heat production in people.
8. What hormones are involved in biochemical heat production?
9. Briefly outline the thermal events that occur during prolonged exercise in a moderate environment. Include in your discussion information about changes in core temperature, skin blood flow, sweating, and skin temperature.
10. Calculate the amount of evaporation that must occur to remove 400 kcal of heat from the body.
11. How much heat would be removed from the skin if 520 ml of sweat evaporated during a 30-minute period?
12. List and discuss the physiological adaptations that occur during heat acclimation.
13. How might exercise in a cold environment affect dexterity in such skills as throwing and catching?
14. Discuss the physiological changes that occur in response to chronic exposure to cold.

SUGGESTED READINGS

Bergeron, M. et al. 2005. Youth football: Heat stress and injury risk. *Medicine and Science in Sports and Exercise* 37: 1421–30.

Blatteis, C. 2001. *Physiology and Pathophysiology of Temperature Regulation*. River Ridge, NJ: World Scientific.

Cheuvront, S. N., R. W. Kenefick, S. J. Montain, and M. N. Sawka. 2010. Mechanisms of aerobic performance impairment with heat stress and dehydration. *J Appl Physiol* 109: 1989–95.

Crandall, C. G., and J. Gonzalez-Alonso. 2010. Cardiovascular function in the heat-stressed human. *Acta Physiol (Oxf)* 199:407–23.

Lorenzo, S., J. R. Halliwill, M. N. Sawka, and C. T. Minson. 2010. Heat acclimation improves exercise performance. *J Appl Physiol* 109: 1140–47.

Maughan, R., S. Shirreffs, and P. Watson. 2007. Exercise, heat, hydration and the brain. *Journal of the American College of Nutrition* 26(5 Suppl):604S–612S.

Maughan, R. J., and S. M. Shirreffs. 2010. Dehydration and rehydration in competetive sport. *Scand J Med Sci Sports* 20 Suppl 3: 40–47.

REFERENCES

1. **Armstrong LE, Johnson EC, Casa DJ, Ganio MS, McDermott BP, Yamamoto LM, Lopez RM, and Emmanuel H.** The American football uniform: uncompensable heat stress and hyperthermic exhaustion. *J Athl Train* 45: 117–127, 2010.
2. **Armstrong LE, and Maresh CM.** The induction and decay of heat acclimatisation in trained athletes. *Sports Med* 12: 302–312, 1991.
3. **Åstrand P, and Rodahl K.** *Textbook of Work Physiology.* New York: McGraw-Hill, 1986.
4. **Bergeron MF, McKeag DB, Casa DJ, Clarkson PM, Dick RW, Eichner ER, Horswill CA, Luke AC, Mueller F, Munce TA, Roberts WO, and Rowland TW.** Youth football: heat stress and injury risk. *Med Sci Sports Exerc* 37: 1421–1430, 2005.

5. **Blatteis C.** *Physiology and Pathophysiology of Temperature Regulation.* River Ridge, NJ: World Scientific 2001.
6. **Brengelmann G.** Control of sweating and skin blood flow during exercise. In: *Problems with Temperature Regulation During Exercise*, edited by Nadel E. New York: Academic Press, 1977.
7. **Cabanac M.** Temperature regulation. *Annu Rev Physiol* 37: 415–439, 1975.
8. **Casa DJ, Armstrong LE, Hillman SK, Montain SJ, Reiff RV, Rich BS, Roberts WO, and Stone JA.** National athletic trainers' association position statement: fluid replacement for athletes. *J Athl Train* 35: 212–224, 2000.
9. **Casa DJ, Becker SM, Ganio MS, Brown CM, Yeargin SW, Roti MW, Siegler J, Blowers JA, Glaviano NR, Huggins RA, Armstrong LE, and Maresh CM.** Validity of devices that assess body temperature during outdoor exercise in the heat. *J Athl Train* 42: 333–342, 2007.
10. **Cheuvront SN, Kenefick RW, Montain SJ, and Sawka MN.** Mechanisms of aerobic performance impairment with heat stress and dehydration. *J Appl Physiol* 109: 1989–1995, 2010.
11. **Chinevere TD, Kenefick RW, Cheuvront SN, Lukaski HC, and Sawka MN.** Effect of heat acclimation on sweat minerals. *Med Sci Sports Exerc* 40: 886–891, 2008.
12. **Crandall CG, and Gonzalez-Alonso J.** Cardiovascular function in the heat-stressed human. *Acta Physiol (Oxf)* 199: 407–423, 2010.
13. **Dawson B.** Exercise training in sweat clothing in cool conditions to improve heat tolerance. *Sports Med* 17: 233–244, 1994.
14. **Delamarche P, Bittel J, Lacour JR, and Flandrois R.** Thermoregulation at rest and during exercise in prepubertal boys. *Eur J Appl Physiol Occup Physiol* 60: 436–440, 1990.
15. **Ely BR, Cheuvront SN, Kenefick RW, and Sawka MN.** Aerobic performance is degraded, despite modest hyperthermia, in hot environments. *Med Sci Sports Exerc* 42: 135–141, 2010.
16. **Fox S.** *Human Physiology.* New York: McGraw-Hill, 2010.
17. **Gisolfi C, and Cohen J.** Relationships among training, heat acclimation, and heat tolerance in men and women: the controversy revisited. *Medicine and Science in Sports* 11: 56–59, 1979.
18. **Gisolfi C, and Wenger C.** Temperature regulation during exercise: old concepts, new ideas. *Exerc Sport Sci Rev* 12: 339–372, 1984.
19. **Godek SF, Bartolozzi AR, and Godek JJ.** Sweat rate and fluid turnover in American football players compared with runners in a hot and humid environment. *Br J Sports Med* 39: 205–211; discussion 205–211, 2005.
20. **Gordon CJ.** *Temperature Regulation in Laboratory Rodents.* New York: Oxford Press, 2009.
21. **Hargreaves M.** Physiological limits to exercise performance in the heat. *J Sci Med Sport* 11: 66–71, 2008.
22. **Hong S, Rennie D, and Park Y.** Humans can acclimatize to cold: a lesson from Korean divers. *News in Physiological Sciences* 2: 79–82, 1987.
23. **Horvath SM.** Exercise in a cold environment. *Exerc Sport Sci Rev* 9: 221–263, 1981.
24. **Johnson EC, Ganio MS, Lee EC, Lopez RM, McDermott BP, Casa DJ, Maresh CM, and Armstrong LE.** Perceptual responses while wearing an American football uniform in the heat. *J Athl Train* 45: 107–116, 2010.
25. **Johnson JM.** Exercise and the cutaneous circulation. *Exerc Sport Sci Rev* 20: 59–97, 1992.
26. **Kenefick RW, Ely BR, Cheuvront SN, Palombo LJ, Goodman DA, and Sawka MN.** Prior heat stress: effect on subsequent 15-min time trial performance in the heat. *Med Sci Sports Exerc* 41: 1311–1316, 2009.
27. **Kenney WL.** Control of heat-induced cutaneous vasodilatation in relation to age. *Eur J Appl Physiol Occup Physiol* 57: 120–125, 1988.
28. **Kenney WL.** Thermoregulation at rest and during exercise in healthy older adults. *Exerc Sport Sci Rev* 25: 41–76, 1997.
29. **Kenney WL, and Johnson JM.** Control of skin blood flow during exercise. *Med Sci Sports Exerc* 24: 303–312, 1992.
30. **Kenney WL, and Munce TA.** Invited review: aging and human temperature regulation. *J Appl Physiol* 95: 2598–2603, 2003.
31. **Kruk B, Pekkarinen H, Manninen K, and Hanninen O.** Comparison in men of physiological responses to exercise of increasing intensity at low and moderate ambient temperatures. *Eur J Appl Physiol Occup Physiol* 62: 353–357, 1991.
32. **Lee SM, Williams WJ, and Schneider SM.** Role of skin blood flow and sweating rate in exercise thermoregulation after bed rest. *J Appl Physiol* 92: 2026–2034, 2002.
33. **Lim CL, Byrne C, and Lee JK.** Human thermoregulation and measurement of body temperature in exercise and clinical settings. *Ann Acad Med Singapore* 37: 347–353, 2008.
34. **Lorenzo S, Halliwill JR, Sawka MN, and Minson CT.** Heat acclimation improves exercise performance. *J Appl Physiol* 109: 1140–1147, 2010.
35. **Makinen TM.** Different types of cold adaptation in humans. *Front Biosci (Schol Ed)* 2: 1047–1067, 2010.
36. **Makinen TM.** Human cold exposure, adaptation, and performance in high latitude environments. *Am J Hum Biol* 19: 155–164, 2007.
37. **Maughan R, and Murray R.** *Sports Drinks: Basic Science and Practical Aspects.* Boca Raton: CRC Press, 2000.
38. **Maughan RJ.** Distance running in hot environments: a thermal challenge to the elite runner. *Scand J Med Sci Sports* 20 Suppl 3: 95–102, 2010.
39. **Maughan RJ, and Shirreffs SM.** Dehydration and rehydration in competitive sport. *Scand J Med Sci Sports* 20 Suppl 3: 40–47, 2010.
40. **Maughan RJ, Shirreffs SM, and Watson P.** Exercise, heat, hydration and the brain. *J Am Coll Nutr* 26: 604S–612S, 2007.
41. **McKenzie J, and Osgood D.** Validation of a new telemetric core temperature monitor. *Journal of Thermal Biology* 29: 605–611, 2004.
42. **Morton JP, Kayani AC, McArdle A, and Drust B.** The exercise-induced stress response of skeletal muscle, with specific emphasis on humans. *Sports Med* 39: 643–662, 2009.
43. **Nadel E.** Temperature regulation. In: *Sports Medicine and Physiology*, edited by Strauss R. Philadelphia: W. B. Saunders, 1979.
44. **Nadel E.** Temperature regulation during prolonged exercise. In: *Perspectives in Exercise Science and Sports Medicine: Prolonged Exercise*, edited by Lamb D, and Murray R. Indianapolis: Benchmark Press, 1988, p. 125–152.
45. **Nielsen B, Savard G, Richter EA, Hargreaves M, and Saltin B.** Muscle blood flow and muscle metabolism during exercise and heat stress. *J Appl Physiol* 69: 1040–1046, 1990.
46. **Nielson B.** Thermoregulation during exercise. *Acta Physiologica Scandinavica* 323 (Suppl.): 10–73, 1969.
47. **Nielson M.** Die regulation der korpertemperatur bei muskelarbeit. *Scandinavica Archives Physiology* 79: 193, 1938.
48. **Noble B.** *Physiology of Exercise and Sport.* St. Louis: C. V. Mosby, 1986.

49. **Nunneley SA.** Physiological responses of women to thermal stress: a review. *Med Sci Sports* 10: 250–255, 1978.

50. **Pandolf KB.** Effects of physical training and cardiorespiratory physical fitness on exercise-heat tolerance: recent observations. *Med Sci Sports* 11: 60–65, 1979.

51. **Pandolf KB.** Time course of heat acclimation and its decay. *Int J Sports Med* 19 Suppl 2: S157–160, 1998.

52. **Pandolf KB, Cadarette BS, Sawka MN, Young AJ, Francesconi RP, and Gonzalez RR.** Thermoregulatory responses of middle-aged and young men during dry-heat acclimation. *J Appl Physiol* 65: 65–71, 1988.

53. **Powers SK, Howley ET, and Cox R.** Blood lactate concentrations during submaximal work under differing environmental conditions. *J Sports Med Phys Fitness* 25: 84–89, 1985.

54. **Powers SK, Howley ET, and Cox R.** A differential catecholamine response during prolonged exercise and passive heating. *Med Sci Sports Exerc* 14: 435–439, 1982.

55. **Powers SK, Howley ET, and Cox R.** Ventilatory and metabolic reactions to heat stress during prolonged exercise. *J Sports Med Phys Fitness* 22: 32–36, 1982.

56. **Powers SK, and Jackson MJ.** Exercise-induced oxidative stress: cellular mechanisms and impact on muscle force production. *Physiol Rev* 88: 1243–1276, 2008.

57. **Rasch W, Samson P, Cote J, and Cabanac M.** Heat loss from the human head during exercise. *J Appl Physiol* 71: 590–595, 1991.

58. **Robinson S.** Temperature regulation in exercise. *Pediatrics* 32: Suppl 691–702, 1963.

59. **Sato F, Owen M, Matthes R, Sato K, and Gisolfi CV.** Functional and morphological changes in the eccrine sweat gland with heat acclimation. *J Appl Physiol* 69: 232–236, 1990.

60. **Shirreffs SM.** Hydration: special issues for playing football in warm and hot environments. *Scand J Med Sci Sports* 20 Suppl 3: 90–94, 2010.

61. **Shirreffs SM.** The importance of good hydration for work and exercise performance. *Nutr Rev* 63: S14–21, 2005.

62. **Shirreffs SM, Armstrong LE, and Cheuvront SN.** Fluid and electrolyte needs for preparation and recovery from training and competition. *J Sports Sci* 22: 57–63, 2004.

63. **Stolwijk JA, Saltin B, and Gagge AP.** Physiological factors associated with sweating during exercise. *Aerosp Med* 39: 1101–1105, 1968.

64. **Thomas CM, Pierzga JM, and Kenney WL.** Aerobic training and cutaneous vasodilation in young and older men. *J Appl Physiol* 86: 1676–1686, 1999.

65. **Tikuisis P, Bell DG, and Jacobs I.** Shivering onset, metabolic response, and convective heat transfer during cold air exposure. *J Appl Physiol* 70: 1996–2002, 1991.

66. **Wanner SP, Guimaraes JB, Rodrigues LO, Marubayashi U, Coimbra CC, and Lima NR.** Muscarinic cholinoceptors in the ventromedial hypothalamic nucleus facilitate tail heat loss during physical exercise. *Brain Res Bull* 73: 28–33, 2007.

67. **Wendt D, van Loon LJ, and Lichtenbelt WD.** Thermoregulation during exercise in the heat: strategies for maintaining health and performance. *Sports Med* 37: 669–682, 2007.

68. **Wenger CB.** Heat of evaporation of sweat: thermodynamic considerations. *J Appl Physiol* 32: 456–459, 1972.

69. **Williams CG, Wyndham CH, and Morrison JF.** Rate of loss of acclimatization in summer and winter. *J Appl Physiol* 22: 21–26, 1967.

70. **Wyndham CH.** The physiology of exercise under heat stress. *Annu Rev Physiol* 35: 193–220, 1973.

71. **Yanagimoto S, Aoki K, Horikawa N, Shibasaki M, Inoue Y, Nishiyasu T, and Kondo N.** Sweating response in physically trained men to sustained handgrip exercise in mildly hyperthermic conditions. *Acta Physiol Scand* 174: 31–39, 2002.

72. **Zuo L, Christofi FL, Wright VP, Liu CY, Merola AJ, Berliner LJ, and Clanton TL.** Intra- and extracellular measurement of reactive oxygen species produced during heat stress in diaphragm muscle. *Am J Physiol Cell Physiol* 279: C1058–1066, 2000.

13

The Physiology of Training: Effect on $\dot{V}O_2$ Max, Performance, Homeostasis, and Strength

■ Objectives

By studying this chapter, you should be able to do the following:

1. Explain the basic principles of training: overload, reversibility, and specificity.

2. Discuss the role that genetics plays in determining $\dot{V}O_2$ max.

3. Indicate the typical change in $\dot{V}O_2$ max with endurance-training programs and the effect of the initial (pretraining) value on the magnitude of the increase.

4. State typical $\dot{V}O_2$ max values for various sedentary, active, and athletic populations.

5. Understand the contribution of heart rate, stroke volume, and the a-$\bar{v}$ O_2 difference in determining $\dot{V}O_2$ max.

6. Discuss how training increases $\dot{V}O_2$ max.

7. Define preload, afterload, and contractility, and discuss the role of each in the increase in the maximal stroke volume that occurs with endurance training.

8. Describe the changes in muscle structure that are responsible for the increase in the maximal a-$\bar{v}$ O_2 difference with endurance training.

9. List and discuss the primary changes that occur in skeletal muscle as a result of endurance training.

10. Explain how endurance training improves acid-base balance during exercise.

11. Outline the "big picture" changes that occur in skeletal muscle as a result of exercise training and discuss the specificity of exercise training responses.

12. List the four primary signal transduction pathways in skeletal muscle.

13. List and define the function of six important secondary messengers in skeletal muscle.

14. Outline the signaling events that lead to endurance training-induced muscle adaptation.

15. Discuss how changes in "central command" and "peripheral feedback" following an endurance training program can lower the heart rate, ventilation, and catecholamine responses to a submaximal exercise bout.

16. Describe the underlying causes of the decrease in $\dot{V}O_2$ max that occurs with cessation of endurance training.

17. Contrast the role of neural adaptations with hypertrophy in the increase in strength that occurs with resistance training.

18. Identify the primary changes that occur in skeletal muscle fibers in response to resistance training.

19. Outline the signaling events that lead to resistance training-induced increases in muscle growth.

20. Discuss how detraining following strength training impacts muscle fiber size and strength. Explain how retraining impacts muscle fiber size and strength.

21. Explain why concurrent strength and endurance training can impair strength gains.

A theme throughout this book is that there are regulatory mechanisms (i.e., control systems) operating at rest and during exercise to maintain homeostasis. It is clear that participation in regular endurance exercise increases the cardiovascular system's ability to deliver blood to the working muscles and increases the muscle's capacity to produce ATP aerobically. These parallel changes result in less disruption of the internal environment during exercise. This, of course, leads to improved performance. Further, regular bouts of resistance exercise result in muscular adaptation that increases the muscle's ability to exert force and also improves performance in power events (e.g., weight lifting).

The purpose of this chapter is to discuss the physiological adaptations that occur in response to both endurance exercise training and resistance training. A major objective of this chapter is to tie together much of the physiology that has been presented previously, because most tissues and organ systems are either directly or indirectly affected by training programs. In the discussion of endurance training, we consider separately those physiological changes that promote an increase in $\dot{V}O_2$ max from those adaptations associated with improvements in prolonged submaximal performance. This is because $\dot{V}O_2$ max is closely linked to the maximal capacity of the cardiovascular system to deliver blood to the working muscles. The ability to sustain long-term, submaximal exercise is linked more to the maintenance of muscle fiber homeostasis due to specific biochemical properties of the working muscles.

This chapter also explores the physiology of strength development. Further, because endurance training causes adaptations in muscle that may conflict with those adaptations associated with strength training programs, we discuss the issue of whether concurrent resistance and endurance training results in a compromised increase in muscular strength compared to resistance training alone. Let's begin with an introduction to the principles of training.

PRINCIPLES OF TRAINING

The three principles of training are overload, specificity, and reversibility. These principles are introduced here and applied in chapters 16 and 17 (training for fitness), and in chapter 21 (training for performance).

Overload

The **overload** principle refers to the fact that a system (e.g., cardiovascular) or tissue (e.g., skeletal muscle) must be exercised at a level beyond which it is accustomed in order for a training effect to occur. The system or tissue gradually adapts to this overload. This pattern of progressively and systematically overloading a system or tissue as adaptations occur results in improved function over time. The typical variables that constitute the overload include the intensity, duration, and frequency (days per week) of exercise. The corollary of the overload principle is the principle of reversibility. The principle of **reversibility** indicates that the fitness gains by exercising at an overload are quickly lost when training is stopped and the overload is removed.

Specificity

The principle of **specificity** refers to the effect that exercise training is specific to the muscles involved in that activity, the fiber types recruited, the principal energy system involved (aerobic versus anaerobic), the velocity of contraction, and the type of muscle contraction (eccentric, concentric, or isometric). This may seem like an obvious statement in that one should not expect the arms to become trained during a ten-week jogging program. However, this also means that if an individual participates in a long, slow, distance running program that utilizes the slow-twitch muscle fibers, there is little or no training effect taking place in those fast-twitch fibers in the same muscle.

Specificity also refers to the types of adaptations occurring in muscle as a result of training. If a muscle is engaged in endurance types of exercise, the primary adaptations are in capillary and mitochondria number, which increase the capacity of the muscle to produce energy aerobically. If a muscle is engaged in heavy resistance training, the primary adaptation is an increase in the quantity of the contractile proteins; the mitochondrial and capillary densities may actually decrease (59).

IN SUMMARY

- The overload principle states that for a training effect to occur, a system or tissue must be challenged with an intensity, duration, or frequency of exercise to which it is unaccustomed. Over time the tissue or system adapts to this load. The reversibility principle is a corollary to the overload principle.
- The principle of specificity indicates that the training effect is limited to the muscle fibers involved in the activity. In addition, the muscle fiber adapts specifically to the type of activity: mitochondrial and capillary adaptations to endurance training, and contractile protein adaptations to resistive weight training.

ENDURANCE TRAINING AND $\dot{V}O_2$ MAX

Maximal aerobic power, $\dot{V}O_2$ max, is a reproducible measure of the capacity of the cardiovascular system to deliver oxygenated blood to a large muscle mass involved in dynamic work (80). Chapter 4 introduced this concept, and chapters 9 and 10 showed how specific cardiovascular and pulmonary variables respond to graded exercise up to $\dot{V}O_2$ max. The following sections discuss the effect of endurance exercise programs on the increase in $\dot{V}O_2$ max and the physiological changes that are responsible for this increase.

Training Programs and Changes in $\dot{V}O_2$ Max

Endurance training programs that increase $\dot{V}O_2$ max involve dynamic exercise using a large muscle mass (e.g., running, cycling, or swimming) for 20–60 minutes per session, three to five times per week at an intensity between 50% to 85% $\dot{V}O_2$ max (3). Details about how to design a training program for the average individual and the athlete are presented in chapters 16 and 21, respectively. While endurance training programs of 2 to 3 months' duration typically cause an increase in $\dot{V}O_2$ max between 15–20%, the range of improvement can be as low as 2% to 3% for those who start the program with high $\dot{V}O_2$ max values (23), and as high as 50% for individuals with low initial $\dot{V}O_2$ max values (23, 29, 41, 80, 84). In addition, individuals with a low $\dot{V}O_2$ max prior to training can experience improvements with relatively low training intensities (e.g., 40–50% $\dot{V}O_2$ max), whereas individuals with high $\dot{V}O_2$ max values may require higher training intensities (e.g., >70% $\dot{V}O_2$ max) (66).

Relative $\dot{V}O_2$ max (i.e., normalized to body weight) can vary widely in adults depending upon their health and training status. For example, $\dot{V}O_2$ max can be less than 20 ml · kg^{-1} · min^{-1} in patients with severe cardiovascular and pulmonary disease, and more than 80 ml · kg^{-1} · min^{-1} in world-class distance runners and cross-country skiers (table 13.1). The extremely high $\dot{V}O_2$ max values possessed by elite male and female endurance athletes are likely the genetic gift of a large cardiovascular capacity and high percentage of slow muscle fibers (5). Early work by Klissouras et al. (53) suggested that 93% of the variation in $\dot{V}O_2$ max values in the general population was due to genetics. However, more recent work has questioned this conclusion, and it is now accepted that heritability of $\dot{V}O_2$ max in the untrained state is approximately 50% (13). Nonetheless, it remains clear that a genetic predisposition for possessing a high $\dot{V}O_2$ max is still a prerequisite to become an elite endurance athlete with a large $\dot{V}O_2$ max.

Research indicates that the response of the individual to the effect of a training program is also genetically determined (14). For example, following a standardized training program, there is a wide variation in the level of $\dot{V}O_2$ max improvement among individuals (12). It is currently believed that the heritability of training gains in $\dot{V}O_2$ max is approximately 47% (14). Evidence points to differences in mitochondrial DNA as being important in both the individual differences in initial (i.e., untrained) $\dot{V}O_2$ max and the training-induced improvements in $\dot{V}O_2$ max (14). See A Closer Look 13.1 for more information on this topic.

In addition to genetic factors, both the intensity and duration of endurance training have an important impact on the magnitude in training-induced changes in $\dot{V}O_2$ max. For example, prolonged periods of endurance training (i.e., 2 to 3 years) can produce large improvements (e.g., 40–50% increases) in $\dot{V}O_2$ max (29). Also, high-intensity endurance training can also increase $\dot{V}O_2$ max by as much as 50% (14, 41). For example, one high-intensity study revealed a large (e.g. 30–50% improvement) and linear increase in $\dot{V}O_2$ max over 10 weeks of training (41). These results are in contrast with many training studies that show a leveling off of the $\dot{V}O_2$ max values after only a few weeks of training. The much larger increase in $\dot{V}O_2$ max with this 10-week training program was due to a higher intensity, frequency, and duration of training than are commonly employed in endurance exercise programs. We next discuss the physiological adaptations that are responsible for endurance training-induced improvements in $\dot{V}O_2$ max.

TABLE 13.1	$\dot{V}O_2$ Max Values Measured in Healthy and Diseased Populations	
Population	Males	Females
Healthy		
Cross-country skiers	84	72
Distance runners	83	62
Sedentary: young	45	38
Sedentary: middle-aged adults	35	30
Diseased		
Post-myocardial infarction patients	22	18
Severe pulmonary disease patients	13	13

Values are expressed in ml · kg^{-1} · min^{-1}.

Taken from Saltin and Åstrand (102), Åtrand and Rodahl (5), and Howley and Franks (58).

IN SUMMARY

- Endurance training programs that increase $\dot{V}O_2$ max involve a large muscle mass in dynamic activity for 20 to 60 minutes per session, three to five times per week, at an intensity of 50% to 85% $\dot{V}O_2$ max.
- Although $\dot{V}O_2$ max increases an average of about 15–20% as a result of an endurance training program, the largest increases are associated with deconditioned or patient populations having very low pretraining $\dot{V}O_2$ max values.
- Genetic predisposition accounts for about 50% of one's $\dot{V}O_2$ max value. Very strenuous and/or prolonged endurance training can increase $\dot{V}O_2$ max in normal sedentary individuals by up to 50%.

The HERITAGE Family Study

The HERITAGE Family Study was designed "to study the role of the genotype in cardiovascular, metabolic, and hormonal responses to aerobic exercise training and the contribution of regular exercise to changes in several cardiovascular disease and diabetes risk factors." Two-generational families of Caucasian and African American descent were recruited for the study. Although this is an ongoing investigation, many of the findings have been reported in the literature, and some of the key outcomes relative to the role of genotype on $\dot{V}O_2$ max are highlighted below.

1. The maximum heritability estimate for $\dot{V}O_2$ max among sedentary adults is approximately 50% (13).

2. The authors found considerable variation in the changes in $\dot{V}O_2$ max to a carefully controlled, 20-week endurance exercise program, even though the average improvement in $\dot{V}O_2$ max was 15–20%. At one extreme, some subjects showed little or no improvement in $\dot{V}O_2$ max in response to exercise training, while at the other extreme, some subjects experienced an improvement in $\dot{V}O_2$ max of about 50%. This large difference in the training response among families indicated the presence of a genetic factor in the training response.

Using these results, the investigators estimate that the maximal heritability of exercise-induced improvements in $\dot{V}O_2$ max due to training is 47%, with a substantial part of that due to maternal transmission (11).

3. A recent HERITAGE Family study has revealed that the large variation in human adaptive capacity to endurance training is due to a group of twenty-one different genes that play important roles in training adaptation (14). Given the focus on the human genome as it relates to health and disease, we are sure to hear more on this topic in the near future.

WHY DOES EXERCISE TRAINING IMPROVE $\dot{V}O_2$ MAX?

Because maximal oxygen uptake is the product of systemic blood flow (cardiac output) and systemic oxygen extraction (arteriovenous [a-$\bar{v}$] oxygen difference), training-induced changes in $\dot{V}O_2$ max must be due to an increase in maximal cardiac output or an increase in the a-$\bar{v}$ O_2 difference, or some combination of both. Details of this story follow. The calculation of oxygen consumption via the Fick equation is illustrated below:

$$\dot{V}O_2 \text{ max} = \text{Maximal cardiac output} \times (\text{maximal a-}\bar{v}\text{ }O_2\text{ difference})$$

Recall from chapter 9 that cardiac output is determined by the product of heart rate times stroke volume (i.e., amount of blood ejected per heart beat). Also, remember that the a-$\bar{v}$ O_2 difference is a measure of how much oxygen is removed from arterial blood and used by the tissues. Again, the Fick equation dictates that training-induced increases in $\dot{V}O_2$ max can be due to increased cardiac output, increased a-$\bar{v}$ O_2 difference, or an increase in both cardiac output and the a-$\bar{v}$ O_2 difference. Many studies indicate that endurance exercise training improves $\dot{V}O_2$ by both increasing maximal cardiac output and increasing the a-$\bar{v}$ O_2 difference. In this regard, endurance training studies using young sedentary subjects suggest that approximately half the gain of $\dot{V}O_2$ max is due to SV increases and half to increased oxygen extraction (i.e., increased a-$\bar{v}$ O_2 difference) (84). However, the size of the contribution of each factor in training-induced improvements in $\dot{V}O_2$ max varies as a function of training duration. This point is illustrated in table 13.2. Notice in table 13.2 that following 4 months of endurance training, the subjects increased their $\dot{V}O_2$ max by 26%. This training-induced increase in $\dot{V}O_2$ max was accompanied by a 10% increase in maximal cardiac output (due to increased stroke volume) and a 4% increase in the a-$\bar{v}$ O_2 difference. Therefore, although changes occurred in both cardiac output and the a-$\bar{v}$ O_2 difference, the exercise-mediated increase in maximal cardiac output made a larger contribution to the improvement in $\dot{V}O_2$ max. Increasing the duration of the training program provides a slightly different picture of how training causes an increase in $\dot{V}O_2$ max. In this case, an additional 28 months of endurance training resulted in a small additional increase (5%) in maximal cardiac output, but there was larger increase (20%) in the a-$\bar{v}$ O_2 difference (table 13.2). Also notice in table 13.2 that a training-induced increase in stroke volume was solely responsible for the exercise-induced increase in maximal cardiac output. What causes the maximal stroke volume and the maximal arteriovenous oxygen difference to increase as a result of endurance training? The answers are provided in the next two sections.

TABLE 13.2	Training-Induced Changes in Maximal Oxygen Uptake in a Healthy and Sedentary Young Adult				
	$\dot{V}O_2$ max (liters · min^{-1})	HR max (b · min^{-1})	Stroke Volume (ml · beat^{-1})	Cardiac Output (Liters · min^{-1})	a-$\bar{v}$ O_2 Difference (ml · liter^{-1})
Before training	3.07	205	122	23.9	126
4 months of training	3.87	205	134	26.2	131
32 months of training	4.36	185	151	27.6	158

From B. Ekblom, "Effect of Physical Training on Oxygen Transport System in Man," in *Acta Physiologica Scandinavica*. Supplement 328. Copyright © 1969 Blackwell Scientific Publications, Ltd., Oxford, England. Reprinted by permission.

Stroke Volume

As you recall from chapter 9, stroke volume is the amount of blood ejected from the heart with each beat and is equal to the difference between end diastolic volume (EDV) and end systolic volume (ESV). Note in table 13.2 that exercise training does not increase maximal heart rate and, in fact, months of training can often result in a small decrease in maximal heart rate. Therefore, all training-induced increases in maximal cardiac output must come from increases in stroke volume. Figure 13.1 summarizes the factors that can increase stroke volume. In brief, an increase in end diastolic volume (preload), increased cardiac contractility, or a decrease in total peripheral resistance (afterload) can increase stroke volume. Let's briefly discuss each of these factors relative to the increase in the maximal stroke volume that occurs with endurance training.

End Diastolic Volume (EDV) One of the key factors responsible for training-induced increases in maximal stroke volume is an increase in EDV. An increase in EDV results in stretch of the left ventricle and a corresponding increase in cardiac contractility via the Frank-Starling mechanism (chapter 9). This increase in EDV in the endurance-trained heart is likely a result of several training-induced changes.

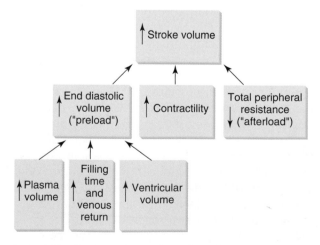

Figure 13.1   Factors increasing stroke volume.

A primary mechanism is that plasma volume increases with endurance training, and this contributes to augmented venous return and increased EDV. These training-induced changes in plasma volume and increased stroke volume changes can occur rapidly. For example, a 6-day training program (2 hr/day at 65% $\dot{V}O_2$ max) can promote a 7% increase in $\dot{V}O_2$ max, 11% increase in plasma volume, and a 10% increase in stroke volume. This training-induced increase in stroke volume is likely due to an increase in end diastolic volume (34).

Also, note that prolonged endurance training increases the size of the left ventricle with little change in ventricular wall thickness. This increase in ventricular size will accommodate a larger EDV and therefore could be a factor in contributing to the training-induced increase in stroke volume (28, 69, 79).

Finally, endurance training not only increases stroke volume during maximal exercise but also increases stroke volume at rest. The increase in resting stroke volume in endurance-trained athletes is likely due to the increased EDV at rest that results from increased stretch of the myocardium because of the increased ventricular filling time associated with the slower resting heart rate (**bradycardia**) that occurs following endurance training.

Cardiac Contractility Cardiac contractility refers to the strength of the cardiac muscle contraction when the fiber length (EDV), afterload (peripheral resistance), and heart rate remain constant. Although an acute exercise bout increases cardiac contractility due to the action of the sympathetic nervous system on the ventricle, it is difficult to determine whether the inherent contractility of the human heart changes with endurance training. This is because the factors that affect contractility (EDV, heart rate, and afterload) are themselves affected by endurance training (80). Nonetheless, animal studies indicate that high-intensity exercise training increases cardiac pumping ability by increasing the force of ventricular contraction (50, 51, 103). These findings imply that high-intensity exercise also improves ventricular contractility in humans (51).

Afterload The term *afterload* refers to the peripheral resistance against which the ventricle is contracting as it tries to push blood into the aorta. Afterload is important because when the heart contracts against a high peripheral resistance, stroke volume will be reduced (compared to a lower peripheral resistance). Following an endurance-training program, trained muscles offer less resistance to blood flow during maximal exercise due to a reduction in the sympathetic vasoconstrictor activity to the arterioles of the trained muscles. This decrease in resistance parallels the increase in maximal cardiac output so that mean arterial blood pressure during exercise remains unchanged.

Arteriovenous O_2 Difference

Again, endurance training-induced increases in $\dot{V}O_2$ are due to increases in both cardiac output (i.e., stroke volume increases) and the a-$\bar{v}$ O_2 difference. The training-induced increase in the a-$\bar{v}$ O_2 difference is due to increased O_2 extraction from the blood. The increased capacity of the muscle to extract O_2 following training is primarily due to the increase in capillary density, with an increase in mitochondrial number being of secondary importance (9, 42). The increase in capillary density in trained muscle accommodates the increase in muscle blood flow during maximal exercise, decreases the diffusion distance to the mitochondria, and slows the rate of blood flow to allow more time for oxygen diffusion from the capillary to the muscle fiber to occur. Changes in capillary density parallel changes in leg blood flow and $\dot{V}O_2$ max with training (80). The increases in mitochondrial number following endurance training increase the muscle fiber's ability to consume oxygen and also contribute to the expanded a-$\bar{v}$ O_2 differences. Note, however, the capacity of the mitochondria to use O_2 exceeds the capability of the heart to deliver O_2, making mitochondrial number not the key factor limiting $\dot{V}O_2$ max (9, 42, 80). Figure 13.2 provides a summary of the factors responsible for the increase in $\dot{V}O_2$ max associated with an endurance training program.

Finally, two individuals that have made major contributions to our understanding of the physiological effects of exercise training are John O. Holloszy and Bengt Saltin. See A Look Back—Important People in Science for more on these outstanding scientists.

IN SUMMARY

- In young sedentary subjects, approximately 50% of the increase in $\dot{V}O_2$ max due to training is related to an increase in maximal stroke volume (maximal heart rate remains the same), and 50% is due to an increase in the a-$\bar{v}$ O_2 difference.

Figure 13.2 Summary of factors causing an increase in $\dot{V}O_2$ max with endurance training.

- The training-induced increase in maximal stroke volume is due to both an increase in preload and a decrease in afterload.
  a. The increased preload is primarily due to an increase in end diastolic ventricular volume and the associated increase in plasma volume.
  b. The decreased afterload is due to a decrease in the arteriolar constriction in the trained muscles, increasing maximal muscle blood flow with no change in the mean arterial blood pressure.
- In young, sedentary subjects, 50% of the increase in $\dot{V}O_2$ max is due to an increase in the systemic a-$\bar{v}$ O_2 difference. The increased a-$\bar{v}$ O_2 difference is due to an increase in the capillary density of the trained muscles, which is needed to accept the increase in maximal muscle blood flow. The greater capillary density allows for a sufficiently slow red blood cell transit time through the muscle, providing enough time for oxygen diffusion, which is facilitated by the increase in the number of mitochondria.

ENDURANCE TRAINING: EFFECTS ON PERFORMANCE AND HOMEOSTASIS

The ability to perform prolonged, submaximal work is dependent on the maintenance of homeostasis during the activity. Endurance training results in a more rapid transition from rest to steady-state exercise, a reduced reliance on the limited liver and muscle

Dr. John O. Holloszy, M.D., and Dr. Bengt Saltin, M.D., Ph.D.—Olympic Prize Winners

The International Olympic Committee (IOC) established the IOC Olympic Prize in Sports Sciences to recognize international leaders in research in the sport sciences. The awardee receives $500,000 and an Olympic medal. The prize is awarded every two years.

In 2000, the International Olympic Committee awarded its IOC Prize in Sport Sciences to **Dr. John O. Holloszy.** He received his medical degree from Washington University School of Medicine in 1957. After serving in the United States Public Health Service, he returned to Washington University School of Medicine as a National Institutes of Health Research Fellow in 1963 and began his prolific career. The prize recognizes his outstanding contributions to our understanding of the effects of endurance training on muscle and metabolism, and how they affect endurance performance, heart disease, diabetes, and aging. That simple sentence cannot do justice to the more than 360 studies he has published in the very best research journals or the impact he has had on the broad areas of exercise science and preventive medicine. Throughout his career, Dr. Holloszy has trained several generations of scientists to follow in his footsteps. His list of postdoctoral fellows, beginning in the 1960s, reads like the who's who in exercise science; the research contributions of his postdoctoral fellows multiply many times over the effect Dr. Holloszy has had on the field of exercise science. Dr. Holloszy continues his active research career at Washington University School of Medicine in the areas of caloric restriction and aging and carbohydrate and fat metabolism.

In 2002. the International Olympic Committee awarded its IOC Prize in Sport Sciences to **Dr. Bengt Saltin,** Director of the Copenhagen Muscle Research Center in Denmark. He received his medical degree in 1962 and his Ph.D. in 1964, and held faculty positions at the Karolinska Institute in Stockholm and the August Krogh Institute in Copenhagen. Dr. Saltin has made major contributions to our understanding of maximal oxygen uptake; how genetics and exercise affect muscle; carbohydrate utilization during intense exercise; and based on his classic bed-rest studies, the importance of physical activity when recovering from accident or disease. Dr. Saltin's research has used unique experimental models to study the roles of the heart and skeletal muscle as factors limiting maximal aerobic power. His Knee Extensor Model allowed him to study a small muscle mass during exercise of various intensities through maximum levels and examine the factors limiting endurance exercise and the mechanisms of adaptations to training. It is clear that the impact of his research is felt throughout society, from the medical field to the elite athlete. He has published more than 400 research articles and many reviews and book chapters. He continues to perform research in Denmark at the Copenhagen Muscle Research Center.

---

glycogen stores, and numerous cardiovascular and thermoregulatory adaptations that assist in maintaining homeostasis. Many of these training-induced adaptations are due to structural and biochemical changes in muscle, and we will discuss those in detail in the next few pages. However, a portion of these adaptations is related to factors external to the muscle. This needs to be stated at the beginning of this section because, while we focus on the link between changes in skeletal muscle and performance, there is clear evidence that some improvements in performance occur rapidly and might precede structural or biochemical changes in skeletal muscle (36). This suggests that the initial metabolic adaptations to endurance training might consist of neural, or neural-hormonal-receptor, adaptations, which are followed by biochemical adaptations in muscle fibers.

In the introduction to this chapter, we mentioned that the increase in submaximal performance following an endurance training program was due more to biochemical and structural changes in the trained skeletal muscle than to an increase in $\dot{V}O_2$ max. The typical changes include increases in the percentage of slow muscle fibers, number of mitochondria in fibers,

added ability for muscle to metabolize fat, improved muscle antioxidant capacity, and increased capillary density (39). It is the changes in these characteristics of muscle that "drive" or determine the overall physiological responses to a given submaximal exercise bout. Let's begin our discussion with an overview of endurance training-induced changes in muscle fiber types and capillary number in skeletal muscle.

Endurance Training-Induced Changes in Fiber Type and Capillarity

It is well known that endurance training results in a shift in fast-to-slow muscle fiber type. Recall from chapter 8 that this exercise-induced shift in muscle fiber type involves a reduction in the amount of fast myosin in the muscle and an increase in slow myosin isoforms. This is significant because slow myosin isoforms have lower myosin ATPase activity but are able to perform more work with less ATP utilization (i.e., more efficient). This fast-to-slow shift in myosin isoforms is physiologically important because it increases mechanical efficiency and therefore can potentially improve endurance performance.

The magnitude of this exercise-induced fiber type shift is dependent upon both the intensity and duration of training sessions along with the total years of endurance training. For example, the number of type I (slow) fibers in leg muscles of distance runners is correlated to the number of years of training. This suggests that the training-induced increase in the number of type I fibers is progressive and could possibly continue during several years of training. Note, however, that most human and animal training studies indicate that although endurance training promotes a fast-to-slow fiber shift in the active muscles, this shift does not result in a complete shift from fast fibers to slow fibers. Therefore, as mentioned earlier in the chapter, the extremely high aerobic capacity possessed by elite male and female endurance athletes is likely the genetic gift of a high percentage of slow muscle fibers.

Endurance training increases the capillary supply to skeletal muscle fibers of trained individuals. In fact, a strong correlation exists between a subject's $\dot{V}O_2$ max and the number of capillaries surrounding muscle fibers in the trained limbs. This exercise-induced capillarization in the skeletal muscle is advantageous because diffusion distances for oxygen and substrate delivery to muscle fibers is reduced. Similarly, the diffusion distance for the removal of metabolic waste from the fiber is also decreased.

Endurance Training Increases Mitochondrial Content in Skeletal Muscle Fibers

Two subpopulations of mitochondria exist in skeletal muscle. One population rests immediately beneath the sarcolemma (subsarcolemmal mitochondria), and the second and larger group of mitochondria (i.e., 80% of total mitochondria) is dispersed around the contractile proteins (intermyofibrillar mitochondria). Endurance training can rapidly increase the density of both mitochondrial subpopulations in the active skeletal muscle fibers. For example, mitochondrial density can increase in muscle fibers within the first 5 days of a training program (102). Prolonged endurance training can typically increase muscle mitochondrial protein by 50–100% within the first 6 weeks of training (16). However, the magnitude of the exercise-induced increase in mitochondria in muscle is dependent upon both the exercise intensity and duration (see A Closer Look 13.2). The increased endurance performance that results from mitochondrial biogenesis is due to changes in muscle metabolism during exercise. Let's briefly examine some of these key changes.

At the onset of exercise, ATP is converted to ADP and P_i in the muscle fibers in order to develop tension. The increase in the ADP concentration in the cytoplasm is the immediate stimulus for ATP-producing systems to meet the ATP demands of the cross-bridges. Phosphocreatine responds immediately to this ATP need, followed by glycolysis, and finally mitochondrial oxidative phosphorylation. The latter process becomes the primary source of ATP during the steady-state phase of exercise. How does endurance training affect these oxygen uptake responses at the onset of submaximal steady-state work?

The steady-state $\dot{V}O_2$ measured during a submaximal work test is not affected by endurance training. The mitochondria are still consuming the same number of O_2 molecules per minute. What is different, due to the large increase in mitochondria, is how the ATP-producing chore is shared among the mitochondria. This point is illustrated in the following example. Suppose an untrained muscle cell has only one mitochondrion, and a breakdown of 100 units of ATP per minute is needed for the muscle to consume 2.0 liters of O_2 per minute to sustain a constant level of exercise. The breakdown of 100 units of ATP/minute results in the formation of 100 units of ADP/minute in the cytosol of the fiber (see figure 13.3). Remember that aerobic formation of ATP requires ADP to be transported into the mitochondria to be combined with P_i to form ATP. After training, when the number of mitochondria in the cell has doubled, the rate of ADP transportation into the mitochondria has also doubled. Therefore, the ADP concentration in the cytosol increases only half as much because of the additional mitochondria present to take up the ADP. This is important for two reasons.

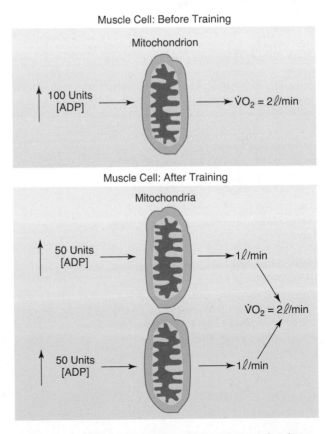

Figure 13.3 Influence of mitochondria number on the change in the ADP concentration needed to increase the $\dot{V}O_2$.

Chapter Thirteen The Physiology of Training **289**

First, the lower ADP concentration results in less phosphocreatine depletion because the reaction for this is $[ADP] + [PC] \rightarrow [ATP] + [C]$. Second, the lower ADP concentration in the cell also results in less stimulation of glycolysis and, therefore, a reduced production of lactate and H^+. Collectively, the reduced stimulation of glycolysis due to the lower ADP and higher PC concentrations following endurance training results in less reliance on anaerobic glycolysis to provide ATP at the onset of exercise (30, 37). The net result is a lower oxygen deficit, less depletion of phosphocreatine, and a reduction in lactate and H^+ formation. Figure 13.4 shows that the biochemical adaptations following endurance training result in a faster rise in the oxygen uptake curve at the onset of work, with less disruption of homeostasis.

Figure 13.4 Endurance training reduces the O_2 deficit at the onset of work.

A CLOSER LOOK 13.2

Role of Exercise Intensity and Duration on Mitochondrial Adaptations

A muscle fiber's oxidative capacity can improve only if the muscle fiber is recruited during the exercise session. Figures 13.5a and 13.5b show changes in citrate synthase (CS) activity, a marker of mitochondrial oxidative capacity, due to exercise programs differing in duration (30, 60, and 90 minutes) and intensity (~55%, ~65%, and ~75% $\dot{V}O_2$ max). Figure 13.5a shows that CS activity increased in the red gastrocnemius (primarily type IIa fibers) for all treatments, but the magnitude of the change was independent of the intensity and duration of the activity. In contrast, figure 13.5b shows that for the white gastrocnemius (primarily type IIx fibers), CS activity increased due to both intensity and duration of activity. Why the difference? The type IIa fibers were easily recruited by the lowest exercise intensity, while very strenuous exercise was required to recruit the type IIx fibers (75). These observations support our understanding of the specificity of exercise—light to moderate exercise will improve or maintain the oxidative capacity of high oxidative fibers (type I and type IIa), whereas strenuous exercise is needed to change low oxidative (type IIx) fibers (25, 96). Given the rapid loss of a muscle's oxidative capacity with cessation of training, it is no surprise that high-level endurance performances, which require the recruitment of type IIx fibers, fall off quickly when training ceases.

FIGURE 13.5 Changes in citrate synthase activity with different intensities and durations of exercise. Citrate synthase is a Krebs cycle enzyme that is measured as a marker of oxidative capacity in the muscle.

Biochemical Adaptations and Plasma Glucose Concentration

Plasma glucose is the primary fuel of the nervous system and, as described in chapter 5, the majority of hormonal changes associated with fasting or exercise are aimed at maintaining blood glucose levels. How do the biochemical changes in muscle that occur as a result of endurance training help maintain the blood glucose concentration during prolonged submaximal exercise? The answer is found in the increases in mitochondrial number and capillary density that occur with endurance training.

The increased number of mitochondria improves a muscle fiber's capacity to oxidize both carbohydrate and fat. However, the most dramatic change in muscle metabolism following training is a decrease in carbohydrate metabolism and an increase in fat utilization. This is due to an improved capacity to take up FFA from the circulation, an increased ability to transport FFA from the cytoplasm to the mitochondria of the muscle, and an increase in the fatty-acid (β-oxidation) cycle enzymes needed to degrade the FFA to acetyl-CoA units for the Krebs cycle (figure 13.6). Details of how training increases fat metabolism follows.

Transport of FFA into Muscle Intramuscular fat provides about 50% of the lipid oxidized during exercise, and plasma FFA provide the rest (45, 101). The uptake of FFA by muscle is proportional to the FFA concentration in the plasma (74). For FFA to enter the muscle fiber, plasma FFA must be transported across the cell membrane to the cytoplasm and then into the mitochondria before oxidation can occur. Movement of FFA into the muscle cell involves a carrier molecule whose capacity to transport FFA can become saturated at high plasma FFA concentrations (85). However, endurance training increases the capacity to transport FFA across the cell membrane so that a trained individual can transport more FFA at the same plasma FFA concentration, compared to an untrained individual (52). This is due to the dramatic training-induced increase in both fatty acid binding protein and fatty acid translocase (FAT) that transport the fatty acids from outside to inside the sarcolemma (48). This increased ability to transport FFA is facilitated by a greater capillary density in the trained muscle, which slows the rate of blood flow past the cell membrane, allowing more time for the FFA to be transported into the cell (85).

Transport of FFA from the Cytoplasm to the Mitochondria A key step in FFA transport into the mitochondria involves both carnitine palmitoyltransferase I (CPT-I) and fatty acid translocase (FAT). CPT-I and FAT work together to increase FFA entry into the mitochondria, and much of the training-induced

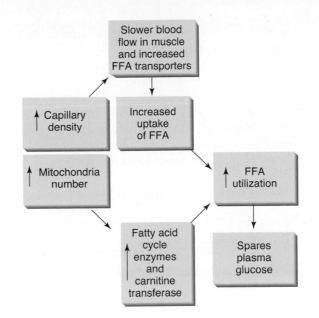

Figure 13.6 Increased mitochondria number and capillary density increase the rate of free-fatty-acid utilization, preserving plasma glucose.

increase in fat oxidation is linked to changes in mitochondrial FAT (87). The increase in the mitochondrial number with endurance training increases the surface area of the mitochondrial membranes and the amount of CPT-I and FAT such that FFA can be transported at a faster rate from the cytoplasm to the mitochondria for oxidation (86). The faster rate of transport from the cytoplasm to the mitochondria favors the movement of more FFA into the muscle cell from the plasma.

Mitochondrial Oxidation of FFA As mentioned previously, endurance training causes an increase in both types of mitochondria—subsarcolemmal and intermyofibrillar (54). These increases in mitochondria number increase the enzymes involved in fatty-acid beta-oxidation. This results in an increased rate at which acetylCoA molecules are formed from FFA for entry to the Krebs cycle, where citrate (the first molecule in the cycle) is formed. The high citrate level inhibits PFK activity in the cytoplasm and therefore reduces carbohydrate metabolism (42). The result of all these adaptations is an increase in lipid oxidation and less reliance on carbohydrate metabolism during exercise, thus preserving the limited liver glycogen store.

IN SUMMARY

- Endurance training improves the ability of muscle fibers to maintain homeostasis during prolonged exercise.
- Regular bouts of endurance training results in a fast-to-slow shift in muscle fiber types and also

increases the number of capillaries surrounding the trained muscle fibers.

- Endurance exercise also increases the number of both subsarcolemmal and intermyofibrillar mitochondria in the exercised muscles.
- The combination of the increase in the density of capillaries and the number of mitochondria per muscle fiber increases the capacity to transport FFA from the plasma → cytoplasm → mitochondria.
- The increase in the enzymes of the fatty acid cycle increases the rate of formation of acetyl-CoA from FFA for oxidation in the Krebs cycle. This increase in fat oxidation in endurance-trained muscle spares both muscle glycogen and plasma glucose. These points are summarized in figure 13.6.

Endurance Training Improves Muscle Antioxidant Capacity

Free radicals are chemical species or molecules that contain an unpaired electron in their outer orbital. Because of this unpaired electron, radicals are highly reactive and can interact with cellular components to promote damage to proteins, membranes, and DNA.

Therefore, it is not surprising that cells contain a network of molecules that neutralize radicals (i.e., antioxidants) and protect against radical-mediated injury. In general, these cellular antioxidants can be divided into two broad groups. The first set of antioxidants is produced within cells of the body (i.e., endogenous antioxidants), whereas the second group is derived from the diet (i.e., exogenous antioxidants). To provide maximum protection against radicals, these two antioxidants groups work as a team to neutralize radicals and maintain a healthy antioxidant/oxidant balance to prevent radical-mediated cellular damage.

Recall from chapter 8 that free radicals are produced during muscular contraction, and radical production can disturb cellular homeostasis, promote oxidative damage to muscle contractile proteins, and contribute to muscle fatigue during prolonged endurance events (77, 78). Nonetheless, endurance training can protect muscle fibers against free radical-mediated damage by increasing the levels of endogenous antioxidants in the trained muscles (77). This increase in muscle antioxidant capacity neutralizes free radicals produced during exercise and protects the fiber against free radical-mediated damage during exercise. This protection against exercise-induced oxidative damage can, in turn, protect against radical-mediated muscle fatigue.

Exercise Training Improves Acid-Base Balance During Exercise

The pH of blood is maintained near 7.40 ± 0.02 at rest. As described in chapter 11, acute and long-term challenges to the pH are met by intracellular buffers and responses of both the pulmonary and renal systems. There is evidence that muscle buffering capacity can be increased by performing high-intensity interval training (27). Although endurance training does not increase muscle buffering capacity, regular endurance training results in less disruption of the blood pH during submaximal work. How is this achieved? The answer relates to the fact that endurance-trained muscles produce less lactate and H^+. Here's the story:

Lactate formation occurs when there is an accumulation of NADH and pyruvate in the cytoplasm of the cell where lactate dehydrogenase (LDH) is present:

$$[pyruvate] + [NADH] \rightarrow [lactate] + [NAD]$$
$$LDH$$

Anything that affects the concentration of pyruvate, NADH, or the type of LDH in the cell will affect the rate of lactate formation. We have already seen that the increased number of mitochondria can have a dramatic effect on pyruvate formation: the lower ADP concentration stimulates PFK less at the onset of work, and the increased capacity to use fats reduces the need for carbohydrate oxidation during prolonged work. If less carbohydrate is used, less pyruvate is formed. In addition, the increase in mitochondria number increases the chance that pyruvate will be taken up by the mitochondria for oxidation in the Krebs cycle, rather than being converted to lactate in the cytoplasm. All of these adaptations favor a lower pyruvate concentration and a reduction in lactate formation.

Two additional biochemical changes in muscle occur due to endurance training that reduces lactate and, consequently, H^+ formation. The NADH produced during glycolysis can react with pyruvate, as shown in the previous equation, or it can be transported into the mitochondrion to be oxidized in the electron transport chain to form ATP (see chapter 3). Endurance training increases the number of "shuttles" used to transport NADH from the cytoplasm into the mitochondrion (42). If the NADH formed in glycolysis is more quickly transported to the mitochondria, there will be less lactate and H^+ formation. Last, endurance training causes a change in the type of LDH present in the muscle cell. This enzyme exists in five forms (isozymes): M_4, M_3H, M_2H_2, MH_3, and H_4. The H_4, or heart form of LDH, has a low affinity for the available pyruvate; therefore, the likelihood of lactate production is diminished. Endurance training shifts the LDH toward

Figure 13.7 Increased mitochondria number decreases lactate and H^+ formation to maintain the blood pH.

the H4 form, making lactate formation less likely and the uptake of pyruvate by the mitochondria more likely. Figure 13.7 summarizes the effects these biochemical changes have on lactate formation and the production of H^+ during submaximal work.

IN SUMMARY

- Endurance training increases endogenous antioxidants in trained muscles and these changes protect muscle fibers against free-radical mediated damage and fatigue during prolonged endurance exercise.
- High intensity (interval) exercise training can increase the buffering capacity of the exercised muscles.
- Endurance training does not increase muscle buffering capacity, but regular endurance training results in less disruption of the blood pH during submaximal work because endurance trained muscles produce less lactate and H^+.

MOLECULAR BASES OF EXERCISE TRAINING ADAPTATION

In the previous segments, we have discussed numerous biochemical changes that occur in skeletal muscle following weeks to months of endurance training. These cellular changes are initiated from an "exercise stimulus" within the active muscles and the end result is an increased synthesis of specific proteins within muscle fibers. This process of exercise-induced

adaptation in skeletal muscle fibers involves many signaling pathways that promote protein synthesis and the formation of new mitochondria (i.e., mitochondrial biogenesis). In the next sections, we present a brief overview of the signaling processes that contribute to exercise-induced muscle adaptation. We begin with a "big picture" view of exercise-induced muscle adaptation to training. This is followed by a brief introduction to both the primary and secondary signaling molecules that participate in muscle adaptation in response to endurance and resistance training. We then highlight the specific signals leading to muscle adaptation due to endurance exercise. Later, we discuss the signaling molecules responsible for muscle adaptation to resistance training.

Training Adaptation—Big Picture

Regardless of whether the training program is endurance exercise or resistance exercise, the exercise-induced adaptation that occurs in muscle fibers is the result of an increase in the amount of specific proteins (39). The process of exercise-induced synthesis of cellular proteins was first introduced in chapter 2. Recall that the "stress" of exercise stimulates cell signaling pathways in contracting muscle fibers that "switch on" transcriptional activators. These transcriptional activators are responsible for "turning on" specific genes to synthesize new proteins. This gene activation results in transcription of messenger RNA (mRNA) which contains the genetic information for a specific protein's amino acid sequence. The newly synthesized mRNA leaves the nucleus and travels to the ribosome where the mRNA message is translated into a specific protein. Remember that individual proteins differ in structure and function and that the specific types of proteins contained in a muscle fiber determine the muscle characteristics and its ability to perform specific types of exercise.

A single bout of endurance exercise is insufficient to produce large changes in proteins within a muscle fiber. Nonetheless, one exercise session promotes transient disturbances in cellular homeostasis that, when repeated over time, result in the specific exercise-induced adaptation associated with long-term training (16, 17). The "big picture" process of exercise-induced training adaptation is as follows. Muscle contraction during a training session generates a signal that promotes muscle adaptation by increasing primary and secondary messengers. These messengers initiate a cascade of coordinated signaling events, resulting in increased expression of specific genes and synthesis of specific proteins. In short, a bout of exercise generates a transient increase in the quantity of specific mRNAs, which typically peaks during the first four to eight hours post-exercise and returns to basal levels within 24 hours (figure 13.8a). Also, notice that mRNA levels for specific muscle proteins increase at different rates and peak at varying time periods following an exercise session. This exercise-induced increase in mRNA results in the increased synthesis of specific muscle proteins. Therefore, exercise repeated on a daily basis has a cumulative effect, leading to a progressive increase in specific muscle proteins that improve muscle function (figure 13.8b). This explains why maintaining a constant level of fitness requires regular bouts of exercise. Further, observe that the training-induced increases in muscle proteins is a gradual process, with large increases in muscle protein levels during the first weeks of training followed by a slower rate of protein accumulation as the training progresses (figure 13.8b).

Specificity of Exercise Training Responses

As we have seen, skeletal muscle is a very adaptable tissue that responds to exercise training by increasing the expression of multiple genes. The features of exercise-induced muscle adaptation are specific to the training volume, intensity, and frequency. That is, the specific adaptations that occur in skeletal muscle fibers result from the type of exercise stimulus (i.e., resistance vs. endurance exercise). Indeed, dissimilar modes of exercise promote the expression of different genes in the active muscle fibers. Specifically, resistance exercise and endurance exercise promote the activation of different cell signaling pathways; therefore, different genes are activated, resulting in the expression of diverse proteins. For example, prolonged endurance training results in a variety of metabolic adaptations (e.g., increased mitochondrial volume)

Figure 13.8 (a) An example illustrating of the rise and decline of mRNA for three different muscle proteins following an acute bout of exercise. (b) Illustration of the training-induced increase in three different muscle proteins during a 12-week training period.

with little change in muscle fiber size. In contrast, heavy resistance exercise results in increased synthesis of contractile proteins and muscle hypertrophy. Consistent with these different functional outcomes induced by these different exercise modes, the signaling pathways and molecular mechanisms responsible for these adaptations are distinct. In the next segment we introduce the general "primary" signaling pathways that produced exercise-induced training adaptations to both endurance and resistance exercise. This will be followed by a discussion of the secondary signals that are responsible for the increased protein synthesis following different types of exercise training.

Primary Signal Transduction Pathways in Skeletal Muscle

Our understanding of the precise mechanisms that enable skeletal muscle to interpret and respond to different types of exercise is currently incomplete. Nonetheless, several primary messengers participate in the exercise-induced adaptation that occurs in skeletal muscle. The four primary signals for muscle adaptation during exercise include muscle stretch, increases in cellular calcium, elevated free radicals, and decreases in muscle phosphate/energy levels.

Mechanical Stretch When muscles contract, the mechanical force placed on the muscle fiber can trigger signaling processes to promote adaptation. For example, passive stretching of a muscle fiber stimulates several biochemical signaling pathways, such as activation of protein kinases and insulin-like growth factor signaling cascades (44). The activation of these signaling pathways can then trigger secondary signaling pathways to turn on specific genes to express more protein. Therefore, the signaling events initiated by mechanical load with exercise can participate in the exercise-induced adaptation of muscle fibers. Importantly, it also appears that muscle fibers can sense differences in the intensity and duration of mechanical stimuli (i.e., resistance exercise vs. endurance exercise) to contribute to the specificity of exercise-induced adaptation (16).

Calcium Calcium is an important signaling mechanism in cells. Indeed, free calcium in the cytoplasm can activate numerous enzymes and proteins. For example, calcium can activate an important kinase called *calmodulin-dependent kinase*. Calmodulin-dependent kinase is one member of a family of enzymes that promote phosphorylation of various protein substrates. Once activated, calmodulin-dependent kinase can initiate a signaling cascade in muscle fibers that contributes to muscle adaptation to exercise training. How does exercise alter muscle calcium levels and control calcium signaling?

What is the source of intracellular calcium in muscle fibers? Remember from chapter 8 that neural activation of skeletal muscle contraction promotes calcium release from the sarcoplasmic reticulum, and stoppage of the neural stimulation initiates the re-uptake of this calcium from the cytosol back to the sarcoplasmic reticulum via active transport calcium pumps. The level of free calcium in the muscle cytosol is determined by the mode, intensity, and volume of exercise (16).

Free radicals It is clear that exercise results in the production of free radicals and other oxidants in active skeletal muscles (77). This is important because growing evidence indicates that radicals are important signals for muscle adaptation to exercise training (76, 78). For example, free radical production during exercise can activate nuclear factor kappa B (NFκB) and mitogen-activated kinase p38 (p38). NFκB is an important transcriptional activator that plays a key role in the expression of several muscle proteins, including antioxidant enzymes that protect muscle fibers against exercise-induced oxidative stress (77). p38 is an intracellular kinase that plays a key signaling role in production of new mitochondria.

Phosphate/Muscle Energy Levels Muscular exercise accelerates ATP consumption in the working muscle and increases the ratio of AMP/ATP in muscle fibers. Increasing the AMP/ATP ratio can initiate numerous downstream signaling events in skeletal muscle fibers (16). This exercise-induced change in cellular energy state has the potential to activate numerous signaling molecules, but one of the most important in exercise-induced muscle adaptation is activation of a secondary messenger called **5'adenosine monophosphate activated protein kinase (AMPK).** Indeed, AMPK is a key downstream signaling molecule that senses the energy state of the muscle and is activated by exercise. This important kinase regulates numerous muscle signaling processes and will be discussed in more detail in the next segment.

Secondary Messengers in Skeletal Muscle

Following the initiation of the primary signal, additional (secondary) signaling pathways are activated to mediate the exercise-induced signal to promote muscle adaptation. Indeed, numerous secondary-signaling pathways exist in skeletal muscle and are regulated at multiple levels. Next we will provide a "big-picture" overview of five secondary signaling pathways that play major roles in exercise-induced muscle adaptation. Specifically, we highlight the roles that AMPK, p38, peroxisome proliferator-activated receptor-gamma coactivator 1α (PGC-1α), calmodulin/calcineurin, insulin-like growth factor-1/Akt, and NFκB play in muscle adaptation to exercise training.

AMPK AMPK is an important signaling molecule that is activated during exercise due to changes in muscle fiber phosphate/energy levels. This key molecule regulates numerous energy-producing pathways in muscle by stimulating glucose uptake and fatty acid oxidation during exercise. AMPK is also linked to the control of muscle gene expression by activating transcription factors associated with fatty acid oxidation and mitochondrial biogenesis. Interestingly, AMPK can inhibit components of the IGF signaling pathway; the importance of this fact will be discussed later.

P38 Mitogen activated kinase p38 (**p38**) is an important signaling molecule that is activated in muscle fibers during endurance exercise. Although several cellular stresses can activate p38, it seems likely that exercise-induced production of free radicals is a major signal to activate p38 in muscle fibers. Once activated, p38 can contribute to mitochondrial biogenesis by activating PGC-1α.

PGC-1α This key molecule is activated by endurance exercise and is considered the master regulator of mitochondrial biogenesis in cells (72). Indeed, **PGC-1α** assists transcriptional activators that promote mitochondrial biogenesis in skeletal muscle following endurance training. Furthermore, PGC-1α regulates many other endurance exercise-mediated changes in skeletal muscle, including the formation of new capillaries (angiogenesis), a fast-to-slow muscle fiber type shift, and synthesis of antioxidant enzymes (72). PGC-1α also plays a role in exercise-induced increases in muscle's ability to metabolize fat and to take up glucose into the muscle fiber. Several factors activate PCG-1α during exercise, including AMPK and another cellular kinase, p38.

Calmodulin Calmodulin-dependent kinase (**CaMK**) is activated during exercise in an intensity-related manner (16). This vital kinase exerts influence on exercise-induced muscle adaptation by contributing to the activation of PCG-1α. The primary upstream signal to activate CaMK is increased cytosolic calcium levels.

Calciuneurin Calciuneurin is a phosphatase activated by increases in cytosolic calcium and participates in several adaptive responses in muscle, including fiber growth/regeneration and the fast-to-slow fiber type transition that occurs as a result of exercise training.

IGF-1/Akt/mTOR The **IGF-1/Akt/mTOR signaling pathway** plays a very important role in the regulation of muscle growth resulting from resistance training. Contractile activity (i.e., muscle stretch) stimulates the secretion of IGF-1 from the active muscle fibers. IGF-1 then acts as an autocrine/paracrine signaling molecule, binding to its membrane receptor and initiating a cascade of molecular events to promote muscle protein synthesis. Briefly, the binding of IGF-1 to its receptor on the muscle membrane activates the important signaling kinase, Akt. Active Akt then activates another downstream kinase called mammalian target of rapamycin (mTOR), which then initiates a series of molecular events to increase protein synthesis by improving translation.

NFκB As mentioned previously, **NFκB** is a transcriptional activator that can be activated by free radicals that are produced in contracting muscles. Active NFκB promotes the expression of several antioxidant enzymes that protect muscle fibers against free radical-mediated injury.

IN SUMMARY

- Independent of the type of exercise stimulus (i.e., endurance or resistance exercise) the training-induced adaptation that occurs in muscle fibers is the result of an increase in the amount of specific proteins.
- The exercise-induced adaptations in skeletal muscle fibers are specific to the type of exercise stimulus (i.e., resistance vs. endurance exercise).
- Exercise-induced muscle adaptation occurs due to the coordination between primary and secondary signaling pathways in muscle fibers.
- Four primary signals for exercise-induced muscle adaptation include muscle stretch, increases in cellular free calcium, elevated free radicals, and decreases in muscle phosphate/energy levels. These primary signals then activate downstream secondary signaling pathways to promote gene expression.
- Seven secondary signaling molecules that contribute to exercise-induced muscle adaptation include AMPK, PGC-1α, calmodulin/calcineurin, IGF-1/Akt/mTOR, p38, and NFκB. These signaling molecules are activated via one of four primary signaling pathways and act directly or indirectly to increase gene expression of specific muscle proteins.

SIGNALING EVENTS LEADING TO ENDURANCE TRAINING-INDUCED MUSCLE ADAPTATION

As we have discussed, endurance training can increase $\dot{V}O_2$ max by 20–50% and also improve performance in submaximal endurance events (39). This training-induced improvement is achieved by alterations at the cellular level in both cardiac and skeletal muscle fibers. In this section we highlight the major exercise-induced signaling events that promote molecular adaptations in skeletal muscle fibers following endurance exercise training.

Repeated muscle contractions during submaximal endurance exercise triggers a signaling cascade within the active muscle fibers leading to mitochondrial biogenesis, a shift in muscle fiber type from fast-to-slow,

Figure 13.9 Illustration of the intracellular signaling network mediated exercise-induced skeletal muscle responses to endurance exercise training. Take note that both primary and secondary signals are involved in muscle adaptation to endurance exercise training. See text for more details.

and increased expression of important antioxidant enzymes. As illustrated in figure 13.9, calcium release, increased AMP/ATP ratio, and production of free radicals are primary signaling events responsible for activation of the downstream, secondary signaling events (i.e., activation of AMPK, CaMK, p38, calcineurin, PGC-1α, and NFκB) that lead to mitochondrial biogenesis, fiber type transformation, and increased expression of antioxidant enzymes.

Note in figure 13.9 that contraction-induced increases in the AMP/ATP ratio activates AMPK in the muscle, whereas increased cellular levels of free calcium are required to activate both CaMK and calcineurin. Active calcineurin acts as a signaling molecule to promote fast-to-slow fiber type transformation. Further, notice that muscle contractions promote an increase in free radicals that serve as the primary signal to activate both p38 and NFκB. Activation of three secondary signals (AMPK, CaMK, and p38) all promote mitochondrial biogenesis by activation of the master regulator of mitochondrial biogenesis, PCG-1α. PCG-1α also contributes to the exercise-induced fast-to-slow fiber type transformation. Finally, note that activation of both PCG-1α and NFκB promote exercise-induced expression of important muscle antioxidant enzymes (76, 77).

IN SUMMARY

- Three primary signals involved in endurance exercise-induced muscle adaptation are increases in cellular free calcium, elevated free radicals, and decreases in muscle phosphate/energy levels. These primary signals then activate one or more of the downstream secondary signaling pathways to promote gene expression.

- Six secondary signaling molecules that contribute to endurance exercise-induced muscle adaptation include AMPK, PGC-1α, calmodulin/calcineurin, p38, and NFκB.

- Both active calcineurin and PGC-1α play important roles in endurance exercise-induced fast-to-slow fiber transformations.

- Collectively, active CaMK, AMPK, and p38 all participate in activation of PGC-1α. Active PGC-1α is the master regulator for mitochondrial biogenesis.

- Both active PGC-1α and NFκB contribute to the exercise-induced increase in muscle antioxidants.

ENDURANCE TRAINING: LINKS BETWEEN MUSCLE AND SYSTEMIC PHYSIOLOGY

The first portions of this chapter described the importance of the local changes occurring in endurance-trained muscle on the maintenance of homeostasis during prolonged submaximal work. However, these same changes are also related to the lower heart rate, ventilation, and catecholamine responses measured during submaximal work following an endurance training program. What is the link between the changes in muscle and the improved heart rate and ventilation responses to exercise?

The following endurance training study illustrates the importance of the trained muscle in the body's overall response to a submaximal work bout. In this study, each subject's left and right legs were tested separately on a cycle ergometer at a submaximal work rate prior to and during an endurance training program. Heart rate and ventilation were measured at the end of the submaximal exercise test, and a blood sample was obtained to monitor changes in lactate, epinephrine, and norepinephrine. During the study, each subject trained only one leg for thirteen endurance training sessions. At the end of each week of training, the subject was tested at the same submaximal work rate. Figure 13.10 shows that heart rate, ventilation, blood lactate, and plasma epinephrine and norepinephrine responses decreased throughout the study. At the end of this training program, the "untrained" leg was then trained for 5 consecutive days at the same submaximal work rate used for the "trained" leg. Physiological measurements were obtained during the exercise session on the first, third, and fifth days. Figure 13.10 shows that all the systems responded as if they had never been exposed to exercise training (15). Therefore, there was no transfer of the training effect from one leg to the other. This example shows that the heart rate, ventilation, and plasma catecholamine responses to prolonged submaximal exercise are determined, not by the specific adaptation of each organ or system, but by the training state of the specific muscle groups engaged in the exercise. How is this possible?

In chapter 10, the control of ventilation during exercise required a discussion of central and peripheral neural influences that could help explain the precise matching of ventilation to the increased oxygen demands of incremental exercise. This same approach will be taken here to explain how endurance training of specific muscle groups results in the decrease in cardiorespiratory and sympathetic nervous system responses to the same submaximal work rate. The output of the cardiovascular and respiratory control centers is influenced by input from higher brain centers, where the motor task originates, as well as from the muscles carrying out the task. A decrease in motor unit recruitment or a reduction in output from the receptors in the working muscles to the brain reduces these physiological responses to the work task. This issue is explained in detail in the next two sections.

Peripheral Feedback

The idea that reflexes in working muscles might control or "drive" cardiovascular or pulmonary systems in proportion to the metabolic rate originated in the early 1900s. Numerous muscle receptors respond to chemical changes in muscle, and these receptors can provide information to the central nervous system regarding muscle work rate. In particular, small-diameter nerve fibers (group III and group IV fibers) are responsive to tension, temperature, and chemical changes in muscle, and these nerve fibers increase their rate of firing in proportion to changes in muscle metabolic rate. Figure 13.11 illustrates how group III and group IV nerve fibers in skeletal muscle provide a peripheral feedback mechanism that contributes to the regulation of the cardiovascular and respiratory responses during exercise.

Central Command

The concept of central control of the physiological response to exercise is presented in figure 13.12. Higher brain centers (motor cortex, basal ganglia, cerebellum—see chapter 7) prepare to execute a motor task and send action potentials through lower brain centers and spinal nuclei to influence the cardiorespiratory and sympathetic nervous system responses to exercise. As more motor units are recruited to develop the greater tension needed to accomplish a work task, larger physiological responses are required to sustain the metabolic rate of the muscles (68, 80). For example, if some muscle fibers are prevented from contracting, additional muscle fibers must be recruited to maintain tension. This generates higher heart-rate responses to the work task (4). How are these peripheral and central controls related to the decreases in sympathetic nervous system activity, heart rate, and ventilation observed during submaximal exercise following an endurance training program?

The ability to perform a constant submaximal exercise bout for a prolonged period is dependent on the recruitment of a sufficient number of motor units to meet the tension (work) requirements to perform the exercise. Prior to endurance training, more mitochondria-poor motor units must be recruited to carry out a work task at a given $\dot{V}O_2$. This results in a greater "central" drive to the cardiorespiratory control centers, which causes higher sympathetic nervous system, heart rate, and ventilation responses. The feedback from chemoreceptors at the untrained muscle would

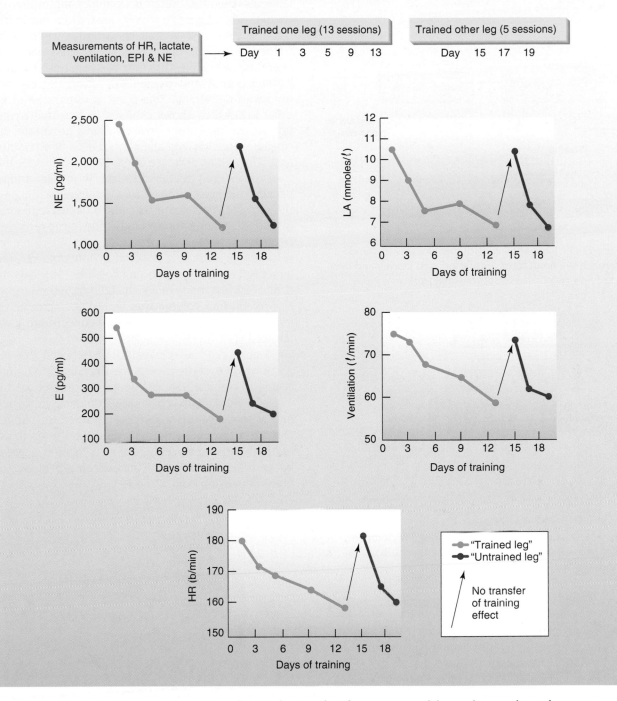

Figure 13.10 The lack of transfer of a training effect, indicating that the responses of the cardiovascular, pulmonary, and sympathetic nervous systems are more dependent on the trained state of the muscles involved in the activity than on some specific adaptation in those systems.

also stimulate the cardiorespiratory control center. With the increase in mitochondrial number following endurance training, the concentration of the local factors (H^+, adenosine compounds, etc.) that stimulate type III and IV afferent nerve fibers do not increase as much. This leads to less chemoreceptor input to the cardiorespiratory centers. In addition, the higher number of mitochondria allows the muscle tension to be maintained with fewer motor units involved in the activity. This reduced "feed forward" input from the higher brain centers and reduced "feedback" from the muscle results in lower sympathetic nervous system output, heart rate, and ventilation responses to exercise (68, 80, 81).

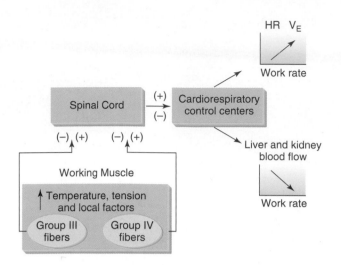

Figure 13.11 Peripheral control mechanisms in muscle influence the heart rate, ventilation, and kidney and liver blood flow responses to submaximal work.

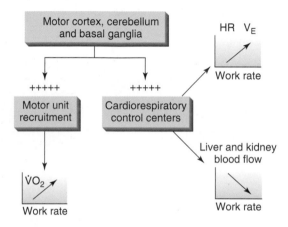

Figure 13.12 Central control of motor unit recruitment, heart rate, ventilation, and liver and kidney blood flow responses to submaximal work.

IN SUMMARY

■ The biochemical changes in muscle due to endurance training influence the heart rate and ventilatory responses to exercise.

■ The reduction in "feedback" from chemoreceptors in the trained muscle and a decreased need to recruit motor units to accomplish an exercise task results in reduced sympathetic nervous system, heart rate, and ventilation responses to submaximal exercise.

DETRAINING FOLLOWING ENDURANCE TRAINING

In the previous sections we discussed the effects of endurance training on both $\dot{V}O_2$ max and the cellular adaptations that occur in the trained muscle fibers.

Let's shift our attention from training adaptations and discuss what happens to $\dot{V}O_2$ max when endurance training ceases. It is well known that when highly trained individuals stop training, $\dot{V}O_2$ max decreases over time. Why? The answer is because both maximal cardiac output and oxygen extraction decline over time with detraining. This point is illustrated in figure 13.13, which shows changes in maximal oxygen uptake, cardiac output, stroke volume, heart rate, and oxygen extraction over an 84-day period of no training (21). The initial decrease (first 12 days) in $\dot{V}O_2$ max was due entirely to the decrease in stroke volume, because the heart rate and a-$\bar{v}$ O_2 difference remained the same or increased. This sudden decrease in maximal stroke volume appears to be due to the rapid loss of plasma volume with detraining (18). When plasma volume was artificially restored by infusion, $\dot{V}O_2$ max increased toward pre-detraining values (18). This was confirmed in a study in which a 200 to 300 ml expansion of plasma volume was shown to increase $\dot{V}O_2$ max, even though the hemoglobin concentration was reduced (19).

Figure 13.13 also reveals that between the 21st and 84th days of detraining, the decrease in $\dot{V}O_2$ max is due to the decrease in the a-$\bar{v}$ O_2 difference. This was associated with a decrease in muscle mitochondria, whereas capillary density remained unchanged. The overall oxidative capacity of skeletal muscle was reduced, with the percentage of type IIa fibers decreasing from 43% to 26% and the percentage of type IIx fibers increasing from 5% to 19% (20, 21).

Figure 13.13 Time course of changes in $\dot{V}O_2$ max and associated cardiovascular variables with detraining. From E. F. Coyle et al., 1984, "Time Course of Loss of Adaptation after Stopping Prolonged Intense Endurance Training" in *Journal of Applied Physiology*, 57:1857–64. Copyright © 1984 American Physiological Society, Bethesda, MD. Reprinted by permission.

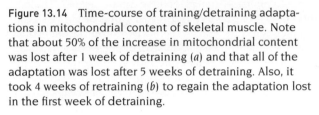

Figure 13.14 Time-course of training/detraining adaptations in mitochondrial content of skeletal muscle. Note that about 50% of the increase in mitochondrial content was lost after 1 week of detraining (*a*) and that all of the adaptation was lost after 5 weeks of detraining. Also, it took 4 weeks of retraining (*b*) to regain the adaptation lost in the first week of detraining.

Detraining not only decreases $\dot{V}O_2$, inactivity can also impact submaximal endurance performance. For example, it is a common experience for most individuals who do run, swim, or cycle training to notice that a break of only 14 days can negatively impact submaximal performance. This is due primarily to a decrease in muscle mitochondria (46, 63, 104). Indeed, muscle mitochondrial oxidative capacity undergoes rapid changes at both the onset and termination of exercise training. Figure 13.14 shows how quickly muscle mitochondria increase at the onset of training, doubling in about 5 weeks of training. However, only 1 week of detraining (shown by the letter "a") results in a loss of about 50% of what was gained during the 5 weeks of training (10, 90). Then 3 to 4 weeks of retraining were required to achieve the former levels (shown by the letter "b" in figure 13.14).

IN SUMMARY

- After stoppage of exercise training, $\dot{V}O_2$ max begins to decline quickly and can decrease by ~8% within 12 days after cessation of training, and decline by almost 20% following 84 days of detraining.
- The decrease in $\dot{V}O_2$ max with cessation of training is due to both a decrease in maximal stroke volume and a decrease in oxygen extraction, the reverse of what happens with training.
- Exercise performance during submaximal exercise tasks also declines rapidly following detraining, due primarily to a decline in the number of mitochondria in muscle fibers.

PHYSIOLOGICAL EFFECTS OF STRENGTH TRAINING

The basic principles of training related to improving strength have been around for thousands of years, and Morpurgo's observation that gains in strength were associated with increases in muscle size was made more than one hundred years ago (6). Despite this history, most recent research on the effects of training has focused on $\dot{V}O_2$ max and endurance performance, possibly because of their link to the prevention and treatment of heart disease. However, it is now recognized that resistance training has many health benefits and becomes even more important with advancing age. See A Closer Look 13.3 for background on why strength training is important as we age.

Before we begin, some terms and basic principles need to be introduced. Muscular strength refers to the maximal force that a muscle or muscle group can generate and is commonly expressed as the one-repetition maximum, or 1-RM, the maximum load that can be moved through a full range of motion. Muscular endurance refers to the ability to make repeated contractions against a submaximal load. Consistent with our earlier discussion of training and $\dot{V}O_2$ max, large individual differences exist in the response to strength-training programs, and the percent gain in strength is inversely related to the initial strength (55). These observations imply a genetic limitation to the gains that can be achieved with training, similar to those observed for training-induced increases in $\dot{V}O_2$ max. Finally, the basic principles of training, overload, and specificity apply here as well. For example, high-resistance training (8–12 reps/set) results primarily in gains in muscular strength; in contrast, low-resistance training (>20 reps/set) results in gains in muscular endurance, with less of a change in strength (55). What physiological changes occur with resistance training that result in improvements in muscular strength?

MECHANISMS RESPONSIBLE FOR RESISTANCE TRAINING-INDUCED INCREASES IN STRENGTH

Chapters 7 and 8 described the roles that motor unit recruitment, stimulus frequency, and synchronous firing of motor units play in the development of muscle tension, as well as the fact that type II motor units develop more tension than type I motor units. These factors are very much involved in the improvement of strength with training. That is, resistance training increases muscular strength by changes in both the

Aging, Strength, and Training

Aging is associated with a decline in strength, with most of the decline occurring after age fifty. The loss of strength is due, in part, to a loss of muscle mass (sarcopenia), which is related to the loss of both type I and II fibers, atrophy of existing type II fibers, and an increase in intramuscular fat and connective tissue (47). The loss of muscle fibers is a result of loss of their motor neurons, so whole motor units are lost with aging. In addition, the remaining type I or type II muscle fibers cluster in homogeneous groups, in contrast to the heterogeneous distribution of fiber types seen in a muscle cross-section from younger individuals (24, 47).

That is the bad news. The good news is that a progressive resistance-training

program causes muscle hypertrophy and very large gains in strength in older individuals, including those in their 90s (31, 32). Such strength training programs are important, not only for being able to carry out activities of daily living, but also for improved balance and reducing the risk of falls (43, 47).

Also, it is common for many older adults to use over-the-counter nonsteroidal anti-inflammatory drugs (e.g., ibuprofen and acetaminophen) to combat both arthritis and sore muscles. Both of these drugs inhibit the activity of cyclooxygenase, which is an enzyme that produces prostaglandins and is involved in inflammatory processes in cells. However, several animal studies suggest that these cyclooxygenase inhibitors can inter-

fere with resistance training-induced muscle hypertrophy (71, 89). These findings suggest that use of these drugs concurrently with strength training would be counterproductive. Nonetheless, two recent human studies have demonstrated that these commonly used pain killers do not impede strength gains in older people engaged in resistance exercise training (57, 99). In fact, one of these studies suggests that concurrent strength training and use of either ibuprofen or acetaminophen may actually enhance muscle hypertrophy and suggests that the cyclooxygenase pathways may be involved in the regulation of muscle protein content in humans (99). These findings are good news for older adults engaged in regular strength training.

nervous system and an increase in muscle mass. In the next two segments, we will discuss the roles both the nervous system and muscular growth play in the development of strength resulting from a resistance training program. Figure 13.15 provides a schematic to follow that will facilitate our discussion of both neural and muscular factors related to gains in strength (33, 82). In training studies of short duration

(8 to 20 weeks), neural adaptations related to learning, coordination, and the ability to recruit the primary muscles (i.e., prime movers) play a major role in the gain in strength. In contrast, in long-term training programs, an increase in muscle size plays the major role in strength development. Let's discuss these resistance training-induced changes in the nervous system and muscle in more detail.

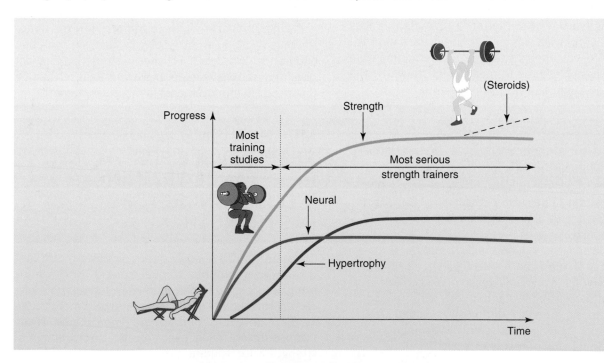

Figure 13.15   Relative roles of neural and muscular adaptations to resistance training.

Resistance Training-Induced Changes in the Nervous System

A significant portion of the gains in strength that occur with resistance training, especially early in a program, is due to neural adaptations and not an enlargement of muscle (82). This concept is illustrated in figure 13.15. Also, note that the neural adaptations to strength training are different from those that occur with endurance exercise training. Recall that figure 13.10 illustrated the point that when one leg was trained on a cycle ergometer, the endurance training effect did not "carry over" to the untrained leg. In contrast, when one arm is exposed to resistance training, a portion of the training effect is "transferred" to the other arm. In this case, the gain in strength in the trained arm was due to both muscle hypertrophy and an increased ability to activate motor units, whereas an improvement in the untrained arm was due solely to neural adaptation (82). Similar results have been reported in a study using a one-leg resistance-training model. In this study, one leg was exposed to resistance training and the gains of muscular strength and endurance of the trained leg were also partially realized in the untrained leg (49). These neural adaptations that occur in response to resistance training result in an improved ability to recruit motor units, alter motor neuron firing rates, enhance motor unit synchronization during a particular movement pattern, and result in the removal of neural inhibition (33, 82). Collectively, these changes result in an increase in muscle force production.

Resistance Training-Induced Increases in Skeletal Muscle Size

Recall from chapter 8 that the amount of force produced by a muscle is directly linked to the amount of actin and myosin within the muscle fibers. The explanation for this observation is that the more myosin cross-bridges that are attached to actin and engaged in the power stroke, the more force produced. This simple principle explains why larger muscles containing more actin and myosin generate more force than smaller muscles. In response to resistance training, skeletal muscles can increase their size by increasing the size of existing fibers (hypertrophy) or increasing their number of total fibers (hyperplasia) in the muscle. Let's discuss these two types of muscle growth separately.

Hyperplasia As mentioned previously, hyperplasia refers to an increase in the total number of muscle fibers within a specific muscle (e.g., biceps brachii). The question of whether resistance training-induced increases in muscle size is achieved by hyperplasia has been raised by animal studies indicating that resistance training can promote an increased number of fibers in the trained muscles (67, 93). However, whether resistance training promotes the generation of new muscle fibers in humans remains controversial as studies that both support (64) and deny this concept exist in the literature (61). Nonetheless, even if hyperplasia does occur in humans, current evidence indicates that most (90–95%) of the increase in muscle size following resistance training occurs due to an increase in muscle fiber size (hypertrophy) and not hyperplasia (22, 33).

Hypertrophy As discussed previously, an increase in muscle fiber cross-sectional area (fiber hypertrophy) is regarded as the primary means to increase muscle size during long-term strength training (33). In general, the resistance training-induced increase in muscle fiber size is a gradual process that occurs during months to years of training. However, there is evidence that with high-intensity resistance training, changes in muscle size are detectable by 3 weeks (~10 sessions) of training (88). Further, although resistance training increases the size of both type I and II fibers, weight training elicits a greater degree of hypertrophy in type II fibers (55, 97). This is physiologically significant because type II fibers generate a greater specific force (i.e., force per cross-sectional area) than type I fibers. The mechanisms to explain why type II fibers are more prone to hypertrophy than type I fibers remains unclear, and additional research is needed to resolve this issue.

This resistance training-induced increase in fiber cross-sectional area results from an increase in myofibrillar proteins (i.e., actin and myosin). This increase in actin/myosin filaments in the fiber occurs due to the addition of sarcomeres in parallel to the existing sarcomeres, resulting in muscle fiber hypertrophy (33). The addition of additional contractile proteins increases the number of myosin cross-bridges in the fiber and therefore increases the fiber's ability to generate force.

Resistance Training-Induced Changes in Muscle Fiber Type

Similar to endurance training, prolonged periods of resistance training have also been shown to promote a fast-to-slow shift in muscle fiber types within the trained muscles (91, 92). However, strength training-induced shifts in muscle fiber types appear to be less prominent than endurance training-induced transformations because all of the change in fiber type is a movement from type IIx to type IIa, with no increase in the percentage of type I fibers. For example, it has been reported that 20 weeks of resistance training can decrease the percentage of type IIx fibers by 5–11%, with a corresponding rise in type IIa fibers in the trained muscles (92). At present, there are no long-term (i.e., several years) resistance-training studies, so it is unknown if this type IIx to IIa fiber transformation will continue over a prolonged period.

Can Resistance Training Improve Muscle Oxidative Capacity and Increase Capillary Number?

As discussed earlier in this chapter, endurance exercise training increases the oxidative capacity (i.e., mitochondrial number increases) and the antioxidant capacity in the exercised muscle fibers. Endurance training also promotes the formation of new capillaries and therefore increases muscle capillarization. Does resistance training also promote these changes in the trained muscle? The answer to this question remains unclear because longitudinal investigations of the effect of resistance training on muscle oxidative capacity have been inconsistent with studies reporting that resistance training decreases mitochondrial content in muscle (62); other studies indicate no change in muscle oxidative capacity (98), and still other investigations conclude that resistance training can promote small increases in muscle oxidative capacity (94). Similarly, investigations about the effect of resistance training on muscle capillarization have failed to provide consistent results, with some studies reporting no formation of new capillaries with training and other reports indicating that strength training can promote small increases in capillary number. What is the explanation for these divergent results? Numerous factors could explain these divergent findings, including the frequency of training, the duration of training, and the number of repetitions performed during training. In fact, studies that incorporated long-duration resistance training programs and high frequencies of training (three days/week) and high volume (i.e., high number of repetitions) of exercise reported small improvements in muscle oxidative capacity and capillarization. Therefore, it appears that whether resistance training improves muscle oxidative properties is dependent upon the duration of the training period and the volume of exercise performed.

Resistance Training Improves Muscle Antioxidant Enzyme Activity

Although limited evidence exists, it appears that resistance exercise training can improve muscle antioxidant capacity. Indeed, a recent study investigated the effects of 12 weeks of strength training on the activities of key antioxidant enzymes in the trained muscles. The results revealed that resistance training increased the activities of two important muscle antioxidant enzymes by almost 100 percent (73). The potential long-term benefits of these adaptations remain unclear. Nonetheless, similar to endurance exercise, resistance exercise training improves the muscle's antioxidant capacity, which should provide cellular protection against the oxidative damage associated with exercise-induced production of free radicals.

IN SUMMARY

- Increases in strength due to short-term (8 to 20 weeks) resistance training are largely the result of changes in the nervous system, whereas gains in strength during long-term training programs are due to an increase in the size of the muscle.
- Current evidence suggests that hyperplasia may occur in humans. Nonetheless, most (90–95%) of the increase in muscle size following resistance training occurs due to an increase in muscle hypertrophy and not hyperplasia.
- Prolonged periods of resistance training can promote a fast-to-slow shift in muscle fiber types. Most of this training-induced fiber shift is the conversion of type IIx to type IIa fibers, with no increase in the number of type I fibers.
- Whether resistance training improves muscle oxidative properties remains controversial. However, it is possible that long-term and high-volume resistance training programs can improve muscle oxidative capacity and increase capillary number around the trained fibers.
- Resistance training improves the antioxidant capacity of the trained muscle fibers.

SIGNALING EVENTS LEADING TO RESISTANCE TRAINING-INDUCED MUSCLE GROWTH

An increase in muscle fiber size (hypertrophy) occurs when the rate of protein synthesis in muscle fibers is greater than the rate of protein breakdown. In general, resistance training-induced muscular hypertrophy is a slow process because protein synthesis must exceed breakdown for several weeks to achieve significant muscle growth. However, a single bout of resistance exercise can elevate the rate of muscle protein synthesis for up to 24 hours. For example, one resistance-training session can increase the rate of muscle protein synthesis by 50% at 4 hours post-exercise and by 100% at 24 hours after the exercise bout (60, 95). Obviously, this exercise-induced increase in muscle protein synthesis is not permanent, and muscle protein synthesis returns to resting levels by 36 hours after exercise (60, 95). These changes in protein synthesis are primarily due to an increase in the amount of protein synthesized per molecule of

Resistance Training

Muscle stretch ↑ — **Primary Signal**

IGF-1 ↑

Akt ↑ — **Secondary Signals**

mTOR ↑

Protein synthesis

Muscle Fiber

Muscle hypertrophy

Figure 13.16 Illustration of the intracellular signaling network mediating exercise-induced skeletal muscle responses to resistance training. Notice that both primary and secondary signals are involved in muscle adaptation to resistance exercise training. See text for more details.

mRNA rather than simply an increase in total mRNA (39). Therefore, resistance exercise promotes muscle protein synthesis, in part, by improving translational efficiency.

What are the molecular signals to stimulate muscle protein synthesis following resistance exercise? The intracellular signaling pathway that regulates protein synthesis is illustrated in figure 13.16. Notice that the primary signal for resistance exercise-induced protein synthesis is the mechanical stretch (i.e., force) applied to the muscle during weight lifting. This resistance exercise-induced mechanical stretch then triggers the secondary signal of IGF-1 synthesis and the cascade of downstream signaling events leading to increased protein synthesis. In brief, the resistance training-induced synthesis of IGF-1 results in the activation of the important signaling molecule Akt. Following activation, active Akt then activates another downstream signaling molecule, mTOR, which promotes protein synthesis by increasing translation and building more proteins (39). Further, it is important to appreciate that resistance training-induced increased protein synthesis requires that all essential amino acids be present in the muscle in order for protein synthesis to occur. Therefore, adequate ingestion of protein prior to or following a workout is essential to optimize muscle growth during resistance training (see Phillips (2009) in the Suggested Readings for more details).

Finally, as muscle fibers increase in size in response to resistance training, these growing fibers add new nuclei (myonuclei) within the fiber. This pro-

cess is illustrated in figure 13.17. Recall from chapter 8 that the source of these additional myonuclei is the satellite cell, which is a type of adult stem cell located between the sarcolemma and the outer layer of connective tissue (i.e., basal lamina) around the fiber (8). Resistance training activates satellite cells to divide and fuse with the adjacent muscle fiber to increase the number of nuclei in the fiber (1). This increase in the number of myonuclei in growing fibers results in a constant ratio between the number of myonuclei and the size of the fiber. Importantly, the addition of these myonuclei to a growing fiber appear to be a requirement to support the increased size and

Muscle fibers

Myonucleus

Hypertrophy

Resistance training

Myonuclear Addition
Myofibrillar proteins ↑
Myofiber CSA ↑

Figure 13.17 Resistance training-induced fiber hypertrophy results in a parallel increase in myonuclei, myofibrillar proteins, and fiber cross-sectional area (CSA).

continued growth of muscle fibers in response to strength training. In fact, evidence indicates that removal of satellite cells from skeletal muscle limits the fibers' ability to grow in response to overload (1, 2). Why are additional myonuclei required to achieve the maximal level of muscle hypertrophy in response to resistance training? A potential explanation is that the addition of myonuclei to growing muscle fibers is a requirement to maintain the high level of translational capacity required to synthesize muscle proteins at a high rate following a strength-training session (1). That is, it appears that a single myonucleus can only manage a specific volume of muscle area; therefore, as the muscle fiber increases in size, the addition of new myonuclei is required to manage the new growth. To conclude, satellite cells are the source for additional nuclei in muscle fibers, and the addition of myonuclei to growing fibers is essential to optimize fiber hypertrophy in response to resistance training (2).

IN SUMMARY

- Resistance training increases the synthesis of contractile proteins in muscle; this results in an increase in the cross-sectional area of the fiber.
- Resistance training-induced increases in protein synthesis occur via an increase in translation, which is controlled by the IGF-1/Akt/mTOR signaling pathway.
- Resistance training results in parallel increases in muscle fiber cross-sectional area and increased numbers of myonuclei.
- Satellite cells are the source for additional nuclei in muscle fibers, and the supplement of myonuclei to muscle fibers is required to achieve maximal fiber hypertrophy in response to resistance training.

DETRAINING FOLLOWING STRENGTH TRAINING

Similar to detraining following endurance training, the "use it or lose it" adage also applies to a resistance training program. Indeed, it is well established that stoppage of resistance training results in a loss of muscular strength and in muscle atrophy. However, compared to endurance training, the rate of detraining (i.e., loss of strength) after a resistance training program is slower. This point is illustrated in figure 13.18a. Specifically, figure 13.18a illustrates the impact of 30 weeks of detraining on muscle strength and muscle fiber size and also shows the impact of 6 weeks of retraining after the prolonged period of detraining (91). In this study, subjects engaged in a 20-week program of resistance training. This rigorous

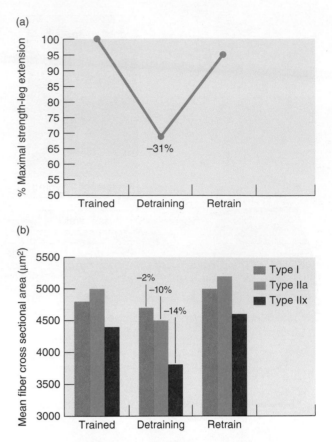

Figure 13.18 (a) Changes in dynamic muscle strength following 30 weeks of detraining and at the completion of 6 weeks of resistance exercise retraining. (b) Changes in muscle fiber cross-sectional area following 30 weeks of detraining followed by 6 weeks of resistance exercise retraining.

training program resulted in a 60% increase in maximal dynamic strength (leg extension) and hypertrophy in all three major fiber types in the extensor muscles of the legs. Following 30 weeks of detraining, the subjects experienced a 31% decrease in maximal dynamic muscle strength. However, this detraining-induced loss of dynamic strength was associated with a relatively small degree of muscle atrophy. For example, type I fibers atrophied approximately −2%, type IIa fibers atrophied −10%, and type IIx fibers atrophied −13% (figure 13.18b). This finding suggests that much of the loss of strength associated with detraining is associated with changes in the nervous system. Collectively, these data indicate that resistance training-induced muscular adaptations (i.e., dynamic strength and muscle hypertrophy) can be retained for long periods during detraining.

Also, notice that 6 weeks of retraining resulted in a rapid regaining of dynamic muscular strength and a complete restoration of muscle fiber size back to post-training levels (figure 13.18) (91). These results reveal that rapid muscular adaptations occur as a result of the reinstatement of strength training in previously trained individuals. This speedy improvement in muscle strength during retraining explains how power athletes can often return to "competitive form" quickly after long periods of detraining.

Finally, studies also reveal that after dynamic muscular strength has been increased by strength training, a reduced-frequency maintenance program of weight lifting can sustain strength for an extended period. For instance, it has been shown that following a 12-week period of rigorous strength training (3 days/week), as few as 1 training day per week can maintain maximal dynamic strength for up to 12 weeks (35). Further, another study reported that maximal dynamic strength of lower back (lumbar extension) muscles can be maintained for 12 weeks by only 1 training day every 2 weeks (100). Collectively, these studies indicate that strength can be maintained for up to 12 weeks with reduced training frequency.

IN SUMMARY

- The stoppage of resistance training results in a loss of muscular strength and muscle atrophy. However, compared to the rate of detraining following endurance exercise, the rate of detraining from resistance exercise is considerably slower.
- Rapid muscular adaptations occur as a result of strength training in previously trained individuals.
- Maximal dynamic strength can be maintained for up to 12 weeks with reduced training frequency.

CONCURRENT STRENGTH AND ENDURANCE TRAINING

At this point in the chapter, it may have occurred to you that strength training might interfere with the adaptations associated with endurance training. For example, endurance training increases mitochondrial proteins, whereas strength training increases the synthesis of contractile proteins. Does one type of training really interfere with the effects of the other? To date, this remains controversial; nonetheless, let's examine studies on this issue.

In 1980, Hickson reported that a 10-week combined strength and endurance training program resulted in similar gains in $\dot{V}O_2$ max compared to an endurance-only group, but concurrent training (strength + endurance) results in an interference with the gains in strength (40). The strength-only group increased strength throughout the entire 10 weeks, but the combined strength and endurance group showed a leveling off and a decrease in strength at 9 and 10 weeks.

Since this early study of Hickson and colleagues, numerous other investigations have supported or disagreed with notion that strength development is impaired during concurrent training. Many of the differences in these studies appear to arise from differences in training programs between the studies. For example, Sale et al. suggests that the effectiveness of concurrent training may depend on a variety of factors, such as the intensity, volume, and frequency of training, and how the training modes are integrated (83). Indeed, clearly the frequency and intensity of training has an impact on the potential for one type of training to interfere with the other (65). That is, studies that combine frequent training sessions and high-intensity endurance exercise often report that concurrent training impairs strength gains (26, 56). Potential mechanisms to explain why concurrent training may impair strength gains are addressed in the next section.

Mechanisms Responsible for the Impairment of Strength Development During Concurrent Strength and Endurance Training

Over the years, several mechanisms have been proposed to explain why concurrent endurance and strength training appears to impede strength development compared to strength training alone. These include neural components, glycogen depletion, fiber-type transition, overtraining, and impaired protein synthesis. A brief discussion of each of these possibilities follows.

Neural Factors It has been proposed that concurrent strength and endurance training impairs strength development because of neural factors. Specifically, some investigators have suggested that concurrent training impairs motor unit recruitment and therefore decreases muscle force production (26, 58). However, limited evidence exists to support this possibility (38). Therefore, it is currently unclear if changes in motor unit recruitment contribute to the impairment of strength gains when concurrent resistance and endurance training is performed.

Low Muscle Glycogen Content Successive bouts of either strength or endurance training can produce chronically low levels of muscle glycogen (70). That is, repeated endurance training and/or repeated bouts of resistance exercise can result in low resting levels of muscle glycogen. Therefore, beginning a training session with low muscle glycogen can reduce the ability to perform subsequent resistance training sessions and impair the magnitude of the strength-training adaptations.

Overtraining Overtraining is often defined as an imbalance between training and recovery. At least one review has concluded that overtraining can contribute to the inability to attain optimal strength gains when concurrent strength and endurance exercise training is performed (58). Nonetheless, no experimental studies provide direct evidence that overtraining is a major factor that contributes to the inhibition of strength gains when both resistance and endurance exercise are performed.

Depressed Protein Synthesis In theory, concurrent resistance and endurance exercise bouts could result in impaired protein synthesis following resistance exercise training (7, 39, 70). The science behind this concept is as follows. Recall that resistance exercise training increases muscle contractile protein synthesis by activation of the IGF-1/Akt/mTOR signaling pathway (figure 13.19). In contrast, endurance exercise training increases AMPK activation and promotes mitochondrial biogenesis. Further, active AMPK can activate a signaling molecule called tuberous sclerosis complex 1/2 (TSC1/2). Active TSC 1/2 inhibits mTOR activity and therefore impairs protein

synthesis (39). Hence, the AMPK/TSC 1/2 pathway provides a biochemical link to explain why concurrent endurance/resistance training may impair strength gains. Nonetheless, additional research is needed to determine if this biochemical signaling path is the sole explanation for why concurrent training impairs strength gains.

IN SUMMARY

- Individuals who engage in concurrent resistance training and high-intensity endurance exercise training often report that concurrent training impairs strength gains.
- Several mechanisms can potentially explain why concurrent training may impair strength gains. These include neural factors, low muscle glycogen content, overtraining, and depressed proteins synthesis.
- Concurrent resistance and endurance exercise bouts can theoretically impair protein synthesis following resistance exercise training. The science behind this prediction is illustrated in figure 13.19.

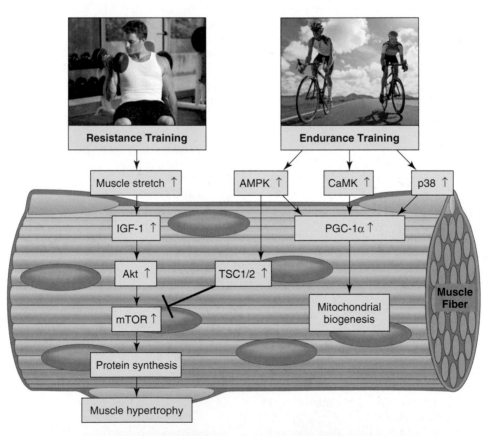

Figure 13.19 Intracellular signaling networks mediating exercise-induced skeletal muscle responses to resistance and endurance exercise training programs. Resistance exercise training activates the IGF-1/Akt/MTOR pathway that promotes protein synthesis by increasing translation. Endurance exercise training activates several secondary signals to promote an increase in PGC-1α and increased mitochondrial biogenesis. Note that activation of AMPK by endurance training can inhibit mTOR signaling via the tuberous sclerosis complex 1/2 (TSC 1/2) and suppress resistance training-induced protein synthesis. The interaction between these two intracellular signaling networks can potentially explain why concurrent resistance and endurance training programs can reduce strength gains observed with resistance training alone.

STUDY QUESTIONS

1. Explain the basic principles of training: *overload, specificity,* and *reversibility.*
2. Discuss the role that genetics plays in determining $\dot{V}O_2$ max.
3. Indicate the typical change in $\dot{V}O_2$ max with endurance-training programs and the effect of the initial (pretraining) value on the magnitude of the increase.
4. State typical $\dot{V}O_2$ max values for various sedentary, active, and athletic populations.
5. Understand the contribution of heart rate, stroke volume, and the a-$\bar{v}$ O_2 difference in determining $\dot{V}O_2$ max.
6. Discuss how training increases $\dot{V}O_2$ max.
7. Define *preload, afterload,* and *contractility,* and discuss the role of each in the increase in the maximal stroke volume that occurs with endurance training.
8. Describe the changes in muscle structure that are responsible for the increase in the maximal a-$\bar{v}$ O_2 difference with endurance training.
9. List and discuss the primary changes that occur in skeletal muscle as a result of endurance training.
10. Explain how endurance training improves acid-base balance during exercise.
11. Outline the "big picture" changes that occur in skeletal muscle as a result of exercise training and discuss the specificity of exercise-training responses.
12. List the four primary signal transduction pathways in skeletal muscle.
13. List and define the function of six important secondary messengers in skeletal muscle.
14. Outline the signaling events that lead to endurance training-induced muscle adaptation.
15. Discuss how changes in "central command" and "peripheral feedback" following an endurance training program can lower the heart rate, ventilation, and catecholamine responses to a submaximal exercise bout.
16. Describe the underlying causes of the decrease in $\dot{V}O_2$ max that occurs with cessation of endurance training.
17. Contrast the role of neural adaptations with hypertrophy in the increase in strength that occurs with resistance training.
18. Identify the primary changes that occur in skeletal muscle fibers in response to resistance training.
19. Outline the signaling events that lead to resistance training-induced increases in muscle growth.
20. Discuss how detraining following strength training impacts muscle fiber size and strength.
21. How does retraining influence muscle fiber size and strength?
22. Explain why concurrent strength and endurance training can impair strength gains.

SUGGESTED READINGS

Coffey, V. G, and J. A. Hawley. 2007. The molecular bases of training adaptation. *Sports Med* 37: 737–63.

Folland, J. P., and A. G. Williams. 2007. The adaptations to strength training: Methodological and neurological contributions to increased strength. *Sports Med* 37: 145–68.

Gabriel, D. A., G. Kamen, and G. Frost. 2006. Neural adaptations to resistance exercise: Mechanisms and recommendations for training practices. *Sports Med* 36: 133–49.

Hawley, J. A. 2009. Molecular responses to strength and endurance training: Are they incompatible? *App. Physiol. Nutr. Metab.* 34:355–61.

Lee, M., and T. J. Carroll. 2007. Cross education: Possible mechanisms for the contralateral effects of unilateral resistance training. *Sports Med* 37:1–14.

Olesen J., K. Kiilerich, and H. Pilegaard. 2010. PGC-1alpha-mediated adaptations in skeletal muscle. *Pflugers Arch* 460: 153–62.

Phillips, S. M. 2009. Physiologic and molecular bases of muscle hypertrophy and atrophy: Impact of resistance exercise on human skeletal muscle (protein and exercise dose effects). *App. Physiol. Nutr. Metab.* 34:403–10.

Powers, S. K., E. E. Talbert, and P. J. Adhihetty. 2011. Reactive oxygen and nitrogen species as intracellular signals in skeletal muscle. *J Physiol* 589:2129–2138.

REFERENCES

1. **Adams GR.** Satellite cell proliferation and skeletal muscle hypertrophy. *Appl Physiol Nutr Metab* 31: 782–790, 2006.
2. **Adams GR, Caiozzo VJ, Haddad F, and Baldwin KM.** Cellular and molecular responses to increased skeletal muscle loading after irradiation. *Am J Physiol Cell Physiol* 283: C1182–1195, 2002.
3. **American College of Sports Medicine.** American College of Sports Medicine Position Stand. The recommended quantity and quality of exercise for developing and maintaining cardiorespiratory and muscular fitness, and flexibility in healthy adults. *Med Sci Sports Exerc* 30: 975–991, 1998.
4. **Asmussen E, Johansen SH, Jorgensen M, and Nielsen M.** On the nervous factors controlling respiration and circulation during exercise. Experiments with curarization. *Acta Physiol Scand* 63: 343–350, 1965.
5. **Åstrand P, and Rodahl K.** *Textbook of Work Physiology.* New York: McGraw-Hill, 1986.
6. **Atha J.** Strengthening muscle. In: *Exercise and Sport Science Reviews,* edited by Miller D. Philadelphia: The Franklin Institute Press, 1981, p. 1–73.
7. **Baar K.** Training for endurance and strength: lessons from cell signaling. *Med Sci Sports Exerc* 38: 1939–1944, 2006.
8. **Biressi S, and Rando TA.** Heterogeneity in the muscle satellite cell population. *Semin Cell Dev Biol* 21: 845–854, 2010.
9. **Blomqvist CG, and Saltin B.** Cardiovascular adaptations to physical training. *Annu Rev Physiol* 45: 169–189, 1983.
10. **Booth F.** Effects of endurance exercise on cytochrome C turnover in skeletal muscle. *Ann N Y Acad Sci* 301: 431–439, 1977.

11. **Bouchard C, An P, Rice T, Skinner JS, Wilmore JH, Gagnon J, Perusse L, Leon AS, and Rao DC.** Familial aggregation of V̇O(2max) response to exercise training: results from the HERITAGE Family Study. J Appl Physiol 87: 1003–1008, 1999.

12. **Bouchard C, Boulay MR, Simoneau JA, Lortie G, and Perusse L.** Heredity and trainability of aerobic and anaerobic performances: an update. Sports Med 5: 69–73, 1988.

13. **Bouchard C, Daw EW, Rice T, Perusse L, Gagnon J, Province MA, Leon AS, Rao DC, Skinner JS, and Wilmore JH.** Familial resemblance for V̇O₂ max in the sedentary state: the HERITAGE family study. Med Sci Sports Exerc 30: 252–258, 1998.

14. **Bouchard C, Sarzynski MA, Rice TK, Kraus WE, Church TS, Sung YJ, Rao DC, and Rankinen T.** Genomic predictors of maximal oxygen uptake response to standardized exercise training programs. J Appl Physiol 2010.

15. **Claytor R.** Selected cardiovascular, sympatho-adrenal, and metabolic responses to one-leg exercise training. The University of Tennessee, Knoxville, 1985.

16. **Coffey VG, and Hawley JA.** The molecular bases of training adaptation. Sports Med 37: 737–763, 2007.

17. **Coffey VG, Pilegaard H, Garnham AP, O'Brien BJ, and Hawley JA.** Consecutive bouts of diverse contractile activity alter acute responses in human skeletal muscle. J Appl Physiol 106: 1187–1197, 2009.

18. **Coyle EF, Hemmert MK, and Coggan AR.** Effects of detraining on cardiovascular responses to exercise: role of blood volume. J Appl Physiol 60: 95–99, 1986.

19. **Coyle EF, Hopper MK, and Coggan AR.** Maximal oxygen uptake relative to plasma volume expansion. Int J Sports Med 11: 116–119, 1990.

20. **Coyle EF, Martin WH, III, Bloomfield SA, Lowry OH, and Holloszy JO.** Effects of detraining on responses to submaximal exercise. J Appl Physiol 59: 853–859, 1985.

21. **Coyle EF, Martin WH, III, Sinacore DR, Joyner MJ, Hagberg JM, and Holloszy JO.** Time course of loss of adaptations after stopping prolonged intense endurance training. J Appl Physiol 57: 1857–1864, 1984.

22. **Craig B.** Hyperplasia: Scientific fact or fiction? National Strength & Conditioning Association 23: 42–44, 2001.

23. **Cronan TL, III, and Howley ET.** The effect of training on epinephrine and norepinephrine excretion. Med Sci Sports 6: 122–125, 1974.

24. **Deschenes MR.** Effects of aging on muscle fibre type and size. Sports Med 34: 809–824, 2004.

25. **Dudley GA, Abraham WM, and Terjung RL.** Influence of exercise intensity and duration on biochemical adaptations in skeletal muscle. J Appl Physiol 53: 844–850, 1982.

26. **Dudley GA, and Djamil R.** Incompatibility of endurance- and strength-training modes of exercise. J Appl Physiol 59: 1446–1451, 1985.

27. **Edge J, Bishop D, and Goodman C.** The effects of training intensity on muscle buffer capacity in females. Eur J Appl Physiol 96: 97–105, 2006.

28. **Ehsani AA, Hagberg JM, and Hickson RC.** Rapid changes in left ventricular dimensions and mass in response to physical conditioning and deconditioning. Am J Cardiol 42: 52–56, 1978.

29. **Ekblom B.** Effect of physical training in adolescent boys. J Appl Physiol 27: 350–355, 1969.

30. **Favier RJ, Constable SH, Chen M, and Holloszy JO.** Endurance exercise training reduces lactate production. J Appl Physiol 61: 885–889, 1986.

31. **Fiatarone MA, Marks EC, Ryan ND, Meredith CN, Lipsitz LA, and Evans WJ.** High-intensity strength training in nonagenarians: effects on skeletal muscle. Jama 263: 3029–3034, 1990.

32. **Fiatarone MA, O'Neill EF, Ryan ND, Clements KM, Solares GR, Nelson ME, Roberts SB, Kehayias JJ, Lipsitz LA, and Evans WJ.** Exercise training and nutritional supplementation for physical frailty in very elderly people. N Engl J Med 330: 1769–1775, 1994.

33. **Folland JP, and Williams AG.** The adaptations to strength training: morphological and neurological contributions to increased strength. Sports Med 37: 145–168, 2007.

34. **Goodman JM, Liu PP, and Green HJ.** Left ventricular adaptations following short-term endurance training. J Appl Physiol 98: 454–460, 2005.

35. **Graves JE, Pollock ML, Leggett SH, Braith RW, Carpenter DM, and Bishop LE.** Effect of reduced training frequency on muscular strength. Int J Sports Med 9: 316–319, 1988.

36. **Green HJ, Jones S, Ball-Burnett ME, Smith D, Livesey J, and Farrance BW.** Early muscular and metabolic adaptations to prolonged exercise training in humans. J Appl Physiol 70: 2032–2038, 1991.

37. **Hagberg JM, Hickson RC, Ehsani AA, and Holloszy JO.** Faster adjustment to and recovery from submaximal exercise in the trained state. J Appl Physiol 48: 218–224, 1980.

38. **Hakkinen K, Alen M, Kraemer WJ, Gorostiaga E, Izquierdo M, Rusko H, Mikkola J, Hakkinen A, Valkeinen H, Kaarakainen E, Romu S, Erola V, Ahtiainen J, and Paavolainen L.** Neuromuscular adaptations during concurrent strength and endurance training versus strength training. Eur J Appl Physiol 89: 42–52, 2003.

39. **Hawley JA.** Molecular responses to strength and endurance training: are they incompatible? Appl Physiol Nutr Metab 34: 355–361, 2009.

40. **Hickson RC.** Interference of strength development by simultaneously training for strength and endurance. Eur J Appl Physiol Occup Physiol 45: 255–263, 1980.

41. **Hickson RC, Dvorak BA, Gorostiaga EM, Kurowski TT, and Foster C.** Potential for strength and endurance training to amplify endurance performance. J Appl Physiol 65: 2285–2290, 1988.

42. **Holloszy JO, and Coyle EF.** Adaptations of skeletal muscle to endurance exercise and their metabolic consequences. J Appl Physiol 56: 831–838, 1984.

43. **Holviala JH, Sallinen JM, Kraemer WJ, Alen MJ, and Hakkinen KK.** Effects of strength training on muscle strength characteristics, functional capabilities, and balance in middle-aged and older women. J Strength Cond Res 20: 336–344, 2006.

44. **Hornberger TA, Armstrong DD, Koh TJ, Burkholder TJ, and Esser KA.** Intracellular signaling specificity in response to uniaxial vs. multiaxial stretch: implications for mechanotransduction. Am J Physiol Cell Physiol 288: C185–194, 2005.

45. **Horowitz JF.** Fatty acid mobilization from adipose tissue during exercise. Trends Endocrinol Metab 14: 386–392, 2003.

46. **Houmard JA, Hortobagyi T, Johns RA, Bruno NJ, Nute CC, Shinebarger MH, and Welborn JW.** Effect of short-term training cessation on performance measures in distance runners. Int J Sports Med 13: 572–576, 1992.

47. **Hunter GR, McCarthy JP, and Bamman MM.** Effects of resistance training on older adults. Sports Med 34: 329–348, 2004.

48. **Juel C.** Training-induced changes in membrane transport proteins of human skeletal muscle. *Eur J Appl Physiol* 96: 627–635, 2006.

49. **Kannus P, Alosa D, Cook L, Johnson RJ, Renstrom P, Pope M, Beynnon B, Yasuda K, Nichols C, and Kaplan M.** Effect of one-legged exercise on the strength, power and endurance of the contralateral leg: a randomized, controlled study using isometric and concentric isokinetic training. *Eur J Appl Physiol Occup Physiol* 64: 117–126, 1992.

50. **Kemi OJ, Hoydal MA, Macquaide N, Haram PM, Koch LG, Britton SL, Ellingsen O, Smith GL, and Wisloff U.** The effect of exercise training on transverse tubules in normal, remodeled, and reverse remodeled hearts. *J Cell Physiol* 2010.

51. **Kemi OJ, and Wisloff U.** Mechanisms of exercise-induced improvements in the contractile apparatus of the mammalian myocardium. *Acta Physiol (Oxf)* 199: 425–439, 2010.

52. **Kiens B, Essen-Gustavsson B, Christensen NJ, and Saltin B.** Skeletal muscle substrate utilization during submaximal exercise in man: effect of endurance training. *J Physiol* 469: 459–478, 1993.

53. **Klissouras V.** Heritability of adaptive variation. *J Appl Physiol* 31: 338–344, 1971.

54. **Koves TR, Noland RC, Bates AL, Henes ST, Muoio DM, and Cortright RN.** Subsarcolemmal and intermyofibrillar mitochondria play distinct roles in regulating skeletal muscle fatty acid metabolism. *Am J Physiol Cell Physiol* 288: C1074–1082, 2005.

55. **Kraemer WJ, Deschenes MR, and Fleck SJ.** Physiological adaptations to resistance exercise:implications for athletic conditioning. *Sports Med* 6: 246–256, 1988.

56. **Kraemer WJ, Patton JF, Gordon SE, Harman EA, Deschenes MR, Reynolds K, Newton RU, Triplett NT, and Dziados JE.** Compatibility of high-intensity strength and endurance training on hormonal and skeletal muscle adaptations. *J Appl Physiol* 78: 976–989, 1995.

57. **Krentz JR, Quest B, Farthing JP, Quest DW, and Chilibeck PD.** The effects of ibuprofen on muscle hypertrophy, strength, and soreness during resistance training. *Appl Physiol Nutr Metab* 33: 470–475, 2008.

58. **Leveritt M, Abernethy PJ, Barry BK, and Logan PA.** Concurrent strength and endurance training: a review. *Sports Med* 28: 413–427, 1999.

59. **MacDougall JD.** Morphological changes in human skeletal muscle following strength training and immobilization. In: *Human Muscle Power*, edited by Jones N, McCartney N, and McComas A. Champaign: Human Kinetics, 1986, p. 269–285.

60. **MacDougall JD, Gibala MJ, Tarnopolsky MA, MacDonald JR, Interisano SA, and Yarasheski KE.** The time course for elevated muscle protein synthesis following heavy resistance exercise. *Can J Appl Physiol* 20: 480–486, 1995.

61. **MacDougall JD, Sale DG, Alway SE, and Sutton JR.** Muscle fiber number in biceps brachii in bodybuilders and control subjects. *J Appl Physiol* 57: 1399–1403, 1984.

62. **MacDougall JD, Sale DG, Elder GC, and Sutton JR.** Muscle ultrastructural characteristics of elite powerlifters and bodybuilders. *Eur J Appl Physiol Occup Physiol* 48: 117–126, 1982.

63. **Madsen K, Pedersen PK, Djurhuus MS, and Klitgaard NA.** Effects of detraining on endurance capacity and metabolic changes during prolonged exhaustive exercise. *J Appl Physiol* 75: 1444–1451, 1993.

64. **McCall GE, Byrnes WC, Dickinson A, Pattany PM, and Fleck SJ.** Muscle fiber hypertrophy, hyperplasia, and capillary density in college men after resistance training. *J Appl Physiol* 81: 2004–2012, 1996.

65. **McCarthy JP, Pozniak MA, and Agre JC.** Neuromuscular adaptations to concurrent strength and endurance training. *Med Sci Sports Exerc* 34: 511–519, 2002.

66. **Midgley AW, McNaughton LR, and Wilkinson M.** Is there an optimal training intensity for enhancing the maximal oxygen uptake of distance runners?: empirical research findings, current opinions, physiological rationale and practical recommendations. *Sports Med* 36: 117–132, 2006.

67. **Mikesky AE, Giddings CJ, Matthews W, and Gonyea WJ.** Changes in muscle fiber size and composition in response to heavy-resistance exercise. *Med Sci Sports Exerc* 23: 1042–1049, 1991.

68. **Mitchell JH.** J.B. Wolffe memorial lecture. Neural control of the circulation during exercise. *Med Sci Sports Exerc* 22: 141–154, 1990.

69. **Morganroth J, Maron BJ, Henry WL, and Epstein SE.** Comparative left ventricular dimensions in trained athletes. *Ann Intern Med* 82: 521–524, 1975.

70. **Nader GA.** Concurrent strength and endurance training: from molecules to man. *Med Sci Sports Exerc* 38: 1965–1970, 2006.

71. **Novak ML, Billich W, Smith SM, Sukhija KB, McLoughlin TJ, Hornberger TA, and Koh TJ.** COX-2 inhibitor reduces skeletal muscle hypertrophy in mice. *Am J Physiol Regul Integr Comp Physiol* 296: R1132–1139, 2009.

72. **Olesen J, Kiilerich K, and Pilegaard H.** PGC-1alpha-mediated adaptations in skeletal muscle. *Pflugers Arch* 460: 153–162, 2010.

73. **Parise G, Phillips SM, Kaczor JJ, and Tarnopolsky MA.** Antioxidant enzyme activity is up-regulated after unilateral resistance exercise training in older adults. *Free Radic Biol Med* 39: 289–295, 2005.

74. **Paul P.** Effects of long-lasting physical exercise and training on lipid metabolism. In: *Metabolic Adaptation to Prolonged Physical Exercise*, edited by Howald H, and Poortmans J. Basel, Switzerland: Birkhauser Verlag Basel, 1975, p. 156–187.

75. **Powers SK, Criswell D, Lawler J, Ji LL, Martin D, Herb RA, and Dudley G.** Influence of exercise and fiber type on antioxidant enzyme activity in rat skeletal muscle. *Am J Physiol* 266: R375–380, 1994.

76. **Powers SK, Duarte J, Kavazis AN, and Talbert EE.** Reactive oxygen species are signalling molecules for skeletal muscle adaptation. *Exp Physiol* 95: 1–9, 2010.

77. **Powers SK, Nelson WB, and Hudson MB.** Exercise-induced oxidative stress in humans: cause and consequences. *Free Radic Biol Med* 2010.

78. **Powers SK, Talbert EE, and Adhihetty PJ.** Reactive oxygen and nitrogen species as intracellular signals in skeletal muscle. *J Physiol* 2011.

79. **Rerych SK, Scholz PM, Sabiston DC, Jr., and Jones RH.** Effects of exercise training on left ventricular function in normal subjects: a longitudinal study by radionuclide angiography. *Am J Cardiol* 45: 244–252, 1980.

80. **Rowell LB.** *Human Circulation-Regulation During Physical Stress.* New York: Oxford University Press, 1986.

81. **Rowell LB, and O'Leary DS.** Reflex control of the circulation during exercise: chemoreflexes and mechanoreflexes. *J Appl Physiol* 69: 407–418, 1990.

82. **Sale DG.** Neural adaptation to resistance training. *Med Sci Sports Exerc* 20: S135–145, 1988.

83. **Sale DG, Jacobs I, MacDougall JD, and Garner S.** Comparison of two regimens of concurrent strength and endurance training. *Med Sci Sports Exerc* 22: 348–356, 1990.

84. **Saltin B.** Physiological effects of physical conditioning. *Medicine and Science in Sports* 1: 50–56, 1969.

85. **Saltin B, and Astrand PO.** Free fatty acids and exercise. *Am J Clin Nutr* 57: 752S–757S; discussion 757S–758S, 1993.

86. **Saltin B, and Gollnick P.** Skeletal muscle adaptability: Significance for metabolism and performance. In: *Handbook of Physiology*, edited by Peachey L, Adrian R, and Geiger S. Baltimore: Lippincott Williams & Wilkins, 1983.

87. **Schenk S, and Horowitz JF.** Coimmunoprecipitation of FAT/CD36 and CPT I in skeletal muscle increases proportionally with fat oxidation after endurance exercise training. *Am J Physiol Endocrinol Metab* 291: E254–260, 2006.

88. **Seynnes OR, de Boer M, and Narici MV.** Early skeletal muscle hypertrophy and architectural changes in response to high-intensity resistance training. *J Appl Physiol* 102: 368–373, 2007.

89. **Soltow QA, Betters JL, Sellman JE, Lira VA, Long JH, and Criswell DS.** Ibuprofen inhibits skeletal muscle hypertrophy in rats. *Med Sci Sports Exerc* 38: 840–846, 2006.

90. **Spina RJ, Ogawa T, Kohrt WM, Martin WH, III, Holloszy JO, and Ehsani AA.** Differences in cardiovascular adaptations to endurance exercise training between older men and women. *J Appl Physiol* 75: 849–855, 1993.

91. **Staron RS, Leonardi MJ, Karapondo DL, Malicky ES, Falkel JE, Hagerman FC, and Hikida RS.** Strength and skeletal muscle adaptations in heavy-resistance-trained women after detraining and retraining. *J Appl Physiol* 70: 631–640, 1991.

92. **Staron RS, Malicky ES, Leonardi MJ, Falkel JE, Hagerman FC, and Dudley GA.** Muscle hypertrophy and fast fiber type conversions in heavy resistance-trained women. *Eur J Appl Physiol Occup Physiol* 60: 71–79, 1990.

93. **Tamaki T, Uchiyama S, and Nakano S.** A weight-lifting exercise model for inducing hypertrophy in the hindlimb muscles of rats. *Med Sci Sports Exerc* 24: 881–886, 1992.

94. **Tang JE, Hartman JW, and Phillips SM.** Increased muscle oxidative potential following resistance training induced fibre hypertrophy in young men. *Appl Physiol Nutr Metab* 31: 495–501, 2006.

95. **Tang JE, Perco JG, Moore DR, Wilkinson SB, and Phillips SM.** Resistance training alters the response of fed state mixed muscle protein synthesis in young men. *Am J Physiol Regul Integr Comp Physiol* 294: R172–178, 2008.

96. **Terjung RL.** Muscle adaptations to aerobic training. In: *Sports Science Exchange*. Barrington: Gatorade Sports Science Institute, 1995.

97. **Tesch PA.** Skeletal muscle adaptations consequent to long-term heavy resistance exercise. *Med Sci Sports Exerc* 20: S132–134, 1988.

98. **Tesch PA, Komi PV, and Hakkinen K.** Enzymatic adaptations consequent to long-term strength training. *Int J Sports Med* 8 Suppl 1: 66–69, 1987.

99. **Trappe TA, Carroll CC, Dickinson JM, LeMoine JK, Haus JM, Sullivan BE, Lee JD, Jemiolo B, Weinheimer EM, and Hollon CJ.** Influence of acetaminophen and ibuprofen on skeletal muscle adaptations to resistance exercise in older adults. *Am J Physiol Regul Integr Comp Physiol* 300: R655–662, 2011.

100. **Tucci JT, Carpenter DM, Pollock ML, Graves JE, and Leggett SH.** Effect of reduced frequency of training and detraining on lumbar extension strength. *Spine* (Phila Pa 1976) 17: 1497–1501, 1992.

101. **Van Loon L.** Use of intramuscular triacylglycerol as a substrate source during exercise in humans. *Journal of Applied Physiology* 97: 1170–1187, 2004.

102. **Vincent HK, Powers SK, Stewart DJ, Demirel HA, Shanely RA, and Naito H.** Short-term exercise training improves diaphragm antioxidant capacity and endurance. *Eur J Appl Physiol* 81: 67–74, 2000.

103. **Wang Y, Wisloff U, and Kemi OJ.** Animal models in the study of exercise-induced cardiac hypertrophy. *Physiol Res* 59: 633–644, 2010.

104. **Wibom R, Hultman E, Johansson M, Matherei K, Constantin-Teodosiu D, and Schantz PG.** Adaptation of mitochondrial ATP production in human skeletal muscle to endurance training and detraining. *J Appl Physiol* 73: 2004–2010, 1992.

14

Risk Factors and Inflammation: Links to Chronic Disease

In this section of the text, we introduce the roles of physical activity and diet in reducing the risks of chronic diseases. To set that up, in this chapter we begin with a discussion of risk factors for chronic diseases that examines the environmental, genetic, and behavioral links to health and disease. These risk factors direct public health interventions to reduce the overall risk to the population (e.g., stop-smoking campaigns). However, although risk factors describe the causes of disease from a macro level, they don't address the underlying physiological causes of these chronic diseases. We will try to do that by exploring the proposition that it is a low-level systemic inflammation (see chapter 6) that is causing many of these chronic diseases. Finally, we will briefly touch on the roles of physical activity and diet related to these chronic diseases, which are addressed in more detail in chapters 16, 17, and 18.

RISK FACTORS FOR HEART DISEASE

Over the past 100 years, attention has shifted from **infectious diseases** (e.g., tuberculosis and pneumonia) as the major causes of death to chronic degenerative diseases, such as cancer and cardiovascular diseases. The five leading causes of death in the United States in 2007 were cardiovascular diseases (31.0%), cancers (23.2%), chronic lower respiratory diseases (5.3%), accidents (5.1%), and Alzheimer's disease (3.1%) (58). The onset of most of the leading causes of death can be delayed or prevented by addressing the risk factors for these diseases. Epidemiologists are the scientists who play a major role in exploring the distribution of diseases in the population and the factors that have an impact on those diseases. Figure 14.1 shows that risk factors associated with chronic diseases can be divided into three categories (60).

Inherited/Biological

These factors include the following:

- Age—older individuals have more chronic diseases than younger individuals.

- Gender—men develop cardiovascular disease at an earlier age than women, but women experience more strokes than men (4).
- Race—African Americans develop about 30% more heart disease than non-Hispanic whites (59).
- Susceptibility to disease—several diseases have a genetic component that increases the potential for having a disease.

Environmental

Environmental factors that impact health and disease include the following:

- physical factors (e.g., climate, water, altitude, pollution),
- socioeconomic factors (e.g., income, housing, education, workplace characteristics), and
- family (e.g., parental values, divorce, and extended family and friends).

Behaviors

To address the behaviors that influence health and disease, let's look at the top three actual causes of death, rather than the leading causes of death (see the right side of figure 14.1). That smoking is at the top of the list should be no surprise given its connection to both lung cancer and cardiovascular diseases. In fact, it is the number one actual cause of deaths, accounting for 18% of all deaths. The existence of smoking-cessation programs and laws that restrict areas in which one can smoke speak to the seriousness with which our society takes that risk to our health. The number two actual cause of death is poor diet and physical inactivity (15.2%), with alcohol consumption being number three (3.5%) (35, 36). The emphasis on healthy eating at work and in schools, the creation of new parks and bike trails to enhance opportunities to be physically active, and "don't drink and drive" campaigns are examples of some systematic attempts to help alter these behaviors.

Figure 14.1 Major categories of risk factors with examples of each.
From U.S. Department of Health, Education, and Welfare, 1979, *Healthy People: The Surgeon General's Report on Health Promotion and Disease Prevention.*

In contrast to infectious disease, in which a single pathogen may be the cause of a disease, establishing the cause of a disease is much more difficult when dealing with chronic, degenerative diseases such as cardiovascular disease. The reason is that genetic, environmental, and behavioral factors interact in a very complex manner to cause the disease. The difficulty of establishing "cause" for these complex diseases is best described by an epidemiologic model called the **web of causation** (33, 55).

In an oversimplification, Figure 14.2 shows links among three major classes of risk factors: genetic (e.g., gender, race), environmental (e.g., access to inexpensive high-fat foods; access to convenient places to walk, cycle, and play), and behavioral (e.g., diet, smoking, inadequate physical activity, too much physical inactivity (TV, video, computer) (55, 56). They act alone and interact with each other to cause **atherosclerosis,** a condition in which a fatty plaque builds up in (not on) the inner wall of an artery. Many of the risk factors interact to cause overweight, obesity, and type 2 diabetes—problems that are connected to cardiovascular disease. Trying to tease out the effect that one factor has on another

and on the final disease process is a difficult task that makes work in epidemiology interesting and challenging. The factors in the web of causation are positively associated with the development of cardiovascular diseases, but are not sufficient in and of themselves to cause them. These are called risk factors, and they play a major role in developing prevention programs aimed at reducing disease and premature death associated with **degenerative diseases.** To expand on this risk factor concept, we will focus on coronary heart disease.

CORONARY HEART DISEASE

Coronary heart disease (CHD) is associated with a gradual narrowing of the arteries serving the heart due to a thickening of the inner lining of the artery. This process, atherosclerosis, is the leading contributor to heart attack and stroke deaths (2, 16). It is now widely accepted that some people are at a greater risk of developing CHD than others. Our understanding of the risks associated with atherosclerotic disease is based primarily on the epidemiological investigation

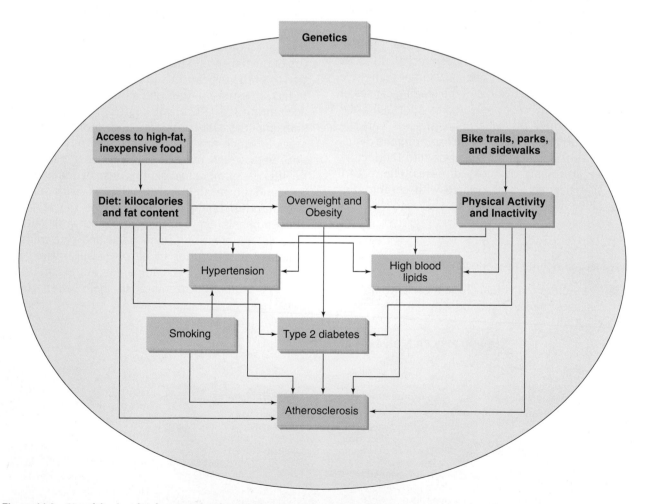

Figure 14.2 Simplified web of causation showing how genetic, environmental, and behavioral factors interact to cause artherosclerosis.

conducted in Framingham, Massachusetts (16). When this study began in 1949, cardiovascular disease already accounted for 50% of all deaths in the United States. The Framingham Study is an observational prospective (longitudinal) study designed to determine how those who develop cardiovascular disease differ from those who do not. Approximately 5,000 men and women were examined every other year, and measures such as blood pressure, electrocardiographic abnormalities, serum cholesterol, smoking, and body weight were obtained. The investigators were then able to relate the different measures to the progression of the coronary heart disease (16). Early in the study, investigators found that about 20% of the population experienced a heart attack before 60 years of age, and of them, 20% resulted in sudden death. The natural history of this disease indicated that prevention was an important goal, and the Framingham Study is recognized for identifying the risk factors to predict subsequent disease and allow early intervention (27). Consistent with the emphasis on prevention, we would like to direct the reader to *Healthy People* 2020, a comprehensive set of goals and objectives with 10-year targets to help guide efforts on health promotion and disease prevention in the United States (see Suggested Readings).

The Framingham Study found that the risk of CHD increases with the number of cigarettes smoked, the degree to which the blood pressure is elevated, and the quantity of cholesterol in the blood (27). In addition, the overall risk of CHD increases with the number of risk factors; that is, a person who has a systolic blood pressure of 160 mm Hg, has a serum cholesterol of 250 mg/dl, and smokes more than a pack of cigarettes a day has about six times the risk of CHD as a person who has only one of these risk factors (14). It is important to remember that risk factors interact with each other to increase the overall risk of CHD. This has implications for prevention as well as treatment. In this regard, getting a hypertensive patient to quit smoking confers more immediate benefit than any antihypertensive drug (27). Further, regular physical activity reduces the risk of CHD, even in those who smoke and are hypertensive (see chapter 16). See A Closer Look 14.1 for more on risk factors and heart disease.

IN SUMMARY

- Risk factors can be divided into three categories: genetic/biological, environmental, and behavioral.
- The risk factors of smoking, high cholesterol, and hypertension interact to magnify the risk of CHD. Similarly, elimination of one of them causes a disproportionate reduction in the risk of CHD.

A CLOSER LOOK 14.1

Risk Factors for Coronary Heart Disease (CHD)

Historically, **risk factors** for CHD were divided into **primary** or major and **secondary** or contributing. *Primary* meant that a factor in and of itself increased the risk of CHD, and *secondary* meant that a certain factor increased the risk of CHD only if one of the primary factors was already present, or that its significance had not been precisely determined (15). Lists of risk factors have evolved over time as more epidemiological evidence has accumulated, showing the association between various behaviors (e.g., physical inactivity) or characteristics (e.g., obesity) and CHD. Consequently, a practical approach used to classify risk factors is to list those that can be changed and those that can't, no matter whether they are primary or secondary.

It should be noted that the American College of Sports Medicine (ACSM) (1) lists one of the subfractions of cholesterol (high-density lipoprotein cholesterol [HDL-C]) as an additional risk factor. There is good evidence that the risk of CHD is lower for those with higher concentrations of HDL-C, and the ratio of total cholesterol to HDL-C is viewed by some as a better index of risk than total cholesterol alone (27). In fact, the ACSM considers HDL-C to be a "negative risk factor" when levels exceed 60 mg/dl. Further, over the years evidence accumulated showing that obesity may be a major risk factor (13, 26, 49), and now both the ACSM and the American Heart Association list it as such. Last, you may have noticed that a high-fat diet is not even cited on the list of risk factors for CHD. The reason is that the detrimental effect of a high-fat diet is already represented in the obesity and serum cholesterol risk factors. However, it is generally believed that controlling the type and amount of dietary fat would reduce the risk of CHD in the American population (see chapter 18).

As we have come to understand that physical inactivity, diet, and stress are risk factors for obesity, glucose intolerance (diabetes), hypertension, and high serum cholesterol, we have developed a new and potent view of how to intervene. Health promotion programs deal directly with physical inactivity, diet, and stress to prevent other risk factors from occurring. In addition, the primary nonpharmacological treatment of these primary risk factors revolves around recommendations for a low-fat diet (see chapter 18), regular physical activity (see chapter 16), and stress reduction (6, 10, 12). To estimate your or your parent's 10-year risk of having a heart attack, go to http://hp2010.nhlbihin.net/atpiii/calculator.asp?usertype=prof.

Physical Inactivity as a Risk Factor

After looking at the web of causation for cardiovascular disease in figure 14.2, one can understand how difficult it is to determine whether an observed association between a risk factor and a disease is a causal one or is due simply to chance. To facilitate the process of determining cause, epidemiologists apply the following guidelines (7):

- Temporal association—Does the cause precede the effect?

- Plausibility—Is the association consistent with other knowledge?

- Consistency—Have similar results been shown in other studies?

- Strength—What is the strength of the association (relative risk) between the cause and the effect? Relative risk is sometimes expressed as the ratio of the risk of disease among those exposed to the factor to the risk of those unexposed. The greater the ratio, the stronger the association.

- Dose-response relationship—Is increased exposure to the possible cause associated with increased effect?

- Reversibility—Does the removal of the possible cause lead to a reduction of the disease risk?

- Study design—Is the evidence based on strong study design?

- Judging the evidence—How many lines of evidence lead to the conclusion?

The concern about whether a risk factor is causally related to cardiovascular disease has special significance for physical activity. For many years, physical inactivity was believed to be only weakly associated with heart disease and was not given much attention as a public health concern. However, in the late 1980s and early 1990s, that view changed rather dramatically. In 1987, Powell et al. (48) did a systematic review of the literature dealing with the role of physical activity in the primary prevention of coronary heart disease, applying the just-listed guidelines to establish causation. They found that the majority of studies indicated that the level of physical inactivity predated the onset of CHD, thus meeting the temporal requirement. They also found a dose-response relationship in that as physical activity increased, the risk of CHD decreased, and the association was stronger in the better studies. The latter results met the consistency and study design criteria for causality. The review found the association to be plausible given the role of physical activity in improving glucose tolerance, increasing fibrinolysis (breaking of

clots), and reducing blood pressure. The investigators calculated the relative risk of CHD due to inactivity to be about 1.9, meaning that sedentary people had about twice the chance of experiencing CHD that physically active people had. The relative risk was similar to smoking (2.5), high serum cholesterol (2.4), and high blood pressure (2.1). When the authors controlled for smoking, blood pressure, cholesterol, age, and sex (all of which are associated with CHD), the association of physical activity and CHD remained, indicating that physical activity was an independent risk factor for CHD (3).

To estimate the real impact a risk factor may have on a population, epidemiologists try to balance the relative risk with the number of people in the population that have the risk factor. This balancing act is summed up in the calculation of the population attributable risk for each risk factor (12). Figure 14.3 describes the relative risk for selected risk factors and the percentage of the population affected. Given the large number of people who are inactive, changes in physical activity habits have a great potential to reduce CHD (see chapter 16). The publication of *Physical Activity and Health: A Report of the Surgeon General* emphasized the critical need to address these issues now (57). See A Look Back—Important People in Science for information on two individuals who have had a major impact on our understanding of physical activity and heart disease.

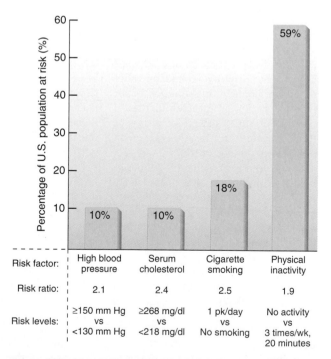

Figure 14.3 Percentages of U.S. population at risk for recognized risk factors related to coronary heart disease and risk ratio for each risk factor.

A LOOK BACK—IMPORTANT PEOPLE IN SCIENCE

Jeremy N. Morris and Ralph S. Paffenbarger, Jr.—Olympic Prize Winners

In 1996, the International Olympic Committee (IOC) awarded its first IOC Olympic Prize in Sport Sciences to Drs. Jeremy N. Morris and Ralph S. Paffenbarger, Jr., for their pioneering studies showing how exercise reduces the risk of heart disease.

Dr. Jeremy N. Morris, D.Sc., D.P.H, Fellow of the Royal College of Physicians, was professor of public health at the University of London, England. He was one of the first epidemiologists to provide scientific support showing the impact of occupational and leisure-time physical activity on the risk of heart disease. In one study, he compared conductors on London's double-decker buses who climbed 500–750 stairs per work day with drivers who sat for 90% of their shift. In another study, postal letter carriers who walked or cycled their routes were compared to sedentary telephonists and clerks. In both cases, those in the more active occupations had fewer heart attacks (39). In another set of studies he examined the effect of different amounts and types of leisure-time physical activities on the risk of coronary heart disease (CHD) in those who held naturally sedentary jobs. He found that only those doing vigorous activity during their leisure time experienced protection against CHD (38). For more information on Dr. Morris, see Paffenbarger, Blair, and Lee (42).

Dr. Ralph S. Paffenbarger, Jr., received his medical degree from Northwestern University in Chicago in 1947 and became a commissioned officer in the U.S. Public Health Service. During this time he completed his M.P.H. and Dr. P.H. degrees at Johns Hopkins. He worked on the polio epidemic until the first vaccine became available in 1955, and then shifted his attention to issues related to physical activity and health. The findings of one of Dr. Paffenbarger's studies on longshoremen (44) confirmed the findings of Dr. Morris, showing that strenuous occupational physical activity was associated with a lower risk of CHD. However, Dr. Paffenbarger is best known for the Harvard Alumni Study (begun in 1960), which tracked alumni who matriculated between 1916 and 1950. The investigators had access to medical and other records when the alumni were students, and they were able to follow the alumni over the years with questionnaires to obtain information about current behaviors (e.g., physical activity, diet, smoking) and examine the link between those behaviors and health problems (e.g., heart disease, hypertension, stroke), and cause of death. More than 100 publications have resulted from this study.

Dr. Paffenbarger's research showed that alumni who participated in greater amounts of physical activity had a lower risk of heart attack (45). In addition, he was able to show that those who increased physical activity from one time period to the next had a 23% reduction in death from all causes—showing that it is never too late to begin an exercise program (43).

Dr. Paffenbarger practiced what he preached, being a successful marathon and ultra-marathon runner. He had a major impact on the 1995 public health physical activity recommendation from the Centers for Disease Control and Prevention (46), and in the development of Physical Activity and Health: A Report of the Surgeon General (57). Dr. Paffenbarger died in 2007 and Dr. Morris in 2009, but their legacies as scientists, mentors, and role models will live on for years to come.

Information for this biographical sketch is taken from cited articles and publicly available curriculum vita.

IN SUMMARY

- Physical inactivity is an independent risk factor for CHD.
- The relative risk of CHD due to inactivity (1.9) is similar to that of hypertension (2.1) and high cholesterol (2.4). The fact that about 59% of the population is inactive indicates the enormous impact a change in physical activity habits can have on the nation's risk for CHD.

INFLAMMATION AND CORONARY HEART DISEASE

We have just seen that a wide variety of risk factors are linked to heart disease. But how are these risk factors connected, physiologically, to the actual appearance of the disease? In atherosclerosis, the narrowing of the coronary artery can result in a reduction in blood flow that may ultimately lead to a heart attack. The decrease in the diameter of the lumen is due to a build-up of lipid and fibrous materials (plaque) in the inner lining of the artery, called the *intima* (see figure 14.4). In many ways, atherosclerosis has been viewed as a plumbing issue, and procedures to flatten the plaque back to the arterial wall (angioplasty) or change out the pipe (coronary artery bypass graft) have been used to correct the problem (see chapter 17 for more on those procedures). However, most of the heart attacks and many strokes occur, not from a gradual occlusion of an artery, but from a sudden rupture of the plaque that triggers a blood clot and blocks blood flow. Let's look at this in more detail (31, 32).

It has become clear that atherosclerosis is caused by the process of inflammation initiated in the inner

Figure 14.4 Process of inflammation leading to the rupture of an atherosclerotic plaque. Adapted from P. Libby, Atherosclerosis: the new view. *Scientific American*, November 10, 2002: 46–55, 2002.

lining of the artery (30, 31). Inflammation is a response of a tissue to injury that involves the recruitment of white blood cells (leukocytes) to the site of the injury (see chapter 6). Normally, the endothelial cells (endothelium) that line the inner surface of the artery do not support the binding of leukocytes; however, when the endothelium is activated by risk factors such as smoking, high blood pressure, a high-fat diet, or obesity, the endothelium generates adhesion molecules on its surface that can bind readily to leukocytes (especially monocytes and T cells) in the blood as they pass by (see figure 14.4) (30–32).

■ Once bound to the adhesion molecules, the endothelial cells secrete chemokines that attract the monocytes to enter the intima, where they mature into macrophages.

■ The macrophages develop scavenger receptors on their surface that help them ingest large amounts of modified LDL-cholesterol.

■ The macrophages become loaded with fatty droplets and develop into foam cells. These foam cells and the T cells make up the "fatty streak," the earliest form of atherosclerotic plaque.

■ As the process continues, the macrophages multiply due to growth factors they produce, and the size of the plaque increases.

■ As this is developing, some of the smooth muscle cells in the middle layer (media) of the artery move to the top layer of the intima (near the lumen) where they multiply and, with connective tissue, form a fibrous matrix cap over the fatty core of the plaque.

At some point the foam cells release inflammatory signals that lead to the digestion and weakening of the fibrous matrix cap. If the cap ruptures, the chemicals from the foam cell interact with factors in the blood to form a clot that might be large enough to completely block an artery. It is this process that causes most of the heart attacks (30, 31).

Obesity, Inflammation, and Chronic Disease

It is now recognized that a chronic low-grade systemic inflammation is linked to a wide variety of chronic diseases, including hypertension, heart disease and stroke, some cancers, respiratory conditions, type 2 diabetes, and the Metabolic Syndrome (to be discussed in more detail in the next section) (34, 53). The chronic low-grade inflammation is characterized by a two- to three-fold increase in inflammatory cytokines (e.g., tumor necrosis factor alpha [TNF-α] and Interleukin-6 [IL-6] and C-reactive protein [CRP]).

Of interest to the readers of this text is the impact of obesity on inflammation and chronic disease. Currently in the United States, 32.3% of men and 35.5% of women are obese, with the combined overweight and obesity prevalence being 68% and 72.3%, respectively (20). Obesity is linked to a variety of chronic diseases, including coronary heart disease, hypertension, and type 2 diabetes, to name a few. The physiological connection between having too much adipose tissue and the inflammation related to chronic disease includes the hormones and inflammatory cytokines released by adipose tissue (24, 61).

Under normal conditions, adipocytes synthesize and store lipids and release anti-inflammatory hormones (e.g., adiponectin—see chapter 5). However, they have the capacity to secrete a variety of inflammatory cytokines (e.g., IL-6). When the adipocytes, especially those in the visceral area, increase in size as seen in obesity, they secrete more IL-6 and less adiponectin (24). In addition, macrophages infiltrate the enlarged visceral adipose tissue, promote a local inflammation, and secrete TNF-α, a potent inflammatory cytokine (61). Increased amounts of free fatty acids (FFA), IL-6, and TNF-α (and reduced amounts of adiponectin) are released from the visceral adipose tissue into the liver and then the general circulation. In combination, they interfere with the action of insulin (causing insulin resistance), which is linked to type 2 diabetes, cardiovascular disease and the Metabolic Syndrome (24, 53, 61).

C-reactive protein (CRP), an acute phase reactant to the presence of inflammation, is released from the liver in response to these inflammatory factors, and the concentration of CRP in the blood is used as a marker of inflammation (30, 31). Although CRP may (61) or may not (31) be directly involved in the atherosclerotic process, there is no question that it is a risk factor for heart disease, independent of the many introduced earlier in the chapter. Investigators have used it and other inflammatory markers to evaluate the impact of different strategies on the low-grade systemic inflammation associated with chronic diseases. Both pharmacological (i.e., drugs) and non-pharmacological (i.e., diet and exercise) interventions have been used to try to reduce this systemic inflammation.

Drugs, Diet, and Physical Activity

One of the most common classes of drugs used to lower LDL-cholesterol (LDL-C) are the statins that block the synthesis of cholesterol in the liver. These medications lower cholesterol and CRP, and therefore the risk of heart disease. In an attempt to understand better the role of statins in reducing the risk of heart disease, subjects were recruited who had normal levels of LDL-C, but elevated levels of CRP. Half the subjects were given a placebo and the other half a statin,

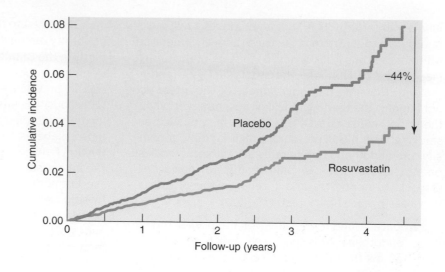

Figure 14.5 A statin (Rosuvastatin) caused a dramatic reduction in the number of patients experiencing one of the study's primary endpoints: myocardial infarction, stroke, angina/revascularization, or death due to cardiovascular disease. From P. M. Ridker et al., Rosuvastatin to prevent vascular events in men and women with elevated C-reactive protein. *New England Journal of Medicine* 359: 2195–2207, 2008.

and they were followed over time to track morbidity and mortality. The statin had such a dramatic impact on the reduction of CRP and in the risk of cardiovascular disease and death that the study was ended early (see figure 14.5) (52). This showed that even in those who had normal cholesterol levels, these drugs could lower inflammation and with it, the risk of cardiovascular disease.

In terms of diet, Esposito et al. showed that eating a Mediterranean-style diet (high in fruits, vegetables, legumes, whole grains, olive oil) for two years resulted in a dramatic reduction in CRP and IL-6, with no changes observed in the control group (18). We will see more on healthy diets in chapter 18.

There is no question that regular participation in physical activity reduces the risk of many chronic diseases (see chapter 16). Related to the systemic inflammation, the evidence is generally positive. There are prospective longitudinal studies (in which individuals are followed over time, with measurements made at different time points) showing, convincingly, that higher levels of physical activity and/or cardiorespiratory fitness are associated with lower levels of inflammation. Intervention studies confirm these findings, but not without exception (8, 9). Paradoxically, the exercise-induced reduction in inflammation appears to be due to the muscle's production of IL-6, which can be transiently elevated in the blood 100-fold as a result of exercise (11, 34, 47). It turns out that the IL-6 can act as both an inflammatory and anti-inflammatory cytokine, depending on the circumstances. In contrast to what happens in adipose tissue, TNF-α is not released from muscle with IL-6; in fact, IL-6 inhibits the effects of some inflammatory cytokines and increases the concentration of other anti-inflammatory cytokines (11, 34, 47). The end result is that exercise reduces the systemic inflammation that is associated with many chronic diseases.

THE METABOLIC SYNDROME

We end this chapter with a discussion of the Metabolic Syndrome as a way of pulling together all of what we have seen and emphasizing, again, the importance of diet and physical activity in the prevention and treatment of chronic diseases. Epidemiologists are not the only scientists interested in looking at potential relationships between variables in an attempt to have a greater understanding of what causes chronic diseases. Physiologists study how tissues and organs function to maintain homeostasis and try to uncover the source of a problem when homeostasis is not maintained. A good example of a failure to maintain homeostasis is hypertension, a problem that affects more than 68 million Americans (21). Interestingly, investigators have found that hypertension does not generally occur in isolation. It is not uncommon for hypertensive individuals to also have multiple metabolic abnormalities such as:

- obesity—especially abdominal obesity
- insulin resistance—a condition in which tissues do not take up glucose easily when stimulated with insulin; muscle is the primary site of the insulin resistance
- dyslipidemia—abnormal levels of triglycerides and other lipids

The fact that these abnormalities often occur as a group suggests a common, underlying cause that might give us a better understanding of the disease processes associated with hypertension. The coexistence of insulin resistance, dyslipidemia, and hypertension has been called Syndrome X (51); those who add obesity to the model call it the Deadly Quartet (28). However, Metabolic Syndrome is currently the preferred term. To establish the prevalence of the Metabolic Syndrome in the population, scientists first established an operational definition of the syndrome—a person has to have three or more of the following to be considered as having the syndrome (40):

- abdominal obesity: waist circumference >102 cm in men and >88 cm in women
- hypertriglyceridemia: ≥150 mg/dl
- low high-density lipoprotein (HDL) cholesterol: <40 mg/dl in men and <50 mg/dl in women
- high blood pressure: ≥130/85 mm Hg
- high fasting blood glucose: ≥100 mg/dl

The prevalence of the Metabolic Syndrome increases from 20.3% in those 20 to 39 years of age to more than 51.5% in those over 60 years. Adjusting for age, 34% of the population has this syndrome, with non-Hispanic whites having the highest age-adjusted prevalence, 37.2% (17).

Figure 14.6 shows hypothesized connections between and among these abnormalities. The central focus of the model is on insulin resistance, with skeletal muscle being the predominant tissue involved. Insulin resistance is commonly associated with obesity, especially upper body (abdominal) obesity (28). However, as the arrows in figure 14.6 indicate, insulin resistance can be caused by a combination of genetic and environmental influences independent of obesity (19, 51). For example, it has been demonstrated that a high-fat, refined-sugar diet can cause insulin resistance (5). Insulin resistance is characterized by a reduced ability to take up glucose at a given insulin concentration. In response to this resistance, the pancreas secretes more insulin to promote blood glucose uptake into tissues to return the blood glucose concentration to normal. If the pancreas cannot secrete enough insulin, the blood glucose remains elevated and a condition known as type 2 diabetes results. A drug may be required to stimulate the pancreas to secrete additional insulin to correct the problem (see chapter 17).

When the pancreas secretes additional insulin to deal with the insulin resistance, the plasma insulin level becomes elevated (hyperinsulinemia); this can elevate blood pressure and lead to hypertension. Figure 14.6 shows that elevated insulin levels can:

- increase sympathetic nervous system (SNS) activity leading to elevation of epinephrine and norepinephrine levels, which can increase heart rate, stroke volume, and blood pressure. The elevated E and NE levels can also interfere with insulin release from the pancreas and interfere with glucose uptake at the tissue, which aggravates the problem (see chapter 5);
- increase sodium and water retention, which increases plasma volume and blood pressure, and
- increase the proliferation of smooth muscle cells in small blood vessels, which can increase resistance to blood flow and drive up blood pressure.

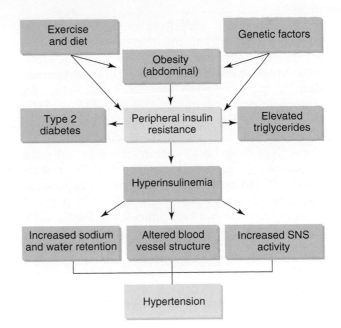

Figure 14.6 The insulin-resistance and hypertension hypothesis: Syndrome X.

Figure 14.6 also shows the connection between insulin resistance and altered blood lipids. Individuals with insulin resistance and/or abdominal obesity tend to have a higher free fatty acid (FFA) level, which can lead to an increase in plasma triglycerides. The higher FFA level could be due to the inability of insulin to suppress FFA release from adipose tissue (51) or abdominal obesity, which is associated with an increased ability to mobilize FFA (28).

In this model, scientists hypothesized that the cause of the hypertension is the insulin resistance, with skeletal muscle being the primary tissue involved. However, alternative hypotheses have been offered in what may be viewed as a chicken-and-egg question; that is, "Which came first?" For example, the following have been proposed:

- Hypertension causes the insulin resistance and not the reverse. The hypertension is believed to cause a decrease in the small blood vessels in muscle, leading to a reduction in the delivery of glucose and insulin, both of which are needed for normal glucose uptake (25).
- The increased level of sympathetic nervous system activity increases the blood pressure and blood glucose by increasing cardiac output (see chapter 9) and the mobilization of blood glucose (see chapter 5), respectively (22).
- Obesity is the cause, given adipose tissue's role as an endocrine gland (see chapter 5), whose secretions can have a direct effect on insulin resistance (41, 62).

These hypotheses, while giving some insight into potential causes of the insulin resistance and other manifestations of the Metabolic Syndrome, don't address the underlying cause. Two theories have been advanced, and they are not mutually exclusive. One theory is that the cause of the Metabolic Syndrome is a **low-grade chronic inflammation,** similar to what we have just seen for atherosclerosis. Figure 14.7 shows the complex interrelationships of the various metabolic disorders that these authors call the Cardiovascular Metabolic Syndrome, because of its obvious connection to cardiovascular disease (50). The double arrows in the figure indicate that each of the disorders can affect the others. The sheer complexity of this web of causation makes it very difficult to identify a single cause of the Metabolic Syndrome. Two potential interpretations include the following:

■ The increased levels of inflammatory cytokines (e.g., TNF-α, IL-6, CRP) cause the insulin resistance that leads to obesity and type 2 diabetes (50).

■ The central obesity leads to an increase in inflammatory cytokines and free fatty acids that, in turn, cause the insulin resistance (37).

Obviously, there are other interpretations, and the inflammation theory is not alone in suggesting cause. The other theory is that an elevated level of oxidative stress causes the Metabolic Syndrome. Oxidative stress exists when free radicals (highly reactive molecules that are missing an electron) accumulate because they are being produced faster than our antioxidant systems can neutralize them, or because the level of antioxidants is inadequate, or both. These highly reactive free radicals react with and can damage lipids, enzymes, and DNA. This can lead, in turn, to altered cellular function and to an

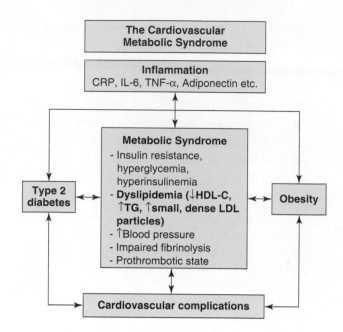

Figure 14.7   The cardiovascular metabolic syndrome. The figure shows the complex interrelationships of the various metabolic disorders. The double arrows indicate that each disorder can affect the others, creating a very complex web of causation. From J. S. Rana et al., Cardiovascular metabolic syndrome—an interplay of obesity, inflammation, diabetes and coronary heart disease. *Diabetes, Obesity and Metabolism* 9: 218–232, 2007.

inflammation response to deal with the cell damage. A growing body of evidence links oxidative stress to hypertension, insulin resistance, cardiovascular disease, type 2 diabetes, and the Metabolic Syndrome (23, 54). We are sure to hear more about these theories in the years ahead. What can we do about these chronic diseases?

Figure 14.8   Interventions used to prevent and treat the Metabolic Syndrome, type 2 diabetes, and cardiovascular disease. The focus is on regular physical activity and a healthy diet. From T. A. Lakka and D. E. Laaksonen, Physical activity in prevention and treatment of the metabolic syndrome. *Applied Physiology, Nutrition, and Metabolism* 32: 76–88, 2007.

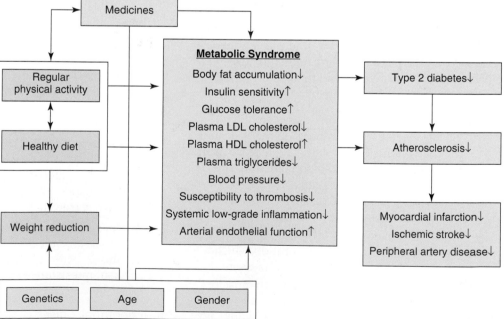

Figure 14.8 provides some clear suggestions that make it a nice wrap-up of what we have just seen and points the way for what is ahead (29). The evidence is clear that exercising on a regular basis (see chapters 16 and 17) and eating a healthy diet to achieve and maintain a healthy weight (see chapter 18) will do much to prevent these chronic diseases. They also are the principal non-pharmacological interventions used to treat those who have these chronic diseases. See the Suggested Readings for the most current guidelines for both diet and physical activity.

IN SUMMARY

- The Metabolic Syndrome model describes potential causative connections between and among obesity, peripheral insulin resistance, hypertension, and dyslipidemia.
- Potential underlying causes of the Metabolic Syndrome include a low-grade chronic inflammation and an increase in oxidative stress.
- Exercising, eating a healthy diet, and maintaining a healthy weight are strategies to both prevent and treat these chronic diseases.

STUDY QUESTIONS

1. What are the leading causes of death? How about the top three actual causes of death?
2. List the major categories of risk factors, and give examples of some in each category.
3. In the web of causation for atherosclerosis, are the various risk factors directly linked to the disease? How do the risk factors interact?
4. Physical inactivity was long considered only a secondary risk factor. What "proof" did investigators have to offer to convince the scientific community otherwise?
5. List the steps (beginning with activation of epithelial cells on the intima) leading to the rupture of plaque that can result in a clot that can cause a heart attack.
6. Discuss the role that enlarged adipose tissue cells (seen in obesity) play in the inflammation response related to numerous chronic diseases.
7. What is the Metabolic Syndrome and what are its potential underlying causes?
8. What two behaviors should be the focus of attention to minimize the systemic inflammation that is linked to chronic disease?

SUGGESTED READINGS

U.S. Department of Agriculture. 2010. *Dietary Guidelines for Americans*. http://www.cnpp.usda.gov/dietaryguidelines.htm

U.S. Department of Health and Human Services. 2010. *Healthy People 2020*. http://www.healthypeople.gov/2020/default.aspx

U.S. Department of Health and Human Services. 2008. 2008 *Physical Activity Guidelines for Americans*. http://www.health.gov/PAGuidelines/

REFERENCES

1. **American College of Sports Medicine.** ACSM's *Guidelines for Exercise Testing and Prescription*. Philadelphia: Lippincott Williams & Wilkins, 2010.
2. **American Heart Association.** *Heart Disease and Stroke Statistics-2010 Update at-a-Glance*. Dallas: AHA, 2010.
3. **American Heart Association.** Statement on exercise. Benefits and recommendations for physical activity programs for all Americans. A statement for health professionals by the Committee on Exercise and Cardiac Rehabilitation of the Council on Clinical Cardiology, American Heart Association. *Circulation* 86: 340–344, 1992.
4. **American Heart Association.** Women and cardiovascular diseases—statistics http://americanheart.org/presenter.jhtml?identifier=3000941. 2010].
5. **Barnard RJ, Roberts CK, Varon SM, and Berger JJ.** Diet-induced insulin resistance precedes other aspects of the metabolic syndrome. J *Appl Physiol* 84: 1311–1315, 1998.
6. **Bassett D, and Zweifler A.** Risk factors and risk factor management. In: *Clinical Ischemic Syndromes*, edited by Zelenock G, D'Alecy L, Fantone III J, Shalfer M, and Stanley J. St. Louis: Mosby, 1990, p. 15–46.
7. **Beaglehole R, Bonita R, and Kjellström T.** *Basic Epidemiology*. Geneva: World Health Organization, 1993.
8. **Beavers KM, Brinkly TE, and Nicklas BJ.** Effect of exercise training on chronic inflammation. *Clinica Chemica Acta* 411: 785–793, 2010.
9. **Beavers KM, Hsu F-C, Isom S, Kritchevsky SB, Church T, Goodpaster B, Pahor M, and Nicklas BJ.** Long-term physical activity and inflammatory biomarkers in older adults. *Medicine and Science in Sports and Exercise* 42: 2189–2196, 2010.
10. **Bouchard C, Shephard R, Stevens T, Sutton J, and McPherson B.** Exercise, fitness, and health: The consensus statement. In: *Exercise, Fitness, and Health*, edited by C. Bouchard RJS, T. Stevens, J. R. Sutton, and B. D. McPherson. Champaign: Human Kinetics, 1990, p. 3–28.
11. **Brandt C, and Pedersen BK.** The role of exercise-induced myokines in muscle homeostasis and the defense against chronic disease. *Journal of Biomedicine and Biotechnology* 2010: Article ID: 520258, 2010.
12. **Brown D.** Exercise, fitness, and mental health. In: *Exercise, Fitness, and Health*, edited by Bouchard C, Shephard R, Stevens T, Sutton J, and McPherson B. Champaign: Human Kinetics, 1990.

13. **Calle EE, Thun MJ, Petrelli JM, Rodriguez C, and Heath CW, Jr.** Body-mass index and mortality in a prospective cohort of U.S. adults. N Engl J Med 341: 1097–1105, 1999.

14. **Caspersen C, and Heath G.** The risk factor concept of coronary heart disease. In: *Resource Manual for Guidelines for Graded Exercise Testing and Prescription*, edited by Blair SN, Painter P, Pate R, Smith L, and Taylor C. Philadelphia: Lea & Febiger, 1988, p. 111–125.

15. **Caspersen CJ.** Physical activity epidemiology: concepts, methods, and applications to exercise science. *Exerc Sport Sci Rev* 17: 423–473, 1989.

16. **Dawber T.** *The Framingham Study*. Cambridge: Harvard University Press, 1980.

17. **Ervin RB.** Prevalence of metabolic syndrome among adults 20 years of age and over, by sex, age, race and ethnicity, and body mass index: United States 2003–2006. In: *National Health Statistics Reports*. Hyattsville, MD: National Center for Health Statistics, 2009.

18. **Esposito K, Marfella R, Ciotola M, Di Palo C, Giugliano F, Giugliano G, D'Armiento M, D'Andrea F, and Giugliano D.** Effect of a Mediterranean-style diet on endothelial dysfunction and markers of vascular inflammation in the metabolic syndrome. JAMA 292: 1440–1446, 2004.

19. **Ferrannini E, Haffner SM, and Stern MP.** Essential hypertension: an insulin-resistant state. J *Cardiovasc Pharmacol* 15 Suppl 5: S18–25, 1990.

20. **Flegal KM, Carroll MD, Ogden CL, and Curtin LR.** Prevalence and trends in obesity among US adults, 1999–2008. JAMA 303: 235–241, 2010.

21. **Gillespie C, Kuklina EV, Briss PA, Blair NA, and Hong Y.** Vital signs: prevalence, treatment, and control of hypertension—United States, 1999–2002 and 2005–2008. *Morbidity and Mortality Weekly Report* 60: 103–108, 2011.

22. **Grassi G, Quarti-Trevano F, Seravalle G, and Dell'Oro R.** Cardiovascular risk and adrenergic overdrive in the metabolic syndrome. *Nutr Metab Cardiovasc Dis* 17: 473–481, 2007.

23. **Grattagliano I, Palmiere VO, Portincasa, Moschetta A, and Palasciano G.** Oxidative stress-induced risk factors associated with the metabolic syndrome: a unifying hypothesis. *Journal of Nutritional Biochemistry* 19: 491–504, 2008.

24. **Gustafson B.** Adipose tissue, inflammation and atherosclerosis. *Journal of Atherosclerosis and Thrombosis* 17: 332–341, 2010.

25. **Julius S, Gudbrandsson T, Jamerson K, and Andersson O.** The interconnection between sympathetics, microcirculation, and insulin resistance in hypertension. *Blood Press* 1: 9–19, 1992.

26. **Kannel W, and Gordon T.** Physiological and medical concomitants of obesity: The Framingham Study. In *Obesity in America*. edited by U.S. Department of Health Education, and WelfareNIH Publication No. 79–359, 1979, p. 125–143.

27. **Kannel WB.** Bishop lecture. Contribution of the Framingham Study to preventive cardiology. J *Am Coll Cardiol* 15: 206–211, 1990.

28. **Kaplan NM.** The deadly quartet: upper-body obesity, glucose intolerance, hypertriglyceridemia, and hypertension. *Arch Intern Med* 149: 1514–1520, 1989.

29. **Lakka TA, and Laaksonen DE.** Physical activity in prevention and treatment of the metabolic syndrome. *Applied Physiology, Nutrition, and Metabolism* 32: 76–88, 2007.

30. **Libby P.** Atherosclerosis: the new view. *Scientific American* November 10, 2002: 46–55, 2002.

31. **Libby P, Okamoto Y, Rocha VZ, and Folco E.** Inflammation in atherosclerosis. *Circulation Journal* 74: 213–220, 2010.

32. **Libby P, Ridker PM, and Maseri A.** Inflammation and atherosclerosis. *Circulation Journal* 105: 1135–1143, 2002.

33. **MacMahon B, and Pugh T.** *Epidemiology*. Boston: Little, Brown, 1970.

34. **Mathur N, and Pedersen BK.** Exercise as a means to control low-grade systemic inflammation. *Mediators of Inflammation* 2008: 1–6, 2008.

35. **Mokdad AH, Marks JS, Stroup DF, and Gerberding JL.** Actual causes of death in the United States, 2000. *Jama* 291: 1238–1245, 2004.

36. **Mokdad AH, Marks JS, Stroup DF, and Gerberding JL.** Correction: actual causes of death in the United States, 2000. *Jama* 293: 293–294, 2005.

37. **Monteiro R, and Azavedo I.** Chronic inflammation in obesity and the metabolic syndrome. *Mediators of Inflammation* 2010: ID 289645, 2010.

38. **Morris JN, Chave SP, Adam C, Sirey C, Epstein L, and Sheehan DJ.** Vigorous exercise in leisure-time and the incidence of coronary heart-disease. *Lancet* 1: 333–339, 1973.

39. **Morris JN, Heady JA, Raffle PA, Roberts CG, and Parks JW.** Coronary heart-disease and physical activity of work. *Lancet* 265: 1111–1120; concl, 1953.

40. **National Heart Blood and Lung Institute.** *Third Report of the National Cholesterol Education Program (NCEP) Expert Panel.* Detection, evaluation, and treatment of high blood cholesterol in adults (Adult Treatment Panel III) executive summary. NIH Publication No. 02–5285, 2002.

41. **Nunes JP.** The risk factor association syndrome as a barisystemic syndrome: a view on obesity and the metabolic syndrome. *Med Hypotheses* 68: 541–545, 2007.

42. **Paffenbarger RS, Jr., Blair SN, and Lee I-M.** A history of physical activity, cardiovascular health and longevity: the scientific contributions of Jeremy N. Morris, DSc, DPH, FRCP. *International J Epidemiol* 30: 1184–1192, 2001.

43. **Paffenbarger RS, Jr., Hyde RT, Wing AL, Lee IM, Jung DL, and Kampert JB.** The association of changes in physical-activity level and other lifestyle characteristics with mortality among men. N *Engl J Med* 328: 538–545, 1993.

44. **Paffenbarger RS, Jr., Laughlin ME, Gima AS, and Black RA.** Work activity of longshoremen as related to death from coronary heart disease and stroke. N *Engl J Med* 282: 1109–1114, 1970.

45. **Paffenbarger RS, Jr., Wing AL, and Hyde RT.** Physical activity as an index of heart attack risk in college alumni. *Am J Epidemiol* 108: 161–175, 1978.

46. **Pate RR, Pratt M, Blair SN, Haskell WL, Macera CA, Bouchard C, Buchner D, Ettinger W, Heath GW, King AC, et al.** Physical activity and public health. A recommendation from the Centers for Disease Control and Prevention and the American College of Sports Medicine. *Jama* 273: 402–407, 1995.

47. **Pedersen BK.** Edward F. Adolph Distinguished Lecture: muscle as an endocrine organ: IL-6 and other myokines. J *Appl Physiol* 107: 1006–1014, 2009.

48. **Powell KE, Thompson PD, Caspersen CJ, and Kendrick JS.** Physical activity and the incidence of coronary heart disease. *Annu Rev Public Health* 8: 253–287, 1987.

49. **Rabkin SW, Mathewson FA, and Hsu PH.** Relation of body weight to development of ischemic heart disease in a cohort of young North American men after a 26 year observation period: the Manitoba Study. *Am J Cardiol* 39: 452–458, 1977.

50. **Rana JS, Nieuwdorp M, Jukema JW, and Kastelein JJP.** Cardiovascular metabolic syndrome—an interplay of obesity, inflammation, diabetes and coronary heart disease. *Diabetes, Obesity and Metabolism* 9: 218–232, 2007.

51. **Reaven GM.** Banting lecture 1988. Role of insulin resistance in human disease. *Diabetes* 37: 1595–1607, 1988.

52. **Ridker PM, Danielson E, Fonseca FAH, Genest J, Gotto AM, Kastelein JJP, Koenig W, Libby P, Lorenxatti AJ, MacFadyen JG, Nordestgaard BG, Shepherd J, Willerson JT, and Glynn RJ.** Rosuvastatin to prevent vascular events in men and women with elevated C-reactive protein. *New England Journal of Medicine* 359: 2008.

53. **Rizvi AA.** Hypertension, obesity, and inflammation: the complex designs of the deadly trio. *Metabolic Syndrome and Related Disorders* 8: 287–294, 2010.

54. **Roberts CK, and Sindhu KK.** Oxidative stress and the metabolic syndrome. *Life Sciences* 84: 705–712, 2009.

55. **Rockett I.** Population and health: an introduction to epidemiology. *Population Bulletin* 49: 1–48, 1994.

56. **Stallones R.** Public Health Monograph 76. U.S. Government Printing Office, 1966.

57. **U. S. Department of Health and Human Services.** *Physical Activity and Health: A Report of the Surgeon General.* Washington, DC: U.S. Government Printing Office, 1996.

58. **U.S. Department of Health and Human Services.** Deaths: final data for 2007. *National Vital Statistics Reports* 58: 1–136, 2010.

59. **U.S. Department of Health and Human Services.** Heart disease and African Americans. http://minority-healthhhsgov/templates/contentaspx?ID=3018 2010.

60. **U.S. Department of Health Education and Welfare.** *Healthy People: The Surgeon General's Report on Health Promotion and Disease Prevention.* Washington, DC: U.S. Government Printing Office, 1979.

61. **Wang Z, and Nakayama T.** Inflammation, a link between obesity and cardiovascular disease. *Mediators of Inflammation* 2010: article ID 535918, 2010.

62. **Wassink AM, Olijhoek JK, and Visseren FL.** The metabolic syndrome: metabolic changes with vascular consequences. *Eur J Clin Invest* 37: 8–17, 2007.

Work Tests to Evaluate Cardiorespiratory Fitness

Objectives

By studying this chapter, you should be able to do the following:

1. Identify the sequence of steps in the procedures for evaluating cardiorespiratory fitness (CRF).
2. Describe one maximal and one submaximal field test used to evaluate CRF.
3. Explain the rationale underlying the use of distance runs as estimates of CRF.
4. Identify the common measures taken during a graded exercise test (GXT).
5. Describe changes in the ECG that may take place during a GXT in subjects with ischemic heart disease.
6. List three criteria for having achieved $\dot{V}O_2$ max.
7. Estimate $\dot{V}O_2$ max from the last stage of a GXT and list the concerns about the protocol that may affect that estimate.
8. Estimate $\dot{V}O_2$ max by extrapolating the HR/$\dot{V}O_2$ relationship to the person's age-predicted maximal HR.
9. Describe the problems with the assumptions made in the extrapolation procedure used in objective 8, and name the environmental and subject variables that must be controlled to improve such estimates.
10. Identify the criteria used to terminate the GXT.
11. Explain why there are so many different GXT protocols and why the rate of progression through the test is of concern.
12. Describe the YMCA's procedure to set the rate of progression on a cycle ergometer test.
13. Estimate $\dot{V}O_2$ max with the Åstrand and Ryhming nomogram given a data set for the cycle ergometer or step.

Outline

Key Terms

angina pectoris
arrhythmia
conduction disturbances
double product
dyspnea
field test
myocardial ischemia
ST segment depression

In chapter 14 we discussed the risk factors that limit health and contribute to coronary heart disease (CHD). One of those risk factors was a sedentary lifestyle. There is no question that by increasing our physical activity and cardiorespiratory function (fitness) (CRF), we can reduce the risk of many chronic diseases and death from all causes (105). This implies that changes in CRF can be measured. Although most scientists believe that the function of the cardiorespiratory system is represented best by the measurement of $\dot{V}O_2$ max, others feel that the monitoring of heart rate (HR) and blood pressure (BP) at several submaximal work rates provides a more sensitive indicator of changes in CRF (50). You are already familiar with the use of a graded exercise test (GXT) to measure $\dot{V}O_2$ max; this chapter picks up on that theme and discusses the types of tests used to evaluate CRF. The type of test used depends on the fitness of the person being tested, the purpose of the test (experimental or epidemiological investigation), and the facilities, equipment, and personnel available to conduct the test. The choice of the GXT would be different for a young healthy child as compared to a 60-year-old person with CHD risk factors. The GXT might be used as a CRF test prior to entry into a fitness program, or it could be used as a diagnostic test by a cardiologist who evaluates a twelve-lead electrocardiogram for evidence of heart disease. Clearly, the type of personnel and equipment, and of course the cost, would be very different in these two situations.

Part of the reason for such diversity in exercise testing procedures is the risk associated with exercise testing. The risk of cardiac events during exercise testing is low in apparently healthy individuals, but increases as the number of risk factors increases. In general, the overall risk of severe cardiovascular complications or death is about 6/10,000 symptom-limited tests in a mixed population (2). The risk is lower for submaximal tests.

TESTING PROCEDURES

Figure 15.1 shows a sequence of steps in a "decision tree" to identify those who might need a physician's clearance prior to taking an exercise test or participating in an exercise program. These procedures begin with a review of the person's health history to identify known diseases, sign and symptoms of disease, and risk factors. On the basis of this risk stratification procedure, decisions are made relative to the need for physician referral, the level of supervision needed for an exercise test, and the type of physical activity program (moderate vs. vigorous intensity; supervised or unsupervised).

Screening

In chapter 14 we indicated the role that risk factors play in an overall profile of health status with regard to CHD. The health histories used to screen people for GXTs or fitness programs can be as simple as the Physical Activity Readiness Questionnaire (PAR-Q) shown in figure 15.2, or a detailed form such as the $PAR_{med} - X$, which highlights absolute and relative contraindications for participating in exercise (see appendix C). An additional question added to various modifications of the PAR-Q asks about medications that might affect a person's response to exercise (e.g., an insulin-dependent diabetic or a cardiac patient taking a beta-adrenergic blocker) (84, 95). Based on known disease, signs or symptoms of specific diseases, and risk-factor information (see figure 15.1), subjects are classified into the following risk categories (2):

- Low risk: asymptomatic men <45 yrs. and women <55 yrs. who have ≤1 risk factor,
- Moderate risk: asymptomatic men ≥45 and women ≥55 who have ≥2 risk-factors, and
- High risk: individuals with known cardiovascular, pulmonary, or metabolic disease or having one or more signs or symptoms listed in figure 15.1.

On the basis of this risk stratification, the American College of Sports Medicine recommends the following (2):

- Low risk: A medical exam and GXT is not needed before beginning an exercise program, and physician supervision is not needed during the GXT.
- Moderate-risk: A medical exam and GXT is recommended prior to beginning a vigorous-intensity exercise program, but not before beginning a moderate-intensity exercise program. Physician supervision is needed during a maximal GXT exercise test, but not during a submaximal GXT.
- High risk: A medical exam and GXT is recommended before exercise of any type, and physician supervision is recommended during either a submaximal or maximal GXT.

Resting and Exercise Measures

Following the screening, measurements of heart rate and blood pressure are taken at rest prior to the exercise test. Additional measurements, such as a blood sample for serum cholesterol and an electrocardiogram (ECG), may also be obtained, with the latter one a necessity if the GXT is to be a diagnostic test. The exercise tests used to evaluate CRF may require

Figure 15.1 Decision tree in the evaluation of cardiorespiratory fitness. From American College of Sports Medicine. ACSM's *Guidelines for Exercise Testing and Prescription*, p. 24. Baltimore: Lippincott, Williams & Wilkins, 2010.

a submaximal or maximal effort by the subject. They may be conducted in a lab containing sophisticated equipment or on a running track with nothing more complicated than a stopwatch. In a submaximal GXT, HR is measured at each stage of the test that progresses from light work (~3 METs) to a predetermined end point such as 70% to 85% of predicted maximal heart rate. A treadmill, cycle ergometer, or a bench can be used to impose the work rates, and these tests will be described in detail in subsequent sections. Instead of stopping the submaximal GXT at some predetermined end point (70% to 85% maximal HR), the GXT can be taken to the point of volitional exhaustion, or to where specific signs (ECG or BP changes) or symptoms such as chest pain (**angina pectoris**) or breathlessness (**dyspnea**) occur. In these cases, CRF is based on the last work rate achieved. However, there are some maximal tests of CRF that are not "graded" and for which physiological

measurements are not made during the test [e.g., Cooper's 12-minute or 1.5-mile run (24), and the FITNESSGRAM's 1-mile run (107)]. These latter **field tests** will now be considered in more detail, along with the Canadian Home (Aerobic) Fitness Test (96) and a one-mile walk test (60). This will be followed by a discussion of GXTs using the treadmill, cycle ergometer, and bench step.

IN SUMMARY

The steps to follow before conducting an exercise test to evaluate CRF include the following:

- Review the health history for known diseases, signs and symptoms, and risk factors.
- Stratify the level of risk.
- Determine the type of test and level of supervision needed.

Physical Activity Readiness
Questionnaire - PAR-Q
(revised 2002)

PAR-Q & YOU

Regular physical activity is fun and healthy, and increasingly more people are starting to become more active every day. Being more active is very safe for most people. However, some people should check with their doctor before they start becoming much more physically active.

If you are planning to become much more physically active than you are now, start by answering the seven questions in the box below. If you are between the ages of 15 and 69, the PAR-Q will tell you if you should check with your doctor before you start. If you are over 69 years of age, and you are not used to being very active, check with your doctor.

Common sense is your best guide when you answer these questions. Please read the questions carefully and answer each one honestly: check YES or NO.

YES	NO		
☐	☐	1.	Has your doctor ever said that you have a heart condition <u>and</u> that you should only do physical activity recommended by a doctor?
☐	☐	2.	Do you feel pain in your chest when you do physical activity?
☐	☐	3.	In the past month, have you had chest pain when you were not doing physical activity?
☐	☐	4.	Do you lose your balance because of dizziness or do you ever lose consciousness?
☐	☐	5.	Do you have a bone or joint problem (for example, back, knee or hip) that could be made worse by a change in your physical activity?
☐	☐	6.	Is your doctor currently prescribing drugs (for example, water pills) for your blood pressure or heart condition?
☐	☐	7.	Do you know of <u>any other reason</u> why you should not do physical activity?

If you answered

YES to one or more questions

Talk with your doctor by phone or in person BEFORE you start becoming much more physically active or BEFORE you have a fitness appraisal. Tell your doctor about the PAR-Q and which questions you answered YES.

- You may be able to do any activity you want — as long as you start slowly and build up gradually. Or, you may need to restrict your activities to those which are safe for you. Talk with your doctor about the kinds of activities you wish to participate in and follow his/her advice.
- Find out which community programs are safe and helpful for you.

NO to all questions

If you answered NO honestly to all PAR-Q questions, you can be reasonably sure that you can:
- start becoming much more physically active — begin slowly and build up gradually. This is the safest and easiest way to go.
- take part in a fitness appraisal — this is an excellent way to determine your basic fitness so that you can plan the best way for you to live actively. It is also highly recommended that you have your blood pressure evaluated. If your reading is over 144/94, talk with your doctor before you start becoming much more physically active.

DELAY BECOMING MUCH MORE ACTIVE:
- if you are not feeling well because of a temporary illness such as a cold or a fever — wait until you feel better; or
- if you are or may be pregnant — talk to your doctor before you start becoming more active.

PLEASE NOTE: If your health changes so that you then answer YES to any of the above questions, tell your fitness or health professional. Ask whether you should change your physical activity plan.

<u>Informed Use of the PAR-Q</u>: The Canadian Society for Exercise Physiology, Health Canada, and their agents assume no liability for persons who undertake physical activity, and if in doubt after completing this questionnaire, consult your doctor prior to physical activity.

No changes permitted. You are encouraged to photocopy the PAR-Q but only if you use the entire form.

NOTE: If the PAR-Q is being given to a person before he or she participates in a physical activity program or a fitness appraisal, this section may be used for legal or administrative purposes.

"I have read, understood and completed this questionnaire. Any questions I had were answered to my full satisfaction."

NAME _____

SIGNATURE _____ DATE_____

SIGNATURE OF PARENT _____ WITNESS _____
or GUARDIAN (for participants under the age of majority)

Note: This physical activity clearance is valid for a maximum of 12 months from the date it is completed and becomes invalid if your condition changes so that you would answer YES to any of the seven questions.

CSEP
SCPE © Canadian Society for Exercise Physiology   Supported by: Health Santé
Canada Canada

Figure 15.2   Physical Activity Readiness Questionnaire (PAR-Q). A questionnaire for people aged 15 to 69. The original PAR-Q was developed by the British Columbia Ministry of Health. It has been revised by an Expert Advisory Committee assembled by the Canadian Society of Exercise Physiology and Fitness Canada (2002).

FIELD TESTS FOR ESTIMATING CRF

Maximal Run Tests

Some field tests for CRF involve a measurement of how far a person can run in a set time (12 to 15 minutes), or how fast a person can run a set distance (1 to 2 miles). The advantages of such field tests include their moderately high correlation with $\dot{V}O_2$ max, the use of a natural activity, the large numbers of people who can be tested at one time, and the low cost. The disadvantages of using field tests include the difficulty of monitoring physiological responses, the importance that motivation plays in the outcome, and the fact that the test is not graded but is a maximal effort. These field tests should be used only after a person has progressed through a program of exercise at lower intensities. The most popular field test for adults is Cooper's 12-minute or 1.5-mile run (24), and for school children, the FITNESSGRAM's 1-mile walk/run (107). The aim is to determine the average velocity that can be maintained over the time or distance. These tests represent evolutionary changes from the original work of Balke (10), who showed that running tests of 10 to 20 minutes provide reasonable estimates of $\dot{V}O_2$ max. The basis for the field tests is the linear relationship that exists between $\dot{V}O_2$ (ml $\cdot$ kg^{-1} $\cdot$ min^{-1}) and running speed, as shown in chapter 1. The duration of 10 to 20 minutes represents a compromise that attempts to maximize the chance that the person is running at a speed demanding 90% to 95% $\dot{V}O_2$ max while minimizing the contribution of energy from anaerobic sources. In distance runs of 5 minutes or less, anaerobic sources would provide relatively large amounts of energy, and $\dot{V}O_2$ max would probably be overestimated. An interesting alternative to the 1-mile run test for children is the PACER test that is used in the FITNESS-GRAM® (see A Closer Look 15.1).

The method of calculating the $\dot{V}O_2$ when the running speed is known was described in detail in A Closer Look 1.2, and the formula is presented here again:

$$\dot{V}O_2 = 0.2 \ (\text{ml} \cdot \text{kg}^{-1} \cdot \text{min}^{-1} \text{ per } \text{m} \cdot \text{min}^{-1})$$
$$+ \ 3.5 \ (\text{ml} \cdot \text{kg}^{-1} \cdot \text{min}^{-1})$$

This formula provides reasonable estimates of $\dot{V}O_2$ max for adults, but would underestimate values for young children because of their relatively poor economy of running (29). On the other hand, this formula would overestimate the value for $\dot{V}O_2$ max for those who walk, because the net cost of walking is half that of running (see A Closer Look 1.1):

$$\dot{V}O_2 = 0.1 \ (\text{ml} \cdot \text{kg}^{-1} \cdot \text{min}^{-1} \text{ per } \text{m} \cdot \text{min}^{-1})$$
$$+ \ 3.5 \ (\text{ml} \cdot \text{kg}^{-1} \cdot \text{min}^{-1})$$

Although percentile rankings of $\dot{V}O_2$ max by age and sex are available (see table 15.1), estimates of $\dot{V}O_2$ max based on distance runs are most useful when compared over time for the same individual, rather than between individuals. Variation in economy of running, motivation, and other factors makes such comparisons of estimated $\dot{V}O_2$ max values between individuals unreasonable (6, 96). In this light, distance swim and bicycle riding tests provide useful information about changes in an individual's CRF over time, even though estimates of $\dot{V}O_2$ max are not available (23, 25).

The formulas used for estimating $\dot{V}O_2$ max from a 12-minute run are not very useful for prepubescent children because their economy of running is less than that of an adult (29). Investigators (62) worked around this problem by testing first-, second-, and third-grade boys and girls with 800-, 1,200-, and 1,600-meter runs, and related performance to the

A CLOSER LOOK 15.1

Progressive Aerobic Cardiovascular Endurance Run (PACER)

An alternative test of aerobic fitness for schoolchildren is the Progressive Aerobic Cardiovascular Endurance Run, or PACER. This test, developed by Leger et al. (64, 65), is a 20-meter shuttle run test done to the sound of a "beep" as the student moves between the boundary lines. The speed required at the start is 5.3 mph (8.5 km/hr), and it increases 0.3 mph (0.5 km/hr) with each level. Three rapid beeps signal progression to the next level, where the time between beeps becomes shorter. The test is terminated when the student cannot keep up with the beeps, and the number of 20-meter laps completed is used to estimate aerobic fitness. Verbal feedback during the test appears to improve performance (76). Criterion-referenced standards for aerobic fitness (see A Closer Look 15.2) have been validated for this test (22).

The PACER test is part of the fitness testing battery in the FITNESSGRAM®, developed by the Cooper Institute (107). This protocol has also been used as a field test to estimate $\dot{V}O_2$ max in adults (75, 103). A recent study showed a "learning curve" when adult subjects were tested multiple times. This suggests that a practice test, to acquaint the subjects with the protocol, would be appropriate (63).

TABLE 15.1   Percentile Rankings for $\dot{V}O_2$ max by Age and Gender

Age	20–29		30–39		40–49		50–59		60–69		70–79	
Rating—Percentile	M	W	M	W	M	W	M	W	M	W	M	W
Superior—95th	56	50	54	47	53	45	50	40	46	37	42	37
Excellent—80th	51	44	48	41	47	39	43	35	40	32	36	30
Good—60th	46	40	44	37	42	35	38	31	35	29	31	27
Average—50th	44	37	42	35	40	33	37	30	33	28	29	25
Fair—40th	42	36	41	34	38	32	35	29	31	27	28	24
Poor—20th	38	32	37	30	35	28	31	26	27	24	24	21

Values are in $ml \cdot kg^{-1} \cdot min^{-1}$ and are rounded to nearest whole number.

Adapted from American College of Sports Medicine. *ACSM's Guidelines for Exercise Testing and Prescription*, pp. 84–89. Baltimore: Lippincott, Williams & Wilkins, 2010. Original data from Cooper Institute, Dallas, TX.

measured $\dot{V}O_2$ max scores. They found the 1,600-meter run was the best predictor with good test/retest reliability (r = 0.82 to 0.92) in children who were given instruction on paced running (62). Although performance in a run test is obviously a function of $\dot{V}O_2$ max, both running economy and the ability to run at a high % $\dot{V}O_2$ max also play a role (12, 13). It has been shown in young children of 6 to 11 years of age that % $\dot{V}O_2$ max is more closely related to performance of the 1-mile walk/run than is $\dot{V}O_2$ max (74). (See A Closer Look 15.2.)

$\dot{V}O_2$ max ($ml \cdot kg^{-1} \cdot min^{-1}$) estimated in an endurance run test is influenced by cardiovascular function and body fatness. It has been shown that differences in estimated $\dot{V}O_2$ max values between males and females can be explained, in part, by differences in % body fat (26, 29, 101). In a 12-minute run test, performance was decreased 89 meters when body weight was experimentally increased to simulate an additional 5% fat (27). One should expect, then, that with a combined exercise and weight reduction program, CRF will increase due to both an increase in cardiovascular function and a decrease in % body fat. In table 15.1, categories for $\dot{V}O_2$ max values are adjusted for age due to the observation that in the general population $\dot{V}O_2$ max decreases with age. However, studies

A CLOSER LOOK 15.2

Cardiovascular Fitness Standards for Children

The best way to evaluate fitness in children has been a concern for educators and scientists for the past century (87). The most recent controversy has revolved around the question of what kind of standards to use in making judgments about a child's level of fitness. Normative standards such as percentile scores have traditionally been used to describe where a child stands relative to his or her peers. (e.g., 75th percentile). The current thinking, especially for health-related fitness tests (1-mile walk/run test and the skinfold test) is that criterion-reference standards might be more appropriate. Criterion-reference standards attempt to describe the minimum level of fitness consistent with good health, independent of what percentile that might be in a normative data set. For example, Blair

(16) showed that in adults, $\dot{V}O_2$ max values associated with a low risk of disease were not that high; e.g., $\geq 35 \ ml \cdot kg^{-1} \cdot min^{-1}$ for men and $\geq 30 \ ml \cdot kg^{-1} \cdot min^{-1}$ for women 20 to 39 years of age. This information was used in setting the criterion-reference standards for the FITNESSGRAM, the fitness evaluation program developed by the Cooper Institute (107). $\dot{V}O_2$ max standards were set at $42 \ ml \cdot kg^{-1} \cdot min^{-1}$ for boys 5 to 17 years of age. For girls, the values were set at $40 \ ml \cdot kg^{-1} \cdot min^{-1}$ for ages 5 to 9 years of age, with a decrease of $1 \ ml \cdot kg^{-1} \cdot min^{-1}$ per year until age 14, where the $35 \ ml \cdot kg^{-1} \cdot min^{-1}$ value held until age 17 years. After the criterion-reference standards were set, the designers of the test had to translate those $ml \cdot kg^{-1} \cdot min^{-1}$ values into equivalent 1-mile run times—the

actual test the children would take. The test designers had to consider the % $\dot{V}O_2$ max at which the children would perform during the run, and the fact that economy of running improves with age. These steps, although complicated, have led to standards that are now used nationwide to classify children as to whether they have a sufficient level of cardiorespiratory fitness consistent with a low risk of disease (28). A recent study (66) and a major review (20) confirmed the validity of the criterion-referenced standards. In addition, the FITNESSGRAM® was shown to be valid and reliable when administered by teachers in a typical school setting (80). For those interested in the history of the FITNESSGRAM®, see the article by Plowman et al. in the Suggested Readings.

(50, 106) have shown that $\dot{V}O_2$ max does not decrease as fast in males who maintain their physical activity program and body weight. This observation provides additional rationale for a regular evaluation of CRF to keep track of small changes before they become big changes.

Walk Tests

An alternative to the maximal run tests used to evaluate CRF is a 1-mile walk test in which the HR is monitored during the test (60). The equation used to predict $\dot{V}O_2$ max was based on one population of men and women, aged 30 to 69, and was then validated on another comparable population. The subject walks as fast as possible for 1 mile on a flat, measured track, and HR is measured at the end of the last lap. The following equation can be used to estimate $\dot{V}O_2$ max $(ml \cdot kg^{-1} \cdot min^{-1})$:

$$\dot{V}O_2 \text{ max} = 132.853 - 0.0769 \text{ (wt)}$$
$$- 0.3877 \text{ (age)} + 6.315 \text{ (sex)}$$
$$- 3.2649 \text{ (time)} - 0.1565 \text{ (HR)}$$

where (wt) is body weight in pounds, (age) is in years, (sex) equals 0 for female and 1 for male, (time) is in minutes and hundredths of minutes, and (HR) is in beats $\cdot$ min^{-1} measured at the end of the last quarter mile.

This test appears to fill a void in the field tests available to estimate $\dot{V}O_2$ max, because it uses a common activity and requires the simple measurement of HR. As a participant's fitness improves, the time required for the mile and/or the HR response decreases, increasing the estimated $\dot{V}O_2$ max. A similar study using a 2-kilometer walk test supports this proposition (85).

Canadian Home Fitness Test

In contrast to the Cooper 1.5-mile run test and the 1-mile walk test, which require an all-out effort, the Canadian Home Fitness Test (CHFT) is a submaximal step test that uses the lowest two 8-inch steps found in a conventional staircase (97). The stepping cadence in this test is maintained by an audiotape. Prior to the test, the person completes the Physical Activity Readiness Questionnaire (PAR-Q) (figure 15.2) to determine if he or she should proceed. The first stage of the test requires the individual to step for 3 minutes at a rate equivalent to 65% to 70% of the average $\dot{V}O_2$ max of the next oldest age group (remember that $\dot{V}O_2$ max generally decreases with age). An immediate 10-second recovery pulse is counted, and if it does not exceed the maximum allowable, another 3-minute step test at 65% to 70% of the average $\dot{V}O_2$ max of the person's own age group is completed. Another pulse rate is then taken. Table 15.2 shows how physical fitness can be estimated as "undesirable, minimum, or

recommended" (97). $\dot{V}O_2$ max can be estimated from the CHFT results (14, 56, 98). A modified version of this test, which provides an improved estimate of $\dot{V}O_2$ max, is available (106, 108).

IN SUMMARY

- Field tests for CRF use natural activities such as walking, running, and stepping, in which large numbers of people can be tested at low cost. However, for some, physiological responses are difficult to measure, and motivation plays an important role in the outcome.
- $\dot{V}O_2$ max estimates from all-out run tests are based on the linear relationship between running speed and the oxygen cost of running.
- The Canadian Home Fitness Test is a step test that uses conventional 8-inch steps to evaluate cardiorespiratory fitness.
- Criterion-referenced standards for $\dot{V}O_2$ max are available. They are preferable to percentile rankings because they focus attention on health-related goals rather than comparisons with others.

GRADED EXERCISE TESTS: MEASUREMENTS

Cardiorespiratory fitness is commonly measured using a treadmill, a cycle ergometer, or a stepping bench. These tests are usually incremental, in which the work rate changes every 2 to 3 minutes until the subject reaches some predetermined end point or when some pathological sign or symptom occurs. These GXTs can be maximal or submaximal, and the variables measured during the test can be as simple as HR and BP, or as complex as $\dot{V}O_2$; it depends on the purpose of the test and the facilities, equipment, and personnel involved (49). What follows is a brief summary of common measurements made during a GXT.

Heart Rate

Heart rate can be measured by palpation of the radial or carotid artery, using a stethoscope with the microphone on the chest wall, by using surface electrodes that transmit the signal to an oscilloscope, an electrocardiograph, or a monitor that can display heart rate directly, or by using a heart watch. In palpating the carotid artery, care must be taken not to use too much pressure because this could slow the HR by way of the baroreceptor reflex. However, when people are trained in this procedure, reliable measurements can be obtained (86, 94). Heart rate is measured over

TABLE 15.2 Physical Fitness Evaluation Chart for the Canadian Home Fitness Test

TEN-SECOND PULSE RATE

Age (yr)	After First Three Minutes of Exercise	After Second Three Minutes of Exercise
15–19	If 30 or more, stop. You have an undesirable personal fitness level.	If 27 or more, you have a minimum personal fitness level. If 26 or less, you have the recommended personal fitness level.
20–29	If 29 or more, stop. You have an undesirable personal fitness level.	If 26 or more, you have a minimum personal fitness level. If 25 or less, you have the recommended personal fitness level.
30–39	If 28 or more, stop. You have an undesirable personal fitness level.	If 25 or more, you have a minimum personal fitness level. If 24 or less, you have the recommended personal fitness level.
40–49	If 26 or more, stop. You have an undesirable personal fitness level.	If 24 or more, you have a minimum personal fitness level. If 23 or less, you have the recommended personal fitness level.
50–59	If 25 or more, stop. You have an undesirable personal fitness level.	If 23 or more, you have a minimum personal fitness level. If 22 or less, you have the recommended personal fitness level.
60–69	If 24 or more, stop. You have an undesirable personal fitness level.	If 23 or more, you have a minimum personal fitness level. If 22 or less, you have the recommended personal fitness level.

From R. J. Shephard et al., "Development of the Canadian Home Fitness Test," originally published in *Canadian Medical Association Journal,* 114:675–79, 1976. Copyright © 1976 Canadian Medical Association, Ottawa, Canada. Reprinted by permission.

a 15- to 30-second time period *during* steady-state exercise to obtain a reliable estimate of the HR. If using a *post-exercise* HR as an indication of the HR during exercise, the HR should be measured for 10 seconds within the first 15 seconds after stopping exercise, because the HR changes rapidly at this time. The 10-second count is multiplied by 6 to express the HR in beats · min^{-1} (94).

Blood Pressure

Blood pressure is measured by auscultation as described in chapter 9. It is important to use the proper cuff size and a sensitive stethoscope to obtain correct values at rest and during work. In addition, if using an aneroid sphygmomanometer, it is important to calibrate it on a regular basis against the mercury sphygmomanometer (58). During the walking or cycling exercise test (BP cannot be reliably measured during a running test), the microphone of the stethoscope is placed below the cuff and over an area where the sound is the loudest (in many cases this will be in the intramuscular space on the medial side of the arm). The subject should not be holding onto the handlebar of the cycle or the railings of the treadmill during the measurement. The first Korotkoff sound is taken as systolic BP, and the fourth sound (change in tone or muffling) is taken as diastolic BP (89).

ECG

GXTs are used to diagnose CHD because exercise causes the heart to work harder and challenges the coronary arteries' ability to deliver sufficient blood to meet the oxygen demand of the myocardium. An estimate of the work (and O_2 demand) of the heart is the **double product**—the product of the HR and the systolic BP (59, 83). As you already know, HR and systolic BP increase with exercise intensity such that myocardial oxygen demand increases throughout the test. The ECG is used as an indicator of the ability of the heart to function normally during these times of imposed work. During exercise the ECG can be measured with a single bipolar lead (e.g., CM_5), but a full twelve-lead arrangement is preferred (2). The ECG is evaluated for arrhythmias, conduction disturbances, and myocardial ischemia. **Arrhythmias** are irregularities in the normal electrical rhythm of the heart that can be localized to the atria (e.g., atrial fibrillation), the AV node (e.g., premature junctional contraction), or in the ventricles (e.g., premature ventricular contractions—PVCs). **Conduction disturbances** describe a defect in which depolarization is slowed or completely blocked (e.g., first-degree AV block, or bundle branch block). **Myocardial ischemia** is defined as an inadequate perfusion of the myocardium relative to the metabolic demand of the heart. Because oxygen uptake by the myocardium

Upsloping ST segment depression   Horizontal ST segment depression   Downsloping ST segment depression

Figure 15.3 Three types of ST segment depression. From A. D. Martin, "ECG and Medications" in E. T. Howley and B. D. Franks, *Health/Fitness Instructor's Handbook.* Copyright © 1986 Human Kinetics Publishers, Inc., Champaign, IL. Used by permission.

is almost completely flow dependent, a flow limitation causes an oxygen insufficiency. A *symptom* of myocardial ischemia is angina pectoris, which is pain or discomfort caused by a temporary ischemia; the pain could be located in the center of the chest, neck, jaw, or shoulders, or could radiate to the arms and hands (69). A *sign* associated with myocardial ischemia is a depression of the ST segment on the electrocardiogram (see chapter 9). Figure 15.3 shows three types of **ST segment depression.** People with upsloping or horizontal ST segment depression have similar life expectancies, but the prognosis for those with downsloping ST segment is worse (33). Interested readers are referred to Dubin's introductory text on ECG analysis (see Suggested Readings), and Ellestad's text on exercise electrocardiography (33). For individuals who cannot perform an exercise test to evaluate cardiovascular function, a pharmacologic stress test may be substituted (see Ask the Expert 15.1).

Rating of Perceived Exertion

Another common measurement made at each stage of the GXT is Borg's (17) Rating of Perceived Exertion (RPE). Table 15.3 lists his original and revised scales. The original scale used the rankings 6 to 20 to approximate the HR values from rest to maximum (60–200). The revised scale represents an attempt to provide a ratio scale of the RPE values. The RPE scores can be used as indicators of subjective effort and provide a quantitative way to track a person's progress through a GXT or an exercise session (19, 21, 42). This is helpful in knowing when a subject is approaching exhaustion, and the values can be used to predict $\dot{V}O_2$ max (34) and prescribe exercise intensity (see chapter 16). However, large between-subject variability in RPE ratings have been noted at the same heart rate, suggesting caution in using the scales (2). What follows is

TABLE 15.3 Rating of Perceived Exertion Scales

Original Rating Scale		Revised Rating Scale	
6		0	Nothing at all
7	Very, very light	0.5	Very, very light (just noticeable)
8		1	Very light
9	Very light	2	Light (weak)
10		3	Moderate
11	Fairly light	4	Somewhat hard
12		5	Heavy (strong)
13	Somewhat hard	6	
14		7	Very heavy
15	Hard	8	
16		9	
17	Very hard	10	Very, very heavy (almost max)
18		•	Maximal
19	Very, very hard		
20			

From: G. A. U. Borg, "Psychological Bases of Physical Exertion" in *Medicine and Science in Sports and Exercise,* 14:377–81, 1982. Copyright ©1982 American College of Sports Medicine, Indianapolis, IN. Reprinted by permission.

a suggested statement from the ACSM Guidelines to read to the subject before testing (3) (p. 78):

> During the exercise test we want you to pay close attention to how hard you feel the exercise work rate is. This feeling should reflect your total amount of exertion and fatigue, combining all sensations and feelings of physical stress, effort, and fatigue. Don't concern yourself with any one factor such as leg pain, shortness of breath or exercise intensity, but try to concentrate on your total, inner feeling of exertion. Try not to underestimate or overestimate your feeling of exertion; be as accurate as you can.

Termination Criteria

The reasons for stopping a GXT vary with the type of population being tested and the purpose of the test. Table 15.4, from the ACSM's *Guidelines for Exercise Testing and Prescription,* is appropriate for nondiagnostic GXTs in apparently healthy adults (2).

IN SUMMARY

- Typical measurements obtained during a graded exercise test include heart rate, blood pressure, ECG, and rating of perceived exertion.
- Specific signs (e.g., fall in systolic pressure with an increase in work rate) and symptoms (e.g., dizziness) are used to stop GXTs.

Pharmacologic Testing to Diagnose Heart Disease
Questions and Answers with Dr. Barry Franklin

*Since 1985, **Barry A. Franklin, Ph.D.,** has been Director of the Cardiac Rehabilitation and Exercise Laboratories, William Beaumont Hospital, Royal Oak, Michigan. He is a past president of the American Association of Cardiovascular and Pulmonary Rehabilitation (AACVPR) and the American College of Sports Medicine (ACSM). He served as editor of the sixth edition of the ACSM's Guidelines for Exercise Testing and Prescription and is an internationally known speaker on topics related to cardiac rehabilitation. Recently, Dr. Franklin received the ACSM's Honor Award, the highest honor bestowed by that organization on a scientist in recognition of his many contributions to the profession.*

QUESTION: Could you briefly describe what a pharmacologic stress test is, what kinds of drugs are used, and likely candidates for such testing?

ANSWER: The need for noninvasive assessments of cardiac function for patients who are unable to exercise has led to the development of pharmacologic stress test for identifying coronary artery disease.

During these medically supervised tests, the patient lies quietly on a padded stretcher or table. Cardiac perfusion imaging (with technetium 99-m sestamibi [Cardiolite] or thallium chloride–201) is obtained with a gamma camera after intravenous dipyridamole or adenosine infusion. These potent vasodilators enhance blood flow to normally perfused heart tissue, whereas heart muscle fed by obstructed coronary arteries demonstrates relative hypoperfusion.

Another popular pharmacologic test uses dobutamine, which, in contrast to dipyridamole or adenosine stress, causes cardiac ischemia by modestly increasing heart rate and myocardial contractility. Echocardiographic images, which involve a recording sensor to bounce ultrasound waves off the heart to create an image of the muscle at work, are obtained throughout the infusion. A new or worsening wall motion abnormality suggests underlying coronary artery disease.

QUESTION: What kinds of measurements are obtained to evaluate cardiac function?

ANSWER: Heart rate, blood pressure, and electrocardiographic measurements are routinely made every minute during these drug infusions, which generally last about 6 minutes. Perfusion imaging under resting conditions is then compared with imaging obtained after coronary vasodilation. Patients are also queried regarding adverse side effects, which may include light-headedness, chest pain or pressure, and nausea. Echocardiographic images (in contrast to perfusion images) are made during dobutamine infusions. In some cases, like exercise stress tests, pharmacologic studies may be prematurely terminated due to the development of worsening symptoms or significant heart rhythm irregularities.

QUESTION: Can the results of these tests be used to develop an exercise prescription?

ANSWER: It is difficult to use the results of these tests to develop an exercise prescription. This is primarily because the rises in heart rate and oxygen consumption during pharmacologic testing are far lower than those achieved with exercise stress. These tests simply suggest whether there is underlying myocardial ischemia and coronary artery disease. Consequently, many clinicians recommend an initial exercise heart rate that is twenty to thirty beats above standing rest, as the prescribed training intensity, using perceived exertion as an adjunctive intensity modulator.

TABLE 15.4	**General Indications for Stopping an Exercise Test in Low-Risk Adults***

- Onset of angina or angina-like symptoms
- Drop in systolic blood pressure of >10 mm Hg from baseline blood pressure despite an increase in workload
- Excessive rise in blood pressure: systolic pressure >250 mm Hg or diastolic pressure >115 mm Hg
- Shortness of breath, wheezing, leg cramps, or claudication
- Signs of poor perfusion: light-headedness, confusion, ataxia, pallor, cyanosis, nausea, or cold and clammy skin
- Failure of heart rate to increase with increased exercise intensity
- Noticeable change in heart rhythm
- Subject requests to stop
- Physical or verbal manifestations of severe fatigue
- Failure of the testing equipment

*Assumes that testing is nondiagnostic and is being performed without direct physician involvement or ECG monitoring.
From American College of Sports Medicine. *ACSM's Guidelines for Exercise Testing and Prescription.* Baltimore: Lippincott, Williams & Wilkins, 2010.

$\dot{V}O_2$ MAX

The measurement of $\dot{V}O_2$ max represents the standard against which any estimate of CRF is compared (see chapters 4 and 20 for procedures). $\dot{V}O_2$ increases with increasing loads on a GXT until the maximal capacity of the cardiorespiratory system is reached; attention to detail is crucial if one is to obtain accurate values (72). Commonly used criteria for having achieved $\dot{V}O_2$ max include a leveling off of the $\dot{V}O_2$ (<150 ml $\cdot$ kg^{-1} $\cdot$ min^{-1} or <2.1 ml $\cdot$ kg^{-1} $\cdot$ min^{-1}) even though a higher work rate is achieved (99), a post-exercise blood lactate level of >8 mmoles $\cdot$ liter^{-1} (5), and the R exceeding 1.15 (54). Some investigators use heart rate (e.g., a value within 10 b/min of age-predicted maximal heart rate) as a criterion for having achieved $\dot{V}O_2$ max. However, due to the relatively large potential error (1 SD = 10–12 b/min) in estimating maximal heart rate with the age-predicted formulas (e.g., 220 − age), its usefulness as a criterion for having achieved $\dot{V}O_2$ max has been questioned (51). Although many subjects will meet these criteria, some, especially the elderly (100), children (5), and postcoronary subjects (57), will not. In addition, one should not expect a subject to meet all of these standards (57, 100). For example, in one study (100), 20 percent of the women subjects who met the "leveling off" criterion did not even achieve an R of 1.00! The R values have been shown to vary with age and the training status of the subjects (1). In general, these criteria are useful because they give the investigator an objective indicator of the subject's effort. However, subjects should not be expected to meet all the criteria on any single test (31, 51). (See A Closer Look 15.3 for an update on the plateau or leveling-off criterion.)

A CLOSER LOOK 15.3

$\dot{V}O_2$ Max and the Plateau—Needed or Not?

The concept of $\dot{V}O_2$ max and its dependence on cardiac output was described by Hill and Lupton in 1923 (48). Over the following decades investigators had to deal with a central issue in the measurement of $\dot{V}O_2$ max: How can one be certain that a true $\dot{V}O_2$ max had actually been obtained? The concept of a plateau in oxygen uptake with increasing intensities of exercise (using a discontinuous format) was central to Hill and Lupton's description of $\dot{V}O_2$ max. However, in practice, great variation exists in the percentage of subjects who achieve a plateau. This led to the development of a variety of secondary criteria for having achieved $\dot{V}O_2$ max (e.g., post-exercise blood lactate >8 mM; respiratory exchange ratio >1.15) as mentioned in the text. The fact that continuous (incremental) exercise tests have become the most common protocol complicates the issue.

In a recent paper, Hawkins et al. (45) used 52 well-trained distance runners as subjects to reevaluate the issue of the plateau. The investigators showed clearly that the $\dot{V}O_2$ max achieved in an incremental running test was not different from that achieved in a subsequent running test requiring a $\dot{V}O_2$ 30% higher than that measured in the incremental test. This study clearly supported the underlying proposition of

Hill and Lupton—that is, there really is an upper limit to oxygen uptake.

In contrast to the clarity of the results of this study by Hawkins et al. (45), most investigators are continuously faced with the dilemma of finding only a small percentage of subjects experiencing a plateau in $\dot{V}O_2$ during a continuous incremental exercise test. Work by Day et al. (30) offers some relief from this problem. They measured $\dot{V}O_2$ on 71 subjects during an incremental ramp-type protocol taken to the point of fatigue. At test termination, only 12 of 71 subjects had demonstrated a plateau in $\dot{V}O_2$ (relative to a $\dot{V}O_2$ max value extrapolated from submaximal $\dot{V}O_2$ measurements). Thirty-eight of the 71 subjects subsequently completed a constant load test at a power output ~90% of the peak power attained in the incremental test. Subjects terminated the test due to fatigue in 4 to 10 minutes. The $\dot{V}O_2$ max achieved in the constant load test was not different from that measured during the incremental test. Additional tests on six subjects were conducted at a variety of higher power outputs and confirmed the $\dot{V}O_2$ max values. The central point was that even though a plateau was not observed in the vast majority of the cases in the incremental test, the $\dot{V}O_2$ max was not different

from that obtained in a follow-up constant load test. Even though the power output in the follow-up test was lower than that achieved in the incremental test, the oxygen demand of the peak power achieved in a ramp protocol is well above the measured $\dot{V}O_2$ as shown by the subjects fatiguing in 4 to 10 minutes at a load ~90% of peak power.

Another study (91) from the same group used a follow-up constant load test 5 minutes after the subjects had fatigued in a standard incremental ramp protocol test. The follow-up tests were done at 95% and 105% of the peak power achieved on the incremental test. For five subjects, who completed both constant load protocols, fatigue occurred at an average of 130 and 89 seconds, respectively. The $\dot{V}O_2$ max achieved in each constant load test was the same as that measured at the end of the incremental ramp protocol in which no subject had demonstrated a plateau. This study showed that one could obtain confirmation of $\dot{V}O_2$ max within the same testing session. Foster et al. (38) supported these findings.

The issue of "being sure" about the $\dot{V}O_2$ max value will be with us for some time; however, Day et al. (30) and Rossiter et al. (91) showed that a plateau is not a prerequisite for being able to measure a true $\dot{V}O_2$ max (50).

$\dot{V}O_2$ max is a very reproducible measure on subjects tested with the same test protocol on the same piece of equipment. The value for $\dot{V}O_2$ max does not seem to be dependent on whether the test is a continuous GXT or a discontinuous GXT, as long as it is conducted with the same work instrument (31, 35, 71, 102). However, when $\dot{V}O_2$ max values are compared across protocols, some systematic differences appear (9). The highest value for $\dot{V}O_2$ max is usually measured with a running test up a grade on a treadmill, followed by a walking test up a grade on a treadmill, and then on a cycle ergometer. In American populations, walk test protocols yield values about 6% lower than those for a run test (71), while cycle test protocols yield values about 10% to 11% lower than those for a run test (31, 36, 61). Europeans show only a 5% to 7% difference in this latter comparison (9, 47). An arm ergometer test will yield values equal to about 70% of the $\dot{V}O_2$ max measured with the legs (39, 93). It is important to recognize these differences when comparing one test to another, or when comparing the same subject over time with different modes of exercise. These differences among tests have led to the convention to call $\dot{V}O_2$ *max* the value measured on a graded running test; $\dot{V}O_2$ *peak* is the term used to describe the highest $\dot{V}O_2$ achieved on walk, cycle, or arm ergometer protocol (92). However, these terms can cause confusion when applied to highly trained athletes, such as cyclists, because they have higher $\dot{V}O_2$ max values when measured on a cycle, compared to a treadmill (104). The actual measurement of $\dot{V}O_2$ max is crucial for research studies and in some clinical settings. However, it is unreasonable to expect the actual measurement of $\dot{V}O_2$ max to be used as the CRF standard in fitness programs.

Estimation of $\dot{V}O_2$ Max from Last Work Rate

Given the complexity and cost of the procedures involved in the measurement of $\dot{V}O_2$ max, it is no surprise that in many fitness and clinical settings $\dot{V}O_2$ max is estimated with equations that allow the calculation of $\dot{V}O_2$ max from the last work rate achieved on the GXT. The equations for estimating the oxygen cost of running and walking outlined in chapter 1 allow such calculations and, in general, the estimates are reasonable (78, 79). What is important in the use of these equations is that the work test is suited to the individual. If the increments in the GXT from one stage to the next are too large relative to a person's CRF, or if the time for each stage is so short that a person might not be able to achieve the steady-state oxygen requirement for that stage, then the equations will overestimate the person's $\dot{V}O_2$ max (37, 44, 78). As described in chapter 4, poorly fit individuals take longer to achieve the steady state at moderate to heavy work rates, and this increases the chance of an overestimation of

$\dot{V}O_2$ max when using these formulas. This suggests that a more conservative protocol be used for low-fit individuals to allow them to reach a steady state at each stage. A recommended procedure is to use only the last completed stage of a test. However, independent of the proper matching of the protocol with the individual, it must be remembered that these are only estimations (see A Closer Look 15.4).

Estimation of $\dot{V}O_2$ Max from Submaximal HR Response

Another common procedure used with GXT protocols is to estimate $\dot{V}O_2$ max on the basis of the subject's HR response to a variety of submaximal work rates (41). In these tests the HR is plotted against work rate (or estimated $\dot{V}O_2$) until the termination criterion of 70% to 85% of age-predicted maximal HR is reached. Figure 15.4 shows the HR response for a 20-year-old who has taken a submaximal GXT on a cycle ergometer. Heart rate was measured at each work rate until a value equal to 85% of estimated maximal HR was reached (170 b · min^{-1}). A line was drawn through the HR points and extrapolated to the estimated maximal HR, which is calculated by subtracting age from 220. Another line is dropped from that point to the x-axis, and the work rate or $\dot{V}O_2$ (in this case, 2.7 L · min^{-1}) that would have been achieved if the individual had worked until maximal HR was reached is recorded (41). Although this is a simple and commonly used procedure to estimate $\dot{V}O_2$ max, it has several potential problems.

The first problem relates to the formula used for estimating the maximal HR. These estimates have a standard deviation (SD) of about ±11 b · min^{-1} (67). A 20-year-old's maximal HR might be estimated to be 200 b · min^{-1}, but if a person were out at ±2 SD, the value would be 178 or 222 b · min^{-1}. For those who do maximal testing, one will occasionally observe subjects having *measured* maximal HRs ±20 b · min^{-1} away from their age-predicted estimate of maximal heart rate. Taking this as an example, what if the subject in figure 15.4 had a true maximal HR of only 180 b · min^{-1} instead of the estimated 200 b · min^{-1}? The estimated $\dot{V}O_2$ max would be an overestimation of the correct value.

Further, a submaximal end point such as 85% of estimated maximal heart rate may be very light work for one person and maximal work for another. The reason for this is related to the estimate of maximal heart rate (220 — age) mentioned earlier. If a 30-year-old has a real maximum heart rate of 160 b min^{-1} and the GXT takes the person to 85% of estimated maximal HR (220 − 30 = 190; 85% of 190 = 161 b · min^{-1}), then the person would be taken to maximal HR.

Another problem with submaximal GXT protocols using the HR response as the primary indicator of fitness is that any variable that affects submaximal heart rate will affect the slope of the HR/$\dot{V}O_2$ line and,

Error in Estimating V̇O₂ Max

It is important to remember that the estimation of $\dot{V}O_2$ max by any of the methods described in this chapter is associated with an inherent "error" compared to the directly measured $\dot{V}O_2$ max value. When investigators try to determine the validity of an exercise test to estimate $\dot{V}O_2$ max, they must first test large numbers of subjects in the laboratory to actually measure each subject's $\dot{V}O_2$ max. On another day, the investigators may have the subjects complete a distance run for time, or a standardized graded treadmill or cycle ergometer test to determine the highest percent grade/speed or work rate that the subject can achieve. That information is then used to develop an equation to predict the measured $\dot{V}O_2$ max value from the time of the distance run, the last grade/speed achieved on a treadmill test, or the final work rate on the cycle ergometer test.

The predicted value will not usually equal the measured $\dot{V}O_2$ max value, and a term called the standard error (SE) is used to describe how far off (higher or lower) the predicted value might be from the true value when using the prediction equation. One standard error (±SE) describes where 68% of the estimates are compared to the true value. If the SE were ± 1 ml · kg^{-1} · min^{-1}, then 68% of the predicted $\dot{V}O_2$ max values would fall within ± 1 ml · kg^{-1} · min^{-1} of the true value. Typically, the SE is larger than that (2, 89). For example:

- If $\dot{V}O_2$ max is estimated from the last stage of a maximal test, the SE = ± 3 ml · kg^{-1} · min^{-1}.

- If $\dot{V}O_2$ max is estimated from heart rate values measured during a submaximal test, the SE = ± 4–5 ml · kg^{-1} · min^{-1}.

- If $\dot{V}O_2$ max is estimated from the 1-mile walk test or the 12-minute run test described earlier, the SE = ± 5 ml · kg^{-1} · min^{-1}.

The relatively large standard errors might suggest that these tests have little value, but that is not the case. The tests are reliable, and when the same individual takes the same test over time, the change in estimated $\dot{V}O_2$ max monitored by the test is a reasonable reflection of improvements in cardiorespiratory fitness. This can serve as both a motivational and educational tool when working with fitness clients.

Figure 15.4 Estimation of $\dot{V}O_2$ max from heart rate values measured during a series of submaximal work rates on a cycle ergometer. The test was stopped when the subject reached 85% of maximal HR. A line is drawn through the HR points measured during the test and is extrapolated to the age-predicted estimate of maximal HR. Another line is dropped from that point to the x-axis, and the $\dot{V}O_2$ max is identified.

of course, the estimate of $\dot{V}O_2$ max. These variables include eating prior to the test, dehydration, elevated body temperature, temperature and humidity of the testing area, emotional state of the subject, medications that affect HR, and previous physical activity (7, 96). Clearly, many environmental variables must be controlled if one is to use such protocols to estimate $\dot{V}O_2$ max.

Despite these problems, this estimate of $\dot{V}O_2$ max is useful in providing appropriate feedback to participants in fitness programs. Following training, the HR response to any fixed submaximal work rate is lower, suggesting an increase in $\dot{V}O_2$ max when the HR/$\dot{V}O_2$ line is drawn through those HR points to the age-predicted maximal HR. In this case, because the same individual is being tested over time, the 220 − age formula introduces only a constant and unknown error that will not affect the projection of the HR/$\dot{V}O_2$ line. Further, the low cost, ease of measurement, and high reliability make it a good test that can be used for education and motivation (95).

IN SUMMARY

- The measurement of $\dot{V}O_2$ max is the gold standard measure of cardiorespiratory fitness.
- $\dot{V}O_2$ max can be estimated based on the final work rate achieved in a graded exercise test.
- $\dot{V}O_2$ max can be estimated from heart rate responses to submaximal exercise by extrapolating the relationship to the subject's age-predicted estimate of maximal heart rate. Careful attention to environmental factors that can affect the heart rate response to submaximal exercise is an important aspect of the procedures for these tests.

GRADED EXERCISE TEST: PROTOCOLS

The GXT protocols can be either submaximal or maximal, depending on the end points used to stop the test. The choice of the GXT should be based on the population (athletes, cardiac patients, children), purpose (estimate CRF, measure $\dot{V}O_2$ max, diagnose CHD), and cost (equipment and personnel) (49, 53). This section will discuss the selection of the test based on these factors and provide examples of common GXT protocols.

When choosing a GXT protocol, the population being tested must be considered, given that the last stage in a GXT for cardiac patients might not even be a warm-up for a young, athletic subject. Test protocols should vary in terms of the initial work rate, how large the increment in work rate will be between stages, and the duration of each stage. In general, the GXT for a sedentary subject might start at 2 to 3 METs (1 MET = 3.5 ml $\cdot$ kg^{-1} $\cdot$ min^{-1}) and progress at about 1 MET per stage, with each stage lasting 2 to 3 minutes to allow enough time for a steady state to be reached. For young, active subjects, the initial work rate might be 5 METs, with increments of 2 to 3 METs per stage (89). Table 15.5 shows four well-known treadmill protocols and the populations for which they are suited. The National Exercise and Heart Disease protocol (82) is usually used with poorly fit subjects, with the work rate increasing only 1 MET each 3 minutes. The Standard Balke protocol (11) starts at about 4 METs and progresses 1 MET each 2 minutes, and is suitable for most average sedentary adults. The Bruce protocol for young, active subjects (18) starts at about 5 METs and progresses at 2 to 3 METs per stage. This protocol includes walking and running up a grade, and may not be suitable for those at the low end of the fitness continuum. The last protocol shown is used by the fit and athletic populations, with the speed dependent on the fitness of the subject (7).

As mentioned earlier, one of the most common approaches used in estimating $\dot{V}O_2$ max is to take the final stage in the test and apply the formula for converting grade and speed to $\dot{V}O_2$ in ml $\cdot$ kg^{-1} $\cdot$ min^{-1}. Nagle et al. (81) and Montoye et al. (78) have shown that apparently healthy individuals reach the new steady-state requirement by approximately 1.5 minutes of each stage up to moderately heavy work. These formulas give reasonable estimates of CRF if the test has been suited to the individual (44, 78). However, if the increments in the stages are too large, or if the time at each stage is too short, the person might not be able to reach the oxygen requirement associated with that stage of the GXT. In these cases the formulas will overestimate the subject's $\dot{V}O_2$ max.

TABLE 15.5 Treadmill Protocols

A—NATIONAL EXERCISE AND HEART DISEASE PROTOCOL FOR POORLY FIT SUBJECTS (82)

Stage*	METs	Speed (mph)	% Grade
1	2.5	2	0
2	3.5	2	3.5
3	4.5	2	7.0
4	5.5	2	10.5
5	6.5	2	14.0
6	7.5	2	17.5
7	8.5	3	12.5
8	9.5	3	15.0
9	10.5	3	17.5

*Stage lasts three minutes.

B—STANDARD BALKE PROTOCOL FOR NORMAL SEDENTARY SUBJECTS (11)

Stage*	METs	Speed (mph)	% Grade
1	4.3	3	2.5
2	5.4	3	5.0
3	6.4	3	7.5
4	7.4	3	10.0
5	8.5	3	12.5
6	9.5	3	15.0
7	10.5	3	17.5
8	11.6	3	20.0
9	12.6	3	22.5

*Stage lasts two minutes.

C—BRUCE PROTOCOL FOR YOUNG, ACTIVE SUBJECTS (18)

Stage*	METs	Speed (mph)	% Grade
1	5	1.7	10
2	7	2.5	12
3	9.5	3.4	14
4	13	4.2	16
5	16	5.0	18

*Stage lasts three minutes.

D—ÅSTRAND AND RODAHL PROTOCOL FOR VERY FIT SUBJECTS (7)

Stage*	METs	Speed (mph)	% Grade
1	12.9/18	7/10	2.5
2	14.1/19.8	7/10	5.0
3	15.3/21.5	7/10	7.5
4	16.5/23.2	7/10	10.0
5	17.7/24.9	7/10	12.5

*Stage lasts two minutes; vigorous warm-up precedes test.

IN SUMMARY

- When selecting a GXT, the population being tested must be considered. The initial work rate and the rate of change of work rate need to accommodate the capabilities of the population.

Treadmill

Treadmill GXT protocols can accommodate most people, from those least fit to those most fit, and use the natural activities of walking and running. Treadmills set the pace for the subject and provide the greatest potential load on the cardiovascular system. However, they are expensive, not portable, and make some measurements (BP and blood sampling) difficult (96). As mentioned previously, the type of treadmill test does influence the magnitude of the measured $\dot{V}O_2$ max, with the graded running test giving the highest value, the running test at 0% grade the next highest, and the walking test protocols the lowest (9, 71). There are also some limitations in the types of measurements that can be made, depending on whether walking or running is used. For example, during running tests, the measurement of BP is not convenient and may be less accurate, and there is more potential for artifact in the ECG tracing.

For estimates of $\dot{V}O_2$ to be obtained from grade and speed considerations, the grade and speed settings must be correct (49). In addition, the subject must follow instructions carefully and not hold onto the treadmill railing during the test. If this is not done, estimates of $\dot{V}O_2$ max based on either the HR/$\dot{V}O_2$ extrapolation procedure or the formula that uses the last speed/grade combination achieved will not be accurate (6, 90). For example, when a subject who was walking on a treadmill at 3.4 mph and 14% grade held onto the railing, the HR decreased 17 b · min^{-1} (6). This would result in an overestimation of the $\dot{V}O_2$ max using either of the submaximal procedures just mentioned, and special equations would have to be developed if holding onto the handrail were allowed (73). Finally, with the treadmill there is no need to make adjustments to the $\dot{V}O_2$ calculation due to differences in body weight. Treadmill tests require the subject to carry his or her own weight, and the $\dot{V}O_2$ is therefore proportional to body weight (77).

In the following example of a submaximal GXT, a 45-year-old male takes a Balke Standard Protocol (3 mph, 2.5% each 2 minutes), and the test is terminated at 85% of age-predicted maximal HR (149 b · min^{-1}). Heart rate was measured in the last 30 seconds of each stage, and $\dot{V}O_2$ max was estimated by the HR/$\dot{V}O_2$ extrapolation to age-predicted maximal HR (175 b · min^{-1}). Figure 15.5 shows the plot of the HR response at each stage, and the extrapolation to the person's estimated maximal heart rate. In the early stages of the test, the HR did not increase in a predictable manner with increasing grade. This may be due to the changes in stroke volume that occur early in upright work (see chapter 9). The beginning stages also act as a warm-up and adjustment period for the subject. The HR response is usually quite linear between 110 b · min^{-1} and 85% maximal HR (8). The HR/$\dot{V}O_2$ line is extrapolated

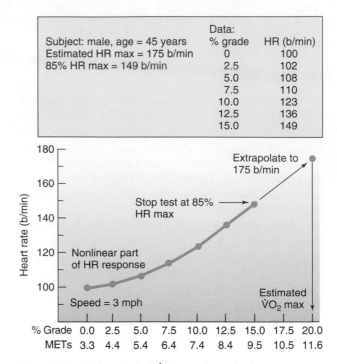

Subject: male, age = 45 years	Data: % grade	HR (b/min)
Estimated HR max = 175 b/min	0	100
85% HR max = 149 b/min	2.5	102
	5.0	108
	7.5	110
	10.0	123
	12.5	136
	15.0	149

Figure 15.5 Estimation of $\dot{V}O_2$ max from the heart rate values measured during different stages of a treadmill test. From E. T. Howley and B. D. Franks, *Health/Fitness Instructor's Handbook*. Copyright © 1986 Human Kinetics Publishers, Inc., Champaign, IL. Used by permission.

to 175 b · min^{-1}, and a vertical line is dropped to the x-axis where the estimated $\dot{V}O_2$ max is identified: 11.6 METs, or 40.6 ml · kg^{-1} · min^{-1}.

A single-stage submaximal treadmill test has been validated for use with low-risk subjects who are likely to have average values for $\dot{V}O_2$ max (32). In this test the treadmill is set at 0% grade, and a walking speed is set between 2 and 4.5 mph to elicit a heart rate between 50% and 70% of age-predicted maximal HR. Following this 4-minute warm-up, the grade is elevated to 5% for 4 minutes. HR is measured in the last minute and used with speed (S in mph), age (A in years), and gender (G, with female = 0 and male = 1) in the following regression equation to predict $\dot{V}O_2$ max:

$$\dot{V}O_2 \text{ max} = 15.1 + 21.8 \text{ (S)} - 0.327 \text{ (HR)} - 0.263$$
$$(S \times A) + 0.00504 \text{ (HR} \times A) + 5.98 \text{ (G)}$$

Finally, investigators have adapted the 1-mile walk test mentioned earlier under "field test" so it could be done on a treadmill. Subjects completed a questionnaire to rate their level of physical activity and then walked on the treadmill at a self-selected speed that they classified as "brisk." The investigators had to develop a new prediction equation, different from the outdoor test, and it was shown to provide a valid estimate of $\dot{V}O_2$ max (88). To learn more about an individual who had a major impact on fitness testing, see A Look Back—Important People in Science.

A LOOK BACK—IMPORTANT PEOPLE IN SCIENCE

Bruno Balke, M.D., Ph.D.—The "Father" of ACSM Certification Programs

As we mentioned in chapter 0, the history of exercise physiology in the United States during the twentieth century had a very strong European flavor. This was certainly the case for the development of fitness testing and cardiac rehabilitation. **Dr. Bruno Balke** (1907–1999) received his training in physical education, medicine, and physiology in Germany and was invited to this country by Dr. Ulrich Luft in 1950.

During the 1950s, Dr. Balke conducted research on high-altitude tolerance and high-speed flight for the U.S. Air Force at the School of Aviation Medicine in San Antonio, Texas, and later, for the Federal Aviation Agency in Oklahoma City. His research on work-capacity testing on the treadmill led to the development of the exercise test protocols that bear his name (discussed earlier in this chapter). In addi-

tion, his distance-run field test to evaluate cardiovascular fitness (maximal aerobic power) was modified by Dr. Ken Cooper for use in his well-known aerobics books (see Field Tests for Estimating CRF in this chapter).

Dr. Balke left government service in 1963 to create the Biodynamics Laboratory at the University of Wisconsin, Madison. Francis J. Nagle, Ph.D., whom he had worked with in Oklahoma City, followed in 1964, and both had joint appointments with the physical education and physiology departments. Dr. Balke's quantitative approach to exercise physiology questions, especially as they related to fitness and performance, set the standard for other graduate exercise physiology programs. He regarded his time in Madison as the most productive in his career.

Dr. Balke left Wisconsin for Aspen, Colorado, in 1973. During this time he invested himself in the development of American College of Sports Medicine

(ACSM) certification programs for exercise leaders of fitness and cardiac rehabilitation programs. Special meetings were held in Aspen to develop the certification programs and ACSM's *Guidelines for Exercise Testing and Prescription.* The first workshops associated with these certification programs were held in Aspen as well. Many consider him the "father" of ACSM certification programs.

Dr. Balke was active in the early days of the ACSM and served as its president in 1966. Balke also took the lead in the creation of ACSM's research journal, then known as *Medicine and Science in Sports,* and was its first editor-in-chief. He enjoyed teaching others how to do things, and he viewed as his greatest accomplishment the graduation of the Ph.D. students from his lab who would now teach others. Dr. Balke died in 1999 at the age of 92, but his legacy will live on for years to come. For more on this interesting man, see his autobiography in the Suggested Readings.

Cycle Ergometer

Cycle ergometers are portable, moderately priced work instruments that allow measurements to be made easily. However, they are self-paced and result in some localized fatigue (96). On mechanically braked cycle ergometers (e.g., Monark), the work rate can be increased by increasing the pedal rate or the resistance on the flywheel. Generally, the pedal rate is maintained constant during a GXT at a rate suitable to the populations being tested: 50 to 60 rpm for the low to average fit, and 70 to 100 for the highly fit and competitive cyclists (43). The pedal rate is maintained by having the subject pedal to a metronome, or by providing some other source of feedback (visual analog or digital display of the rpm). The load on the wheel is increased in a sequential fashion to systematically overload the cardiovascular system. The starting work rate and the increment from one stage to the next depend on the fitness of the subject and the purpose of the test. The $\dot{V}O_2$ can be estimated from an equation that gives reasonable estimates of the $\dot{V}O_2$ up to work rates of about 1,200 kgm · min^{-1} (2):

$$\dot{V}O_2 \text{ (ml · min}^{-1}) = 1.8 \text{ ml · kgm}^{-1} \times \text{kgm · min}^{-1}$$
$$+ (7 \text{ ml · kg}^{-1} · \text{min}^{-1} \times \text{kg body wt.)}$$

The cycle ergometer is different from the treadmill in that the body weight is supported by the seat, and the work rate is dependent primarily on the crank speed and the load on the wheel. This means that for a small person, the relative $\dot{V}O_2$ at any work rate is higher than that for a big person. For example, if a work rate requires a $\dot{V}O_2$ of 2,100 ml · min^{-1}, this represents a relative $\dot{V}O_2$ of 35 ml · kg^{-1} · min^{-1} for a 60-kg person, and only 23 ml · kg^{-1} · min^{-1} for a 90-kg person. In addition, the increments in the work rate, by demanding a fixed increase in the $\dot{V}O_2$ (e.g., an increment of 150 kgm · min^{-1} is equal to a $\dot{V}O_2$ change of 270 ml · min^{-1}), force a small and unfit subject to make larger cardiovascular adjustments than a large or high-fit subject. These factors have been taken into consideration by the YMCA (41) in recommending submaximal GXT protocols. The idea is to provide a means of obtaining a variety of HR responses to several submaximal work rates in a way that reduces the duration of the test.

Figure 15.6 shows the different "routes" followed in the YMCA protocol depending on the subject's HR response to a work rate of 150 kgm · min^{-1}. The YMCA protocol makes use of the observation that the relationship between $\dot{V}O_2$ and HR is a linear one between 110 and 150 b · min^{-1}. For this reason the YMCA protocol

First work load — 150 kgm / 0.5 kp

HR<86 | HR 86-100 | HR>100

Second work load
600 kgm 2.0 kp | 450 kgm 1.5 kp | 300 kgm 1.0 kp

Third work load
750 kgm 2.5 kp | 600 kgm 2.0 kp | 450 kgm 1.5 kp

Fourth work load
900 kgm 3.0 kp | 750 kgm 2.5 kp | 600 kgm 2.0 kp

Directions:

1. Set the first work load at 25 W or 150 kgm · min^{-1} (0.5 kp).
2. If the HR in the 3rd minute is
   - less than (<) 86, set the second load at 100 W or 600 kgm · min^{-1} (2 kp);
   - 86 to 100, set the second load at 75 W or 450 kgm · min^{-1} (1.5 kp);
   - greater than (>) 100, set the second load at 50 W or 300 kgm · min^{-1} (1 kp).
3. Set the third and fourth (if required) loads according to the loads in the columns below the second loads.

Figure 15.6   YMCA protocol used to select work rates for submaximal cycle ergometer tests. From the YMCA *Fitness Testing and Assessment Manual.* Copyright © 2000 YMCA of the USA. Reprinted by permission.

requires the subject to exercise at only one more work rate past the one that yields an HR ≥ 110 b · min^{-1}. As a general recommendation for all cycle ergometer tests, seat height is adjusted so that the knee is slightly bent when the foot is at the bottom of the pedal swing and parallel to the floor; the seat height is recorded for later testing. In the YMCA protocol, each stage lasts 3 minutes and heart rate values are obtained in the last 30 seconds of the second and third minutes. If the difference in HR is <5 b · min^{-1} between the two time periods, a steady state is assumed; if not, an additional minute is added to that stage. A line then connects the two HR values and is extrapolated to the subject's estimated maximal HR. A vertical line is dropped to the x-axis and the estimated $\dot{V}O_2$ max value is obtained as described for the submaximal treadmill protocol.

Figure15.7 shows the YMCA protocol for a 30-year-old female who weighs 60 kg. The first work rate chosen was 150 kgm · min^{-1}, and a heart rate of 103 b · min^{-1} was measured. Following the YMCA protocol, the next loads were 300 and then 450 kgm · min^{-1}, and the measured HR values were 115 and 128 b · min^{-1}, respectively. A line was drawn through the two HR points greater than 110 b · min^{-1} and extrapolated to age-predicted max HR (190 b · min^{-1}). The estimated $\dot{V}O_2$ max for this woman

Data:
Subject: female, age = 30 years	Work rate (kpm/min)	Heart rate (b/min)
Estimated HR max = 190 b/min	150	103
85% HR max = 162 b/min	300	115
Body weight = 60 kg	450	128

Figure 15.7   Example of the YMCA protocol used to estimate $\dot{V}O_2$ max. From E. T. Howley and B. D. Franks, *Health/Fitness Instructor's Handbook.* Copyright © 1986 Human Kinetics Publishers, Inc., Champaign, IL. Used by permission.

was approximately 2.58 liters · min^{-1} or 43 ml · kg^{-1} · min^{-1}, using the previous equation.

In addition to this extrapolation procedure for estimating $\dot{V}O_2$ max, Åstrand and Ryhming (8) provide a method that requires the subject to complete one work bout of approximately 6 minutes, demanding an HR between 125 and 170 b · min^{-1}. These investigators observed that at 50% $\dot{V}O_2$ max, males had an average HR of 128, and females, 138 b · min^{-1}, and at 70% $\dot{V}O_2$ max the average HRs were 154 and 164 b · min^{-1}, respectively. These data were collected on young men and women, ages 18 to 30. The basis for the test is that if you know from an HR response that a person is at 50% $\dot{V}O_2$ max at a work rate equal to 1.5 L · min^{-1}, then the estimated $\dot{V}O_2$ max would be twice that, or 3.0 L · min^{-1}. A nomogram (see figure 15.8) is used to estimate the $\dot{V}O_2$ max based on the subject's HR response to one 6-minute work bout. Because maximal HR decreases with increasing age, and the data were collected on young subjects, Åstrand (4) established correction factors to multiply the estimated $\dot{V}O_2$ max values taken from the nomogram in order to correct for the lower maximal HR.

Siconolfi et al. (99) developed a submaximal cycle ergometer test for epidemiological investigations that is a modification of the YMCA protocol that uses the Åstrand and Ryhming (8) nomogram. It is presented here because the advantages of this test include (1) the requirement that the subject achieve only 70% of the estimated maximal HR, and (2) the procedure was validated on men and women of ages 20 to 70 years. Men over age 35 and all women start the

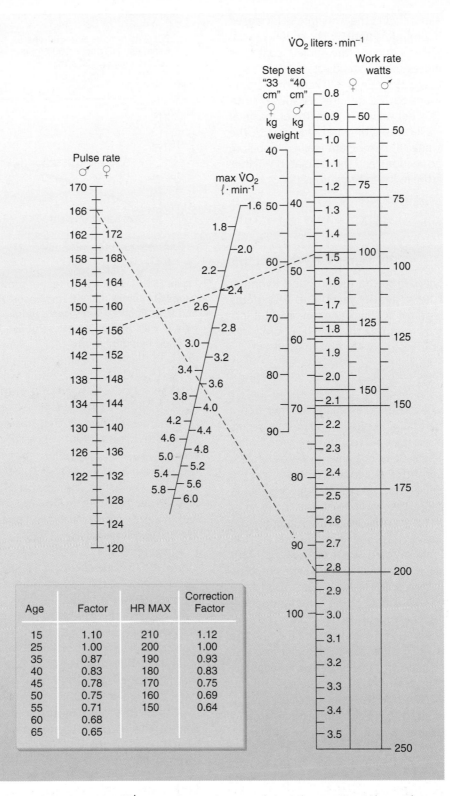

Figure 15.8 Nomogram for the estimation of $\dot{V}O_2$ max from submaximal HR values measured on either a cycle ergometer or step test. For the cycle ergometer, the work rate in watts (1 watt = 6.1 kgm · min⁻¹) is shown on the two rightmost columns, one for men and one for women. The results of a cycle ergometer test for a man who worked at 200 watts is shown. A dashed line is drawn between the 200-watt work rate and the HR value of 166 measured during the test. The estimated $\dot{V}O_2$ max is 3.6 liters · min⁻¹. The step test uses a rate of 22.5 lifts · min⁻¹, and two different step heights, 33 cm for women and 40 cm for men. The step test scale lists body weight for the subject, and the results of a test on a 61-kg woman are shown. A dashed line is drawn between the 61 kg on the 33-cm scale and the HR value of 156 b · min⁻¹ measured during the test. The estimated $\dot{V}O_2$ max is 2.4 liters · min⁻¹. These estimates of $\dot{V}O_2$ max are influenced by the person's maximal HR, which is known to decrease with age. A correction factor chosen from the accompanying table corrects these $\dot{V}O_2$ max values when either the maximal HR or age is known. Simply multiply the $\dot{V}O_2$ value by the correction factor.

test at 150 kgm · min⁻¹, and the work rate is increased that amount each 2 minutes until an HR ≥ 70% of estimated maximal HR is achieved; the subject continues for 2 or more minutes until a steady-state HR is measured. Men under age 35 begin at 300 kgm · min⁻¹ and increase that amount each 2 minutes as above. However, when the HR is between 60% and 70% of maximal HR, the work rate is increased only 150 kgm · min⁻¹. The Åstrand and Ryhming (8) nomogram is used as before (without the age correction), and the estimated $\dot{V}O_2$ max values are used in the following equations (99):

For males:
$$\dot{V}O_2 \text{ (liters} \cdot \text{min}^{-1}) = 0.348 (X_1) - 0.035 (X_2) + 3.011$$
For females:
$$\dot{V}O_2 \text{ (liters} \cdot \text{min}^{-1}) = 0.302 (X_1) - 0.019 (X_2) + 1.593$$

where $X_1 = \dot{V}O_2$ max from the Åstrand and Ryhming nomogram, and $X_2 =$ age in years. The test yields acceptable estimates of $\dot{V}O_2$ max and puts the subject under less stress by requiring that an HR of only 70% of the age-predicted maximal HR be achieved.

Step Test

A step-test protocol is used to estimate $\dot{V}O_2$ max in the same way that treadmill and cycle ergometer protocols are used. The step test does not require expensive equipment, the step height does not have to be calibrated, everyone is familiar with the stepping exercise, and the energy requirement is proportional to body weight, as with the treadmill (68). The work rate can be increased by increasing the step height while keeping the cadence the same, or by increasing the cadence while keeping the step height the same. The step height can be varied with a hand-cranking device (81) or by using a series of steps with increments in step height of 10 cm. The rate of stepping is established with a metronome, and the stepping cadence has four counts: up, up, down, down. The subjects must step all the way up and down in time with the metronome. Figure 15.9 shows the results of a step test on a 60-year-old female. In this step test the height of the step was kept constant at 16 centimeters and the rate of stepping increased 6 lifts · min⁻¹ each 2 minutes. The line drawn through the HR points is extrapolated to the estimated maximal HR, 160 b · min⁻¹, and a line is dropped to the horizontal axis to estimate the $\dot{V}O_2$ max using the following equation (2):

$$\dot{V}O_2 = 0.2 \text{ (step rate)} + [1.33 \times 1.8$$
$$\times \text{ (step height [m])} \times \text{(step rate)]} + 3.5$$

The equation yields values in ml · kg⁻¹ · min⁻¹, which are converted to METs by dividing by 3.5.

The Åstrand and Ryhming (8) nomogram (figure 5.8) also accommodates a step test, using a rate of 22.5 lifts per minute (metronome = 90) and step heights of 40 cm for men and 33 cm for women. The principle is the same as described for their cycle ergometer protocol.

Figure 15.9 Use of a step test to predict $\dot{V}O_2$ max from a series of submaximal HR responses. From E. T. Howley and B. D. Franks, *Health/Fitness Instructor's Handbook.* Copyright © 1986 Human Kinetics Publishers, Inc., Champaign, IL. Used by permission.

The introduction of step ergometers (i.e., StairMaster) allows a graded exercise test to be conducted in a manner similar to that of a treadmill. The work rates are independent of step rate, and the HR responses are slightly higher than those measured on the treadmill at any $\dot{V}O_2$ (52). Such a test has been shown to measure changes in $\dot{V}O_2$ max that result from either treadmill or step-ergometer training, indicating more commonality than specificity among step and treadmill tests (15).

In summary, a variety of tests can be used to estimate CRF. The usefulness of a test is a function of both the accuracy of the measurement and the ability to repeat the test on a routine basis to evaluate changes in CRF over time. It is this latter point that decreases the need that the test be able to estimate the true $\dot{V}O_2$ max to the nearest ml · kg⁻¹ · min⁻¹. In effect, if a person is taking a submaximal GXT on a regular basis and the HR response to a fixed work rate is decreasing over time, one can reasonably conclude that the person is making progress in the intended direction, independent of how accurate the estimate of $\dot{V}O_2$ max is. But what if a person did not have to take an exercise test to estimate $\dot{V}O_2$ max? See A Closer Look 15.5.

IN SUMMARY

- $\dot{V}O_2$ max can be estimated with the extrapolation procedure using the treadmill, cycle ergometer, or step.
- The subject must follow directions carefully and environmental conditions must be controlled if the estimate of $\dot{V}O_2$ max is to be reasonable and reproducible.

A CLOSER LOOK 15.5

Can $\dot{V}O_2$ Max Be Estimated Without Doing an Exercise Test?

This may seem like a strange question given the focus of this chapter on exercise testing. However, if it were possible, investigators (e.g., epidemiologists) could easily classify large numbers of individuals into levels of cardiorespiratory fitness (e.g., bottom 20%, middle 20% and top 20%), and determine if cardiorespiratory fitness is linked to various chronic diseases. Doing exercise testing on large populations of individuals is impossible due to time, cost, personnel, etc.

In one of the earliest investigations, Jackson et al. (55) showed that by using the simple variables of age, gender, body fatness or body mass index, and self-reported physical activity, $\dot{V}O_2$ max could be estimated with a SE of $\sim \pm 5 \ ml \cdot kg^{-1} \cdot min^{-1}$, an error similar to what we observe with our field tests and submaximal GXT estimates of $\dot{V}O_2$ max. The accuracy of the prediction (SE $\sim \pm 4$–$6 \ ml/kg^{-1} \cdot min^{-1}$) has been confirmed in several other studies (40, 46, 70, 109–111). These models have been useful in placing subjects into different fitness categories; however, the accuracy of the prediction is less in the most and least fit subjects (110).

What does this say about doing exercise tests—the focus of this chapter? As we mentioned at the outset, even though the SE is relatively large for field tests and submaximal GXTs, the tests are reliable, and when the same individual takes the same test over time, the change in estimated $\dot{V}O_2$ max monitored by the test is a reasonable reflection of improvements in cardiorespiratory fitness. This can serve as both a motivational and educational tool when working with fitness clients.

STUDY QUESTIONS

1. What is the sequence of steps used in evaluating cardiorespiratory fitness?
2. What is the PAR-Q? What does risk stratification mean?
3. Name one maximal and one submaximal field test to estimate $\dot{V}O_2$ max.
4. A 40-year-old man runs 1.5 miles (2,415 meters) in 10 minutes. What is his estimated $\dot{V}O_2$ max? Is his value "normal"?
5. Because many subjects do not exhibit a plateau in oxygen consumption in the last stages of a maximal GXT, what other criteria could be used to show that the person was exercising maximally when the highest $\dot{V}O_2$ was measured?
6. Given the following information collected during a treadmill test on a 50-year-old man, estimate his $\dot{V}O_2$ max.

Work Rate	Heart Rate
3 METs	110
5 METs	125
7 METs	140

7. Given the assumption that the formula 220 – age can be used to estimate maximal heart rate, how far off could you be in your estimate of $\dot{V}O_2$ max in question 6?
8. What information do you gain by monitoring the RPE during a GXT?
9. List five reasons for stopping a GXT for low-risk adults.
10. Should you use the same GXT protocol on all subjects? Why or why not?

SUGGESTED READINGS

Balke, B. 2007. *Matters of the Heart: Adventures in Sports Medicine* (H. Marg, ed.). Monterey, CA: Healthy Learning.

Dubin, D. 2000. *Rapid Interpretation of EKGs: A Programmed Course*, 6th ed. Tampa, FL: Cover.

Heyward, V. H. 2006. *Advanced Fitness Assessment and Exercise Prescription*, 5th ed. Champaign, IL: Human Kinetics.

Plowman, S. A., C. L. Sterling, C. B. Corbin, M. D. Meredith, G. J. Welk, and J. R. Morrow. 2006. The history of the FITNESSGRAM®. *Journal of Physical Activity and Health*. 3 (Supple 2): S5–S20.

REFERENCES

1. **Aitken JC, and Thompson J.** The respiratory $\dot{V}CO_2/\dot{V}O_2$ exchange ratio during maximum exercise and its use as a predictor of maximum oxygen uptake. *European Journal of Applied Physiology and Occupational Physiology* 57: 714–719, 1988.
2. **American College of Sports Medicine.** *ACSM's Guidelines for Exercise Testing and Prescription*. Baltimore: Lippincott Williams & Wilkins, 2010.
3. **American College of Sports Medicine.** *Guidelines for Exercise Testing and Prescription*. Baltimore: Lippincott Williams & Wilkins, 2006.
4. **Astrand I.** Aerobic work capacity in men and women with special reference to age. *Acta Physiologica Scandinavica* 49: 1–92, 1960.
5. **Åstrand PO.** *Experimental Studies of Physical Working Capacity in Relation to Sex and Age*. Copenhagen: Manksgaard, 1952.
6. **Åstrand PO.** Principles of ergometry and their implications in sports practice. *International Journal of Sports Medicine* 5: 102–105, 1984.
7. **Åstrand PO, and Rodahl K.** *Textbook of Work Physiology*. New York: McGraw-Hill, 1986.

8. **Astrand PO, and Ryhming I.** A nomogram for calculation of aerobic capacity (physical fitness) from pulse rate during sub-maximal work. *Journal of Applied Physiology* 7: 218–221, 1954.

9. **Astrand PO, and Saltin B.** Maximal oxygen uptake and heart rate in various types of muscular activity. *Journal of Applied Physiology* 16: 977–981, 1961.

10. **Balke B.** *A Simple Feld Test for Assessment of Physical Fitness.* Civil Aeromedical Research Institute Report 63–66, 1963.

11. **Balke B.** *Advanced Exercise Procedures for Evaluation of the Cardiovascular System. Monograph.* Milton: The Burdick Corporation, 1970.

12. **Bassett DR, Jr., and Howley ET.** Limiting factors for maximum oxygen uptake and determinants of endurance performance. *Medicine and Science in Sports and Exercise* 32: 70–84, 2000.

13. **Bassett DR, Jr., and Howley ET.** Maximal oxygen uptake: "classical" versus "contemporary" viewpoints. *Medicine and Science in Sports and Exercise* 29: 591–603, 1997.

14. **Bell DG, Jacobs I, and Lee SW.** Blood lactate response to the Canadian Aerobic Fitness Test (CAFT). *Canadian Journal of Sport Sciences = Journal Canadien des Sciences du Sport* 17: 14–18, 1992.

15. **Ben-Ezra V, and Verstraete R.** Step ergometry: is it task-specific training? *European Journal of Applied Physiology and Occupational Physiology* 63: 261–264, 1991.

16. **Blair SN, Kohl HW, III, Paffenbarger RS, Jr., Clark DG, Cooper KH, and Gibbons LW.** Physical fitness and all-cause mortality: a prospective study of healthy men and women. *JAMA* 262: 2395–2401, 1989.

17. **Borg GA.** Psychophysical bases of perceived exertion. *Medicine and Science in Sports and Exercise* 14: 377–381, 1982.

18. **Bruce RA.** Multi-stage treadmill tests of maximal and submaximal exercise. In: *Exercise Testing and Training of Apparently Healthy Individuals: A Handbook for Physicians.* New York: American Heart Association, 1972, p. 32–34.

19. **Carton RL, and Rhodes EC.** A critical review of the literature on ratings scales for perceived exertion. *Sports Medicine (Auckland, NZ)* 2: 198–222, 1985.

20. **Castro-Piñero J, Artero EG, España-Romero V, Ortega FB, Sjöström M, Suni J, and Ruiz JR.** Criterion-related validity of field-based fitness tests in youth: a systematic review. *British Journal of Sports Medicine* 44: 934–943, 2010.

21. **Chow RJ, and Wilmore JH.** The regulation of exercise intensity by ratings of perceived exertion. *Journal of Cardiac Rehabilitation* 4: 382–387, 1984.

22. **Chun DM, Corbin CB, and Pangrazi RP.** Validation of criterion-referenced standards for the mile run and progressive aerobic cardiovascular endurance tests. *Research Quarterly for Exercise and Sport* 71: 125–134, 2000.

23. **Conley DS, Cureton KJ, Dengel DR, and Weyand PG.** Validation of the 12-min swim as a field test of peak aerobic power in young men. *Medicine and Science in Sports and Exercise* 23: 766–773, 1991.

24. **Cooper KH.** *The Aerobics Way.* New York: Bantam, 1977.

25. **Cooper M, and Cooper KH.** *Aerobics for Women.* New York: Evans, 1972.

26. **Cureton KJ, Hensley LD, and Tiburzi A.** Body fatness and performance differences between men and women. *Research Quarterly* 50: 333–340, 1979.

27. **Cureton KJ, Sparling PB, Evans BW, Johnson SM, Kong UD, and Purvis JW.** Effect of experimental alterations in excess weight on aerobic capacity and distance running performance. *Medicine and Science in Sports* 10: 194–199, 1978.

28. **Cureton KJ, and Warren GL.** Criterion-referenced standards for youth health-related fitness tests: a tutorial. *Research Quarterly for Exercise and Sport* 61: 7–19, 1990.

29. **Daniels J, Oldridge N, Nagle F, and White B.** Differences and changes in $\dot{V}O_2$ among young runners 10 to 18 years of age. *Medicine and Science in Sports* 10: 200–203, 1978.

30. **Day JR, Rossiter HB, Coats EM, Skasick A, and Whipp BJ.** The maximally attainable $\dot{V}O_2$ during exercise in humans: the peak vs. maximum issue. *Journal of Applied Physiology* 95: 1901–1907, 2003.

31. **Duncan GE, Howley ET, and Johnson BN.** Applicability of $\dot{V}O_2$ max criteria: discontinuous versus continuous protocols. *Medicine and Science in Sports and Exercise* 29: 273–278, 1997.

32. **Ebbeling CB, Ward A, Puleo EM, Widrick J, and Rippe JM.** Development of a single-stage submaximal treadmill walking test. *Medicine and Science in Sports and Exercise* 23: 966–973, 1991.

33. **Ellestad M.** *Stress Testing: Principles and Practice.* Philadelphia: F. A. Davis, 2003.

34. **Eston RG, Faulkner JA, Mason EA, and Parfitt G.** The validity of predicting maximal oxygen uptake from perceptually regulated graded exercise tests of different durations. *European Journal of Applied Physiology* 97: 535–541, 2006.

35. **Falls HB, and Humphrey LD.** A comparison of methods for eliciting maximum oxygen uptake from college women during treadmill walking. *Medicine and Science in Sports* 5: 239–241, 1973.

36. **Faulkner JA, Roberts DE, Elk RL, and Conway J.** Cardiovascular responses to submaximum and maximum effort cycling and running. *Journal of Applied Physiology* 30: 457–461, 1971.

37. **Foster C.** Prediction of oxygen uptake during exercise testing in cardiac patients and health volunteers. *Journal of Cardiac Rehabilitation* 4: 537–542, 1984.

38. **Foster C, Kuffel E, Bradley N, Battista RA, Wright G, Porcari JP, Lucia A, and deKoning JJ.** $\dot{V}O_2$ max during successive maximal efforts. *European Journal of Applied Physiology* 102: 67–72, 2007.

39. **Franklin BA.** Exercise testing, training and arm ergometry. *Sports Medicine (Auckland, NZ)* 2: 100–119, 1985.

40. **George JD, Stone WJ, and Burkett LN.** Non-exercise $\dot{V}O_2$ max estimation for physcially active college students. *Med Sci Sports Exercise* 29: 415–423, 1997.

41. **Golding LA.** YMCA *Fitness Testing and Assessment Manual.* Champaign: Human Kinetics, 2000.

42. **Gutmann M.** Perceived exertion-heart rate relationship during exercise testing and training of cardiac patients. *Journal of Cardiac Rehabilitation* 1: 52–59, 1981.

43. **Hagberg JM, Mullin JP, Giese MD, and Spitznagel E.** Effect of pedaling rate on submaximal exercise responses of competitive cyclists. *Journal of Applied Physiology* 51: 447–451, 1981.

44. **Haskell WL, Savin W, Oldridge N, and DeBusk R.** Factors influencing estimated oxygen uptake during exercise testing soon after myocardial infarction. *The American Journal of Cardiology* 50: 299–304, 1982.

45. **Hawkins MN, Raven PB, Snell PG, Stray-Gundersen J, and Levine BD.** Maximal oxygen uptake as a parametric measure of cardiorespiratory capacity. *Medicine and Science in Sports and Exercise* 39: 103–107, 2007.

46. **Heil DP, Freedson PS, Ahlquist LE, Price J, and Rippe JM.** Nonexercise regression models to estimate peak oxygen consumption. *Med Sci Sports Exercise* 27: 599–606, 1995.

47. **Hermansen L, and Saltin B.** Oxygen uptake during maximal treadmill and bicycle exercise. *Journal of Applied Physiology* 26: 31–37, 1969.

48. **Hill A, and Lupton H.** Muscular exercise, lactic acid, and the supply and utilization of oxygen. *Q J Med* 16: 135–171, 1923.

49. **Howley ET.** Exercise testing laboratory. In: *Resource Manual for Guidelines for Exercise Testing and Prescription*, edited by Blair SN. Philadelphia: Lea & Febiger, 1988.

50. **Howley ET.** $\dot{V}O_2$ max and the plateau—needed or not? *Medicine and Science in Sports and Exercise* 39: 101–102, 2007.

51. **Howley ET, Bassett DR, Jr., and Welch HG.** Criteria for maximal oxygen uptake: review and commentary. *Medicine and Science in Sports and Exercise* 27: 1292–1301, 1995.

52. **Howley ET, Colacino DL, and Swensen TC.** Factors affecting the oxygen cost of stepping on an electronic stepping ergometer. *Medicine and Science in Sports and Exercise* 24: 1055–1058, 1992.

53. **Howley ET, and Franks BD.** *Health Fitness Instructor's Handbook.* Champaign: Human Kinetics, 2007.

54. **Issekutz B, Birkhead NC, and Rodahl K.** The use of respiratory quotients in assessment of aerobic power capacity. *Journal of Applied Physiology* 17: 47–50, 1962.

55. **Jackson AS, Blair SN, Mahar MT, Wier LT, Ross RM, and Stuteville JE.** Prediction of functional aerobic capacity without exercise testing. *Medicine and Science in Sports and Exercise* 22: 863–870, 1990.

56. **Jette M, Campbell J, Mongeon J, and Routhier R.** The Canadian Home Fitness Test as a predictor for aerobic capacity. *Canadian Medical Association Journal* 114: 680–682, 1976.

57. **Kavanagh T, and Shephard RJ.** Maximum exercise tests on "postcoronary" patients. *Journal of Applied Physiology* 40: 611–618, 1976.

58. **Kirkendall WM, Feinleib M, Freis ED, and Mark AL.** Recommendations for human blood pressure determination by sphygmomanometers: subcommittee of the AHA Postgraduate Education Committee. *Circulation* 62: 1146A–1155A, 1980.

59. **Kitamura K, Jorgensen CR, Gobel FL, Taylor HL, and Wang Y.** Hemodynamic correlates of myocardial oxygen consumption during upright exercise. *Journal of Applied Physiology* 32: 516–522, 1972.

60. **Kline GM, Porcari JP, Hintermeister R, Freedson PS, Ward A, McCarron RF, Ross J, and Rippe JM.** Estimation of $\dot{V}O_2$ max from a one-mile track walk, gender, age, and body weight. *Medicine and Science in Sports and Exercise* 19: 253–259, 1987.

61. **Kohl HW, Gibbons LW, Gordon NF, and Blair SN.** An empirical evaluation of the ACSM guidelines for exercise testing. *Medicine and Science in Sports and Exercise* 22: 533–539, 1990.

62. **Krahenbuhl GS, Pangrazi RP, Petersen GW, Burkett LN, and Schneider MJ.** Field testing of cardiorespiratory fitness in primary school children. *Medicine and Science in Sports* 10: 208–213, 1978.

63. **Lamb KL, and Rogers L.** A re-appraisal of the reliability of the 20 m multi-stage shuttle run test. *European Journal of Applied Physiology* 100: 287–292, 2007.

64. **Leger LA, and Lambert J.** A maximal multistage 20-m shuttle run test to predict $\dot{V}O_2$ max. *European Journal of Applied Physiology and Occupational Physiology* 49: 1–12, 1982.

65. **Leger LA, Mercier D, Gadoury C, and Lambert J.** The multistage 20 metre shuttle run test for aerobic fitness. *Journal of Sports Sciences* 6: 93–101, 1988.

66. **Lobelo F, Pate RR, Dowda M, Liese AD, and Ruiz JR.** Validity of cardiorespiratory fitness criterion-referenced standards for adolescents. *Medicine and Science in Sports and Exercise* 41: 1222–1229, 2009.

67. **Londeree BR, and Moeschberger ML.** influence of age and other factors on maximal heart rate. *Journal of Cardiac Rehabilitation* 4: 44–49, 1984.

68. **Margaria R, Aghemo P, and Rovelli E.** Indirect determination of maximal O_2 consumption in man. *Journal of Applied Physiology* 20: 1070–1073, 1965.

69. **Martin AD.** ECG and medications. In: *Health/Fitness Instructor's Handbook*, edited by Howley ET, and Franks BD. Champaign: Human Kinetics, 1986.

70. **Matthews CE, Heil DP, Freedson PS, and Pastides H.** Classification of cardiorespiratory fitness without exercise testing. *Medicine and Science in Sports and Exercise* 31: 486–493, 1999.

71. **McArdle WD, Katch FI, and Pechar GS.** Comparison of continuous and discontinuous treadmill and bicycle tests for max $\dot{V}O_2$. *Medicine and Science in Sports* 5: 156–160, 1973.

72. **McConnell TR.** Practical considerations in the testing of $\dot{V}O_2$ max in runners. *Sports Medicine* (Auckland, NZ) 5: 57–68, 1988.

73. **McConnell TR, and Clark BA.** Prediction of maximal oxygen consumption during handrailsup ported treadmill exercise. *Journal of Cardiopulmonary Rehabilitation* 7: 324–331, 1987.

74. **McCormack WP, Cureton KJ, Bullock TA, and Weyand PG.** Metabolic determinants of 1-mile run/walk performance in children. *Medicine and Science in Sports and Exercise* 23: 611–617, 1991.

75. **McNaughton L, Hall P, and Coolcy D.** Validation of several methods of estimating maximal oxygen uptake in young men. *Perceptual and Motor Skills* 87: 575–584, 1998.

76. **Metsios GS, Flouris AD, Koutedakis Y, and Theodorakis Y.** The effect of performance feedback on cardiorespiratory fitness field tests. *Journal of Science and Medicine in Sport/Sports Medicine Australia* 9: 263–266, 2006.

77. **Montoye HJ, and Ayen T.** Body size adjustment for oxygen requirement in treadmill walking. *Research Quarterly for Exercise and Sport* 57: 82–84, 1986.

78. **Montoye HJ, Ayen T, Nagle F, and Howley ET.** The oxygen requirement for horizontal and grade walking on a motor-driven treadmill. *Medicine and Science in Sports and Exercise* 17: 640–645, 1985.

79. **Montoye HJ, Ayen T, and Washburn RA.** The estimation of $\dot{V}O_2$ max from maximal and sub-maximal measurements in males, age 10–39. *Research Quarterly for Exercise and Sport* 57: 250–253, 1986.

80. **Morrow Jr. JR, Martin SB, and Jackson AW.** Reliability and validity of the FITNESSGRAM®: quality of teacher-collected health-related fitness surveillance data. *Research Quarterly for Exercise and Sport* 81: S24–S30, 2010.

81. **Nagle FJ, Balke B, and Naughton JP.** Gradational step tests for assessing work capacity. *Journal of Applied Physiology* 20: 745–748, 1965.

82. **Naughton JP, and Haider R.** Methods of exercise testing. In: *Exercise Testing and Exercise Training in Coronary Heart Disease*, edited by J. P. Naughton HKH, and L. C. Mohler. New York: Academic Press, 1973, p. 79–91.

83. **Nelson RR, Gobel FL, Jorgensen CR, Wang K, Wang Y, and Taylor HL.** Hemodynamic predictors of myocardial oxygen consumption during static and dynamic exercise. *Circulation* 50: 1179–1189, 1974.

84. **NIH.** *Exercise and Your Heart:* Publication, No. 81–1677. edited by U.S. Department of Health and Human Services 1981.

85. **Oja P, Laukkanen R, Pasanen M, Tyry T, and Vuori I.** A 2-km walking test for assessing the cardiorespiratory fitness of healthy adults. *Int J Sports Med* 12: 356–362, 1991.

86. **Oldridge NB, Haskell WL, and Single P.** Carotid palpation, coronary heart disease and exercise rehabilitation. *Medicine and Science in Sports and Exercise* 13: 6–8, 1981.

87. **Park RJ.** Measurement of physical fitness: a historical perspective. edited by U.S. Department of Health and Human Services, Public Health Service, 1989.

88. **Pober DM, Freedson PS, Kline GM, McInnis KJ, and Rippe JM.** Development and validation of a one-mile treadmill walk test to predict peak oxygen uptake in healthy adults ages 40 to 79 years. *Canadian Journal of Applied Physiology = Revue Canadienne de Physiologie Appliquee* 27: 575–589, 2002.

89. **Pollock ML, and Wilmore JH.** *Exercise in Health and Disease.* Philadelphia: W. B. Saunders, 1990.

90. **Ragg KE, Murray TP, Karbonit LM, and Jump DA.** Errors in predicting functional capacity from a treadmill exercise stress test. *American Heart Journal* 100: 581–583, 1980.

91. **Rossiter HB, Kowalchuk JM, and Whipp BJ.** A test to establish maximum O_2 uptake despite no plateau in the O_2 uptake response to ramp incremental exercise. *Journal of Applied Physiology* 100: 764–770, 2006.

92. **Rowell LB.** Human cardiovascular adjustments to exercise and thermal stress. *Physiological Reviews* 54: 75–159, 1974.

93. **Sawka MN, Foley ME, Pimental NA, Toner MM, and Pandolf KB.** Determination of maximal aerobic power during upper-body exercise. *Journal of Applied Physiology* 54: 113–117, 1983.

94. **Sedlock D.** Accuracy of subject-palpated carotid pulse after exercise. *The Physician and Sportsmedicine* 11: 106–116, 1983.

95. **Sharkey BJ.** *Physiology of Fitness.* Champaign: Human Kinetics, 1984.

96. **Shephard RJ.** Tests of maximum oxygen intake: a critical review. *Sports Medicine* (Auckland, NZ) 1: 99–124, 1984.

97. **Shephard RJ, Bailey DA, and Mirwald RL.** Development of the Canadian Home Fitness Test. *Canadian Medical Association Journal* 114: 675–679, 1976.

98. **Shephard RJ, Thomas S, and Weller I.** The Canadian Home Fitness Test: 1991 update. *Sports Medicine* (Auckland, NZ) 11: 358–366, 1991.

99. **Siconolfi SF, Cullinane EM, Carleton RA, and Thompson PD.** Assessing $\dot{V}O_2$ max in epidemiologic studies: modification of the Astrand-Rhyming test. *Medicine and Science in Sports and Exercise* 14: 335–338, 1982.

100. **Sidney KH, and Shephard RJ.** Maximum and submaximum exercise tests in men and women in the seventh, eighth, and ninth decades of life. *Journal of Applied Physiology* 43: 280–287, 1977.

101. **Sparling PB, and Cureton KJ.** Biological determinants of the sex difference in 12-min run performance. *Medicine and Science in Sports and Exercise* 15: 218–223, 1983.

102. **Stamford BA.** Step increment versus constant load tests for determination of maximal oxygen uptake. *European Journal of Applied Physiology and Occupational Physiology* 35: 89–93, 1976.

103. **Stickland MK, Petersen SR, and Bouffard M.** Prediction of maximal aerobic power from the 20-m multi-stage shuttle run test. *Canadian Journal of Applied Physiology = Revue Canadienne de Physiologie Appliquee* 28: 272–282, 2003.

104. **Stromme SB, Ingjer F, and Meen HD.** Assessment of maximal aerobic power in specifically trained athletes. *Journal of Applied Physiology* 42: 833–837, 1977.

105. **U.S. Department of Health and Human Services.** 2008 Physcial activity guidelines for Americans. http://wwwhealthgov/paguidelines/guidelines/defaultaspx 2008.

106. **Wallace JP.** Physical conditioning: intervention in aging cardiovascular function: part A: quantitation, epidemiology, and clinical research. In: *Intervention in the Aging Process,* edited by Liss AR1983, p. 307–323.

107. **Welk GJ, and Meredith MD.** FITNESSGRAM/ACTIVITYGRAM *Reference Guide.* Dallas, TX: The Cooper Institute, 2008.

108. **Weller IM, Thomas SG, Corey PN, and Cox MH.** Prediction of maximal oxygen uptake from a modified Canadian aerobic fitness test. *Canadian Journal of Applied Physiology = Revue Canadienne de Physiologie Appliquee* 18: 175–188, 1993.

109. **Whaley MH, Kaminsky LA, SDwyer GB, and Getchell LH.** Failure of predicted $\dot{V}O_2$ peak to discriminate physical fitness in epidemiological studies. *Medicine and Science in Sports and Exercise* 27: 85–91, 1995.

110. **Wier LT, Jackson AS, Ayers GW, and Arenare B.** Nonexercise models for estimating $\dot{V}O_2$ max with waist girth, percent fat, or BMI. *Medicine and Science in Sports and Exercise* 38: 555–561, 2006.

111. **Williford HN, Scharff-Olson M, Wang N, Blessing DL, Smith FH, and Duey WJ.** Cross-validation of nonexercise predictions of $\dot{V}O_2$ peak in women. *Med Sci Sports Exercise* 28: 926–930, 1996.

Exercise Prescriptions for Health and Fitness

■ Objectives

By studying this chapter, you should be able to do the following:

1. Characterize physical inactivity as a coronary heart disease risk factor comparable to smoking, hypertension, and high serum cholesterol.

2. Contrast exercise with physical activity; explain how both relate to a lower risk of CHD and improvement in cardiorespiratory fitness (CRF).

3. Describe the current public health physical activity recommendation from the U.S. *Physical Activity Guidelines* to improve the health status of sedentary U.S. adults.

4. Explain what screening and progression mean for a person wanting to initiate an exercise program.

5. Identify the optimal range of frequency, intensity, and duration of activity associated with improvements in CRF.

6. Calculate a target heart rate range by either the heart rate reserve or percent of maximal HR methods.

7. Explain why the appropriate sequence of physical activity for sedentary persons is walk → walk/jog → jog → games.

8. Explain how the target heart rate (THR) helps adjust exercise intensity in times of high heat, humidity, or while at altitude.

9. Describe the recommended resistance-training program for adults.

■ Outline

■ Key Terms

dose
effect (response)
exercise
physical activity (PA)
physical fitness
target heart rate (THR) range

In chapter 14 we discussed a variety of risk factors related to cardiovascular and other diseases. Physical inactivity had long been considered only a secondary risk factor in the development of CHD—that is, an inactive lifestyle would increase a person's risk for CHD only if other primary risk factors were present. However, as explained in chapter 14, this is no longer the case. Numerous studies (43, 45, 55, 65) suggest that physical inactivity is a primary risk factor for coronary heart disease (CHD), similar to smoking, hypertension, and high serum cholesterol. These studies also show that regular vigorous physical activity is instrumental in reducing the risk of CHD in those who smoke or are hypertensive (38, 44). Based on this growing body of evidence, the American Heart Association (AHA) recognized physical inactivity as a primary or major risk factor (6). Finally, epidemiological studies show that increases in physical activity (46) and fitness (8) are associated with a reduced death rate from all causes as well as from CHD. This means that physical activity should be used along with other therapies to reduce the risk of CHD in those possessing other risk factors. Consequently, there is little disagreement that regular physical activity is a necessary part of a healthy lifestyle (74). The only question is, how much?

Before we answer this question we need to distinguish among the terms *physical activity*, *exercise*, and *physical fitness*. **Physical activity (PA)** is defined as any form of muscular activity. Therefore physical activity results in the expenditure of energy proportional to muscular work and is related to physical fitness. **Physical fitness** is defined as a set of attributes that people have or develop that relate to the ability to perform physical activity. **Exercise** represents a subset of physical activity that is planned, with a goal of improving or maintaining fitness (12). These distinctions, while subtle, are important to understand in our discussion of the role of physical activity as a part of a healthy lifestyle. For example, there is no question that a planned exercise program will improve $\dot{V}O_2$ max, and that a higher $\dot{V}O_2$ max is associated with a lower death rate (9). However, we must emphasize that physical activity, including that done at a moderate intensity, is beneficial. The reduction in the risks of CHD due to the latter types of activity may be mediated through changes in the distribution of cholesterol or an increase in fibrinolysis (clot dissolving) activity (24). It should be no surprise that the American College of Sports Medicine, in the ACSM's *Guidelines for Exercise Testing and Prescription*, and *Physical Activity and Health: A Report of the Surgeon General*, state the need for increased participation in moderate-intensity exercise (e.g., brisk walking) throughout the life span (2, 74). Such a recommendation is consistent with exposing the general population to low-risk physical activity to achieve health-related benefits aimed at reducing cardiovascular and metabolic diseases. In contrast to this general recommendation for everyone, there is a need to follow a variety of guidelines in prescribing moderate to strenuous exercise that is aimed at improving $\dot{V}O_2$ max. We will address both concerns in this chapter. For information on training for performance, see chapter 21.

IN SUMMARY

- Physical inactivity has been classified as a primary risk factor for coronary heart disease.
- Regular participation in physical activity can reduce the overall risk for those who smoke or who are hypertensive.
- Those who increase their physical activity and/or cardiorespiratory fitness have a lower death rate from all causes compared to those who remain sedentary.

PRESCRIPTION OF EXERCISE

The concern about the proper **dose** of exercise needed to bring about a desired **effect (response)** is similar to the physician's need to know the type and quantity of a drug, as well as the time frame over which it must be taken, to cure a disease. Clearly, there is a difference in what is needed to cure a headache compared to what is needed to cure tuberculosis. In the same way there is no question that the dose of physical activity needed to achieve high-level running performance is different from that required to improve a health-related outcome (e.g., lower blood pressure) or fitness (e.g., an increase in $\dot{V}O_2$ max). This dose-response relationship for medications is described in figure 16.1 (20).

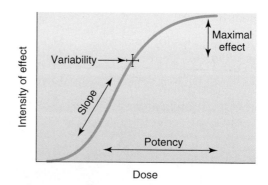

Figure 16.1 The relationship between the dose of a drug (expressed as the log of the dose) and the effect. Data from L. S. Goodman and A. Gilman, eds., 1975, *The Pharmacological Basis of Therapeutics*. New York: Macmillan Publishing Company.

- *Potency.* The potency of a drug is a relatively unimportant characteristic of a drug in that it makes little difference whether the effective dose of a drug is 1 μg or 100 mg as long as it can be administered in an appropriate dosage. Applied to exercise, walking 4 miles is as effective in expending calories as running 2 miles.

- *Slope.* The slope of the curve gives some information about how much of a change in effect is obtained from a change in dose. Some physiological measures change quickly for a given dose of exercise, while some health-related effects require the application of exercise over many months to see a desired outcome.

- *Maximal effect.* The maximal effect (efficacy) of a drug varies with the type of drug. For example, morphine can relieve pain of all intensities, while aspirin is effective against only mild to moderate pain. Similarly, strenuous exercise can cause an increase in $\dot{V}O_2$ max as well as modify risk factors, while light-to-moderate exercise can change risk factors with a smaller impact on $\dot{V}O_2$ max (an important point we will return to later).

- *Variability.* The effect of a drug varies between individuals—and within individuals, depending on the circumstances. The intersecting brackets in figure 16.1 indicate the variability in the dose required to bring about a particular effect, and the variability in the effect associated with a given dose. For example, gains in $\dot{V}O_2$ max due to endurance training show considerable variation, even when the initial $\dot{V}O_2$ max value is controlled for (17). See A Closer Look 13.1 for more on the issue of variability.

- *Side effect.* A last point worth mentioning that can also be applied to our discussion of exercise prescription is that no drug produces a single effect. The spectrum of effects might include adverse (side) effects that limit the usefulness of the drug. For exercise, the side effects might include increased risk of injury.

In contrast to drugs that individuals stop taking when a disease is cured, there is a need to engage in some form of physical activity throughout one's life to experience the health-related and fitness effects.

Dose-Response

The exercise dose is usually characterized by the intensity, frequency, duration, and type of activity. The intensity can be described in terms of:

- % $\dot{V}O_2$ max,
- % maximal heart rate,

- rating of perceived exertion, and
- the lactate threshold.

The frequency could include:

- the number of days per week and
- the number of times per day.

The duration of exercise for each exercise session can be given as the:

- number of minutes of exercise,
- total kilocalories (kcal) expended, and
- total kcal expended per kilogram body weight.

The type of exercise relates to whether resistance exercises or cardiovascular endurance exercises are used in the training program. For the latter, we would also distinguish among the effects of walking vs. jogging/running vs. swimming. Although we know a considerable amount about the role that each of these variables may play in a gain in $\dot{V}O_2$ max, we are learning more each year about the minimum or optimal quantities of each variable related to health outcomes (37, 72, 73).

The response (effect) generated by a particular dose of exercise can include changes in $\dot{V}O_2$ max, resting blood pressure, insulin sensitivity, body weight (percent fat), and depression. Haskell (23, 24) provided an important insight into how we should rethink our understanding of cause and effect when we study how a dose of physical activity is related to the responses, physical fitness and health. Physical activity could bring about favorable changes by:

- improving fitness (especially cardiovascular fitness), thereby improving health, or
- improving fitness and health simultaneously and separately, or
- improving fitness, but not a specific health outcome, or
- improving some specific health outcome, but not fitness.

It has become clear that improvements in a variety of health-related concerns are not dependent on an increase in $\dot{V}O_2$ max. This is important and provides a transition to our next section.

IN SUMMARY

- An exercise dose reflects the interaction of the intensity, frequency, and duration of exercise.
- The cause of the health-related response may be related to an improvement in $\dot{V}O_2$ max or may act through some other mechanism, making health-related outcomes and gains in $\dot{V}O_2$ max independent of each other.

Physical Activity and Health

The issue of the proper dose of exercise to bring about a desired effect is a crucial one in the prescription of exercise for both prevention and rehabilitation. Over the past two decades we have learned that the proper dose differs greatly, depending on the outcome. For example, an improvement in some health-related variable (e.g., resting blood pressure) might be accomplished with an exercise intensity lower than that required to achieve an increase in $\dot{V}O_2$ max. In addition, the frequency with which the exercise must be taken to have the desired effect varies with the intensity and the duration of the session (see later discussion).

Certain physiological variables respond very quickly to a "dose" of exercise. For example, we have shown how rapidly the sympathetic nervous system, blood lactate, and heart rate (see chapter 13) adapt to exercise training, taking only days to see changes in response. In contrast to these rapid responses to exercise training, a variety of physiological variables, such as the capillary number, change more slowly (62). Similarly, when Haskell describes the potential association between physical activity and health, he distinguishes between short-term (acute) and long-term (training) responses (23). The following terms are used to describe the patterns of responses in the weeks following the initiation of a dose of exercise:

- acute responses—occur with one or several exercise bouts but do not improve further
- rapid responses—benefits occur early and plateau
- linear—gains are made continuously over time
- delayed—occur only after weeks of training

The need for such distinctions can be seen in figure 16.2, which shows proposed dose-response relationships between physical activity, defined as minutes of exercise per week at 60% to 70% of maximal work capacity, and a variety of physiological responses (34): (1) blood pressure and insulin sensitivity are most responsive to exercise, (2) changes in $\dot{V}O_2$ max and resting heart rate are intermediate, and (3) serum lipid changes such as high-density lipoprotein (HDL) are delayed. For an update on dose-response issues, see Clinical Applications 16.1.

By this time it should be clear that it is difficult to provide a single exercise prescription that addresses all issues related to prevention and/or treatment of various diseases. However, in spite of this difficulty, there was a pressing need to spell out a general public health physical activity recommendation to improve the health status of all U.S. adults. In 1995 the American College of Sports Medicine and the Centers for Disease Control and Prevention (CDC) responded to this need. Their guidelines were based on a comprehensive review of the literature dealing

Figure 16.2 Proposed dose-response relationships between amount of exercise performed per week at 60% to 70% maximum work capacity and changes in several variables. Blood pressure (BP) and insulin sensitivity (curve to the left side) appear to be most sensitive to exercise. Maximum oxygen consumption ($\dot{V}O_2$ max) and resting heart rate, which are parameters of physical fitness (middle curve), are next in sensitivity, and lipid changes such as high-density lipoprotein (HDL) (right-hand curve) are least sensitive.

with the health-related aspects of physical activity (47). Their recommendation was that every U.S. adult should accumulate 30 minutes or more of moderate-intensity (3–6 METs) physical activity on most, preferably all, days of the week. This recommendation was based on the finding that caloric expenditure and total time of physical activity are associated with reduced cardiovascular disease and mortality. Further, doing the activity in intermittent bouts as short as 10 minutes was a suitable way of meeting the 30-minute goal (5, 47, 74).

In 2007 the ACSM and AHA released an update to this 1995 public health physical activity guideline, and in 2008 the first edition of the U.S. *Physical Activity Guidelines* was released (2008). Both guidelines supported the original statement, but attempted to provide more clarity about the roles of moderate versus strenuous physical activity in meeting the recommendation (25, 72). Because of the similarity between the two, we will present only the U.S. *Physical Activity Guidelines*.

- Individuals can realize the health-related benefits of physical activity by doing between 150 and 300 minutes of moderate-intensity physical activity per week, or 75 to 150 minutes of vigorous intensity physical activity per week, or some combination of the two.
  - 150 minutes of moderate-intensity physical activity or 75 minutes of vigorous intensity physical activity is the minimum goal.

Dose-Response: Physical Activity and Health

In 2001 the results of a special symposium that examined whether a dose-response relationship existed between physical activity and a variety of health outcomes were published (37). At the end of the decade, another systematic review of the literature (73) was conducted on this same topic prior to the publication of the first set of national physical activity guidelines (2008 U.S. *Physical Activity Guidelines*). The more recent review supported the vast majority of the findings in the earlier report. Regular participation in physical activity was associated with:

- lower rates of all-cause mortality, total cardiovascular disease (CVD), and coronary heart disease incidence and mortality;
- increased weight loss, and reduced amount of weight regain after weight loss;
- a lower incidence of obesity, type 2 diabetes, and metabolic syndrome;
- a lower risk of colon and breast cancer;
- an improvement in the ability of older adults to do activities of daily living;
- reduced risk of falls in older adults at risk of falling;
- a reduction in depression and cognitive decline in adults and older adults; and
- favorable changes in cardiovascular risk factors, including blood pressure and blood lipid profile.

In general, the review found that:

- the volume of physical activity done was the most important

FIGURE 16.3 Dose-response of physical activity related to all-cause mortality. From: U.S. Department of Health and Human Services. Physical Activity Guidelines Advisory Committee Report 2008, Fig. G1.3, p. G1-19. http://www.health.gov/paguidelines/committeereport.aspx.

variable tied to health outcomes;
- the risk of many chronic diseases was reduced about 20% to 40% by regular participation in physical activity (see later discussion for how much physical activity); and
- a dose-response relationship existed for most health outcomes, meaning that "more is better." See figure 16.3 as an example for the health outcome, death from all causes.

That last finding, "more is better," had to be balanced by the increased risk of adverse outcomes when too much was done or when the exercise was a major change from what was currently being done. See more on this in Exercise Prescription for CRF.

The inability to establish a clear dose-response relationship between physical activity and some health outcomes was linked to lack of appropriate studies; methods of measuring physical activity not being sensitive enough to accurately characterize the "dose"; the small effect of physical activity on some health outcomes; uncontrolled factors such as genetic variability; and simultaneous changes in body weight, which confounded the data analysis. Clearly, there is a great need for additional, well-designed studies that use more sophisticated measurements of physical activity on a larger and more diverse population to be able to describe whether a dose-response relationship exists between physical activity and a specific health outcome.

- The range of physical activity (150–300 minutes) indicates that more health-related benefits are realized by doing additional activity (i.e., more is better).
- Physical activity can be done in multiple intermittent bouts (e.g., 10 minutes each) to meet the goal.

The health-related gains associated with physical activity are realized when the volume of PA is between about 500 and 1000 MET-min per week (72). Moderate-intensity PA is defined as absolute intensities of 3.0 to 5.9 METs, and vigorous intensity PA is defined as intensities of 6.0 METs or more.

- For example, walking at 3 mph requires ~3.3 METs, an activity at the low end of the moderate-intensity range. If the person walks at this speed for 30 minutes, an energy expenditure of 99 MET-min (3.3 METs times

30 min) is achieved. If done 5 days per week, the volume of PA is 495 MET-min per week.

- If an individual were to jog at 5 mph (~8 METs) for 25 minutes, the PA volume would be 200 MET-min. If done 3 days per week, the energy expenditure would be 600 MET-min per week.
- The fact that it takes about twice the time when doing moderate-intensity PA to achieve the same energy expenditure as when doing vigorous-intensity PA leads to the 2:1 ratio when comparing the time it takes to meet the PA guidelines for these different intensities (150 vs. 75 min).

In addition, the new guidelines recommended resistance training (at least 1 set, or 8–12 reps, of 8–10 exercises) on two or more days per week to improve or maintain muscular strength and endurance (25, 72). These new guidelines only spell out the number of minutes per week, without listing the number of days per week to exercise. That does not mean that one should do the 150 minutes of moderate-intensity physical activity on one day and rest for 6 days. For reasons that will be discussed later, spreading out the physical activity and exercise over the course of the week makes it easier to schedule and reduces the risk of adverse events (72). Even though there is an emphasis on moderate-intensity PA, because this is the type of activity most frequently done by adults (e.g., a brisk walk), much can be gained from participation in vigorous-intensity PA (see Clinical Applications 16.2).

IN SUMMARY

- To realize the health-related benefits of physical activity, adults should do between 150 and 300 minutes of moderate-intensity physical activity per week, or 75 to 150 minutes of vigorous intensity physical activity per week, or some combination of the two.
- Resistance training (8–10 exercises, 8–12 reps) should be done on 2 or more nonconsecutive days per week).

GENERAL GUIDELINES FOR IMPROVING FITNESS

An increase in moderate-intensity physical activity is an important goal for reducing health-related problems in sedentary individuals. These benefits occur at a point where the overall risk associated with physical activity is relatively small. However, even though the risk of cardiac arrest in habitually active men is higher during vigorous activity, the overall (rest + exercise) risk of cardiac arrest in vigorously active men is only

40% of the risk in sedentary men (64). A growing body of evidence indicates that achievement of an average-to-high level of cardiorespiratory fitness ($\dot{V}O_2$ max) confers additional health benefits, as well as increasing one's ability to engage in a broad range of recreational activities. The purpose of this section is to review the general guidelines for exercise programs aimed at increasing $\dot{V}O_2$ max. In chapter 13 the concepts of overload and specificity were presented relative to the adaptations that take place with different training programs. Although these principles apply here, it is important to remember that little exercise is needed to achieve a health-related effect. This stands in marked contrast to the intensity of exercise needed to achieve performance goals (see chapter 21).

IN SUMMARY

- In previously sedentary subjects, small changes in physical activity result in a large number of health benefits with only minimal risk.
- Strenuous exercise increases the risk of a heart attack during the activity, but reduces the overall (rest + exercise) risk of such an event.
- Moderate to high levels of cardiorespiratory fitness confers additional health benefits and increases one's ability to engage in recreational activities.

Screening

The first thing to do, if not already done in the evaluation of CRF, is to carry out some form of health status screening to decide who should begin an exercise program and who should obtain further consultation with a physician (see chapter 15 for details). The risk of cardiovascular complications during exercise is directly related to the degree of pre-existing cardiac disease. In young people the risk of sudden death is about 1/133,000 and 1/769,000 per year in men and women, respectively, due primarily to congenital or acquired heart disease. In adults the risk is one per year for every 15,000 to 18,000 individuals (2).

Progression

The emphasis in any health-related exercise program, for those who are sedentary, is to do too little rather than too much. By starting slowly and progressing from the easily accomplished activities to those that are more difficult, the chance of causing muscle soreness and of aggravating old injuries is reduced (72). The emphasis on moderate-intensity activities, such as walking at 3 to 4 mph, early in the fitness program is consistent with this recommendation, and the participant must be educated not to move too quickly

CLINICAL APPLICATIONS 16.2

Achieving Health-Related Outcomes: Is Vigorous Exercise Better than Moderate Activity?

There has been an ongoing debate over this question since the ACSM/CDC released their public health PA recommendation in 1995, with its emphasis on moderate-intensity PA. Prior to that, the emphasis was on vigorous-intensity exercise as described in the classic position stands of the ACSM (1). It must be noted that although moderate-intensity PA was emphasized, the 1995 statement also indicated that more exercise was better and encouraged vigorous exercise. Therefore, the question remains, is vigorous-intensity PA better than moderate-intensity PA for health-related outcomes?

Swain and Franklin (67) addressed this question in a systematic review of the literature examining the relationship of PA to the incidence of coronary heart disease (CHD) and risk factors for CHD. It was important in this review that the total energy expenditure associated with the PA was controlled for to allow a fair comparison of moderate-intensity versus vigorous-intensity PA (since for any duration of vigorous PA, more energy would be expended compared to moderate-intensity PA). Their findings follow:

- The vast majority of epidemiological studies observed a greater reduction in the risk of cardiovascular disease with vigorous-intensity PA ($\geq$6 METs) than with moderate-intensity PA (3–5.9 METs). In addition, more favorable risk factor profiles were found for those doing vigorous-intensity vs. moderate-intensity PA.

- Clinical intervention studies showed, generally, greater improvements in diastolic blood pressure, glucose control, and cardiorespiratory fitness after vigorous-intensity PA, compared to moderate-intensity PA. However, there was no difference between the two intensity

categories for improvements in systolic blood pressure, the blood lipid profile, or loss of body fat.

Clearly, more health-related benefits are realized, independent of the larger gains in $\dot{V}O_2$ max, through participating in vigorous-intensity exercise. O'Donovan et al. (42) supported these findings by showing that even when training groups are doing vigorous-intensity exercise, the higher the intensity the better the impact on CHD risk factors. In addition, regular participation in vigorous-intensity PA was shown to be associated with less sick leave, whereas moderate-intensity PA appeared to have no effect (56). This raises other questions: What is moderate-intensity PA? Vigorous-intensity PA?

Public health PA recommendations define moderate-intensity PA as being equal to an energy expenditure of 3–5.9 METs, but surprising as it may seem, moderate-intensity exercise may actually be vigorous-intensity PA for a large segment of the population.

Figure 16.4 shows the relative intensity for two fixed exercises (walking at 3 or 4 mph) to vary considerably across the range of $\dot{V}O_2$ max values (31, 73). Consequently, individuals with low $\dot{V}O_2$ max values who are doing moderate-intensity physical activity (3–5.9 METs) may actually be working at a relative intensity equivalent to vigorous exercise (60–84% $\dot{V}O_2$ max), consistent with achieving gains in $\dot{V}O_2$ max. This example emphasizes the need to consider measures of the relative exercise intensity (e.g., % HR max, %$\dot{V}O_2$ max) when developing PA programs, rather than relying solely on the absolute intensities (e.g., METs). Therefore, "moderate" activities, coupled with the lower threshold of training in deconditioned individuals, may be sufficient to elevate the metabolic rate and heart rate to the appropriate levels needed to achieve the various fitness ($\dot{V}O_2$ max) and health benefits that were a part of the original ACSM fitness recommendation.

FIGURE 16.4 The relative exercise intensity for walking at 3.0 mph (3.3 METs) and 4.0 mph (5.0 METs) expressed as a percent of $\dot{V}O_2$ max for adults with an exercise capacity ranging from 4 to 14 METs. From: U.S. Department of Health and Human Services. Physical Activity Guidelines Advisory Committee Report 2008. Figure D.1; p. D-7. http://www.health.gov/paguidelines/committeereport.aspx.

www.mhhe.com/powers8e   Chapter Sixteen   Exercise Prescriptions for Health and Fitness   **357** into the more demanding activities. When the person can walk about two miles without fatigue, the progression to a walk-jog and jogging program is a reasonable recommendation (32).

Warm-Up, Stretch, and Cool-Down, Stretch

Prior to the actual activity used in the exercise session, a variety of very light exercises and stretches are done to improve the transition from rest to the exercise state. The emphasis at the onset of an exercise session is to gradually increase the level of activity until the proper intensity is reached. Stretching exercises to increase the range of motion of the joints involved in the activity, as well as specific stretches to increase the flexibility of the lower back, are included in the warm-up. At the end of the activity session, about 5 minutes of cool-down activities—slow walking and stretching exercises—are recommended to gradually return HR and BP toward normal. This part of the exercise session is viewed as important in reducing the chance of a hypotensive episode after the exercise session (32).

EXERCISE PRESCRIPTION FOR CRF

The exercise program includes dynamic, large muscle activities such as walking, jogging, running, swimming, cycling, rowing, and dancing. The CRF training effect of exercise programs is dependent on the proper frequency, duration, and intensity of the exercise sessions. The ACSM recommends three to five sessions per week, for 20 to 60 minutes per session, at an intensity of about 40/50% to 84% heart rate reserve (HRR) or oxygen uptake reserve ($\dot{V}O_2R$) (2). This relative intensity range accommodates both moderate intensity (40–59% HRR) and vigorous intensity (60–84% HRR). The term, % $\dot{V}O_2R$, is being used in place of the traditional % $\dot{V}O_2$ max, but for those of average to high fitness, the terms are quite similar (see later discussion). The combination of duration and intensity should result in the expenditure of about 200 to 300 kcal per session. A 75-kg person accumulating 600 MET-min/week of PA expends about 750 kcal/week, indicating a consistency between the U.S. *Physical Activity Guidelines* recommendation and the older ACSM position stands (1) and their *Guidelines* (2). This program is consistent with achieving weight-loss goals and reducing the risk factors associated with CHD (2, 26, 49-51, 74). See A Look Back—Important People in Science for information on someone who had a major impact on exercise testing and prescription.

Frequency

Improvements in CRF increase with the frequency of exercise sessions, with two sessions being the minimum, and the gains in CRF leveling off after three to four sessions per week (2, 75). Gains in CRF can be achieved with a 2-day-per-week program, but the intensity has to be higher than the 3-day-per-week program, and participants might not achieve weight-loss goals (50). In addition, the high-intensity exercise associated with a 2-day-per-week frequency may not be appropriate for previously sedentary individuals. The schedule of 3 to 4 days per week includes a day off between sessions and reduces the scheduling problems associated with planned exercise programs. Figure 16.5 shows that higher frequencies are associated with higher rates of injuries (16, 52).

Duration

The duration has to be viewed together with intensity, in that the total work accomplished per session (200–300 kcal) is an important variable associated with improvements in CRF after the minimal threshold of intensity is achieved (2). A good example showing the role that duration plays (at constant exercise intensity) in the increase in CRF is a recent study by Church et al. (16). Sedentary, postmenopausal overweight or obese women were randomly assigned into either a control group or one of three moderate-intensity (~50% $\dot{V}O_2$ peak) physical activity groups to achieve an energy expenditure of 4, 8, or 12 kcal/kg per week. The increase in $\dot{V}O_2$ peak was 4.2%, 6%, and 8.2% in these groups, respectively, indicating a dose-response relationship with exercise duration (16). This is important, given that many sedentary persons can more easily accomplish an exercise session of low intensity and long duration than the reverse, and achieve the health-related benefits of physical activity with minimal risk. Obviously, if the participants choose to exercise at higher intensities, it would take less time to achieve an energy expenditure goal. For example, an 80-kg (176-lb) person walking at about 3.5 mph would consume O_2 at the rate of 1 liter per minute. Given 5 kcal per liter of O_2, the person is using 5 kcal · min^{-1}, and 60 minutes of walking would be required to expend 300 kcal. As the intensity of exercise increases, the duration needed to expend 300 kcal decreases. Given that "lack of time" is often cited as a principal reason for not exercising, doing vigorous-intensity PA would help address that problem. Figure 16.5 shows that doing strenuous exercise (75% $\dot{V}O_2$ max) for more than 30 minutes per session increases the risk of orthopedic problems.

Michael L. Pollock, Ph.D., Laid the Foundation for Exercise Prescription

Michael L. Pollock received his Ph.D. at the University of Illinois under the direction of Dr. Thomas K. Cureton (see chapter 0's A Look Back—Important People in Science). In so many ways, Dr. Pollock built on Dr. Cureton's commitment to fitness, but raised it to a much higher level. Mike Pollock's research laid the foundation for much of the quantitative aspects of exercise prescription that were established in the 1970s and are little changed today. When we read about the optimal intensity, frequency, and duration of exercise to achieve fitness goals and health benefits, we have Dr. Pollock to thank for providing the foundation for much of that. In 1972 he published a chapter, "Quantification of Endurance Training Programs," in the first volume of *Exercise and Sports Sciences Reviews*. This chapter led the way for the American College of Sports Medicine's first position stand in 1978: "Recommended Quantity and Quality of Exercise for Developing and Maintaining Fitness," of which Dr. Pollock was the lead author. His research on the importance of strength training was instrumental in including resistance training in a later revision of that position stand. In addition, Mike Pollock's name is attached to one of the most popular equations for converting the sum of skinfolds into percentage of body fat. The fact that these equations are still used on a daily basis, many years after their development, speaks well of the quality of his work in so many areas.

Dr. Pollock also had a major impact on the development, maturation, and recognition of cardiopulmonary exercise testing and training. His research publications and textbooks (*Heart Disease and Rehabilitation* and *Exercise in Health and Disease*) in this area provided clear guidance for the delivery of safe and effective exercise programs in the cardiopulmonary rehabilitation environment (see Suggested Readings for a textbook written in his honor: *Pollock's Textbook of Cardiovascular Disease and Rehabilitation*). He was a founding member of the American Association of Cardiovascular and Pulmonary Rehabilitation (AACVPR) and was the founder of the *Journal of Cardiopulmonary Rehabilitation*. In addition to these valuable contributions, Dr. Pollock served as President of the American College of Sports Medicine.

Mike Pollock accomplished all this work while suffering (quietly) from ankylosing spondylitis—a degenerative inflammatory disease that impairs the mobility of the spinal column. He died of a stroke in 1998, but his legacy is with us each day we do exercise testing, write an exercise prescription, and talk about "how much exercise is enough?"

Note: Special thanks to Barry Franklin and William Haskell for information for this box.

Figure 16.5 Effects of increasing the frequency, duration, and intensity of exercise on the increase in $\dot{V}O_2$ max in a training program. This figure demonstrates the increasing risk of orthopedic problems due to exercise sessions that are too long or conducted too many times per week. The probability of cardiac complications increases with exercise intensity beyond that recommended for improvements in cardiorespiratory fitness.

Intensity

Intensity describes the overload on the cardiovascular system that is needed to bring about a training effect. It should be no surprise that the intensity threshold for a CRF training effect is lower for the less fit and higher for the more fit. Swain and Franklin (68) found that the threshold for an improvement in $\dot{V}O_2$ max was only 30% of oxygen uptake reserve ($\dot{V}O_2R$) for those with $\dot{V}O_2$ max values less than 40 ml · kg^{-1} · min^{-1}, and only 46% $\dot{V}O_2R$ for those with a $\dot{V}O_2$ max greater than 40 ml · kg^{-1} · min^{-1}. However, in general, they found that higher-intensity exercise was better for increasing $\dot{V}O_2$ max. As mentioned at the beginning of this section, the range of exercise intensities associated with an increase in $\dot{V}O_2$ max is 40/50% to 84% $\dot{V}O_2R$, which is similar to 40/50% to 84% $\dot{V}O_2$ max for people of average or better fitness (see Clinical Applications 16.3). However, for most people, 60% to 80% $\dot{V}O_2$ max seems to be a range sufficient to achieve CRF goals (32). It appears that for this information to be useful, the exercise leader has to know the energy requirements ($\dot{V}O_2$) of all the fitness activities so that a correct match can be made between the activity and

Prescribing Exercise Intensity by the $\dot{V}O_2$ Reserve ($\dot{V}O_2R$) Method

Historically, the intensity portion of an exercise prescription was given as a % $\dot{V}O_2$ max, percent of maximal HR, or percent of the HR reserve (HRR). The linear relationship between HR and $\dot{V}O_2$ allowed the former to predict the latter. In this regard, some preferred the use of the HRR method because the percent values used in the calculation of the target heart rates were believed to be similar to the % $\dot{V}O_2$ max values (i.e., 60% HRR = 60% $\dot{V}O_2$ max). Research by Swain and colleagues (69, 70) questioned that close association, especially for subjects at the low end of the fitness scale. They found that the % HRR was more closely linked to the % $\dot{V}O_2R$ (the difference between maximal $\dot{V}O_2$ and

resting $\dot{V}O_2$) than to % $\dot{V}O_2$ max. This approach has been adopted in all of ACSM's position stands on the quantity and quality of exercise needed for fitness (1), and their *Guidelines for Exercise Testing and Prescription* (2). As Swain points out (66), the calculation of the % $\dot{V}O_2R$ is similar to that of the HHR. For example, the target $\dot{V}O_2$ of a person with a $\dot{V}O_2$ max of 35 ml $\cdot$ kg$^{-1}\cdot$ min^{-1} who works at 60% HRR is:

$$\text{Target } \dot{V}O_2 = (0.60)(35 \text{ ml} \cdot \text{kg}^{-1} \cdot \text{min}^{-1}$$
$$- 3.5 \text{ ml} \cdot \text{kg}^{-1} \cdot \text{min}^{-1})$$
$$+ 3.5 \text{ ml} \cdot \text{kg}^{-1} \cdot \text{min}^{-1}$$
$$\text{Target } \dot{V}O_2 = 18.9 \text{ ml} \cdot \text{kg}^{-1} \cdot \text{min}^{-1}$$
$$+ 3.5 \text{ ml} \cdot \text{kg}^{-1} \cdot \text{min}^{-1}$$
$$\text{Target } \dot{V}O_2 = 22.4 \text{ ml} \cdot \text{kg}^{-1} \cdot \text{min}^{-1}$$

The advantage of this approach is that the % HRR and % $\dot{V}O_2R$ values are directly coupled over the entire range of fitness ($\dot{V}O_2$ max values) and exercise intensities, but it is most useful for those at the low end of the scale, where large discrepancies exist between % HRR and % $\dot{V}O_2$ max (66, 69, 70). On the other hand, for those with average to high fitness levels, the difference between the % $\dot{V}O_2$ max and % $\dot{V}O_2R$ is not very great. The following table gives a brief summary of the expected % $\dot{V}O_2$ max values across a broad range of $\dot{V}O_2$ max values (in METs) when exercise intensities are set at a % HRR:

$\dot{V}O_2$ max (METs)	40% HRR	50% HRR	60% HRR	70% HRR	80% HRR
18	43.3	52.8	62.2	71.7	81.1
16	43.8	53.1	62.5	71.9	81.3
14	44.3	53.6	62.9	72.1	81.4
12	45.0	54.2	63.3	72.5	81.7
10	46.0	55.2	64.3	73.0	82.5
8	47.5	56.3	65.0	73.8	82.5
6	50.0	58.3	66.7	75.0	83.3

Percent $\dot{V}O_2$ Max at Different Percent Heart Rate Reserve (HRR) and Cardiorespiratory Fitness ($\dot{V}O_2$ Max) Values

As you can see, for those at the high end of the fitness spectrum and at higher intensities of exercise, the difference between the % HRR and % $\dot{V}O_2$ max is not too great. This was recently shown to be the case for the elite cyclist, where for intensities greater than 75% of maximum, there was no difference between % HRR, % $\dot{V}O_2R$ or % $\dot{V}O_2$ max (40). However, for those at the low end of the fitness scale (e.g., 6

METs), there is a large (e.g., 10%) difference between the % $\dot{V}O_2$ max and % HRR at 40% HRR.

Special Notes

■ When using an exercise heart rate value to estimate the % $\dot{V}O_2$ max or % $\dot{V}O_2R$ at which the individual is working, the error is about ±6% (i.e., 60% HRR = 60 ± 6% $\dot{V}O_2R$)

for two-thirds of the population when the measured maximal heart rate is known.

■ If we use an age-predicted maximal heart rate to set the target heart rate range, the error involved in estimating the maximal heart rate value (one standard deviation is ± 11 b $\cdot$ min^{-1}) adds to the error in estimating % $\dot{V}O_2$ max or % $\dot{V}O_2R$.

---

the participant. Fortunately, because of the linear relationship between exercise intensity and HR, the exercise intensity can be set by using the HR values equivalent to 60% to 80% $\dot{V}O_2$ max. The range of heart rate values associated with the exercise intensity needed to have a CRF training effect is called the **target heart rate (THR) range.** How do you determine the THR range?

Direct Method Figure 16.6 shows the HR response of a twenty-year-old subject during a maximal GXT on a treadmill. The subject's $\dot{V}O_2$ max was 12 METs, so that 60% and 80% $\dot{V}O_2$ max is equal to about 7.2 and 9.6 METs, respectively. A line is drawn from each of these work rates up to the HR/$\dot{V}O_2$ line, and over to the y-axis where the HR values equivalent to these work rates are obtained. These HR values, 138

Figure 16.6 Target heart rate range determined from the results of an exercise stress test. The heart rate values measured at work rates equal to 60% and 80% $\dot{V}O_2$ max constitute the THR range.

to 164 b · min⁻¹, represent the THR range, the proper intensity for a CRF training effect (1, 32).

Indirect Methods The THR range can also be estimated by some simple calculations, knowing that the relationship between HR and $\dot{V}O_2$ is linear. The heart rate reserve, or Karvonen, method of calculating a THR range has three simple steps (35, 36):

1. Subtract resting HR from maximal HR to obtain HR reserve (HRR).
2. Take 60% and 80% of the HRR.
3. Add each HRR value to resting HR to obtain the THR range.

For example:

1. If a subject has a maximal HR of 200 b · min⁻¹ and a resting HR of 60 b · min⁻¹, then the HRR is 140 b · min⁻¹ (200 − 60).
2. 60% × 140 b · min⁻¹ = 84 b · min⁻¹ and 80% × 140 b · min⁻¹ = 112 b · min⁻¹
3. 84 b · min⁻¹ + 60 b · min⁻¹ = 144 b · min⁻¹
   112 b · min⁻¹ + 60 b · min⁻¹ = 172 b · min⁻¹
   The THR range is 144 to 172 b · min⁻¹.

This method gives reasonable estimates of the exercise intensity because 60% to 80% of the HRR is equal to about 60% to 80% $\dot{V}O_2$ max for those with average or high fitness (see Clinical Applications 16.3).

The other indirect method of calculating the THR range is the *percentage of maximal* HR method. In this method you simply take 70% and 85% of maximal HR to obtain the THR range. In the following example, the subject has a maximal HR of 200 b · min⁻¹. The THR range for this person is 140 to 170 b · min⁻¹ (70% × 200 = 140 b · min⁻¹; 85% × 200 = 170 b · min⁻¹). Seventy percent of maximal HR is equal to

about 55% $\dot{V}O_2$ max, and 85% of maximal HR is equal to about 75% $\dot{V}O_2$ max, both within the intensity range needed for CRF gains (27–29, 39).

The intensity of exercise can be prescribed by the direct method or by either of the indirect methods. Both of the indirect methods require knowledge of the maximal HR. If the maximal HR is measured during a maximal GXT, use it in the calculations. However, if you have to use the age-adjusted estimate of maximal HR (220 − age), remember the potential error, with the standard deviation of the estimate equal to ±11 b · min⁻¹. Tanaka, Monahan, and Seals (71) evaluated the validity of the classic "220 − age" equation to estimate maximal heart rate. They carried out an analysis of 351 published studies and cross-validated the findings with a well-controlled laboratory study. They found almost identical results using both approaches: HR max = 208 − 0.7 × age. This new equation yields maximal heart rate values that are 6 b · min⁻¹ lower for 20-year-olds and 6 b · min⁻¹ higher for 60-year-olds. A recent longitudinal study confirmed the above, with their equation being HR max = 207 − 0.7 × age (19). Although the new formulas yield better estimates of HR max *on average*, the investigators emphasize the fact that the estimated HR max for a given individual is still associated with a standard deviation of ±10 b · min⁻¹. Consequently, the estimated THR range is a guideline for exercise intensity and is meant to be used with other information (abnormal symptoms or signs) to determine if the exercise intensity is reasonable.

In this regard, Borg's RPE scale can be used as an adjunct to HR in prescribing exercise intensity for apparently healthy individuals. The RPE range of 12 to 16 on the original Borg scale covers the range of exercise intensities similar to 40/50% to 84% HRR (1, 2, 7, 15, 21, 22, 53). The RPE scale is helpful because the participant learns to associate the THR range with a certain whole-body perception of effort, decreasing the need for frequent pulse rate measurements. The RPE scale has been shown to have a high test-retest reliability (14), and it is closely linked to the % $\dot{V}O_2$ max and lactate threshold, independent of the mode of exercise and fitness of the subject (30, 59, 63). Remember, the intensity threshold needed to achieve CRF goals is lower for the less fit, and vice versa.

IN SUMMARY

■ A sedentary person needs to go through a health status screening before participating in exercise.
■ Exercise programs for previously sedentary persons should start with moderate-intensity activities (walking), and the person should not progress until he or she can walk briskly for about 2 miles.

- The optimal characteristics of an exercise program to increase $\dot{V}O_2$ max are intensity = 60% to 80% $\dot{V}O_2$ max; frequency = three to four times per week; duration = minutes needed to expend about 200 to 300 kcal.
- The THR range, taken as 60% to 80% HRR, or 70% to 85% of maximal HR, is a reasonable estimate of the proper exercise intensity.

To determine if the subject is in the THR range during the activity, HR should be checked immediately after stopping, taking a 10-second pulse count within the first 15 seconds. The pulse can be taken at the radial artery or the carotid artery; if the latter is used, the participant should use only light pressure, since heavy pressure can actually slow the HR (32, 53).

The proper intensity, frequency, and duration of exercise needed to have a CRF training effect were discussed in the previous section. It is important that sedentary individuals start slowly before exercising at the recommended intensities specified in the THR range. The next section provides some directions on how to make that transition.

SEQUENCE OF PHYSICAL ACTIVITY

The old adage that you should "walk before you run" is consistent with the way exercise should be recommended to sedentary persons, be they young or old (72). After the person demonstrates an ability to do prolonged walking without fatigue, then controlled fitness exercises conducted at a reasonable intensity (THR) can be introduced. After that, and depending on the interest of the participant, a variety of fitness activities that are more game-like can be included. This section will deal with this sequence of activities that can lead to a fit life (32).

Walking

The primary activity to recommend to someone who has been sedentary for a long period of time is walking, or its equivalent if orthopedic problems exist. This recommendation is consistent with the introductory material on health benefits, and it deals with the issue of injuries associated with more strenuous physical activity. In addition, there is good reason to believe that some (many) individuals may use walking as their primary form of exercise. The emphasis at this stage is to simply get people active by providing an activity that can be done anywhere, anytime, and with anyone, young or old. In this way, the number of

possible interfering factors that can result in the discontinuance of the exercise is reduced.

The person should choose comfortable shoes that are flexible, offer a wide base of support, and have a fitted heel cup. There are a great number of "walking" shoes available, but a special pair of shoes is not usually required. The emphasis is on getting started; if walking becomes a "serious" activity, or leads to hiking, then the investment would be reasonable. If weather is not to interfere with the activity, then proper selection of clothing is necessary. The participant should wear light, loose-fitting clothing in warm weather, and layers of wool or polypropylene in cold weather. For those who cannot bear the extremes in temperature and humidity out of doors, various shopping malls provide a controlled environment with a smooth surface. Walkers should choose the areas in which they walk with care in order to avoid damaged streets, high traffic zones, and poorly lighted areas. Safety is important in any health-related exercise program (32, 72). A walking program is presented in table 16.1 (32). The steps are rather simple in that progression to the next stage does not occur unless the individual feels comfortable at the current stage. The HR should be recorded as described previously, but the emphasis is not on achieving the THR. Later on in the walking program if higher walking speeds are used, the THR zone will be attained. Remember that walking, in spite of not being very strenuous by the THR zone scale, when combined with long duration is an effective part of a weight-control and CHD risk factor reduction program (45, 54). Walking is an activity that many people find they can do every day, providing many opportunities to expend calories.

Jogging

Jogging begins when a person moves at a speed and form that results in a period of flight between foot strikes; this may be 3 or 4 mph, or 6 or 7 mph, depending on the fitness of the individual. As described in chapter 1, the net energy cost of jogging/running is about twice that of walking (at slow to moderate speeds) and requires a greater cardiovascular response. This is not the only reason for the jogging program to follow a walking program; there is also more stress on joints and muscles due to the impact forces that must be tolerated during the push off and landing while jogging (13).

The emphasis at the start of a jogging program is to make the transition from the walking program in such a way as to minimize the discomfort associated with the introduction of any new activity. This is accomplished by beginning with a jog-walk-jog program that eases the person into jogging by mixing in the lower energy cost and trauma associated with walking. The jogging speed is set according to the

TABLE 16.1 Walking Program

Rules	Stage	Duration	Heart Rate	Comments
1. Start at a level that is	1	15 min	_____	_____
comfortable for you.	2	20 min	_____	_____
2. Be aware of new aches	3	25 min	_____	_____
or pains.	4	30 min	_____	_____
3. Don't progress to the next	5	30 min	_____	_____
level if you are not	6	30 min	_____	_____
comfortable.	7	35 min	_____	_____
4. Monitor your heart rate and	8	40 min	_____	_____
record it.	9	45 min	_____	_____
5. It would be healthful to walk	10	45 min	_____	_____
at least every other day.	11	45 min	_____	_____
	12	50 min	_____	_____
	13	55 min	_____	_____
	14	60 min	_____	_____

Reprinted, by permission, from B. D. Franks and E. T. Howley, 1989, *Fitness Leader's Handbook*, Champaign, IL: Human Kinetics Publishers, 136. This form may be copied by the fitness leader for distribution to participants.

THR, with the aim to stay at the low end of the THR zone at the beginning of the program. As the participant adapts to jogging, the HR response for any jogging speed will decrease, and jogging speed will have to be increased to stay in the THR zone. This is the primary marker that a training effect is taking place. Table 16.2 presents a jogging program with some simple rules to follow. Special attention is made to completing the walking program first, staying in the THR zone, and not progressing to the next level if the participant is not comfortable with the current level. Jogging is not for everyone, and for those who are obese, or have ankle, knee, or hip problems, it might be a good activity to avoid. Two activities that reduce such stress are cycling (stationary or outdoor) and swimming (32). More on exercise for special populations will be presented in chapter 17.

Games and Sports

As a person becomes accustomed to exercising in the THR range while jogging, swimming, or cycling, more uncontrolled activities can be introduced that require higher levels of energy expenditure, but do so in a more intermittent fashion. Games (paddleball, racquetball, squash), sports (basketball, soccer), and various forms of group exercise can keep a person's interest and make it more likely that the person will maintain a physically active life. These activities should be built on a walk-and-jogging base to reduce the chance that the participant will make poor adjustments to the activity. In addition, by having the habit of walking or jogging (swimming or cycling), the participant will still be able to maintain his or her habit of physical activity when there is no one to play with or lead the class. In contrast to jogging, cycling, or swimming, it will be more difficult to stay in the THR range with these intermittent activities. It is more likely that the HR will move from below the threshold value to above the top end of the THR from time to time. This is a normal response to activities that are intermittent in nature. It must be stressed, however, that when playing games it is important that the participants have some degree of skill and be reasonably well matched. If one is much better than the other, neither will have a good workout (41).

STRENGTH AND FLEXIBILITY TRAINING

The focus in this chapter has been on training to improve cardiorespiratory fitness. However, both the ACSM position stand on fitness (1) and the recent update on the public health PA guidelines (25) recommend both strength and flexibility exercises as part of the complete fitness program. There is a growing body of evidence showing that resistance training has a variety of health benefits in addition to increasing or maintaining strength:

- Increases bone density and reduces risk of fractures
- Increases fat free mass and reduces percent fat
- Improves functional health
- Improves glucose metabolism, and
- Reduces risk of falls in seniors at risk of falling

TABLE 16.2 Jogging Program

Rules

1. Complete the Walking Program before starting this program.
2. Begin each session with walking and stretching.
3. Be aware of new aches and pains.
4. Don't progress to the next level if you are not comfortable.
5. Stay at the low end of your THR zone; record your heart rate for each session.
6. Do the program on a work-a-day, rest-a-day basis.

Stage 1 Jog 10 steps, walk 10 steps. Repeat five times and take your heart rate. Stay within THR zone by increasing or decreasing walking phase. Do 20–30 minutes of activity.

Stage 2 Jog 20 steps, walk 10 steps. Repeat five times and take your heart rate. Stay within THR zone by increasing or decreasing walking phase. Do 20–30 minutes of activity.

Stage 3 Jog 30 steps, walk 10 steps. Repeat five times and take your heart rate. Stay within THR zone by increasing or decreasing walking phase. Do 20–30 minutes of activity.

Stage 4 Jog 1 minute, walk 10 steps. Repeat three times and take your heart rate. Stay within THR zone by increasing or decreasing walking phase. Do 20–30 minutes of activity.

Stage 5 Jog 2 minutes, walk 10 steps. Repeat two times and take your heart rate. Stay within THR zone by increasing or decreasing walking phase. Do 30 minutes of activity.

Stage 6 Jog 1 lap (400 meters, or 440 yards) and check heart rate. Adjust pace during run to stay within the THR zone. If heart rate is still too high, go back to the Stage 5 schedule. Do 6 laps with a brief walk between each.

Stage 7 Jog 2 laps and check heart rate. Adjust pace during run to stay within the THR zone. If heart rate is still too high, go back to Stage 6 activity. Do 6 laps with a brief walk between each.

Stage 8 Jog 1 mile and check heart rate. Adjust pace during the run to stay within THR zone. Do 2 miles.

Stage 9 Jog 2 to 3 miles continuously. Check heart rate at the end to ensure that you were within THR zone.

Reprinted, by permission, from B. D. Franks and E. T. Howley, 1989, *Fitness Leader's Handbook*, Champaign, IL: Human Kinetics Publishers, 137. This form may be copied by the fitness leader for distribution to participants.

In a recent study (61), muscular strength was associated with a lower cancer mortality risk in men, even after controlling for both adiposity and cardiorespiratory fitness. Collectively, these health-related findings point to the need for resistance training to be a part of a regular exercise program. Further, the combination of adequate flexibility and strength allows individuals to do the activities of daily living comfortably and safely. The ACSM recommendation emphasizes dynamic exercises done on a routine basis, but there is some debate about how much is enough (see Clinical Applications 16.4).

The Activity Pyramid provides a nice summary of the overall recommendations for health and fitness (see figure 16.7). It is beyond the scope of this text to go into detail regarding strength and flexibility programs aimed at improving or maintaining these fitness components. We recommend the Suggested Readings by Faigenbaum and McInnis, for muscular strength and endurance, and by Liemohn, for flexibility and low-back function, as good starting points.

IN SUMMARY

- A logical progression of physical activities is from walking to jogging to games. The progression addresses issues of intensity, as well as the risk of injury. For many, walking may be their only aerobic activity.
- Strength and flexibility activities should be included as a regular part of an exercise program.

ENVIRONMENTAL CONCERNS

It is important that the participant be educated about the effects of extreme heat and humidity, altitude, and cold on the adaptation to exercise. The THR range acts as a guide in that it provides feedback to the participant about the interaction of the environment and the exercise intensity. As the heat and humidity increase, there

Strength Training: Single Versus Multiple Sets

In 1998 the ACSM recommended resistance training as a part of a well-rounded fitness program. The goals were to increase or maintain muscular strength and endurance, the fat-free mass, and bone mineral density (1). To accomplish this, the ACSM recommended:

- A minimum of one set of eight to ten exercises that conditions the major muscle groups,
- eight to twelve reps per set (ten to fifteen for older individuals), and
- two or more nonconsecutive sessions per week.

Although the position stand acknowledges that "multiple-set regimes may provide greater benefits," the review of literature supported the use of one set to achieve the health-related and fitness goals. This conclusion received additional support from a comprehensive review by Carpinelli and Otto (11), but not without reaction and reply to that reaction (10).

The debate was raised to a higher level when the ACSM published a second Position Stand in 2002 with a focus on progression models of resistance training for improving strength (4). This position stand recommended a variety of approaches to achieve strength goals, including using multiple sets. Since the appearance of that position stand, a number of systematic analyses of the research literature dealing with the issue of single set versus multiple sets have been published. They revealed the following:

- Prior to 1998 the evidence was split, and suggested that there was no difference in strength gains when a single set was compared to multiple sets. However, the use of small sample sizes, very short duration studies, and different methods

for measuring strength gains complicated the interpretation of the data. After 1998 most studies showed that multiple sets were better than single sets relative to strength gains, in both short- and long-term studies (18).

- Scientists re-examined all the literature on this topic by pooling the data from the various studies (to deal with the issues of small sample sizes and short duration studies). This analysis showed that multiple sets were better than single sets, and in the better-controlled studies the differences between the two were greater (57).
- Multiple sets were shown to be more effective in increasing strength in trained individuals and over long-duration training programs (76).

These review articles, as well as the most recent studies (33, 60), indicate that multiple sets are better than one set at increasing strength. However, "when maximal strength gain is not the principal goal of the training program, a single-set protocol may be sufficient to significantly improve upper- and lower-body strength as well as being time efficient" (18). This would appear to support both the "one-set" recommendation for improving and maintaining muscular fitness in the average individual as well as the "multiple set" recommendation for those interested in achieving higher strength goals.

The issue of dose-response was discussed earlier in this chapter relative to health-related outcomes and increases in $\dot{V}O_2$ max. For strength and conditioning programs, two recent comprehensive analyses of the literature suggest the following for *maximal gains* in strength:

- For untrained subjects: do four sets at 60% 1-RM, 3 days a week (58).
- For trained subjects: do four sets at 80% 1-RM, 2 days a week (58).
- For athletes: do eight sets at 85% 1-RM, 2 days a week (48).

This growing body of research prompted the American College of Sports Medicine to update its 2002 position standing on progression models in resistance training for healthy adults (3). What follows is a very brief summary of the position stand for gains in strength. Additional guidelines are provided in the position stand for gains in hypertrophy, power, and local muscular endurance.

- For novice (untrained individuals): loads should correspond to 60%–70% of 1-RM for 8–12 repetitions; do 1–3 sets at slow and moderate velocities of contraction, with at least 2–3 min rest between sets; train 2–3 days per week.
- For intermediate (~6 months training) individuals: loads should correspond to 60%–70% of 1-RM for 8–12 repetitions; use multiple sets with variations in volume and intensity over time; do at moderate velocities of contraction with 3–5 min rest between sets; train 3–4 days a week.
- For advanced (years of training) individuals: loads should correspond to 80%–100% of 1-RM; do multiple sets with variations in volume and intensity over time, using variable velocities of contraction (relative to intensity), with at least 2–3 min rest between sets; train 4–6 days a week.

---

is an increased need to circulate additional blood to the skin to dissipate the heat. As altitude increases, there is less oxygen bound to hemoglobin, and the person must pump more blood to the muscles to have the same

oxygen delivery. In both of these situations the HR response to a fixed work bout will be higher. To counter this tendency and stay in the THR range, the subject should decrease the work rate. Exercise in most cold

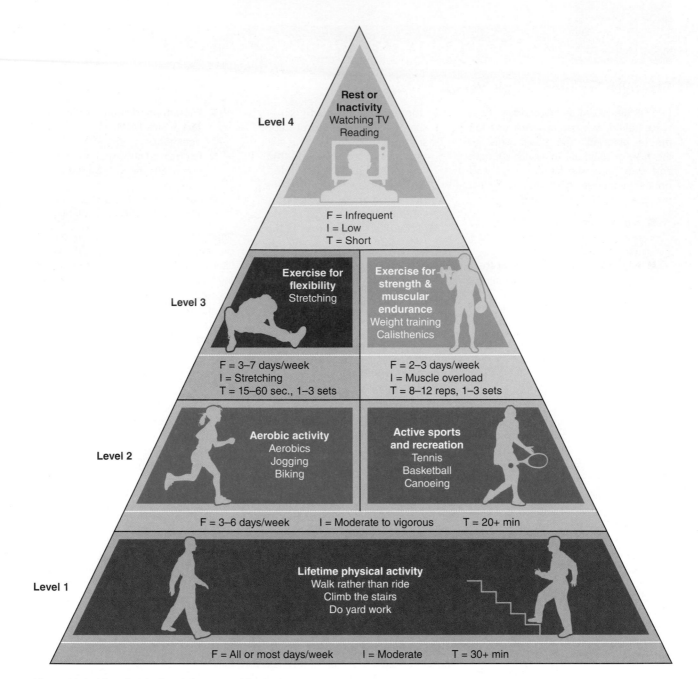

Figure 16.7 The physical activity pyramid.

environments can be refreshing and safe if a person plans in advance and dresses accordingly. However, there are some temperature/wind combinations that should be avoided because of the inability to adapt to them. As mentioned previously, some people simply plan exercise indoors (shopping malls, health spas, home exercise) during those occasions so that their routine is not interrupted. These environmental factors will be considered in more detail in chapter 24.

IN SUMMARY

■ The THR acts as a guide to adjust exercise intensity in adverse environments such as high temperature and humidity, or altitude.
■ A decrease in exercise intensity will counter the effects of high environmental temperature and humidity to allow one to stay in the target HR zone.

STUDY QUESTIONS

1. What are the practical implications of classifying physical inactivity as a primary risk factor?
2. From a public health standpoint, why is there so much attention paid to increasing a sedentary person's physical activity by a small amount rather than recommending strenuous exercise?
3. What is the risk of cardiac arrest for someone who participates in a regular physical activity program?
4. What is the difference between "exercise" and "physical activity"?
5. List the optimal frequency, intensity, and duration of exercise needed to achieve an increase in cardiorespiratory function.

6. For a person with a maximal heart rate of 180 b · min⁻¹ and a resting heart rate of 70 b · min⁻¹, calculate a target heart rate range by the Karvonen method and the percent of maximal HR method.
7. Recommend an appropriate progression of activities for a sedentary person wanting to become fit.
8. Why is it important to monitor heart rate frequently during exercise in heat, in humidity, and at altitude?
9. What is the recommended resistance-training program for untrained adults?

SUGGESTED READINGS

American College of Sports Medicine. 2010. ACSM's *Resource Manual for Guidelines for Exercise Testing and Prescription*. 6th ed. Baltimore: Lippincott Williams & Wilkins.

Baechle, T. R., and R. W. Earle. 2008. *Essentials of Strength Training and Conditioning*. 3rd ed. Champaign, IL: Human Kinetics.

Durstine, J. L., G. E. Moore, M. J. LaMonte, and B. A. Franklin. 2008. *Pollock's Textbook of Cardiovascular Disease and Rehabilitation*. Champaign, IL: Human Kinetics.

Faigenbaum, A. D., and K. J. McInnis. 2007. Guidelines for muscular strength and endurance training. In *Health Fitness Instructor's Handbook*, 5th ed. E. T. Howley and B. D. Franks (eds). Champaign, IL: Human Kinetics.

Howley, E. T., and B. D. Franks. 2007. *Health Fitness Instructor's Handbook*. 5th ed. Champaign, IL: Human Kinetics.

Liemohn, W. P. 2007. Exercise prescription for flexibility and low-back function. In *Health Fitness Instructor's Handbook*. 5th ed. E. T. Howley and B. D. Franks (eds). Champaign, IL: Human Kinetics.

U.S. Department of Health and Human Services. 1996. *Physical Activity and Health: A Report of the Surgeon General*. Atlanta, GA: U.S. Department of Health and Human Services, Centers for Disease Control and Prevention, National Center for Chronic Disease Prevention and Health Promotion.

REFERENCES

1. **American College of Sports Medicine.** American College of Sports Medicine position stand: the recommended quantity and quality of exercise for developing and maintaining cardiorespiratory and muscular fitness, and flexibility in healthy adults. *Medicine and Science in Sports and Exercise* 30: 975–991, 1998.
2. **American College of Sports Medicine.** *Guidelines for Exercise Testing and Prescription*. Baltimore: Lippincott Williams & Wilkins, 2010.
3. **American College of Sports Medicine.** Progression models in resistance training for healthy adults. *Medicine and Science in Sports and Exercise* 41: 1510–1530, 2009.
4. **American College of Sports Medicine.** Progression models in resistance training for healthy adults. *Medicine and Science in Sports and Exercise* 34: 364–380, 2002.
5. **American College of Sports Medicine.** Summary statement: workshop on physical activity and public health. *Sports Medicine Bulletin* 28:7: 1993.
6. **American Heart Association.** Statement on exercise: benefits and recommendations for physical activity programs for all Americans. A statement for health professionals by the Committee on Exercise and Cardiac Rehabilitation of the Council on Clinical Cardiology, American Heart Association. *Circulation* 86: 340–344, 1992.
7. **Birk TJ, and Birk CA.** Use of ratings of perceived exertion for exercise prescription. *Sports Medicine* (Auckland, NZ) 4: 1–8, 1987.
8. **Blair SN, Kohl HW, III, Barlow CE, Paffenbarger RS, Jr., Gibbons LW, and Macera CA.** Changes in physical fitness and all-cause mortality: a prospective study of healthy and unhealthy men. *JAMA 273*: 1093–1098, 1995.

9. **Blair SN, Kohl HW, III, Paffenbarger RS, Jr., Clark DG, Cooper KH, and Gibbons LW.** Physical fitness and all-cause mortality: a prospective study of healthy men and women. *JAMA 262*: 2395–2401, 1989.
10. **Byrd R, Chandler TJ, Conley MS, Fry AC, Haff GG, Koch A, Hatfield F, Kirksey KB, McBride J, McBride T, Newton H, HS OB, Stone MH, Pierce KC, Plisk S, Ritchie-Stone M, and Wathen D.** Strength training: single versus multiple sets. *Sports Medicine* (Auckland, NZ) 27: 409–416, 1999.
11. **Carpinelli RN, and Otto RM.** Strength training: single versus multiple sets. *Sports Medicine* (Auckland, NZ) 26: 73–84, 1998.
12. **Caspersen CJ, Powell KE, and Christenson GM.** Physical activity, exercise, and physical fitness: definitions and distinctions for health-related research. *Public Health Reports* 100: 126–131, 1985.
13. **Cavanagh PR.** *The Running Shoe Book*. Mountain View: Anderson World, 1980.
14. **Ceci R, and Hassmen P.** Self-monitored exercise at three different RPE intensities in treadmill vs field running. *Medicine and Science in Sports and Exercise* 23: 732–738, 1991.
15. **Chow RJ, and Wilmore JH.** The regulation of exercise intensity by ratings of perceived exertion. *Journal of Cardiac Rehabilitation* 4: 382–387, 1984.
16. **Church TS, Earnest CP, Skinner JS, and Blair SN.** Effects of different doses of physical activity on cardiorespiratory fitness among sedentary, overweight or obese postmenopausal women with elevated blood pressure: a randomized controlled trial. *JAMA 297*: 2081–2091, 2007.

17. **Dionne FT, Turcotte L, Thibault MC, Boulay MR, Skinner JS, and Bouchard C.** Mitochondrial DNA sequence polymorphism, $\dot{V}O_2$ max, and response to endurance training. *Medicine and Science in Sports and Exercise* 23: 177–185, 1991.

18. **Galvao DA, and Taaffe DR.** Single- vs. multiple-set resistance training: recent developments in the controversy. *Journal of Strength and Conditioning Research / National Strength & Conditioning Association* 18: 660–667, 2004.

19. **Gellish RL, Goslin BR, Olson RE, McDonald A, Russi GD, and Moudgil VK.** Longitudinal modeling of the relationship between age and maximal heart rate. *Medicine and Science in Sports and Exercise* 39: 822–829, 2007.

20. **Goodman LS, and Gilman A.** *The Pharmacological Basis of Therapeutics.* New York: Macmillan Publishing Company, Inc, 1975.

21. **Gutmann M.** Perceived exertion-heart rate relationship during exercise testing and training in cardiac patients. *Journal of Cardiac Rehabilitation* 1: 52–59, 1981.

22. **Hage P.** Perceived exertion: One measure of exercise intensity. *The Physician and Sportsmedicine* 9: 136–143, 1981.

23. **Haskell WL.** Dose-response issues from a biological perspective. In: *Physical Activity, Fitness, and Health,* edited by Bouchard C, Shephard RJ, and Stevens T. Champaign: Human Kinetics, 1994, p. 1030–1039.

24. **Haskell WL.** Physical activity and health: need to define the required stimulus. *The American Journal of Cardiology* 55: 4D–9D, 1985.

25. **Haskell WL, Lee IM, Pate RR, Powell KE, Blair SN, Franklin BA, Macera CA, Heath GW, Thompson PD, and Bauman A.** Physical activity and public health: updated recommendation for adults from the American College of Sports Medicine and the American Heart Association. *Medicine and Science in Sports and Exercise* 39: 1423–1434, 2007.

26. **Haskell WL, Montoye HJ, and Orenstein D.** Physical activity and exercise to achieve health-related physical fitness components. *Public Health Rep* 100: 202–212, 1985.

27. **Hellerstein H.** Principles of exercise prescription for normals and cardiac subjects. In: *Exercise Training in Coronary Heart Disease,* edited by Naughton JP, and Hellerstein HK. New York: Academic Press, 1973, p. 129–167.

28. **Hellerstein HK, and Ader R.** Relationship between percent maximal oxygen uptake (% max $\dot{V}O_2$) and percent maximal heart rate (% MHR) in normals and cardiacs (ASHD). *Circulation* 43–44 (Suppl. II): 76, 1971.

29. **Hellerstein HK, and Franklin BA.** Exercise testing and prescription. In: *Rehabilitation of the Coronary Patient,* edited by Wenger NK, and Hellerstein HK. New York: Wiley, 1984, p. 197–284.

30. **Hetzler RK, Seip RL, Boutcher SH, Pierce E, Snead D, and Weltman A.** Effect of exercise modality on ratings of perceived exertion at various lactate concentrations. *Medicine and Science in Sports and Exercise* 23: 88–92, 1991.

31. **Howley ET.** Type of activity: resistance, aerobic and leisure versus occupational physical activity. *Medicine and Science in Sports and Exercise* 33: S364–369; discussion S419–320, 2001.

32. **Howley ET, and Franks BD.** *Health Fitness Instructor's Handbook.* Champaign: Human Kinetics, 2007.

33. **Humburg H, Baars H, Schroder J, Reer R, and Braumann KM.** 1-set vs. 3-set resistance training: a crossover study. *Journal of Strength and Conditioning Research/National Strength & Conditioning Association* 21: 578–582, 2007.

34. **Jennings GL, Deakin G, Korner P, Meredith I, Kingwell B, and Nelson L.** What is the dose-response relationship between exercise training and blood pressure? *Annals of Medicine* 23: 313–318, 1991.

35. **Karvonen J, and Vuorimaa T.** Heart rate and exercise intensity during sports activities: practical application. *Sports Medicine* (Auckland, NZ) 5: 303–311, 1988.

36. **Karvonen MJ, Kentala E, and Mustala O.** The effects of training on heart rate; a longitudinal study. *Annales Medicinae Experimentalis et Biologiae Fenniae* 35: 307–315, 1957.

37. **Kasaniemi YA, Danforth J, E., Jensen MD, Kopelman PG, Lefebvre P, and Reeder BA.** Dose-response issues concerning physical activity and health: an evidenced-based symposium. *Medicine and Science in Sports and Exercise* 33 (Supp): S351–358, 2001.

38. **Lee IM, Hsieh CC, and Paffenbarger RS, Jr.** Exercise intensity and longevity in men. The Harvard alumni health study. *JAMA* 273: 1179–1184, 1995.

39. **Londeree BR, and Ames SA.** Trend analysis of the % $\dot{V}O_{2\ max}$-HR regression. *Medicine and Science in Sports* 8: 123–125, 1976.

40. **Lounana J, Campion F, Noakes TD, and Medelli J.** Relationship between %HRmax, %HR reserve, % $\dot{V}O_2$ max, and %$\dot{V}O_2$ reserve in elite cyclists. *Medicine and Science in Sports and Exercise* 39: 350–357, 2007.

41. **Morgans L.** Heart rate responses during singles and doubles tennis competition. *The Physician and Sportsmedicine* 15: 67–74, 1987.

42. **O'Donovan G, Owen A, Bird SR, Kearney EM, Nevill AM, Jones DW, and Woolf-May K.** Changes in cardiorespiratory fitness and coronary heart disease risk factors following 24 wk of moderate- or high-intensity exercise of equal energy cost. *J Appl Physiol* 98: 1619–1625, 2005.

43. **Paffenbarger RS, and Hale WE.** Work activity and coronary heart mortality. *The New England Journal of Medicine* 292: 545–550, 1975.

44. **Paffenbarger RS, Hyde RT, and Wing AL.** Physical activity and physical fitness as determinants of health and longevity. In: *Exercise, Fitness and Health,* edited by Bouchard C, Shephard RJ, Stevens T, Sutton JR, and McPherson BD. Champaign: Human Kinetics, 1990, p. 33–48.

45. **Paffenbarger RS, Jr., Hyde RT, Wing AL, and Hsieh CC.** Physical activity, all-cause mortality, and longevity of college alumni. *The New England Journal of Medicine* 314: 605–613, 1986.

46. **Paffenbarger RS, Jr., Hyde RT, Wing AL, Lee IM, Jung DL, and Kampert JB.** The association of changes in physical-activity level and other lifestyle characteristics with mortality among men. *The New England Journal of Medicine* 328: 538–545, 1993.

47. **Pate RR, Pratt M, Blair SN, Haskell WL, Macera CA, Bouchard C, Buchner D, Ettinger W, Heath GW, King AC, et al.** Physical activity and public health: a recommendation from the Centers for Disease Control and Prevention and the American College of Sports Medicine. *JAMA* 273: 402–407, 1995.

48. **Peterson MD, Rhea MR, and Alvar BA.** Maximizing strength development in athletes: a meta-analysis to determine the dose-response relationship. *Journal of Strength and Conditioning Research / National Strength & Conditioning Association* 18: 377–382, 2004.

49. **Pollock ML.** How much exercise is enough? *The Physician and Sportsmedicine* 6: 50–64, 1978.

50. **Pollock ML, Broida J, Kendrick Z, Miller HS, Jr., Janeway R, and Linnerud AC.** Effects of training two days per week at different intensities on middle-aged men. *Medicine and Science in Sports* 4: 192–197, 1972.

51. **Pollock ML, Dimmick J, Miller HS, Jr., Kendrick Z, and Linnerud AC.** Effects of mode of training on cardiovascular function and body composition of adult men. *Medicine and Science in Sports* 7: 139–145, 1975.

52. **Pollock ML, Gettman LR, Milesis CA, Bah MD, Durstine L, and Johnson RB.** Effects of frequency and duration of training on attrition and incidence of injury. *Medicine and Science in Sports* 9: 31–36, 1977.

53. **Pollock ML, and Wilmore JH.** *Exercise in Health and Disease.* Philadelphia: W. B. Saunders, 1990.

54. **Porcari JP, Ebbeling CB, Ward A, Freedson PS, and Rippe JM.** Walking for exercise testing and training. *Sports Medicine (Auckland, NZ)* 8: 189–200, 1989.

55. **Powell KE, Thompson PD, Caspersen CJ, and Kendrick JS.** Physical activity and the incidence of coronary heart disease. *Annual Review of Public Health* 8: 253–287, 1987.

56. **Proper KI, van den Heuvel SG, De Vroome EM, Hildebrandt VH, and Van der Beek AJ.** Dose-response relation between physical activity and sick leave. *British Journal of Sports Medicine* 40: 173–178, 2006.

57. **Rhea MR, Alvar BA, and Burkett LN.** Single versus multiple sets for strength: a meta-analysis to address the controversy. *Research Quarterly for Exercise and Sport* 73: 485–488, 2002.

58. **Rhea MR, Alvar BA, Burkett LN, and Ball SD.** A meta-analysis to determine the dose response for strength development. *Medicine and Science in Sports and Exercise* 35: 456–464, 2003.

59. **Robertson RJ, Goss FL, Auble TE, Cassinelli DA, Spina RJ, Glickman EL, Galbreath RW, Silberman RM, and Metz KF.** Cross-modal exercise prescription at absolute and relative oxygen uptake using perceived exertion. *Medicine and Science in Sports and Exercise* 22: 653–659, 1990.

60. **Ronnestad BR, Egeland W, Kvamme NH, Refsnes PE, Kadi F, and Raastad T.** Dissimilar effects of one- and three-set strength training on strength and muscle mass gains in upper and lower body in untrained subjects. *Journal of Strength and Conditioning Research / National Strength & Conditioning Association* 21: 157–163, 2007.

61. **Ruiz JR, Sui X, Lobelo F, Lee D-C, Morrow JR, Jackson AW, Hébert JR, Mathews CE, Sjöström M, and Blair SN.** Muscular strength and adiposity as predictors of adulthood cancer mortality in men. *Cancer Epidemiology, Biomarkers & Prevention* 18: 1468–1476, 2009.

62. **Saltin B, and Gollnick PD.** Skeletal muscle adaptability: significance for metabolism and performance. In: *Handbook of Physiology-Section 10: Skeletal Muscle,* edited by Peachey LD, Adrian RH, and Geiger SR. Baltimore: Lippincott Williams & Wilkins, 1983.

63. **Seip RL, Snead D, Pierce EF, Stein P, and Weltman A.** Perceptual responses and blood lactate concentration: effect of training state. *Medicine and Science in Sports and Exercise* 23: 80–87, 1991.

64. **Siscovick DS, Weiss NS, Fletcher RH, and Lasky T.** The incidence of primary cardiac arrest during vigorous exercise. *The New England Journal of Medicine* 311: 874–877, 1984.

65. **Siscovick DS, Weiss NS, Fletcher RH, Schoenbach VJ, and Wagner EH.** Habitual vigorous exercise and primary cardiac arrest: effect of other risk factors on the relationship. *Journal of Chronic Diseases* 37: 625–631, 1984.

66. **Swain DP.** $\dot{V}O_2$ reserve-a new method for exercise prescription. *ACSM's Health and Fitness Journal* 3: 10–14, 1999.

67. **Swain DP, and Franklin BA.** Comparison of cardioprotective benefits of vigorous versus moderate intensity aerobic exercise. *The American Journal of Cardiology* 97: 141–147, 2006.

68. **Swain DP, and Franklin BA.** $\dot{V}O_{(2)}$ reserve and the minimal intensity for improving cardiorespiratory fitness. *Medicine and Science in Sports and Exercise* 34: 152–157, 2002.

69. **Swain DP, and Leutholtz BC.** Heart rate reserve is equivalent to %$\dot{V}O_2$ reserve, not to % $\dot{V}O_2$ max. *Medicine and Science in Sports and Exercise* 29: 410–414, 1997.

70. **Swain DP, Leutholtz BC, King ME, Haas LA, and Branch JD.** Relationship between % heart rate reserve and % $\dot{V}O_2$ reserve in treadmill exercise. *Medicine and Science in Sports and Exercise* 30: 318–321, 1998.

71. **Tanaka H, Monahan KD, and Seals DR.** Age-predicted maximal heart rate revisited. *Journal of the American College of Cardiology* 37: 153–156, 2001.

72. **U.S. Department of Health and Human Services.** 2008 Physcial activity guidelines for Americans. http://wwwhealthgov/paguidelines/guidelines/defaultaspx 2008.

73. **U.S. Department of Health and Human Services.** Physical Activity Guidelines Advisory Committee Report 2008. http://wwwhealthgov/paguidelines/committeereportaspx 2008.

74. **U.S. Department of Health and Human Services.** *Healthy People 2000: National Health Promotion and Disease Prevention Objectives.* U.S. Government Printing Office, 1990.

75. **Wenger HA, and Bell GJ.** The interactions of intensity, frequency and duration of exercise training in altering cardiorespiratory fitness. *Sports Medicine (Auckland, NZ)* 3: 346–356, 1986.

76. **Wolfe BL, LeMura LM, and Cole PJ.** Quantitative analysis of single- vs. multiple-set programs in resistance training. *Journal of Strength and Conditioning Research/ National Strength & Conditioning Association* 18: 35–47, 2004.

Exercise for Special Populations

■ Objectives

By studying this chapter, you should be able to do the following:

1. Describe the difference between type 1 and type 2 diabetes.

2. Contrast how a diabetic responds to exercise when blood glucose is "in control," compared to when it is not.

3. Explain why exercise may complicate the life of a type 1 diabetic, while being a recommended and primary part of a type 2 diabetic's lifestyle.

4. Describe the changes in diet and insulin that might be made prior to a diabetic undertaking an exercise program.

5. Describe the sequence of events leading to an asthma attack, and how cromolyn sodium and β-adrenergic agonists act to prevent and/or relieve an attack.

6. Describe the cause of exercise-induced asthma, and how one may deal with this problem.

7. Contrast chronic obstructive pulmonary disease (COPD) with asthma in terms of causes, prognosis, and the role of rehabilitation programs in a return to "normal" function.

8. Identify the types of patient populations that one might see in a cardiac rehabilitation program, and the types of medications that these individuals may be taking.

9. Contrast the type of exercise test used for cardiac populations with the test used for the apparently healthy population.

10. Describe the physiological changes in the elderly that result from an endurance-training program.

11. Describe the guidelines for exercise programs for pregnant women.

■ Outline

■ Key Terms

arrhythmias
beta-receptor agonist
   (β_2-agonist)
coronary artery bypass graft
   surgery (CABGS)
cromolyn sodium
diabetic coma
immunotherapy
insulin shock
ketosis
mast cell
myocardial infarction (MI)
nitroglycerin
percutaneous transluminal
   coronary angioplasty (PTCA)

Chapter 16 presented some recommendations for planning an appropriate exercise program for the apparently healthy individual. Exercise has also been used as a primary nonpharmacological intervention for a variety of problems, such as obesity and mild hypertension, and as a normal part of therapy for the treatment of diabetes and coronary heart disease. This chapter discusses the special concerns that must be addressed when exercise is used for populations with specific diseases, disabilities, or limitations. However, the student of exercise science should recognize that this information is introductory in nature. More detailed accounts are cited throughout the chapter.

DIABETES

Diabetes is a disease characterized by hyperglycemia (elevated blood glucose) resulting from inadequate insulin secretion (type 1), reduced insulin action (type 2), or both (7). Diabetes is a major health problem and leading cause of death in the United States, representing a total (direct and indirect) annual cost of $174 billion in 2007. Of the more than 25.8 million individuals with diabetes, only 18.8 million are diagnosed, and the disease is not evenly distributed in the population. The prevalence of diabetes is greater in older (26.9% in those over age 60) than younger (11.3% in those age 20 and older) individuals, and is more common in Native Americans, African Americans, Hispanic Americans, and Asian and Pacific Island Americans. Diabetes injures and kills indirectly by causing blindness, kidney disease, heart disease, stroke, and peripheral vascular disease (30). Diabetics are divided into two distinct groups on the basis of whether the diabetes is caused by lack of insulin (type 1) or a resistance to insulin (type 2). Type 1, insulin-dependent diabetes, develops primarily in young persons and is associated with viral (flu-like) infections. The warning signs, which develop quickly, consist of (25):

- frequent urination/unusual thirst,
- extreme hunger,
- rapid weight loss, weakness, and fatigue, and
- irritability, nausea, and vomiting.

Because type 1 diabetics do not produce insulin, they are dependent on exogenous (injected) insulin to maintain the blood glucose concentration within normal limits. Type 2, noninsulin-dependent, diabetes typically develops more slowly and later in life than does type 1 diabetes; however, some overweight children are diagnosed with this disease. Type 2 diabetes represents about 90% to 95% of all diabetics (7), and it is linked to upper-body or android obesity and physical inactivity. The increased mass of fat tissue results in a resistance to insulin, which is usually available in adequate amounts within the body. However, some type 2 diabetics may require injectable insulin or an oral medication that stimulates the pancreas to produce additional insulin. Not surprisingly, the treatment of type 2 diabetics includes diet (8) and exercise (6, 10) to reduce body weight and to help control plasma glucose. Table 17.1 summarizes the differences between type 1 and type 2 diabetics (16, 26).

IN SUMMARY

- Type 1, or insulin-dependent, diabetes develops early in life and represents 5% to 10% of the diabetic population.
- Type 2, or insulin-resistant, diabetes occurs later in life and is associated with upper-body or android obesity and physical inactivity. Diet and exercise are important parts of the treatment program for type 2 diabetes to achieve weight loss and improved insulin sensitivity.

TABLE 17.1 Summary of the Differences Between Type 1 and Type 2 Diabetes

Characteristics	Type 1 Insulin-Dependent	Type 2 Noninsulin-Dependent
Another name	Juvenile-onset	Adult-onset
Proportion of all diabetics	5–10%	90–95%
Age at onset	<20	>40
Development of disease	Rapid	Slow
Family history	Uncommon	Common
Insulin required	Always	Common, but not always
Pancreatic insulin	None, or very little	Normal or higher
Ketoacidosis	Common	Rare
Body fatness	Normal/lean	Generally obese

From Berg (16) and Cantu (26).

Figure 17.1 Effect of prolonged exercise on blood glucose and ketone body levels in normal subjects, diabetics in "control," and diabetics taking an inadequate amount of insulin (ketosis). From M. Berger et al., 1977, "Metabolic and Hormonal Effects of Muscular Exercise in Juvenile Type Diabetics" in Diabetologia, 13:355–65. Copyright © 1977 Springer-Verlag, New York, NY. Reprinted by permission.

Exercise and the Diabetic

In chapter 5 we described how exercise increases the rate at which muscle removes glucose from the blood to provide energy for contraction. This effect makes exercise a useful part of the treatment of diabetes because it helps regulate the blood glucose concentration. However, this beneficial effect of exercise is dependent on whether the diabetic is in reasonable "control" before exercise begins. Control means that the blood glucose concentration is close to normal. Figure 17.1 shows the effect of a prolonged exercise bout on diabetics who were in control versus those who had not taken an adequate amount of insulin. A lack of insulin causes **ketosis,** a metabolic acidosis resulting from the accumulation of too many ketone bodies (due to excessive fat metabolism). A type 1 diabetic who is in control shows a decrease in plasma glucose toward normal values during exercise, suggesting better control. On the other hand, those type 1 diabetics who do not inject an adequate amount of insulin before exercise show an increase in the plasma glucose concentration (6, 9). Why the difference in response? The controlled diabetic has sufficient insulin such that glucose can be taken up into muscle during exercise and can counter the normal increase in glucose release from the liver due to the action of catecholamines and glucagon (see chapter 5). In contrast, the diabetic with inadequate insulin experiences

Figure 17.2 Effect of varied plasma insulin levels in type 1 diabetics on glucose homeostasis during exercise.

only a small increase in glucose utilization by muscle, but has the normal increase in glucose release from the liver. This, of course, causes an elevation of the plasma glucose, resulting in hyperglycemia.

Figure 17.2 summarizes these effects and adds one more (64). If an insulin-dependent diabetic starts exercise with too much insulin, the rate at which plasma glucose is used by muscle is accelerated, while glucose release from the liver is decreased. This causes a very dangerous hypoglycemic response. This information is crucial to understanding how to prescribe exercise for diabetics. Because the importance of exercise as a part of a treatment plan is different for type 1 and type 2 diabetics, we will discuss each type separately.

Type 1 Diabetes For many years, exercise was one part of the treatment for type 1 diabetes, with insulin and diet being the other two (66). However, as mentioned earlier, if a diabetic is not in control prior to exercise, the ability to maintain a reasonable plasma glucose concentration may be compromised. Further, exercise programs, by themselves, have not been shown to improve control of blood glucose (8). The greatest concern is not the hyperglycemia and ketosis that can lead to **diabetic coma** when too little insulin is present; rather, it is the possibility of hypoglycemia, which can lead to **insulin shock.** Richter and Galbo (90) and Kemmer and Berger (66) point out the difficulties a type 1 diabetic has starting an exercise program: The person must maintain a regular exercise schedule in terms of intensity, frequency, and duration, as well as altering diet and insulin. Such regimentation is difficult for some to follow, and given the variability in how a diabetic's blood glucose might respond to exercise on a day-to-day basis, the use of exercise as a primary tool in maintaining metabolic control has been diminished (8). Because metabolic control can be achieved by altering insulin and diet based on self-monitored blood glucose, exercise complicates this picture (66, 92). However, considering the importance of physical activity in an individual's life, and the effect of regular activity on CHD risk factors, a type 1 diabetic should not be discouraged from participation in regular exercise—if there are no complications (8).

An ECG monitored stress test may be needed for those individuals meeting one or more of the following (6):

- Age >40 years
- Age >30 and
  - Type 1 or 2 diabetes of >10 years' duration
  - Hypertension
  - Cigarette smoking
  - Dyslipidemia
  - Proliferative or preproliferative retinopathy
  - Nephropathy, including microalbuminuria
- Any of the following, regardless of age
  - Known or suspected coronary artery disease, cerebrovascular disease, and/or peripheral artery disease
  - Autonomic neuropathy
  - Advanced nephropathy with renal failure

These recommendations are based on the elevated risk individuals with diabetes have and the observation that strenuous exercise may accelerate or worsen retina, kidney, or peripheral nerve damage that is already present. The concern for the retina is related to the higher blood pressures developed during exercise, whereas the concern for the kidney is related to the decrease in blood flow to that organ with increasing intensities of exercise. The peripheral nerve damage may block signals coming from the foot such that serious damage may occur before it is perceived. Proper shoes for exercise, as well as the choice of the activity, are important (9, 69, 105).

The primary concern to address when exercise is prescribed for the type 1 diabetic is the avoidance of hypoglycemia. This is achieved through careful self-monitoring of the blood glucose concentration before, during, and after exercise, and varying carbohydrate intake and insulin depending on the exercise intensity and duration, and the fitness of the individual (9):

- Metabolic control before physical activity
  - Avoid physical activity if fasting glucose levels are >250 mg/dl and ketosis is present. Use caution if glucose levels are >300 mg/dl without ketosis.
  - Ingest added carbohydrate if glucose levels are <100 mg/dl.

- Blood glucose monitoring before and after physical activity
  - Identify when changes in insulin or food intake are needed.
  - Learn how blood glucose responds to different types of physical activity.

- Food intake
  - Consume added carbohydrate as needed to prevent hypoglycemia.
  - Carbohydrate-based foods should be readily available during and after physical activity.

Variability exists in how a type 1 diabetic responds to exercise and hypoglycemia (21). Consequently, frequent and consistent monitoring of blood glucose and fine-tuning of the insulin dose and carbohydrate intake are essential for long-term success in preventing hypoglycemia.

The exercise prescription for the type 1 diabetic must also consider other problems associated with this disease: autonomic neuropathy, peripheral neuropathy, retinopathy, and nephropathy. Individuals with autonomic nervous system dysfunction may have abnormal heart rate and blood pressure responses to exercise. Those with peripheral nerve damage may experience pain, impaired balance, weakness, and decreased proprioception. Damage to the retina is common in diabetics and is aggravated by increased blood pressure or any jarring action directed at the head. Finally, kidney damage is also a common experience for those with type 1 diabetes. This can lead to altered blood pressure responses that can affect the retina (9, 69, 106). It should be no surprise that the exercise prescription for the diabetic must address these problems if they are present. Recommendations from the American College of Sports Medicine include the following (4, 6, 105):

Aerobic Exercise Training:

- exercise 3 to 7 days per week;
- work at 50% to 80% heart rate reserve or 12–16 on the 6–20 RPE scale;
- do 20 to 60 minutes per session to accumulate at least 150 min of moderate-intensity or 75 min of vigorous-intensity physical activity per week; and
- use nonweight-bearing, low-impact activities (bicycle or stationary cycle, swimming, water exercise), if weight-bearing activities are contraindicated.

Resistance Exercise Training:

- exercise 2 to 3 days per week;
- work at 60%–80% 1-RM; ~14–16 on 6–20 RPE scale; and
- do two to three sets of 8–12 exercises for major muscle groups, avoiding the Valsalva maneuver.

Other:

- follow a progression schedule for both aerobic and resistance training programs;
- drink more fluid and carry a readily available form of carbohydrate and adequate identification; and
- exercise with someone who can help in an emergency.

In conclusion, although exercise may not be viewed as a primary factor in maintaining the blood glucose concentration in the normal range, the fact that type 1 diabetics who stay physically active have fewer diabetic complications is reason enough to pursue the active life.

IN SUMMARY

- A sedentary type 1 diabetic has to juggle diet and insulin to achieve control of the blood glucose concentration. An exercise program may complicate matters, and therefore exercise is not viewed as a primary means of achieving "control." In spite of this, the diabetic is encouraged to participate in a regular exercise program to experience its health-related benefits.
- The diabetic may have to increase carbohydrate intake and/or decrease the amount of insulin prior to activity to maintain the glucose concentration close to normal during the exercise. The extent of these alterations is dependent on a number of factors, including the intensity and duration of the physical activity, the blood glucose concentration prior to the exercise, and the physical fitness of the individual.

Type 2 Diabetes As mentioned earlier, type 2 diabetes occurs later in life, and the patients have a variety of risk factors in addition to their diabetes: hypertension, high cholesterol, obesity, and inactivity. Given the magnitude of this problem, more attention is being paid to identifying persons early in the disease process to delay or prevent the problem (see Research Focus 17.1). There is convincing evidence that type 2 diabetes is linked to a lack of physical activity, independent of obesity (6). In addition, current research supports the benefits of exercise training in the prevention and treatment of insulin resistance and type 2 diabetes (4, 6, 10). In contrast to the insulin-dependent diabetic whose life may be more complicated (in terms of blood glucose control) at the start of an exercise program, exercise is a primary recommendation for the type 2 diabetic, both to

help deal with the obesity that is usually present and to help control blood glucose. The combination of exercise and diet may be sufficient and eliminate the need for insulin or the oral medication used to stimulate insulin secretion (6, 10). Because type 2 diabetics represent about 90% of the whole population of diabetics, and because type 2 diabetes occurs later in life (after 40 years of age), it is not uncommon to see such individuals in adult fitness programs. It is important for clear communication to exist between the participant and the exercise leader to reduce the chance of a "surprise" hypoglycemic response.

Noninsulin-dependent diabetics do not experience the same fluctuations in blood glucose during exercise as do the type 1 diabetics; however, those taking oral medication to stimulate insulin secretion may have to decrease their dosage to maintain a normal blood glucose concentration during exercise (6). The exercise prescription for the type 2 diabetic is similar to what was just presented for the type 1 diabetic (4, 105), including the resistance training, which, when combined with aerobic training, results in benefits greater than either type alone. However, given that many individuals with type 2 diabetes are also overweight or obese (6):

- The focus should be on moderate-intensity physical activity (e.g., brisk walking), in which individuals can begin with 10-minute bouts, with the goal of at least 150 minutes per week. More is gained by walking for longer periods of time.
- The frequency of aerobic activity should be as high as four to seven times per week to promote a sustained increase in insulin sensitivity and to facilitate weight loss and weight maintenance.

As with all exercise programs for deconditioned individuals, it is more important to do too little than too much at the start of a program. By starting with moderate activity and gradually increasing the duration, exercise can be done each day. This will provide an opportunity to learn how to maintain adequate control of blood glucose while minimizing the chance of a hypoglycemic response. In addition, a "habit" of exercise will develop that is crucial if one is to realize the benefits, because the exercise-induced increase in insulin sensitivity does not last long (6). Further, the combination of intensity, frequency, and duration mentioned previously has been shown to directly benefit those with borderline hypertension, a condition often associated with type 2 diabetes. Consistent with the recommendations for the type 1 diabetic, clear identification and a readily available source of carbohydrate should be carried along in any exercise session. In addition, it would be much safer for a

RESEARCH FOCUS 17.1

Prevention or Delay of Type 2 Diabetes

Over the past decade, there has been an increase in the prevalence of type 2 diabetes that is linked to the increased prevalence of obesity. A great deal of activity has been under way to try to understand how to prevent or slow down the development of type 2 diabetes. One of the first things is earlier identification of people at risk of type 2 diabetes with the use of the fasting blood glucose and the oral glucose tolerance test (person drinks 75 g of glucose and blood samples are taken at 30 minutes and 1, 2, and 3 hours to track how fast glucose is taken up into tissues). These tests are used to identify those with:

- impaired fasting glucose (IFG): if fasting blood glucose values are

≥100 mg/dl (5.6 mmol/l) but <126 mg/dl (7.0 mmol/l), and

- impaired glucose tolerance (IGT): 2-hour value in an oral glucose tolerance test is ≥140 mg/dl (7.8 mmol/l) but <200 mg/dl (11.1 mmol/l).

Those with IFG or IGT are said to be "prediabetic" (7). Between 2005–2008 approximately 79 million Americans age 20 or older were classified as being prediabetic (30). Studies have shown that both drugs and lifestyle modifications can slow down or prevent the development of type 2 diabetes. However, lifestyle changes—increasing physical activity by 150 minutes per week and losing 5% to 10% of body weight—seem to be a better approach

than using drugs. In a now classic study, lifestyle modifications reduced the risk of type 2 diabetes by 58%, better than Metformin, one of the best drugs available (68). A recent review of all of the clinical trials in this area confirmed the findings that nonpharmacological therapy is a crucial part of the prevention process (103). In addition to dealing with the prediabetes problems, the loss of weight and increased physical activity reduce the risk of several cardiovascular risk factors (9). This "good news" must be balanced by the reality that we need better and cheaper ways to change the eating and physical activity behaviors of the average person.

---

diabetic to exercise with someone who could help out if a problem occurred.

Exercise is only one part of the treatment; diet is the other. The American Diabetes Association (8) states that there are four goals related to nutrition therapy for all diabetics:

- Achieve and maintain
  - Blood glucose levels in the normal range or as close to normal as is safely possible.
  - A lipid and lipoprotein profile that reduces the risk for vascular disease.
  - Blood pressure levels in the normal range or as close to normal as is safely possible.

- To prevent, or at least slow, the rate of development of the chronic complications of diabetes by modifying nutrient intake and lifestyle.

- To address individual nutrition needs, taking into account personal and cultural preferences and willingness to change.

- To maintain the pleasure of eating by limiting food choices only when indicated by scientific evidence.

The emphasis in achieving optimal nutrition is through a high-carbohydrate diet (with little processed sugars) to achieve nutrient goals for protein,

vitamins, and minerals. The low-fat diet has been shown to be useful in achieving weight-loss and blood lipid goals as well as diabetic control (8). The type 2 diabetic secures a variety of benefits from proper exercise and dietary practices: lower body fat and weight (see chapter 18), increased HDL cholesterol, increased sensitivity to insulin (decreasing the need), improved capacity for work, and an improved self-concept (6). These changes should not only improve the prognosis of the type 2 diabetic as far as control of blood glucose is concerned, but should also reduce the overall risk of coronary heart disease.

IN SUMMARY

- Type 2 diabetics have a variety of risk factors in addition to their diabetes, including hypertension, high cholesterol, obesity, and inactivity.
- An exercise prescription emphasizing low-intensity, long-duration activity that is done almost every day will maximize the benefits related to insulin sensitivity and weight loss.
- The dietary recommendation is for a low-fat diet, similar to what is recommended for all Americans for good health, with the additional goals of achieving normal serum glucose and lipid levels.

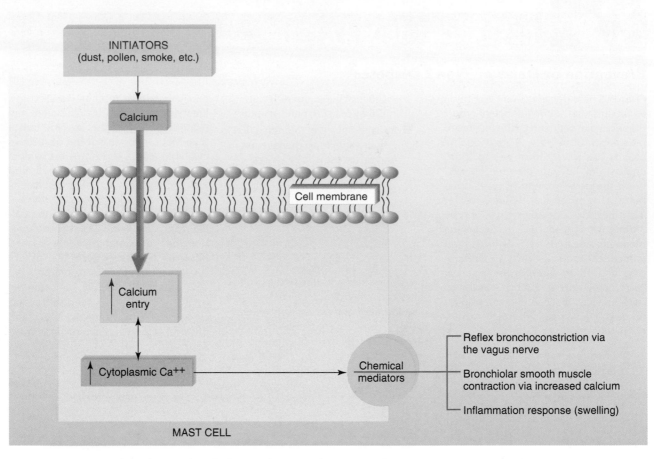

Figure 17.3 Proposed mechanism by which an asthma attack is initiated.

ASTHMA

Asthma is a respiratory problem characterized by a chronic inflammation of the airways and a reversible airway obstruction. An asthma attack is associated with a shortness of breath accompanied by a wheezing sound. It is due to a contraction of the smooth muscle around the airways, a swelling of the mucosal cells, and a hypersecretion of mucus. The asthma can be caused by an allergic reaction, exercise, aspirin, dust, pollutants, and emotion (84).

Asthma is a very common disease in the United States. In 2008, 23.3 million American adults were affected, resulting in 1.7 million emergency room visits and more than 3,600 deaths. Estimated direct and indirect costs were $20.7 billion. The large increase in the prevalence of asthma over the past 20 years appears to be leveling off, perhaps due to better management of the problem (**http://www.lungusa.org**).

Diagnosis and Causes

The diagnosis of asthma is made using pulmonary-function testing. If an obstruction to airflow (e.g., low maximal expiratory flow rate) is corrected by administration of a bronchodilator, then asthma is suspected. An asthma attack is the result of an orderly sequence of events that can be initiated by a variety of factors. These events are important if we are to understand how certain medications prevent or relieve the asthma attack. Figure 17.3 summarizes these events. The focus of attention is on the **mast cell,** one of the cells that is part of tissue in the bronchial tubes. It is believed that a variety of factors such as dust, chemicals, antibodies, and exercise initiate an asthma attack by increasing Ca^{++} influx into the mast cell, causing a release of chemical mediators such as histamine, prostaglandins, leukotrienes, and a special chemical that attracts white blood cells. The mediators, in turn, trigger the following effects:

- increase smooth muscle contraction (via an elevation of Ca^{++} in the muscle cell) leading to bronchoconstriction,
- initiate a bronchoconstrictor reflex via the vagus nerve, and
- cause an inflammation response (swelling of tissue).

Given that the vast majority of people do not experience an asthma attack while being exposed to these factors, a "sensitivity" or hyperirritability of the respiratory tract is a necessary prerequisite (84).

Prevention/Relief of Asthma

A variety of steps can be taken to prevent the occurrence of an asthma attack and to provide relief should one occur. If a person is sensitive (allergic) to something, then simple avoidance of the allergen will prevent the problem. If a person cannot avoid contact with the allergen, **immunotherapy** may be helpful in making the person less sensitive to the allergen while being treated.

Drugs have been developed to deal with the mast cell, which is a focal point in the asthmatic response, as well as the bronchiolar smooth muscle that causes the decrease in airway diameter. **Cromolyn sodium** inhibits the chemical mediator release from the mast cell, probably by interfering with Ca^{++} influx into the cell. **Beta-receptor agonists (β_2-agonists)** decrease chemical mediator release and cause the relaxation of bronchiolar smooth muscle by decreasing the Ca^{++} concentration in mast and smooth muscle cells. These effects are brought about through increased adenylate cyclase activity leading to an elevation of cytoplasmic cyclic AMP (see chapter 5). Daily use of β_2-agonists should be avoided because a desensitization of the β_2-receptor on the mast cells may occur (less of a response for the same level of drug). A physician can change the medication to achieve better control (11, 89). Corticosteroids and leukotriene antagonists are used to reduce the inflammation response, which is central to dealing with the long-term management of asthma (33, 78, 84, 89). Treatment with corticosteroids has been shown to increase arterial blood oxygenation and time to exhaustion from 9.9 minutes to 14.8 minutes in a treadmill test done at 90% of $\dot{V}O_2$ max (57). The net result of the medications is that both the inflammation response and the constriction of bronchiolar smooth muscle are blocked.

Exercise-Induced Asthma

A form of asthma that may be of particular interest to the reader is exercise-induced asthma (EIA). The asthma attack is caused by exercise and can occur 5 to 15 minutes (Early Phase) or 4 to 6 hours (Late Phase) after exercise. The prevalence of EIA varies from 7% to 20% in the general population, to 30% to 70% in elite winter athletes and elite athletes in summer endurance sports, and 70% to 90% in individuals with persistent asthma (89, 109). What is interesting is that 61% of the 1984 U.S. Olympic team members with EIA won an Olympic medal (107). Furthermore, if one compares 1988 Olympic athletes who experienced EIA with the athletes who did not, one finds no difference in the percentage who won medals (78). Similar

success was noted through the 2008 Olympics (89). Clearly, if anyone wondered whether EIA can be controlled, those results should dispel any doubts.

Many causes of EIA have been identified over the past 100 years. These include cold air, hypocapnia (low PCO_2), respiratory alkalosis, and specific intensities and durations of exercise. The focus of attention is now on the *cooling and drying* of the respiratory tract that occurs when large volumes of dry air are breathed during the exercise session (44, 73, 97). Respiratory heat loss is related primarily to the rate of ventilation, with the humidity and the temperature of the inspired air being of secondary and tertiary importance. As you remember from chapter 10, when dry air is taken into the lungs it is moistened and warmed as it moves through the respiratory airways. In this way moisture is evaporated from the surface of the airways, which is therefore cooled.

The proposed mechanism for how EIA is initiated takes us back to the mast cell mentioned earlier. When dry air removes water from the surface of the mast cell, an increase in osmolarity occurs. This increase in osmolarity triggers the influx of Ca^{++} that leads to the increased release of chemical mediators and the narrowing of the airways (78, 84, 89). Although the temperature of the air was believed to contribute to the problem, recent evidence suggests otherwise (47). What kind of circumstances bring on EIA?

The probability of an exercise-induced bronchospasm is related to the type of exercise, the time since the previous bout of exercise, the interval since medication was taken, and the temperature and humidity of the inspired air. It has been known since the late 1600s that certain types of exercise cause an attack more readily than others. Running was observed to cause more attacks than cycling or walking, which, in turn, caused more than swimming (78, 84, 89). However, in elite athletes, asthma is diagnosed more frequently in swimmers than in other sports. It may be that these elite swimmers self-selected the sport which is less likely to trigger EIA (89).

Generally, EIA is precipitated more with strenuous, long-duration exercise compared to short-term moderate-intensity exercise. One way to deal with this is to do short-duration exercise (<5 min) at low to moderate intensities. Further, when an exercise session occurs within 60 minutes of a previous EIA attack, the degree of bronchospasm is reduced. This suggests that a warm-up within an hour of more strenuous exercise would reduce the severity of an attack, and there is good evidence to support that proposition (75, 78, 84, 89).

There was special concern for the athletes of the 1984 Olympic Games, given the pollution in Los Angeles, which can aggravate an EIA attack (87). As mentioned before, the fact that 61% of the athletes who experienced EIA won Olympic medals

A CLOSER LOOK 17.1

Screening for Asthma in Children

Asthma is the leading cause of chronic illness and the most common respiratory disorder in children (38). Concern has been expressed about the need for screening programs early in life to identify those with a high risk of developing asthma. Jones and Bowen (60) measured peak expiratory flow rate before and after an all-out run in children from ten primary schools. Over a 6-year follow-up period, they compared children who had a negative result with those who had a positive result (a decrease in peak expiratory flow rate of $\geq 15\%$) due to the exercise test. Of the 864 children not known to have asthma, 60 had a positive test result. A follow-up of 55 of these 60 children showed 32 had developed clinically recognizable asthma 6 years later. These children also had a significantly higher prevalence of respiratory illnesses. Such field tests have much to offer in gaining control over this disease. In addition to screening, there is strong support to not back away from physical activity for asthmatic children. Most studies show that asthmatics can exercise safely and increase their cardiorespiratory fitness. Some scientists believe that the decrease in physical activity in children may have played a role in the recent increase in the prevalence and severity of asthma (71, 94). Finally, schoolchildren should have their medication available in the gym area, rather than in a central administrator's office (78).

---

suggests that procedures for preventing EIA with medication are generally established. Voy (107) reports that a simple questionnaire identified 90% of the athletes with EIA, even though only 52% were receiving treatment prior to the Olympics. However, there is abundant evidence that self-reported symptoms of asthma and/or EIA are not reliable for evaluating EIA in competitive athletes (89, 109). Typically, a strenuous exercise challenge (e.g., running at 85–90% of maximal heart rate on a treadmill) lasting 6 to 8 minutes is used to evaluate the presence of EIA (4). Some recommend that the air they breathe should be cool and dry during the test, or have the athlete perform the exercise challenge in the environment that triggers it (109). In addition, a non-exercise test can be used in which the subject breathes cool, dry air containing 5% CO_2 (to maintain the blood's CO_2 level) for 6 minutes at 85% of predicted maximum voluntary ventilation. It is a test of choice for screening elite athletes (42, 109), but it is much too complicated to use on a general basis, especially for children where a field test may be sufficient (see A Closer Look 17.1). In any case, a 10% or greater decrease in forced expiratory flow rate in one second (FEV_1) is classified as a positive test (109). The medications mentioned earlier are used to manage the condition to allow the athletes to go "all out." Some non-asthmatic athletes want to be identified as having EIA, believing that the medications might give them an edge. In a recent review, inhaled β_2-agonists were shown to not improve performance; however, ingested salbutamol (a β_2-agonist) did improve strength, anaerobic power, and endurance performance, but only at a dose 10–20 times that of what is inhaled (67).

A growing body of evidence suggests that specific nutritional factors may be helpful in managing EIA. The strategies include (76):

■ Reducing dietary salt intake to reduce smooth muscle constriction (as in hypertension—see later discussion). This approach has been shown to reduce asthma symptoms and medication use.
  ● The lower salt use is linked to lower calcium levels in smooth muscle, a lower osmolarity, and reduced release of proinflammatory factors.

■ Increasing intake of antioxidants such as vitamin C, vitamin E, lycopene, β-carotene, and selenium. These nutrients may desensitize the cell to proinflammatory mediators.

■ Taking fish oil supplement. This supplement is used for its therapeutic potential for a variety of inflammatory diseases. Relative to asthma, fish oil may act both prophylactically and/or by interacting with the medications being used.

As more research supports these findings, the message will be clear to those with asthma, as it has been for those with high blood pressure, blood lipid abnormalities, and diabetes—that diet really does matter.

In a majority of cases, EIA can be prevented with the medications mentioned earlier, used alone or in combination (23, 72, 84, 89, 100). The asthmatic who is participating in a fitness program should also follow a medication plan to *prevent* the occurrence of an EIA attack. The exercise session should include the conventional warm-up, with mild to moderate activity planned in 5-minute segments. Swimming is better than other types of exercise, given that air above the water contains more moisture. A scarf or face mask can be used when exercising outdoors in cold weather to help trap moisture. The participant should carry an inhaler with a β_2-agonist and use it at the first sign of wheezing (78, 84). As with the diabetic, the buddy system is a good plan to follow in case a major attack occurs.

IN SUMMARY

- An asthma attack is brought on when an agent causes an increased influx of Ca^{++} into a mast cell in the respiratory tract, which, in turn, triggers the release of chemical mediators. These chemical mediators cause a reflex and calcium-mediated constriction of bronchiolar smooth muscle along with an increase in secretions into the airways.
- Cromolyn sodium and β_2-adrenergic agonists act to prevent this by preventing the entry of Ca^{++} into the mast cell and by increasing the level of cyclic AMP in the mast and smooth muscle cells, respectively.
- Drying of the respiratory tract leads to an increase in the osmolarity of the fluid on the surface of a mast cell. This event is believed to be the central factor in the initiation of the asthma attack during exercise. Exercise of short duration, preceded by a warm-up, appears to reduce the chance of an attack. Drugs should be used prior to exercise to prevent an attack, and β_2-adrenergic agonists should be carried along in case one occurs.

CHRONIC OBSTRUCTIVE PULMONARY DISEASE

Chronic obstructive pulmonary diseases (COPD) cause a reduction in airflow that can have a dramatic effect on daily activities. These diseases include chronic bronchitis, emphysema, and bronchial asthma, either alone or in combination. These diseases are distinct from the exercise-induced asthma discussed earlier in that the airway obstruction remains in spite of continuous medication (36). Chronic bronchitis is characterized by a persistent production of sputum due primarily to a thickened bronchial wall with excess secretions. In emphysema, the elastic recoil of alveoli and bronchioles is reduced and those pulmonary structures are enlarged (17, 35, 95). The patient with developing COPD cannot perform normal activities without experiencing dyspnea, but, tragically, by the time this occurs the disease is

already well advanced (17). COPD is characterized by a decreased ability to exhale, and because of the narrowed airways, a "wheezing" sound is made. The person with COPD experiences a decreased capacity for work, which may influence employment, but he/she may also experience an increase in psychological problems, including anxiety (regarding the simple act of breathing) and depression (related to a loss of sense of self-worth).

It should be no surprise then that treatment of COPD includes more than simple medication and oxygen-inhalation therapy. A typical COPD rehabilitation program focuses on the goal of the patient's ability for self-care. To achieve that goal, a number of medical and support personnel are recruited to deal with the various manifestations of the disease process (77, 99). The COPD patient receives education about the different ways to deal with the disease, including breathing exercises, ways to approach the activities of daily living at home, and how to handle work-related problems. The latter can be so affected that new on-the-job responsibilities may have to be assigned, or if the person cannot meet the requirements, retirement may be the only outcome. To help deal with these problems, counseling by psychologists and clergy may be needed for patient and family. The extent of these problems is directly related to the severity of the disease. Those with minimal disease may require the help of only a few of the professionals just mentioned, whereas others with severe disease may require the assistance of all. It is therefore important to understand that the rehabilitation program is very individualized (34, 35).

Testing and Training

The consistent recommendation for anyone with known disease is to have a complete medical exam, including exercise testing, prior to beginning an exercise program (4). This is especially true for COPD patients because the severity of the disease varies greatly. A common test used to classify COPD patients is the FEV_1. Because the FEV_1 test is not a good predictor of exercise performance, Cooper (34) emphasizes a need to focus on the hyperinflation of the lung, which results from air trapping due to the person's inability to exhale completely. Hyperinflation is linked more directly to patients' outcomes, including exercise performance (34, 35). A graded exercise test to evaluate $\dot{V}O_2$ max, maximum exercise ventilation, and changes in the arterial blood gases, PO_2 and PCO_2, is also recommended. The results of this GXT are very helpful in developing the exercise prescription, especially when selecting the appropriate exercise intensity (35). However, because the FEV_1 test is the most common, guidelines have been established to screen patients with this test. The Global Initiatives for Chronic Obstructive

Lung Disease (www.goldcopd.org) provides guidelines to use in working with patients with COPD. They classify patients into the following four categories:

- Stage I: Mild COPD—$FEV_1 \geq 80\%$ predicted
- Stage II: Moderate COPD—$50\% \leq FEV_1 < 80\%$ predicted
- Stage III: Severe COPD—$30\% \leq FEV_1 < 50\%$ predicted
- Stage IV: Very severe COPD—$FEV_1 < 30\%$ predicted, or $< 50\%$ of FEV_1 plus chronic respiratory failure

Individuals in Stage I are usually unaware that their lung function is abnormal. In contrast, those in Stage III experience such a shortness of breath and fatigue that quality of life is affected, and by Stage IV, the patients may be in respiratory failure (54).

Even though exercise training does not reverse the disease process, it can interrupt the steady increase in symptoms of fatigue and breathlessness and the decline in quality of life. As mentioned above, the pulmonary rehabilitation program is very individualized. The program should include aerobic training using various modes (e.g., walking, cycling, arm ergometry, swimming), and be done 3–5 days per week (4, 35). In addition, resistance training is recommended to deal with local muscle fatigue in both the upper and lower body. The recommended intensity can be similar to what is recommended for healthy older adults (see later) for those in Stage I COPD. In contrast, for those with severe or very severe limitations, the GXT results can be most helpful. During the GXT the O_2 saturation of arterial blood is monitored, and the patient is asked to rate the level of breathlessness using a scale similar to the RPE scale. These results can help define an appropriate intensity to use in the aerobic portion of the exercise program and determine whether supplemental oxygen is needed (4, 35). Both moderate-intensity and high-intensity exercises are used, depending on patient status. Interval training allows the patient to work at a higher intensity (for a shorter duration) than conventional continuous training. There appear to be clear benefits to this approach, including a reduction in the respiratory load due to the short duration of the activity (24). Respiratory muscle training may be used, depending on the patient, but it is not a standard part of pulmonary rehabilitation (35).

Generally, COPD patients achieve an increase in exercise tolerance without dyspnea and an increase in the sense of well-being, but without a reversal of the disease process (29, 35, 65, 110). The changes in the psychological variables are very important in the long run, given that the person's willingness to continue the exercise program is a major factor in determining the rate of decline during the course of the disease (19).

IN SUMMARY

- Chronic obstructive pulmonary disease (COPD) includes chronic asthma, emphysema, and bronchitis. These latter two diseases create changes in the lung that are irreversible and result in a gradual deterioration of function.
- Rehabilitation is a multidisciplinary approach involving medication, breathing exercises, dietary therapy, exercise, and counseling. The programs are individually designed due to the severity of the illness, and the goals are very pragmatic in terms of the events of daily living and work.

HYPERTENSION

As mentioned in chapter 14, the risk of coronary heart disease (CHD) increases with increases in resting values of systolic and diastolic blood pressure (61). Blood pressure (BP) classifications have changed over the years, with normal BP being $<120/<80$ mm Hg. Prehypertension exists when either the systolic BP is 120 to 139 mm Hg or the diastolic BP is 80 to 89 mm Hg. The prehypertension category is not unlike the prediabetic category mentioned earlier in the chapter. The idea is to identify potential problems early and try to prevent or delay the development of hypertension. Stage 1 hypertension is a systolic BP of 140 to 159 mm Hg or a diastolic BP of 90 to 99 mm Hg. Approximately 68 million U.S. adults have hypertension (53). These stage 1 individuals represent the majority of all hypertensives, and they account for most of the morbidity and mortality associated with hypertension (55). Although there is little disagreement that medication should be used to treat hypertension, many believe that nonpharmacological approaches should be used for those with mild or borderline hypertension (4, 15, 56, 61, 62, 114). The reasons nonpharmacological approaches are recommended include the possibility of side effects due to medication and the counterproductive behavioral changes associated with classifying a person as a "patient" (56).

Generally, the person with mild hypertension should have a physical exam to identify potential underlying problems, as well as the presence of other risk factors. Kannel (61) indicates that while medication might be used to control blood pressure when multiple risk factors (smoking, high cholesterol, inactivity, etc.) are present, the simple act of stopping smoking confers more immediate benefit against the overall risk of CHD than any medication. It is within this context that a nonpharmacological intervention program focuses on the use of exercise and diet to control blood pressure and establish behaviors that favorably influence other aspects of health (15, 56).

Dietary recommendations to control blood pressure include a reduction in sodium intake for those sensitive to excess sodium, and in caloric intake for those who are overweight (31). Kaplan's (62) review indicates that salt restriction results in an average reduction in systolic and diastolic blood pressures of 5 and 3 mm Hg, and a 1-kg weight loss is associated with a 1.6 and 1.3 mm Hg reduction, respectively. Both fitness and physical activity are inversely related to the development of hypertension (27). Endurance exercise is associated with a 5–7 mm Hg reduction in resting blood pressure in hypertensive individuals; however, the magnitude of the reduction is inversely related to the pretraining blood pressure (4, 55). Although not all hypertensive individuals respond to endurance exercise in this way, exercise is recommended for all because other changes occur to reduce the risk of CHD, even if blood pressure is not reduced (55).

The standard American College of Sports Medicine exercise prescription for improving $\dot{V}O_2$ max (see chapter 16) is also effective in reducing blood pressure in hypertensive individuals. However, exercise in the moderate-intensity range (i.e., 40–59% of heart rate reserve) is effective and can be accomplished with lifestyle activities and structured exercise programs. The recommendation is to do at least 30 minutes on most, preferably all, days of the week, supplemented by resistance training at 60% to 80% 1-RM (2, 4, 55, 96, 108). Gordon (55) indicates that the combination of intensity, frequency, and duration should result in a weekly physical activity energy expenditure of 700 (initially) to 2,000 (goal) kcal. In addition to using exercise to lower elevated blood pressure, Gordon recommends that individuals:

- lose weight if overweight,
- limit alcohol intake (<1 ounce per day of ethanol—24 ounces of beer, 8 ounces of wine, or 2 ounces of 100-proof whiskey),
- reduce sodium intake,
- eat a diet rich in fruits, vegetables, low-fat dairy products, and reduced in saturated fat and cholesterol, and
- stop smoking.

For recreational athletes who need medication to control blood pressure, the preferred drugs are the angiotensin converting enzyme (ACE) inhibitors and calcium channel blockers (2, 4, 108). Blood pressure should be checked frequently so that the medication regime can be altered by the physician, if necessary.

IN SUMMARY

- Exercise can be used as a nonpharmacological intervention for those with hypertension. Exercise recommendations include moderate-intensity physical activity (40–59% $\dot{V}O_2$ max), done most days per week, and for 30 minutes per session. For those on medication, blood pressure should be checked frequently.

CARDIAC REHABILITATION

Exercise training is now an accepted part of the therapy used to restore an individual who has some form of coronary heart disease (CHD). The details of how to structure such programs, from the first steps taken after being confined to a bed to the time of returning to work and beyond, are spelled out clearly in books such as ACSM's *Guidelines for Exercise Testing and Prescription* (4), ACSM's *Exercise Management for Persons with Chronic Diseases and Disabilities*, and ACSM's *Resource Manual for Guidelines for Exercise Testing and Prescription* (see the Suggested Readings). This brief section will comment on various aspects of such programs.

Population

The persons served by cardiac rehabilitation programs include those who have experienced angina pectoris, myocardial infarctions (MI), coronary artery bypass graft surgery (CABGS), and angioplasty (51, 52). Angina pectoris is the chest pain related to ischemia of the ventricle due to occlusion of one or more of the coronary arteries. The symptoms occur when the work of the heart (estimated by the double product: systolic blood pressure × HR) exceeds a certain value. **Nitroglycerin** is used to prevent an attack and/or relieve the pain by relaxing the smooth muscle in veins to reduce venous return and the work of the heart. Angina patients may also be treated with a beta blocker to reduce the HR and/or blood pressure so that the angina symptoms occur at a later stage into work. Exercise training supports this drug effect: As the person becomes trained, the HR response at any work rate is reduced. This allows the individual to take on more tasks without experiencing the chest pain.

Myocardial infarction (MI) patients have actual heart damage (loss of ventricular muscle) due to a prolonged occlusion of one or more of the coronary arteries. The degree to which left ventricular function is compromised is dependent on the mass of the ventricle permanently damaged. These patients are usually on medications to reduce the work of the heart (β-blockers) and control the irritability of the heart tissue so that dangerous **arrhythmias** (irregular heart rhythms) do not occur. Generally, these patients experience a training effect similar to those who do not have an MI (51).

Coronary artery bypass graft surgery (CABGS) patients have had surgery to bypass one or more blocked coronary arteries. In this procedure, either a saphenous vein or an internal mammary artery from the patient is sutured onto the existing coronary arteries above and below the blockage. Sixty percent of those with saphenous vein grafts experience an occlusion by year 11, while the mammary artery graft is still patent in 93% of patients by year 10 (52). The success of the surgery is dependent on the amount of heart damage that existed prior to surgery, as well as the success of the revascularization itself. In those who had chronic angina pectoris prior to CABGS, most find a relief of symptoms, with 70% having no more pain at 5-year follow-up. Generally, with an increased blood flow to the ventricle there is an improvement in both left-ventricular function and the capacity for work (52). These patients benefit from systematic exercise training because most are deconditioned prior to surgery as a result of activity restrictions related to chest pain. In addition, exercise improves the chance that the blood vessel graft will remain open (88). Finally, the cardiac rehabilitation program helps the patient to differentiate angina pain from chest wall pain related to the surgery. The overall result is a smoother and less traumatic transition back to normal function.

Some CHD patients undergo **percutaneous transluminal coronary angioplasty (PTCA)** to open occluded arteries. In this procedure the chest is not opened; instead, a balloon-tipped catheter (a long, slender tube) is inserted into the coronary artery, where the balloon is inflated to push the plaque back toward the arterial wall (52, 102). "Stents" may be used in the PTCA procedure to help keep the artery open. Unfortunately, 30% of clients undergoing a PTCA will show an occlusion within 6 months, versus only 5–8% of those receiving a drug-eluting stent that reduces the chance of inflammation of the blood vessel (52). For more on who should and should not be referred to cardiac rehabilitation programs, see Thomas et al. in Suggested Readings.

Testing

The testing of patients with CHD is much more involved than that presented for the apparently healthy person in chapter 15 (45). There are classes of CHD patients for whom exercise or exercise testing is inappropriate and dangerous (4). The PARmed-X screening form in appendix C lists some absolute and relative contraindications for exercise. For those who can be tested, a twelve-lead ECG is monitored at discrete intervals during the GXT, while a variety of leads are displayed continuously on an oscilloscope. Blood pressure, RPE, and various signs or symptoms are also noted. The criteria for terminating the GXT go well beyond achieving a certain percentage of maximal HR, focusing instead on various pathological signs (e.g., ST-segment depression) and symptoms, such as angina pectoris. On the basis of the response to the GXT, the person may be referred for additional testing, such as the use of radioactive molecules (e.g., [99m]technetium sestamibi) to evaluate heart function at rest and during exercise, or direct angiography, in which a dye that is opaque to X-rays is injected into the coronary arteries to determine the blockage directly (74). The results of all the tests are used to classify the individual as a low-, intermediate-, or high-risk patient. The resulting classification has a major impact on deciding whether to use exercise as a part of the rehabilitation process and, if exercise is appropriate, determines the type and format of the exercise program (4).

Exercise Programs

Cardiac rehabilitation includes a "Phase I" inpatient exercise program that is used to help the patients make the transition from the cardiovascular event (e.g., a myocardial infarction that put them in the hospital) to the time of discharge from the hospital. The specific signs and symptoms exhibited by the patient are used to determine whether the patient should be placed in an exercise program, and if so, when to terminate the exercise session (4). After the patient is discharged from the hospital, a "Phase II" program can be started. This program resembles the one mentioned earlier for apparently healthy persons in that warm-up with stretching, endurance, and strengthening exercises, and cool-down activities are included. However, the CHD patients, who are generally very deconditioned ($\dot{V}O_2$ max of ~20 ml · kg^{-1} · min^{-1}), require only light exercise to achieve their target heart rate (THR). In addition, because these patients are on a variety of medications that may decrease maximal heart rate, the THR zone is determined from their GXT results; the 220 − age formula cannot be used. The patients usually begin with intermittent low-intensity exercise (1 minute on, 1 minute off) using a variety of exercises to distribute the total work output over a larger muscle mass. In time, the patient increases the duration of the work period for each exercise. The strengthening exercises emphasize a low resistance and high repetition format to involve the major muscle groups; free and machine weights, bands, and wall pulleys can be used in a circuit program format. Initial loads should allow 12–15 reps that can be done comfortably. Loads should be gradually increased as strength increases. A series of 8–10 exercises should be done to involve the major muscle groups on two to three days a week (4). Given that CABGS and post-MI patients have had direct damage to their hearts, the exercise should facilitate, not interfere with, the healing process. As you might guess, given the nature of the patient and the risk involved, cardiac rehabilitation programs take place in hospitals and clinics where there is direct medical supervision and the capacity to deal with emergencies, should they occur. After a patient completes an 8- to 12-week "Phase II" program, the person may continue in a "Phase III" program away from the hospital where there is less supervision, except for the ability to respond to an emergency (4). The frequency of major cardiovascular complications associated with doing exercise in cardiac rehabilitation programs is quite low (83, 101). What are the benefits of such programs to the patient with CHD?

Effects There is no question that CHD patients have improved cardiovascular function as a result of an exercise program. This is shown in higher $\dot{V}O_2$ max values, higher work rates achieved without ischemia as shown by angina pectoris or ST-segment changes, and an increased capacity for prolonged submaximal work (51, 52, 94). The improved lipid profile (lower total cholesterol and higher HDL cholesterol) is a function of more than the exercise alone, given that weight loss and the saturated fat content of the diet can modify these variables (see chapter 18). There is evidence that home-based cardiac rehabilitation programs for low-risk patients generate outcomes similar to hospital-based programs, but because only a limited number of patients have been involved in these home-based programs, more work needs to be done (59). It must be mentioned that a cardiac rehabilitation program should not be viewed simply as an exercise program. It is a multi-intervention effort involving exercise, medication, diet, and counseling. The latter characteristics are what make these programs "secondary prevention programs" aimed at reducing the risk of a subsequent cardiac event in high-risk patient populations. See Hamm et al. in the Suggested Readings for information on the core competencies of cardiac rehabilitation/secondary prevention professionals.

What is surprising, given the documented success of cardiac rehabilitation programs, is that they are underutilized. In a study of 72,817 patients from 156 hospitals who were discharged after treatment for an MI, PCTA, or CABG surgery, only 56% (40, 974) were referred to cardiac rehabilitation (22). There was considerable variability in response, with some hospitals referring 20% and others, 80%. However, referral is only part of the picture because more than 50% of patients referred to the program do not enroll (20). Clearly, more needs to be done to increase the use of cardiac rehabilitation programs—the patients would be the winners.

IN SUMMARY

- Cardiac rehabilitation programs serve a variety of patients, including those having angina pectoris, bypass surgery, myocardial infarctions, and angioplasty. These patients may be taking nitroglycerin to control angina symptoms, β-blockers to reduce the work of the heart, or anti-arrhythmia medications to control dangerous heart rhythms.
- The exercise tests for CHD patients include a twelve-lead ECG and are used for referral to other tests. Exercise programs bring about large changes in functional capacity in these populations due to their low starting point. The programs are gradual and are based on their entry-level exercise tests and other clinical findings.

EXERCISE FOR OLDER ADULTS

The number of older individuals (over age 65) in the United States will double between 2000 and 2030 as the "baby boom" generation comes to full maturity. Older individuals are a special challenge from the standpoint of exercise prescription due to the usual presence of chronic disease and physical activity limitations. However, participation in physical activity and exercise will go a long way in preventing the progress of diseases and in extending the years of independent living (3, 80, 104).

Maximal Aerobic Power

Maximal aerobic power decreases at the rate of about 1% per year from its peak value, which occurs at age 20 to 40 years, depending on the population (58). A report by Kasch et al. (63) shows that not only can this decline be interrupted by a physical activity program, but middle-aged men who maintain their activity and body weight show half the expected decrease in $\dot{V}O_2$ max over a 20-year period. The same is apparently not the case for women (see A Closer Look 17.2). Consistent with Kasch et al. (63), cross-sectional and longitudinal data show that the decrease in $\dot{V}O_2$ max with age is influenced by decreases in physical activity and increases in percent body fat, as well as any true "aging" effect (58). Because the vast majority of people experience a steady decline in $\dot{V}O_2$ max over time, by 60 years of age their ability to engage comfortably in normal activities is reduced. This initiates a vicious cycle that leads to lower and lower levels of cardiorespiratory fitness, which may not allow them to perform daily tasks. In turn, this affects quality of

Changes in $\dot{V}O_2$ Max with Age in Women

A study (50) has called into question some of our accepted wisdom about the change in $\dot{V}O_2$ max with age and the effect of fitness on that response. The authors' systematic and analytical review of the literature (a meta-analysis) showed that in endurance-trained women, $\dot{V}O_2$ max fell 6.2 ml $\cdot$ kg^{-1} $\cdot$ min^{-1} per decade, in contrast to 4.4 ml $\cdot$ kg^{-1} $\cdot$ min^{-1} and 3.5 ml $\cdot$ kg^{-1} $\cdot$ min^{-1} for active and sedentary women, respectively. This was different from what had been observed in men, and about whom most of the "accepted wisdom" had been based. It must be noted, however, that when these absolute changes (ml $\cdot$ kg^{-1} $\cdot$ min^{-1}) were expressed as a percentage of their respective $\dot{V}O_2$ max values, the percent decline was about 10% per decade for all groups, which is similar to what has been measured in sedentary men. Why did the most highly fit female subjects experience the largest change in $\dot{V}O_2$ max with age?

The investigators examined the decreases in maximal heart rate with age in these three groups to see if it might help explain why $\dot{V}O_2$ max decreased fastest in the most-fit group. It didn't. The decline in maximal heart rate was very similar across the three groups (7.0 to 7.9 b $\cdot$ min^{-1} per decade) and could not explain why the most-fit group had the fastest decline in $\dot{V}O_2$ max. The authors suggested the following possibilities:

- Baseline effect. Those with the highest $\dot{V}O_2$ max values had the greatest decline. A parallel observation was found in comparisons between men and women. On average, young men have higher $\dot{V}O_2$ max values than young women; the men also have a greater decrease in $\dot{V}O_2$ max with age. However, the percent decline is about 10% per decade for both genders, similar to what has been observed for the three groups of women.

- The most-fit women were found to have a greater decrease in their training stimulus with age, compared with sedentary women (since the sedentary women were just that, sedentary, their "change" would have been modest at best). The large reduction in training volume as they aged would help explain why the most-fit women had the greatest loss in $\dot{V}O_2$ max.

- An increase in body weight in adults with age is associated with a decline in $\dot{V}O_2$ max (ml $\cdot$ kg^{-1} $\cdot$ min^{-1}). The authors wondered if a difference in weight gain could help explain why the most-fit (least-fat) subjects had the greatest decrease in $\dot{V}O_2$ max. Interestingly, they found no support for this in their data analysis.

The authors remind us that, in spite of these observations, men and women of any age who participate regularly in endurance training have higher $\dot{V}O_2$ max values than their less-active counterparts.

---

life and independence, which may necessitate reliance on others (4). See A Look Back—Important People in Science for an individual who helped shape our understanding of the role of exercise in slowing the physiological changes we typically see with aging. A physical activity program is useful in dealing not only with this downward spiral of cardiorespiratory fitness but also with the osteoporosis that is related to the sudden hip fractures that can lead to more inactivity and death (3, 5, 80, 104).

Osteoporosis

Osteoporosis is a loss of bone mass that primarily affects women over 50 years of age and is responsible for 1.5 million fractures annually (86). Type I osteoporosis is related to vertebral and distal radius fractures in 50- to 65-year-olds and is eight times more common in women than men. Type II osteoporosis, found in those aged 70 and above, results in hip, pelvic, and distal humerus fractures and is twice as common in women (18). The problem is more common in women over age 50 due to menopause and the lack of estrogen. Hormone replacement therapy (HRT) initiated early in menopause prevents bone loss and can increase bone mineral density and reduce fracture risk (18, 86). However, such treatments are not without risks. HRT has been associated with an increase in cardiovascular disease and mortality and an increased risk of certain cancers (81). Given that prevention is better than treatment, attention is focused on adequate dietary calcium and vitamin D and exercise throughout life (5, 86).

Dietary calcium and vitamin D are important in preventing and treating osteoporosis. Although dietary intake of calcium for females is inadequate, when supplements are included and the average intake of calcium is considered, only adolescent girls fell dramatically short of achieving the recommendation (13). This is a major concern for the latter age group because it is during this time that bone mass should be built up. Vitamin D intakes were better across the board for all but the oldest age group, in part because their vitamin D requirement is higher than for other age groups (see chapter 18) (13).

A LOOK BACK—IMPORTANT PEOPLE IN SCIENCE

Dr. Fred W. Kasch's Adult Fitness Program Studied Patients Over 40 years

Dr. Fred W. Kasch received his B.S. and M.S. degrees at the University of Illinois, Urbana, and his Ph.D. at New York University. Dr. Kasch was hired at San Diego State University in 1948 and within 10 years established one of the first adult fitness programs in the country—a unique thing to do at a time when the medical community did not view the combination of exercise and adults as anything but risky business. His adult fitness program recruited cardiac patients—those with high blood pressure and those who simply wanted to become fit. Dr. John Boyer, a cardiologist, began to work with Dr. Kasch in the early 1960s and together, with their students, they collected data on the participants at regular intervals over the next 40 years to allow them to study changes over time. Measurements included an EKG,

blood pressure, weight, body fatness, and measured $\dot{V}O_2$ max (using classical techniques that involved a Douglas Bag and Scholander gas analyzer). At regular intervals over the 40 years, Dr. Kasch and his colleagues published research papers updating the changes (or lack thereof) that occurred in the program's participants. These reports showed that, compared with sedentary adults, regular participation in Kasch's program resulted in:

■ Decreases in blood pressure in those who were hypertensive
■ Maintenance of normal resting blood pressure over the years when inactive peers were experiencing an "age-related" increase in resting blood pressure values
■ Decreases in body fatness and the maintenance of lower percent fat values over time
■ A much slower decrease in $\dot{V}O_2$ max over the years

Dr. Kasch's reports provided clear evidence to the medical community that regular participation in exercise provided excellent health-related benefits in adults of various ages, including those with diagnosed disease. His adult fitness program became a model that was emulated by others throughout the 1970s and beyond. Dr. Kasch published more than 100 articles over his career. For an update on his participants, see *Age and Ageing* 28:531–536, 1999.

Dr. Kasch practiced what he preached throughout his entire life, remaining active as an archer and deer hunter into his nineties. He made his own long bow and arrows and began each day with a regime of exercise that each of us would do well to follow. Dr. Kasch passed away on April 8, 2008, a few days short of his ninety-fifth birthday. His memory and influence will live on.

Bone structure is maintained by the force of gravity (upright posture) and the lateral forces associated with muscle contraction. Even though the best exercise prescription for bone health in adults is a work in progress, we have guidance from both the ACSM and the U.S. *Physical Activity Guidelines* (3, 5, 80, 86, 104):

■ Modes: weight-bearing endurance activities (tennis, stair climbing, jogging, at least intermittently during walking); activities that involve jumping (volleyball, basketball); and resistance exercise.

■ Intensity: moderate to high, in terms of bone loading

■ Frequency: weight-bearing activities 3–5 times/week; resistance exercise 2–3 times/week

■ Duration: 30–60 min/day of a combination of weight-bearing endurance activities, activities that involve jumping, and resistance exercise that targets all the muscle groups.

Clearly, as age increases, one would have to use additional care to ensure that exercises can be done

safely. For some special insights into what is needed for bone health, see Ask the Expert 17.1.

Strength

Strength declines only about 10% between 20 and 50 years of age, but decreases at a much faster rate after that. The loss of strength is due, in part, to the lower level of physical activity in older individuals, but the large decrease in strength between 60 and 80 years of age is due to the actual loss of muscle mass, a condition known as sarcopenia. Chapter 8 (Clinical Applications, p. 183) provides a good overview of this problem and is worth rereading at this point. The good news is that strength training can increase strength in older individuals by about 30%, much like that seen in younger individuals (3, 85).

As is true for any special population, a complete medical exam is a reasonable recommendation to help discover problems or the presence of a combination of risk factors that might affect decisions about entry into an exercise program (4). There is no question that older adults, like their younger counterparts, exhibit a specificity and an adaptability to training, be

Exercise and Bone Health
Questions and Answers with Dr. Susan A. Bloomfield

Dr. Susan Bloomfield is Professor in the Department of Health and Kinesiology and a member of the Intercollegiate Faculty of Nutrition at Texas A&M University. Her current research utilizes animal models to study the integrative physiology driving bone adaptation to modeled microgravity, prolonged caloric restriction, and exercise, as well as functional relationships of bone and muscle in these models. She also serves as Associate Lead for the Bone Loss Team at the National Space Biomedical Research Institute, whose mission is finding effective countermeasures for spaceflight-induced bone loss. She lives in College Station with her youngest daughter, a rowdy Lab mix, and a cat, and can be found competing at U.S. Masters swim meets several times each year.

QUESTION: What are the primary factors affecting bone health?

ANSWER: Optimal bone health depends on adequate nutritional intake of calcium as well as regular exercise in the context of a normal hormonal profile. If serum levels of estrogen or testosterone are low, bone mass (usually measured by bone mineral density, or BMD) tends to decline. Interestingly, the primary effect of estrogen is to suppress activity of osteoclasts (bone-resorbing cells). Hence, estrogen deficiency, whether occurring at menopause or after prolonged amenorrhea in a young woman, "takes the brakes off" bone resorption and bone loss results. Glucocorticoids, be it endogenous cortisol or prescribed anti-inflammatory medications taken for chronic medical conditions, can directly stimulate bone resorption activity, thereby causing a loss of BMD. But if the endocrine milieu is reasonably normal, then calcium intake and physical activity patterns are the two most important determinants of bone mass and resistance to fracture.

QUESTION: Is exercise and good nutrition more important later in life when bone loss most often occurs?

ANSWER: Important as exercise and good nutrition are after the age of 50, when age-related or menopause-induced bone loss becomes more apparent, the most critical years from a public health viewpoint actually fall right around puberty. We gain an incredible 30% of our eventual peak bone mass in the 3 years surrounding puberty; further increases in BMD occur until at least the age of 25. The greatest impact of exercise on BMD and optimal bone geometry occurs during these years of rapid growth, with the result that the active child grows into an adult with a high peak bone mass before age-related loss begins. High calcium intakes (1,200–1,500 mg/d) at this age help ensure the maximal benefit. However, calcium intake is declining among American children and, ironically, most dramatically in adolescent girls who stand to benefit the most in terms of reducing their risk of osteoporotic fractures later in life. The clear public health message here is that we need to promote more consumption of calcium-rich foods (especially milk!) and more physical activity for American children and teens. In my mind this translates to the removal of soda machines from our schools' hallways and the promotion of regular physical education classes through high school. On a population-wide basis, the prevention of osteoporosis, rather than attention to treating established bone loss, is likely to be far more effective. A final caveat: It is important to encourage calcium intake of 1,200 to 1,500 mg/d and regular weight-bearing activity in older individuals, too. There is reasonably good evidence that age-related bone loss can be substantially slowed by adopting these habits.

QUESTION: What are the general characteristics of exercise programs that produce increments in bone mass and decrease the risk of osteoporotic fractures later in life?

ANSWER: There are important lessons to learn from key experiments done in animal models, with results being more frequently applied to the human condition. For example, experiments by Rubin and Lanyon (93) on the ulnas of turkeys revealed the importance of the magnitude of force applied to bone (as opposed to many loading cycles) as well as a unique distribution of loading. Hence, we have the current emphasis on either weight-training or weight-bearing activities that involve impact forces to provide adequate stimulus to the skeleton. In addition, a diversified exercise program that uses a wide variety of muscle groups with frequent and varied movement patterns is better than a monotonous signal to bone like running or cycling. The most recent findings from Robling and fellow researchers (91) using external loading of rat tibiae suggest that two to four shorter exercise bouts spread over the day might be more osteogenic (promoting gain in bone mass) than one long bout. Interestingly, this approach agrees well with the recommendations we're hearing from exercise epidemiologists that activity accumulated over the day provides significant health benefits. Incorporating more activity into our daily life (commuting by bicycle, physical work at home, more walking as well as planned exercise) holds much promise for improving bone health across the life span.

it for strength or endurance. Consequently, the exercise program should provide endurance, flexibility, and strength activities within the capacity of the population being served in order to make improvements in these fitness components. A combination of strength training and balance training has been shown to reduce the risk of falls (3, 80, 104). The potential benefits are clearly worth the time and energy invested (see A Closer Look 17.3).

In conclusion, the use of exercise programs for older adults improves cardiorespiratory fitness and strength and helps to maintain the integrity of bone. When this is coupled with the opportunity for socialization, it is easy to see why exercise is an important part of life from youth to old age.

IN SUMMARY

- The "normal" deterioration of physiological function with age can be attenuated or reversed with regular endurance and strength training. The benefits of participation in a regular exercise program include an improved risk factor profile (e.g., higher HDL and lower LDL cholesterol, improved insulin sensitivity, higher $\dot{V}O_2$ max, and lower blood pressure), but the training effects may take longer to realize.

- The guidelines for exercise training programs for older adults are similar to those for younger people, emphasizing the need for a medical exam and screening for risk factors. The effort required to bring about the training effect may be less than for younger individuals.

EXERCISE DURING PREGNANCY

Pregnancy places special demands on a woman due to the developing fetus's needs for calories, protein, minerals, vitamins, and of course, the physiologically stable environment needed to process these nutrients. It is against this background that the implementation of a fitness program must be evaluated. In much the same way that a diabetic, asthmatic, or cardiac patient would initiate an exercise program, the pregnant woman should begin with a thorough medical examination by her physician to rule out complications that would make exercise inappropriate, and to provide specific information about signs or symptoms to watch for during the course of the pregnancy. Absolute contraindications for aerobic exercise during pregnancy include hemodynamically significant heart disease, restrictive lung disease, incompetent cervix/cerclage, multiple gestation at risk for premature labor, persistent second- and third-trimester bleeding, placenta previa after 26 weeks of gestation, premature labor during the current pregnancy, ruptured membranes, and preeclampsia/pregnancy-induced hypertension. Relative contraindications include severe anemia, unevaluated maternal cardiac arrhythmias, chronic bronchitis, poorly controlled type 1 diabetes, extreme morbid obesity, extreme underweight (BMI <12), history of extremely sedentary lifestyle, intrauterine growth restriction in current pregnancy, poorly controlled hypertension, orthopedic limitations, poorly controlled seizure disorder, poorly controlled hyperthyroidism, and heavy smoking (1). Clearly, to protect mother and fetus, a consultation with a physician is a reasonable recommendation prior to the initiation of an exercise program.

Interestingly, compared to our knowledge of how diabetics, asthmatics, and cardiac patients respond to exercise training, we are now only beginning to understand how the mother and fetus respond to such a program (28, 112, 113). In general, the following describe the major cardiovascular and metabolic adaptations to pregnancy compared to the nonpregnant state (111, 112):

- Blood volume increases 40% to 50%.
- Oxygen uptake is slightly higher at rest and during submaximal exercise.
- The oxygen cost of weight-bearing exercise is markedly increased.
- Heart rates are higher at rest and during submaximal exercise.
- Cardiac output is higher at rest and during submaximal exercise for the first two trimesters; in the third trimester, cardiac output is lower and the potential for arterial hypotension is greater.

In spite of all these changes, moderate exercise does not appear to interfere with oxygen delivery to the fetus, and the heart rate response of the fetus shows no signs of distress. The fetal heart rate increases with the intensity and duration of exercise, and it gradually returns to normal during postexercise recovery (111–113). Cardiac output has been shown to be higher at 26 weeks' gestation during submaximal exercise than at 8 weeks following delivery. The fact that the a-$\bar{v}$ O_2 difference was lower suggests that the higher cardiac output was distributed to other vascular beds (e.g., the uterus) and muscle blood flow was

Exercise and Older Individuals: The Training Effect

Over the past 20 years, a substantial body of knowledge has accumulated, documenting the capacity of older individuals to experience a training effect similar to what has been observed in younger men and women (3, 80). This has major ramifications when one considers the increase in the number of older individuals in our population and the need to maintain their health status and independence for as long as possible. Data on the effect of exercise on older individuals have been obtained from cross-sectional studies comparing older athletes to their sedentary counterparts and from longitudinal studies in which training programs have been carried out over many months. A brief summary of each follows (56, 82).

Cross-sectional studies have shown that, in contrast to older sedentary individuals, endurance-trained older athletes have

- higher $\dot{V}O_2$ max values,
- higher HDL cholesterol, and lower triglycerides, total, and LDL cholesterol,
- enhanced glucose tolerance and insulin sensitivity, and
- greater strength, quicker reaction time, and a lower risk of falling.

These comparisons could be biased due to the potential for a strong genetic factor that might drive an individual to pursue an active life. In contrast, longitudinal studies compare a trained group to a control group over many months to see how each changes; this minimizes the concerns raised in the cross-sectional studies. The results from these studies parallel those mentioned previously. Endurance training:

- increases $\dot{V}O_2$ max and the kinetics of oxygen uptake in a manner similar to younger individuals, but more time may be required for the training effect to occur (12). In men, the increase in $\dot{V}O_2$ max is due to both peripheral (skeletal muscle) and central (cardiovascular) adaptations. However, the increase in $\dot{V}O_2$ max in older women is due solely to peripheral adaptations (98).
- causes favorable changes in blood lipids, but the changes seem to be linked to a reduction in body fatness, rather than exercise, per se.
- lowers blood pressure to the same degree as shown for younger hypertensives.
- improves glucose tolerance and insulin sensitivity.
- increases or maintains muscular strength and bone density. It must be added that resistance training results in large increases in strength, which may play an important role in reducing the risk of falls.

We currently have a variety of physical activity recommendations for older adults (3, 80, 104). What follows is a compilation, based primarily on the U.S. *Physical Activity Guidelines*:

- The following PA guidelines are the same for adults and older adults:
  - All older adults should avoid inactivity; some PA is better than none; and older adults who participate in any amount of PA gain some health benefits.
  - For substantial health benefits, older adults should do at least 150 minutes a week of moderate-intensity PA or 75 minutes per week of vigorous-intensity aerobic PA, or an appropriate combination of both. The PA should be done in bouts of at least 10 minutes, and the total amount should be spread throughout the week.
    - On a scale of 0 to 10 for a level of physical exertion, use 5 to 6 for moderate-intensity PA and 7 to 8 for vigorous-intensity PA.
  - For additional and more extensive health benefits, older adults should increase their aerobic physical activity to 300 minutes per week of moderate-intensity PA or 150 minutes per week of vigorous-intensity PA. Additional health benefits can be gained by going beyond this amount.
  - Older adults should also perform 8–10 muscle strengthening exercises on at least 2 days per week using the major muscle groups. A resistance should be used that allows 8–12 repetitions for each exercise. Interestingly, there is evidence in older adults (>65 years) that one day per week of resistance training may be as good as two days per week in terms of strength gains (43). Further, periodized programs offer no advantage compared to standard fixed repetition programs (41).
  - Perform flexibility exercises for at least 10 minutes on at least 2 days per week. Recent evidence shows that flexibility exercise can improve the walking ability of older adults (faster speed, longer stride) (37).

- The following guidelines are just for older adults:
  - If older adults cannot do 150 minutes of moderate-intensity PA per week because of chronic conditions, they should be as active as their abilities and conditions allow.
  - Older adults should determine their level of effort for physical activity relative to their level of fitness.
  - Older adults should do exercises that maintain or improve balance if they are at risk of falling. In that regard, exercise programs using multiple modes appear to have an advantage in fall prevention (14). However, gains are more likely to be realized in the pre-frail older adult than in the frail older adult (49).
  - Older adults with chronic conditions should understand how their conditions affect their ability to do regular PA safely.

An important point made throughout the U.S. *Physical Activity Guidelines* is the importance of progression, and this is certainly the case when working with older adults (104). Visit the following website to see exercise programs for older adults: http://www.nia.nih.gov/HealthInformation/Publications/ExerciseGuide/default.htm.

maintained (94, 113). Since absolute $\dot{V}O_2$ max (L/min) doesn't change much over the course of a pregnancy (70), what happens when exercise training is done during pregnancy?

In general, there is evidence that estimated $\dot{V}O_2$ max (in L/min) is increased as a result of training in previously sedentary pregnant women, while relative $\dot{V}O_2$ max (ml $\cdot$ kg^{-1} $\cdot$ min^{-1}) is maintained or increased slightly, despite the weight gain (113). What is interesting is that when well-conditioned recreational athletes trained throughout and following their pregnancy, absolute $\dot{V}O_2$ max was increased as long as 36 to 44 weeks after delivery compared to a "control" group of women who maintained training and did not become pregnant (32). This suggests that the combination of pregnancy and training resulted in adaptations greater than what could be achieved by training alone. What are reasonable recommendations to follow when a pregnant woman wants to exercise?

Guidelines have been developing over the past two decades. In an earlier set of guidelines from the American College of Obstetricians and Gynecologists, fixed criteria (e.g., don't exercise over an HR of 140 b/min) were provided, with the emphasis on taking a conservative approach to exercise prescription. Current guidelines emphasize the need to avoid doing exercise in the supine position to avoid a reduction in venous return and orthostatic hypotension (1). Weight-supported activities are encouraged due to the lower risk of injury, and attention is focused on the need for hydration to maintain body temperature in the normal range associated with exercise. Research suggests that normal exercise-induced increases in body temperatures carry little risk to the fetus (1, 28, 112).

The American College of Obstetricians and Gynecologists states that in the absence of either medical or obstetric complications, pregnant women can follow the public health recommendation of doing 150 minutes of moderate-intensity physical activity per week.

- Recreational and competitive athletes with uncomplicated pregnancies can remain active during pregnancy, and modify activities as medically indicated. Pregnant women who engage in strenuous exercise require close medical supervision.
- Previously inactive women and those with medical or obstetric complications should be evaluated by a physician before exercise recommendations are made.
- A physically active woman with a history of, or at risk for, preterm labor or fetal growth restriction should reduce her activity in the second and third trimesters.

For those doing structured exercise programs, the Canadian Guidelines (40) suggest using the "talk test" (reduce intensity when conversation cannot be continued without pauses to catch one's breath) or the RPE (12–14 on the original Borg scale) to set exercise intensity. However, the following heart rate ranges were offered for additional guidance:

- less than 20 years old, 140 to 155 b/min,
- 20 to 29 years old, 135 to 150 b/min,
- 30 to 39 years old, 130 to 145 b/min, and
- 40 years or older, 125 to 140 b/min.

A recent study by Mottola et al. (79) examined the heart rate/% $\dot{V}O_2$ peak relationship in pregnant women to validate the preceding heart rate recommendations. Pregnant women who were at 16 to 22 weeks' gestation completed a graded treadmill test to measure the heart rate response and $\dot{V}O_2$ peak (highest $\dot{V}O_2$ achieved in the test). They divided the group into "fit" (top 25th percentile), "unfit" (bottom 25th percentile), and "active" (those in between). For both the 20–29 and 30–39-year-old age groups, the heart rate range equivalent of 60% to 80% $\dot{V}O_2$ peak was similar to the above recommendations for the active group and for the unfit 30–39-year-old group. The fit group's heart rate values were 10 b/min higher than those recommended above. In contrast, for the unfit 20–29-year-olds, the heart rate for 60% $\dot{V}O_2$ peak was 6 b/min lower than the above recommendation. This information will be useful when these recommendations are revised. In the meantime, the authors support the use of the "talk test" and the RPE as additional guides to individualize the exercise prescription. For more on this, see the review article by Melzer, et al. in Suggested Readings.

In spite of the growing body of knowledge supporting the appropriateness of recommending exercise during pregnancy, only about 50% of private/small group practice obstetricians recommend physical activity during pregnancy (46). This is unfortunate given that regular physical activity during pregnancy is associated with a reduced risk of both gestational diabetes and preeclampsia, growing problems in an overweight and obese society (39). A recent study emphasized the need to disseminate current recommendations and information about the risks and benefits of physical activity during pregnancy to obstetricians in order to overcome the gap between science and practice (48).

IN SUMMARY

- A pregnant woman should consult with her physician before starting an exercise program.
- Endurance exercise can be done during pregnancy without complications to mother or fetus.

STUDY QUESTIONS

1. What is the difference between type 1 and type 2 diabetes?
2. If a type 1 diabetic does not take an adequate amount of insulin, what happens to the blood glucose concentration during prolonged exercise? Why?
3. If exercise is helpful in controlling blood glucose, how could it complicate the life of a type 1 diabetic?
4. Provide general recommendations regarding changes in insulin and diet for diabetics who engage in exercise.
5. How is exercise-induced asthma triggered, and how do medications reduce the chance of an attack?
6. Why are exercise and diet recommended as nonpharmacological treatments for those with borderline hypertension?
7. What is COPD, and where does exercise fit in as a part of a rehabilitation program?
8. What are angina pectoris, CABGS, and angioplasty?
9. What additional measurements are made during a GXT of a cardiac patient, as compared to an apparently healthy individual?
10. How do elderly people respond to exercise training compared to younger subjects?
11. What are the concerns about exercise during pregnancy, and what are the guidelines recommended for a pregnant woman who wants to begin an exercise program?

SUGGESTED READINGS

American College of Sports Medicine. 2009. ACSM's *Exercise Management for Persons with Chronic Diseases and Disabilities*. Champaign, IL: Human Kinetics.

American College of Sports Medicine. 2010. ACSM's *Resource Manual for Guidelines for Exercise Testing and Prescription*. 6th ed. Baltimore: Lippincott Williams & Wilkins.

Hamm, L. F., B. K. Sanderson, P. A. Ades, K. Berra, L. A. Kaminsky, J. L. Roitman, M. A. Williams. 2011. Core competencies for cardiac rehabilitation/secondary prevention professionals: 2010 update. *Journal of Cardiopulmonary Rehabilitation and Prevention*. 31:2–10.

Melzer, K., Y. Schutz, M. Boulvain, and B. Kayser. 2010. Physical activity and pregnancy. *Sports Medicine*. 40:493–507.

Thomas, R. J., M. King, K. Lui, N. Oldridge, I. L. Piña, and J. Spertus. 2010. ACC/AHA 2010 update: performance measures on cardiac rehabilitation for referral to cardiac rehabilitation/secondary prevention services. *Journal of the American College of Cardiology*. 56:1159–67.

REFERENCES

1. **American College of Obstetricians and Gynecologists.** Exercise during pregnancy and the postpartum period. (Opinion No. 267). *Obstet Gynecol* 99: 171–173, 2002.
2. **American College of Sports Medicine.** Exercise and hypertension. *Medicine and Science in Sports and Exercise* 25: i–x, 2004.
3. **American College of Sports Medicine.** Exercise and physical activity for the older adult. *Medicine and Science in Sports and Exercise* 41: 1510–1530, 2009.
4. **American College of Sports Medicine.** *Guidelines for Exercise Testing and Prescription*. Baltimore: Lippincott Williams & Wlikins, 2010.
5. **American College of Sports Medicine.** Physcial activity and bone health. *Medicine and Science in Sports and Exercise* 36: 1985–1996, 2004.
6. **American College of Sports Medicine and American Diabetes Association.** Exercise and type 2 diabetes. *Medicine and Science in Sports and Exercise* 42: 2282–2303, 2010.
7. **American Diabetes Association.** Diagnosis and classification of diabetes mellitus. *Diabetes Care* 27: S5–10, 2007.
8. **American Diabetes Association.** Nutrition recommendations and interventions for diabetes. *Diabetes Care* 30 (Supple 1): S48–65, 2007.
9. **American Diabetes Association.** Physical activity/exercise and diabetes. *Diabetes Care* 27: S58–62, 2004.
10. **American Diabetes Association.** Prevention or delay of type 2 diabetes. *Diabetes Care* 27: S47–54, 2004.
11. **Anderson SD, Caillaud C, and Brannan JD.** Beta2-agonists and exercise-induced asthma. *Clinical Reviews in Allergy & Immunology* 31: 163–180, 2006.
12. **Babcock MA, Paterson DH, and Cunningham DA.** Effects of aerobic endurance training on gas exchange kinetics of older men. *Med Sci Sports Exerc* 26: 447–452, 1994.
13. **Bailey RL, Dodd KW, Goldman JA, Gahche JJ, Dwyer JT, Moshfegh AJ, Sempos CT, and Picciano MF.** Estimation of total usual calcium and vitamin D intakes in the United States. *Journal of Nutrition* 140: 817–822, 2010.
14. **Baker MK, Atlantis E, and Fiatarone Singh MA.** Multi-modal exercise programs for older adults. *Age and Ageing* 36: 375–381, 2007.
15. **Bassett DR, and Zweifler AJ.** Risk factors and risk factor management. In: *Clinical Ischemic Syndromes*, edited by Zelenock GB, D'Alecy LG, Fantone III JC, Shlafer M, and Stanley JC. St. Louis: C. V. Mosby, 1990, p. 15–46.
16. **Berg KE.** *Diabetic's Guide to Health and Fitness*. Champaign: Life Enhancement Publications, 1986.
17. **Berman LB, and Sutton JR.** Exercise and the pulmonary patient. *Journal of Cardiopulmonary Rehabilitation* 6: 52–61, 1986.
18. **Bloomfield SA, and Smith SS.** Osteoporosis. In: *ACSM's Exercise Management for Persons with Chronic Diseases and Disabilities*. Champaign: Human Kinetics, 2003, p. 222–229.
19. **Booker R.** Chronic obstructive pulmonary disease: non-pharmacological approaches. *British Journal of Nursing* (Mark Allen Publishing) 14: 14–18, 2005.
20. **Boyden T, Rubenfire M, and Franklin B.** Will increasing referral to cardiac rehabilitatation improve participation? *Preventive Cardiology* 13: 192–201, 2010.
21. **Briscoe VJ, Tate DB, and Davis SN.** Type 1 diabetes: exercise and hypoglycemia. *Applied Physiology, Nutrition, and Metabolism = Physiologie Appliquee, Nutrition et Metabolisme* 32: 576–582, 2007.
22. **Brown TM, Hernandez AF, Bittner V, Cannon CP, Ellrodt G, Liang L, Peterson ED, Pina IL, Safford MM, and Fonarow GC.** Predictors of cardiac rehabilitation

referral in coronary artery disease patients: finding from the American Heart Association Get With the Guidelines Program. *Journal of the American College of Cardiology* 54: 515–521, 200.

23. **Brusasco V, and Crimi E.** Allergy and sports: exercise-induced asthma. *International Journal of Sports Medicine* 15 Suppl 3: S184–186, 1994.

24. **Butcher SJ, and Jones RL.** The impact of exercise training intensity on change in physiological function in patients with chronic obstructive pulmonary disease. *Sports Medicine (Auckland, NZ)* 36: 307–325, 2006.

25. **Campaign BN.** Exercise and diabetes mellitus. In: ACSM's *Resource Manual for Guidelines for Graded Exercise Testing and Prescription*. Baltimore: Lippincott Williams & Wilkins, 2001, p. 277–284.

26. **Cantu DC.** *Diabetes and Exercise.* Ithaca: Movement Publications, 1982.

27. **Carnethon MR, Evans NS, Church TS, Lewis CE, Schreiner PJ, Jacobs DR, Sternfeld B, and Sidney S.** Joint associations of physical activity and aerobic fitness on the development of incident hypertension: coronary artery disease risk development in young adults. *Hypertension* 56: 49–55, 2010.

28. **Carpenter MW.** Physical activity, fitness, and health of the pregnant mother and fetus. In: *Physical Activity, Fitness, and Health*, edited by Bouchard C, Shephard RJ, and Stephens T. Champaign: Human Kinetics, 1994, p. 967–979.

29. **Carter R, Coast JR, and Idell S.** Exercise training in patients with chronic obstructive pulmonary disease. *Med Sci Sports Exerc* 24: 281–291, 1992.

30. **Centers for Disease Control and Prevention.** *National Diabetes Fact Sheet: National Estimates and General Information on Diabetes and Prediabetes in the United States, 2011.* Atlanta, GA: U. S. Department of Health and Human Servcies, Centers for Disease Control and Prevention, 2011.

31. **Chobanian AV, Bakris GL, Black HR, Cushman WC, Green LA, Izzo JL, Jr., Jones DW, Materson BJ, Oparil S, Wright JT, Jr., and Roccella EJ.** Seventh report of the Joint National Committee on Prevention, Detection, Evaluation, and Treatment of High Blood Pressure. *Hypertension* 42: 1206–1252, 2003.

32. **Clapp JF, III, and Capeless E.** The $\dot{V}O_{2max}$ of recreational athletes before and after pregnancy. *Med Sci Sports Exerc* 23: 1128–1133, 1991.

33. **Clark CJ.** Asthma. In: *ACSM's Exercise Management for Persons with Chronic Diseases and Disabilities.* Champaign: Human Kinetics, 2003, p. 105–110.

34. **Cooper CB.** Airflow obstruction and exercise. *Respiratory Medicine* 103: 325–334, 2009.

35. **Cooper CB, and Storer TW.** Exercise prescription in patients with pulmonary disease. In: *ACSM's Resource Manual for Guidelines for Exercise Testing and Prescription*, edited by Ehrman JK. Baltimore: Lippincott Williams & Wilkins, 2010, p. 575–599.

36. **Cox NJ, van Herwaarden CL, Folgering H, and Binkhorst RA.** Exercise and training in patients with chronic obstructive lung disease. *Sports Medicine (Auckland, NZ)* 6: 180–192, 1988.

37. **Cristopoliski F, Barela JA, Leite N, Fowler NE, and Rodacki ALF.** Stretching exercise programs improve gait in the elderly. *Gerontology* 55: 614–620, 2009.

38. **Cypcar D, and Lemanske RF, Jr.** Asthma and exercise. *Clinics in Chest Medicine* 15: 351–368, 1994.

39. **Damm P, Breitowicz B, and Hegaard H.** Exercise, pregnancy, and insulin sensitivity—what is new? *Applied Physiology, Nutrition, and Metabolism = Physiologie Appliquee, Nutrition et Metabolisme* 32: 537–540, 2007.

40. **Davies GA, Wolfe LA, Mottola MF, and MacKinnon C.** Joint SOGC/CSEP clinical practice guideline: exercise in pregnancy and the postpartum period. *Canadian Journal of Applied Physiology = Revue Canadienne de Physiologie Appliquee* 28: 330–341, 2003.

41. **DeBellso M, C. Harris C, and Spitzer-Gibson T.** A comparison of periodised and fixed repetition training protocol on strength in older adults. *J Sci Med Sports* 8: 190–199, 2005.

42. **Dickinson JW, Whyte GP, McConnell AK, and Harries MG.** Screening elite winter athletes for exercise induced asthma: a comparison of three challenge methods. *British Journal of Sports Medicine* 40: 179–182; discussion 179–182, 2006.

43. **DiFrancisco-Donoghue J, Werner W, and Douris PC.** Comparison of once-weekly and twice-weekly strength training in older adults. *British Journal of Sports Medicine* 41: 19–22, 2007.

44. **Eggleston PA.** Pathophysiology of exercise-induced asthma. *Med Sci Sports Exerc* 18: 318–321, 1986.

45. **Ehrman JK, and Schairer JR.** Diagnostic procedures for cardiovascular disease. In: ACSM's *Resource Manual for Guidelines for Exercise Testing and Prescription.* Baltimore: Lippincott Williams & Wilkins, 2006, p. 277–288.

46. **Entin PL, and Munhall KM.** Recommendations regarding exercise during pregnancy made by private/small group practice obstetricians in the USA. *J Sports Sci and Med* 5: 449–458, 2006.

47. **Evans TM, Rundell KW, Beck KC, Levine AM, and Baumann JM.** Cold air inhalation does not affect the severity of EIB after exercise or eucapnic voluntary hyperventilation. *Med Sci Sports Exerc* 37: 544–549, 2005.

48. **Everson KR, and Pompeii LA.** Obstetricians practice patterns and recommednations for physcial activity during pregnancy. *Journal of Women's Health* 19: 1733–1740, 2010.

49. **Faber MJ, Bosscher RJ, Chin APMJ, and van Wieringen PC.** Effects of exercise programs on falls and mobility in frail and pre-frail older adults: a multi-center randomized controlled trial. *Archives of Physical Medicine and Rehabilitation* 87: 885–896, 2006.

50. **Fitzgerald MD, Tanaka H, Tran ZV, and Seals DR.** Age-related declines in maximal aerobic capacity in regularly exercising vs. sedentary women: a meta-analysis. *J Appl Physiol* 83: 160–165, 1997.

51. **Franklin BA.** Myocardial infarction. In: *ACSM's Exercise Management for Persons with Chronic Disease and Disabilities*, edited by Durstine JL, Moore GE, Painter PL, and Roberts SO. Champaign, IL: Human Kinetics, 2009, p. 49–57.

52. **Franklin BA.** Revascularization: CABGS abd PTCA or PCI. In: *ACSM's Exercise Management for Persons with Chronic Disease and Disabilities*, edited by Durstine JL, Moore GE, Painter PL, and Roberts SO. Champaign, IL: 2009.

53. **Gillespie C, Kuklina EV, Briss PA, Blair NA, and Hong Y.** Vital signs: prevalence, treatment, and control of hypertension—United States, 1999–2002 and 2005–2008. *Morbidity and Mortality Weekly Report* 60: 103–108, 2011.

54. **Global Inititive for Chronic Obstructive Lung Disease (GOLD).** *Global Strategy for Diagnosis, Management, and Prevention of COPD.* http://www.goldcopd.org, 2010.

55. **Gordon NF.** Hypertension. In: *ACSM's Exercise Management for Persons with Chronic Disease and Disabilities*, edited by Durstine JL, Moore GE, Painter PL, and Roberts SO. Champaign, IL: Human Kinetics, 2009, p. 107–113.

56. **Hagberg JM.** Exercise, fitness, and hypertension. In: *Exercise, Fitness, and Health,* edited by Bouchard C, Shephard RJ, Stephens T, Sutton JR, and McPherson BD. Champaign: Human Kinetics, 1990, p. 455–466.

57. **Haverkamp HC, Dempsey JA, Pegelow DF, Miller JD, Romer LM, Santana M, and Eldridge MW.** Treatment of airway inflammation improves exercise pulmonary gas exchange and performance in asthmatic subjects. *The Journal of Allergy and Clinical Immunology* 120: 39–47, 2007.

58. **Jackson AS, Sui X, Hebert JR, Church TS, and Blair SN.** Role of lifestyle and aging on the longitudinal change in cardiorespiratory fitness. *Arch. Intern. Med.* 169: 1781–1787, 2009.

59. **Jolly K, Taylor RS, Lip GY, and Stevens A.** Home-based cardiac rehabilitation compared with centre-based rehabilitation and usual care: a systematic review and meta-analysis. *International Journal of Cardiology* 111: 343–351, 2006.

60. **Jones A, and Bowen M.** Screening for childhood asthma using an exercise test. *Br J Gen Pract* 44: 127–131, 1994.

61. **Kannel WB.** Bishop lecture. Contribution of the Framingham Study to preventive cardiology. *Journal of the American College of Cardiology* 15: 206–211, 1990.

62. **Kaplan NM.** *Clinical Hypertension.* Baltimore: Lippincott Williams & Wilkins, 1998.

63. **Kasch FW, Boyer JL, Van Camp SP, Verity LS, and Wallace JP.** The effect of physical activity and inactivity on aerobic power in older men (a longitudinal study). *The Physician and Sportsmedicine* 18: 73–83, 1990.

64. **Katz RM.** Coping with exercise-induced asthma in sports. *The Physician and Sportsmedicine* 15: 100–112, 1987.

65. **Keilty SE, Ponte J, Fleming TA, and Moxham J.** Effect of inspiratory pressure support on exercise tolerance and breathlessness in patients with severe stable chronic obstructive pulmonary disease. *Thorax* 49: 990–994, 1994.

66. **Kemmer FW, and Berger M.** Exercise and diabetes mellitus: physical activity as a part of daily life and its role in the treatment of diabetic patients. *International Journal of Sports Medicine* 4: 77–88, 1983.

67. **Kindermann W.** Do inhaled β_2-agonists have an ergogenic potential in non-asthmatic competitive athletes? *Sports Medicine (Auckland, NZ)* 37: 95–102, 2007.

68. **Knowler WC, Barrett-Connor E, Fowler SE, Hamman RF, Lachin JM, Walker EA, and Nathan DM.** Reduction in the incidence of type 2 diabetes with lifestyle intervention or Metformin. *The New England Journal of Medicine* 346: 393–403, 2002.

69. **Lampman RM, and Campaign BN.** Exercise testing in patients with diabetes. In: ACSM's *Resource Manual for Guidelines for Exercise Testing and Prescription.* Baltimore: Lippincott Williams & Wilkins, 2006, p. 245–254.

70. **Lotgering FK, van Doorn MB, Struijk PC, Pool J, and Wallenburg HC.** Maximal aerobic exercise in pregnant women: heart rate, O_2 consumption, CO_2 production, and ventilation. *J Appl Physiol* 70: 1016–1023, 1991.

71. **Lucas SR, and Platts-Mills TA.** Physical activity and exercise in asthma: relevance to etiology and treatment. *The Journal of Allergy and Clinical Immunology* 115: 928–934, 2005.

72. **Mahler DA.** Exercise-induced asthma. *Med Sci Sports Exerc* 25: 554–561, 1993.

73. **Makker HK, and Holgate ST.** Mechanisms of exercise-induced asthma. *European Journal of Clinical Investigation* 24: 571–585, 1994.

74. **McCullough PA.** Diagnostic procedures for cardiovascular disease. In: ACSM's *Resource Manual for Guidelines for Exercise Testing and Prescription,* edited by Ehrman JK. Baltimore: Lippincott Williams & Wilkins, 2010, p. 360–374.

75. **McKenzie DC, McLuckie SL, and Stirling DR.** The protective effects of continuous and interval exercise in athletes with exercise-induced asthma. *Med Sci Sports Exerc* 26: 951–956, 1994.

76. **Mickleborough TD.** A nutritional approach to managing exercise-induced asthma. *Exercise and Sport Sciences Reviews* 36: 135–144, 2008.

77. **Miracle VA.** Pulmonary exercise program: a model for pulmonary rehabilitation. *Journal of Cardiopulmonary Rehabilitation* 6: 368–371, 1986.

78. **Morton AR, and Fitch KD.** *Exercise Testing and Exercise Prescription for Special Cases.* Baltimore: Lippincott Williams & Wilkins, 2005.

79. **Mottola MF, Davenport MH, Brun CR, Inglis SD, Charlesworth S, and Sopper MM.** $\dot{V}O_{2peak}$ prediction and exercise prescription for pregnant women. *Med Sci Sports Exerc* 38: 1389–1395, 2006.

80. **Nelson ME, Rejeski WJ, Blair SN, Duncan PW, Judge JO, King AC, Macera CA, and Castaneda-Sceppa C.** Physical activity and public health in older adults: recommendations from the American College of Sports Medicine and the American Heart Association. *Medicine and Science in Sports and Exercise* 39: 1435–1445, 2007.

81. **Nichols DL, and Essery EV.** Osteoporosis and exercise. In: ACSM's *Resource Manual for Guidelines for Exercise Testing and Prescription.* Baltimore: Lippincott Williams & Wilkins, 2006, p. 489–499.

82. **Paterson DH, Jones GR, and Rice CL.** Ageing and physical activity: evidence to develop exercise recommendations for older adults. *Canadian Journal of Public Health* 98 Suppl 2: S69–108, 2007.

83. **Pavy B, Iliou MC, Meurin P, Tabet JY, and Corone S.** Safety of exercise training for cardiac patients: results of the French registry of complications during cardiac rehabilitation. *Archives of Internal Medicine* 166: 2329–2334, 2006.

84. **Peno-Green LA, and Cooper CB.** Treatment and rehabilitation of pulmonary diseases. In: ACSM's *Resource Manual for Guidelines for Exercise Testing and Prescription.* Baltimore: Lippincott Williams & Wilkins, 2006, p. 452–469.

85. **Peterson MD, Rhea MR, Sen A, and Gordon PM.** Resistance exercise for muscular strength in older adults: a meta analysis. *Ageing Research Reviews* 9: 226–237, 2010.

86. **Petit MA, Hughes JM, and Warpeha JM.** Exercise prescription for people with osteoporosis. In: ACSM's *Resource Manual for Guidelines for Exercise Testing and Prescription,* edited by Ehrman JK. Baltimore: Lippincott Williams & Wilkins, 2010, p. 635–650.

87. **Pierson WE, Covert DS, Koenig JQ, Namekata T, and Kim YS.** Implications of air pollution effects on athletic performance. *Med Sci Sports Exerc* 18: 322–327, 1986.

88. **Quaglietti S, and Froelicher VF.** Physical activity and cardiac rehabilitation for patients with coronary heart disease. In: *Physical Activity, Fitness, and Health,* edited by Bouchard C, Shephard RJ, and Stephens T. Champaign: Human Kinetics, 1994, p. 591–608.

89. **Randolph C.** An update on exercise-induced bronchoconstriction with and without asthma. *Current Allergy and Asthma Reports* 9: 433–438, 2009.

90. **Richter EA, and Galbo H.** Diabetes, insulin and exercise. *Sports Medicine (Auckland, NZ)* 3: 275–288, 1986.

91. **Robling AG, Burr DB, and Turner CH.** Partitioning a daily mechanical stimulus into discrete loading bouts improves the osteogenic response to loadin. *Journal of Bone and Mineral Research* 15: 1596–1602, 2000.

92. **Rogers MA.** Acute effects of exercise on glucose tolerance in non-insulin-dependent diabetes. *Med Sci Sports Exerc* 21: 362–368, 1989.

93. **Rubin CT, and Lanyon LE.** Regulation of bone mass by mechanical strain magnitude. *Calcified Tissue International* 37: 411–417, 1985.

94. **Schairer JS, and Keteyian SJ.** Exercise testing in patients with cardiovascular disease. In: *ACSM's Resource Manual for Guidelines for Exercise Testing and Prescription.* Baltimore: Lippincott Williams & Wilkins, 2006, p. 439–451.

95. **Shephard RJ.** Exercise and chronic obstructive lung disease. In: *Exercise and Sport Sciences Reviews*, edited by Keogh J, and Hutton RS. Los Angeles: Journal Publishing Affiliates, 1976, p. 263–296.

96. **Skinner JS.** Hypertension. In: *Exercise Testing and Exercise Prescription for Special Cases*, edited by Skinner JS. Baltimore: Lippincott Williams & Wilkins, 2005, p. 305–312.

97. **Sly RM.** History of exercise-induced asthma. *Med Sci Sports Exerc* 18: 314–317, 1986.

98. **Spina RJ.** Cardiovascular adaptations to endurance exercise training in older men and women. *Exercise and Sport Sciences Reviews* 27: 317–332, 1999.

99. **Stockdale-Woolley R, Haggerty MC, and McMahon PM.** The pulmonary rehabilitation program at Norwalk Hospital. *Journal of Cardiopulmonary Rehabilitation* 6: 505–518, 1986.

100. **Storms WW.** Review of exercise-induced asthma. *Med Sci Sports Exerc* 35: 1464–1470, 2003.

101. **Thompson PD, Franklin BA, Balady GJ, Blair SN, Corrado D, Estes NA, III, Fulton JE, Gordon NF, Haskell WL, Link MS, Maron BJ, Mittleman MA, Pelliccia A, Wenger NK, Willich SN, and Costa F.** Exercise and acute cardiovascular events placing the risks into perspective: a scientific statement from the American Heart Association Council on Nutrition, Physical Activity, and Metabolism and the Council on Clinical Cardiology. *Circulation* 115: 2358–2368, 2007.

102. **Tommaso CL, Lesch M, and Sonnenblick EH.** Alterations in cardiac function in coronary heart disease, myocardial infarction, and coronary bypass surgery. In: *Rehabilitation of the Coronary Patient*, edited by Wenger NK, and Hellerstein HK. New York: Wiley, 1984, p. 41–66.

103. **Tuomilehto J.** Nonpharmacoligcal therapy and exercise in the prevention of type 2 diabetes. *Diabetes Care* 32: S189–S193, 2009.

104. **U.S. Department of Health and Human Services.** *2008 Physical Activity Guideliens for Americans.* Washington, DC: Author, 2008.

105. **Verity LS.** Exercise prescription in patients with diabetes. In: ACSM's *Resource Manual for Guidelines for Exercise Testing and Prescription*, edited by Ehrman JK. Baltimore: Lippincott Williams & Wilkins, 2010, p. 600–616.

106. **Verity LS.** Exercise testing in patients with cardiovascular disease. In: *Diabetes and Exercise.* Baltimore: Lippincott Williams & Wilkins, 2006, p. 470–479.

107. **Voy RO.** The U.S. Olympic Committee experience with exercise-induced bronchospasm, 1984. *Med Sci Sports Exerc* 18: 328–330, 1986.

108. **Wallace JP.** Exercise in hypertension: a clinical review. *Sports Medicine* (Auckland, NZ) 33: 585–598, 2003.

109. **Weiler JM, Bonini S, Coifman R, Craig T, Delgado L, Capao-Filipe M, Passali D, Randolph C, and Storms W.** American Academy of Allergy, Asthma & Immunology Work Group report: exercise-induced asthma. *The Journal of Allergy and Clinical Immunology* 119: 1349–1358, 2007.

110. **Wilson CR.** Evidence supporting the use of endurance exercise to decrease dyspnea in COPD. *Cardiopulmonary Physical Therapy Journal* 14: 7–11, 2003.

111. **Wolfe LA.** Pregnancy. In: *Exercise Testing and Exercise Prescription for Special Cases*, edited by Skinner JS. Baltimore: Lippincott Williams & Wilkins, 2005, p. 377–391.

112. **Wolfe LA, Brenner IK, and Mottola MF.** Maternal exercise, fetal well-being and pregnancy outcome. *Exercise and Sport Sciences Reviews* 22: 145–194, 1994.

113. **Wolfe LA, Ohtake PJ, Mottola MF, and McGrath MJ.** Physiological interactions between pregnancy and aerobic exercise. *Exercise and Sport Sciences Reviews* 17: 295–351, 1989.

114. **World Hypertension League.** Physical exercise in the management of hypertension: a consensus statement by the World Hypertension League. *Journal of Hypertension* 9: 283–287, 1991.

18

Body Composition and Nutrition for Health

■ Objectives

By studying this chapter, you should be able to do the following:

1. Describe the recommended range for the dietary intake of carbohydrates, fats, and proteins.

2. Describe what is meant by the terms *Recommended Dietary Allowance* (RDA) and *Dietary Reference Intakes* (DRIs), and how they relate to the Daily Value (DV) used in food labeling.

3. List the classes of nutrients.

4. Identify the fat- and water-soluble vitamins, describe what toxicity is, and identify which class of vitamins is more likely to cause this problem.

5. Contrast major minerals with trace minerals, and describe the role of calcium, iron, and sodium in health and disease.

6. Identify the primary role of carbohydrates, the two major classes, and the recommended changes in the American diet to improve health status.

7. Identify the primary role of fat and the recommended changes in the American diet to improve health status.

8. Describe the common dietary recommendations from the major health-related organizations.

9. Describe the Dietary Approaches to Stop Hypertension (DASH) eating plan.

10. Describe the limitation of height/weight tables and the Body Mass Index in determining overweight and obesity.

11. Provide a brief description of the following methods of measuring body composition: isotope dilution, photon absorptiometry, potassium-40, hydrostatic (underwater weighing), dual energy X-ray absorptiometry,

near infrared interactance, radiography, ultrasound, nuclear magnetic resonance, total body electrical conductivity, bioelectrical impedance analysis, air displacement plethysmography, and skinfold thickness.

12. Describe the two-component model of body composition and the assumptions made about the density values for the fat-free mass and the fat mass; contrast this with the multicomponent model.

13. Explain the principle underlying the measurement of whole-body density with underwater weighing, and why one must correct for residual volume.

14. Explain why there is an error of 2.0% in the calculation of the percentage of body fat with the underwater weighing technique.

15. Explain how a sum of skinfolds can be used to estimate a percentage of body fatness value.

16. List the recommended percentage of body fatness values for health and fitness for males and females, and explain the concern for both high and low values.

17. Explain how deaths from cardiovascular disease have decreased while the prevalence of obesity has increased.

18. Distinguish between obesity due to hyperplasia of fat cells and obesity due to hypertrophy of fat cells.

19. Describe the roles of genetics and environment in the development of obesity.

20. Explain the set point theory of obesity, and give an example of a physiological and behavioral control system.

21. Describe the pattern of change in body weight and caloric intake over the adult years.
22. Discuss the changes in body composition when weight is lost by diet alone versus diet plus exercise.
23. Describe the relationship of the fat-free mass and caloric intake to the BMR.
24. Define thermogenesis and explain how it is affected by both short- and long-term overfeeding.

25. Describe the effect of exercise on appetite and body composition.
26. Explain quantitatively why small differences in energy expenditure and dietary intake are important in weight gain over the years.
27. Describe physical activity recommendations for preventing overweight and obesity, and for the prevention of weight regain in those who were previously obese.

■ Key Terms

Adequate Intake (AI)
anorexia nervosa
basal metabolic rate (BMR)
bulimia nervosa
cholesterol
Daily Value (DV)
deficiency
Dietary Guidelines for Americans
Dietary Reference Intake (DRI)
elements
energy wasteful systems
Estimated Average Requirement (EAR)
Estimated Energy Requirement (EER)
ferritin
food records
HDL cholesterol
high-density lipoproteins (HDLs)
LDL cholesterol
lipoprotein
low-density lipoproteins (LDLs)
major minerals
nutrient density
osteoporosis
provitamin
Recommended Dietary Allowances (RDAs)
resting metabolic rate (RMR)
thermogenesis
tolerable upper intake level (UL)
toxicity
trace elements
transferrin
twenty-four-hour recall
underwater weighing
whole-body density

Chapter 14 described factors that limit health and fitness. These included hypertension, obesity, and elevated serum cholesterol. These three risk factors are linked to an excessive consumption of salt, total calories, and dietary fat, respectively. Clearly, knowledge of nutrition is essential to our understanding of health-related fitness. Whereas chapters 3 and 4 described the metabolism of carbohydrates, fats, and proteins, this chapter focuses on the type of diet that should provide them. The first part of the chapter presents the nutritional guidelines for our nation, the nutrition standards and what they mean, a summary of the six classes of nutrients, and a way to evaluate our present diets and meet our nutritional goals. The second part of the chapter discusses the role of exercise and diet in altering body composition. Nutrition related to athletic performance is covered in chapter 23.

NUTRITIONAL GUIDELINES

We are all familiar with the work of the American Heart Association (AHA), the American Cancer Society (ACS), and the American Diabetes Association (ADA) to bring special attention on the importance of diet in the prevention and treatment of cardiovascular diseases, cancers, and diabetes, respectively. As mentioned in chapter 14, an underlying component associated with these diseases is a chronic low-grade systemic inflammation, which can be altered with diet and physical activity. What are the dietary recommendations associated with good health?

The current recommendations for the distribution of calories in our diet comes from the Institute of Medicine (IOM) (99):

■ Adults should get 45% to 65% of their calories from carbohydrates, 20% to 35% from fat, and 10% to 35% from protein. Acceptable ranges for children are similar to those for adults, except that infants and younger children need a slightly higher proportion of fat (25–40%).

How to best meet those standards, and those associated with vitamins and minerals (see later), is addressed in the **Dietary Guidelines for Americans,** which has been published every 5 years since 1980. The 2005 update of the *Dietary Guidelines for Americans* reflects the work of the Institute of Medicine and provides guidance on how to meet those nutritional standards (219). Excerpts of recommendations from this document follow:

■ Consume a variety of nutrient-dense foods and beverages within and among the basic food groups while choosing foods that limit the intake of saturated and trans fats, cholesterol, added sugars, salt, and alcohol.
  • Choose a variety of fruits and vegetables each day. In particular, select from all five vegetable subgroups (dark green, orange, legumes, starchy vegetables, and other vegetables) several times a week.
  • Consume 3 or more ounce-equivalents of whole-grain products per day, with the rest of the recommended grains coming from enriched or whole-grain products.
  • Consume 3 cups per day of fat-free or lowfat milk or equivalent milk products.
  • Keep total fat intake between 20% and 35% of calories, with most fats coming from sources of polyunsaturated and monounsaturated fatty acids, such as fish, nuts, and vegetable oils.
  • Choose fiber-rich fruits, vegetables, and whole grains often, and prepare foods and beverages with little added sugars or caloric sweeteners.
  • Choose and prepare foods with little salt. At the same time, consume potassium-rich foods, such as fruits and vegetables.
  • Those who choose to drink alcoholic beverages should do so sensibly and in moderation.

■ To maintain body weight in a healthy range, balance calories from foods and beverages with calories expended, engage in regular physical activity, and reduce sedentary activities.

The 2010 *Dietary Guidelines for Americans* (see Suggested Readings) provided direct support for those recommendations by emphasizing the following themes:

■ Balancing calories to manage weight
■ Foods and food components to reduce
■ Foods and nutrients to increase, and
■ Building healthy eating patterns

We will incorporate these new guidelines as we move through the various sections of this chapter.

IN SUMMARY

■ Current recommendations for the distribution of calories in foods include a broad range, rather than a single goal: carbohydrates: 45% to 65%, fats: 20% to 35%, and proteins: 10% to 35%.
■ The *Dietary Guidelines for Americans* has been revised over time to reflect new science and to deal with nutrition (and physical activity) and health-related issues. The 2005 edition provided recommendations to meet the 2002 IOM nutritional standards with special focus on achieving energy balance. The 2010 *Dietary Guidelines for Americans* emphasized what to reduce and add to our diet to improve health.

STANDARDS OF NUTRITION

Food provides the carbohydrates, fats, protein, minerals, vitamins, and water needed for life. The quantity of each nutrient needed for proper function and health is defined in one of the **Dietary Reference Intakes (DRIs),** an umbrella term encompassing specific standards for dietary intake (99).

If you had a nutrition class, or even a few lectures dealing with nutrition, you would have been introduced to the Recommended Dietary Allowance (RDA) standards for nutrients such as protein, vitamins, and minerals. With the expansion of knowledge about the role of specific nutrients in preventing deficiency diseases and reducing the risk of chronic diseases, there was a need for a new approach to setting nutrient standards. In collaboration with Health Canada, the Food and Nutrition Board of the National Academy of Sciences has developed new nutrient standards. The term *Dietary Reference Intakes (DRIs)* is the umbrella term given to these new standards. The following descriptions will help us make the transitions from where we are to where we will be when the full implementation of the standards takes place (233).

■ **Recommended Dietary Allowance (RDA).** The average daily dietary nutrient intake level sufficient to meet the nutrient requirement of nearly all (97–98%) healthy individuals in a particular group.

- **Adequate Intakes (AI).** Formerly the Estimated Safe and Adequate Daily Dietary Intake, the AI describes the recommended average daily intake level based on observed or experimentally determined approximations or estimates of nutrient intake by a group (or groups) of apparently healthy people. Levels are assumed to be adequate and are used when an RDA cannot be determined. (See appendix E.)
- **Tolerable Upper Intake Level (UL).** The highest average daily nutrient intake level that is likely to pose no risk of adverse health effects to almost all individuals in the general population. As intake increases above the UL, the potential risk of adverse effects may increase.
- **Estimated Average Requirement (EAR).** The average daily nutrient intake level estimated to meet the requirement of half the healthy individuals in a particular group. This value is needed to set the RDA values.

The values for each nutrient vary due to gender, body size, whether long-bone growth is taking place, pregnancy, and lactation (149). Given that individuals differ in their need for each nutrient, some requiring more than the average and others less, the standards were set high enough to meet the needs of almost everyone (97.5% of the population) and also account for inefficient utilization by the body (149). Previous RDA tables did not provide recommendations for carbohydrate and fat intake, but that has changed. We will provide recommendations from the Institute of Medicine report (99) when we discuss each.

In the past, RDA tables did not have standards for energy intake set at the same level as for the nutrients like vitamins and minerals (sufficient to meet 97% to 98% of the population). Instead, average values of energy intake were provided, which assumed an average level of physical activity. In the current recommendations, a new standard, the **Estimated Energy Requirement (EER),** is identified: the average dietary energy intake that is predicted to maintain energy balance in a healthy adult of a defined age, gender, weight, height, and level of physical activity, consistent with good health (99). The report provides energy intake recommendations for four levels of physical activity, with the stated purpose of achieving a healthy body weight (see appendix F). When it comes to the RDA for specific nutrients like vitamins and minerals, how do we know how much is contained in the food we eat?

The **Daily Value (DV)** is a standard used in nutritional labeling. For the essential nutrients (protein, vitamins, and minerals), the DVs are based on the nutrition standards (e.g., RDA). In addition, the food label contains important information about the calorie and fat content of the food. For example, if one serving of a product provides 50% of the DV for fat, it contains 50% of the total amount of fat recommended for one day (based on a 2,000-calorie diet). Figure 18.1 provides an example of a food label; the following points are highlighted (233):

- serving size information,
- total calories and fat calories,
- total fat grams, saturated fat grams, trans fat grams, cholesterol, and the percent of DV for each (based on a 2,000-calorie diet),
- total carbohydrate and its sources, and
- the percentage of the DV for certain vitamins (e.g., A and C) and minerals (e.g., calcium and iron); sodium is given special attention.

IN SUMMARY

- The Recommended Dietary Allowance (RDA) is the quantity of a nutrient that will meet the needs of almost all healthy persons.
- The Daily Value (DV) is a standard used in nutritional labeling.

CLASSES OF NUTRIENTS

There are six classes of nutrients: water, vitamins, minerals, carbohydrates, fats, and proteins. In the following sections each nutrient is described briefly, and the primary food sources of each are identified.

Water

Water is absolutely essential for life. Although we can go without food for weeks, we would not survive long without water. The body is 50% to 75% water, depending on age and body fatness, and a loss of more than 2% of body water adversely affects aerobic performance. Larger losses can lead to death (238). Under normal conditions without exercise, water loss equals about 2,500 ml/day, with most lost in urine. However, as higher environmental temperatures and heavy exercise are added, water loss can increase dramatically to 6 to 7 liters per day (84, 238).

Under normal conditions the 2,500 ml of water per day is replaced with beverages (1,500 ml), solid food (750 ml), and the water derived from metabolic processes (250 ml) (233). Most people are surprised

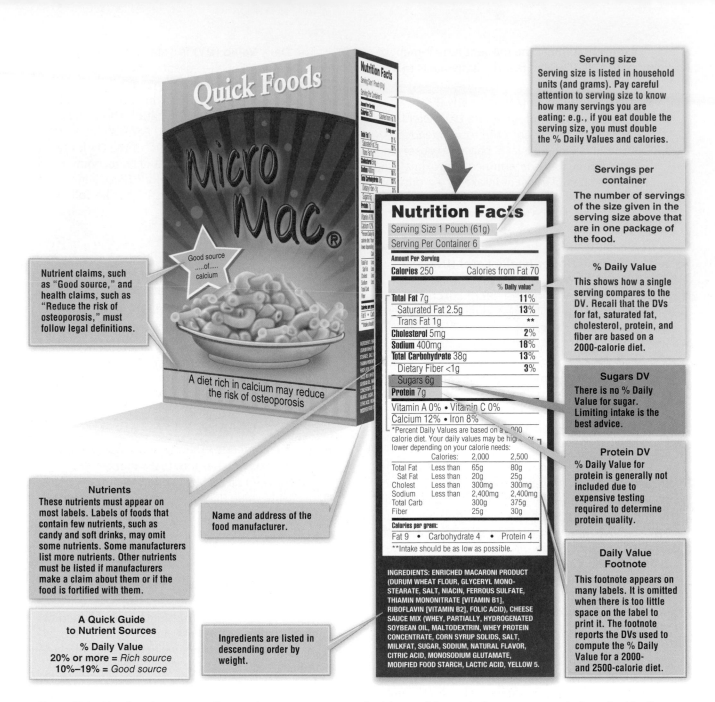

Nutrient claims, such as "Good source," and health claims, such as "Reduce the risk of osteoporosis," must follow legal definitions.

Serving size
Serving size is listed in household units (and grams). Pay careful attention to serving size to know how many servings you are eating: e.g., if you eat double the serving size, you must double the % Daily Values and calories.

Servings per container
The number of servings of the size given in the serving size above that are in one package of the food.

% Daily Value
This shows how a single serving compares to the DV. Recall that the DVs for fat, saturated fat, cholesterol, protein, and fiber are based on a 2000-calorie diet.

Sugars DV
There is no % Daily Value for sugar. Limiting intake is the best advice.

Protein DV
% Daily Value for protein is generally not included due to expensive testing required to determine protein quality.

Daily Value Footnote
This footnote appears on many labels. It is omitted when there is too little space on the label to print it. The footnote reports the DVs used to compute the % Daily Value for a 2000- and 2500-calorie diet.

Nutrients
These nutrients must appear on most labels. Labels of foods that contain few nutrients, such as candy and soft drinks, may omit some nutrients. Some manufacturers list more nutrients. Other nutrients must be listed if manufacturers make a claim about them or if the food is fortified with them.

Name and address of the food manufacturer.

Ingredients are listed in descending order by weight.

A Quick Guide to Nutrient Sources
% Daily Value
20% or more = *Rich source*
10%–19% = *Good source*

Nutrition Facts
Serving Size 1 Pouch (61g)
Serving Per Container 6

Amount Per Serving

Calories 250	Calories from Fat 70

	% Daily value*
Total Fat 7g	**11%**
Saturated Fat 2.5g	**13%**
Trans Fat 1g	**
Cholesterol 5mg	**2%**
Sodium 400mg	**16%**
Total Carbohydrate 38g	**13%**
Dietary Fiber <1g	**3%**
Sugars 6g	
Protein 7g	

Vitamin A 0% • Vitamin C 0%
Calcium 12% • Iron 8%

*Percent Daily Values are based on a 2,000 calorie diet. Your daily values may be higher or lower depending on your calorie needs:

	Calories:	2,000	2,500
Total Fat	Less than	65g	80g
Sat Fat	Less than	20g	25g
Cholest	Less than	300mg	300mg
Sodium	Less than	2,400mg	2,400mg
Total Carb		300g	375g
Fiber		25g	30g

Calories per gram:
Fat 9 • Carbohydrate 4 • Protein 4

**Intake should be as low as possible.

INGREDIENTS: ENRICHED MACARONI PRODUCT (DURUM WHEAT FLOUR, GLYCERYL MONO-STEARATE, SALT, NIACIN, FERROUS SULFATE, THIAMIN MONONITRATE [VITAMIN B1], RIBOFLAVIN [VITAMIN B2], FOLIC ACID), CHEESE SAUCE MIX (WHEY, PARTIALLY, HYDROGENATED SOYBEAN OIL, MALTODEXTRIN, WHEY PROTEIN CONCENTRATE, CORN SYRUP SOLIDS, SALT, MILKFAT, SUGAR, SODIUM, NATURAL FLAVOR, CITRIC ACID, MONOSODIUM GLUTAMATE, MODIFIED FOOD STARCH, LACTIC ACID, YELLOW 5.

Figure 18.1 Food packages must list product name, name and address of the manufacturer, amount of product in the package, and ingredients. The Nutrition Facts panel is required on virtually all packaged food products. The % Daily Value listed on the label is the percent of the amount of a nutrient needed daily that is provided by a single serving of the product.

by the large volume of water contributed by "solid" food until they consider the following percentages of water in solid food: baked potato—75%, apple—75%, lettuce—96% (233). A general recommendation under ordinary circumstances is to consume 1 to 1.5 ml of water per kcal of energy expenditure (149). The AI for total water intake (food + beverages) for women and men 19 to 70 years of age is set at 2.7 L/day and 3.7 L/day, respectively (98). However, to avoid potential problems associated with dehydration, one should drink water before and during exercise; thirst is not an adequate stimulus to achieve water balance (see chapter 23).

Water weight can fluctuate depending on the body stores of carbohydrate and protein. Water is involved in the linkage between glucose molecules in glycogen and amino acid molecules in protein. The ratio is about 2.7 of water per gram of carbohydrate, and if an individual stores 454 g (1 lb) of carbohydrate, body weight would increase by 3.7 lbs. Of course, when one diets and depletes this carbohydrate store, the reverse occurs. This results in an apparent weight loss of 3.7 lbs when only 1,816 kcal (454 g of carbohydrate times 4 kcal/g) have been lost. More on this later.

Vitamins

Vitamins were introduced in chapter 3 as organic catalysts involved in metabolic reactions. They are needed in small amounts and are not "used up" in the metabolic reactions. However, they are degraded (metabolized) like any biological molecule and must be replaced on a regular basis to maintain body stores. Several vitamins are in a precursor, or **provitamin,** form in foods and are converted to the active form in the body. Beta-carotene, the most important of the provitamin A compounds, is a good example. A chronic lack of certain vitamins can lead to **deficiency** diseases, and an excess of others can lead to a **toxicity** condition (233). In our presentation, vitamins will be divided into the fat-soluble and water-soluble groups.

Fat-Soluble Vitamins The fat-soluble vitamins include A, D, E, and K. These vitamins can be stored in large quantities in the body; thus a deficiency state takes longer to develop than for water-soluble vitamins. However, because of their solubility, so much can be stored that a toxicity condition can occur. The Tolerable Upper Intake Level (UL) for vitamin A (3,000 μg), D (4,000 IU), and E (1,000 mg) have been established (97, 149). Toxicity, of course, is far from a health-related goal. Table 18.1 summarizes the information on these vitamins, including the RDA/AI standards, dietary sources, function, and signs associated with deficiency or excess.

Water-Soluble Vitamins The water-soluble vitamins include vitamin C and the B vitamins: thiamin (B_1), riboflavin (B_2), niacin, pyridoxine (B_6), folic acid, B_{12}, pantothenic acid, and biotin. Most are involved in energy metabolism. You have already seen the role of niacin, as NAD, and riboflavin, as FAD, in the transfer of energy in the Krebs cycle and electron transport chain. Thiamin (as thiamine pyrophosphate) is involved in the removal of CO_2 as pyruvate enters the Krebs cycle. Vitamin B_6, folic acid, B_{12}, pantothenic acid, and biotin are also involved as coenzymes in metabolic reactions. Vitamin C is involved in the maintenance of bone, cartilage, and connective tissue. Table 18.1 summarizes the information on these vitamins, including the RDA/AI standards, functions, dietary sources, and signs associated with deficiency or excess.

IN SUMMARY

- The fat-soluble vitamins include A, D, E, and K. These can be stored in the body in large quantities and toxicity can develop.
- The water-soluble vitamins include thiamin, riboflavin, niacin, B_6, folic acid, B_{12}, pantothenic acid, biotin, and C. Most of these are involved in energy metabolism. Vitamin C is involved in the maintenance of bone, cartilage, and connective tissue.

Minerals

Minerals are the chemical **elements,** other than carbon, hydrogen, oxygen, and nitrogen, associated with the structure and function of the body. We have already seen the importance of calcium in bone structure and in the initiation of muscle contraction, iron in O_2 transport by hemoglobin, and phosphorus in ATP. Minerals are important inorganic nutrients and are divided into two classes: (1) **major minerals** and (2) **trace elements.** The major minerals include calcium, phosphorus, magnesium, sulfur, sodium, potassium, and chloride, with whole-body quantities ranging from 35 g for magnesium to 1,200 g for calcium in a 70-kg man (233). The trace elements include iron, iodine, fluoride, zinc, selenium, copper, cobalt, chromium, manganese, molybdenum, arsenic, nickel, and vanadium. There are only 4 g of iron and 0.0009 g of vanadium in a 70-kg man. Like vitamins, some minerals taken in excess (e.g., iron and zinc) can be toxic. The following sections focus attention on calcium, iron, and sodium.

Calcium Calcium (Ca^{++}) and phosphorus combine with organic molecules to form the teeth and bones. The bones are a "store" of calcium that helps to maintain the plasma Ca^{++} concentration when dietary intake is inadequate (see parathyroid hormone in chapter 5). Bone is constantly turning over its calcium and phosphorus, so diet must replace what is lost. If the diet is deficient in calcium for a long period of time, loss of bone, or **osteoporosis,** can occur. This weakening of the bone due to the loss of calcium and phosphorus from its structure is more common in women than in men, is accelerated at menopause, and is directly related to the higher rate of hip fractures in women. Three major factors are implicated: dietary calcium intake, inadequate estrogen, and lack of physical activity (6).

There is concern that the increase in osteoporosis in our society is related to an inadequate calcium intake. The adult RDA for calcium is 1,000 mg/day, and although many men come close to meeting the standard, few women do (233). Given that the RDA is

TABLE 18.1 — Summary of the Vitamins, Their Functions, Deficiency Conditions, and Food Sources

FAT-SOLUBLE

Vitamin	Major Functions	Deficiency Symptoms	People Most at Risk
Vitamin A (retinoids) and provitamin A (carotenoids)	Promote vision: light and color; Promote growth; Prevent drying of skin and eyes; Promote resistance to bacterial infection	Night blindness; Xerophthalmia; Poor growth; Dry skin	People in poverty, especially preschool children (still very rare in the United States); People with alcoholism; People with AIDS
D (chole- and ergocalciferol)	Facilitate absorption of calcium and phosphorus; Maintain optimal calcification of bone	Rickets; Osteomalacia	Breastfed infants not exposed to sunlight, elderly
E (tocopherols)	Act as an antioxidant: prevent breakdown of vitamin A and unsaturated fatty acids	Hemolysis of red blood cells; Nerve destruction	People with poor fat absorption, smokers (still rare as far as we know)
K (phyilo- and menaquinone)	Help form prothrombin and other factors for blood clotting and contribute to bone metabolism	Hemorrhage	People taking antibiotics for months at a time (still quite rare)

WATER-SOLUBLE

Vitamin	Major Functions	Deficiency Symptoms	People Most at Risk
Thiamin	Coenzyme involved in carbohydrate metabolism; nerve function	Beriberi: nervous tingling, poor coordination, edema, heart changes, weakness	People with alcoholism or in poverty
Riboflavin	Coenzyme involved in energy metabolism	Inflammation of mouth and tongue, cracks at corners of the mouth, eye disorders	Possibly people on certain medications if no dairy products consumed
Niacin	Coenzyme involved in energy metabolism, fat synthesis, fat breakdown	Pellagra: diarrhea, dermatitis, dementia	Severe poverty where corn is the dominant food; people with alcoholism
Pantothenic acid	Coenzyme involved in energy metabolism, fat synthesis, fat breakdown	Tingling in hands, fatigue, headache, nausea	People with alcoholism
Biotin	Coenzyme involved in glucose production, fat synthesis	Dermatitis, tongue soreness, anemia, depression	People with alcoholism
Vitamin B_6 pyridoxine, and other forms	Coenzyme involved in protein metabolism, neurotransmitter synthesis, hemoglobin synthesis, many other functions	Headache, anemia, convulsions, nausea, vomiting, flaky skin, sore tongue	Adolescent and adult women; people on certain medications; people with alcoholism
Folate (folic acid)	Coenzyme involved in DNA synthesis, other functions	Megaloblastic anemia, inflammation of tongue, diarrhea, poor growth, depression	People with alcoholism, pregnancy, people on certain medications
Vitamin B_{12} (cobalamins)	Coenzyme involved in folate metabolism, nerve function, other functions	Macrocytic anemia, poor nerve function	Elderly people because of poor absorption, vegans, people with AIDS
Vitamin C (ascorbic acid)	Connective tissue synthesis, hormone synthesis, neurotransmitter synthesis	Scurvy: poor wound healing, pinpoint hemorrhages, bleeding gums	People with alcoholism, elderly who eat poorly

Note: Values are the Recommended Dietary Allowances (RDAs) for adults 19 to 50 years, unless marked by an asterisk (*), in which case they represent the Adequate Intakes (AIs). The Tolerable Upper Intake Levels (ULs) are listed under toxicity; intakes above these values can lead to negative health consequences.

Dietary Sources*	RDA or AI*	Toxicity Symptoms or UL

Vitamin A
  Liver
  Fortified milk
  Fortified breakfast cereals
Provitamin A
  Sweet potatoes, spinach, greens, carrots,
  cantaloupe, apricots, broccoli
	Men: 900 micrograms
	Women: 700 micrograms
		Fetal malformations, hair loss, skin changes, pain in bones (UL = 3,000 micrograms)

Vitamin D-fortified milk Fortified breakfast cereals Fish oils Sardines Salmon	600 IU	Growth retardation, kidney damage, calcium deposits in soft tissue (UL = 4000 IU)
Vegetable oils Some greens Some fruits Fortified breakfast cereals	15 milligrams	Muscle weakness, headaches, fatigue, nausea, inhibition of vitamin K metabolism (UL = 1,000 mg)
Green vegetables Liver	Men: 120 micrograms* Women: 90 micrograms*	Anemia and jaundice (medicinal forms only)

Dietary Sources*	RDA or AI*	Toxicity Symptoms
Sunflower seeds, pork, whole and enriched grains, dried beans, peas, brewers yeast	Men: 1.2 milligrams Women: 1.1 milligrams	None possible from food
Milk, mushrooms, spinach, liver, enriched grains	Men: 1.3 milligrams Women: 1.1 milligrams	None reported
Mushrooms, bran, tuna, salmon, chicken, beef, liver, peanuts, enriched grains	Men: 16 milligrams Women: 14 milligrams	Toxicity can begin at over 35 milligrams (UL) (flushing of skin especially seen at over 100 milligrams per day)
Mushrooms, liver, broccoli, eggs; most foods have some	5 milligrams*	None
Cheese, egg yolks, cauliflower, peanut butter, liver	30 micrograms	Unknown
Animal protein foods, spinach, broccoli, bananas, salmon, sunflower seeds	1.3 milligrams	UL = 100 mg; nerve destruction at doses over 200 milligrams
Green leafy vegetables, orange juice, organ meats, sprouts, sunflower seeds	400 micrograms	UL = 1,000 micrograms
Animal foods, especially organ meats, oysters, clams (not natural in plants)	2.4 micrograms	None
Citrus fruits, strawberries, broccoli, greens	Men: 90 milligrams Women: 75 milligrams	UL = 2,000 mg

higher for 9–18 year olds (1,300 mg/day) and for females 51–70 years of age (1,200 mg/day), the concern is greater for those age groups. Part of the reason for the low intake of calcium is the relatively low caloric intake of women compared to men. One way of dealing with this is to increase energy expenditure through exercise and, in turn, caloric intake; another is to take calcium supplements. The latter has been shown (when combined with dietary intake) to increase the number of individuals meeting the RDA (11). Although menopause is the usual cause of a reduced secretion of estrogen, young, extremely active female athletes are experiencing this problem associated with amenorrhea (7). The decrease in estrogen secretion is associated with the acceleration of osteoporosis. Estrogen therapy, with or without calcium supplementation, has been used successfully in menopausal women to reduce the rate of bone loss, but not without the risk of increasing cardiovascular problems in some women. Because exercise has been shown to slow the rate of bone loss, we now have physical activity recommendations to build bone mass in early childhood and to hold on to it as we age (5, 6, 221) (see Ask the Expert 17.1 in chapter 17).

Iron   The majority of iron is found in hemoglobin in the red blood cells, which is involved with oxygen transport to cells (see chapter 10). Other iron-containing molecules include myoglobin in muscle and the cytochromes in mitochondria, accounting for about 25% of the body's iron. A large portion of the remaining iron is bound to **ferritin** in the liver, with the serum ferritin concentration being a sensitive measure of iron status (233, 238).

Iron is an important part of hemoglobin and myoglobin, as well as the cytochromes of the electron transport chain. To remain in iron balance, the RDA is set at 8 mg/day for an adult male and 18 mg/day for an adult female; the higher amount is needed to replace that which is lost in the menses.

In spite of the higher need for iron, American women take in only 13.7 mg/day, whereas men take in 17.7 mg/day (240). This is due to higher caloric intakes in males than females. Because there are only 6 mg of iron per 1,000 kcal of energy in the American diet, a woman consuming 2,000 kcal/day would take in only 12 mg of iron. The male, consuming about 3,000 kcal/day, takes in 18 mg. The diet provides iron in two forms, heme (ferrous) and nonheme (ferric). Heme iron, found primarily in meats, fish, and organ meats, is absorbed better than nonheme iron, which is found in vegetables. However, the absorption of nonheme iron can be increased by the presence of meat, fish, and vitamin C (87, 233, 238).

Anemia is a condition in which the hemoglobin concentration is low: less than 13 g/dl in men and less than 12 g/dl in women. This can be the result of blood loss (e.g., blood donation or bleeding) or a lack of vitamins or minerals in the diet. The most common cause of anemia in North America is a lack of dietary iron (233, 238). In fact, iron deficiency is the most common nutrient deficiency. In iron deficiency anemia, more than hemoglobin is affected. The iron bound to **transferrin** in the plasma is reduced, and serum ferritin (an indicator of iron stores) is low (87). Although children aged 1 to 5 years, adolescents, young adult women, and the elderly are more apt to develop anemia, it also occurs in competitive athletes. This latter point is discussed in detail in chapter 23. The 2010 *Dietary Guidelines for Americans* call for an increase in iron intake, especially for women capable of becoming pregnant or who are pregnant or breast feeding (220).

Sodium   Sodium is directly involved in the maintenance of the resting membrane potential and the generation of action potential in nerves (see chapter 7) and muscles (see chapter 8). In addition, sodium is the primary electrolyte determining the extracellular fluid volume. If sodium stores fall, the extracellular volume, including plasma, decreases. This could cause major problems with the maintenance of the mean arterial blood pressure (see chapter 9) and body temperature (see chapter 12).

The problem in our society is not with sodium stores that are too small, but just the opposite. The estimated average intake of sodium for Americans ages 2 years and older is about 3,400 mg/day. This is considerably more than the AI for adults (1,500 mg/day) and exceeds the UL for adults (2,300 mg/day) (220). There is no question about the link between sodium intake and blood pressure, with evidence showing that reducing salt intake is feasible and will result in a reduction in cardiovascular morbidity and mortality (109, 234). The *Dietary Guidelines for Americans* have consistently supported the need to reduce sodium intake, and they recommend the Dietary Approaches to Stop Hypertension (DASH) eating plan (see later) to accomplish that goal:

- Use reduced sodium or no-salt-added products. For example, choose low or reduced sodium, or no-salt-added versions of foods and condiments when available.

- Buy fresh, plain frozen, or canned with "no-salt-added" vegetables.

- Use fresh poultry, fish, and lean meat, rather than canned, smoked, or processed types.

- Choose ready-to-eat breakfast cereals that are lower in sodium.

- Limit cured foods (such as bacon and ham), foods packed in brine (such as pickles, pickled vegetables, olives, and sauerkraut), and condiments (such as MSG, mustard, horseradish, catsup, and barbecue sauce). Limit even lower-sodium versions of soy sauce and teriyaki sauce—treat these condiments as you do table salt.

- Use spices instead of salt. In cooking and at the table, flavor foods with herbs, spices, lemon, lime, vinegar, or salt-free seasoning blends. Start by cutting salt in half.

- Cook rice, pasta, and hot cereals without salt. Cut back on instant or flavored rice, pasta, and cereal mixes, which usually have added salt.

- Choose "convenience" foods that are lower in sodium. Cut back on frozen dinners, mixed dishes such as pizza, packaged mixes, canned soups or broths, and salad dressing—these often have a lot of sodium.

- Rinse canned foods, such as tuna, to remove some sodium.

Those involved in athletic competition or strenuous exercise or who work in the heat must be concerned about adequate sodium replacement. Generally, because these individuals consume more kcal of food (containing more sodium), this is usually not a problem. More on this in chapter 23.

The previous sections have focused attention on three minerals—calcium, iron, and sodium—because of their relationship to current medical and health-related problems. A summary of each of the minerals, their functions, and food sources is presented in table 18.2.

IN SUMMARY

- The major minerals include calcium, phosphorus, magnesium, sulfur, sodium, potassium, and chloride. The trace elements include iron, iodine, fluoride, zinc, selenium, copper, cobalt, chromium, manganese, molybdenum, arsenic, nickel, and vanadium.
- Inadequate calcium and iron intake has been linked with osteoporosis and anemia, respectively. The 2010 *Dietary Guidelines for Americans* recommends an increase in calcium and iron intake to address these problems, and a reduction in sodium intake, especially for those at risk of hypertension.

Carbohydrates

Carbohydrates and fats are the primary sources of energy in the average American diet (149) (for recommendations on carbohydrates, fats, and proteins from the Institute of Medicine, see Clinical Applications 18.1). Carbohydrates suffer a bad reputation from those on

diets, especially when you consider that you would have to eat more than twice as much carbohydrate as fat to consume the same number of calories (4 kcal/g versus 9 kcal/g). Carbohydrates can be divided into two classes: those that can be digested and metabolized for energy (sugars and starches), and those that are undigestible (fiber). The sugars are found in jellies, jams, fruits, soft drinks, honey, syrups, and milk, whereas the starches are found in cereals, flour, potatoes, and other vegetables (233).

Sugars and Starches Carbohydrate is a major energy source for all tissues and a crucial source for two: red blood cells and neurons. The red blood cells depend exclusively on anaerobic glycolysis for energy, and the nervous system functions well only on carbohydrate. These two tissues can consume 180 grams of glucose per day (50). Given this need, it is no surprise that the plasma glucose concentration is maintained within narrow limits by hormonal control mechanisms (see chapter 5). During strenuous exercise the muscle can use 180 grams of glucose in less than 1 hour. As a result of these needs, one might expect that carbohydrate would make up a large fraction of our energy intake. Currently about 50% of energy intake is derived from carbohydrate (240), within the range of recommended carbohydrate intakes (99). There is great interest not only in the amount of carbohydrate in the diet, but also in the type of carbohydrate as it relates to the prevention and management of diabetes (see Clinical Applications 18.2). While the goal is to increase carbohydrate intake, one of the *Dietary Guidelines for Americans* is to avoid too much sugar (220). The following are helpful suggestions on how to limit intake of added sugars while meeting the overall carbohydrate goal (219, 220):

- Choose and prepare foods and beverages with little added sugars or caloric sweeteners, such as amounts suggested in the DASH eating plan.
- Replace sweetened beverages with water and unsweetened beverages.

Dietary Fiber Dietary fiber is an important part of the diet. Over the past few years, in an attempt to clarify what is and is not "fiber," fiber has been divided into the following classes (99):

- *Dietary fiber* consists of nondigestible carbohydrates and lignin that are *intrinsic and intact* in plants. Examples of dietary fiber include plant nonstarch polysaccharides such as cellulose, pectin, gums, hemicellulose, β-glucans, and fibers in oat and wheat bran.
- *Functional fiber* consists of *isolated, nondigestible carbohydrates* that have beneficial physiological effects in humans. Examples of functional

TABLE 18.2 A Summary of Minerals

MAJOR MINERALS

Mineral	Major Functions	Deficiency Symptoms	People Most at Risk
Sodium	Functions as a major ion of the extracellular fluid; aids nerve impulse transmission	Muscle cramps	People who severely restrict sodium to lower blood pressure (250–500 milligrams)
Potassium	Functions as a major ion of intracellular fluid; aids nerve impulse transmission	Irregular heartbeat, loss of appetite, muscle cramps	People who use potassium-wasting diuretics or have poor diets, as seen in poverty and alcoholism
Chloride	Functions as a major ion of the extracellular fluid; participates in acid production in stomach; aids nerve transmission	Convulsions in infants	No one, probably
Calcium	Provides bone and tooth strength; helps blood clotting; aids nerve impulse transmission; required for muscle contractions	Inadequate intake increases the risk for osteoporosis	Women, especially those who consume few dairy products
Phosphorus	Required for bone and tooth strength; serves as part of various metabolic compounds; functions as major ion of intracellular fluid	Poor bone maintenance is a possibility	Older people consuming very nutrient-poor diets; people with alcoholism
Magnesium	Provides bone strength; aids enzyme function; aids nerve and heart function	Weakness, muscle pain, poor heart function	Women, and people on certain diuretics

KEY TRACE MINERALS

Mineral	Major Functions	Deficiency Symptoms	People Most at Risk
Iron	Used for hemoglobin and other key compounds used in respiration; used for immune function	Low blood iron; small, pale red blood cells; low blood hemoglobin values	Infants, preschool children, adolescents, women in childbearing years
Zinc	Required for enzymes, involved in growth, immunity, alcohol metabolism, sexual development, and reproduction	Skin rash, diarrhea, decreased appetite and sense of taste, hair loss, poor growth and development, poor wound healing	Vegetarians, elderly people, people with alcoholism
Selenium	Aids antioxidant system	Muscle pain, muscle weakness, form of heart disease	Unknown in healthy Americans
Iodide	Aids thyroid hormone	Goiter; poor growth in infancy when mother is iodide deficient during pregnancy	None in America because salt is usually fortified
Copper	Aids in iron metabolism; works with many enzymes, such as those involved in protein metabolism and hormone synthesis	Anemia, low white blood cell count, poor growth	Infants recovering from semistarvation, people who use overzealous supplementation of zinc
Fluoride	Increases resistance of tooth enamel to dental caries	Increased risk of dental caries	Areas where water is not fluoridated and dental treatments do not make up for a lack of fluoride
Chromium	Enhances blood glucose control	High blood glucose after eating	People on intravenous nutrition, and perhaps elderly people with type 2 diabetes
Manganese	Aids action of some enzymes, such as those involved in carbohydrate metabolism	None in humans	Unknown
Molybdenum	Aids action of some enzymes	None in healthy humans	Unsupplemented intravenous nutrition

Note: Values are the Recommended Dietary Allowances (RDAs) for adults 19 to 50 years, unless marked by an asterisk (*), in which case they represent the Adequate Intakes (AIs). The Tolerable Upper Intake Levels (ULs) are listed under toxicity; intakes above these values can lead to negative health consequences.

RDA or AI*	Rich Dietary Sources	Results of Toxicity or UL
1,500 milligrams*	Table salt, processed foods, condiments, sauces, soups, chips	UL = 2,300 mg; contributes to high blood pressure in susceptible individuals; leads to increased calcium loss in urine
4,700 milligrams*	Spinach, squash, bananas, orange juice, other vegetables and fruits, milk, meat, legumes, whole grains	Results in slowing of the heartbeat; seen in kidney failure
2,300 milligrams*	Table salt, some vegetables, processed foods	UL = 3,600 mg; linked to high blood pressure in susceptible people when combined with sodium
1,000 milligrams	Dairy products, canned fish, leafy vegetables, tofu, fortified orange juice (and other fortified foods)	UL = 2,500 mg; higher intakes may cause kidney stones and other problems in susceptible people; poor mineral absorption in general
700 milligrams	Dairy products, processed foods, fish, soft drinks, bakery products, meats	UL = 4,000 milligrams; impairs bone health in people with kidney failure; results in poor bone mineralization if calcium intakes are low
Men: 420 milligrams Women: 320 milligrams	Wheat bran, green vegetables, nuts, chocolate, legumes	UL = 350 mg, but refers only to pharmacologic agents

RDA or AI*	Rich Dietary Sources	Results of Toxicity
Men: 8 milligrams Women: 18 milligrams	Meats, spinach, seafood, broccoli, peas, bran, enriched breads	UL = 45 mg; toxicity seen when children consume 60 milligrams or more in iron pills; also in people with hemochromatosis
Men: 11 milligrams Women: 8 milligrams	Seafoods, meats, greens, whole grains	UL = 40 milligrams; reduces copper absorption; can cause diarrhea, cramps, and depressed immune function
55 micrograms	Meats, eggs, fish, seafoods, whole grains	UL = 400 micrograms; nausea, vomiting, hair loss, weakness, liver disease
150 micrograms	Iodized salt, white bread, saltwater fish, dairy products	UL = 1,100 micrograms; inhibition of function of the thyroid gland
900 micrograms	Liver, cocoa, beans, nuts, whole grains, dried fruits	UL = 10 milligrams; vomiting; nervous system disorders
Men: 4 milligrams* Women: 3 milligrams*	Fluoridated water, toothpaste, dental treatments, tea, seaweed	UL = 10 mg; stomach upset; mottling (staining) of teeth during development; bone pain
Men: 30–35 micrograms* Women: 20–25 micrograms*	Egg yolks, whole grains, pork, nuts, mushrooms, beer	Liver damage and lung cancer (caused by industrial contamination, not dietary excess)
Men: 2.3 milligrams* Women: 1.8 milligrams*	Nuts, oats, beans, tea	UL = 11 milligrams
45 micrograms	Beans, grains, nuts	UL = 2,000 micrograms

Institute of Medicine Report

At the beginning of the chapter, we indicated that a report from the Institute of Medicine (99) made a series of recommendations that has impacted a variety of existing nutritional recommendations from both federal agencies (e.g., U.S. Department of Agriculture) and professional organizations (e.g., American Heart Association). What follows is a brief summary of information and recommendations related to the intakes of carbohydrate, fat, and protein.

- An RDA for carbohydrate was established for the first time: 130 g/day to meet the glucose needs of the brain.
- An AI for fiber was set at 38 and 25 g/day for men and women, respectively.
- No RDA, AI, or EAR standards were set for saturated fat, mono-saturated fat, and cholesterol because they have no known beneficial role in preventing chronic disease. In addition, because they are synthesized in the body, they are not required in the diet.
- AI values were set for the omega-6 fatty acid, linoleic acid (17 and 12 g/day for young men and women, respectively), and the omega-3 fatty acid, α-linoleic acid (1.6 and 1.1 g/day for men and women, respectively).
- The long-held adult protein requirement of 0.8 g/day per kilogram of body weight was maintained.
- The AI for water was set at 3.7 L/day and 2.7 L/day for men and women, respectively.

The Institute of Medicine's report recommends a new dietary standard, called the Acceptable Macronutrient Distribution Ranges (AMDRs). These are defined as ranges of intakes for a particular energy source that is associated with a reduced risk of chronic disease, while providing adequate intake of essential nutrients. The Institute recommends ranges of 20% to 35% fat, 45% to 65% carbohydrate, and the balance (10–35%), protein. There is evidence that at the *extreme* end of the range, diets low in fat and high in carbohydrate reduce HDL cholesterol and increase the total cholesterol:HDL cholesterol ratio and plasma triglycerides. At the opposite end, when fat intake is high, weight gain occurs and the metabolic consequences of obesity increase, as does the plasma LDL cholesterol. (99)

---

fiber include isolated, nondigestible plants (e.g., resistant starches, pectin, and gums) and animal (e.g., chitin and chitosan) or commercially produced (e.g., resistant starch, inulin, and indigestible dextrins) carbohydrates.

- *Total fiber* is the sum of dietary fiber and functional fiber.

Dietary fiber cannot be digested and metabolized, and consequently it provides a sense of fullness (satiation) during a meal without adding calories (59). This fact has been used by bakeries that lower the number of calories per slice of bread by adding cellulose from wood! Pectin and gum are used in food processing to thicken, stabilize, or emulsify the constituents of various food products (233).

Dietary fiber has long been linked to optimal health. Fiber acts as a hydrated sponge as it moves along the large intestine, making constipation less likely by reducing transit time (8, 59, 233). Vegetarian diets high in soluble fiber have been linked to lower serum cholesterol due to the loss of more bile (cholesterol-containing) acids in the feces. However, the fact that vegetarian diets are also lower in the percentage of calories from fat, which can also lower serum cholesterol, makes the interpretation of the data more complicated (59). Although a high-fiber diet reduces the incidence of diverticulosis, a condition in which outpouchings (diverticula) occur in the colon wall, the role of fiber in preventing colon cancer is mixed (8, 59). A review by the American Dietetic Association (ADA) indicated strong epidemiological evidence that a diet rich in fiber reduces the risk of colon cancer. In contrast, intervention studies (in which individuals received added fiber) did not confirm the epidemiological evidence. However, on balance, the ADA believes that the abundance of evidence supports the promotion of a diet high in fiber to protect against colon cancer (8).

Given the broad role of dietary fiber in normal health, it is no surprise that the *Dietary Guidelines for Americans* recommends that Americans increase their intake of fiber (219). A new AI for total fiber, based on an intake level observed to protect against coronary heart disease, has been set at 38 and 25 g/day for men and women, 19 to 50 years of age, respectively. According to *Dietary Guidelines for Americans*, to increase the intake of fiber and complex carbohydrates, we should choose fiber-rich fruits, vegetables, and whole grains often. This can be accomplished by consuming whole fruit rather than fruit juices, eating dry beans and peas several times per week, and making sure at least half of the grain servings come from whole grains.

Glycemic Index—What Is It and Is It Important?

We all know that when we eat, insulin secretion increases to promote the uptake, use, and storage of carbohydrates. The degree to which the blood glucose concentration increases and remains elevated depends on the kinds and amounts of carbohydrate ingested, as well as the person's insulin response and tissue sensitivity to the insulin (193).

It is well known that certain carbohydrates elicit a more rapid blood glucose response than others. The glycemic index (GI) has been used to describe the magnitude of those differences and help those who have difficulty processing glucose make better decisions in planning meals. The GI quantifies the blood glucose response (above fasting) to an individual carbohydrate food over a 2-hour period following ingestion. This response is compared to a reference food (glucose or white bread) of the same weight. Those foods with a low GI would provide less of a challenge to someone with a reduced capacity to take up and use glucose (e.g., type 2 diabetic). However, because these carbohydrates are compared on a "per gram" basis, the GI does not consider the impact that the actual amount of carbohydrate in the meal has on the response. The "glycemic load (GL)" attempts to do that by multiplying the GI by the amount of carbohydrate in the serving (193).

The simplicity of the GI and GL is complicated by the fact that most meals do not contain a single carbohydrate. Factors such as the amount of protein and fat in the diet will impact the blood glucose response to the carbohydrate ingested. In spite of that, studies support the use of the GI as a tool to help shape the selection of carbohydrate-containing foods to reduce cholesterol and improve the metabolic control of diabetics (154). In addition, there is evidence that diets with a high GI and/or GL contribute to vascular inflammation that is tied to the development of atherosclerosis (115, 167). However, focus on the GI and GL should not ignore the importance of achieving a healthy body weight in the prevention and management of diabetes (193). This is supported in two studies of overweight subjects who were placed on either a low GL or high GL weight-loss diet. Both groups lost similar amounts of weight and experienced similar improvements in insulin dynamics (60, 161). However, there is a new twist to this tale of the GI and GL.

Fructose makes up a substantial part of total carbohydrate intake in the average American's diet. Concern was raised several years ago when it was found that there was a parallel increase in the intake of high-fructose corn syrup and obesity prevalence in this country. The reason for the concern is that, in contrast to glucose, fructose does not increase the insulin and leptin responses as much, and consequently, provides less input to the brain centers associated with feeding and body weight (29). In concert with this, when fructose is administered directly into the brain, food intake actually increases, opposite of the effect of glucose (45, 120). It should be no surprise that some investigators suggest that we examine the role of the "fructose index" (FI) and "fructose load" (FL) on the development of cardiovascular disease and diabetes, rather than limit it to GI and GL alone (189). We are sure to hear more about this in the future.

Fats

Dietary lipids include triglycerides, phospholipids, and **cholesterol.** If solid at room temperature, lipids are fats; if liquid, oils. Lipids contain 9 kcal/g and represent about 33% of the American diet, slightly higher than the dietary goal of 30%, but lower than the 42% recorded in 1977 (47, 83, 149, 222, 233). However, part of the decrease in this percentage was due to an increase in total calorie consumption, primarily from carbohydrate (44).

Fat not only provides fuel for energy, it is important in the absorption of fat-soluble vitamins, and for cell membrane structure, hormone synthesis (steroids), insulation, and the protection of vital organs. Most fat is stored in adipose tissue, for subsequent release into the bloodstream as free fatty acids (see chapter 4). Because of fat's caloric density (9 kcal/g), we are able to carry a large energy reserve, with little weight. In fact, the energy content of one pound of adipose tissue, 3,500 kcal, is sufficient to cover the cost of running a marathon. The other side of this coin is that because of this very high caloric density, it takes a long time to decrease the mass of adipose tissue when on a diet.

The focus of attention in the medical community has been on the role of dietary fat in the development of atherosclerosis, a process in which the arterial wall becomes thickened, leading to a narrowing of the lumen of the artery. This is the underlying problem associated with coronary artery disease and stroke (see chapter 14). In the section on dietary guidelines, two of the recommendations dealt with this problem of atherosclerosis: a reduction in salt intake (see minerals), and a reduction in fat, saturated fat, and cholesterol. A reduction in each of the last three has been shown to reduce serum cholesterol, and with it, the risk of atherosclerosis (3). See Clinical Applications 18.3 for more on the role of diet composition on risk factor development.

Usually the cholesterol concentration in the serum is divided into two classes on the basis of what type of **lipoprotein** is carrying the cholesterol.

Diet Composition and Syndrome X

In chapter 14 we introduced you to "syndrome X" ("the deadly quartet" or the "metabolic syndrome") as an example of how scientists have tried to establish links among various cardiovascular risk factors to better understand how one affects the other. The risk factors included elevated levels of plasma insulin (hyperinsulinemia) and lipids (hyperlipidemia), high blood pressure (hypertension), and obesity. Some suggest that obesity, especially abdominal obesity, is the underlying cause of elevated cardiovascular disease risk, whereas others point to insulin resistance (and the resulting elevated insulin) as the cause. In one of a series of provocative studies, Barnard et al. (12) make a case for diet composition as the underlying cause of the problem. This is an important consideration given the potential to break up the deadly quartet.

These investigators put rats on either a high-fat, refined-sugar (HFS) diet or a low-fat, complex carbohydrate (LFCC) diet for 2 years. Animals were taken from each group beginning at 2 weeks and ending at 2 years to evaluate changes in body fatness and fat cell size, insulin resistance (ability of a tissue to take up glucose), plasma insulin and lipid levels, and blood pressure. They found that:

- Insulin resistance and elevated levels of plasma insulin were present at 2 weeks in the HFS group and, therefore, preceded all other aspects of the syndrome.
- Plasma triglycerides were significantly elevated by the second month in the HFS group.
- Body fatness was not different until 6 months, but fat cell size was already increased in those on the HFS diet by 2 months.
- Blood pressure was not different until 12 months, but by 18 months all the rats on the HFS diet had high blood pressure.

This study showed that the composition of the diet was the cause of the insulin resistance, and that the insulin resistance preceded the other aspects of the syndrome. However, the authors acknowledged that the obesity probably contributed to the gradual worsening of the insulin resistance (demanding higher levels of insulin) over time. Blood pressure was the slowest-responding component of the syndrome and may be linked to the insulin resistance as described in chapter 14. This study confirmed the importance of diet on risk factor development and supports the recommendation of a low-fat, high-complex carbohydrate diet.

Low-density lipoproteins (LDLs) carry more cholesterol than do the **high-density lipoproteins (HDLs)**. High levels of **LDL cholesterol** are directly related to cardiovascular risk, whereas high levels of **HDL cholesterol** offer protection from heart disease (3). The concentration of HDL cholesterol is influenced by heredity, gender, exercise, and diet. Diets high in saturated fats increase LDL cholesterol. A reduction in the sources of saturated fats, including meats, animal fat, palm oil, coconut oil, hydrogenated shortenings, whole milk, cream, butter, ice cream, and cheese would reduce LDL cholesterol. Just substituting unsaturated fats for these saturated fats will lower serum cholesterol. The most recent recommendation for fat intake from the Institute of Medicine provides a range of values (20–35%), with the emphasis on unsaturated fats.

Dietary restriction of cholesterol has been shown to be effective in lowering serum cholesterol (3); however, this effect is influenced by the percentage of saturated fat in the diet and the initial level of serum cholesterol (i.e., those with high serum cholesterol levels benefit the most) (62). Based on currently available evidence, it is reasonable and prudent to recommend a decrease in cholesterol in the diet to 300 mg/day or less (3, 148). In addition, there is a special emphasis on eliminating trans fats from the diet. These fats rival saturated fats as a contributor to heart disease, and substituting polyunsaturated fats should reduce cholesterol levels (118). The following suggestions, provided as part of the 2005 *Dietary Guidelines for Americans*, were emphasized in the 2010 report (219, 220):

- Consume less than 10% of calories from saturated fatty acids and less than 300 mg/day of cholesterol, and keep trans fatty acid consumption as low as possible.

- Keep total fat intake between 20% and 35% of calories, with most fats coming from sources of polyunsaturated and monounsaturated fatty acids, such as fish, nuts, and vegetable oils.

- When selecting and preparing meat, poultry, dry beans, and milk or milk products, make choices that are lean, low fat, or fat free.

- Increase seafood intake in place of some meats and poultry.

- Limit intake of fats and oils high in saturated and/or trans fatty acids, and choose products low in such fats and oils.

- Replace solid fats with oils.

Protein

Even though protein has the same energy density as carbohydrate (4 kcal/g), it is not viewed as a primary energy source, as are fats and carbohydrates. Rather, it is important because it contains the nine essential (indispensable) amino acids, without which the body cannot synthesize all the proteins needed for tissues, enzymes, and hormones. The *quality* of protein in a diet is based on how well these essential amino acids are represented. In terms of quality, the best sources for protein are eggs, milk, and fish, with *good* sources being meat, poultry, cheese, and soybeans. *Fair* sources of protein include grains, vegetables, seeds and nuts, and other legumes. Given that a meal contains a variety of foods, one food of higher-quality protein tends to complement another of lower-quality protein to result in an adequate intake of essential amino acids (233).

The adult RDA protein requirement of 0.8 g/kg is easily met with diets that include a variety of the aforementioned foods. Although the vast majority of Americans meet this recommendation, an athlete's protein requirement is higher than this level. The protein requirement for athletes is discussed in chapter 23.

IN SUMMARY

- Carbohydrate is a primary source of energy in the American diet and is divided into two classes: that which can be metabolized (sugars and starches) and dietary fiber.
- Two recommendations to improve health status in the American population are to consume complex carbohydrates to represent about 45% to 65% of the calories, and to add more dietary fiber.
- Americans consume too much saturated fat, and the recommended change is to reduce this to no more than 10% of the total calories. Trans fat intake should be reduced as much as possible, and most fat intake should come from sources containing polyunsaturated and monounsaturated fatty acids.
- The protein requirement of 0.8 g/kg can be met with low-fat selections to minimize fat intake.

MEETING THE DIETARY GUIDELINES

A good diet would allow an individual to achieve the RDA/AI for protein, minerals, and vitamins, while emphasizing carbohydrates and minimizing fats. The 2005 *Dietary Guidelines for Americans* describes a healthy diet as one that:

- emphasizes fruits, vegetables, whole grains, and fat-free or low-fat milk and milk products;

- includes lean meats, poultry, fish, beans, eggs, and nuts; and
- is low in saturated fats, trans fats, cholesterol, salt (sodium), and added sugars.

A variety of food group plans have been developed to help plan a diet consistent with these guidelines.

Food Group Plans

The 2010 *Dietary Guidelines for Americans* provides some background on the research that helped them recommend specific eating patterns (plans). They considered a variety of eating patterns that have a solid research basis. These included the Dietary Approaches to Stop Hypertension (DASH) eating plan, traditional Mediterranean style diets, and vegetarian diets, including both lacto-ovo and vegan. Some elements common to all included the following:

- Abundant vegetables and fruits
- Whole gains
- Moderate amounts of foods high in protein (seafood, beans and peas, nuts, seeds, soy products, meat, poultry and eggs)
- Limited amounts of foods high in added sugars
- More oils than solid fats
- Most are low in full-fat milk and milk products, with some having substantial amounts of low-fat milk and milk products

These diets have a high unsaturated-to-saturated fat ratio, more fiber, and a high potassium content. At the beginning of this section we indicated that various organizations (e.g., AHA) emphasize the importance of diet in the prevention and treatment of various chronic diseases. Table 18.3 shows the consistency in dietary and physical activity recommendations across these organizations (212). These recommendations are clearly in tune with the *Dietary Guidelines for Americans*. The *Guidelines* recommended two major eating plans.

USDA Food Pattern   This food plan identifies daily amounts of foods with a focus on **nutrient density** from the five major food groups (and *subgroups*):

Vegetables—includes *dark green* (broccoli and spinach) and *red and orange* (carrots and sweet potatoes) vegetables; *beans and peas*, *starchy vegetables* (corn, potatoes), and *others* (onions, iceberg lettuce)

Fruits—fresh, frozen, canned or dried

Grains—including *whole grain* products (whole-wheat bread) and *enriched grains* (white bread and pasta)

TABLE 18.3 — Consistency of Dietary and Physical Activity Recommendations Among Chronic Disease Organizations

Lifestyle Factor	American Diabetes Association	American Heart Association	American Cancer Society/ American Institute for Cancer Research
Weight control	+++	+++	+++
Increase fiber	+	++	++
Increase plant food	+	++	+++
Decrease total fat	NA	+++	+++
Decrease saturated fat	++	++	+
Avoid trans-fatty acids	++	+++	+
Increase omega-3 fatty acids	++	++	++
Alcohol	moderation	moderation	moderation
Daily physical activity	++	+++	++

NA—not addressed

Note: from Thompson and Thompson (212).

Dairy products—with the emphasis on low-fat choices

Protein foods—All meat, poultry, seafood, eggs, nuts, seeds, and processed soy products, with an emphasis on low-fat choices.

The food plan has both a lacto-ovo and vegan adaptations. Details can be found at **http://www.health.gov/dietaryguidelines/**.

Dietary Approaches to Stop Hypertension (DASH) The DASH eating plan (191) was also identified in the *Dietary Guidelines for Americans* as a means to meet DRI/RDA standards and the various recommendations set forth in the document. The DASH plan was developed (as indicated in the title) to deal with hypertension, both to prevent it and to lower blood pressure in those with the problem (see **http://www.nhlbi.nih.gov/health/public/heart/hbp/dash/new_dash.pdf**). The DASH eating plan has been recognized for some time as an excellent approach to healthy eating consistent with reducing cardiovascular risk factors and achieving and maintaining a normal body weight. Those who follow the *Dietary Guidelines for Americans* have a lower risk of the metabolic syndrome (69). In addition, use of the DASH eating plan in a weight-loss program conveys more benefits to patients with the metabolic syndrome than a regular weight-loss diet (10).

The USDA developed a new online resource, *MyPlate*, to promote healthy eating and physical activity to achieve one's body weight goal. We encourage you to log on to this website **(http://www.choosemyplate.gov)** to get a feel for its user-friendly nature.

Evaluating the Diet

Independent of your dietary plan, the question arises as to how well you are achieving the guidelines. How do you analyze your diet? The first thing to do is to determine what you are eating, without fooling yourself. The use of the **twenty-four-hour recall** method relies on your ability to remember, from a specific time in one day, what you ate during the previous 24 hours. You have to judge the size of the portion you have eaten and make a judgment of whether that day was representative of what you normally eat. Other people use **food records,** in which a person records what is eaten throughout the day. It is recommended that a person obtain food records for 3 or 4 days per week to have a better estimate of usual dietary intake. Because the simple act of recording food intake may change our eating habits, one has to try to eat as normally as possible when recording food intake. It is important to remember that the RDA standards are to be met over the long run, and variations from those standards will exist from day to day (233).

IN SUMMARY

- The *Dietary Guidelines for Americans* identified two major approaches to use to meet dietary standards and achieve a healthy body weight: the USDA Food Patterns, with adaptations for vegetarians, and the Dietary Approaches to Stop Hypertension (DASH) food plan.
- The U.S. Department of Agriculture's MyPlate promotes a personalized approach to healthy eating and physical activity.

BODY COMPOSITION

Obesity is a major problem in our society, being related to hypertension, elevated serum cholesterol, and adult onset diabetes (147). In addition, there is growing concern that as the incidence of childhood obesity increases, so will the pool of obese adults. To deal with this problem, we must be able to assess the prevalence of overweight and obesity, as well as describe in more specific terms changes in body composition. This section presents a brief overview on how to do that. For those interested in a thorough discussion of body composition assessment issues, we refer you to Heyward and Wagner's *Applied Body Composition Assessment* and Roche, Heymsfield, and Lohman's *Human Body Composition* in the Suggested Readings, and Ratamess's chapter in the ACSM's *Resource Manual for Guidelines for Exercise Testing and Prescription* (170).

Methods of Assessing Overweight and Obesity

In the latter part of the twentieth century, one of the most common ways of making a judgment about whether a person was overweight was to use the Metropolitan Life Insurance height and weight tables (142). This has been replaced with a measure that has now been universally adopted—the Body Mass Index (BMI)—the ratio of body weight (in kilograms) to height (in meters) squared: $BMI = wt\ [kg] \div ht\ [m^2]$. The BMI is easily calculated, and guidelines for classifying someone as overweight or obese have used percentile rankings or fixed BMI values (127). As these BMI guidelines were developed, some allowances were made for age (higher values), but some scientists felt that the higher values were too generous given their association with higher rates of morbidity and mortality (28, 236, 237). Current BMI standards that have been adopted worldwide include (147):

Underweight	<18.5
Normal	18.5–24.9
Overweight	25.0–29.9
Obesity—Class I	30.0–34.9
Obesity—Class II	35.0–39.9
Extreme Obesity—Class III	≥40

The BMI standards listed previously are for adults. Investigators and clinicians have relied on percentile cutoffs (e.g., 85th and 95th percentile) to classify the fatness of children, without labeling them as overweight or obese. However, there is now agreement to use a BMI >30.0 or the ≥95th percentile (for age and gender) for classifying obesity and a BMI of 30.0 or ≥85th percentile but <95th percentile for classifying overweight in children (116) .

One of the major problems associated with height/weight tables and the BMI is that there is no way to know if the person is heavily muscled or simply overfat. One of the earliest uses of body composition analysis showed that with height/weight tables, "All-American" football players weighing 200 lbs would have been found unfit for military service and would not have received life insurance (14), even though they were lean. Clearly there is a need to distinguish overweight from overfat, and that will be the purpose of the next section of this chapter.

Methods of Measuring Body Composition

The most direct way to measure body composition is to do a chemical analysis of the whole body to determine the amount of water, fat, protein, and minerals. This is a common method used in nutritional studies on rats, but it is useless in providing information for the average person. The following is a brief summary of techniques providing information about (a) the composition of the whole body and (b) the development or change in specific tissues of the body. The error involved in the estimates of percent body fat is given as the standard error of estimates (SEE), which is addressed at the end of this section.

Isotope Dilution   Total body water (TBW) is determined by the isotope dilution method. In this method a subject drinks an isotope of water (tritiated water—^3H_2O), deuterated water (^2H_2O), or ^{18}O labeled water ($H_2^{18}O$) that is distributed throughout the body water. After 3 to 4 hours to allow for distribution of the isotope, a sample of body fluid (serum or saliva) is obtained, and the concentration of the isotope is determined. The volume of TBW is obtained by calculating how much body water would be needed to achieve that concentration. A person with a large amount of body water will dilute the isotope to a greater extent. People with large TBW volumes possess more lean tissue and less fat tissue, so TBW can be used to determine body fatness (63, 182).

Photon Absorptiometry   This method is used to determine the mineral content and density of bones. A beam of photons from iodine-125 is passed over a bone or bones, and the transmission of the photon beam through bone and soft tissue is obtained. There is a very strong positive relationship between the absorption of the photons and the mineral density of the bones (42, 127).

Potassium-40   Potassium is located primarily within the cells, along with a naturally occurring radioactive isotope of potassium: ^{40}K. The ^{40}K can be measured in a whole-body "counter" and is proportional to the mass of lean tissue (32).

Hydrostatic (Underwater) Weighing   Water has a density of about 1 g/ml, and body fat, with a density of about 0.900 g/ml, will float in water. Lean tissue has a density of about 1.100 in adults and will sink in water. Whole-body density provides information about the portion of the body that is lean and fat. Underwater weighing methods are commonly used to determine body density and will be discussed in more detail (127). The SEE is ±2.5% (170).

Dual Energy X-Ray Absorptiometry (DEXA)   In this new technology, a single X-ray source is used to determine whole-body and regional estimates of lean tissue, bone, mineral, and fat with a high degree of accuracy. The software required for this process continues to be refined, and DEXA continues to play a major role in the future of body composition analysis (61, 127, 138, 226). The SEE is approximately ±1.8%, but more research is needed (170).

Near Infrared Interactance (NIR)   This method is based on the absorption of light, reflectance, and near infrared spectroscopy (33). A fiber-optic probe is placed over the biceps and an infrared light beam is emitted. The light passes through subcutaneous fat and muscle and is reflected by bone back to the probe. Generally, there has been little interaction between scientists and the manufacturers in the development and validation of this type of device (127), and as a result there is limited research on this technique. The SEE is about ±5% (170).

Radiography   An X-ray of a limb allows one to measure the widths of fat, muscle, and bone, and has been used extensively in tracing the growth of these tissues over time (108). Fat-width measurements can also be used to estimate total body fat (74, 111).

Ultrasound   Sound waves are transmitted through tissues and the echoes are received and analyzed. This technique has been used to measure the thickness of subcutaneous fat. Present technology allows for whole-body scans and the determination of the volumes of various organs (33).

Nuclear Magnetic Resonance (NMR)   In this method, electromagnetic waves are transmitted through tissues. Select nuclei absorb and then release energy at a particular frequency (resonance). The resonant-frequency characteristics are related to the type of tissue. Computer analysis of the signal can provide detailed images, and the volumes of specific tissues can be calculated (33).

Total Body Electrical Conductivity (TOBEC)   Body composition is analyzed by TOBEC on the basis that lean tissue and water conduct electricity better than does fat. In this method, the subject lies in a large cylindrical coil while an electric current is injected into the coil. The electromagnetic field developed in the space enclosed by the cylindrical coil is affected by the subject's body composition (166, 188, 224).

Bioelectrical Impedance Analysis (BIA)   The basis for BIA is similar to that of TOBEC, but it uses a small portable instrument. An electrical current (50 μA usually set at a frequency of 50 kHz) is applied to an extremity and resistance to that current (due to the specific resistivity and volume of the conductor— the fat-free mass) is measured (127, 188, 224). Total body water is calculated, and the value can be used to estimate the percentage of body fatness, as was mentioned for the isotope dilution procedure. BIA devices using multiple frequencies (7, 54, and 100 kHz) show promise of improved accuracy (127, 186, 227). This technique may be an appropriate field method to use in place of or in addition to skinfolds in testing the elderly (78). However, one has to be careful to standardize hydration status to obtain valid and reliable measurements. The SEE is about ±3.5%–5% (170).

Air Displacement Plethysmography   Body density can also be calculated from body volume measurements obtained via air displacement plethysmography (in contrast to water displacement that is used in hydrostatic weighing). Small changes in pressure, due to the change in volume of air in the chamber, are used to calculate the volume of the individual sitting in the chamber. The Bod Pod uses this technology to simplify the measurement of body volume and therefore the calculation of whole-body density (see figure 18.2). The information obtained is used in the same way as that collected in hydrostatic weighing (54). Although body fat percentage values derived from this method may not be the same as those from hydrostatic weighing, the differences are small (143). The SEE is approximately ±2.2–3.7% (170).

Skinfold Thickness   An estimate of total body fatness is made from a measure of subcutaneous fat. A number of skinfold measurements are obtained and the values used in equations to calculate body density (127, 131). Details on this technique are presented in a later section. The SEE is approximately ±3.5% (170).

Some of these procedures are expensive in terms of personnel and equipment (e.g., potassium-40, TOBEC, radiography, ultrasound, NMR, DEXA, TBW) and are not used on a routine basis for body composition analysis. BIA has gained greater acceptance in the past few years, due in part to a collaborative

Figure 18.2 The Bod Pod system for measuring body volume using air displacement plethysmography.

multi-university research project that showed it to be comparable to skinfold estimates of body fatness in men and women (127, 231). The data from these techniques can be used alone or in combination to provide an assessment of body composition. A variety of models have been proposed for this purpose (94, 127, 133, 159):

- Four-component model—this model uses information on mineral, water, protein, and fat to assess body composition. The careful measurement of each of these components allows one to account for variations in bone density (mineral) and total body water that might vary dramatically in certain populations (e.g., growing children, the elderly). These procedures would give the best estimates of the percentage of fat.

- Three-component model—in this model the body is divided into three components: (a) body water, protein + mineral, and fat, or (b) body water + protein, mineral, and fat. The three-component model also allows one to account for variations in either bone density or body water and improve estimates of body fatness.

- Two-component model—this, the oldest model, divides the body into two components: the fat mass and the fat-free mass. Although it

is still the most commonly used approach to estimate the percentage of fat, the assumptions underlying this model have been questioned. The limitations of the two-component model have been addressed using information collected with the three- and four-component models. The details are provided in the following sections.

When using any of the body composition techniques, it is important to keep in mind that there is an inherent error involved in the estimations of percent body fat. The error is usually given as the standard error of estimate (SEE). If a technique estimates percent body fat as 20% and the SEE is ±2.5% (as it is for hydrostatic weighing), that means the actual percent body fat lies between 22.5% and 17.5% for 68% of subjects being measured as having 20% fat. Given that we don't know where in that range an individual is, caution is needed when interpreting percent body fat values. It is best to compare these estimates of percent body fat over time on the same subject, where the change in percent fat is indicative of changes in the fat mass or fat-free mass (170).

IN SUMMARY

- The BMI uses a simple ratio of weight-to-height squared (kg/m^2) to classify individuals as being normal weight, overweight, or obese. However, just like the old height-weight tables, the BMI does not consider the composition of the body weight (i. e., proportion of muscle tissue vs. fat tissue)
- Body composition can be measured in terms of total body water (isotope dilution, bioelectric impedance analysis), bone density (photon absorptiometry), lean tissue mass (potassium-40), density (underwater weighing, air displacement plethysmography), and thickness of various tissues (ultrasound, radiography, skinfolds).
- Body composition assessment can be based on four-component (mineral, water, protein, and fat), three-component (body water, protein + mineral, and fat, or body water + protein, mineral, and fat), or two-component (fat-free mass and fat mass) models. The four-component model is the most accurate.

Two-Component System of Body Composition

Two approaches that are used extensively to estimate percent fat include the **underwater weighing** and skinfold methods. In both of these methods, the investigator obtains an estimate of **whole-body density,** and from this calculates the percentage of the body that is fat and the percentage that is fat-free. This is the two-component body composition system described by Behnke that is commonly used to describe changes in body composition (14). The conversion of whole-body density values to fat and fat-free tissue components relies on "constants" used for each of those tissue components. Human fat tissue is believed to have a density of 0.900 g/ml, and fat-free tissue a density of 1.100 g/ml. Using these density values, Siri (197) derived an equation to calculate the percentage of body fat from whole-body density:

$$\% \text{ body fat} = \frac{495}{\text{Density}} - 450$$

This equation is correct only if the density values for fat tissue and fat-free tissue are 0.900 and 1.100 g/ml, respectively. Investigators sensed that certain populations might have fat-free tissue densities different from that of 1.100 g/ml when they observed high values for body fatness for children and the elderly, and extremely low values (<0% body fat) in professional football players (78, 134, 239). Children have lower bone mineral contents, less potassium, and more water per unit fat-free mass, yielding a lower density for fat-free mass (134). Lohman (128) reports density values (g/ml) of 1.080 at age 6, 1.084 at age 10, and 1.097 for boys aged 15½. The lower values in the prepubescent child would overestimate percent body fat by 5%. Based on data from the multicomponent models of body composition, Lohman (129) recommends the values found in table 18.4 for Siri's equation when applied to children, youth, and young adults (see table 18.4).

| TABLE 18.4 | Equations for Estimating % Fat from Body Density Based on Age and Gender | | | |

| Age, yrs. | MALE | | FEMALE | |
	C_1	C_2	C_1	C_2
1	572	536	569	533
1–2	564	526	565	526
3–4	553	514	558	520
5–6	543	503	553	514
7–8	538	497	543	503
9–10	530	489	535	495
11–12	523	481	525	484
13–14	507	464	512	469
15–16	503	459	507	464
Young adult	495	450	505	462

Note: C_1 and C_2 are the terms in percent fat equation to substitute for the Siri equation of percent fat = $\left[\dfrac{C_1}{D_b} - C_2 \right]$.

Reprinted, by permission, from T. G. Lohman, 1989, "Assessment of Body Composition in Children," in *Pediatric Exercise Science*, Vol. 1(1):22.

In contrast to children, who have density values below 1.100 for the fat-free mass, African Americans were shown to have a density of 1.113 g/ml (185). The Siri equation would have to be modified as follows:

$$\% \text{ body fat} = \frac{437}{\text{Density}} - 393$$

Although this may appear to be quite complicated, there is good reason to have the correct equation for a specific population. If judgments are to be made about the distribution of obesity in our society, it is important that estimates of body fatness be reasonably accurate. The following sections will discuss how whole-body density values are determined by underwater weighing and skinfold procedures. Heyward and Wagner's text (see the Suggested Readings) provides guidance in choosing the most appropriate equation depending on age, race, gender, or other factors.

Underwater Weighing Density is equal to mass divided by volume (D = M/V). Because we already know body mass (body weight), we only have to determine body volume to calculate whole-body density (80). The underwater weighing method applies Archimedes' principle, which states that when an object is placed in water it is buoyed up by a counterforce equal to the water it displaces. The volume of water displaced (spilled over) would equal the *loss of weight* while the object is completely submerged. Some investigators determine body volume by measuring the actual volume of water displaced; others measure weight while the subject is underwater, and obtain body volume by subtracting the weight measured in water (MW) from that measured in air (MA), or ($M_A - M_W$). Both methods of determining volume are reproducible, but body fat percentage values are slightly but significantly (0.7%) lower with the volume displacement method (232). The weight of water displaced is converted to a volume by dividing by the density of the water (D_W) at the time of measurement:

$$D = \frac{M}{V} = \frac{M_A}{\dfrac{(M_A - M_W)}{D_W}}$$

This denominator must now be corrected for two other volumes: the volume of air in the lungs at the time of measurement [usually residual volume (V_R)], and the volume of gas in the gastrointestinal tract (V_{GI}). It is recommended that $\dot{V}_R$ be measured at the time that underwater weight is measured, but measurement on land with the subject in the same position is a suitable alternative (128). Residual volume can also be estimated with gender-specific regression equations, or by taking 24% (males) or 28% (females) of vital capacity. However, the latter two procedures introduce measurement errors of 2% to 3% fat for a given individual (146). V_{GI} can be quite variable, and although some investigators ignore this measure, others assume a 100 ml volume for all subjects (38, 127).

The density equation can now be rewritten:

$$D = \frac{M}{V} = \frac{M_A}{\dfrac{(M_A - M_W)}{D_W} - V_R - V_{GI}}$$

Figure 18.3 shows the equipment used to measure underwater weight. Water temperature is measured to obtain the correct water density. The subject is weighed on land on a scale accurate to within 100 grams. The subject puts on a diver's belt with sufficient weight to prevent floating during the weighing procedure, and sits on the chair suspended from the precision scale. The scale can be read to 10 grams and it has major divisions of 50 grams. The subject sits on the chair with the water at chin level and as a maximal exhalation is just about completed, the subject bends over and pulls the head under. When a maximal expiration is achieved, the subject holds that position for about 5 to 10 seconds while the investigator reads the scale. This procedure is repeated six to ten times until the values stabilize. The weight of the diver's belt and chair (measured under water) are subtracted from this weight to obtain the true value for M_W. If V_R were to be measured at the time underwater weight is measured, the subject would have to be breathing through a mouthpiece and valve assembly that could be activated at the correct time (165).

Figure 18.3 The underwater weighing technique illustrating two individuals with the same weight and height, but different body composition.

The following data were obtained on a white male, aged 36: $M_A = 75.20$ kg, $M_W = 3.52$ kg, $V_R = 1.43$ liters, $D_W = 0.9944$ at 34°C, $V_{GI} = 0.1$ liter.

$$D = \frac{M}{V} = \frac{75.20}{\dfrac{(75.20 - 3.52)}{0.9944} - 1.43 - 0.1} = \frac{75.20}{70.55} = 1.066$$

This density value is now used in Siri's equation to calculate the percentage of body fat:

$$\% \text{ body fat} = \frac{495}{\text{Density}} - 450$$

$$14.3 = \frac{495}{1.066} - 450$$

The underwater weighing procedure in which V_R is measured (and not estimated) has been used as the "standard" against which other methods are compared. However, remember that due to the normal biological variability in the fat-free mass in a given population, the body fat percentage value is estimated to be within about ±2.0–2.5% of the "true" value (127, 170).

IN SUMMARY

- In the two-component system of body composition analysis, the body is divided into fat-free and fat mass, with densities of 1.100 and 0.900, respectively. The estimate of the density of the fat-free mass must account for differences that exist in various populations (i.e., children and African Americans).
- Body density is equal to mass ÷ volume. Underwater weighing is used to determine body volume using the principle of Archimedes: When an object is placed in water it is buoyed up by a counterforce equal to the water it displaces. One can measure the actual volume of water displaced, or the loss of weight while underwater. The weight of water is divided by the density of water to yield body volume, which must then be corrected for the residual volume and the volume of gas in the GI tract.
- The body fat percentage value has an error of about ±2.0–2.5% due to the normal biological variation of the fat-free mass.

Sum of Skinfolds Underwater weighing, although a good way to obtain a measurement of body density, is time consuming and requires special equipment and personnel. Paralleling the development of the advanced technologies used in body composition analysis, scientists developed equations that predicted body density from a collection of skinfold measurements. The skinfold method relies on the observation that within any population a certain fraction of the total body fat lies just under the skin

(subcutaneous fat), and if one could obtain a representative sample of that fat, overall body fatness (density) could be predicted. Generally, these prediction equations were developed with the underwater weighing method used as the standard. For example, a group of college males and females would have body density measured by underwater weighing, and a variety of skinfold measures would also be obtained. The investigator would then determine what collection of skinfolds would most accurately predict the body density determined by underwater weighing.

Investigators found that subcutaneous fat represents a variable fraction of total fat (20–70%), depending on age, sex, overall fatness, and the measurement technique used. At a specific body fatness, women have less subcutaneous fat than men, and older subjects of the same sex have less than younger subjects (131). Given that these variables could influence an estimate of body density, it is no surprise that of the more than 100 equations developed, most were found to be "population specific" and could not be used for groups of different ages or sex. This obviously creates problems for exercise leaders in adult fitness programs or elementary or high school physical education teachers when they try to find the equation that works best for their particular group. Fortunately, a good deal of progress has been made to reduce these problems.

Jackson and Pollock (102) and Jackson, Pollock, and Ward (104) developed "generalized equations" for men and women—that is, equations that could be used across various age groups. In addition, these equations have been validated for athletic and non-athletic populations, including postpubescent athletes (128, 195, 196). In these equations, specific skinfold measurements are obtained and the values are used along with age to calculate body density. Here are two such equations, one for men and one for women, which can be used to predict body density (103). The body density value obtained is used in the Siri equation presented earlier to calculate body fat percentage.

Men

$$\text{Density} = 1.1125025 - 0.0013125\,(X_1) \\ + 0.0000055\,(X_1)^2 - 0.0002440\,(X_2)$$

where X_1 = sum of chest, triceps, subscapular skinfolds, and X_2 = age in years.

Women

$$\text{Density} = 1.089733 - 0.0009245\,(X_1) \\ + 0.0000025\,(X_1)^2 - 0.0000979\,(X_2)$$

where X_1 = sum of triceps, suprailium, and abdominal skinfolds, and X_2 = age in years.

Jackson and Pollock (103) simplified this procedure by providing tabulated body fatness percentage values for different skinfold thicknesses across age. All that is needed is the sum of skinfolds to obtain a body fatness percentage value. Appendixes G and H show the percent body fat tables for men and women, respectively, using the sum of three skinfolds. For example, a woman, aged 25, with a sum of skinfolds equal to 50 mm has a body fat percentage equal to 22.9% (look to the right of the sum of skinfold column where 48–52 is shown, over to the second column—ages 23–27). Body fatness percentage derived from skinfold measures is estimated to have an error of about ±3.5% relative to the "true" value (130, 170). Recently, concern has been expressed about the need to cross-validate the skinfold equations against the multicomponent models and to clarify the effects that age, gender, ethnicity, and fitness have on the various components of body composition—for example, the density of the fat-free mass (78, 127).

The use of skinfold measurements was extended to children in the schools for early identification of obesity. The American Alliance for Health, Physical Education, Recreation, and Dance (9, 132) developed a health-related fitness test to evaluate cardiorespiratory function, muscular strength, low back function, and body fatness. The body fatness assessment relies on a triceps and subscapular or calf skinfold(s), and percentile norms are provided. When this test was developed, the skinfold values could not be converted to body fatness percentage values because the assumption that the fat-free mass had a density of 1.100 g/cc was known to be false. However, based on recent research with young populations using the four-component model (202), appropriate equations are available to convert skinfolds to body fat for young African American and white girls and boys (127) (see table 18.5).

Body Fatness for Health and Fitness

The previous sections showed how to determine body density by underwater weighing and skinfold procedures. This information on body density is converted to percentage of body fat and can be used to make judgments about one's status relative to health and fitness. Lohman, Houtkooper, and Going (126) recommend the following range of percent fat values for health and fitness for men and women:

Health Standards

	Men	Women
Young adults	8–22	20–35
Middle age	10–25	25–38
Elderly	10–23	25–35

Fitness Standards for Active Individuals

	Men	Women
Young adults	5–15	16–28
Middle age	7–18	20–33
Elderly	9–18	20–33

TABLE 18.5	Prediction Equations of Percent Fat from Triceps and Calf and from Triceps and Subscapular Skinfolds in Children and Youth for Males and Females

Triceps and calf skinfolds
Males, all ages: % Fat = 0.735 ΣSF + 1.0
Females, all ages: % Fat = 0.610 ΣSF + 5.0

Triceps and subscapular skinfolds (>35 mm)
Males: % Fat = 0.783 ΣSF + 1
Females: % Fat = 0.546 ΣSF + 9.7

Triceps and subscapular skinfolds (<35 mm)[a]
Males: % Fat = 1.21 (ΣSF) − 0.008 (ΣSF)^2 + 1
Females: % Fat = 1.33 (ΣSF) − 0.013 (ΣSF)^2 + 2.5
(2.0 African Americans, 3.0 whites)

1 = Intercept varies with maturation level and racial group for males as follows:

Age	African Americans	Whites
Prepubescent	−3.5	−1.7
Pubescent	−5.2	−3.4
Postpubescent	−6.8	−5.5
Adult	−6.8	−5.5

[a]Thus for a white pubescent male with a triceps of 15 and a subscapular of 12, the % fat would be: % Fat = 1.21 (27) − 0.008 (27)^2 − 3.4 = 23.4%

Note. Calculations were derived using the Slaughter et al. (1988) equation. Reprinted, by permission, from T. G. Lohman, 1992, *Advances in Body Composition Assessment* (Champaign, Il : Human Kinetics Publishers), 74.

Now that we know how to obtain a percent body fatness measure, and what the healthy and fitness percent body fat standards are, how can we determine the body weight associated with those values? In the following example, a female college student has 30% body fat and weighs 142 lbs. She wants to be at the low end of the healthy range, so her goal is 20% fat.

Step 1. Calculate fat-free weight:

100% − 30% fat = 70% fat free
70% × 142 lb = 99.4 lb fat-free weight

Step 2. Goal weight = $\dfrac{\text{fat-free weight}}{(1 - \text{goal \% fat})}$, with goal % fat expressed as a fraction:

For 20% = $\dfrac{99.4 \text{ lb}}{(1 - .20)}$ = 124 lb;

Her weight at her 20% goal is 124 lb.

Lohman (130) also provides values for body fat percentages that are below the optimal range: for boys, 6% to 10% is classified as low and <6% as very low. Comparable values for girls are 12% to 15% and

<12%, respectively. There is a great pressure in our society to be thin, and this can be carried to an extreme. A far-too-common problem in our high schools and colleges is an eating disorder known as **anorexia nervosa,** in which young females have an exaggerated fear of getting fat. This fear leads to food restriction and increased exercise in an attempt to stay thin, when they are, in fact, already thin (73). **Bulimia nervosa** is an eating disorder in which large quantities of food are taken in (binging), only to be followed by self-induced vomiting or the use of laxatives to rid the body of the food that was eaten (purging). While anorexia nervosa is characterized by the cessation of the menstrual cycle and the development of an emaciated state, the majority of the bingers/purgers are in the normal weight range (233).

It is clear that to stay in the optimal body fat percentage range, one must balance the dietary consumption of calories with energy expenditure. We will now consider that topic.

IN SUMMARY

- Subcutaneous fat can be "sampled" as skinfold thicknesses, and a sum of skinfolds can be converted to a body fat percentage with formulas derived from the relationship of the sum of skinfolds to a body composition standard based on a two-, three-, or four-component model.
- The recommended range of body fatness for health for young men is 8% to 22%, and for young women is 20% to 35%; values for fitness are 5% to 15% and 16% to 28%, respectively.

OBESITY AND WEIGHT CONTROL

In chapter 14 we discussed the major risk factors associated with degenerative diseases. Although high blood pressure, cigarette smoking, elevated serum cholesterol, and inactivity have been accepted as major risk factors, more and more evidence points to obesity as being a separate and independent risk factor for CHD, and one directly tied to two of the major risk factors. A variety of diseases are linked to obesity: hypertension, type 2 diabetes, coronary heart disease (CHD), stroke, gallbladder disease, osteoarthritis, sleep apnea and respiratory problems, and some types of cancer (endometrial, breast, prostate, and colon). In addition, obesity is also associated with complications of pregnancy, menstrual irregularities, hirsutism, stress incontinence, and psychological disorders (e.g., depression) (40, 147, 169, 172).

It should be no surprise that obesity is linked to an increased morbidity due to cardiovascular disease and some types of cancers. However, being overweight is not. Overweight was associated with a lower mortality from all causes, including cardiovascular disease (68). This information provides special urgency to promote strategies, including doing physical activity on a regular basis, to reduce the chance of a person moving from the overweight to the obese category. Let's take a more detailed look at obesity.

Obesity

If we use a BMI of ≥30 as a classification for obesity, the prevalence of obesity in U.S. adults increased from 15% in the 1976–1980 reporting period, to 23.3% in 1988–1994, to 30.9% in 1999–2000, to 32.2% in 2004 and to 33.8% for 2007–08 (67, 152). When you include those who are classified as overweight (BMI 25.0–29.9), the prevalence of overweight and obesity was 68.0%. Consequently, more than two-thirds of the U.S. adult population is overweight, and one-third is obese. In addition, some ethnic groups were overrepresented. More than half of non-Hispanic Black women aged 40 years and older were obese, and almost 80% were overweight (67). The good news is that the prevalence of obesity is not increasing at the same rate as it was 10 years ago.

All obesity is not the same. Studies suggest that not only is the relative body fatness related to an increased risk of CVD, but the distribution of that fatness must also be considered. Individuals with a large waist circumference compared to hip circumference have a higher risk of CVD and sudden death (200, 201). These data suggest that in addition to skinfold or underwater weighing estimates of body density, measurements of waist and hip circumferences should also be obtained (121, 122). Ratios of waist to hip circumference >0.95 for men and >0.8 for women are associated with the CVD risk factors of insulin resistance, high cholesterol, and hypertension, and such individuals are treated even if they are only borderline obese (19, 36, 43, 200). Given that the risk of these problems is associated with abdominal obesity, the guidelines mentioned previously (147) use only waist circumference and recommend values of 102 cm (40 in) and 88 cm (35 in) to be used for men and women, respectively, when classifying those at high risk. Recent reviews support the continued use of circumference measurements to assess health risk (190), but there is renewed interest in developing appropriate cutoff values for different racial groups since existing standards were derived primarily from Caucasian populations (96, 168, 205).

In addition to fat tissue distribution, there is a need to determine whether the obesity is due to an increase in the amount of fat in each fat cell (hypertrophic obesity), or to an increase in the number of fat

Figure 18.4 Relationship of fat cell size and fat cell number to total kilograms of body fat. Fat cell size is given in μg of fat, and fat cell number in billions of cells. The increase in body fatness beyond about 30 kg of fat is directly related to an increasing fat cell number; fat cell size remains relatively constant.

cells (hyperplastic obesity), or both (16, 17, 20). In moderate obesity where the mass of adipose tissue is less than 30 kg, the increase in fat cell size appears to be the primary means of storing the additional fat. Beyond that, the cell number is the variable most strongly related to the mass of adipose tissue (16, 92). This is shown in figure 18.4, where cell size increases up to about 30 kg of body fat, but does not significantly change thereafter. In contrast, the fat cell number is strongly related to the mass of adipose tissue (198, 199).

There are about 25 billion fat cells in a normal-weight individual versus 60 to 80 billion in the extremely obese (16, 92, 199). When a person undergoes dietary restriction, the size of the fat cells decreases but the number does not (16, 92). This high fat-cell number is believed to be related to the difficulty obese patients have in maintaining body weight after it has been lost (119). For example, a study was conducted to determine the pattern of weight loss, maintenance, and gain of groups classified as having obesity that is hyperplastic, hypertrophic, or both. Those with hyperplastic obesity or combined hyperplastic and hypertrophic obesity lost weight quickly, kept it off for only a short period of time, and regained it at a high rate. At this point we have seen that dieting does not change fat cell number, and that those who possess a high number of fat cells have difficulty maintaining a reduced body weight. The next question to consider is, when does the fat cell number increase?

In a longitudinal study of children during the first 18 months of life, the fat cell number did not increase during the first 12 months; the increase in cell size was entirely responsible for the increase in body fat. In contrast, the gain in body fat from 12 to 18 months was due entirely to an increase in fat cell number with cell size remaining stable (85). When

these data were plotted along with data from other studies, the results indicated that cell number increases throughout growth (85, 92). Given that physical activity and dietary intervention in extremely obese young children (8 years old) can slow the rate of growth in the fat cell number, and that the fat cell number is tied to the inability of obese children to lose their obesity as adults, the emphasis on treatment during childhood is obvious (86, 114). Unfortunately, in spite of our understanding of the problem, the prevalence of overweight and obesity in children and adolescents increased dramatically (from ~6% to ~15%)) between the late 1970s and 2000; however, the rate of increase has slowed between 2000 and 2007–08 for both 6–11 year olds (15.1% to 19.0%) and 12–19 year olds (14.8% to 18.1%) (151, 153). A major concern is that the prevalence of those at the high end of the BMI scale (97th percentile for BMI) continue to increase at a fast rate (151).The increase in overweight and obesity in children over the past 35 years carries with it a disease burden (e.g., type 2 diabetes), formerly reserved for those over age 40 and overweight. What causes obesity?

There is clearly no single cause of obesity. Obesity is related to both genetic and environmental variables. In 1965, Mayer (135) commented on the numerous studies showing that 70% to 80% of obese children had at least one obese parent, but concluded that it was difficult to interpret those data given the way cultural background interacts with genetics. In effect, the need to do hard physical work in some countries, or extreme social pressure against obesity (discussed later), might not allow a genetic predisposition to express itself. Garn and Clark (75) found a strong relationship between parental fatness and the fatness of children. They identified three categories of fatness on the basis of triceps skinfold: lean = <15th percentile; medium = 15th to 85th percentile, and obese = >85th percentile. The triceps skinfold thickness was related to parental fatness, being below average for the lean-dad/lean-mom pair and above average for the obese-dad/obese-mom pair. Although this might imply that a genetic link exists, when the investigators compared husbands to wives (usually no genetic tie), the relationship was similar to that for their children, suggesting either that there was a tendency of like to mate like, or that communal living exerts a major influence.

A slightly different approach to this question was taken when the body mass index of biological and adoptive parents were compared to the values of the adopted child as an adult. On the basis of a health questionnaire, they were classified as thin (≤4th percentile), median (50th percentile), overweight (92nd–96th percentile), and obese (>96th percentile). A stronger relationship existed between the BMI of the adoptee and that of the biological parent (207).

However, a subsequent review of this work pointed out that while the results were consistent with a genetic effect, it was not a very strong one (25). Other observations support the importance of the environment as a cause of obesity. In American women, obesity is inversely related to socioeconomic class: 30% for lower, 18% for middle, and 5% for the upper class (79). Further, women and adolescent girls have been shown to suffer the most direct discrimination because of this obesity (230). Clearly, although we may possess a genetic predisposition for obesity, a variety of social factors influence its appearance. Is there any way to determine the importance of each?

Bouchard (25) and colleagues have determined, on the basis of an analysis of the relationships between and among nine types of relatives (spouses, parent-child, siblings, uncle-nephew, etc.), that 25% of body fat and fat mass is tied to genetic factors, and 30% is due to cultural transmission. What is interesting is the components of energy expenditure that are influenced by genetic factors: (a) the amount of spontaneous physical activity, (b) resting metabolic rate, (c) thermic effect of food, and (d) relative rate of carbohydrate and fat oxidation. Further, when challenged with an excess of calories due to overeating, there is a genetic component related to the amount of weight gained and the proportion of that weight that is stored as fat or lean tissue. Given that information, it should be no surprise that physicians and scientists who work in this area believe that genetic factors are important causes of obesity (30, 89). However, as we will see, there is more to the story.

IN SUMMARY

- Obesity is associated with an increased mortality from cardiovascular disease and some types of cancer, but being overweight is not. Emphasis should be on maintaining or reducing weight in the overweight individual to decrease the chance of migration to the obese category.
- Obesity associated with fat mass in excess of 30 kg is due primarily to an increase in fat cell number, with fat cell hypertrophy being related to smaller degrees of obesity. Those with hyperplasia have a more difficult time losing weight and keeping it off.
- Genetic factors account for about 25% of the transmissible variance for fat mass and percentage of body fat; culture accounts for 30%.

Set Point and Obesity   Obese individuals, as previously mentioned, have a great deal of difficulty maintaining a reduced weight. In fact, the tendency of a person to return to a certain weight suggests that there is a biological set point for body weight much

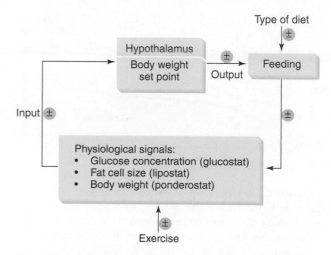

Figure 18.5   Physiological set point model for control of body weight by altering feeding behavior, showing the glucostatic (blood glucose), lipostatic (adipose tissue), and ponderostatic (weight) input to the hypothalamus. The signals from these latter mechanisms are compared against a "set point," and an appropriate increase or decrease in feeding behavior occurs. In this model, exercise can modify the input, and the type of diet can modify feeding behavior.

like the set points for any negative feedback biological control system. Although the hypothalamus contains centers associated with satiety and feeding behavior, we must remember that the *body weight set point is a concept, rather than a reality* (24). Figure 18.5 shows a physiological model of a body weight set point in which biological signals with regard to blood glucose (glucostatic signal), lipid stores (lipostatic signal), or weight on feet (ponderostatic signal) provide input to the hypothalamus (24). If the collective signals indicate low energy stores, food intake is stimulated until the source of the signal is diminished and the energy stores now equal the set point. Like any biological control system, if the set point were to be increased, body weight would increase to meet this new value. Exercise can modify the signals going to the hypothalamus, and the type of diet can also influence feeding behavior. In addition, drugs can be used to directly affect the neurotransmitters in the hypothalamus to alter feeding behavior (see Clinical Applications 18.4).

In contrast to this physiological model, Booth's cognitive set-point model (24) deals with the role the environment (culture, socioeconomic class, etc.) has on body weight. Figure 18.6 shows that relative to a personally selected "ideal" body weight set point, we are constantly receiving a variety of cognitive signals about how we look, body weight, clothing size, perception of effort, and concerns about health. A mismatch between the "ideal" set point and these perceptions leads to appropriate eating behavior. Exercise can modify the signals, and the type of diet can influence the feeding behavior. There is clear

Drugs, Dietary Supplements, and Weight Loss

Obesity is such a big problem in this country that it is not surprising that people seek help wherever they can find it. In response to this need, a variety of dietary supplements and drugs have been offered to help obese people lose weight. A survey of adults regarding beliefs and practices about weight control found that 33.9% used dietary supplements for weight loss, and many thought such products were approved by the Food and Drug Administration (FDA). They aren't (160). In one major review, the following dietary supplements were examined: chitosan, chromium picolinate, *Ephedra sinica*, *Garcinia cambogia*, glucomannan, guar gum, hydroxy-methylbutyrate, plantago psyllium, pyruvate, yerba maté, and yohimbe. Although the authors found some encouraging results, there was simply not enough evidence to recommend any specific dietary supplement for reducing body weight. The only exception was *E. sinica*- and ephedrine-containing supplements, both of which have been associated with adverse events (162).

Currently, only two drugs (orlistat and sibutramine) have been approved by the FDA to treat obesity over the long term, but both have undesirable side effects. Other drugs have been approved for short-term use (e.g., sympathomimetic drugs), but they also have potential adverse effects (82, 174). As of now, the following statement sums up the evidence (46, 162): The focus of any weight-loss (and maintenance) program should be on long-term diet and exercise behaviors.

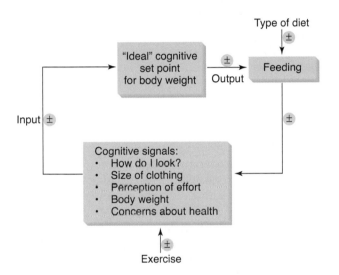

Figure 18.6 Cognitive set point for control of body weight by altering feeding behavior. A person's perception of "ideal" body weight is balanced against signals about how one looks, body weight, clothing size, and so on. Exercise can modify the input, and the type of diet can modify feeding behavior.

evidence that a high-fat diet results in an increase in caloric intake before satiety is reached—leading to weight gain in the long run (215). This set-point model is closely related to the behavior modification approach to diet, exercise, and weight control.

In a review of this topic, Levitsky (124) suggests that we might want to look at this issue as a "settling-point" theory rather than a "set-point" theory. This revision suggests that biology might set a range or zone of body weights, rather than a fixed weight. Within that zone, body weight may "settle" at a value determined by behaviors that are influenced by environmental and cognitive stimuli. In effect, Levitsky's "settling point" theory attempts to integrate aspects of each of the two positions just mentioned. He suggests that if the body weight zone is large enough to allow a person to move between a hypertensive condition and normal blood pressure condition or between a type 2 diabetic and nondiabetic state, then additional attention must be directed at the environmental and cognitive factors that drive eating behavior.

IN SUMMARY

- Investigators have proposed a set-point theory to explain obesity given the tendency for people who diet to return to their former weight. Theories based on weight sensors (ponderostatic), the blood glucose concentration (glucostatic), and the mass of lipid (lipostatic) have been proposed.
- A behavioral set-point theory has been proposed that relies on the person making appropriate activity and dietary judgments when body weight, size, or shape does not match up with that person's ideal.

DIET, EXERCISE, AND WEIGHT CONTROL

The Framingham Heart Study showed that body weight increases as we age. A reasonable question to ask is whether this gain in weight was due to an increase in caloric intake. Interestingly, caloric intake decreased over the same age span (27). We are forced to conclude that energy expenditure decreased faster than the decrease in caloric intake, and as a result, weight gain occurred (22). This weight gain problem can be corrected by understanding and dealing with one or both sides of the energy balance equation. We will deal with the energy balance equation first, and then discuss how modifications in energy intake can affect weight loss. Finally, we will explore the variables on the energy expenditure side of the equation.

Energy and Nutrient Balance

Weight gain occurs when there is a chronic increase in caloric intake, compared to energy expenditure. A net gain of about 3,500 kcal is needed to add 1 lb (454 grams) of adipose tissue. We are all familiar with the energy balance equation:

Change in energy stores = energy intake − energy expenditure

What is implied by this equation is that an excess energy intake of 250 kcal/day will cause body weight to increase 1 pound in 14 days (250 kcal/day × 14 day = 3,500 kcal = 1 pound). At the end of one year the person will have gained about 24 pounds. As reasonable as this equation may appear, we know that a weight gain of that magnitude will not occur. The equation is a "static" energy balance equation that does not consider the effect that the weight gain will have on energy expenditure (208).

The energy balance equation can be expressed in a manner to account for the dynamic nature of energy balance in biological systems:

Rate of change of = rate of change of − rate of change of
energy stores   energy intake   energy
                                          expenditure

When body weight increases as a result of a chronically elevated energy intake, there is a compensatory increase in the amount of energy used at rest, as well as during activity when that heavier body weight is carried about. At some point, then, the additional 250 kcal/d of energy intake will be balanced by a higher rate of energy expenditure brought about by the higher body weight. Body weight will stabilize at a new and higher value, but it will be more like 3.5 pounds, rather than 24 pounds, higher (208).

IN SUMMARY

- The dynamic energy balance equation correctly expresses the dynamic nature of changes in energy intake and body weight. An increase in energy intake leads to an increase in body weight; in turn, energy expenditure increases to eventually match the higher energy intake. Body weight is now stable at a new and higher value.

Nutrient Balance Investigators have taken this issue of energy balance one step further in an attempt to understand the causes of obesity. The dynamic energy balance equation can be subdivided into its components, representing the three major nutrients to generate nutrient-balance equations:

Rate of change of = rate of change of − rate of change of
protein stores   protein intake   protein oxidation

Rate of change of = rate of change of − rate of change of
carbohydrate   carbohydrate   carbohydrate
stores   intake   oxidation

Rate of change of = rate of change of − rate of change of
fat stores   fat intake   fat oxidation

If a person maintains balance for each of these nutrients—that is, what is taken in is expended—then energy balance is achieved. Nutrient balance is not a problem for protein and carbohydrate. The daily protein intake is used to maintain existing tissue protein, hormones, and enzymes. If more is taken in than is needed, the "extra" is oxidized for metabolic needs, and fat mass is not increased. The same is true for carbohydrates. Ingested carbohydrates are used to fill liver and muscle glycogen stores; the excess is oxidized and is not converted to fat (1, 18, 88). Carbohydrate intake promotes its own oxidation. This is a relatively new idea that has major ramifications for our understanding of nutrient and energy balance. The evidence seems to be quite convincing that *de novo* lipogenesis from carbohydrates (the making of new lipids from other nutrients) is of only minor consequence in humans. Simply, carbohydrates are either stored as carbohydrates or oxidized; they do not add *directly* to adipose tissue mass. This leaves fat.

In contrast to carbohydrate and protein, fat intake is not automatically balanced by fat oxidation. When "extra" fat is added to the diet, the same amounts of carbohydrate, fat, and protein are oxidized as before; the extra fat is stored in adipose tissue. Fat intake *does not* promote its own oxidation. Fat oxidation is determined primarily by the difference between total energy expenditure and the amount of energy ingested in the form of carbohydrate and protein. Consequently, if one wishes to keep the size of the adipose tissue stores constant (i.e., maintain body weight), one should not eat more fat than one can oxidize (64–66, 106, 107, 208). In this regard, when individuals are placed on a short-term, high-fat diet, the use of exercise (compared to rest) shortens the time needed to achieve fat balance (48). One last point: Alcohol intake is balanced by its own oxidation, but in the process, it suppresses fat oxidation. In this sense, the calories from alcohol should be included with that provided by fat (66).

In chapter 4 you were introduced to the concept of the respiratory quotient (RQ = $\dot{V}CO_2/\dot{V}O_2$) as an indicator of the fuel oxidized during exercise. An RQ of 1.0 indicates that 100% of the energy is derived from carbohydrates, and an RQ of 0.7 indicates that 100% of the energy comes from fat. An RQ of 0.85 indicates that a 50%/50% mixture of carbohydrate and fat was used. This RQ concept has been extended to the foods we ingest, and it is called the Food Quotient, or FQ. The FQ is defined as the ratio of the CO_2 produced to the O_2 consumed during the oxidation of a representative sample of the diet (65). The following equations are used to calculate FQ:

- O_2 consumption (L/day) = (0.966 × protein intake) + (2.019 × fat intake) + (0.829 × carbohydrate intake), and
- CO_2 production (L/day) = (0.774 × protein intake) + (1.427 × fat intake) + (0.829 × carbohydrate intake),

where intake of protein, fat, and carbohydrate is expressed in grams/day (81). The reason for describing this is that the FQ concept can be used with the RQ concept to determine if an individual is in nutrient balance (106, 107). Figure 18.7 presents this concept, and the following comments summarize its content:

- When RQ = FQ, the person is in nutrient and energy balance; the RQ/FQ ratio is 1.0.
- When RQ > FQ, the person is not oxidizing as much fat as was consumed (positive energy balance), and some fat has been stored in adipose tissue; the RQ/FQ ratio is >1.0.

Figure 18.7 Relationship between respiratory quotient (RQ)-to-food quotient (FQ) ratio and energy balance in humans. Each point represents values for a given subject measured over a 24-hour period. (From E. Jéquier. 1992. Calorie balance versus nutrient balance. In *Energy Metabolism: Tissue Determinants and Cellular Corollaries*, eds. J. M. Kinney and H. N. Tucker, p. 131. New York: Raven.)

- When RQ < FQ, the person used more fat than was consumed (negative energy balance), and some of the fat stores were used; the RQ/FQ ratio is <1.0.

This concept is helpful in discussing weight control, because one could improve nutrient and energy balance with regard to fat by either reducing the amount of fat in the diet (increasing the FQ), or doing exercise to use more fat (decreasing the RQ). We will now discuss both of these options.

IN SUMMARY

- Nutrient balance exists for both protein and carbohydrate. Excess intake is oxidized and is not converted to fat.
- Excess fat intake does not drive its own oxidation; the excess is stored in adipose tissue. Achieving fat balance is an important part of weight control.
- The ratio of the Food Quotient (FQ) to the Respiratory Quotient (RQ) provides good information about the degree to which an individual is in nutrient balance.

Diet and Weight Control

A good diet provides the necessary nutrients and calories to provide for tissue growth and regeneration and to meet the daily energy requirements of work and play. In our society we are fortunate to have a variety of foods to meet these needs. However, we tend to consume more than the recommended amount of fat, which is believed to be related to our country's obesity problem. The focus on dietary fat is twofold:

- Fat contains more than twice the number of calories per gram as carbohydrate and can contribute to a positive energy balance.
- It is difficult to achieve nutrient balance for fat when it represents a large fraction of caloric intake.

The hypothesis that the FQ of the diet is an important aspect of weight control revolves around the factors driving energy intake. There is a mandatory need for carbohydrate oxidation by the nervous system, and we are driven to eat what is used (64, 91). If we eat a high-fat diet, we will take in a considerable amount of fat while consuming the necessary carbohydrates to refill the carbohydrate stores. This fat is stored and body weight will increase. As mentioned earlier, as body weight increases, daily energy expenditure increases until an energy balance is achieved at a new and higher body weight. The fat-balance concept is consistent with this. Flatt (64) proposes that the increase in adipose tissue mass that accompanies weight gain increases the mobilization of free fatty acids, shifting the RQ to a lower value, and bringing it into balance with the FQ. In this sense, the elevation of body weight and fat mass due to a high fat/calorie diet is a compensatory mechanism that results in weight maintenance.

However, while we focus on the FQ/RQ concept, we should not forget that calories count in any weight-loss or weight-maintenance program. For example, studies in which subjects were switched from a high-fat to a low-fat diet, *while maintaining a constant caloric intake*, showed no change in energy expenditure or body weight (91, 123, 180, 215). In addition, in conditions in which a negative caloric balance was imposed to achieve weight loss, the composition of the diet (high-fat vs. low-fat) did not matter (90). In this sense, one should not get carried away with the high-carbohydrate diet and consume calories in excess of what is needed (66). In fact, when a variety of popular diets (Atkins, Ornish, Weight Watchers, and Zone) were compared over the course of one year, each modestly reduced body weight, with no difference between diets. It should be no surprise that the best predictor of weight loss was the degree to which individuals adhered to the diet—no matter which one (52, 71, 150, 181). Given these facts, why should diet composition matter in terms of weight control and obesity?

Quite simply, diets with a high fat-to-carbohydrate ratio are associated with obesity (144). When subjects are given free access to food, more calories are consumed when one eats a high-fat diet than when one eats a high-carbohydrate diet (23, 210). The high-carbohydrate content may contribute to satiety better than the high-fat diet, resulting in an earlier termination of eating (175). The nutrient balance (RQ = FQ) concept helps focus our attention on the need for a high-carbohydrate/low-fat diet to achieve and maintain a healthy level of body fatness. This diet is also consistent with what is needed to have normal cholesterol levels and sufficient carbohydrate for physical performance (see chapter 23). However, there is renewed interest in the diet-composition issue, not just related to weight loss, but also to weight control (maintenance). Three different reviews suggest that a high protein (25% to 30%) diet, coupled with moderate carbohydrate (35% to 50%) and fat (25% to 35%), should be studied in a systematic way to evaluate its effect on risk factors, feelings of satiety and hunger, and the fat-free mass (2, 183, 206). One of the *Dietary Guidelines for Americans* was to balance the food you eat with physical activity—maintain or improve your weight. Recommendations to accomplish this include the following:

- To maintain body weight in a healthy range, balance calories from foods and beverages with calories expended.
- To prevent gradual weight gain over time, make small decreases in food and beverage

calories and increase physical activity. We will see more on physical activity in a later section.

One last point before leaving this topic: As we mentioned earlier in the chapter, data on energy intake is assessed by twenty-four-hour recall or food records. However, one has to be cautious when interpreting these data as part of a weight-loss program. Research suggests that these methods may result in a considerable underestimation of caloric intake, especially in obese individuals (21, 53, 125, 141, 216). This, of course, would create a misdirection in looking for the cause of the obesity problem. It should be no surprise then that careful energy balance studies are done in highly controlled laboratory situations.

In the Institute of Medicine (100) recommendations that set appropriate levels of energy intakes for different levels of physical activity, the experts used data from doubly labeled water (DLW) rather than dietary recall. The DLW method measures total energy expenditure in free-living individuals, without the need for the person to remember what he or she had eaten. In the DLW method, the subject ingests a drink containing two isotopes of water: $H_2^{18}O$ and ^2H_2O. Urine or blood samples are obtained over a period of 7 to 21 days to evaluate the disappearance of ^2H_2O (relates to water flux) and $H_2^{18}O$ (reflects water flux plus the CO_2 production rate). The difference between the two rates gives information about total energy expenditure (rate of CO_2 production) and represents an improvement over earlier approaches that relied solely on dietary recall information.

IN SUMMARY

- Diets with a high fat-to-carbohydrate ratio are linked to obesity. Nutrient balance for fat can be most easily achieved with a low-fat diet (high FQ).
- Calories do count, and they must be considered in any diet aimed at achieving or maintaining a weight-loss goal.

Energy Expenditure and Weight Control

The other side of the energy balance equation involves the expenditure of energy and includes the basal metabolic rate, thermogenesis (shivering and nonshivering), and exercise. We will examine each of these relative to its role in energy balance.

Basal Metabolic Rate Basal metabolic rate **(BMR)** is the rate of energy expenditure measured under standardized conditions (i.e., immediately after rising, 12 to 18 hours after a meal, in a supine position in a thermoneutral environment). Because of the difficulty of achieving these conditions during routine measurements, investigators have measured **resting metabolic rate (RMR)** instead. In this latter procedure, the subject reports to the lab about 4 hours after eating a light meal, and after a period of time (30 to 60 minutes) the metabolic rate is measured (145). Given the low level of oxygen uptake measured for BMR or RMR (200 to 400 ml · min⁻¹), a variation of only ±20 to 40 ml · min⁻¹ represents a potential ±10% error. In the following discussion both BMR and RMR will be discussed interchangeably, except where a specific contrast must be made for clarification.

The BMR is important in the energy balance equation because it represents 60% to 75% of total energy expenditure in the average sedentary person (163). The BMR is proportional to the fat-free mass, and after age 20 it decreases approximately 2% and 3% per decade in women and men, respectively. Women have a significantly lower BMR at all ages, due primarily to their lower fat-free mass (49, 57, 158, 235). Consistent with this, when RMR is expressed per unit of fat-free mass, there is no gender difference. At any body weight the RMR decreases about 0.01 kcal/min for each 1% increase in body fatness (158). Although this may appear to be insignificant, this small difference can become meaningful in the progressive increase in weight gain over time. For example, a 5% difference in body fatness at the same body weight results in a difference of 0.05 kcal · min⁻¹, or 3 kcal · hr⁻¹, which is equal to 72 kcal · d⁻¹. It must be emphasized that the percentage of body fat makes only a small contribution to the BMR. This was confirmed in a study examining the relationship of body composition to BMR; fat mass did not improve the prediction of BMR based on the fat-free mass alone (49).

As mentioned earlier, part of the variation in BMR is due to a genetic predisposition to be higher or lower (25). The range (±3 SD) in normal BMR values is about ±21% from the average value, and such variation helps to explain the observation that some have an easier time at maintaining body weight than others. If an average adult male has a BMR of 1,500 kcal · d⁻¹, those at +3 SD can take in an additional 300 kcal · d⁻¹ (21% of 1,500 kcal) to maintain weight, whereas others at the low end of the range (−3 SD) would have to take in 300 fewer kcals (57, 76).

The fat-free mass is not the only factor influencing the BMR. In 1919, Benedict et al. (15) showed that prolonged dieting (reduction from about 3,100 kcal to 1,950 kcal) was associated with a 20% decrease in the BMR expressed per kilogram of body weight. This observation was confirmed in the famous Minnesota Starvation Experiment (113), and is shown in figure 18.8. In this figure the BMR is expressed as

Figure 18.8 Decrease in basal metabolic rate during 24 weeks of semi-starvation.

a percent of the value measured before the period of semi-starvation. The percent decrease in BMR is larger "per man" because of the loss of lean tissue (as well as fat tissue); however, when the value is expressed per kilogram of body weight or per unit of surface area (m²), the BMR is still shown to be reduced. A decrease in the concentration of one of the thyroid hormones (T₃) and a reduced level of sympathetic nervous system activity have been implicated in this lower BMR due to caloric restriction (26). What these data mean is that during a period of low caloric intake, the energy production of the tissues decreases in an attempt to adapt to the lower caloric intake and reduce the rate of weight loss. This is an appropriate adaptation in periods of semi-starvation, but is counterproductive in weight-reduction programs. This information bears heavily on the use of low-calorie diets as a primary means of weight reduction (56, 70, 225, 228).

The BMR is also responsive to periods of overfeeding. In the dieting experiment of Benedict et al. (15) mentioned earlier, when the subjects were allowed a day of free eating, the BMR was elevated on the following day. Further, in long-term (14 to 20 days) overfeeding to cause obesity, increases in resting and basal metabolic rates have been recorded. In essence, during the dynamic phase of weight gain (going from a lower to a higher weight), more calories are required per kg of body weight to maintain the weight gain than to simply maintain normal body weight (76, 194). This increased heat production due to an excess caloric intake, called **thermogenesis,** will be discussed in the next section. However, before leaving this discussion of the BMR, we need to mention the effect of exercise.

There is no doubt that the resting metabolic rate is elevated following exercise. The questions relate to how much and how long it is elevated, and to what extent it contributes to total daily energy expenditure (31, 164). A review of this topic indicates that controversies still exist even though the questions have been studied for over 100 years (145). At the heart of the matter is the measure of the metabolic rate that is taken as the baseline in these experiments. Should it be the BMR? The RMR? Molé (145) suggests that we need to create a new measurement called the Standard Metabolic Rate that would take into consideration the day-to-day fluctuations in normal physical activity, dietary intake, added exercise, and body composition. In support of these concerns it has been shown that trained subjects had a higher RMR than untrained subjects only when they did heavy exercise and consumed sufficient calories to maintain energy balance (37). This suggests that the higher RMR in trained individuals is not due to chronic adaptations associated with training, but more to the higher energy flux associated with the training and diet. This is consistent with other studies showing that the RMR, expressed per kg of fat-free mass, is similar for trained and untrained individuals, and that resistance and endurance training do not affect the value (34, 35). Aside from helping to maintain or increase the lean body mass and the RMR, exercise training may favorably impact nutrient balance. Two studies, using strength training, showed a significant decrease in the 24-hour (218) and sleeping (223) metabolic rate RQ values, signifying an increased use of fat. This is consistent with achieving nutrient balance and energy balance over time (241).

IN SUMMARY

- The BMR represents the largest fraction of total energy expenditure in sedentary persons. The BMR decreases with age, and women have lower BMR values than men.
- The fat-free mass is related to both the gender difference and to the decline in BMR with age. A reduction in caloric intake by dieting or fasting can reduce the BMR, while physical activity is important in maintaining it.

Thermogenesis Core temperature is maintained at about 37° C by balancing heat production with heat loss. Under thermoneutral conditions, the BMR (RMR) provides the necessary heat, but under cold environmental conditions, the process of shivering is actuated and 100% of the energy required for involuntary muscle contraction appears as heat to maintain core temperature. In addition, some animals (including newborn humans) produce heat by a process called nonshivering thermogenesis, involving brown adipose tissue. This type of adipose tissue is rich in mitochondria and increases heat production in response to norepinephrine (NE). Thyroid hormones, especially T_3, may either directly affect this process or act in a permissive manner to facilitate the action of NE (26, 27, 105). Heat production is increased by

uncoupling oxidative phosphorylation; that is, oxygen is used without ATP formation, so the energy contained in NADH and FADH appears directly as heat. Those individuals with large quantities of brown adipose tissue have a greater capacity to "throw off" calories in the form of heat rather than store them in adipose tissue. It has been hypothesized that variations in brown adipose tissue might be related to the ease or difficulty with which one gains weight.

Thermogenesis involves more than brown adipose tissue. The heat generated due to the food we consume accounts for about 10% to 15% of our total daily energy expenditure; this is called the *thermic effect of food* (27, 163). Generally, this is determined by having a subject ingest a test meal (700–1,000 kcal), and the elevation in the metabolic rate is measured following the meal. This portion of our daily energy expenditure is influenced by genetic factors (25, 163), is lower in obese than in lean individuals (110, 187), and is influenced by the level of spontaneous activity and the degree of insulin resistance (209). However, because it represents such a small part of the overall daily energy expenditure, it is not a good predictor of subsequent obesity.

In individuals who have been on a diet (underfeeding), just one day of overfeeding leads to an increase in the next day's BMR. The BMR then quickly returns to the level consistent with the low-caloric intake specified in the diet (15). It is as if the body is throwing off extra heat to maintain body weight during this period of relative overfeeding. This phenomenon has also been observed in the chronic overfeeding of human subjects. In Garrow's (77) and Danforth's (51) reviews of these overfeeding studies, the subjects showed an unexplained heat production associated with chronic excess caloric intakes. The elevations of the BMR have been explained on the basis of an increase in the mass of brown adipose tissue (mentioned earlier), and the involvement of other **energy wasteful systems.** These latter systems include a change in the Na^+/K^+ pump activity, or "futile cycles" in which the equivalent of one ATP is lost in each turn of the cycle (26, 27). An example of a futile cycle is when an ATP is used to convert fructose 6-phosphate to fructose 1,6-diphosphate, which, in the next step, is converted back to fructose 6-phosphate. In situations in which heat, but no ATP, is produced, the resting oxygen consumption would have to be higher to maintain the normal ATP-consuming systems. Whatever the mechanism by which this dietary thermogenesis is induced, via brown fat or by futile cycles, it must be made clear that, like the BMR, there are marked differences in how individuals respond to an increased dietary intake. Clearly, those who have a normally high BMR and are very responsive to a large caloric excess would have an easier time staying at normal weight than those who do not.

IN SUMMARY

- Thermogenesis (heat generation) is associated with the ingestion of meals (thermic effect of feeding), brown adipose tissue, and "futile cycles."
- The thermic effect of food represents a small part of total energy expenditure and is not predictive of obesity.

Physical Activity and Exercise   Physical activity constitutes the most variable part of the energy expenditure side of the energy balance equation, being 5% to 40% of the daily energy expenditure (41, 163). There are those who have sedentary jobs and who do little physical activity during their leisure time. Others may have strenuous jobs, or expend 300 to 1,000 kcal during their leisure time every day or two. Just how important is physical activity in weight control? Epidemiological evidence suggests an inverse association between physical activity and body weight, with body fat being more favorably distributed in those who are physically active (55). One study examined the relationship of body fatness to the different components of energy expenditure. Figure 18.9 shows that body fatness was inversely related to "nonbasal" (primarily that associated with physical activity) energy expenditure. In this sense, the level of physical activity is a permissive factor for obesity (173, 184). Consistent with this, recent studies showed an inverse relationship between BMI and

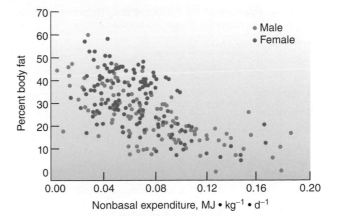

Figure 18.9   Relationship between body fatness and nonbasal energy expenditure is highly significant (P < 0.01); for females it is $r = -0.83$, for males $r = -0.55$.

accumulated daily walking (measured by pedometer). Those accumulating more than 10,000 steps per day were more likely to be in the "normal" BMI range (93, 213). For those wondering if a diet calorie is the same as an exercise calorie, see Clinical Applications 18.5.

Appetite   The classic animal study describing the role of exercise on appetite was conducted by Mayer and colleagues (136). Figure 18.10 shows that when female rats exercised for 20 to 60 minutes per day (sedentary range), the caloric intake actually decreased slightly and the animals lost weight. Over the durations of 1 to 6 hours of activity the caloric

CLINICAL APPLICATIONS 18.5

A Calorie Is a Calorie

From a weight-loss perspective, a caloric deficit that results from an increase in energy expenditure through physical activity is equivalent to that due to a decrease in caloric intake. However, as Ross et al. (178) point out, leading authorities (147) state that the addition of exercise makes only a modest contribution to weight loss. How can this be the case, given the equivalency of the caloric deficit induced by either diet or exercise? Ross et al. (178) show that in the majority of weight-loss studies in which a diet treatment was compared to an exercise treatment, the energy deficit caused by exercise was only a fraction of that caused by diet. In

this situation, it is not surprising that weight loss due to diet was greater than that due to exercise; however, the weight loss due to exercise was as expected. The exercise-induced weight loss, 30% of that due to diet, was equivalent to the caloric deficit associated with the exercise (28% of that due to diet). Ross et al. (177) did a controlled experiment designed to achieve a 700 kcal/day energy deficit due to either exercise alone or diet alone. Both groups lost 16.5 lbs over 12 weeks— exactly what was expected from the 58,800 kcal deficit (700 kcal/day times 84 days). However, the exercise group lost more total fat, thus preserving mus-

cle. These results were supported in a more recent study that compared subjects who underwent a 6-month 25% caloric restriction with those who had a 12.5% caloric restriction plus an exercise intervention equal to a 12.5% reduction in caloric intake (171). Both groups lost the same amount of weight, similar to what was mentioned earlier. There is little question that a calorie of aerobic exercise is really equal to a calorie of diet restriction as far as change in body weight is concerned; however, the exercise intervention yields results (e.g., increase in $\dot{V}O_2$ max) that cannot be realized by a diet-alone approach to weight loss (171).

Figure 18.10 Pattern of caloric intake for rats versus the durations of exercise. When rats do little or no exercise, caloric intake exceeds what is needed and body weight increases (see top-left part of figure). However, over a broad range of physical activity, caloric intake increases proportional to the activity, and body weight (top line) remains constant.

intake increased proportionately and body weight was maintained, but at a level below that of the sedentary rat. Durations in excess of 6 hours were associated with a relative decrease in caloric intake and body weight (exhaustion). Twenty-five years after this study, Katch et al. (112) showed that in male rats accomplishing the same amount of work, those exercising at the higher intensity had a greater depression in appetite and weight gain than those at the lower intensity, with both groups being lower than the sedentary animals. In contrast, female rats tend to respond to increasing exercise intensity with an increase in appetite (156).

Mayer and colleagues (137) also studied the relationship of exercise to caloric intake on mill workers in West Bengal, India. Figure 18.11 shows a pattern of response similar to Mayer et al.'s (136) study on rats. In the activity classifications from light to very heavy work, caloric intake increased proportionately so that body weight was not different among the various groups. However, in the sedentary classification, caloric intake was as high as for the very heavy work classification, and body weight was higher than the other groups. This suggests that a minimal level of exercise is needed to help regulate appetite. This study has been cited over the years as a primary supporting piece of evidence showing exercise to be important in the regulation of appetite. However, in 1978 Garrow (76) questioned the analysis of the data at the sedentary end of the scale where the group called "Clerks I" had a body weight similar to the more active groups, *but consumed about 400 kcal/day more* than those in the light work category. This analysis of the data would support a conclusion opposite that of

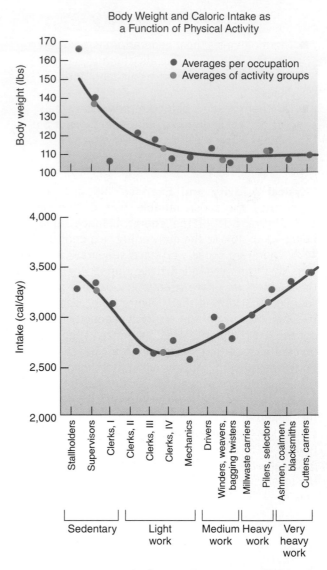

Figure 18.11 Pattern of caloric intake versus occupational activity in humans. For occupations ranging from light work to very heavy work, there is a balance between caloric intake and physical activity such that body weight remains constant. For sedentary occupations, caloric intake (see left side of lower figure) exceeds needs and body weight is higher than expected (see left side of top figure).

Mayer et al. (137). It should be clear that there would have to be some proportional increase in appetite as subjects increased physical activity; otherwise, an athlete would gradually waste away during the course of a competitive season! However, when an exercise program is introduced to obese and/or sedentary individuals, appetite does not appear to increase. In Wilmore's (239) and Titchenal's (214) reviews of such exercise intervention studies, appetite did not increase in proportion to energy expenditure, suggesting a net loss of appetite. In summary, in male animals, exercise decreases appetite in proportion to exercise intensity, whereas in female animals,

A LOOK BACK—IMPORTANT PEOPLE IN SCIENCE

Jean Mayer, Ph.D., D.Sc. Recognized the Problems of Overweight and Obesity

Jean Mayer (pronounced Zhahn my-YAIR) (1920–1993) was one of the most well-known scientists in the twentieth century in the field of nutrition. He received his B.S. and M.S. degrees at the University of Paris in the late 1930s, but his progress to the Ph.D. was interrupted by World War II. He served in the French army, was captured by German troops, and escaped from a prison camp. He then served with distinction in the French underground and fought with the Free French and Allied forces across Europe, for which he was recognized with numerous military decorations. Following the war he studied at Yale University for his Ph.D. in physiological chemistry. He later attended the Sorbonne where he received the D.Sc. in physiology.

Dr. Mayer taught and did research at Harvard University from 1950 to 1975 during which time his classical studies on physical activity, appetite, and body weight (reported in this chapter) were done. During this time he played a major role in the United Nations' fight against hunger and malnutrition in third-world countries in Africa; he also highlighted the problems of hunger and poverty in the United States, which resulted in the food stamp program and an expanded lunch program for schoolchildren.

In 1976 he became the president of Tufts University and was a prime mover in developing the first graduate school in nutrition, New England's only veterinary school, and the USDA Human Nutrition Research Center on Aging at Tufts. He co-founded the Sackler School of Graduate Biomedical Sciences and the Center for Environmental Management.

Dr. Mayer published more than 750 scientific papers and numerous articles for popular magazines, and had a syndicated weekly newspaper column on nutrition that was published in 150 newspapers. He also published numerous books, including *Overweight: Causes, Cost and Control* in 1968. Many might be surprised by the title of that 1968 book given the fact that the late 1960s and early 1970s are used as a "reference point" (for how little obesity there was in the adult and childhood populations) when we talk about the current prevalence of overweight and obesity. However, it is simply a reflection of how far he was ahead of his time in recognizing the overweight and obesity problem and the importance of physical activity. It is unfortunate that we did not listen.

Source: http://www.bookrags.com/biography/jean-mayer/

---

exercise stimulates appetite. Generally, in humans, caloric intake is regulated in proportion to energy expenditure over a broad range of exercise intensities and durations to help maintain body weight, but when exercise is introduced to a formerly sedentary population, a net decrease in appetite results. See A Look Back—Important People in Science for an individual who had a major impact on nutrition and health in the twentieth century.

Body Composition Although exercise may help regulate appetite to maintain body weight, exercise has an independent effect on the composition of that weight. This has been shown in both animal and human studies. In general, male rats that participate in regular exercise have lower body weights, less lean body mass, and very little body fat compared to their sedentary control litter mates. In contrast, female rats tend to respond to exercise training with an increase in appetite such that they are as heavy as the sedentary group, with a lower fat weight and a higher lean weight (155). Oscai et al. (157) have shown that, in addition to these general changes in body composition due to exercise, exercise or food restriction in rats results in fewer and smaller fat cells. This observation is supported by Hager et al.'s (86) finding that

in a group of 8-year-old obese girls, a diet/activity program was instrumental in reducing the rate of gain in fat cell number.

The advantage of using exercise compared to caloric restriction alone in weight-loss programs is that the composition of the weight that is lost is more fat tissue than lean tissue. In both animal (157) and human (36, 39, 58) studies using dietary restriction alone, lean body mass loss can equal 30% to 40% of the weight loss. Exercise plus diet results in less lean body mass loss and a proportionately greater fat loss (157). In addition, the preferential mobilization of fat from visceral adipose tissue results in an improved body fat distribution and risk factor profile (179, 229). However, it must be remembered that body composition changes take place slowly in human exercise studies, and the magnitude of the change is small. Wilmore's 1983 summary (239) of exercise and body composition studies showed the average decrease in percentage of body fat to be only 1.6% with fitness programs ranging in duration from 6 to 104 weeks. This old observation was recently confirmed in a collection of well-designed randomized controlled trials in which subjects participated in various physical activity interventions for a duration of 8 to 12 months. In general, and to no one's surprise, those doing the

Successful Losers—How Much Exercise Is Needed to Keep the Weight Off?

There is general agreement that most U.S. adults need more physical activity. The question is, how much? The systematic increase in the prevalence of obesity over the past 25 years has provided a strong incentive to address this issue and, to some extent, we are making progress.

In chapter 16 we presented the U.S. *Physical Activity Guidelines'* recommendation that all adults should do at least 150 minutes of moderate-intensity or 75 minutes of vigorous-intensity physical activity per week (see Suggested Readings). There is clear evidence that this amount of physical activity results in significant health benefits. This is a minimal recommendation, with clear support that "more is better." So, doing 300 minutes per week of moderate-intensity or 150 minutes per week of vigorous-intensity physical activity results in additional benefits, including maintaining or losing weight. This is consistent with both the 2002 Institute of Medicine (IOM) report (100), and the most recent ACSM position stand on the issue of physical activity and weight (4), in which they recommend:

■ 150–250 min/wk of moderate-intensity physical activity to prevent weight gain

■ >250 min/wk of moderate-intensity physical activity to achieve significant weight loss, and
■ >250 minutes per week of moderate-intensity physical activity may be needed to prevent weight regain after weight lost

Regarding the last point, Dr. Rena Wing of the University of Pittsburgh and Dr. James Hill of the University of Colorado formed the National Weight Control Registry (NWCR) in 1993 to gain some insights into what made "successful losers"—individuals who lost weight and kept it off. To be included in the registry, individuals had to have lost substantial weight (≥13.6 kg [30 lb]) and kept it off for at least one year. Some of the findings follow (211):

■ The average weight loss of the registrants was 33.6 kg, and they kept the weight off for an average of 5.2 years, which placed most in the normal (57.9%) or overweight (29.9%) BMI range.
■ About 88% limit foods high in fat and sugar, 44% limit the amount of food consumed, and 44% count calories.
■ A total of 75% of registrants expend more than 1,000 kcal/week, and 54% expend more

than 2,000 kcal/week (about 200 min/wk of moderate-intensity physical activity).

The NWCR has provided unique and helpful insights into what makes a successful loser. The seven key habits for long-term success at weight loss include (211):

1. High level of physical activity
2. Limit television watching—63% watch less than 10 hours a week
3. Low-calorie, low-fat diet—1,380 kcal/day, with less than 30% fat
4. Consistent diet—eat the same foods regularly
5. Breakfast consumption—at least 78% eat breakfast daily
6. High dietary restraint (good control over eating)
7. Self-monitoring—more than 50% weigh weekly and track their daily food intake

These characteristics are consistent with those in a recent review describing an ideal person who is a successful weight maintainer (60). Clearly, these messages from those who have been successful in maintaining weight loss have great value for both the professional and the client working toward that goal.

---

largest amount of physical activity had the greatest changes in percentage of body fat (101, 139, 203). However, those doing about 180 minutes per week of moderate-intensity aerobic physical activity (similar to current public health physical activity recommendations) experienced a decrease in percentage of fat of only 2.5% over this time period (101, 203).

IN SUMMARY

■ Humans increase appetite over a broad range of energy expenditure to maintain body weight; however, formerly sedentary individuals show a net loss of appetite when they undertake an exercise program.
■ When weight loss occurs with an exercise and diet program, less lean body mass is lost than when the same weight loss is achieved by diet alone.

Weight Loss vs. Weight Maintenance One point that needs to be stated at the outset is that exercise is not required to achieve weight loss. All that is necessary is a caloric deficit, the magnitude of which is easily controlled by diet (90). However, as mentioned previously, the use of exercise as a part of a weight-loss program might maintain a higher lean body mass and RMR, and result in an optimal body fatness at a higher body weight.

Although exercise might not be an essential ingredient in a weight-loss program, it is in a weight-maintenance program (204). A major, unresolved question is, how much? However, some of the general exercise recommendations for health and fitness presented in chapter 16 would be considered reasonable for weight-maintenance programs. The primary factor involved in energy expenditure is the total work accomplished, so low-intensity, long-duration exercise is as good as high-intensity, short-duration exercise in expending calories. For the sedentary, overweight person, moderate-intensity exercise is the proper choice because it can be done for longer periods of time in each exercise session and can be done each day. Recent, well-controlled physical activity interventions showed that regular participation in moderate-intensity physical activity of 180 minutes or more per week (with no dietary restriction) was associated with a weight loss of about 1 to 2 pounds over 8 to 12 months, indicating that the subjects were weight stable over that time (101, 139, 203). Although the magnitude of weight change is small, the message it conveys is very important: only 30 minutes or more of moderate-intensity physical activity per day is enough to prevent migration from one BMI level to the next—an important effect considering the prevalence of overweight and obesity in our society. However, as we saw in chapter 16, "more is better" when it comes to physical activity and health, including maintaining a healthy body weight.

Further, at moderate intensities, free fatty acids are mobilized from the periphery to provide the majority of the fuel used and help with maintaining fat balance (176). This does not mean that "fat-burning" is restricted to low-intensity activities. Individuals interested in more vigorous activity (~65% $\dot{V}O_2$ max) that can increase $\dot{V}O_2$ max can also reap the benefits of high rates of calorie and fat use (176). Finally, even though carbohydrate makes up a large fraction of the energy supply during high-intensity exercise (~85% $\dot{V}O_2$ max) (176), training programs using intermittent high-intensity exercise have been shown to cause a greater reduction in skinfold thickness than programs conducted at the target heart rate range (217). Although there is considerable interest in the role exercise plays in fat oxidation after exercise, results are inconsistent (13, 140). It is clear that virtually any form of exercise contributes to fat loss and the maintenance of body weight. The important thing is to just do it. See Clinical Applications 18.6 for information on "successful losers."

IN SUMMARY

- Moderate-intensity physical activity is an appropriate choice for most Americans to achieve health-related and weight-loss goals.
- Vigorous-intensity physical activity is effective in expending calories and achieving health-related fitness, performance, and weight-loss goals.

For weight-loss considerations, the caloric cost of an activity should be listed as the net cost (that above resting), because the gross cost of the activity includes energy already associated with resting metabolism. Table 18.6 shows the net energy cost per kg for walking and running 1 mile. In chapter 1, the net cost per $m \cdot min^{-1}$ of horizontal travel was $0.1 \ ml \cdot kg^{-1} \cdot min^{-1}$ for walking (up to about 3.75 mph), and $0.2 \ ml \cdot kg^{-1} \cdot min^{-1}$ for jogging or running. This translates to about 0.77 kcal per kg per mile for walking ($0.1 \ ml \cdot kg^{-1} \cdot min^{-1}$ times $1,609 \ m \cdot mile^{-1}$ times .0048 kcal per ml O_2), and 1.53 kcal per kg per mile for jogging or running. If a 60-kg person wished to expend 250 kcal by walking, a distance of 5.4 miles would have to be covered (250 kcal ÷ [60 kg × 0.77 kcal $\cdot kg^{-1} \cdot mile^{-1}$]); the

TABLE 18.6	Net Caloric Cost Per Mile for Walking, Jogging, and Running						
Walking							
Mph	2	2.5	3	3.5	4	4.5	5
Meters/min	54	67	80	94	107	121	134
Net cost kcal $\cdot$ kg^{-1} $\cdot$ mile^{-1}	.77	.77	.77	.77	.96	1.15	1.38
Jogging/Running							
Mph	3	4	5	6	7	8	9
Meters/min	80	107	134	160	188	215	241
Net cost kcal $\cdot$ kg^{-1} $\cdot$ mile^{-1}	1.53	1.53	1.53	1.53	1.53	1.53	1.53

Note: Multiply by body weight in kilograms to obtain the number of kilocalories used per mile.

From E. T. Howley and B. D. Franks, *Health/Fitness Instructor's Handbook*, 2d ed. Copyright © 1992 Human Kinetics Publishers, Inc., Champaign, IL. Used by permission.

$\dot{V}O_2$ Max (METs) ($kcal \cdot kg^{-1} \cdot hr^{-1}$)	Net Energy Expenditure at 70% $\dot{V}O_2$ Max ($kcal \cdot kg^{-1} \cdot min^{-1}$)	BODY WEIGHT (KG)		
		50	70 ($kcal \cdot hr^{-1}$)	90
20	13.0	650	910	1,170
18	11.6	580	812	1,044
16	10.2	510	714	918
14	8.8	440	616	792
10	6.0	300	420	540
8	4.6	230	322	414
6	3.2	160	224	287

From E. T. Howley and B. D. Franks, *Health/Fitness Instructor's Handbook*, 2d ed. Copyright © 1992 Human Kinetics Publishers, Inc., Champaign, IL. Used by permission.

distance would be only 2.7 miles if jogged. If the person walks at relatively high walking speeds, the caloric cost is higher than for the slower walking speeds, and a shorter distance would have to be walked to expend the same number of calories. As mentioned earlier, because it is the total amount of work that is important in weight loss, the total distance walked or jogged does not have to be done at any one time.

In selecting activities to achieve weight-loss goals, one must be careful not to overestimate the energy expenditure. If a table of values of the caloric cost of activities lists climbing stairs as requiring $15 \, kcal \cdot min^{-1}$, one must realize that this is an impossible goal to achieve aerobically for those with a maximal oxygen uptake of less than $3 \, liters \cdot min^{-1}$. Further, while an average value may be stated in such tables, some activities (e.g., swimming) have extreme variations in the energy required for the task. To deal realistically with this problem, Sharkey (192) provides a means of estimating the caloric expenditure associated with exercise for people of different fitness levels. If a person has a $\dot{V}O_2$ max equal to 10 METs, the appropriate range of exercise intensities to be in the THR zone would be 6 to 8 METs (60% to 80% $\dot{V}O_2$ max). Since 1 MET is $1 \, kcal \cdot kg^{-1} \cdot hr^{-1}$ (in addition to

$3.5 \, ml \cdot kg^{-1} \cdot min^{-1}$), this subject would be working in the range of 6 to $8 \, kcal \cdot kg^{-1} \cdot hr^{-1}$. If the person weighs 70 kg and exercises for 30 minutes at $7 \, kcal \cdot kg^{-1} \cdot hr^{-1}$, the person would expend a total of 245 kcal (70 kg × $7 \, kcal \cdot kg^{-1} \cdot hr^{-1}$ × 0.5 hr). The net caloric expenditure would be about 210 kcal. Table 18.7 summarizes the estimated energy expenditure associated with exercise training for those with different $\dot{V}O_2$ max values (95). It should be clear that as the person loses weight, the number of kcal used per fixed workout decreases, along with a decrease in the BMR. The combined effect of these two elements on the expenditure side of the weight-balance equation is that there will be a slowing of the rate of weight loss over time.

IN SUMMARY

- Although 150 minutes/week of moderate-intensity physical activity is associated with clear and significant health gains, more may be necessary to prevent weight gain (150–250 minutes/week) or prevent weight regain after weight loss (>250 minutes/week).

STUDY QUESTIONS

1. Summarize the range of carbohydrate, fat, and protein intakes recommended by the Institute of Medicine.
2. What is the difference between an RDA standard and a Daily Value?
3. Is there any risk in taking fat-soluble vitamins in large quantities? Explain.
4. Which two minerals are believed to be inadequate in women's diets?
5. Relative to coronary heart disease, why is there a major focus on dietary fat?
6. Generate a one-week menu using the MyPlate website. How do the choices compare to those in the DASH eating plan?
7. Identify and describe the following methods of measuring body composition: isotope dilution, potassium-40, ultrasound, bioelectrical impedance analysis, dual energy X-ray absorptiometry, skinfold thickness, and underwater weighing.
8. Contrast the four-component and two-component models of body composition assessment.

9. What is the principle of underwater weighing? Why should a different body density equation be used for children, in contrast to adults?
10. Given: a 20-year-old college male, 180 lb, 28% fat. What is his target body weight to achieve 17% fat?
11. In terms of the resistance to weight reduction, contrast obesity due to hypertrophy with obesity due to hyperplasia of fat cells.
12. Is obesity more related to genetics or the environment?
13. If a person consumes 120 kcal per day in excess of need, what weight gain does the static energy balance equation predict compared to the dynamic energy balance equation?
14. What does nutrient balance mean and how is the ratio of the RQ to FQ used to determine nutrient balance?

15. Contrast a physiological set point with a behavioral set point related to obesity.
16. What happens to the BMR when a person goes on a low-calorie diet?
17. What recommendations would you give about the use of diet alone versus a combination of diet and exercise to achieve a weight-loss goal?
18. What is thermogenesis and how might it be related to a weight gain?
19. What is the effect of exercise on appetite and body composition?
20. In contrast to the general physical activity recommendation for achieving significant health benefits, how much physical activity may be needed to prevent weight gain or maintain weight once it has been lost?

SUGGESTED READINGS

Heyward, V. H., and D. R. Wagner. 2004. *Applied Body Composition Assessment.* 2nd ed. Champaign, IL: Human Kinetics.

Roche, A. F., S. B. Heymsfield, and T. G. Lohman, (eds). 2005. *Human Body Composition.* 2nd ed. Champaign, IL: Human Kinetics.

U.S. Department of Health and Human Services. 2008. *2008 Physical Activity Guidelines for Americans.* Washington, D.C: Author.

U.S. Department of Agriculture, 2010. *2010 Dietary Guidelines for Americans* (http://www.health.gov/dietaryguidelines/)

Wardlaw, G. M. and A. M. Smith. 2011. *Contemporary Nutrition.* 8th ed. New York: McGraw-Hill Companies.

REFERENCES

1. **Acheson KJ, Schutz Y, Bessard T, Flatt JP, and Jequier E.** Carbohydrate metabolism and de novo lipogenesis in human obesity. *The American Journal of Clinical Nutrition* 45: 78–85, 1987.
2. **Adam-Perrot A, Clifton P, and Brouns F.** Low-carbohydrate diets: nutritional and physiological aspects. *Obes Rev* 7: 49–58, 2006.
3. **AHA Committee Report.** Rationale of the diet-heart statement of the American Heart Association. *Nutrition Today* 1982.
4. **American College of Sports Medicine.** Appropriate physcial activity intervention strategies for weight loss and prevention of weight regain for adults. *Medicine and Science in Sports and Exercise* 41: 459–471, 2009.
5. **American College of Sports Medicine.** Exercise and physical activity for the older adult. *Medicine and Science in Sports and Exercise* 41: 1510–1530, 2009.
6. **American College of Sports Medicine.** Physcial activity and bone health. *Medicine and Science in Sports and Exercise* 36: 1985–1996, 2004.
7. **American College of Sports Medicine.** The female athlete triad. *Medicine and Science in Sports and Exercise* 39: 1867–1882, 2007.
8. **American Dietetic Association.** Position of the American Dietetic Association: health implications of dietary fiber. *Journal of the American Dietetic Association* 102: 993–1000, 2002.
9. **American Alliance for Health Physical Education Recreation and Dance.** *Physical Best.* Reston: AAHPERD, 1988.
10. **Azadbakht L, Mirmiran P, Esmaillzadeh A, Azizi T, and Azizi F.** Beneficial effects of dietary approaches to stop hypertension eating plan on features of the metabolic syndrome. *Diabetes Care* 28: 2823–2831, 2005.

11. **Bailey RL, Dodd KW, Goldman JA, Gahche JJ, Dwyer JT, Moshfegh AJ, Sempos CT, and Picciano MF.** Estimation of total usual calcium and vitamin D intakes in the United States. *Journal of Nutrition* 140. 817–822, 2010.
12. **Barnard RJ, Roberts CK, Varon SM, and Berger JJ.** Diet-induced insulin resistance precedes other aspects of the metabolic syndrome. *J Appl Physiol* 84: 1311–1315, 1998.
13. **Barwell ND, Malkova D, Leggate M, and Gill JMR.** Individual responsiveness to exercise-induced fat loss is associated with change in resting substrate utilization. *Metabolism Clinical and Experimental* 58: 1320–1328, 2009.
14. **Behnke AR, Welham WC, and Feen BG.** The specific gravity of healthy men: body weight volume as an index of obesity. *Journal of the American Medical Association* 118: 495–498, 1942.
15. **Benedict F.** *Human Vitality and Efficiency Under Prolonged Restricted Diet.* The Carnegie Institution of Washington, 1919.
16. **Björntorp P.** Number and size of adipose tissue fat cells in relation to metabolism in human obesity. *Metabolism: Clinical and Dxperimental* 20: 703–713, 1971.
17. **Björntorp P, Bengtsson C, Blohme G, Jonsson A, Sjöström L, Tibblin E, Tibblin G, and Wilhelmsen L.** Adipose tissue fat cell size and number in relation to metabolism in randomly selected middle-aged men and women. *Metabolism: Clinical and Experimental* 20: 927–935, 1971.
18. **Björntorp P, and Sjöstrom L.** Carbohydrate storage in man: speculations and some quantitative considerations. *Metabolism: Clinical and Experimental* 27: 1853–1865, 1978.

19. **Björntrop P.** Regional patterns of fat distribution. *Annals of Internal Medicine* 103: 994–995, 1985.

20. **Björntrop P.** The fat cell: a clinical view. In: *Recent Advances in Obesity Research: II*, edited by Bray G. Westport: Technomic, 1978, p. 153–168.

21. **Black AE, Goldberg GR, Jebb SA, Livingstone MB, Cole TJ, and Prentice AM.** Critical evaluation of energy intake data using fundamental principles of energy physiology: evaluating the results of published surveys. *European Journal of Clinical Nutrition* 45: 583–599, 1991.

22. **Blair SN, and Nichaman MZ.** The public health problem of increasing prevalence rates of obesity and what should be done about it. *Mayo Clinic Proceedings* 77: 109–113, 2002.

23. **Blundell JE, Burley VJ, Cotton JR, and Lawton CL.** Dietary fat and the control of energy intake: evaluating the effects of fat on meal size and postmeal satiety. *The American Journal of Clinical Nutrition* 57: 772S–777S; discussion 777S–778S, 1993.

24. **Booth DA.** Acquired behavior controlling energy intake and output. In: *Obesity*, edited by Stunkard AJ. Philadelphia: W. B. Saunders, 1980, p. 101–143.

25. **Bouchard C.** Heredity and the path to overweight and obesity. *Medicine and Science in Sports and Exercise* 23: 285–291, 1991.

26. **Bray GA.** Effect of caloric restriction on energy expenditure in obese patients. *Lancet* 2: 397–398, 1969.

27. **Bray GA.** The energetics of obesity. *Medicine and Science in Sports and Exercise* 15: 32–40, 1983.

28. **Bray GA, and Atkinson RL.** New weight guidelines for Americans. *The American Journal of Clinical Nutrition* 55: 481–483, 1992.

29. **Bray GA, Nielsen SJ, and Popkin BM.** Consumption of high fructose corn syrup in beverages may play a role in the epidemic of obesity. *Amercian Journal of Clinical Nutrition* 79: 537–543, 2004.

30. **Bray GA, York B, and DeLany J.** A survey of the opinions of obesity experts on the causes and treatment of obesity. *The American Journal of Clinical Nutrition* 55: 151S–154S, 1992.

31. **Brehm BA.** Elevation of metabolic rate following exercise: implications for weight loss. *Sports Medicine (Auckland, NZ)* 6: 72–78, 1988.

32. **Brodie DA.** Techniques of measurement of body composition. Part I. *Sports Medicine (Auckland, NZ)* 5: 11–40, 1988.

33. **Brodie DA.** Techniques of measurement of body composition. Part II. *Sports Medicine* (Auckland, NZ) 5: 74–98, 1988.

34. **Broeder CE, Burrhus KA, Svanevik LS, and Wilmore JH.** The effects of aerobic fitness on resting metabolic rate. *The American Journal of Clinical Nutrition* 55: 795–801, 1992.

35. **Broeder CE, Burrhus KA, Svanevik LS, and Wilmore JH.** The effects of either high-intensity resistance or endurance training on resting metabolic rate. *The American Journal of Clinical Nutrition* 55: 802–810, 1992.

36. **Brozek J, Grande F, Anderson JT, and Keys A.** Densitometric analysis of body composition: revision of some quantitative assumptions. *Annals of the New York Academy of Sciences* 110: 113–140, 1963.

37. **Bullough RC, Gillette CA, Harris MA, and Melby CL.** Interaction of acute changes in exercise energy expenditure and energy intake on resting metabolic rate. *The American Journal of Clinical Nutrition* 61: 473–481, 1995.

38. **Buskirk ER.** Underwater weighing and body density: a review of procedures. In: *Techniques for Measuring Body Composition*, edited by J. Brozek J, and Henschel A. National Research Council, 1961.

39. **Buskirk ER, Thompson RH, Lutwak L, and Whedon GD.** Energy balance of obese patients during weight reduction: influence of diet restriction and exercise. *Annals of the New York Academy of Sciences* 110: 918–940, 1963.

40. **Calle EE, Thun MJ, Petrelli JM, Rodriguez C, and Heath CW, Jr.** Body-mass index and mortality in a prospective cohort of U.S. adults. *The New England Journal of Medicine* 341: 1097–1105, 1999.

41. **Calles-Escandon J, and Horton ES.** The thermogenic role of exercise in the treatment of morbid obesity: a critical evaluation. *The American Journal of Clinical Nutrition* 55: 533S–537S, 1992.

42. **Cameron JR, and Sorenson J.** Measurement of bone mineral in vivo: an improved method. *Science* (New York, NY) 142: 230–232, 1963.

43. **Campaigne BN.** Body fat distribution in females: metabolic consequences and implications for weight loss. *Medicine and Science in Sports and Exercise* 22: 291–297, 1990.

44. **Centers for Disease Control and Prevention.** Trends in intake of energy and macronutrients—United States 1971–2000. *Morbidity & Mortality Weekly Report* 53: 80–82, 2004.

45. **Cha SH, Wolfgang M, Tokutake Y, Chohnan S, and Lane MD.** Differential effects of central fructose and glucose on hypothalamic malonyl-CoA and food intake. *Proceedings of the National Academy of Sciences* 105: 16871–16875, 2008.

46. **Clarkson PM.** The skinny on weight loss supplements & drugs. *ACSM's Health and Fitness Journal* 2: 18–55, 1999.

47. **Coniglio JG.** Fat. In: *Nutrition Reviews' Present Knowledge in Nutrition*. Washington, D.C.: The Nutrition Foundation, 1984, p. 79–89.

48. **Cooper JA, Watras AC, Shriver T, Adams AK, and Schoeller DA.** Influence of dietary fatty acid composition and exercise on changes in fat oxidation from a high-fat diet. *Journal of Applied Physiology* 109: 2010.

49. **Cunningham JJ.** Body composition as a determinant of energy expenditure: a synthetic review and a proposed general prediction equation. *The American Journal of Clinical Nutrition* 54: 963–969, 1991.

50. **Dahlquist A.** Carbohydrates. In: *Nutrition Reviews' Present Knowledge in Nutrition*. Washington, D.C.: The Nutrition Foundation, 1984, p. 116–130.

51. **Danforth E.** Undernutrition contrasted to overnutrition. In: *Recent Advances in Obesity Research: II*, edited by Bray G. Westport: Technomic, 1978, p. 229–236.

52. **Dansinger ML, Gleason JA, Griffith JL, Selker HP, and Schaefer EJ.** Comparison of the Atkins, Ornish, Weight Watchers, and Zone diets for weight loss and heart disease risk reduction: a randomized trial. *JAMA* 293: 43–53, 2005.

53. **De Vries JH, Zock PL, Mensink RP, and Katan MB.** Underestimation of energy intake by 3-d records compared with energy intake to maintain body weight in 269 nonobese adults. *The American Journal of Clinical Nutrition* 60: 855–860, 1994.

54. **Dempster P, and Aitkens S.** A new air displacement method for the determination of human body composition. *Medicine and Science in Sports and Exercise* 27: 1692–1697, 1995.

55. **DiPietro L.** Physical activity, body weight, and adiposity: an epidemiologic perspective. *Exercise and Sport Sciences Reviews* 23: 275–303, 1995.

56. **Donnelly JE, Jakicic J, and Gunderson S.** Diet and body composition: effect of very low calorie diets and exercise. *Sports Medicine* (Auckland, NZ) 12: 237–249, 1991.

57. **DuBois EF.** Basal energy, metabolism at various ages: man. In: *Metabolism: Clinical and Experimental*, edited by Altman PL, and Dittmer DS. Bethesda: Federation of American Societies for Experimental Biology, 1968.

58. **Durnin JV.** Possible interaction between physical activity, body composition, and obesity in man. In: *Recent Advances in Obesity Research: II*, edited by Bray G. Westport: Technomic, 1978, p. 237–241.

59. **Eastwood M.** Dietary fiber. In: *Nutrition Reviews' Present Knowledge in Nutrition*. Washington, D.C.: The Nutrition Foundation, 1984, p. 156–175.

60. **Ebbeling CB, Leidig MM, Feldman HA, Lovesky MM, and Ludwig DS.** Effects of a low-glycemic load vs low-fat diet in obese young adults: a randomized trial. JAMA 297: 2092–2102, 2007.

61. **Ellis KJ, Shypailo RJ, Pratt JA, and Pond WG.** Accuracy of dual-energy x-ray absorptiometry for body-composition measurements in children. *The American Journal of Clinical Nutrition* 60: 660–665, 1994.

62. **Ernst ND, and Levy RI.** Diet and cardiovascular disease. In: *Nutrition Reviews' Present Knowledge in Nutrition*. Washington, D.C.: The Nutrition Foundation, 1984, p. 724–739.

63. **Finberg L.** Clinical assessment of total body water. In: *Body-Composition Assessments in Youth and Adults*, edited by Roche AF. Columbus: Ross Laboratories, 1985.

64. **Flatt JP.** Dietary fat, carbohydrate balance, and weight maintenance. *Annals of the New York Academy of Sciences* 683: 122–140, 1993.

65. **Flatt JP.** Importance of nutrient balance in body weight regulation. *Diabetes/Metabolism Reviews* 4: 571–581, 1988.

66. **Flatt JP.** Use and storage of carbohydrate and fat. *American Journal of Clinical Nutrition* Suppl. 61: 952S–959S, 1995.

67. **Flegal KM, Carroll MD, Ogden CL, and Curtin LR.** Prevalence and trends in obesity among US adults, 1999–2008. JAMA 303: 235–241, 2010.

68. **Flegal KM, Graubard BI, Williamson DF, and Gail MH.** Cause-specific excess deaths associated with underweight, overweight, and obesity. JAMA 298: 2028–2037, 2007.

69. **Fogli-Cawley JJ, Dwyer JT, Saltzman E, McCullough ML, Troy LM, Meigs JB, and Jacques PF.** The 2005 Dietary Guidelines for Americans and risk of the metabolic syndrome. *The American Journal of Clinical Nutrition* 86: 1193–1201, 2007.

70. **Foster GD, Wadden TA, Feurer ID, Jennings AS, Stunkard AJ, Crosby LO, Ship J, and Mullen JL.** Controlled trial of the metabolic effects of a very-low-calorie diet: short- and long-term effects. *The American Journal of Clinical Nutrition* 51: 167–172, 1990.

71. **Franz MJ, VanWormer JJ, Crain AL, Boucher JL, Histon T, Caplan W, Bowman JD, and Pronk NP.** Weight-loss outcomes: a systematic review and meta-analysis of weight-loss clinical trials with a minimum 1-year follow-up. J Am Diet Assoc 107: 1755–1767, 2007.

72. **Gao X, Wilde PE, Lichtenstein AH, and Tucker KL.** The 2005 USDA Food Guide Pyramid is associated with more adequate nutrient intakes within energy constraints than the 1992 Pyramid. *The Journal of Nutrition* 136: 1341–1346, 2006.

73. **Garfinkle PE, and Garner DM.** *Anorexia Nervosa*. New York: Brunner/Mazel, 1982.

74. **Garn SM.** Radiographic analysis of body composition. In: *Techniques for Measuring Body Composition*, edited by J. Brozek J, and Henschel A. National Research Council, 1961.

75. **Garn SM, and Clark DC.** Trends in fatness and the origins of obesity ad hoc committee to review the ten-state nutrition survey. *Pediatrics* 57: 443–456, 1976.

76. **Garrow JS.** *Energy Balance and Obesity in Man*. New York: Elsevier North-Holland, 1978.

77. **Garrow JS.** The regulation of energy expenditure in man. In: *Recent Advances in Obesity Research: II*, edited by Bray G. Westport: Technomic, 1978, p. 200–210.

78. **Going S, Williams D, and Lohman T.** Aging and body composition: biological changes and methodological issues. *Exercise and Sport Sciences Reviews* 23: 411–458, 1995.

79. **Goldblatt PB, Moore ME, and Stunkard AJ.** Social factors in obesity. JAMA 192: 1039–1044, 1965.

80. **Goldman RF, and Buskirk ER.** Body volume measurement by underwater weighing: description of a method. In: *Techniques for Measuring Body Composition*, edited by J. Brozek J, and Henschel A. National Research Council, 1961.

81. **Goris AHC, and Westerterp KR.** Postabsorptive respiratory quotient and food quotient-an analysis in lean and obese men and women. *European Journal of Clinical Nutrition* 54: 546–550, 2000.

82. **Greenway FL, and Bray GA.** Combination drugs for treating obesity. *Current Diabetes Reports* 10: 108–115, 2010.

83. **Guthrie HA, and Picciano MF.** *Human Nutrition*. St. Louis: Mosby, 1995.

84. **Guyton AG.** Body fat and adipose tissue cellularity in infants: a longitudinal study. *Metabolism: Clinical and Experimental* 26: 607–614, 1977.

85. **Guyton AG.** *Textbook of Medical Physiology*. Philadelphia: W. B. Saunders, 1981.

86. **Hager A, Sjorstrom L, Arvidsson B, Bjorntorp P, and Smith U.** Adipose tissue cellularity in obese school girls before and after dietary treatment. *The American Journal of Clinical Nutrition* 31: 68–75, 1978.

87. **Hallberg L.** Iron. In: *Nutrition Reviews' Present Knowledge in Nutrition*. Washington, D.C.: The Nutrition Foundation, 1984, p. 459–478.

88. **Hellerstein MK, et al.** Measurement of de novo hepatic lipogenesis in humans using stable isotopes. *The American Society for Clinical Investigation, Inc* 87: 1841–1852, 1991.

89. **Herrera BM, and Lindgren CM.** The genetics of obesity. *Current Diabetes Reports* 10: 498–505, 2010.

90. **Hill J.** Obesity treatment: can diet composition play a role? *American College of Physicians* 119: 694–697, 1993.

91. **Hirsch J.** Role and benefits of carbohydrate in the diet: key issues for future dietary guidelines. *American Journal of Clinical Nutrition* Suppl. 61: 996S–1000S, 1995.

92. **Hirsch J, and Knittle JL.** Cellularity of obese and nonobese human adipose tissue. *Federation Proceedings* 29: 1516–1521, 1970.

93. **Hornbuckle LM, Bassett DR, Jr., and Thompson DL.** Pedometer-determined walking and body composition variables in African-American women. *Medicine and Science in Sports and Exercise* 37: 1069–1074, 2005.

94. **Houtkooper LB, and Going SB.** *Body Composition: How Should It Be Measured? Does It Affect Performance?* Barrington: Gatorade Sports Science Institute, 1994.

95. **Howley ET, and Don Franks B.** *Health/Fitness Instructor's Handbook.* Champaign: Human Kinetics, 1992.

96. **Huxley R, Mendis S, Zheleznyakov E, Reddy S, and Chan J.** Body mass index, waist circumference and waist:hip ratio as predictors of cardiovascular risk—a review of the literature. *European Journal of Clinical Nutrition* 64: 16–22, 2010.

97. **Institute of Medicine.** *Dietary Reference Intakes for Calcium and Vitamin D.* Washington, D.C.: National Academy of Sciences, 2010.

98. **Institute of Medicine.** *Dietary Reference Intakes for Water, Potassium, Sodium, Chloride, and Sulfate.* Washington, D.C.: National Academies Press, 2004.

99. **Institute of Medicine.** *Dietary Reference Intakes for Energy, Carbohydrate, Fiber, Fat, Fatty Acids, Cholesterol, Protein, and Amino Acids.* Washington, D.C.: National Academies Press, 2002.

100. **Institute of Medicine.** *Dietary Reference Intakes for Energy, Carbohydrate, Fiber, Fat, Fatty Acids, Cholesterol, Protein, and Amino Acids.* Washington, D.C.: National Academies Press, 2002.

101. **Irwin ML, Yasui Y, Ulrich CM, Bowen D, Rudolph RE, Schwartz RS, Yukawa M, Aiello E, Potter JD, and McTiernan A.** Effect of exercise on total and intra-abdominal body fat in postmenopausal women: a randomized controlled trial. *JAMA* 289: 323–330, 2003.

102. **Jackson AS, and Pollock ML.** Generalized equations for predicting body density of men. *The British Journal of Nutrition* 40: 497–504, 1978.

103. **Jackson AS, and Pollock ML.** Practical assessment of body composition. *The Physician and Sportsmedicine* 13: 76–90, 1985.

104. **Jackson AS, Pollock ML, and Ward A.** Generalized equations for predicting body density of women. *Medicine and Science in Sports and Exercise* 12: 175–181, 1980.

105. **James WP, and Trayhurn P.** Thermogenesis and obesity. *British Medical Bulletin* 37: 43–48, 1981.

106. **Jéquier E.** Body weight regulation in humans: the importance of nutrient balance. *News in Physiological Sciences* 8: 273–276, 1993.

107. **Jéquier E.** Calorie balance versus nutrient balance. In: *Energy Metabolism: Tissue Determinants and Cellular Corollaries,* edited by Kinney JM, and Tucker HN. New York: Raven, 1992, p. 123–137.

108. **Johnston FE, and Malina RM.** Age changes in the composition of the upper arm in Philadelphia children. *Human Biology: An International Record of Research* 38: 1–21, 1966.

109. **Jones DW.** Dietary sodium and blood pressure. *Hypertension* 43: 932–935, 2004.

110. **Jung RT, Shetty PS, James WP, Barrand MA, and Callingham BA.** Reduced thermogenesis in obesity. *Nature* 279: 322–323, 1979.

111. **Katch FI.** Assessment of lean body tissues by radiography and bioelectrical impedance. In: *Body-Composition Assessment in Youths and Adults,* edited by Roche AF. Columbus: Ross Laboratories, 1985.

112. **Katch VL, Martin R, and Martin J.** Effects of exercise intensity on food consumption in the male rat. *The American Journal of Clinical Nutrition* 32: 1401–1407, 1979.

113. **Keys A.** *The Biology of Human Starvation.* Minneapolis: The University of Minnesota Press, 1950.

114. **Knittle JL.** Obesity in childhood: a problem in adipose tissue cellular development. *The Journal of Pediatrics* 81: 1048–1059, 1972.

115. **Kopp W.** The atherogenic potential of dietary carbohydrate. *Preventive Medicine* 42: 336–342, 2006.

116. **Krebs NF, Himes JH, Jacobson D, Nicklas TA, Guilday P, and Styne D.** Assessment of child and adolescent overweight and obesity. *Pediatrics* 120: S193–S228, 2007.

117. **Krebs-Smith SM, and Kris-Etherton P.** How does MyPyramid compare to other population-based recommendations for controlling chronic disease? *J Am Diet Assoc* 107: 830–837, 2007.

118. **Kris-Etherton P, Daniels SR, Eckel RH, Engler M, Howard BV, Krauss RM, Lichtenstein AH, Sacks F, St Jeor S, Stampfer M, Eckel RH, Grundy SM, Appel LJ, Byers T, Campos H, Cooney G, Denke MA, Howard BV, Kennedy E, Krauss RM, Kris-Etherton P, Lichtenstein AH, Marckmann P, Pearson TA, Riccardi G, Rudel LL, Rudrum M, Sacks F, Stein DT, Tracy RP, Ursin V, Vogel RA, Zock PL, Bazzarre TL, and Clark J.** Summary of the scientific conference on dietary fatty acids and cardiovascular health: conference summary from the nutrition committee of the American Heart Association. *Circulation* 103: 1034–1039, 2001.

119. **Krotkiewski M, Sjostrom L, Bjorntorp P, Carlgren G, Garellick G, and Smith U.** Adipose tissue cellularity in relation to prognosis for weight reduction. *International Journal of Obesity* 1: 395–416, 1977.

120. **Lane MD, and Cha SH.** Effect of glucose and fructose on food intake via malonyl-CoA signaling in the brain. *Biochemical and Biophysical Research Communications* 382: 1–5, 2009.

121. **Lapidus L, Bengtsson C, Larsson B, Pennert K, Rybo E, and Sjostrom L.** Distribution of adipose tissue and risk of cardiovascular disease and death: a 12 year follow up of participants in the population study of women in Gothenburg, Sweden. *British Medical Journal (Clinical Research Ed)* 289: 1257–1261, 1984.

122. **Larsson B, Svardsudd K, Welin L, Wilhelmsen L, Bjorntorp P, and Tibblin G.** Abdominal adipose tissue distribution, obesity, and risk of cardiovascular disease and death: 13 year follow up of participants in the study of men born in 1913. *British Medical Journal (Clinical Research Ed)* 288: 1401–1404, 1984.

123. **Leibel RL, Hirsch J, Appel BE, and Checani GC.** Energy intake required to maintain body weight is not affected by wide variation in diet composition. *The American Journal of Clinical Nutrition* 55: 350–355, 1992.

124. **Levitsky DA.** Putting behavior back into feeding behavior: a tribute to George Collier. *Appetite* 38: 143–148, 2002.

125. **Lichtman SW, Pisarska K, Berman ER, Pestone M, Dowling H, Offenbacher E, Weisel H, Heshka S, Matthews DE, and Heymsfield SB.** Discrepancy between self-reported and actual caloric intake and exercise in obese subjects. *The New England Journal of Medicine* 327: 1893–1898, 1992.

126. **Lohman T, Houtkooper LB, and Going S.** Body fat meaurement goes high-tech. *ACSM's Health & Fitness Journal* 1: 30–35, 1997.

127. **Lohman TG.** *Advances in Body Composition Assessment.* Champaign: Human Kinetics, 1992.

128. **Lohman TG.** Applicability of body composition techniques and constants for children and youths. In: *Exercise and Sport Sciences Reviews,* edited by Pandolf KB. New York: Macmillan, 1986, p. 325–357.

129. **Lohman TG.** Assessment of body composition in children. *Pediatric Exercise Science* 1: 19–30, 1989.

130. **Lohman TG.** Body composition methodology in sports medicine. *The Physician and Sportsmedicine* 10: 47–58, 1982.

131. **Lohman TG.** Skinfolds and body density and their relation to body fatness: a review. *Human Biology: An International Record of Research* 53: 181–225, 1981.

132. **Lohman TG.** The use of skinfold to estimate body fatness in children and youth. *Journal of the Alliance for Health, Physical Education, Recreation and Dance* 58: 98–102, 1987.

133. **Lohman TG, and Going SB.** Multicomponent models in body composition research: Opportunities and pitfalls. In: *Human Body Composition*, edited by Ellis KJ, and Eastman JD. New York: Plenum Press, 1993, p. 53–58.

134. **Lohman TG, Slaughter MH, Boileau RA, Bunt J, and Lussier L.** Bone mineral measurements and their relation to body density in children, youth and adults. *Human Biology: An International Record of Research* 56: 667–679, 1984.

135. **Mayer J.** Genetic factors in human obesity. *Annals of the New York Academy of Sciences* 131: 412–421, 1965.

136. **Mayer J, Marshall NB, Vitale JJ, Christensen JH, Mashayekhi MB, and Stare FJ.** Exercise, food intake and body weight in normal rats and genetically obese adult mice. *The American Journal of Physiology* 177: 544–548, 1954.

137. **Mayer J, Roy P, and Mitra KP.** Relation between caloric intake, body weight, and physical work: studies in an industrial male population in West Bengal. *The American Journal of Clinical Nutrition* 4: 169–175, 1956.

138. **Mazess RB, Barden HS, Bisek JP, and Hanson J.** Dual-energy x-ray absorptiometry for total-body and regional bone-mineral and soft-tissue composition. *The American Journal of Clinical Nutrition* 51: 1106–1112, 1990.

139. **McTiernan A, Sorensen B, Irwin ML, Morgan A, Yasui Y, Rudolph RE, Surawicz C, Lampe JW, Lampe PD, Ayub K, and Potter JD.** Exercise effect on weight and body fat in men and women. *Obesity* (Silver Spring, Md) 15: 1496–1512, 2007.

140. **Melanson EL, Gozansky WS, Barry DW, MacLean PS, Grunwald GK, and Hill JO.** When energy balance is maintained exercise does not induce negative fat balance in lean sedentary, obese sedentary, or lean enduranced-trainined individuals. *Journal of Applied Physiology* 107: 1847–1856, 2009.

141. **Mertz W, Tsui JC, Judd JT, Reiser S, Hallfrisch J, Morris ER, Steele PD, and Lashley E.** What are people really eating? The relation between energy intake derived from estimated diet records and intake determined to maintain body weight. *The American Journal of Clinical Nutrition* 54: 291–295, 1991.

142. **Metropolitan Life Insurance Company.** New weight standards for men and women. *Statistical Bulletin Metropolitan Life Insurance Company.* 40: 1–4, 1959.

143. **Millard-Stafford ML, Collins MA, Evans EM, Snow TK, Cureton KJ, and Rosskopf LB.** Use of air displacement plethysmography for estimating body fat in a four-component model. *Medicine and Science in Sports and Exercise* 33: 1311–1317, 2001.

144. **Miller WC.** Diet composition, energy intake, and nutritional status in relation to obesity in men and women. *Medicine and Science in Sports and Exercise* 23: 280–284, 1991.

145. **Mole PA.** Impact of energy intake and exercise on resting metabolic rate. *Sports Medicine* (Auckland, NZ) 10: 72–87, 1990.

146. **Morrow JR, Jr., Jackson AS, Bradley PW, and Hartung GH.** Accuracy of measured and predicted residual lung volume on body density measurement. *Medicine and Science in Sports and Exercise* 18: 647–652, 1986.

147. **National Institutes of Health.** Clinical guidelines on the identification, evaluation, and treatment of overweight and obesity in adults. *Obesity Research* 6 (Suppl 2): 1998.

148. **National Research Council.** *Diet and Health.* Washington, D.C.: National Academy Press, 1989.

149. **National Research Council.** *Recommended Dietary Allowances.* Washington, D.C.: National Academy Press, 1989.

150. **Nordmann AJ, Nordmann A, Briel M, Keller U, Yancy WS, Jr., Brehm BJ, and Bucher HC.** Effects of low-carbohydrate vs low-fat diets on weight loss and cardiovascular risk factors: a meta-analysis of randomized controlled trials. *Archives of Internal Medicine* 166: 285–293, 2006.

151. **Ogden CL, Carroll MD, Curtin LR, Lamb MM, and Flegal KM.** Prevalence of high body mass index in US children and adolescents, 2007–2008. *JAMA* 303: 242–249, 2010.

152. **Ogden CL, Carroll MD, Curtin LR, McDowell MA, Tabak CJ, and Flegal KM.** Prevalence of overweight and obesity in the United States, 1999–2004. *JAMA* 295: 1549–1555, 2006.

153. **Ogden CL, Flegal KM, Carroll MD, and Johnson CL.** Prevalence and trends in overweight among US children and adolescents, 1999–2000. *JAMA* 288: 1728–1732, 2002.

154. **Opperman AM, Venter CS, Oosthuizen W, Thompson RL, and Vorster HH.** Meta-analysis of the health effects of using the glycaemic index in meal-planning. *The British Journal of Nutrition* 92: 367–381, 2004.

155. **Oscai LB.** The role of exercise in weight control. In: *Exercise and Sport Sciences Reviews*, edited by Wilmore JH. New York: Academic Press, 1973, p. 103–120.

156. **Oscai LB, Mole PA, and Holloszy JO.** Effects of exercise on cardiac weight and mitochondria in male and female rats. *The American Journal of Physiology* 220: 1944–1948, 1971.

157. **Oscai LB, Spirakis CN, Wolff CA, and Beck RJ.** Effects of exercise and of food restriction on adipose tissue cellularity. *Journal of Lipid Research* 13: 588–592, 1972.

158. **Passmore R.** Energy metabolism at various weights: man. part II. resting: adults. In: *Metabolism: Clinical and Experimental*, edited by Altman PL, and Dittmer DS. Bethesda: Federation of American Societies for Experimental Biology, 1968, p. 344–345.

159. **Pietrobelli A, Heymsfield SB, Wang ZM, and Gallagher D.** Multi-component body composition models: recent advances and future directions. *European Journal of Clinical Nutrition* 55: 69–75, 2001.

160. **Pillitteri JL, Shiffman S, Rohay JM, Harkins AM, Burton SL, and Wadden TA.** Use of dietary supplements for weight loss in the United States: results of a national survey. *Obesity* (Silver Spring, Md) 16: 790–796, 2008.

161. **Pittas AG, Roberts SB, Das SK, Gilhooly CH, Saltzman E, Golden J, Stark PC, and Greenberg AS.** The effects of the dietary glycemic load on type 2 diabetes risk factors during weight loss. *Obesity* (Silver Spring, Md) 14: 2200–2209, 2006.

162. **Pittler MH, and Ernst E.** Dietary supplements for body-weight reduction: a systematic review. *American Journal of Clinical Nutrition* 79: 529–536, 2004.

163. **Poehlman ET.** A review: exercise and its influence on resting energy metabolism in man. *Medicine and Science in Sports and Exercise* 21: 515–525, 1989.

164. **Poehlman ET, Melby CL, and Goran MI.** The impact of exercise and diet restriction on daily energy expenditure. *Sports Medicine* (Auckland, NZ) 11: 78–101, 1991.

165. **Pollock ML, and Wilmore JH.** *Exercise in Health and Disease.* Philadelphia: W. B. Saunders, 1990.

166. **Presta E, Casullo AM, Costa R, Slonim A, and Van Itallie TB.** Body composition in adolescents: estimation by total body electrical conductivity. *J Appl Physiol* 63: 937–941, 1987.

167. **Qi L, and Hu FB.** Dietary glycemic load, whole grains, and systemic inflammation in diabetes: the epidemiological evidence. *Current Opinion in Lipidology* 18: 3–8, 2007.

168. **Qiao Q, and Nyamdorj R.** Is the association of type II diabetes with waist circumference or waist:hip ratio stronger than that with body mass index? *European Journal of Clinical Nutrition* 64: 3–34, 2010.

169. **Rabkin SW, Mathewson FA, and Hsu PH.** Relation of body weight to development of ischemic heart disease in a cohort of young North American men after a 26 year observation period: the Manitoba Study. *The American Journal of Cardiology* 39: 452–458, 1977.

170. **Ratamess N.** Body composition status and assessment. In: *ACSM's Resource Manual for Guidelines for Exercise Testing and Prescription,* edited by Ehrman JK. Baltimore: Lippincott Williams & Wilkins, 2010, p. 264–281.

171. **Redman LM, Heilbronn LK, Martin CK, Alfonso A, Smith SR, and Ravussin E.** Effect of calorie restriction with or without exercise on body composition and fat distribution. *The Journal of Clinical Endocrinology and Metabolism* 92: 865–872, 2007.

172. **Rimm AA, and P. L. White.** Obesity: its risks and hazards. In *Obesity in America,* edited by U.S. Department of Health EaWNIH Publication No. 79–359, 1979.

173. **Rising R, Harper IT, Fontvielle AM, Ferraro RT, Spraul M, and Ravussin E.** Determinants of total daily energy expenditure: variability in physical activity. *The American Journal of Clinical Nutrition* 59: 800–804, 1994.

174. **Robinson JR, and Niswender KD.** What are the risks and benefits of current and emerging weight-loss medications? *Current Diabetes Reports* 9: 368–375, 2009.

175. **Rolls BJ.** Carbohydrates, fats, and satiety. *American Journal of Clinical Nutrition* Suppl. 61: 960S–967S, 1995.

176. **Romijn JA, Coyle EF, Sidossis LS, Gastaldelli A, Horowitz JF, Endert E, and Wolfe RR.** Regulation of endogenous fat and carbohydrate metabolism in relation to exercise intensity and duration. *The American Journal of Physiology* 265: E380–391, 1993.

177. **Ross R, Dagnone D, Jones PJ, Smith H, Paddags A, Hudson R, and Janssen I.** Reduction in obesity and related comorbid conditions after diet-induced weight loss or exercise-induced weight loss in men: randomized, controlled trial. *Ann Intern Med* 133: 92–103, 2000.

178. **Ross R, Freeman JA, and Janssen I.** Exercise alone is an effective strategy for reducing obesity and related comorbidities. *Exercise and Sport Sciences Reviews* 28: 165–170, 2000.

179. **Ross R, and Rissanen J.** Mobilization of visceral and subcutaneous adipose tissue in response to energy restriction and exercise. *The American Journal of Clinical Nutrition* 60: 695–703, 1994.

180. **Roust LR, Hammel KD, and Jensen MD.** Effects of isoenergetic, low-fat diets on energy metabolism in lean and obese women. *The American Journal of Clinical Nutrition* 60: 470–475, 1994.

181. **Sacks FM, Bray GA, Carey VJ, Smith SR, Ryan DH, Anton SD, McManus K, Champagne CM, Laranjo LMB, Leboff MS, Rood JC, de Jonge L, Greenway FL, Loria CM, Obarzanek E, and Williamson DA.** Comparison of weight-loss diets with different compositions of fat, protein and carbohydrates. *New England Journal of Medicine* 360: 859–873, 2009.

182. **Schoeller D.** Measurement of total body water: isotope dilution techniques. In: *Body-Composition Assessment in Youths and Adults,* edited by Roche AF. Columbus: Ross Laboratories, 1985, p. 24–29.

183. **Schoeller DA, and Buchholz AC.** Energetics of obesity and weight control: does diet composition matter? *J Am Diet Assoc* 105: S24–28, 2005.

184. **Schulz LO, and Schoeller DA.** A compilation of total daily energy expenditures and body weights in healthy adults. *The American Journal of Clinical Nutrition* 60: 676–681, 1994.

185. **Schutte JE, Townsend EJ, Hugg J, Shoup RF, Malina RM, and Blomqvist CG.** Density of lean body mass is greater in blacks than in whites. *J Appl Physiol* 56: 1647–1649, 1984.

186. **Segal KR, Burastero S, Chun A, Coronel P, Pierson RN, Jr., and Wang J.** Estimation of extracellular and total body water by multiple-frequency bioelectrical-impedance measurement. *The American Journal of Clinical Nutrition* 54: 26–29, 1991.

187. **Segal KR, Edano A, Blando L, and Pi-Sunyer FX.** Comparison of thermic effects of constant and relative caloric loads in lean and obese men. *The American Journal of Clinical Nutrition* 51: 14–21, 1990.

188. **Segal KR, Gutin B, Presta E, Wang J, and Van Itallie TB.** Estimation of human body composition by electrical impedance methods: a comparative study. *J Appl Physiol* 58: 1565–1571, 1985.

189. **Segal MS, Gollub E, and Johnson RJ.** Is the fructose index more relevant with regards to cardiovascular disease than the glycemic index? *European Journal of Nutrition* 46: 406–417, 2007.

190. **Seidell JC.** Waist circumference and waist/hip ratio in relation to all-cause mortality, cancer and sleep apnea. *European Journal of Clinical Nutrition* 64: 35–41, 2010.

191. **Services US Department of Health and Human Services.** DASH Eating Plan. Washington, D.C.: Author, 2006.

192. **Sharkey B.** *The Physiology of Fitness.* Champaign: Human Kinetics, 1984.

193. **Sheard NF, Clark NG, Brand-Miller JC, Franz MJ, Pi-Sunyer FX, Mayer-Davis E, Kulkarni K, and Geil P.** Dietary carbohydrate (amount and type) in the prevention and management of diabetes: a statement by the American Diabetes Association. *Diabetes Care* 27: 2266–2271, 2004.

194. **Sims EA, Danforth E, Jr., Horton ES, Bray GA, Glennon JA, and Salans LB.** Endocrine and metabolic effects of experimental obesity in man. *Recent Progress in Hormone Research* 29: 457–496, 1973.

195. **Sinning WE, Dolny DG, Little KD, Cunningham LN, Racaniello A, Siconolfi SF, and Sholes JL.** Validity of "generalized" equations for body composition analysis in male athletes. *Medicine and Science in Sports and Exercise* 17: 124–130, 1985.

196. **Sinning WE, and Wilson JR.** Validity of "generalized" equations for body composition analysis in women athletes. *Research Quarterly for Exercise Sport* 55: 153–160, 1984.

197. **Siri WE.** Body composition from fluid spaces and density: analysis of methods. In: *Techniques for Measuring Body Composition*, edited by Brozek J, and Henschel A. Washington, D.C.: National Academy of Sciences, 1961, p. 223–244.

198. **Siri WE.** Fat cells and body weight. In: *Obesity*, edited by Strunkard, JA. Philadelphia: W. B. Saunders, 1980, p. 72–100.

199. **Sjöström L, and Björntrop P.** Body composition and adipose tissue cellularity in human obesity. *Acta Media Scandinavica* 195: 201–211, 1974.

200. **Sjöström LV.** Morbidity of severely obese subjects. *The American Journal of Clinical Nutrition* 55: 508S–515S, 1992.

201. **Sjöström LV.** Mortality of severely obese subjects. *The American Journal of Clinical Nutrition* 55: 516S–523S, 1992.

202. **Slaughter MH, Lohman TG, Boileau RA, Horswill CA, Stillman RJ, Van Loan MD, and Bemben DA.** Skinfold equations for estimation of body fatness in children and youth. *Human Biology: An International Record of Research* 60: 709–723, 1988.

203. **Slentz CA, Duscha BD, Johnson JL, Ketchum K, Aiken LB, Samsa GP, Houmard JA, Bales CW, and Kraus WE.** Effects of the amount of exercise on body weight, body composition, and measures of central obesity: STRRIDE—a randomized controlled study. *Archives of Internal Medicine* 164: 31–39, 2004.

204. **Stefanick ML.** Exercise and weight control. *Exercise and Sport Sciences Reviews* 21: 363–396, 1993.

205. **Stevens J, Katz EG, and Huxley RR.** Associations between gender, age and waist circumference. *European Journal of Clinical Nutrition* 64: 6–15, 2010.

206. **Stiegler P, and Cunliffe A.** The role of diet and exercise for the maintenance of fat-free mass and resting metabolic rate during weight loss. *Sports Medicine (Auckland, NZ)* 36: 239-262, 2006.

207. **Stunkard AJ, Sorensen TI, Hanis C, Teasdale TW, Chakraborty R, Schull WJ, and Schulsinger F.** An adoption study of human obesity. *The New England Journal of Medicine* 314: 193–198, 1986.

208. **Swinburn B, and Ravussin E.** Energy balance or fat balance? *The American Journal of Clinical Nutrition* 57: 766S–770S; discussion 770S–771S, 1993.

209. **Tataranni PA, Larson DE, Snitker S, and Ravussin E.** Thermic effect of food in humans: methods and results from use of a respiratory chamber. *The American Journal of Clinical Nutrition* 61: 1013–1019, 1995.

210. **Thomas CD, Peters JC, Reed GW, Abumrad NN, Sun M, and Hill JO.** Nutrient balance and energy expenditure during ad libitum feeding of high-fat and high-carbohydrate diets in humans. *The American Journal of Clinical Nutrition* 55: 934–942, 1992.

211. **Thomas JG, Bond DS, Hill JO, and Wing RR.** The national weight control registry. *ACSM's Health & Fitness Journal* 15: 8–12, 2011.

212. **Thompson CA, and Thompson PA.** Healthy lifestyle and cancer prevention. *ACSM's Health & Fitness Journal* 12: 18–26, 2008.

213. **Thompson DL, Rakow J, and Perdue SM.** Relationship between accumulated walking and body composition in middle-aged women. *Medicine and Science in Sports and Exercise* 36: 911–914, 2004.

214. **Titchenal CA.** Exercise and food intake:what is the relationship? *Sports Medicine* (Auckland, NZ) 6: 135–145, 1988.

215. **Tremblay A.** Dietary fat and body weight set point. *Nutrition Reviews* 62: S75–77, 2004.

216. **Tremblay A, Seale J, Almeras N, Conway J, and Moe P.** Energy requirements of a post obese man reporting a low energy intake at weight maintenance. *The American Journal of Clinical Nutrition* 54: 506–508, 1991.

217. **Tremblay A, Simoneau JA, and Bouchard C.** Impact of exercise intensity on body fatness and skeletal muscle metabolism. *Metabolism: Clinical and Experimental* 43: 814–818, 1994.

218. **Treuth MS, Hunter GR, Weinsier RL, and Kell SH.** Energy expenditure and substrate utilization in older women after strength training: 24-h calorimeter results. *J Appl Physiol* 78: 2140–2146, 1995.

219. **U.S. Department of Agriculture.** *Dietary Guidelines for Americans.* Washington, D.C.: Author, 2005.

220. **U.S. Department of Agriculture.** *Dietary Guidelines for Americans.* Washington, D.C.: Author, 2010.

221. **U.S. Department of Health and Human Services.** *2008 Physical Activity Guidelines for Americans.* Washington, D.C.: Author, 2008.

222. **U.S. Senate Select Committee on Nutrition and Human Needs.** *Eating in America: Dietary Goals for the U.S.* Washington, D.C.: U.S. Government Printing Office, 1977.

223. **Van Etten LM, Westerterp KR, and Verstappen FT.** Effect of weight-training on energy expenditure and substrate utilization during sleep. *Medicine and Science in Sports and Exercise* 27: 188–193, 1995.

224. **Van Itallie T.** Clinical assessment of body fat content in adults: potential role of electrical impedance methods. In: *Body-Composition Assessment in Youths and Adults*, edited by Roche AF. Columbus: Ross Laboratories, 1985, p. 5–8.

225. **Van Itallie TB.** Conservative approaches to treatment. In: *Obesity in America*, edited by Bray G. Department of Health, Education, and Welfare. NIH Publication No. 79–359, 1979.

226. **Van Loan MD, Keim NL, Berg K, and Mayclin PL.** Evaluation of body composition by dual energy x-ray absorptiometry and two different software packages. *Medicine and Science in Sports and Exercise* 27: 587–591, 1995.

227. **Van Marken Lichtenbelt WD, et al.** Validation of bio-electrical-impedance measurements as a method to estimate body-water compartments. *American Journal of Clinical Nutrition* 60: 159–166, 1994.

228. **Vasselli JR, Cleary MP, and Van Itallie TB.** Obesity. In: *Nutrition Reviews' Present Knowledge in Nutrition.* Washington, D.C.: The Nutrition Foundation, 1984, p. 35–36.

229. **Wabitsch M, Hauner H, Heinze E, Muche R, Bockmann A, Parthon W, Mayer H, and Teller W.** Body-fat distribution and changes in the atherogenic risk-factor profile in obese adolescent girls during weight reduction. *The American Journal of Clinical Nutrition* 60: 54–60, 1994.

230. **Wadden TA, and Stunkard AJ.** Social and psychological consequences of obesity. *Ann Intern Med* 103: 1062–1067, 1985.

231. **Wagner DR, and Heyward VH.** Techniques of body composition assessment: a review of laboratory and field methods. *Research Quarterly for Exercise and Sport* 70: 135–149, 1999.

232. **Ward A, Pollock ML, Jackson AS, Ayres JJ, and Pape G.** A comparison of body fat determined by underwater weighing and volume displacement. *The American Journal of Physiology* 234: E94–96, 1978.

233. **Wardlaw GM, and Smith AM.** *Contemporary Nutrition.* New York: McGraw-Hill, 2011.

234. **Weinberger MH.** Sodium and blood pressure 2003. *Current Opinion in Cardiology* 19: 353–356, 2004.

235. **Weinsier RL, Schutz Y, and Bracco D.** Reexamination of the relationship of resting metabolic rate to fat-free mass and to the metabolically active components of fat-free mass in humans. *The American Journal of Clinical Nutrition* 55: 790–794, 1992.

236. **Willett WC, Stampfer M, Manson J, and VanItallie T.** New weight guidelines for Americans: justified or injudicious? *The American Journal of Clinical Nutrition* 53: 1102–1103, 1991.

237. **Willett WC, Stampfer M, Manson J, and VanItallie T.** Reply to G. A. Bray and R. L. Atlinson. *American Journal of Clinical Nutrition* 55: 482–483, 1992.

238. **Williams MH.** *Nutrition for Health, Fitness, & Sport.* New York: McGraw-Hill, 2010.

239. **Wilmore JH.** Body composition in sport and exercise: directions for future research. *Medicine and Science in Sports and Exercise* 15: 21–31, 1983.

240. **Wright J.** Dietary intake of ten key nutrients for public health, United States: 1999–2000. Advance data from vital and health statistics. No. 334. National Center for Health Statistics, 2003.

241. **Zurlo F, Lillioja S, Esposito-Del Puente A, Nyomba BL, Raz I, Saad MF, Swinburn BA, Knowler WC, Bogardus C, and Ravussin E.** Low ratio of fat to carbohydrate oxidation as predictor of weight gain: study of 24-h RQ. *The American Journal of Physiology* 259: E650–657, 1990.

Physiology of Performance

19

Factors Affecting Performance

■ Objectives

By studying this chapter, you should be able to do the following:

1. Identify factors affecting maximal performance.
2. Provide evidence for and against the central nervous system being a site of fatigue.
3. Identify potential neural factors in the periphery that may be linked to fatigue.
4. Explain the role of cross-bridge cycling in fatigue.
5. Summarize the evidence on the order of recruitment of muscle fibers with increasing intensities of activity, and the type of metabolism upon which each is dependent.
6. Describe the factors limiting performance in all-out activities lasting less than 10 seconds.
7. Describe the factors limiting performance in all-out activities lasting 10 to 180 seconds.
8. Discuss the subtle changes in the factors affecting optimal performance as the duration of a maximal performance increases from 3 minutes to 4 hours.

■ Key Terms

central fatigue
peripheral fatigue
free radicals

In the last few chapters we have focused on proper exercise and nutrition for health and fitness. The emphasis was on *moderation* in both to reduce the risk factors associated with a variety of diseases. We must now change that focus to discuss the factors limiting physical performance.

Performance goals require much more time, effort, and risk of injury than fitness goals. What are the requirements for optimal performance? To answer this question we must ask another: What kind of performance? It is clear that the requirements for the best performance in the 400-meter run are different from those associated with the marathon. Figure 19.1 shows a diagram of factors influencing performance (5). Every performance requires a certain amount of strength, as well as the "skill" to apply that strength in the best way. Further, energy must be supplied in the manner needed or performance will suffer. Different activities require differing amounts of energy from aerobic and anaerobic processes. Both the environment (altitude and heat) and diet (carbohydrate and water intake) play a role in endurance performance. In addition, best performances require a psychological commitment to "go for the gold." The purpose of this chapter is to expand on this diagram and discuss the factors limiting performance in a variety of activities, which will point the way to the remaining chapters. However, before we discuss these factors, we will summarize the potential sites of fatigue that would clearly affect performance.

SITES OF FATIGUE

Fatigue is simply defined as an inability to maintain a power output or force during repeated muscle contractions (23). As the two examples of the 400-meter run and the marathon suggest, the causes of fatigue vary and are usually specific to the type of physical activity. Figure 19.2 provides a summary of potential sites of fatigue (23). The discussion of mechanisms starts at the brain, where a variety of factors can influence the "will to win," and continues to the cross-bridges of the muscles themselves. There is evidence to support many of the sites listed in figure 19.2 as "weak links" in the development of the muscle tension needed for optimal performance. However, there is far from perfect agreement among scientists about the exact causes of fatigue. The reasons for this include (a) the fiber type and training state of the subject, (b) whether the muscle was stimulated voluntarily or electrically, (c) the use of both amphibian and mammalian muscle preparations, with some isolated from the body, and (d) the intensity and duration of the exercise, and whether it was continuous or intermittent activity (54, 55). Table 19.1 provides a summary of the advantages and disadvantages of the various approaches scientists use to study fatigue (1). Clearly, depending on the nature of the exercise, the subject, and the experimental approach used to study fatigue, different results may be obtained. Within the scope of these limitations, we now provide a summary of the evidence about each weak link and apply the information to specific types of performances.

Central Fatigue

The central nervous system (CNS) would be implicated in fatigue if there were (a) a reduction in the number of functioning motor units involved in the activity or (b) a reduction in motor unit firing frequency (18). There is evidence both for and against the concept of "**central fatigue**"—that is, that fatigue originates in the CNS.

Figure 19.1 Factors affecting performance.

Possible Fatigue Mechanisms

"Psyche"/brain

Impaired:

Motivation (arousal)
(i.e., motor unit recruitment)

Spinal cord

Reflex drive

Peripheral
nerve

Neuromuscular transmission

Muscle
sarcolemma

Muscle action potential

Transverse
tubular
system

K^+, Na^+

Excitation

Ca^{++}
release

Activation
Energy supply

Actin-
myosin
interaction

Cross-bridge
tension + heat

Force/power
output

Figure 19.2 Possible sites of fatigue.

Merton's classic experiments showed no difference in tension development when a *voluntary* maximal contraction was compared to an *electrically induced* maximal contraction. When the muscle was fatigued by voluntary contractions, electrical stimulation could not restore tension (41). This suggested that the CNS was not limiting performance, and that the "periphery" was the site of fatigue.

In contrast, the early work of Ikai and Steinhaus (27) showed that a simple shout during exertion could increase what was formerly believed to be "maximal" strength. Later work showed that electrical stimulation of a muscle fatigued by voluntary contractions resulted in an increase in tension development (28).

These studies suggest that the upper limit of voluntary strength is "psychologically" set, given that certain motivational or arousal factors are needed to achieve a physiological limit (28). In agreement with these results (that the CNS can limit performance) are two studies by Asmussen and Mazin (5, 6). Their subjects lifted weights 30 times a minute, causing fatigue in 2 to 3 minutes. Following a 2-minute pause, the lifting continued. These investigators showed that when either a physical diversion, consisting of the contraction of nonfatigued muscles, or a mental diversion, consisting of doing mental arithmetic, was used between fatiguing bouts of exercise, work output was greater than when nothing was done during the pause. They also found that if a person did a series of muscle contractions to the point of fatigue with the eyes closed, simply opening the eyes restored tension (5). These studies suggest that alterations in central nervous system "arousal" can facilitate motor unit recruitment to increase strength and alter the state of fatigue.

Excessive endurance training (overtraining) has been associated with symptoms such as reduced performance capacity, prolonged fatigue, altered mood states, sleep disturbance, loss of appetite, and increased anxiety (16, 60, 61). Over the past decade, a considerable amount of attention has been directed at brain serotonin (5-hydroxytryptamine) as a factor in fatigue due to its links to depression, sleepiness, and mood (60, 61). There is evidence that increases and decreases in brain serotonin activity during prolonged exercise hasten and delay fatigue, respectively (15). Although regular, moderate exercise has been shown to improve the mood states of depressive patients, excessive exercise seems to have an opposite effect. Numerous experiments have been conducted over the past decade to try to understand the connection between serotonin and fatigue, but the answer remains elusive (60, 61). However, recent studies indicate that it is not the serotonin alone, but the ratio of serotonin to dopamine that contributes to tiredness on the one hand and arousal on the other, and that brain levels of norepinephrine also contribute to the picture (39, 40).

The CNS is intimately involved in exercise, including the psyching-up prior to exercise (63), the recruitment of motor units, and the continual feedback from a host of receptors sensing tension, temperature, blood gases, blood pressure, and other variables. The brain integrates these various signals and generates commands that automatically reduce power output to protect the organism. In this sense, exercise begins and ends in the brain (30). Noakes and others (32, 46–48, 58) have developed the "central governor" model of central fatigue that focuses primarily on the conscious and subconscious brain and does not involve the spinal cord or motor unit. This model has many novel aspects, but it has attracted some

Muscle in vivo	Advantages	All physiological mechanisms present
		Fatigue can be central or peripheral
		All types of fatigue can be studied
		Stimulation patterns appropriate for fiber types and stage of fatigue
	Disadvantages	Mixture of fiber types
		Complex activation patterns
		Produces correlative data; hard to identify mechanisms
		Experimental interventions very limited
Isolated muscle	Advantages	Central fatigue eliminated
		Dissection simple
	Disadvantages	Mixture of fiber types
		Inevitable extracellular gradients of O_2, CO_2, K^+, lactic acid
		Mechanisms of fatigue biased by presence of extracellular gradients
		Drugs cannot be applied rapidly because of diffusion gradients
Isolated single fiber	Advantages	Only one fiber type present
		Force and other changes (ionic, metabolic) can be unequivocally correlated
		Fluorescent measurements of ions, metabolites, membrane potential, etc. possible
		Easy and rapid application of extracellular drugs, ions, metabolites, etc.
	Disadvantages	Dissection difficult
		Environment different to in vivo
		K^+ accumulation and other in vivo changes absent
		Prone to damage at physiological temperatures
		Small size makes analysis of metabolites difficult
Skinned fiber	Advantages	Precise solutions can be applied
		Possible to study myofibrillar properties, SR release and uptake, AP/Ca^{2+} release coupling
		Metabolic and ionic changes associated with fatigue can be studied in isolation
	Disadvantages	Relevance to fatigue can be questionable
		May lose important intracellular constituents
		Relevant metabolites to study must be identified in other systems

criticism (66). Let us now look at some of the events outside the CNS that are tied to the fatigue process.

Peripheral Fatigue

Although evidence exists both for and against the CNS being a site of fatigue, the vast majority of evidence points to the periphery (**peripheral fatigue**), where neural, mechanical, or energetic events can hamper tension development (19, 67).

Neural Factors If you are looking for potential sites of fatigue, you might track the movement of the action potential from the nerve to the muscle, and within the muscle, its progress along the sarcolemma and t-tubule to the sarcoplasmic reticulum (SR) where Ca^{++} is stored. When the Ca^{++} is released it interacts with regulatory proteins (e.g., troponin) that causes movement of the cross-bridges to generate tension. Finally, the Ca^{++} must be pumped back into the SR to allow the muscle to relax before the next contraction. Let's take a look at the evidence to see if any of these sites is implicated in the fatigue process.

Neuromuscular Junction The action potential appears to reach the neuromuscular junction even when fatigue occurs (41). In addition, evidence based on simultaneous measurements of electrical activity at the neuromuscular junction and in the individual muscle fibers suggests that the neuromuscular junction is not the site of fatigue (10).

Sarcolemma and Transverse Tubules It has been hypothesized that the sarcolemma might be the site of fatigue due to its inability to maintain Na^+ and K^+ concentrations during repeated stimulation. When the Na^+/K^+ pump cannot keep up, K^+ accumulates outside the membrane and decreases inside the cell. This results in a depolarization of the cell and a reduction in action potential amplitude (56). The gradual depolarization of the sarcolemma could result in altered t-tubule function, including a block of the t-tubule action potential. If the latter occurs, Ca^{++} release from the SR will be affected, as will muscle contraction (3). However, the evidence indicates that the typical reduction in the size of the action potential amplitude has little effect on force output by the muscle. In addition, the lower frequency of action potential firing with repeated stimulation of muscle seems to protect the muscle from further fatigue (rather than cause fatigue) by shifting the activation to a lower, more optimal, rate of firing (19). This does not mean that the t-tubule is not involved in the fatigue process. Under certain stimulation conditions an action potential block can occur in the t-tubule, leading to a reduction in Ca^{++} release from the SR (19, 24). As a result, myosin cross-bridge activation would be adversely affected. One of the beneficial effects of training is an increase in the capacity of the Na^+/K^+ pump, which may contribute to the maintenance of the Na^+/K^+ gradient and reduce the potential for fatigue via this mechanism (24).

IN SUMMARY

- Increases in CNS arousal facilitate motor unit recruitment to increase strength and alter the state of fatigue.
- Repeated stimulation of the sarcolemma can result in a reduction in the size and frequency of action potentials; however, shifts in the optimal frequency needed for muscle activation preserve force output.
- Under certain conditions, an action potential block can occur in the t-tubule to result in a reduction in Ca^{++} release from the SR.

Mechanical Factors The primary mechanical factor that may be related to fatigue is cross-bridge "cycling." The action of the cross-bridge depends on (a) the functional arrangement of actin and myosin, (b) Ca^{++} being available to bind with troponin to allow the cross-bridge to bind with the active site on actin, and (c) ATP, which is needed for both the activation of the cross-bridge to cause movement, and the dissociation of the cross-bridge from actin. Exercise, especially eccentric exercise, can cause a physical disruption of the sarcomere and reduce the capacity of the muscle to produce tension (4). However, a high H^+ concentration, which generally occurs with heavy exercise, may contribute to fatigue in a variety of ways (19, 20, 22, 54, 55):

- reduce the force per cross-bridge,
- reduce the force generated at a given Ca^{++} concentration (related to H^+ ion interference with Ca^{++} binding to troponin), and
- inhibit SR Ca^+ release.

Consistent with this, data from skinned muscle fibers studied at room temperature ($\sim$20 °C) showed that an increase in the H^+ concentration was linked to a decrease in force and the maximal velocity of shortening. However, when experiments in both skinned and intact muscle fibers were done at 30 °C (a more physiological temperature), the acidosis decreased force by only 10% and did not accelerate the rate of fatigue. The latter results are consistent with data from exercising humans in which force recovered before the H^+ concentration did (50).

One sign of fatigue in isometric contractions is a longer "relaxation time"—the time from peak tension development to baseline tension. This appears to be an important aspect of fatigue in fast-twitch fibers. This longer relaxation time could be due to a slowing of the SR's ability to pump Ca^{++} and/or to slowing of cross-bridge cycling, but the latter appears to be most important (50). This longer relaxation time would result in a reduction in stride rate, a feature of fatigue in 400-m races (50). Although H^+ is implicated in this longer relaxation time, the accumulation of inorganic phosphate (P_i) from the breakdown of ATP is also involved. That is where we will now turn our attention.

IN SUMMARY

- The cross-bridge's ability to "cycle" is important in continued tension development. Fatigue may be related, in part, to the effect of a high H^+ concentration and the inability of the sarcoplasmic reticulum to rapidly take up Ca^{++}. The end result may be a longer relaxation time, which affects the rate of muscle contraction.

Energetics of Contraction Fatigue can be viewed as the result of a simple imbalance between the ATP requirements of a muscle and its ATP-generating capacity (55). As described in chapter 3, when exercise begins and the need for ATP accelerates, a series of ATP-generating reactions occur to replenish the ATP.

- As the cross-bridges use ATP and generate ADP, phosphocreatine provides for the immediate resynthesis of the ATP ($PC + ADP \rightarrow ATP + C$).
- As the phosphocreatine becomes depleted, ADP begins to accumulate and the myokinase reaction occurs to generate ATP ($ADP + ADP \rightarrow ATP + AMP$).
- The accumulation of all these products stimulates glycolysis to generate additional ATP, which may result in an H^+ accumulation (7).

A CLOSER LOOK 19.1

Radical Production During Exercise Contributes to Muscle Fatigue

Free radicals (radicals) are highly reactive molecules that contain an unpaired electron in their outer orbital. This unpaired electron results in molecular instability; therefore, radicals are highly reactive and capable of damaging proteins, lipids, and DNA in the cell (25). Radical-mediated damage to cellular constituents is called oxidative stress, and high levels of oxidative stress can lead to cellular damage and dysfunction.

Interestingly, although regular exercise provides many health benefits, exercise promotes the production of radicals in skeletal muscles and prolonged and/or intense exercise can lead to oxidative stress in the exercising muscle. Importantly, this exercise-induced oxidative damage is a key contributor to muscle fatigue during prolonged exercise (i.e., >30 minutes' duration) (33, 34, 38).

The mechanism(s) to explain why radicals promote muscle fatigue remains an active topic of research. Current evidence indicates that radical production can contribute to muscle fatigue in at least two important ways. First, radicals can damage key contractile proteins including myosin and troponin (11). Damage to these muscle proteins reduces the calcium sensitivity of myofilaments and limits the number of myosin cross-bridges in the strong binding state (57). It follows that when fewer myosin cross-bridges are bound to actin, muscle force production is reduced (i.e., fatigue occurs). A second mechanism to explain how radicals may contribute to muscle fatigue is that high radical production can depress sodium/potassium pump activity in skeletal muscle (34). Impaired sodium/potassium pump function results in disturbances in muscle potassium levels, and this disruption in potassium homeostasis has been linked to muscle fatigue during exercise (34).

Because radicals contribute to muscle fatigue, it is feasible that antioxidant supplementation can retard exercise-induced muscle fatigue. To date, studies using antioxidant vitamins (e.g., vitamins E and C) do not support the concept that dietary antioxidants can improve human performance (51). Nonetheless, experiments using the powerful antioxidant N-acetyl-cysteine reveal that this unique antioxidant can delay fatigue during prolonged submaximal exercise (34, 37). Although optimal levels of antioxidants can postpone fatigue, high doses of antioxidants (i.e., above the optimal dose) can impair muscle performance (12). Therefore, indiscriminant antioxidant supplementation could be detrimental to athletic performance.

However, as ATP demand continues to exceed supply, a variety of reactions occur in the cell that limit work and protect the cell from damage. Remember that ATP is needed to pump ions and maintain cell structure. In this sense, fatigue serves a protective function. What are the signals to the muscle cell that energy utilization must slow down? When ATP-generating mechanisms cannot keep up with ATP use, inorganic phosphate (P_i) begins to accumulate in the cell (P_i and ADP are not being converted to ATP). An increase in P_i in the muscle has been shown to inhibit maximal force, and the higher the P_i concentration, the lower the force measured during recovery from fatigue. The P_i seems to act directly on the cross-bridges to reduce its binding to actin (19, 20, 36, 50, 65) and also inhibits calcium release from the sarcoplasmic reticulum (2, 17, 50). However, the accumulation of P_i reduces the total ATP cost per unit of force, suggesting an improvement in efficiency (45). What is interesting is that the cell does not run out of ATP, even in cases of extreme fatigue. Typically, the ATP concentration falls to only 70% of its pre-exercise level. The factors that cause fatigue reduce the rate of ATP utilization faster than ATP generation so that ATP concentration is maintained. This is believed to be a protective function aimed at minimizing changes in cellular homeostasis with continued stimulation. See Fitts in the Suggested Readings for an excellent review of this topic. Other novel factors may be related to fatigue (see A Closer Look 19.1).

IN SUMMARY

- Fatigue is directly associated with a mismatch between the rate at which the muscle uses ATP and the rate at which ATP can be supplied.
- Cellular fatigue mechanisms slow down the rate of ATP utilization faster than the rate of ATP generation to preserve the ATP concentration and cellular homeostasis.

In chapter 8 we linked the different methods of ATP production to the different muscle fiber types that are recruited during activity. We will briefly summarize this information as it relates to our discussion of fatigue. Figure 19.3 shows the pattern of recruitment of muscle fiber types with increasing intensities of exercise. Up to about 40% of $\dot{V}O_2$ max, the type I slow-twitch oxidative muscle fiber is recruited to provide tension development (55). This fiber type is dependent on a continuous supply of blood to provide the oxygen needed for the generation of ATP from carbohydrates and fats. Any factor limiting the

Figure 19.3 Order of muscle fiber type recruitment in exercise of increasing intensity. From D. G. Sale, "Influence of Exercise and Training in Motor Unit Activation" in Kent B. Pandolf, ed., *Exercise and Sport Sciences Reviews*, vol. 15. Copyright © 1987 McGraw-Hill, Inc., New York. Reprinted by permission.

oxygen supply to this fiber type (e.g., altitude, dehydration, blood loss, or anemia) would cause a reduction in tension development in these fibers and necessitate the recruitment of type IIa fibers to generate tension.

Between 40% and 75% $\dot{V}O_2$ max type IIa fast-twitch, fatigue-resistant fibers are recruited, in addition to the type I fibers (55). These fast-twitch fibers are rich in mitochondria, as are the type I fibers, making them dependent on oxygen delivery for tension development. They also have a great capacity to produce ATP via anaerobic glycolysis. The mitochondrial content of type IIa fibers is sensitive to endurance training, so that with detraining, more of the ATP supply would be provided by glycolysis, leading to lactate production (see chapter 13). If oxygen delivery to this fiber type is decreased, or the ability of the fiber to use oxygen is decreased (due to low mitochondrial number), tension development will fall, requiring type IIx fiber recruitment to maintain tension.

Type IIx is the fast-twitch muscle fiber with a low mitochondrial content. This fiber can generate great tension via anaerobic sources of energy, but it fatigues quickly. It is recruited at about 75% $\dot{V}O_2$ max, adding to the tension from type I and type IIa fibers and making heavy exercise dependent upon its ability to develop tension (56).

Although the primary focus of this text has been on the fitness and performance of individuals stuck (by gravity) on the earth, we are all familiar with the weakness and instability of astronauts as they emerge from the space shuttle after returning from space. With the

space station now in orbit and crews rotating on a regular basis, it should be no surprise that physiologists have been studying the impact of prolonged weightlessness on muscle function (21). Ask the Expert 19.1 provides some insights into why astronauts are weaker when they return to earth.

IN SUMMARY

■ Muscle fibers are recruited in the following order with increasing intensities of exercise: type I → type IIa → type IIx.
■ The progression moves from the most to the least oxidative muscle fiber type. Intense exercise (>75% $\dot{V}O_2$ max) demands that type IIx fibers (in addition to the type I and type IIa fibers) be recruited, resulting in an increase in H^+ production.

FACTORS LIMITING ALL-OUT ANAEROBIC PERFORMANCES

As exercise intensity increases, muscle fiber recruitment progresses from type I → type IIa → type IIx. This means that the ATP supply needed for tension development becomes more and more dependent upon anaerobic metabolism (55). In this way, fatigue is specific to the type of task undertaken. If a task requires only type I fiber recruitment, then the factors limiting performance will be very different from those associated with tasks requiring type IIx fibers. With this review and summary in mind, let's now examine the factors limiting performance.

Ultra Short-Term Performances (10 Seconds or Less)

The events that fit into this category include the shot put, high jump, long jump, and 50- and 100-meter sprints. These events require that tremendous amounts of energy be produced in a short period of time (high-power events), and type II muscle fibers must be recruited. Figure 19.4 shows that maximal performance is limited by the fiber type distribution (type I versus type II) and by the number of muscle fibers recruited, which is influenced by the level of motivation and arousal (27). Optimal performance is also affected by skill and technique, which are dependent on practice. It should be no surprise that the anaerobic sources of ATP—the ATP-PC system and glycolysis—provide the energy. Chapter 20 provides tests for anaerobic power, and chapter 21 provides a

ASK THE EXPERT 19.1

Muscle Adaptations to Space Travel: Questions and Answers with Dr. Robert H. Fitts

Dr. Fitts is Professor and Chairman of the Department of Biological Sciences at Marquette University. His primary research interests include excitation contraction coupling and muscle mechanics, and the mechanism of muscle adaptation to space flight and programs of regular exercise. His research also focuses on elucidating the cellular causes of muscle fatigue. He was awarded the American College of Sports Medicine's Citation Award in 1999 for his research accomplishments and received the Researcher of the Year Award from Marquette University in 2000.

QUESTION: What changes occur in skeletal muscle due to space travel?

ANSWER: The primary change in skeletal muscle with space travel is fiber atrophy due to a selective loss in the myofilaments. The antigravity muscles of the legs are more affected than arm muscles, and primarily slow muscles like the soleus are more affected than fast-twitch muscles such as the gastrocnemius. Due to the loss of myofilaments, muscle fibers generate less force and power. Following short-duration (≤3 weeks) space flight, slow type I fibers show an elevated maximal shortening velocity, which is not caused by an expression of fast-type myosin. It has been hypothesized that the increased velocity results from a selective loss of the thin filament actin, which increases the space between the filaments, causing the myosin cross-bridge to

detach sooner at the end of the power stroke. Recent results from International Space Station experiments have shown the elevated velocity to be a transient change, with slow fiber velocity showing a significant decline following long-duration flights. This change, plus additional fiber atrophy, contributes to the considerably greater loss in slow fiber power after long-duration, compared to short duration, flights. Space flight appears to increase the muscle's reliance on carbohydrates and reduce its ability to oxidize fats. This metabolic change is not caused by a reduced activity of any of the enzymes of the β-oxidative pathway or the Krebs cycle. The loss in fiber power and increased reliance on carbohydrates cause a reduced work capacity. Additionally, post-flight crew members experience muscle soreness due to an increased susceptibility to eccentric contraction-induced fiber damage.

QUESTION: Do animal studies mimic the changes experienced by humans?

ANSWER: Many of the space flight Induced changes in skeletal muscle are observed in rodents, nonhuman primates, and humans. Fiber atrophy caused by the selective loss of myofilaments has been observed in all species. There are species differences in the time course of the adaptive process. For example, rats flown in space show a faster rate of fiber atrophy than do humans. Flights as short as 2 or 3 weeks have been

shown to increase soleus muscle velocity in both rats and humans, but in rats the increase was in part due to a conversion of approximately 20% of the slow type I fibers to fast-twitch fibers containing fast myosin isozymes. In humans, short-duration space flight does not cause fiber type conversion. However, recent data suggest that such conversions (slow-twitch to fast-twitch) do occur in humans following long-duration (6 months) space flight.

QUESTION: Are there any intervention (training) strategies being employed to reduce the impact of space flight on skeletal muscle?

ANSWER: The primary countermeasure used to protect skeletal muscle from microgravity-induced loss has employed endurance exercise on either a bicycle or treadmill. This type of modality has not been completely successful, as crew members still lose up to 20% of their leg muscle mass following 6 months in space. High-intensity exercise has been incorporated into the countermeasure program on the ISS, but the loads have been insufficient to adequately protect limb muscle size or power. Recently, a new high-resistance device has been installed on the ISS, but its effectiveness has not yet been established. (Readers are directed to Dr. Fitts's major review on the effects of space flight on muscle structure and function in Suggested Readings.)

---

detailed list of the activities dependent upon such power. There is evidence that ingestion of creatine can influence performance in high-power exercise; see chapter 25 for details.

IN SUMMARY

- In events lasting 10 seconds or less, optimal performance is dependent on the recruitment of appropriate type II fibers to generate the great forces that are needed.

- Motivation and arousal are required, as well as the skill needed to direct the force.
- The primary energy sources are anaerobic, with the focus on phosphocreatine.

Short-Term Performances (10 to 180 Seconds)

Maximal performances in the 10- to 60-second range are still predominantly (>70%) anaerobic, using the high force, fast-twitch fiber, but when a maximal

Figure 19.4 Factors affecting fatigue in ultra short-term events.

Figure 19.5 Factors affecting fatigue in short-term events.

IN SUMMARY

- In short-term performances lasting 10 to 180 seconds, there is a shift from 70% of the energy supplied anaerobically at 10 seconds to 60% being supplied aerobically at 180 seconds.
- Anaerobic glycolysis provides a substantial portion of the energy, resulting in elevated lactate levels.

performance is extended to 3 minutes, about 60% of the energy comes from the slower aerobic, ATP-generating processes. As a result of this transition from anaerobic to aerobic energy production, maximal running speed decreases as the duration of the race increases from 10 to 180 seconds. Given that the ATP-PC system can supply ATP for only several seconds, the vast majority of the ATP will be derived from anaerobic glycolysis (see chapter 3). Figure 19.5 shows that this will cause an accumulation of H^+ in muscle as well as blood. The elevated H^+ concentration may actually interfere with the continued production of ATP via glycolysis, or the contractile machinery itself, by interfering with troponin's ability to bind with Ca^{++}. However, it must be added that following exhausting exercise, muscle tension recovers before the H^+ concentration does, indicating the complex nature of the fatigue process (22, 53, 54, 63). In an effort to slow H^+ accumulation, some athletes have attempted to ingest buffers prior to a race. This procedure is discussed in detail in chapter 25, which deals with ergogenic aids and performance.

FACTORS LIMITING ALL-OUT AEROBIC PERFORMANCES

As the duration of an all-out performance increases, more demand is placed on the aerobic sources of energy. In addition, environmental factors such as heat and humidity, and dietary factors such as water and carbohydrate ingestion, play a role in fatigue.

Moderate-Length Performances (3 to 20 Minutes)

Although 60% of ATP production is derived from aerobic processes in a 3-minute maximal effort, the value jumps to 90% in a 20-minute all-out performance. Given this dependence on oxidative energy production, the factors limiting performance include both the cardiovascular system, which delivers oxygen-rich blood to the muscles, and the mitochondrial content of the muscles involved in the activity. Because speed is a prerequisite in races lasting fewer than 20 minutes, type IIa fibers, which are rich in mitochondria, are involved in supplying the ATP aerobically (in addition to the already recruited type I fibers). Races lasting fewer than 20 minutes are run at 90% to 100% of maximal aerobic power, so the athlete

Figure 19.6 Factors affecting fatigue in aerobic performances lasting 3 to 20 minutes.

with the highest $\dot{V}O_2$ max has a distinct advantage. However, because type IIx fibers are also recruited, lactate and H^+ production are increased, and H^+ accumulation would affect tension development as previously described (22, 53, 54, 64). Figure 19.6 summarizes the factors affecting performances requiring a high maximal oxygen uptake. The maximal stroke volume is the crucial key to a high cardiac output (see chapter 13) and is influenced by both genetics and training. The arterial oxygen content (CaO_2) is influenced by the arterial hemoglobin content [Hb], the fraction of inspired oxygen (FIO_2), and PO_2 of the inspired air. Chapter 24 discusses the effect of altitude (low PO_2) on $\dot{V}O_2$ max, and chapter 25 discusses the use of blood doping (to raise the [Hb]) and oxygen breathing on aerobic performance. Training programs are discussed in chapter 21.

IN SUMMARY

- In moderate-length performances lasting 3 to 20 minutes, aerobic metabolism provides 60% to 90% of the ATP, respectively.
- These activities require an energy expenditure near $\dot{V}O_2$ max, with type II fibers being recruited, in addition to the type I fibers.
- Any factor interfering with oxygen delivery (e.g., altitude or anemia) would decrease performance, because it is so dependent on aerobic energy production. High levels of H^+ accompany these types of activities.

Intermediate-Length Performances (21 to 60 Minutes)

In all-out performances lasting 21 to 60 minutes, the athlete will generally work at <90% $\dot{V}O_2$ max. A high $\dot{V}O_2$ max is certainly a prerequisite for success, but now other factors come into play. For example, an individual who is an "economical" runner can move at a higher speed for the same amount of oxygen compared to a runner who is not economical. The importance of both $\dot{V}O_2$ max and running economy in predicting distance running performance was recently confirmed (35), and evidence exists that both are important in shorter (e.g., 1,500 m) races (29). Differences in running economy are due to biomechanical and/or bioenergetic factors. In this case, measurements of both $\dot{V}O_2$ max and running economy would be needed to predict performance (see chapter 20). However, another variable must be considered. Because races of this duration are not run at $\dot{V}O_2$ max, a person who can run at a high percentage of $\dot{V}O_2$ max would have an advantage. The ability to run at a high percentage of $\dot{V}O_2$ max is related to the concentration of lactate in the blood, and one of the best predictors of race pace is the lactate threshold (8, 9). See The Winning Edge 19.1 for more on this. Interestingly, a high percentage of type I muscle fibers is associated with both a greater lactate threshold and a higher mechanical efficiency (14). Chronic severe training over many years has been linked to improvements in delta and gross efficiencies (+1.75% and +1.87%, respectively—an 8% and 9% change) that contributed to the consecutive victories of the Tour de France champion Lance Armstrong (13). The procedures to follow in estimating the maximal running speed for long-distance races are presented in chapter 20. Factors limiting performance in runs of 21 to 60 minutes are summarized in figure 19.7. Note that we must now consider the environmental factors of heat and humidity, as well as the state of hydration of the runner. The heat load will require that a portion of the cardiac output be directed to the skin, pushing the cardiovascular system closer to maximum at any running speed. Chapters 23 and 24 deal with the effects of dehydration and environmental heat loads on performance. See A Look Back—Important People in Science for a physiologist who had a major role in discovering the factors linked to endurance performance.

IN SUMMARY

- Intermediate-length activities lasting 21 to 60 minutes are usually conducted at less than 90% $\dot{V}O_2$ max and are predominantly aerobic.
- Given the length of the activity, environmental factors such as heat, humidity, and the state of hydration of the subject play a role in the outcome.

Is Maximal Oxygen Uptake Important in Distance-Running Performance?

$\dot{V}O_2$ max is directly related to the rate of ATP generation that can be maintained during a distance race, even though it is not run at 100% $\dot{V}O_2$ max. The rate of ATP generation is dependent on the actual $\dot{V}O_2$ that can be maintained during the run (ml · kg^{-1} · min^{-1}), which is a function of the runner's $\dot{V}O_2$ max and the percent $\dot{V}O_2$ max at which the runner can perform. To run a 2:15 marathon, the runner would have to maintain a $\dot{V}O_2$ of about 60 ml · kg^{-1} · min^{-1} throughout the race. A runner working at 80% $\dot{V}O_2$ max would need a $\dot{V}O_2$ max of 75 ml · kg^{-1} · min^{-1}. In this way the $\dot{V}O_2$ max sets the upper limit for energy production in endurance events but does not determine the final performance. It is clear that both the percent of $\dot{V}O_2$ max that can be maintained over the course of the run (estimated by the lactate threshold) and running economy have a dramatic impact on the speed that can be maintained over distance (8, 9, 35). Interestingly, the progressive reduction in $\dot{V}O_2$ max with age appears to be the primary physiological mechanism associated with a reduction in the endurance performance of Master athletes, along with the reduction in the velocity at the lactate threshold (62).

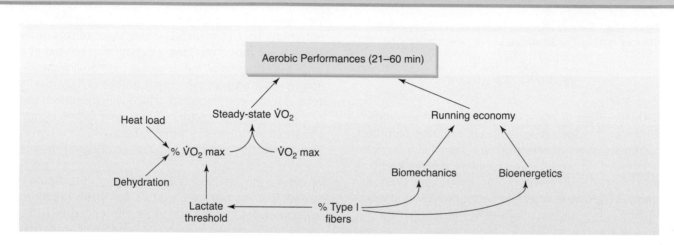

Figure 19.7 Factors affecting fatigue in aerobic performances lasting 21 to 60 minutes.

Long-Term Performances (1 to 4 Hours)

Performances of 1 to 4 hours are clearly aerobic performances involving little anaerobic energy production. Using the shorter aerobic performances (sixty minutes or less) as a lead-in, the longer the performance, the greater the chance that environmental factors will play a role in the outcome. In addition, for performances greater than 1 hour, the ability of the muscle and liver carbohydrate stores to supply glucose may be exceeded (see chapter 23). Glucose supplementation during long-term performances provides the fuel needed not only for ATP generation for the cross-bridges, but also for the protection of muscle membrane excitability (59). As pointed out in chapter 4, fatty acids can provide substantial fuel during prolonged muscular work at intensities <60% $\dot{V}O_2$ max. However, for the many endurance activities that are performed at higher exercise intensities (e.g., marathon running), muscle fibers must have carbohydrate to oxidize or performance will decline. Some have wondered if this same model could be used for predicting performance in "ultra" type performances (see A Closer Look 19.2). Chapter 23 provides information about the optimal dietary strategies for performance in long-term events, including the consumption of fluids and carbohydrates during the run. Figure 19.8 summarizes the factors limiting performance in long-distance running events (see Joyner and Coyle in Suggested Readings for a recent update on this topic, with a list of questions that still need attention). If we were to address long-term cycling performance, a variety of other variables (e.g., minimizing air resistance and rolling resistance) would have to be considered. See Faria, Parker, and Faria in the Suggested Readings for a recent review on factors affecting cycling performance.

IN SUMMARY

- In long-term performances of 1 to 4 hours' duration, environmental factors play a more important role as the muscle and liver glycogen stores try to keep up with the rate at which carbohydrate is used.
- Diet, fluid ingestion, and the ability of the athlete to deal with heat and humidity all influence the final outcome.

A LOOK BACK—IMPORTANT PEOPLE IN SCIENCE

Dr. David L. Costill, Ph.D., Advanced the Study of Endurance Performance

Dr. David Costill has had a major impact on our understanding of the factors affecting endurance performance. Dr. Costill completed his Ph.D. at The Ohio State University and, after a two-year appointment at the State University of New York at Cortland, assumed a position at Ball State University. He directed the Human Performance Laboratory at Ball State throughout his entire career and made it *the* place to be if you wanted to study the factors affecting performance. Dr. Costill and his students addressed a variety of variables influencing endurance performance:

- Role of $\dot{V}O_2$ max
- Contribution of the percent of $\dot{V}O_2$ max
- Importance of running economy
- How blood/plasma lactate concentration is linked to performance
- Strategies for loading muscle glycogen (see chapter 23)

- Fluid replacement—with emphasis on characteristics of sports drinks (see chapter 23)
- Role of muscle fiber type (see chapter 8)
- Whether ergogenic aids work (e.g., caffeine; L-carnitine—see chapter 25).

Many of the studies dealing with these variables have become "classics" that investigators cite decades after they were done. Dr. Costill was not just interested in discovering the science behind endurance performance; he also committed his time and energy to getting the message out to athletes and coaches to help them develop better methods to improve performances based on scientific principles. Dr. Costill's work went well beyond studying distance running. Both early and later in his career, he focused attention on how to improve swimming performance, and he is currently involved in studies designed to improve our understanding of how to prevent deleterious changes in the muscles of astronauts who spend long

periods of time on the International Space Station. He has always practiced what he preached, being involved in distance running early in his career, and now Master's swimming—where he is swimming faster than he did when he was in college!

Dr. Costill provided exemplary service to the American College of Sports Medicine over his career, including serving as its president. His research has been recognized with numerous awards over the past 30 years, including the Honor Award from the American College of Sports Medicine. The impact of his research has reached all corners of the globe, not just by publications (more than 400), but by being invited to speak about his research in more than 30 countries. His personal impact, like that of most scientists, is multiplied many times over by the students he trained—a list that reads like a "who's who" of scientists interested in muscle, metabolism, and performance. He continues to maintain an active research program at Ball State University, where he holds the John and Janis Fisher Chair in Exercise Science.

A CLOSER LOOK 19.2

Factors Affecting Performance in Ultra-endurance Events

In contrast to the duration of endurance performances just mentioned, ultra-endurance events are in a class of their own. Examples include: 166-km mountain runs (44), Triple Iron Triathlons (11.6 km swim, 540 km bike, 126.6 km run) (31), and a Paris to Beijing run (8,500 km in 161 days) (43). In a recent study to evaluate the factors related to ultra-endurance performance, fourteen subjects ran as many kilometers as possible in 24 hours on a treadmill. They covered an average of 149.2 km in 18 h 39 min of actual treadmill running

in the 24 hours. Two of the most important variables related to performance included $\dot{V}O_2$ max and the percentage of $\dot{V}O_2$ max that they could maintain over the 24 hours (42), two of the three variables linked to the regular endurance performances we just discussed.

Studies that have tracked metabolic responses before and after ultra-endurance events find that fat oxidation is markedly elevated after an ultra-endurance race, with plasma free fatty acids being 3.5 times higher (26). Given the low % $\dot{V}O_2$ max

maintained in many of these events (<60%), the metabolic response is not surprising (see chapter 4). However, it doesn't mean that carbohydrate is not important, as some studies have shown a 50% reduction in muscle glycogen stores (26). Although ultra-endurance runs increase the potential for hyponatremia (a dangerous condition in which the body's sodium store is diluted because of the ingestion of too much water—see chapter 23), only 4% of the runners experienced a mild form of the condition (49).

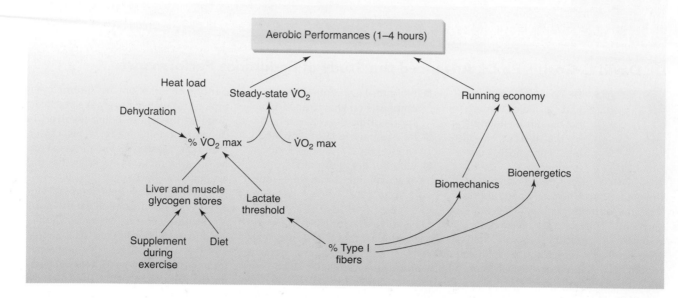

Figure 19.8 Factors affecting fatigue in aerobic performances lasting 1 to 4 hours.

In conclusion, the factors limiting performance are specific to the type of performance. Short-term explosive performances are dependent on type IIx fibers that can generate great power through anaerobic processes. In contrast, longer-duration aerobic events require a cardiovascular system that can deliver oxygen at a high rate to muscle fibers with many mitochondria. It is clear that the testing and training of athletes must focus on the factors limiting performance for the specific event. For example, dietary carbohydrate and fluid ingestion are more crucial for the long-distance runner than for the high jumper. A recent review article by Abbiss and Laursen in the Suggested Readings pulls together the various models of fatigue into a single diagram. This is worth reading now that you have a general feel for the factors affecting performance. The following chapters will explore how to appropriately test, train, and feed athletes for optimal performance.

ATHLETE AS MACHINE

One question we might keep in mind as we explore the details of how to improve performance is whether we might exceed what are regarded as reasonable and ethical boundaries for scientists and treat the elite athlete as a machine rather than as a person. Are elite athletes being treated like racing cars in which engineers and mechanics (scientists and coaches) try to spot weaknesses that compromise performance, and then recommend solutions? Some may say yes, and indicate the worthiness of such an enterprise. Others may suggest that this has the potential to be dehumanizing if the athlete is reduced to no more than a collection of working parts that are evaluated by a variety of specialists. Much would appear to depend on the goal of the research. If we are trying to understand how we function, and we develop healthy and safe methods that allow us to overcome personal limitations, we would appear to be on the right track. In contrast, if we use an athlete as a tool, that would be a different story. We are all familiar with the use of athletes by some countries to advance a particular political doctrine, and the complicity of scientists who were recruited to make athletes run faster and longer and jump higher. Fortunately, universities, hospitals, and research centers have Institutional Review Boards (IRBs) to approve research proposals so that the rights of the subject are protected. This process also forces the investigator to provide a strong rationale showing that the risk to the subject (however small) is worth the benefits that might occur. Consistent with this, research journals require authors to follow IRB guidelines if they want their work to be considered for publication. In this way we can move forward in our understanding of the physiological mechanisms underlying fatigue while protecting the rights of the subject.

STUDY QUESTIONS

1. List the factors influencing performance.
2. Is the limiting factor for strength development located in the CNS or out in the periphery? Support your position.
3. Tracing the path the action potential takes from the time it leaves the motor end plate, where might the "weak link" be in the mechanisms coupling excitation to contraction?
4. When fatigue occurs there is still ATP present in the cell. What is the explanation for this?
5. Describe the pattern of recruitment of muscle fiber types during aerobic activities of progressively greater intensity.

6. As the duration of a maximal effort increases from 10 seconds or less to between 10 to 180 seconds, what factor becomes limiting in terms of energy production?
7. Draw a diagram of the factors limiting maximal running performances of 1,500 m to 5 km.
8. Although a high $\dot{V}O_2$ max is essential to world-class performance, what role does running economy play in a winning performance?

9. Given that lactate accumulation will adversely affect endurance, what test might be an indicator of maximal sustained running (swimming, cycling) speed?
10. What is the role of environmental factors, such as altitude and heat, in very long-distance performances lasting 1 to 4 hours?

SUGGESTED READINGS

Abbiss, C. R., and P. B. Laursen. 2005. Models to explain fatigue during prolonged endurance cycling. *Sports Medicine* 35:865–98.

Daniels, J. T. 2005. *Daniels' Running Formula*, 2d ed. Champaign, IL: Human Kinetics.

Faria, E. W., D. L. Parker, and I. Faria. 2005. The science of cycling: Factors affecting performance—Part 2. *Sports Medicine* 35:313–37.

Fitts, R. H. 2006. The muscular system: Fatigue processes. In ACSM's *Advanced Exercise Physiology*. Edited by C. M. Tipton,

M. N. Sawka, C. A. Tate, and R. L. Terjung. Baltimore: Lippincott Williams & Wilkins. pp. 178–196.

Fitts R. H. et al. 2010. Prolonged space flight-induced alterations in the structure and function of human skeletal muscle fibres. *Journal of Physiology* 588: 3567–92.

Joyner, M. J., and E. F. Coyle. 2008. Endurance exercise performance: The physiology of champions. J. *Physiol.* 586:35–44.

REFERENCES

1. **Allen DG, Lamb GD, and Westerblad H.** Skeletal muscle fatigue: cellular mechanisms. *Physiological Reviews* 88: 287–332, 2008.
2. **Allen DG, and Westerblad H.** Role of phosphate and calcium stores in muscle fatigue. *The Journal of Physiology* 536: 657–665, 2001.
3. **Allen DG, Westerblad H, Lee JA, and Lannergren J.** Role of excitation-contraction coupling in muscle fatigue. *Sports Medicine (Auckland, NZ)* 13: 116–126, 1992.
4. **Appell HJ, Soares JM, and Duarte JA.** Exercise, muscle damage and fatigue. *Sports Medicine (Auckland, NZ)* 13: 108–115, 1992.
5. **Asmussen E, and Mazin B.** A central nervous component in local muscular fatigue. *European Journal of Applied Physiology and Occupational Physiology* 38: 9–15, 1978.
6. **Asmussen E, and Mazin B.** Recuperation after muscular fatigue by "diverting activities." *European Journal of Applied Physiology and Occupational Physiology* 38: 1–7, 1978.
7. **Banister EW, and Cameron BJ.** Exercise-induced hyperammonemia: peripheral and central effects. *International Journal of Sports Medicine* 11 Suppl 2: S129–142, 1990.
8. **Bassett DR, Jr., and Howley ET.** Limiting factors for maximum oxygen uptake and determinants of endurance performance. *Medicine and Science in Sports and Exercise* 32: 70–84, 2000.
9. **Bassett DR, Jr., and Howley ET.** Maximal oxygen uptake: "classical" versus "contemporary" viewpoints. *Medicine and Science in Sports and Exercise* 29: 591–603, 1997.
10. **Bigland-Ritchie B.** EMG and fatigue of human voluntary and stimulated contractions. In: *Human Muscle Fatigue: Physiological Mechanisms*. London: Pitman Medical, 1981, p. 130–156.
11. **Coirault C, Guellich A, Barbry T, Samuel JL, Riou B, and Lecarpentier Y.** Oxidative stress of myosin contributes to skeletal muscle dysfunction in rats with chronic heart failure. *American Journal of Physiology* 292: H1009–1017, 2007.
12. **Coombes JS, Powers SK, Rowell B, Hamilton KL, Dodd SL, Shanely RA, Sen CK, and Packer L.** Effects of vitamin E and alpha-lipoic acid on skeletal muscle contractile properties. J *Appl Physiol* 90: 1424–1430, 2001.
13. **Coyle EF.** Improved muscular efficiency displayed as Tour de France champion matures. J *Appl Physiol* 98: 2191–2196, 2005.
14. **Coyle EF.** Integration of the physiological factors determining endurance performance ability. *Exercise and Sport Sciences Reviews* 23: 25–63, 1995.
15. **Davis JM, Alderson NL, and Welsh RS.** Serotonin and central nervous system fatigue: nutritional considerations. *The American Journal of Clinical Nutrition* 72: 573S–578S, 2000.
16. **Davis JM, and Bailey SP.** Possible mechanisms of central nervous system fatigue during exercise. *Medicine and Science in Sports and Exercise* 29: 45–57, 1997.
17. **Duke AM, and Steele DS.** Mechanisms of reduced SR Ca^{+2} release induced by inorganic phosphate in rat skeletal muscle fibers. *Am J Physiol Cell Physiol* 281: C418–429, 2001.
18. **Edwards R.** Human muscle function and fatigue. In: *Human Muscle Fatigue: Physiological Mechanisms*. London: Pitman Medical, 1981.
19. **Fitts RH.** Cellular mechanisms of muscle fatigue. *Physiological Reviews* 74: 49–94, 1994.
20. **Fitts RH.** The cross-bridge cycle and skeletal muscle fatigue. J *Appl Physiol* 104: 551–558, 2008.
21. **Fitts RH, Riley DR, and Widrick JJ.** Functional and structural adaptations of skeletal muscle to microgravity. *The Journal of Experimental Biology* 204: 3201–3208, 2001.
22. **Fuchs F, Reddy Y, and Briggs FN.** The interaction of cations with the calcium-binding site of troponin. *Biochimica et Biophysica Acta* 221: 407–409, 1970.
23. **Gibson H, and Edwards RH.** Muscular exercise and fatigue. *Sports Medicine (Auckland, NZ)* 2: 120–132, 1985.
24. **Green HJ.** Membrane excitability, weakness, and fatigue. *Canadian Journal of Applied Physiology = Revue Canadienne de Physiologie Appliquee* 29: 291–307, 2004.

25. **Halliwell B, and Gutteridge J.** *Free Radicals in Biology and Medicine.* Oxford: Oxford Press, 2007.

26. **Helge JW, Rehrer NJ, Pilegaard H, Manning P, Lucas SJE, Gerrard DF, and Cotter JD.** Increased fat oxidation and regulation of metabolic genes with ultraendurance exercise. *Acta Physiologica* 191: 77–86, 2007.

27. **Ikai M, and Steinhaus AH.** Some factors modifying the expression of human strength. *J Appl Physiol* 16: 157–163, 1961.

28. **Ikai M, and Yabe K.** Training effect of muscular endurance by means by voluntary and electrical stimulation. *Internationale Zeitschrift Fur Angewandte Physiologie, Einschliesslich Arbeitsphysiologie* 28: 55–60, 1969.

29. **Ingham SA, Whyte GP, Pedlar C, Bailey DM, Dunman N, and Nevill AM.** Determinants of 800-m and 1500-m running performance using allometric models. *Medicine and Science in Sports and Exercise* 40: 345–350, 2008.

30. **Kayser B.** Exercise starts and ends in the brain. *European Journal of Applied Physiology* 90: 411–419, 2003.

31. **Knechtle B, and Kohler G.** Running performance, not anthropometric factors, is associated with race success in a triple iron triathlon. *British Journal of Sports Medicine* 43: 437–441, 2009.

32. **Lambert EV, St Clair Gibson A, and Noakes TD.** Complex systems model of fatigue: integrative homeostatic control of peripheral physiological systems during exercise in humans. *British Journal of Sports Medicine* 39: 52–62, 2005.

33. **Matuszczak Y, Farid M, Jones J, Lansdowne S, Smith MA, Taylor AA, and Reid MB.** Effects of N-acetylcysteine on glutathione oxidation and fatigue during handgrip exercise. *Muscle & Nerve* 32: 633–638, 2005.

34. **McKenna MJ, Medved I, Goodman CA, Brown MJ, Bjorksten AR, Murphy KT, Petersen AC, Sostaric S, and Gong X.** N-acetylcysteine attenuates the decline in muscle Na^+, K^+-pump activity and delays fatigue during prolonged exercise in humans. *The Journal of Physiology* 576: 279–288, 2006.

35. **McLaughlin JE, Howley ET, Bassett Jr DR, Thompson DL, and Fitzhugh EC.** Test of the classic model for predicting endurance running performance. *Medicine and Science in Sports and Exercise* 42: 991–997, 2010.

36. **McLester JR, Jr.** Muscle contraction and fatigue. The role of adenosine 5'-diphosphate and inorganic phosphate. *Sports Medicine (Auckland, NZ)* 23: 287–305, 1997.

37. **Medved I, Brown MJ, Bjorksten AR, and McKenna MJ.** Effects of intravenous N-acetylcysteine infusion on time to fatigue and potassium regulation during prolonged cycling exercise. *J Appl Physiol* 96: 211–217, 2004.

38. **Medved I, Brown MJ, Bjorksten AR, Murphy KT, Petersen AC, Sostaric S, Gong X, and McKenna MJ.** N-acetylcysteine enhances muscle cysteine and glutathione availability and attenuates fatigue during prolonged exercise in endurance-trained individuals. *J Appl Physiol* 97: 1477–1485, 2004.

39. **Meeusen R, and Watson P.** Amino acids and the brain: do they play a role in "central fatigue"? *International Journal of Sport Nutrition and Exercise Metabolism* 17: S37–S46, 2007.

40. **Meeusen R, Watson P, Hasegawa H, Roelands B, and Piacentini MF.** Central fatigue: the serotonin hypothesis and beyond. *Sports Medicine (Auckland, NZ)* 36: 881–909, 2006.

41. **Merton PA.** Voluntary strength and fatigue. *The Journal of Physiology* 123: 553–564, 1954.

42. **Millet GY, Banfi JC, Kerherve H, Morin JB, Vincent L, Estrade C, Geyssant A, and Feasson L.** Physiological and biological factors associated with a 24 h treadmill ultra-marathon performance. *Scandinavian Journal of Medicine & Science in Sports* 21: 54–61, 2011.

43. **Millet GY, Morin JB, Degache F, Edouard P, Feasson L, Verney J, and Oullion R.** Running from Paris to Neijing: biomechanical and physiological consequences. *European Journal of Applied Physiology* 107: 731–738, 2009.

44. **Millet GY, Tomazin K, Verges S, Vincent C, Bonnefoy R, Boisson RC, Gergele L, Feasson L, and Martin V.** Neuromuscular consequences of an extreme mountain ultra-marathon. *PLOS ONE* 6: No. e17059, 2011.

45. **Nielsen B, and Nybo L.** Cerebral changes during exercise in the heat. *Sports Medicine (Auckland, NZ)* 33: 1–11, 2003.

46. **Noakes TD, and St Clair Gibson A.** Logical limitations to the "catastrophe" models of fatigue during exercise in humans. *British Journal of Sports Medicine* 38: 648–649, 2004.

47. **Noakes TD, St Clair Gibson A, and Lambert EV.** From catastrophe to complexity: a novel model of integrative central neural regulation of effort and fatigue during exercise in humans. *British Journal of Sports Medicine* 38: 511–514, 2004.

48. **Noakes TD, St Clair Gibson A, and Lambert EV.** From catastrophe to complexity: a novel model of integrative central neural regulation of effort and fatigue during exercise in humans: summary and conclusions. *British Journal of Sports Medicine* 39: 120–124, 2005.

49. **Page AJ, Reid SA, Speedy DB, Mulligan GP, and Thompson J.** Exercise-associated hyponatremia, renal function, and nonsteroidal antiinflammatory drug use in an ultraendurance mountain run. *Clinical Journal of Sport Medicine* 17: 43–48, 2007.

50. **Place N, Yamada T, Bruton JD, and Westerblad H.** Muscle fatigue: from observations in humans to underlying mechanisms studies in intact single muscle fibers. *European Journal of Applied Physiology* 110: 1–15, 2010.

51. **Powers S, and Jackson M.** Exercise-induced oxidative stress: cellular mechanisms and impact on skeletal muscle force production. *Physiological Reviews* 88: 1243–1276, 2008.

52. **Powers SK, DeRuisseau KC, Quindry J, and Hamilton KL.** Dietary antioxidants and exercise. *Journal of Sports Sciences* 22: 81–94, 2004.

53. **Roberts D, and Smith DJ.** Biochemical aspects of peripheral muscle fatigue. A review. *Sports Medicine (Auckland, NZ)* 7: 125–138, 1989.

54. **Sahlin K.** Metabolic factors in fatigue. *Sports Medicine (Auckland, NZ)* 13: 99–107, 1992.

55. **Sale D.** Influence of exercise and training on motor unit activation. In: *Exercise and Sport Sciences Reviews*, edited by Pandolf K. New York: Macmillan, 1987, p. 95–151.

56. **Sejersted OM, and Sjogaard G.** Dynamics and consequences of potassium shifts in skeletal muscle and heart during exercise. *Physiological Reviews* 80: 1411–1481, 2000.

57. **Smith MA, and Reid MB.** Redox modulation of contractile function in respiratory and limb skeletal muscle. *Respiratory Physiology & Neurobiology* 151: 229–241, 2006.

58. **St Clair Gibson A, and Noakes TD.** Evidence for complex system integration and dynamic neural regulation of skeletal muscle recruitment during exercise in humans. *British Journal of Sports Medicine* 38: 797–806, 2004.

59. **Stewart RD, Duhamel TA, Foley KP, Ouyang J, Smith IC, and Green HJ.** Protection of muscle membrane excitability during prolonged cycle exercise with glucose supplementation. *J Appl Physiol* 103: 331–339, 2007.

60. **Struder HK, and Weicker H.** Physiology and pathophysiology of the serotonergic system and its implications on mental and physical performance. Part I. *International Journal of Sports Medicine* 22: 467–481, 2001.

61. **Struder HK, and Weicker H.** Physiology and pathophysiology of the serotonergic system and its implications on mental and physical performance. Part II. *International Journal of Sports Medicine* 22: 482–497, 2001.

62. **Tod D, Iredale F, and Gill N.** 'Psyching-up' and muscular force production. *Sports Medicine (Auckland, NZ)* 33: 47–58, 2003.

63. **Trivedi B, and Danforth WH.** Effect of pH on the kinetics of frog muscle phosphofructokinase. *The Journal of Biological Chemistry* 241: 4110–4112, 1966.

64. **Tupling AR.** The sarcoplasmic reticulum in muscle fatigue and disease: role of the sarco(endo)plasmic reticulum Ca^{2+}-ATPase. *Canadian Journal of Applied Physiology = Revue Canadienne de Physiologie Appliquee* 29: 308–329, 2004.

65. **Vandenboom R.** The myofibrillar complex and fatigue: a review. *Canadian Journal of Applied Physiology = Revue Canadienne de Physiologie Appliquee* 29: 330–356, 2004.

66. **Weir JP, Beck TW, Cramer JT, and Housh TJ.** Is fatigue all in your head? A critical review of the central governor model. *British Journal of Sports Medicine* 40: 573–586; discussion 586, 2006.

67. **Westerblad H, Lee JA, Lannergren J, and Allen DG.** Cellular mechanisms of fatigue in skeletal muscle. *The American Journal of Physiology* 261: C195–209, 1991.

Laboratory Assessment
of Human Performance

■ Objectives

By studying this chapter, you should be able to do the following:

1. Discuss the factors that determine the effectiveness of a physiological test of athletic performance.
2. Define "specificity of $\dot{V}O_2$ max."
3. Explain the difference between $\dot{V}O_2$ max and $\dot{V}O_2$ peak.
4. Discuss the physiological rationale for the assessment of the lactate threshold in the endurance athlete.
5. Describe methods for the assessment of anaerobic power.
6. Discuss the techniques used to evaluate muscular strength.

■ Outline

■ Key Terms

critical power
dynamic
dynamometer

isokinetic
power test

Quebec 10-second test
Wingate test

In general, there have been two principal approaches to the assessment of physical performance: (1) field tests of general physical fitness, which include a variety of measurements requiring basic performance demands, and (2) laboratory assessments of physiological capacities such as maximal aerobic power ($\dot{V}O_2$ max), anaerobic power, and exercise economy. It can be argued that physical fitness testing is important for an overall assessment of general conditioning, particularly in terms of evaluating student progress in a physical education conditioning class (1, 68). However, the use of these test batteries does not provide the detailed physiological information needed to assess an athlete's current level of conditioning or potential weaknesses. Therefore, more specific laboratory tests are required to provide detailed physiological information about performance in specific athletic events. This chapter will discuss tests designed to measure physical work capacity and performance in athletes. Specifically, much of this chapter will focus on both laboratory and field tests to evaluate the maximum energy transfer capacities discussed in chapters 3 and 4. The performance tests described in this chapter differ from the exercise tests described in chapter 15 in several ways. Recall that the exercise tests described in chapter 15 were targeted toward assessing cardiorespiratory fitness in healthy adults entering or actively engaged in a regular "health-related" exercise program. In contrast, the exercise tests described in this chapter are targeted toward measurement of performance in athletes actively engaged in competitive sports. Let's begin with a discussion of the theory and ethics of laboratory assessment of performance.

LABORATORY ASSESSMENT OF PHYSICAL PERFORMANCE

Physiological Testing: Theory and Ethics

Designing laboratory tests to assess physical performance requires an understanding of those factors that contribute to success in a particular sport or athletic event. In general, physical performance is determined by the individual's capacity for maximal energy output (i.e., maximal aerobic and anaerobic processes), muscular strength, coordination/economy of movement, and psychological factors (e.g., motivation and tactics) (32, 79). Figure 20.1 illustrates a simple model of the components that interact to determine the quality of physical performance. Many types of athletic events require a combination of several of these factors for an outstanding performance to occur. However, often one or more of these factors plays a dominant role in determining ath-

Figure 20.1 Factors that contribute to physical performance. See text for details.

letic success. In golf, there is little need for a high-energy output, but proper coordination is essential. Sprinting 100 meters requires not only good technique, but a high anaerobic power output. In distance running, cycling, or swimming, a high capacity for aerobic energy-yielding processes is essential for success. Again, laboratory evaluation of performance requires an understanding of those factors that are important for optimal performance in a particular athletic event. Thus, a test that stresses the same physiological systems required by a particular sport or athletic event would be a valid means of assessing physical performance.

A key concern in the performance of "athletic" laboratory testing is maintaining respect for the athlete's human rights. Therefore, laboratory testing should be performed only on athletes who are volunteers and have given written consent prior to testing. Further, prior to testing, the exercise scientist has the responsibility of informing the athlete about the purpose of the tests and the potential risks or discomfort associated with laboratory testing.

WHAT THE ATHLETE GAINS BY PHYSIOLOGICAL TESTING

Laboratory measurement of physical performance can be expensive and time consuming. An obvious question arises: What does the athlete gain by laboratory testing? A testing program can benefit the athlete and coach in at least three major ways:

1. Physiological testing can provide information regarding an athlete's strengths and weaknesses in his/her sport; this information can be used as baseline data to plan individual exercise training programs. As discussed above, athletic success in

most sports involves the interaction of several physiological components (Figure 20.1). In the laboratory, the exercise scientist can often measure these physiological components separately and provide the athlete with information about which physiological components require improvement in order for the athlete to raise his/her level of athletic performance. This information becomes the foundation for an individual exercise prescription that concentrates on the identified areas of weakness (53).

2. Laboratory testing provides feedback to the athlete about the effectiveness of a training program (53). For example, comparing the results of physiological tests performed before and after a training program provides a basis for evaluating the success of the training program (5).

3. Laboratory testing educates the athlete about the physiology of exercise (53). By participation in laboratory testing, the athlete learns more about those physiological parameters that are important to success in his/her sport. This is important because athletes with a basic understanding of elementary exercise physiology will likely make better personal decisions concerning the design of both exercise training and nutritional programs.

WHAT PHYSIOLOGICAL TESTING WILL NOT DO

Laboratory testing of the athlete is not a magical aid for the identification of future Olympic gold medalists (53). Although laboratory testing can provide valuable information concerning an athlete's strengths and weaknesses, this type of testing has limitations in that it is difficult to simulate in the laboratory the physiological and psychological demands of many sports. Therefore, it is difficult to predict athletic performance from any single battery of laboratory measurements. Performance in the field is the ultimate test of athletic success, and laboratory testing should be considered primarily a training aid for coach and athlete (53).

COMPONENTS OF EFFECTIVE PHYSIOLOGICAL TESTING

For laboratory testing to be effective, several key factors need consideration (53):

1. The physiological variables to be tested should be relevant to the sport. For example, measurement of maximal handgrip strength in a distance

runner would not be relevant to the athlete's event. Therefore, only those physiological components that are important for a particular sport should be measured.

2. Physiological tests should be valid and reliable. Valid tests are tests that measure what they are supposed to measure. Reliable tests are tests that are reproducible. Based on these definitions, the need for tests that are both valid and reproducible is clear (20). (See A Closer Look 20.1.)

3. Tests should be as sport-specific as possible. For instance, the distance runner should be tested while running (i.e., treadmill), and the cyclist should be tested while cycling.

4. Tests should be repeated at regular intervals. One of the main purposes of laboratory testing is to provide the athlete with systematic feedback concerning training effectiveness. To meet this objective, tests should be performed on a regular basis.

5. Testing procedures should be carefully controlled. The need to rigidly administer the laboratory test relates to the reliability of tests. For tests to be reliable, the testing protocol should be standardized. Factors to be controlled include the instructions given to the athletes prior to testing, the testing protocol itself, the calibration of instruments involved in testing, the time of the day for testing, prior exercise, diet standardization, and other factors such as sleep, illness, hydration status, or injury.

6. Test results should be interpreted to the coach and athlete clearly. This final step is a key goal of effective laboratory testing.

IN SUMMARY

- Designing laboratory tests to assess physical performance requires an understanding of those factors that contribute to success in a particular sport. Physical performance is determined by the interaction of the following factors: (a) maximal energy output, (b) muscular strength, (c) coordination/economy of movement, and (d) psychological factors such as motivation and tactics.
- To be effective, physiological tests should be (a) relevant to the sport; (b) valid and reliable; (c) sport specific; (d) repeated at regular intervals; (e) standardized; and (f) interpreted to the coach and athlete.

Reliability of Physiological Performance Tests

For a physiological test of human performance to be useful, the test must be reliable. That is, the test results must be reproducible. Several factors influence the reliability of physiological performance tests. These include the caliber of athletes tested, the type of ergometer used during the test, and the specificity of the test.

Physiological tests of performance are more reliable when highly trained and experienced athletes are tested (38). The explanation for this observation appears to be that these athletes are highly motivated to perform and that they are better able to pace themselves in a reproducible manner during a performance test. That is, high-caliber athletes may have a better "feel" for pace, and their perceptions of fatigue are less variable than those of less-experienced athletes (38).

It is clear that some ergometers are more unvarying than others in providing a constant resistance. For instance, an ergometer that maintains its calibration and delivers a constant power output during a test would result in a more reproducible test of human performance than an ergometer that provides variable power outputs during the test.

Although controversy exists, it is believed that exercise tests with a movement pattern and exercise intensity that mimics the actual sporting event are more reliable than tests that do not imitate the event (38, 39). For example, testing racing cyclists on a cycle ergometer at an exercise intensity close to the intensity of competition should be a more reliable performance test than testing these athletes on other types of ergometers, such as treadmills.

DIRECT TESTING OF MAXIMAL AEROBIC POWER

Let's begin our discussion of the laboratory assessment of human performance by describing tests to measure the maximal oxygen uptake ($\dot{V}O_2$ max) of athletes. Exercise testing to determine $\dot{V}O_2$ max dates back to studies conducted more than 80 years ago by the British scientist A.V. Hill. Indeed, A.V. Hill coined the term "$\dot{V}O_2$ max" in the early 1920s (3). *Maximal oxygen uptake* was first mentioned in chapter 4 and is defined as the highest oxygen uptake that an individual can obtain during exercise using large muscle groups (1). By necessity, the type of exercise performed to determine $\dot{V}O_2$ max must use large muscle groups (e.g., legs). Although several tests to estimate $\dot{V}O_2$ max exist (12, 24, 89), the most accurate means of determination is by direct laboratory measurement. Direct measurement of $\dot{V}O_2$ max is generally performed using a motorized treadmill or cycle ergometer, and open-circuit spirometry is used to measure pulmonary gas exchange (see chapter 1). However, $\dot{V}O_2$ max has also been measured during both free and tethered swimming, cross-country skiing, bench stepping, ice skating, and rowing (8, 12, 54, 57, 64, 95).

Historically, the measurement of $\dot{V}O_2$ max has been considered the test of choice for predicting success in endurance events such as distance running (11, 16, 27, 28, 34, 45, 53, 63, 101). For example, relative $\dot{V}O_2$ max (i.e., $\dot{V}O_2$ max expressed in ml $\cdot$ kg^{-1} $\cdot$ min^{-1}) has been shown to be the single most important factor in predicting distance running success in a heterogeneous (i.e., different $\dot{V}O_2$ max) group of athletes (17, 18, 28). The logical explanation for this finding is that because distance running is largely an aerobic event (see chapters 4 and 19), those individuals with a high $\dot{V}O_2$ max should have an advantage over individuals with lower aerobic capacities. However, as one would expect, the correlation between $\dot{V}O_2$ max and distance running performance is low in a homogeneous (i.e., similar $\dot{V}O_2$ max) group of runners (15, 75). These observations suggest that although a high $\dot{V}O_2$ max is important in determining distance running success, other variables are important as well. Therefore, measurement of $\dot{V}O_2$ max is only one in a battery of tests that should be used in evaluating physical work capacity in endurance athletes.

Specificity of Testing

As stated previously, running on a treadmill and pedaling a cycle ergometer are the two most common forms of exercise used to determine $\dot{V}O_2$ max. However, much evidence exists to suggest that a test to determine $\dot{V}O_2$ max should involve the specific movement used by the athlete in his or her event (7, 8, 69). For example, if the athlete being tested is a runner, it is important that $\dot{V}O_2$ max be assessed during running. Likewise, if the athlete being evaluated is a trained cyclist, the exercise test should be performed on the cycle ergometer. Further, specific testing procedures have been established for cross-country skiers and swimmers as well (54, 57, 64).

A LOOK BACK—IMPORTANT PEOPLE IN SCIENCE

Robert Bruce Was a Pioneer in the Development of the Graded Exercise Test

Robert Arthur Bruce (1916–2004) was born in the Boston suburb of Somerville, Massachusetts. He earned his B.S degree from Boston College and completed his medical school training in 1943 at the University of Rochester. After finishing his medical residency in 1946, he joined the faculty at the University of Rochester. Dr. Bruce later (1950) became the chief of cardiology at the University of Washington Medical School, where he remained until his retirement from academic medicine in 1987.

Early in his career, Dr. Bruce recognized that an exercise test could play an important role in the clinical evaluation of cardiac patients. He published his first paper on exercise testing in 1949 and concluded that a standardized exercise test provides key diagnostic information about cardiac patients. Dr. Bruce continued to explore exercise testing protocols for patient testing, and in 1963 he conceived and validated a multistage exercise protocol that was designed to evaluate the patient's exercise performance and provide important diagnostic information from the measurement of heart rate, blood pressure, and ECG changes during exercise. Subsequently the standard Bruce Exercise Test evolved into its present form with seven 3-minute stages. This test became known as the "Bruce Protocol" and is one of the most widely used treadmill protocols in North America to evaluate cardiac patients.

Dr. Bruce developed his exercise test for patient populations in the clinical laboratory. Nonetheless, the Bruce graded exercise test was the conceptual model behind many of the current graded exercise tests that are used in the exercise physiology laboratory to evaluate both $\dot{V}O_2$ max and the lactate threshold in athletes. Because of his research accomplishments in the area of clinical exercise testing, Dr. Bruce has been labeled as a pioneer of the cardiac stress test.

Exercise Test Protocol

Although the first exercise tests to determine $\dot{V}O_2$ max were performed in the 1920s, rigorous studies to optimize laboratory exercise tests were not performed until the 1940s and 1950s. An early leader in the development of graded exercise tests was Dr. Robert Bruce, a cardiologist at the University of Washington (See A Look Back—Important People in Science).

A test to determine $\dot{V}O_2$ max generally begins with a submaximal "warm-up" load that may last 3 to 5 minutes. After the warm-up period, the power output can be increased in several ways: (1) the work rate may be increased to a load that in preliminary experiments has been shown to represent a load near the predicted maximal load for the subject, (2) the load may be increased stepwise each minute until the subject reaches a point at which the power output cannot be maintained, or (3) the load may be increased stepwise every 2 to 4 minutes until the subject cannot maintain the desired work rate. When any one of these procedures is carefully followed, it yields approximately the same $\dot{V}O_2$ max as the others (1, 49, 73, 104), although an exercise protocol that does not exceed 10 to 12 minutes seems preferable (10, 49).

The criteria to determine if $\dot{V}O_2$ max has been obtained were discussed in chapter 15. Because of the importance of this measure, some important issues will be reviewed here. The primary criterion to determine if $\dot{V}O_2$ max has been reached during an

Figure 20.2 Changes in oxygen uptake during an incremental cycle ergometer test designed to determine $\dot{V}O_2$ max. The observed plateau in $\dot{V}O_2$ with an increase in work rate is considered to be the "gold standard" for validation of $\dot{V}O_2$ max.

incremental exercise test is a plateau in oxygen uptake with a further increase in work rate (94). This concept is illustrated in figure 20.2. Unfortunately, when testing untrained subjects, a plateau in $\dot{V}O_2$ is rarely observed during an incremental exercise test. Does this mean that the subject did not reach his or her $\dot{V}O_2$ max? This possibility exists, but it is also possible that the subject reached his or her $\dot{V}O_2$ max at the last work rate but could not complete another exercise stage; therefore, a plateau in $\dot{V}O_2$ was not observed. In light of this possibility, several investigators have suggested that the validity of a $\dot{V}O_2$ max test be determined from not one but several criteria. In chapter 15 it was discussed that a blood lactate concentration of >8 mmoles $\cdot$ liter^{-1} during the last stage of exercise could be used as one of the criteria to determine if $\dot{V}O_2$ max had been obtained. However, to avoid the difficulty of taking blood samples and subsequent analysis for lactate levels, investigators have proposed additional criteria that do not involve blood sampling. For example, Williams et al. (100) and McMiken and Daniels (58) have proposed that a $\dot{V}O_2$ max test be judged as valid if any two of the following criteria are met: (1) a respiratory exchange ratio of ≥ 1.15, (2) a heart rate during the last exercise stage that is ± 10 beats per minute within the subject's predicted maximum heart rate, or (3) a plateau in $\dot{V}O_2$ with an increase in work rate.

Determination of Peak $\dot{V}O_2$ in Paraplegic Athletes

Again, by definition, $\dot{V}O_2$ max is the highest $\dot{V}O_2$ that can be attained during exercise using large muscle groups (1). However, subjects with injuries to or paralysis of their lower limbs can have their aerobic fitness evaluated through arm ergometry, which substitutes arm cranking for cycling or running. Given the aforementioned definition of $\dot{V}O_2$ max, the highest $\dot{V}O_2$ obtained during an incremental arm ergometry test is not referred to as $\dot{V}O_2$ max, but is called the peak $\dot{V}O_2$ for arm exercise.

The protocols used to determine peak $\dot{V}O_2$ during arm ergometry are similar in design to the previously mentioned treadmill and cycle ergometer protocols (84, 86). Evidence suggests that in subjects who are not specifically arm trained, a higher peak $\dot{V}O_2$ is obtained during arm ergometry if the test begins at some predetermined load that represents approximately 50% to 60% of peak $\dot{V}O_2$ during arm work (97). A logical explanation for these findings is that an "accelerated" incremental arm testing protocol that rapidly reaches a high power output might limit muscular fatigue early in the test, allowing the subject to reach a higher power output and therefore obtain a higher peak $\dot{V}O_2$.

In an effort to provide a more specific form of testing for paraplegics who are wheelchair racing athletes, some laboratories have modified a wheelchair by connecting the wheels to a cycle ergometer in such a way that the resistance to turn the wheels can be adjusted in the same manner as the load is altered on the cycle ergometer (81). This allows wheelchair athletes to be tested using the exact movement that they use during a race; therefore, it is superior to using arm ergometry to evaluate peak $\dot{V}O_2$ in this population.

IN SUMMARY

- The measurement of $\dot{V}O_2$ max requires the use of large muscle groups and should be specific to the movement required by the athlete in his or her event or sport.
- A $\dot{V}O_2$ max test can be judged to be valid if two of the following criteria are met: (a) respiratory exchange ratio $>1:15$, (b) HR during the last test stage that is ± 10 beats per minute within the predicted HR max, and/or (c) plateau in $\dot{V}O_2$ with an increase in work rate.
- Arm crank ergometry and wheelchair ergometry are commonly used to determine the peak $\dot{V}O_2$ in paraplegic athletes.

LABORATORY TESTS TO PREDICT ENDURANCE PERFORMANCE

Exercise physiologists, coaches, and athletes have actively searched for a single laboratory test that can predict success in endurance events. Numerous tests have been developed in an effort to predict athletic performance. In this section, we describe two well-developed laboratory tests—lactate threshold and critical power—that are useful in predicting endurance performance. Also, another laboratory test to predict performance, called "peak running velocity," is introduced in Research Focus 20.1. Let's begin with a discussion of the lactate threshold.

Use of the Lactate Threshold to Evaluate Performance

Numerous studies have provided evidence that some measure of the maximal steady-state running speed is useful in predicting success in distance running events from 2 miles to the marathon (19, 25, 26, 48–50, 52, 74, 91, 92). The most common laboratory measurement to estimate this maximal steady-state speed is the determination of the lactate threshold. Recall that the lactate threshold represents an exercise intensity wherein blood lactate levels begin to systematically increase. Because fatigue is associated with high levels of blood and muscle lactate, it is logical that the lactate threshold would be related to endurance performance in events lasting longer than 12 to 15 minutes (51). Although much of the research examining the role of the lactate threshold in predicting endurance performance has centered around distance running, the same principles apply to predicting performance in endurance cycling, swimming, and cross-country skiing.

RESEARCH FOCUS 20.1

Measurement of Peak Running Velocity to Predict Performance in Distance Running

The lactate threshold and critical power measurements have generally been used to predict performance in endurance events lasting longer than 20 minutes (e.g., 10-kilometer run). In an effort to develop a laboratory or field test to predict performance in endurance events lasting fewer than 20 minutes (e.g., 5-kilometer run), researchers have developed a test called "peak running velocity" (42, 66, 67, 85). The test is easy to administer and can be performed on a treadmill or track. For example, the measurement of peak running velocity on a treadmill involves a short test of progressively increasing the treadmill speed every 30 seconds (0% grade) until volitional fatigue. Peak running velocity (meters · second^{-1}) is defined as the highest speed that can be maintained for more than 5 seconds' duration (85).

How well does peak running velocity predict performance? In a well-designed study, researchers demonstrated that peak running velocity was an excellent predictor of success in a 5-kilometer run (85). This point is illustrated by the strong correlation between peak running velocity and 5-kilometer race time (see figure 20.3). Surprisingly, similar findings have been reported for longer running events (e.g., 10–90 kilometer) as well (46, 67). Although additional research is required to fully investigate the application of this test to athletic performance, peak running velocity appears to be a promising laboratory or field test to predict endurance performance.

FIGURE 20.3 Relationship between running peak velocity and finish time of a 5-kilometer (km) race. Data from reference (77).

Direct Determination of Lactate Threshold

Similar to the assessment of $\dot{V}O_2$ max, the determination of the lactate threshold requires athletes to be tested in a manner that simulates their competitive movements (i.e., specificity of testing). Testing protocols to determine the lactate threshold generally begin with a 2- to 5-minute warm-up at a low work rate followed by a stepwise increase in the power output every 1 to 3 minutes (76, 92, 95, 98, 99, 104). In general, the stepwise increases in work rate are small in order to provide better resolution in the determination of the lactate threshold (104).

To determine the blood concentration of lactate, blood samples are obtained at each work rate from a catheter (an indwelling tube) placed in an artery or vein in the subject's arm or from a small puncture of the fingertip. After the test, these blood samples are chemically analyzed for lactate, and the concentration at each exercise stage is then graphed against the oxygen consumption at the time the sample is removed. This concept is illustrated in figure 20.4. How is the lactate threshold determined? Recall that the formal definition of the lactate threshold is the point after which there is a systematic and continuous rise in blood lactate concentration. Although several techniques are available, the simplest and most common

Figure 20.4 Typical graph of the changes in blood lactic acid concentrations during an incremental exercise test. The sudden rise in blood lactic acid is called the "lactate threshold."

procedure is to allow two independent investigators to subjectively pick the lactate "breakpoint" by visual inspection of the lactate/$\dot{V}O_2$ plot (22, 76, 98). If the two investigators disagree as to where the threshold occurs, a third investigator is used to arbitrate.

In practice, the lactate "break point" can often be chosen by using a ruler and drawing a straight line through the lactate concentrations at the first several

Section Three Physiology of Performance

work rates. The last point on the line is considered the lactate threshold (figure 20.4). The obvious advantage of this technique is its simplicity. The disadvantage is that not all investigators agree that this procedure yields valid and reliable results (76). In light of this concern, several researchers have proposed that complex computer programs be used to more accurately predict the lactate threshold, or that an arbitrary lactate value (e.g., 4 mM) be used as an indication of the lactate threshold (31, 51).

Prediction of the Lactate Threshold by Ventilatory Alterations

A technique to estimate the lactate threshold that does not require blood withdrawal has obvious appeal to both investigators and experimental subjects. This need for a noninvasive method to determine the lactate threshold has led to the widespread use of ventilatory and gas exchange measures to estimate the lactate threshold. Recall from chapter 10 that the rationale for the use of the "ventilatory threshold" as a "marker" of the lactate threshold is linked to the belief that the increase in blood lactate concentration at the lactate threshold stimulates ventilation via hydrogen ion influence on the carotid bodies. Although there are several noninvasive techniques in use today (4, 13, 87), the least complex procedure to estimate the lactate threshold by gas exchange is to perform an incremental exercise similar to the previously discussed test used to determine the lactate threshold. Upon completion of the test, the minute ventilation at each work rate during the test is graphed as a function of the oxygen uptake. Figure 20.5 illustrates this procedure. Similar to the determination

of the lactate threshold, the usual procedure is to allow two independent researchers to visually inspect the graph and subjectively determine the point where there is a sudden increase in ventilation (figure 20.5). The point at which ventilation increases rapidly is considered the ventilatory threshold and is used as an estimate of the lactate threshold. The error in predicting the lactate threshold from the ventilator threshold is estimated to range from 12–17% (36). Therefore, some authors have criticized this technique for a lack of precision (36, 76). Nonetheless, this procedure has been shown to be useful in predicting success in endurance events (29, 75).

Measurement of Critical Power

Another laboratory measurement that can be used to predict performance in endurance events is critical power. The concept of **critical power** is based upon the notion that athletes can maintain a specific submaximal power output without fatigue (35, 42, 46). Figure 20.6 illustrates the critical power concept for running performance. In this illustration, running speed is plotted on the y-axis, and the time that the athlete can run at this speed prior to exhaustion is plotted on the x-axis. Critical power is defined as the running speed (i.e., power output) at which the running speed/time curve reaches a plateau. Therefore, in theory, the critical power is considered the power output that can be maintained indefinitely (44). In practice, however, this is not the case. In fact, most athletes fatigue within 30 to 60 minutes when exercising at their critical power (35).

Critical power can be determined in the laboratory by having subjects perform a series of five to seven timed exercise trials to exhaustion. This is

Figure 20.5 Example of the ventilatory threshold determination. Note the linear rise in ventilation up to an oxygen uptake of 2.0 liters/minute—above which ventilation begins to increase in an alinear fashion. This break in linearity of ventilation is termed the "ventilatory threshold" and can be used as an estimate of the lactate threshold.

Figure 20.6 Concept of critical power.

generally accomplished over several days of testing. The results are graphed, and critical power is determined by subjective assessment of the point where the power/time curve begins to plateau or by using a mathematical technique (see references (35, 41, 46) for details). Although figure 20.6 illustrates the critical power measurement for running, the same principle of measurement can be applied to other endurance sports (e.g., cycling, rowing, etc.) (35, 40).

How well does critical power predict performance? Several studies have shown that critical power is significantly correlated with performance in endurance events lasting 3 to 100 minutes (e.g., r = 0.67 − 0.85) (35, 40, 42, 46). Therefore, critical power is a useful laboratory predictor of success in endurance sports.

Is critical power a better predictor of success in endurance events than other laboratory measures such as the lactate threshold or $\dot{V}O_2$ max? The answer remains controversial because many investigators report that $\dot{V}O_2$ max is the best single predictor of endurance performance success (17, 18, 28). However, in events lasting approximately 30 minutes, the lactate threshold, $\dot{V}O_2$ max, and critical power appear to be similar in their abilities to predict performance (46). This is not surprising, considering that critical power is dependent upon both $\dot{V}O_2$ max and the lactate threshold. Indeed, critical power is highly correlated to both $\dot{V}O_2$ max and the lactate threshold (46, 62). In other words, a subject with a high $\dot{V}O_2$ max and lactate threshold will also possess a high critical power. See Jones et al. (2010) in the Suggested Readings for more details on the critical power concept.

IN SUMMARY

- Common laboratory tests to predict endurance performance include measurement of the lactate threshold, critical power, and peak running velocity. All these measurements have been proven useful in predicting performance in endurance events.
- The lactate threshold can be determined during an incremental exercise test using any one of several exercise modalities (e.g., treadmill, cycle ergometer, etc.). The lactate threshold represents an exercise intensity at which blood lactate levels begin to systematically increase.
- Critical power is defined as the running speed (i.e., power output) at which the running speed/ time curve reaches a plateau.
- Peak running velocity (meters · second^{-1}) can be determined on a treadmill or track and is defined as the highest speed that can be maintained for more than 5 seconds.

TESTS TO DETERMINE EXERCISE ECONOMY

The topic of exercise economy was first introduced in chapter 1. The economy of a particular sport movement (e.g., running or cycling) has a major influence on the energy cost of the sport and consequently interacts with $\dot{V}O_2$ max in determining endurance performance (15, 21, 51, 61). For example, a runner who is uneconomical will expend a greater amount of energy to run at a given speed than will an economical runner. With all other variables being equal, the more economical runner would likely defeat the less economical runner in head-to-head competition. Therefore, the measurement of exercise economy would seem appropriate when performing a battery of laboratory tests to evaluate an athlete's performance potential.

How is exercise economy evaluated? Conceptually, exercise economy is assessed by graphing energy expenditure during a particular activity (e.g., running, cycling, etc.) at several speeds. In general, the energy costs of running, cycling, or swimming can be determined using similar methods. Let's use running as an example to illustrate this procedure. The economy of running is quantified by measuring the steady-state oxygen cost of running on a horizontal treadmill at several speeds. The oxygen requirement of running is then graphed as a function of running speed (9, 37). Figure 20.7 illustrates the change in $\dot{V}O_2$ in two runners at a variety of running speeds. Notice that at any given speed, runner B requires less oxygen and therefore expends less energy than runner A (i.e., runner B is more economical than runner A). A marked difference in running economy between athletes can have an important impact on performance.

Figure 20.7 An oxygen cost-of-running curve for two subjects. Note the higher $\dot{V}O_2$ cost of running at any given running speed for subject A when compared to subject B. See text for details.

ESTIMATING SUCCESS IN DISTANCE RUNNING USING THE LACTATE THRESHOLD AND RUNNING ECONOMY

Over the past 15 to 20 years, many investigators have tried to apply laboratory tests to predict performance in a variety of sports [see reference (71) for examples]. The sport that has received the most attention is distance running. Theoretically, the prediction of potential performance in any endurance sport involves the use of similar laboratory measurements ($\dot{V}O_2$ max, economy of movement, etc.). We will use distance running as an example of how a sport scientist or coach might use laboratory measurements to estimate an athlete's performance in a particular event. Let's begin our discussion with a brief overview of the physiological factors that contribute to distance running success. As previously mentioned, the best test for determining an endurance runner's potential is $\dot{V}O_2$ max. However, other factors modify the pace that can be maintained for races of different lengths. For example, anaerobic energy contributes significantly to the ability to maintain a specified pace during shorter distance runs (e.g., 1,500 meters) (11, 51). In longer runs (5,000 to 10,000 meters), running economy and the lactate threshold may play important roles in determining success (25, 75, 92). To predict endurance performance, we must determine the athlete's maximal race pace that can be maintained for a particular racing distance.

To illustrate how performance in distance running might be estimated, consider an example of predicting performance in a 10,000-meter race. We begin with an assessment of the athlete's running economy and then perform an incremental treadmill test to determine $\dot{V}O_2$ max and the lactate threshold. The test results for our runner are graphed in figure 20.8. How do we determine the maximal race pace from the laboratory data? Numerous studies have shown that a close relationship exists between the lactate or ventilatory threshold and the maximal pace that can be maintained during a 10,000-meter race (25, 75, 92). For instance, it appears that well-trained runners can run 10,000 meters at a pace that exceeds their lactate threshold by approximately 5 m · min⁻¹ (37, 72). With this information and the data from figure 20.8, we can now predict a finish time for an athlete. First, we examine figure 20.8, part b, to determine the $\dot{V}O_2$ at the lactate threshold. The lactate threshold occurred at a $\dot{V}O_2$ of 40 ml · kg⁻¹ · min⁻¹, which corresponds to a running speed of 200 m · min⁻¹ (part a of figure 20.8). Assuming that the athlete can exceed this speed by 5 m · min⁻¹, the projected average race pace for a 10,000-meter run would be 205 m · min⁻¹. Therefore, an estimate of the athlete's finish time could

Figure 20.8 Incremental exercise test results for a hypothetical runner. These test results can be used to predict performance in an endurance race. See text for details.

be obtained by dividing 10,000 meters by his predicted running speed (m · min⁻¹):

$$\text{Estimated finish time} = 10{,}000 \text{ m} \div 205 \text{ m} \cdot \text{min}^{-1}$$
$$= 48.78 \text{ min}$$

Although theoretical predictions of performance, such as the example presented here, can generally estimate performance with a reasonable degree of precision, a number of outside factors can influence racing performance. For example, motivation and race tactics play an important role in distance running success. Environmental conditions (heat/humidity, altitude, etc.) also influence an athlete's ultimate performance (see chapters 19 and 24). For information on the ability of laboratory testing to predict future champions, see The Winning Edge 20.1.

IN SUMMARY

- Success in an endurance event can be predicted by a laboratory assessment of the athlete's movement economy, $\dot{V}O_2$ max, and lactate threshold. These parameters can be used to determine the maximal race pace that an athlete can maintain for a given racing distance.

Exercise Physiology Applied to Sports—Can Laboratory Testing of Young Athletes Predict Future Champions?

Numerous articles in popular magazines have proclaimed the ability of laboratory testing in children to predict future athletic champions. For example, it has been argued that determination of skeletal muscle fiber type (via a muscle biopsy) in youth athletes can be used to predict the future athletic success of these individuals. The truth is that there are no laboratory measurements that accurately predict the "ultimate" athletic ability of anyone. Indeed, athletic success depends on numerous physiological and psychological factors, many of which are difficult, if not impossible, to measure in the laboratory. As mentioned earlier, the primary benefits of laboratory testing of athletes are to provide the individual with information about his or her strengths and weaknesses in a sport, to offer feedback about the effectiveness of the conditioning program, and to educate the athlete about the physiology of exercise (2). For more details on testing elite young athletes see Barker et al. (2011) in the Suggested Readings.

DETERMINATION OF ANAEROBIC POWER

For the assessment of anaerobic power, it is essential that the test employed use the muscle groups involved in the sport (i.e., specificity) and involve the energy pathways used in the performance of the event. Although several classification schemes have been proposed (6, 33), tests to assess maximal anaerobic power can be generally classified into (1) ultra short-term tests designed to test the maximal capacity of the "ATP-PC system," and (2) short-term tests to evaluate the overall anaerobic capacity, which measures the maximal capacity for ATP production by both the ATP-PC system and anaerobic glycolysis. Remember that events lasting fewer than 10 seconds are believed to principally use the ATP-PC system to produce ATP, while events lasting 30 to 60 seconds utilize anaerobic glycolysis as the major bioenergetic pathway to synthesize ATP. This principle is illustrated in figure 20.9 and should be remembered when designing tests to evaluate an athlete's anaerobic power for a specific sport.

Tests of Ultra Short-Term Maximal Anaerobic Power

Several practical "field tests" have been developed to assess the maximal capacity of the ATP-PC system to produce ATP over a very short time period (e.g., 1 to 10 seconds) (55). These tests are generally referred to as **power tests.** Recall from chapter 1 that power is defined as:

$$\text{Power} = (F \times D) \div T$$

where F is the force generated, D is the distance over which the force is applied, and T is the time required to perform the work.

Figure 20.9 The percent contribution of the ATP-PC system, anaerobic glycolysis, and aerobic metabolism as a function of time during a maximal effort.

Jumping Power Tests For many years, tests such as the standing broad jump and vertical jump have been used as field tests to evaluate an individual's explosive anaerobic power. The standing broad jump is the distance covered in a horizontal leap from a crouched position, whereas the vertical jump is the distance between the standing reach height and the maximum jump-and-touch height. Both tests probably fail to adequately assess an individual's maximal ATP-PC system capacity because of their brief duration. Moreover, neither test is considered a good predictor of running success in a short dash (e.g., 40–100 yards) (80, 88). Nonetheless, the vertical jump test is considered valuable in predicting vertical leaping ability of athletes and is widely used by coaches in professional football, soccer, and basketball as one of the many performance tests used to evaluate athletic potential.

Running Power Tests for American Football The 40-yard dash has been a popular test to evaluate power output in football players for many years. The athlete generally performs two to three timed 40-yard dashes with full recovery between efforts. The fastest time recorded is considered an indication of the individual's power output. Although a 40-yard dash is a rather specific test of power output for football players, there is little evidence that a 40-yard run in a straight line is a reliable predictor of an athlete's success at a particular position. Perhaps a shorter run (e.g., 10–20 yards), with several changes in direction, might provide a more specific test of power output in football players (57).

Stuart and colleagues (90) have proposed a fitness test for football players that is designed to evaluate the athlete's ability to perform repeated short bursts of power. The test is conducted in the following way. After a brief warm-up, the athlete performs a series of ten timed 40-yard dashes (maximum effort), with a 25-second recovery between dashes. The 25-second recovery period is designed to simulate the elapsed time between plays in a football game. The athletes' time for each 40-yard dash is graphed as a function of the trial number. This procedure is illustrated in figure 20.10 where line A represents data from a well-conditioned athlete and line B is data from a less-fit athlete. Notice that both lines A and B have negative slopes (fatigue slope). This demonstrates that each of the two athletes is slowing down with each succeeding 40-yard trial. Athletes who are highly conditioned will be able to maintain faster 40-yard dash times over the ten trials when compared to less-conditioned athletes, and therefore will have a less-negative fatigue slope. In an effort to establish a set of standards for this test, Stuart and co-workers have proposed that athletes be classified into one of four groups on the basis of the maximal

TABLE 20.1	Classification of Fitness Levels for Football Players on the Basis of a Series of 40-Yard Dash Times	
Level	Category	Percentage of Maximal Velocity Maintained*
1	Superior	>90%
2	Good	85%–89%
3	Sub-par	80%–84%
4	Poor	<79%

*The "percentage of the maximal velocity maintained" is calculated by averaging the velocity of the last three trials and dividing by the average velocity over the first three trials. This ratio is then expressed as a percentage. See text for further details.

running velocity percentage that can be maintained over the final three 40-yard dash trials (see table 20.1). At present, levels 1 and 2 are considered acceptable levels of fitness for football players of any position, whereas levels 3 and 4 are labeled as subpar and poor fitness standards, respectively.

Running Tests for Soccer Soccer (called football outside of North America) remains the most popular sport in many countries around the world. Therefore, it is not surprising that numerous performance tests have been developed for soccer players (14, 60, 77, 78). Included in these performance tests are both tests of motor skills required for soccer and fitness tests. The design of a fitness test for soccer is complicated by the fact that soccer is a complex game requiring intermittent bursts of maximal running followed by periods of walking and/or running slowly. Therefore, soccer is a sport that utilizes both anaerobic and aerobic bioenergetic pathways to produce the required ATP. One of the most widely used field tests to determine both performance and metabolic responses of soccer athletes is the Loughborough Intermittent Shuttle Test developed at Loughborough University in England (65). This shuttle run test is designed to simulate the activity pattern of soccer players during a 90-minute match and consists of intermittent shuttle running (i.e., running back and forth) between markers placed 20 meters apart. The Loughborough intermittent shuttle test is performed with the subjects completing the following runs:

- 3 × 20 meters at walking pace
- 1 × 20 meters at maximal running speed with 4-second recovery
- 3 × 20 meters at a running speed corresponding to 55% of individual $\dot{V}O_2$ max
- 3 × 20 meters at a running speed corresponding to 95% of individual $\dot{V}O_2$ max

Figure 20.10 Illustration of the use of a series of timed 40-yard dashes to determine the anaerobic fitness of football players. In this illustration, athlete A shows a small but constant decline in running speed with each additional dash. In contrast, athlete B shows a large systematic decline in speed across dash trials. Therefore, athlete A is considered to be in better condition than athlete B. See text for details.

This block of exercise is repeated continuously for 90 minutes. In practice, the 20-meter distance is marked on the ground (or floor), and walking and running speeds are dictated by audio signals produced from a computer. Sprint times for the maximal 20-meter runs are recorded throughout the test by infrared photoelectric cells and represent one of the measured performance variables. That is, soccer players with the highest fitness levels will be able to maintain a higher percentage of their maximal sprint speed throughout the shuttle test. Further, the total distance covered during the test is also measured as a performance variable. During this shuttle test, it is estimated that 22% of the total exercise time is spent at or above 95% $\dot{V}O_2$ max, whereas the activity level for the remainder of the test is 55% $\dot{V}O_2$ max or below (65). Complete details of the numerous tests used to evaluate soccer performance are beyond the scope of this chapter, and the reader is referred to Castagna et al. (2010), Mirkov et al. (2008), and Psotta et al. (2011) in the Suggested Readings for more details about performance testing of soccer players.

Cycling Power Tests The **Quebec 10-second test** was developed to assess ultra short-term anaerobic power in cyclists (88). The technical error of this test is small, and the procedure is highly reliable (6). The test is performed on a friction-braked cycle ergometer that contains a photocell capable of measuring flywheel revolutions; the number of flywheel revolutions and resistance against the flywheel are electrically relayed to a microcomputer for analysis. The design of the test is simple. After a brief warm-up, the subject performs two all-out 10-second cycling trials separated by a rest period. The initial resistance on the cycle flywheel is determined by the subject's weight (about 0.09 kg per kg of body weight). Upon a verbal start command by the investigator, the subject begins pedaling at 80 rpm, and the load is rapidly adjusted within 2 to 3 seconds of the desired load. The subject then pedals as fast as possible for 10 seconds. Strong verbal encouragement is provided throughout the test. After a 10-minute rest period, a second test is performed and the results of the two tests averaged. The test results are reported in peak joules per kg of body weight and total joules per kg of body weight.

In addition to the evaluation of cyclists, the Quebec 10-second test has been used to test ultra short-term anaerobic power in nonathletes, runners, speed skaters, biathletes, and body builders. For complete details of these results, see Bouchard et al. (6).

Tests of Short-Term Anaerobic Power

As illustrated in figure 20.9, the ATP-PC system for production of ATP during intense exercise is important for short bursts of exercise (1 to 10 seconds),

whereas glycolysis becomes an important metabolic pathway for energy production in events lasting longer than 15 seconds. In an effort to evaluate the maximal capacity for anaerobic glycolysis to produce ATP during exercise, several short-term anaerobic power tests have been developed. Like other performance tests, anaerobic power tests should involve the specific muscles used in a particular sport.

Cycling Anaerobic Power Tests Researchers at the Wingate Institute in Israel have developed a maximal effort cycling test **(Wingate test)** designed to determine both peak anaerobic power and mean power output over the 30-second test. This test has been shown to be highly reproducible (43) and offers an excellent means of evaluating anaerobic power output in cyclists. The test is administered in the following manner. The subject performs a short, 2- to 4-minute warm-up on the cycle ergometer at an exercise intensity sufficient to elevate heart rate to 150 to 160 beats · min^{-1}. After a 3- to 5-minute rest interval, the test begins with the subject pedaling the cycle ergometer as fast as possible without resistance on the flywheel. After the subject reaches full pedaling speed (e.g., 2 to 3 seconds), the test administrator quickly increases the flywheel resistance to a predetermined load. This predetermined load is an estimate (based on body weight) of a workload that would exceed the subject's $\dot{V}O_2$ max by 20% to 60% (see table 20.2). The subject continues to pedal as

TABLE 20.2	The Resistance Setting for the Wingate Test Is Based on the Subject's Body Weight
Subject's Body Weight (kg)	Resistance Setting on the Flywheel (kg)
20–24.9	1.75
25–29.9	2.0
30–34.9	2.5
35–39.9	3.0
40–44.9	3.25
45–49.9	3.5
50–54.9	4.0
55–59.9	4.25
60–64.9	4.75
65–69.9	5.0
70–74.9	5.5
75–79.9	5.75
80–84.9	6.25
>85	6.5

From B. Noble, *Physiology of Exercise and Sport.* Copyright © 1986. The C. V. Mosby Company, St. Louis MO. Reprinted by permission.

rapidly as possible, and the pedal rate is recorded every 5 seconds during the test. The highest power output over the first few seconds is considered the peak power output and is indicative of the maximum rate of the ATP-PC system to produce ATP during this type of exercise. The decline in power output during the test is used as an index of anaerobic endurance and presumably represents the maximal capacity to produce ATP via a combination of the ATP-PC system and glycolysis. The decrease in power output is expressed as the percentage of peak power decline. The peak power output obtained during a Wingate test occurs near the beginning of the test, and the lowest power output is recorded during the last 5 seconds of the test. The difference in these two power outputs (i.e., highest power output minus lowest power output) is then divided by the peak power output and expressed as a percentage. For instance, if the peak power output was 600 watts and the lowest power output during the test was 200 watts, then the decline in power output would be computed as:

$$(600 - 200) \div 600 = .666 \times 100\% = 67\%$$

The 67% decline in power output means that the athlete decreases his or her peak power output by 67% over the 30-second exercise period.

Since the introduction of the Wingate test in the early 1970s, a number of modifications to the original protocol have been proposed (23, 30, 43, 70, 82). An Australian team of sport scientists (30) has developed a new test for the measurement of anaerobic power on a cycle ergometer that involves 60 seconds of maximal exercise and uses a variable resistance loading. The test design permits the measurement of both peak anaerobic power (i.e., peak ATP-PC system power) and mean (glycolytic) power output over the 60-second maximal exercise bout. The test is designed as follows. The subject performs a 5-minute warm-up at a low work rate (e.g., 120 watts). After a 2-minute recovery, the subject begins pedaling as fast as possible with no load against the cycle flywheel. When peak pedaling speed is obtained (i.e., 3 seconds), the investigator quickly increases the load on the flywheel to 0.095 kg resistance per kg of body weight. The subject continues to pedal as fast as possible at this load for 30 seconds; at the 30-second point, the load on the flywheel is reduced to 0.075 kg resistance per kg of body weight for the remainder of the test. The subject's power output during the test is continuously monitored electronically and work output is recorded as peak power output (joules per kg per second) and mean power output (joules per kg per second) during the entire test.

The rationale for the variable load is that although a high resistance is required to elicit maximal anaerobic power, such a resistance is too great for a supramaximal test of 60 seconds' duration (30). By reducing the resistance midway through the test, the workload becomes more manageable, which enables the subject to complete a maximal effort test for the entire 60-second period. The advantage of this test over the Wingate test is that the variable resistance design permits the measurement of peak anaerobic power and maximal anaerobic power over 60 seconds' duration. This type of test would be useful for athletes who compete in events lasting between 45 and 60 seconds. Note that while this test maximally taxes both the ATP-PC system and glycolysis, because of the test duration, the aerobic system is also activated (see chapters 3 and 4). Therefore, although the energy required to perform 60 seconds of maximal exercise comes primarily (e.g., 70%) from anaerobic pathways, the aerobic energy contribution may reach 30%.

Running Anaerobic Power Tests Maximal distance runs from 35 to 800 meters have been used to evaluate anaerobic power output in runners (83, 93, 103). Because such factors as running technique and motivation influence the performance of these types of power tests, the development of appropriate norms has been difficult. Nevertheless, this type of test can be used effectively to determine improvement within individuals as a result of a training regimen. One example of a valid and reliable running anaerobic test is the "running anaerobic sprint test" (RAST) (102). This running anaerobic sprint test is easy to administer and has been reported to be reliable and a good predictor of success in sprint races (103). A brief overview of the test is as follows. Subjects perform a series of six 35-meter maximal sprints with a 10-second recovery between run. Each sprint is timed, and peak power is calculated (power = (body mass $\times$ distance^2)/time^3) for each of the individual sprints. Mean power is then calculated as the average of the peak power of the six runs. The mean power output from this test has been shown to be a moderately good predictor of running performance at 100, 200, and 400 meters (103).

Sport-specific Tests Ultra short-term and short-term sport-specific anaerobic tests can be developed to meet the needs of team sports or individual athletic events not previously discussed here. The tests could attempt to measure the peak power output in a few seconds or measure mean power output during a period of 10 to 60 seconds, depending upon the energy demands of the sport.

Tests could be developed for tennis, basketball, ice skating, swimming, and so on. In some cases, time or distance covered would be the dependent variable measured rather than a direct measurement of power output (6). This type of sport-specific test provides the coach and athlete with direct feedback about the athlete's present level of fitness; subsequent periodic testing can be used to evaluate the success of training programs.

IN SUMMARY

- Anaerobic power tests are classified as (a) ultra short-term tests to determine the maximal capacity of the ATP-PC system and (b) short-term tests to evaluate the maximal capacity for anaerobic glycolysis.
- Ultra short-term and short-term power tests should be sport-specific in an effort to provide the athlete and coach with feedback about the athlete's current fitness level.

EVALUATION OF MUSCULAR STRENGTH

Muscular strength is defined as the maximum force that can be generated by a muscle or muscle group (1). The measurement of muscular strength is a common practice in the evaluation of training programs for football players, shot-putters, weight lifters, and other power athletes. Strength testing can be used to monitor training progress or the rehabilitation of injuries (56). Muscular strength can be assessed by using one of four methods: (1) isometric testing, (2) free-weight testing, (3) isokinetic testing, and (4) variable resistance testing. Before we discuss these methods of strength measurement, let's consider some general guidelines for the selection of a strength-testing method.

Criteria for Selection of a Strength-Testing Method

The criteria for selecting a method of strength testing include the following factors (80): specificity, ease of data acquisition and analysis, cost, and safety. Given the importance of proper strength-test selection, a brief discussion of each of these factors is warranted.

Specificity of strength testing considers the muscles involved in the sport movement, the movement pattern and contraction type, and the velocity of the contraction. For example, the measurement of sport-specific strength should use the muscle groups involved in the activity. Further, the testing mode should simulate the type of contraction used in the sport (isometric vs. dynamic). If the contraction used in the sport is dynamic, further consideration should

be given to whether the contraction is concentric or eccentric. A final level of specificity is the velocity of shortening. There is a degree of velocity specificity in strength training; speed and power athletes perform better on high-velocity power tests than on low (96). Therefore, there is a justification for trying to make the velocity of test contractions similar to those used in the sport.

Factors such as convenience and time required for strength measurements are important considerations when measurements are made on a large number of athletes (47). Currently, a number of companies market strength measurement devices that are interfaced with computer analysis packages. These devices greatly reduce the time required for strength measurement and analysis.

Much of the commercially available computerized equipment for strength measurement is expensive. The high cost of this equipment may prevent its purchase by physical therapy, exercise science, or athletic programs with small budgets. In these cases, the physical therapist, exercise scientist, or coach must choose the best available option within his/her budget.

A final concern for the selection of a strength-testing method is the safety of the technique. Safety should be a key concern for any measurement of strength. Clearly, strength-measurement techniques that put the athlete at high risk of injury should be avoided.

Isometric Measurement of Strength

Measurement of isometric strength requires a device that permits testing of the sport-specific muscle groups. These devices are commercially available from numerous sources. Most of the isometric testing devices available today are computerized instruments that are capable of measuring isometric force in a variety of muscle groups. Figure 20.11 illustrates one of these devices being used to measure leg strength during a knee extension. As the subject generates maximal isometric force, the computerized tensiometer (tension-measuring device) measures the force produced, and this information is recorded and displayed on an electronic panel on the instrument.

The measurement of isometric strength is typically performed at several joint angles. Isometric testing at each joint angle usually consists of two or more trials of maximal contractions (contraction duration of approximately 5 seconds), and the best of these trials is considered to be the measure of strength.

Advantages of isometric testing using computerized equipment include the fact that these tests are generally simple and safe to administer. For example, computerized measurement of isometric strength has been used in physical therapy to evaluate training progress in injured limbs. It has been argued that

Figure 20.11 Use of a commercially available tensiometer to measure static force during a knee extension. Photo courtesy of Biodex Medical Systems, Inc.

The one-repetition maximum (1-RM) method of evaluating muscular strength involves the performance of a single, maximal lift. This refers to the maximal amount of weight that can be lifted during one complete dynamic repetition of a particular movement (e.g., bench press). To test the 1-RM for any given muscle group, the subject selects a beginning weight that is close to the anticipated 1-RM weight. If one repetition is completed, the weight is increased by a small increment and the trial repeated. This process is continued until the maximum lifting capacity is obtained. The highest weight moved during one repetition is considered the 1-RM. The 1-RM test can be performed using free weights (barbells) or an adjustable resistance exercise machine. For more details of the 1-RM test, see Powers et al. (2006) in the Suggested Readings.

Because of safety concerns, some physical therapists and exercise scientists have recommended that a dynamic test consisting of three or six repetitions be substituted for the 1-RM test. The rationale is that the incidence of injury may be less with a weight that can be lifted a maximum of three or six times compared to the heavier weight that can be lifted during a 1-RM contraction.

In addition to the use of free weights or machines, maximal dynamic strength can be measured using dynamometers. A **dynamometer** is a device capable of measuring force. Hand-grip dynamometers have been used to evaluate grip strength for many years. Dynamometers operate in the following way. When force is applied to the dynamometer, a steel spring is compressed and moves a pointer along a scale. By calibrating the dynamometer with known weights, one can determine how much force is required to move the pointer a specified distance on the scale. Figure 20.12 illustrates the use of a hand-grip dynamometer to assess grip strength.

The advantages of dynamic strength testing include low cost of equipment and the fact that force is dynamically applied, which may simulate sport-specific movements. The disadvantages of free-weight testing using a 1-RM technique include the possibility of subject injury and the fact that it does not provide information concerning the force application over the full range of motion. This point will be discussed again in the next section.

since the isometric tensiometer can be used to measure static strength at many different joint angles with a low risk of injury, this technique might be more effective in evaluating strength gains during therapeutic training than conventional weight-lifting tests (57). Disadvantages of isometric testing include the high cost of some commercial devices and the fact that many sport activities involve dynamic movements. Further, because strength differs over the full range of joint movement, isometric measurements must be made at numerous joint angles; this increases the amount of time required to perform a test.

Free-Weight Testing of Strength

The term *isotonic* means constant tension. This term is often applied to conventional weight-lifting exercise because the weight of the barbell or dumbbell remains constant as the weight is lifted over the range of movement. In a strict sense, application of the term *isotonic* to weight lifting is not appropriate because the actual force or torque applied to the weight does not remain constant over the full range of movement. Acceleration and deceleration of the limbs during a weight-lifting movement often cause variation in the force applied. Therefore, in place of the term isotonic, the term **dynamic** is now commonly used to describe this type of muscle activity when exercising with a constant external resistance, such as free weights or weight stacks on machines where the resistance remains constant throughout the range of motion. The most common measure of dynamic strength is the one-repetition maximum, but tests involving three to six repetitions have been employed.

Isokinetic Assessment of Strength

Over the past several years, many commercial computer-assisted devices to assess dynamic muscular force have been developed. The most common type of computerized strength measurement device on the market is an isokinetic dynamometer, which provides variable resistance. The term **isokinetic** means moving at a constant rate of speed. A variable-resistance isokinetic dynamometer is an electronic-mechanical

Figure 20.12 Use of the typical hand-grip dynamometer. Photo courtesy of Lafayette Instrument Company.

Figure 20.13 Use of a commercially available computer-assisted isokinetic dynamometer to measure strength during a knee extension. Photo courtesy of Biodex Medical Systems, Inc.

instrument that maintains a constant speed of movement while varying the resistance during a particular movement. The resistance offered by the instrument is an accommodating resistance, which is designed to match the force generated by the muscle. A force transducer inside the instrument constantly monitors the muscular force generated at a constant speed and relays this information to a computer, which calculates the average force generated over each time period and joint angle during the movement. An example of this type of instrument is pictured in figure 20.13.

A typical computer printout of data obtained during a maximum-effort leg extension on a computerized isokinetic dynamometer is illustrated in figure 20.14. This type of strength assessment provides a great deal more information than that supplied by a 1-RM test. The force curve pictured in figure 20.14 illustrates that the subject generates the smallest amount of force early in the movement pattern and the greatest amount of force during the middle portion of the movement. The 1-RM test provides only the final outcome, which is the maximum amount of weight lifted during this particular movement. That is, a 1-RM test does not provide information about the differences in force generation over the full range of movement. Therefore, a computer-assisted isokinetic instrument appears to offer advantages over the more

traditional 1-RM test. Further, isokinetic strength testing has been shown to be highly reliable (59).

Variable-Resistance Measurement of Strength

Several commercial companies market weight machines that vary the resistance (weight) during dynamic muscular contractions. The measurement of strength using a variable-resistance device is similar in principle to isotonic tests using 1-RM or three to six repetitions, with the exception that the variable-resistance machine creates a variable resistance over the range of movement. This variable resistance is typically achieved via a "cam," which in theory is designed to vary the resistance according to physiological and mechanical factors that determine force generation by muscles over the normal range of movement.

Figure 20.14 Example of a computer printout from a computer-assisted isokinetic dynamometer during a maximal-effort knee extension.

Potential advantages of these devices include the fact that most sport movement patterns are performed using variable forces, and the design of these machines makes adjustment of weight easy; therefore, little time is required for measurement. A disadvantage of these machines is the high cost; this is compounded by the fact that several individual machines are often required to measure strength in different muscle groups. For more details on the evaluation of muscular strength, see Baechle and Earle (2008) in the Suggested Readings.

IN SUMMARY

- Muscular strength is defined as the maximum force that can be generated by a muscle or muscle group.
- Evaluation of muscular strength is useful in assessing training programs for athletes involved in power sports or events.
- Muscular strength can be evaluated using any one of the following techniques: (a) isometric, (b) free-weight testing, (c) isokinetic, or (d) variable-resistance devices.

STUDY QUESTIONS

1. Discuss the rationale behind laboratory tests designed to assess physical performance in athletes. How do these tests differ from general physical fitness tests?
2. Define maximal oxygen uptake. Why might relative $\dot{V}O_2$ max be the single most important factor in predicting distance running success in a heterogeneous group of runners?
3. Discuss the concept of "specificity of testing" for the determination of $\dot{V}O_2$ max. Give a brief overview of the design of an incremental test to determine $\dot{V}O_2$ max. What criteria can be used to determine the validity of a $\dot{V}O_2$ max test?
4. Briefly, explain the technique employed to determine the lactate threshold and the ventilatory threshold.
5. Describe how the economy of running might be evaluated in the laboratory.
6. Discuss the theory and procedures involved in predicting success in distance running.
7. Explain how short-term maximal anaerobic power can be evaluated by field tests.
8. Describe how the Wingate test is used to assess medium-term anaerobic power.
9. Provide an overview of the 1-RM technique to evaluate muscular strength. Why might a computer-assisted dynamometer be superior to the 1-RM technique in assessing strength changes?
10. Discuss the advantages and disadvantages of each of the following types of strength measurement: (1) dynamic, (2) free weights, (3) isokinetic, and (4) variable resistance.

SUGGESTED READINGS

Baechle, T. R., and R. W. Earle, 2000 *Essentials of Strength Training and Conditioning*. Champaign, IL: Human Kinetics.

Bentley, D.J., J. Newell, and D. Bishop. 2007. Incremental exercise test design and analysis: Implications for performance diagnostics in endurance athletes. *Sports Medicine*. 37(7):575–86.

Castagna C., V. Manzi, F. Impellizzeri, M. Weston, and J. C. Barbero Alvarez. 2010. Relationship between endurance field tests and match performance in young soccer players. *J Strength Cond Res* 24:3227–33.

Currell K., and A. E. Jeukendrup. 2008. Validity, reliability and sensitivity of measures of sporting performance. *Sports Med* 38:297–316.

Mirkov D., A. Nedeljkovic, M. Kukolj, D. Ugarkovic, and S. Jaric. 2008. Evaluation of the reliability of soccer-specific field tests. *J Strength Cond Res* 22:1046–50.

Powers, S., S. Dodd, and E. Jackson. 2009. *Total Fitness and Wellness*. San Francisco:Pearson.

Reiman, M., and R. Manske. 2009. *Functional Testing in Human Performance*. Champaign: Human Kinetics.

Van Praagh, E. Anaerobic fitness tests: What are we measuring? *Medicine and Science in Sports and Exercise* 50:26–45, 2007.

Zagatto A. M., W. R. Beck, and C. A. Gobatto. 2009. Validity of the running anaerobic sprint test for assessing anaerobic power and predicting short-distance performances. *J Strength Cond Res* 23:1820–27.

REFERENCES

1. **Åstrand P, and Rodahl K.** *Textbook of Work Physiology.* New York: McGraw-Hill, 1986.
2. **Barker AR, and Armstrong N.** Exercise testing elite young athletes. *Med Sport Sci* 56: 106–125, 2011.
3. **Bassett DR, Jr., and Howley ET.** Limiting factors for maximum oxygen uptake and determinants of endurance performance. *Med Sci Sports Exerc* 32: 70–84, 2000.
4. **Beaver WL, Wasserman K, and Whipp BJ.** A new method for detecting anaerobic threshold by gas exchange. *J Appl Physiol* 60: 2020–2027, 1986.
5. **Bentley DJ, Newell J, and Bishop D.** Incremental exercise test design and analysis: implications for performance diagnostics in endurance athletes. *Sports Med* 37: 575–586, 2007.
6. **Bouchard C.** Testing anaerobic power and capacity. In: *Physiological Testing of the High Performance Athlete*, edited by MacDougall J, Wenger H, and Green H. Champaign: Human Kinetics, 1991, p. 175–222.
7. **Bouckaert J, and Pannier J.** Specificity of $\dot{V}O_{2\ max}$ and blood lactate determinations in runners and cyclists. *International Archives of Physiology and Biochemistry* 93: 30–31, 1984.
8. **Bouckaert J, Pannier JL, and Vrijens J.** Cardiorespiratory response to bicycle and rowing ergometer exercise in oarsmen. *Eur J Appl Physiol Occup Physiol* 51: 51–59, 1983.
9. **Bransford DR, and Howley ET.** Oxygen cost of running in trained and untrained men and women. *Med Sci Sports* 9: 41–44, 1977.

10. **Buchfuhrer MJ, Hansen JE, Robinson TE, Sue DY, Wasserman K, and Whipp BJ.** Optimizing the exercise protocol for cardiopulmonary assessment. J Appl Physiol 55: 1558–1564, 1983.

11. **Bulbulian R, Wilcox AR, and Darabos BL.** Anaerobic contribution to distance running performance of trained cross-country athletes. Med Sci Sports Exerc 18: 107–113, 1986.

12. **Burke EJ.** Validity of selected laboratory and field tests of physical working capacity. Res Q 47: 95–104, 1976.

13. **Caiozzo VJ, Davis JA, Ellis JF, Azus JL, Vandagriff R, Prietto CA, and McMaster WC.** A comparison of gas exchange indices used to detect the anaerobic threshold. J Appl Physiol 53: 1184–1189, 1982.

14. **Castagna C, Manzi V, Impellizzeri F, Weston M, and Barbero Alvarez JC.** Relationship between endurance field tests and match performance in young soccer players. J Strength Cond Res 24: 3227–3233, 2010.

15. **Conley DL, and Krahenbuhl GS.** Running economy and distance running performance of highly trained athletes. Med Sci Sports Exerc 12: 357–360, 1980.

16. **Costill D.** A scientific approach to distance running. Los Altos: Track and Field News Press 1979.

17. **Costill DL.** Metabolic responses during distance running. J Appl Physiol 28: 251–255, 1970.

18. **Costill DL.** The relationship between selected physiological variables and distance running performance. J Sports Med Phys Fitness 7: 61–66, 1967.

19. **Costill DL, Thomason H, and Roberts E.** Fractional utilization of the aerobic capacity during distance running. Med Sci Sports 5: 248–252, 1973.

20. **Currell K, and Jeukendrup AE.** Validity, reliability and sensitivity of measures of sporting performance. Sports Med 38: 297–316, 2008.

21. **Daniels J, and Daniels N.** Running economy of elite male and elite female runners. Med Sci Sports Exerc 24: 483–489, 1992.

22. **Davis JA, Rozenek R, DeCicco DM, Carizzi MT, and Pham PH.** Comparison of three methods for detection of the lactate threshold. Clin Physiol Funct Imaging 27: 381–384, 2007.

23. **Dotan R, and Bar-Or O.** Load optimization for the Wingate Anaerobic Test. Eur J Appl Physiol Occup Physiol 51: 409–417, 1983.

24. **Ebbeling CB, Ward A, Puleo EM, Widrick J, and Rippe JM.** Development of a single-stage submaximal treadmill walking test. Med Sci Sports Exerc 23: 966–973, 1991.

25. **Farrell PA, Wilmore JH, Coyle EF, Billing JE, and Costill DL.** Plasma lactate accumulation and distance running performance. Med Sci Sports 11: 338–344, 1979.

26. **Foster C.** Blood lactate and respiratory measurement of the capacity for sustained exercise. In: Physiological Assessment of Human Fitness, edited by Maud P, and Foster C. Champaign: Human Kinetics, 1995, p. 57–72.

27. **Foster C.** $\dot{V}O_{2\,max}$ and training indices as determinants of competitive running performance. Journal of Sports Sciences 1: 13–27, 1983.

28. **Foster C, Daniels J, and Yarbough R.** Physiological correlates of marathon running and performance. Australian Journal of Sports Medicine 9: 58–61, 1977.

29. **Gaskill SE, Ruby BC, Walker AJ, Sanchez OA, Serfass RC, and Leon AS.** Validity and reliability of combining three methods to determine ventilatory threshold. Med Sci Sports Exerc 33: 1841–1848, 2001.

30. **Gastin P, Lawson D, Hargreaves M, Carey M, and Fairweather I.** Variable resistance loadings in anaerobic power testing. Int J Sports Med 12: 513–518, 1991.

31. **Grant S, McMillan K, Newell J, Wood L, Keatley S, Simpson D, Leslie K, and Fairlie-Clark S.** Reproducibility of the blood lactate threshold, 4 mmol.l(-1) marker, heart rate and ratings of perceived exertion during incremental treadmill exercise in humans. Eur J Appl Physiol 87: 159–166, 2002.

32. **Green H.** What do tests measure? In: Physiological Testing of the High Performance Athlete, edited by MacDougall J, Wenger H, and Green H. Champaign: Human Kinetics, 1991.

33. **Green S.** Measurement of anaerobic work capacities in humans. Sports Med 19: 32–42, 1995.

34. **Hagan RD, Smith MG, and Gettman LR.** Marathon performance in relation to maximal aerobic power and training indices. Med Sci Sports Exerc 13: 185–189, 1981.

35. **Hill DW.** The critical power concept: a review. Sports Med 16: 237–254, 1993.

36. **Hopker JG, Jobson SA, and Pandit JJ.** Controversies in the physiological basis of the 'anaerobic threshold' and their implications for clinical cardiopulmonary exercise testing. Anaesthesia 66: 111–123, 2011.

37. **Hopkins P, and Powers SK.** Oxygen uptake during submaximal running in highly trained men and women. Am Correct Ther J 36: 130–132, 1982.

38. **Hopkins WG, Hawley JA, and Burke LM.** Design and analysis of research on sport performance enhancement. Med Sci Sports Exerc 31: 472–485, 1999.

39. **Hopkins WG, Schabort EJ, and Hawley JA.** Reliability of power in physical performance tests. Sports Med 31: 211–234, 2001.

40. **Housh DJ, Housh TJ, and Bauge SM.** The accuracy of the critical power test for predicting time to exhaustion during cycle ergometry. Ergonomics 32: 997–1004, 1989.

41. **Housh TJ, Cramer JT, Bull AJ, Johnson GO, and Housh DJ.** The effect of mathematical modeling on critical velocity. Eur J Appl Physiol 84: 469–475, 2001.

42. **Hughson RL, Orok CJ, and Staudt LE.** A high velocity treadmill running test to assess endurance running potential. Int J Sports Med 5: 23–25, 1984.

43. **Jacobs I.** The effects of thermal dehydration on performance of the Wingate Anaerobic Test. International Journal of Sports Medicine 1: 21–24, 1980.

44. **Jones AM, Vanhatalo A, Burnley M, Morton RH, and Poole DC.** Critical power: implications for determination of $\dot{V}O_2$ max and exercise tolerance. Med Sci Sports Exerc 42: 1876–1890, 2010.

45. **Kenney WL, and Hodgson JL.** Variables predictive of performance in elite middle-distance runners. Br J Sports Med 19: 207–209, 1985.

46. **Kolbe T, Dennis SC, Selley E, Noakes TD, and Lambert MI.** The relationship between critical power and running performance. J Sports Sci 13: 265–269, 1995.

47. **Kraemer W, and Fry A.** Physiological Assessment of Human Fitness, edited by Maud P, and Foster C. Champaign, IL: Human Kinetics, 1995, p. 115–138.

48. **LaFontaine TP, Londeree BR, and Spath WK.** The maximal steady state versus selected running events. Med Sci Sports Exerc 13: 190–193, 1981.

49. **Lawler J, Powers SK, and Dodd S.** A time-saving incremental cycle ergometer protocol to determine peak oxygen consumption. Br J Sports Med 21: 171–173, 1987.

50. **Lehmann M.** Correlations between laboratory testing and distance running performance in marathoners of similar ability. International Journal of Sports Medicine 4: 226–230, 1983.

51. **Londeree B.** The use of laboratory test results with long distance runners. Sports Medicine 3: 201–213, 1986.

52. **Lorenzo S, Minson CT, Babb TG, and Halliwill JR.** Lactate threshold predicting time trial performance: impact of heat and acclimation. *Journal of Applied Physiology* In press: 2011.

53. **MacDougall J, and Wenger H.** The purpose of physiological testing. In: *Physiological Testing of the High Performance Athlete*, edited by MacDougall J, Wenger H, and Green H. Champaign: Human Kinetics, 1991.

54. **Magel JR, and Faulkner JA.** Maximum oxygen uptakes of college swimmers. *J Appl Physiol* 22: 929–933, 1967.

55. **Margaria R, Aghemo P, and Rovelli E.** Measurement of muscular power (anaerobic) in man. *J Appl Physiol* 21: 1662–1664, 1966.

56. **Mayhew T, and Rothstein J.** Measurement of muscle performance with instruments. In: *Measurement of Muscle Performance with Instruments*, edited by Rothstein J. New York: Churchill Livingstone, 1985, p. 57–102.

57. **McArdle W, Katch F, and Katch V.** *Exercise Physiology: Energy, Nutrition, and Human Performance.* Baltimore: Lippincott Williams & Wilkins, 2001.

58. **McMiken DF, and Daniels JT.** Aerobic requirements and maximum aerobic power in treadmill and track running. *Med Sci Sports* 8: 14–17, 1976.

59. **Meeteren J, Roebroeck ME, and Stam HJ.** Test-retest reliability in isokinetic muscle strength measurements of the shoulder. *J Rehabil Med* 34: 91–95, 2002.

60. **Mirkov D, Nedeljkovic A, Kukolj M, Ugarkovic D, and Jaric S.** Evaluation of the reliability of soccer-specific field tests. *J Strength Cond Res* 22: 1046–1050, 2008.

61. **Morgan DW, and Craib M.** Physiological aspects of running economy. *Med Sci Sports Exerc* 24: 456–461, 1992.

62. **Moritani T, Nagata A, deVries HA, and Muro M.** Critical power as a measure of physical work capacity and anaerobic threshold. *Ergonomics* 24: 339–350, 1981.

63. **Murase Y, Kobayashi K, Kamei S, and Matsui H.** Longitudinal study of aerobic power in superior junior athletes. *Med Sci Sports Exerc* 13: 180–184, 1981.

64. **Mygind E, Larsson B, and Klausen T.** Evaluation of a specific test in cross-country skiing. *J Sports Sci* 9: 249–257, 1991.

65. **Nicholas CW, Nuttall FE, and Williams C.** The Loughborough Intermittent Shuttle Test: a field test that simulates the activity pattern of soccer. *J Sports Sci* 18: 97–104, 2000.

66. **Noakes TD.** Implications of exercise testing for prediction of athletic performance: a contemporary perspective. *Med Sci Sports Exerc* 20: 319–330, 1988.

67. **Noakes TD, Myburgh KH, and Schall R.** Peak treadmill running velocity during the $\dot{V}O_2$ max test predicts running performance. *J Sports Sci* 8: 35–45, 1990.

68. **Noble B.** *Physiology of Exercise and Sport.* St. Louis: C. V. Mosby, 1986.

69. **Pannier JL, Vrijens J, and Van Cauter C.** Cardiorespiratory response to treadmill and bicycle exercise in runners. *Eur J Appl Physiol Occup Physiol* 43: 243–251, 1980.

70. **Parry-Billings M.** The measurement of anaerobic power and capacity: studies on the Wingate Anaerobic Test. *Snipes* J9: 48–58, 1986.

71. **Peronnet F, and Thibault G.** Mathematical analysis of running performance and world running records. *J Appl Physiol* 67: 453–465, 1989.

72. **Pollock ML.** Submaximal and maximal working capacity of elite distance runners. Part I: cardiorespiratory aspects. *Ann N Y Acad Sci* 301: 310–322, 1977.

73. **Pollock ML, Bohannon RL, Cooper KH, Ayres JJ, Ward A, White SR, and Linnerud AC.** A comparative analysis of four protocols for maximal treadmill stress testing. *Am Heart J* 92: 39–46, 1976.

74. **Pollock ML, Jackson AS, and Pate RR.** Discriminant analysis of physiological differences between good and elite distance runners. *Res Q Exerc Sport* 51: 521–532, 1980.

75. **Powers S.** Ventilatory threshold, running economy, and distance running performance of trained athletes. *Research Quarterly for Exercise and Sport* 54: 179–182, 1983.

76. **Powers SK, Dodd S, and Garner R.** Precision of ventilatory and gas exchange alterations as a predictor of the anaerobic threshold. *Eur J Appl Physiol Occup Physiol* 52: 173–177, 1984.

77. **Psotta R, Bunc V, Hendl J, Tenney D, and Heller J.** Is repeated-sprint ability of soccer players predictable from field-based or laboratory physiological tests? *J Sports Med Phys Fitness* 51: 18–25, 2011.

78. **Rampinini E, Bishop D, Marcora SM, Ferrari Bravo D, Sassi R, and Impellizzeri FM.** Validity of simple field tests as indicators of match-related physical performance in top-level professional soccer players. *Int J Sports Med* 28: 228–235, 2007.

79. **Reiman M, and Manske R.** *Functional Testing in Human Performance.* Champaign: Human Kinetics, 2009.

80. **Sale D.** Testing strength and power. In: *Physiological Testing of the High Performance Athlete*, edited by MacDougall J, Wenger H, and Green H. Champaign: Human Kinetics, 1991, p. 21–106.

81. **Sawka MN, Foley ME, Pimental NA, Toner MM, and Pandolf KB.** Determination of maximal aerobic power during upper-body exercise. *J Appl Physiol* 54: 113–117, 1983.

82. **Schenau G.** Can cycle power output predict sprint running performance? *European Journal of Applied Physiology* 63: 255–260, 1991.

83. **Schnabel A, and Kindermann W.** Assessment of anaerobic capacity in runners. *Eur J Appl Physiol Occup Physiol* 52: 42–46, 1983.

84. **Schwade J, Blomqvist CG, and Shapiro W.** A comparison of the response to arm and leg work in patients with ischemic heart disease. *Am Heart J* 94: 203–208, 1977.

85. **Scott BK, and Houmard JA.** Peak running velocity is highly related to distance running performance. *Int J Sports Med* 15. 504–507, 1994.

86. **Shaw DJ, Crawford MH, Karliner JS, DiDonna G, Carleton RM, Ross J, Jr., and O'Rourke RA.** Arm-crank ergometry: a new method for the evaluation of coronary artery disease. *Am J Cardiol* 33: 801–805, 1974.

87. **Sherrill DL, Anderson SJ, and Swanson G.** Using smoothing splines for detecting ventilatory thresholds. *Med Sci Sports Exerc* 22: 684–689, 1990.

88. **Simoneau JA, Lortie G, Boulay MR, and Bouchard C.** Tests of anaerobic alactacid and lactacid capacities: description and reliability. *Can J Appl Sport Sci* 8: 266–270, 1983.

89. **Storer TW, Davis JA, and Caiozzo VJ.** Accurate prediction of $\dot{V}O_2$ max in cycle ergometry. *Med Sci Sports Exerc* 22: 704–712, 1990.

90. **Stuart M, Powers S, and Nelson J.** Development of an anaerobic fitness test for football players. In: Unpublished observations.

91. **Tanaka K, and Matsuura Y.** Marathon performance, anaerobic threshold, and onset of blood lactate accumulation. *J Appl Physiol* 57: 640–643, 1984.

92. **Tanaka K, Matsuura Y, Kumagai S, Matsuzaka A, Hirakoba K, and Asano K.** Relationships of anaerobic threshold and onset of blood lactate accumulation with endurance performance. *Eur J Appl Physiol Occup Physiol* 52: 51–56, 1983.

93. **Taunton JE, Maron H, and Wilkinson JG.** Anaerobic performance in middle and long distance runners. *Can J Appl Sport Sci* 6: 109–113, 1981.

94. **Taylor HL, Buskirk E, and Henschel A.** Maximal oxygen intake as an objective measure of cardio-respiratory performance. *J Appl Physiol* 8: 73–80, 1955.

95. **Thoden J.** Testing aerobic power. In: *Physiological Testing of the High Performance Athlete*, edited by MacDougall J, Wenger H, and Green H. Champaign: Human Kinetics, 1991, p. 107–174.

96. **Thorland WG, Johnson GO, Cisar CJ, Housh TJ, and Tharp GD.** Strength and anaerobic responses of elite young female sprint and distance runners. *Med Sci Sports Exerc* 19: 56–61, 1987.

97. **Walker R, Powers S, and Stuart MK.** Peak oxygen uptake in arm ergometry: effects of testing protocol. *Br J Sports Med* 20: 25–26, 1986.

98. **Wasserman K, Whipp BJ, Koyl SN, and Beaver WL.** Anaerobic threshold and respiratory gas exchange during exercise. *J Appl Physiol* 35: 236–243, 1973.

99. **Weltman A, Snead D, Stein P, Seip R, Schurrer R, Rutt R, and Weltman J.** Reliability and validity of a continuous incremental treadmill protocol for the determination of lactate threshold, fixed blood lactate concentrations, and $\dot{V}O_{2max}$. *Int J Sports Med* 11: 26–32, 1990.

100. **Williams JH, Powers SK, and Stuart MK.** Hemoglobin desaturation in highly trained athletes during heavy exercise. *Med Sci Sports Exerc* 18: 168–173, 1986.

101. **Wyndham CH, Strydom NB, van Rensburg AJ, and Benade AJ.** Physiological requirements for world-class performances in endurance running. *S Afr Med J* 43: 996–1002, 1969.

102. **Zacharogiannis E, Pardisis G, and Tziortzis S.** An evaluation of tests of anaerobic power and capacity. *Med Sci Sports Exerc* 36: S116, 2004.

103. **Zagatto AM, Beck WR, and Gobatto CA.** Validity of the running anaerobic sprint test for assessing anaerobic power and predicting short-distance performances. *J Strength Cond Res* 23: 1820–1827, 2009.

104. **Zhang YY, Johnson MC, II, Chow N, and Wasserman K.** Effect of exercise testing protocol on parameters of aerobic function. *Med Sci Sports Exerc* 23: 625–630, 1991.

21

Training for Performance

■ Objectives

By studying this chapter, you should be able to do the following:

1. Design a sport-specific training program based on an analysis of the energy systems utilized by the activity.
2. Define the terms *overload*, *specificity*, and *reversibility*.
3. Compare and contrast the use of interval training and continuous training in the improvement of the maximal aerobic power in athletes.
4. Discuss the differences between training for anaerobic power and training for the improvement of strength.
5. Discuss the advantages and disadvantages of different equipment types in weight training.
6. Define delayed-onset muscle soreness (DOMS). List the factors that contribute to its development.
7. Discuss the use of static and ballistic stretching to improve flexibility.
8. Discuss the differences between conditioning goals during (1) the off-season, (2) the preseason, and (3) in-season.
9. List and discuss several common training errors.

■ Key Terms

delayed-onset muscle soreness (DOMS)
dynamic stretching
hyperplasia
hypertrophy
overtraining
progressive resistance exercise (PRE)
proprioceptive neuromuscular facilitation (PNF)
repetition
rest interval
set
static stretching
tapering
variable-resistance exercise
work interval

Traditionally, coaches and trainers have planned conditioning programs for their teams by following regimens used by teams that have successful win-loss records. This type of reasoning is not sound because win-loss records alone do not scientifically validate the conditioning programs used by the successful teams. In fact, the successful team might be victorious by virtue of its superior athletes and not its outstanding conditioning program. Without question, the planning of an effective athletic conditioning program can best be achieved by the application of proven physiological training principles. Optimizing training programs for athletes is important because failure to properly condition an athletic team results in a poor performance and often defeat. This chapter presents an overview of how to apply scientific principles to the development of an athletic conditioning program.

TRAINING PRINCIPLES

The overall objective of a sport conditioning program is to improve performance. Depending upon the specific sport, this can be achieved by increasing the muscle's ability to generate force and power, improving muscular efficiency, and/or improving muscular endurance (8, 70). Recall that throughout this book (e.g., chapters 3, 4, and 20), emphasis has been placed on the fact that dissimilar sport activities use different metabolic pathways or "energy systems" to produce the ATP needed for movement. An understanding of exercise metabolism is important to the coach or trainer because the design of a conditioning program to optimize athletic performance requires knowledge of the principal energy systems utilized by the sport. Consider a few examples. The performance of a 60-meter dash uses the ATP-PC system almost exclusively to produce the needed ATP. In contrast, a marathon runner depends on aerobic metabolism to provide the energy needed to complete the race. However, most sport activities use multiple energy pathways. For instance, soccer uses a combination of metabolic pathways to provide the needed ATP. Knowledge of the relative anaerobic-aerobic contributions to ATP production during an activity is the cornerstone of planning a conditioning program. A well-designed conditioning program allocates the appropriate amount of aerobic and anaerobic conditioning time to match the energy demand of the sport. For instance, if an activity derives 40% of its ATP from anaerobic pathways and 60% from aerobic pathways (e.g., 1,500-meter run), the training program should be divided 40%/60% between anaerobic/aerobic training (8). Table 21.1 contains a list of various sports and an estimation of their predominant energy systems. The

TABLE 21.1 The Predominant Energy Systems for Selected Sports

Sport/ Activity	% ATP CONTRIBUTION BY ENERGY SYSTEM		
	ATP-PC	Glycolysis	Aerobic
Baseball	80	15	5
Basketball	80	10	10
Field hockey	60	20	20
Football	90	10	—
Golf (swing)	100	—	—
Gymnastics	90	10	—
Ice hockey:			
Forwards/ defense	80	20	—
Goalie	95	5	—
Rowing	20	30	50
Soccer:			
Goalie/wings/ strikers	80	20	—
Halfbacks	60	20	20
Swimming:			
Diving	98	2	—
50 meters	95	5	—
100 meters	80	15	—
200 meters	30	65	5
400 meters	20	40	40
1,500 meters	10	20	70
Tennis	70	20	10
Track and field:			
100/200 meters	98	2	—
Field events	90	10	—
400 meters	40	55	5
800 meters	10	60	30
1,500 meters	5	35	60
5,000 meters	2	28	70
Marathon	—	2	98
Volleyball	90	10	—
Wrestling	45	55	—

From E. L. Fox and D. K. Mathews, *Interval Training: Conditioning for Sports and General Fitness*. Copyright © 1974 Saunders College Publishing, Orlando FL. Reprinted by permission of the author.

coach or trainer can use this information to allocate the appropriate amount of time to training each energy system.

This discussion does not necessarily imply that power athletes (e.g., sprinters) should not perform aerobic training. On the contrary, aerobic activity during the preseason to strengthen tendons and ligaments is generally recommended for all athletes (90).

Overload, Specificity, and Reversibility

The terms *overload*, *specificity*, and *reversibility* were introduced in chapter 13 and are repeated here only briefly. Recall that an organ system (e.g., cardiovascular, skeletal muscle, etc.) increases its capacity in response to a training overload. That is, the training program must stress the system above the level to which it is accustomed. While a training overload is required to achieve improvements in performance, too much overload can result in overtraining. **Overtraining** is defined as an accumulation of training stress that impairs an athlete's ability to perform training sessions and results in long-term decrements of performance (45). Overtraining is commonly associated with both physiological and psychological symptoms (e.g., chronic fatigue, mood disturbance, etc.). Recovery from overtraining can restore performance capacity but may require several weeks or months of reduced exercise training. A related term, *overreaching*, is also commonly used in the exercise training literature. The definition of overreaching is an accumulation of training stress that results in a short-term decrement in performance capacity with/without reaching the physiological signs and symptoms of overtraining (45). As you can see, these two terms are very similar and it has been argued that overreaching and overtraining studies should be viewed with caution because it is difficult to distinguish between these two terms (45). Therefore, this chapter will refer to an extreme accumulation of training stress as overtraining, and the term overreaching will not be used (23, 24, 86).

The concept of specificity refers not only to the specific muscles involved in a particular movement, but also to the energy systems that provide the ATP required to complete the movement under competitive conditions. Therefore, training programs need to deal with specificity by using not only those muscle groups engaged during competition, but also the energy systems that will be providing the ATP. For instance, specific training for a sprinter would involve running high-intensity dashes. Similarly, specific training for a marathoner would involve long, slow-paced runs in which virtually all the ATP needed by the working muscles would be derived from aerobic metabolism.

When an athlete stops training, the training effect is quickly lost (reversibility). Studies have demonstrated that within 2 weeks after the cessation of training, significant reductions in $\dot{V}O_2$ max can occur (23, 24). A classic study by Saltin and colleagues (86) demonstrated that after 20 days of bed rest, a group of subjects showed a 25% reduction in $\dot{V}O_2$ max and maximal cardiac output. These dramatic decrements in working capacity as a result of inactivity clearly demonstrate the rapid reversibility of training.

Influence of Gender and Initial Fitness Level

At one time, it was believed that conditioning programs for women had special requirements that differed from those used to train men. Today, however, much evidence exists to demonstrate that men and women respond to training programs in a similar fashion (7, 89). Therefore, the same general approach to physiological conditioning can be used in planning programs for men and women. This does not mean that men and women should perform identical exercise training sessions (e.g., same volume and intensity). Indeed, individual training programs should be designed appropriately to match the level of fitness and maturation of the athlete, regardless of gender. Individual "exercise prescriptions" is an important concern in the design of training programs and is discussed in further detail in the next several paragraphs.

It is a common observation that individuals differ greatly in the degree to which their performance benefits from training programs. Many factors contribute to the observed individual variations in the training response. One of the most important influences is the athlete's beginning level of fitness. In general, the amount of training improvement is always greater in those who are less conditioned at the beginning of the training program. It has been demonstrated that sedentary, middle-aged men with heart disease may improve their $\dot{V}O_2$ max by as much as 50%, whereas the same training program in normal, active adults improves $\dot{V}O_2$ max by only 10% to 20% (51). Similarly, conditioned athletes may improve their level of conditioning by only 3% to 5% following an increase in training intensity. However, this 3% to 5% improvement in the trained athlete may be the difference between winning an Olympic gold medal and failing to place in the event.

Influence of Genetics

As discussed in chapter 13, it is clear that genetics plays an important role in how an individual responds to a training program (4, 10, 48, 83). For instance, a person with a high genetic endowment for endurance sports responds differently to endurance training than one with a markedly different genetic profile. Indeed, recent research has provided genetic clues as to why some individuals are "high responders" to training and improve their fitness levels quickly to a greater extent than "low responders" (10). For this reason, and the fact that athletes begin conditioning programs at different levels of fitness, training programs should be individualized. It is unrealistic to expect each athlete on the team to perform the same amount of work or to exercise at the same work rate during training sessions.

Note that while training can greatly improve performance, there is no substitute for genetically inherited athletic talent if the individual is to compete at a world-class level. For example, there is a limit to how much training can improve aerobic power. Therefore, those individuals with a low genetic endowment for aerobic power cannot, under any training program, increase their $\dot{V}O_2$ max to world-class levels. Åstrand and Rodahl (8) have commented that if you want to become a world-class athlete, you must choose your parents wisely.

Similar to aerobic exercise, research indicates that genetics plays a key role in determining the performance level that can be achieved in anaerobic sports (e.g., sprinting in track and field) (13, 67). Indeed, it is well known that training can only improve anaerobic performance to a small degree. The primary reason is that the type of skeletal muscle fiber that is best suited for anaerobic performance (i.e., fast fibers, type IIx) is determined early in development, and the relative percentage of muscle fiber types does not vary widely over the lifetime. Therefore, anaerobic capacity appears to be largely genetically determined because the percentage of fast/anaerobic fibers is a primary determinant of anaerobic capacity.

IN SUMMARY

- The general objective of sport conditioning is to improve performance by increasing muscle force/power output, improving muscular efficiency, and/or improving muscle endurance.
- A conditioning program should allocate the appropriate amount of training time to match the aerobic and anaerobic energy demands of the sport.
- Muscles respond to training as a result of a progressive overload. When an athlete stops training, a rapid decline in fitness occurs due to detraining (reversibility).
- In general, men and women respond to conditioning in a similar fashion. The amount of training improvement is always greater in those individuals who are less conditioned at the onset of the training program.

COMPONENTS OF A TRAINING SESSION: WARM-UP, WORKOUT, AND COOL DOWN

Every training session should consist of three components: (1) warm-up, (2) workout, and (3) cool down. This idea was first introduced in chapter 16 and is mentioned only briefly here. The warm-up prior to a training workout has several important objectives. First, warm-up exercises increase cardiac output and blood flow to the skeletal muscles to be used during the training session. Second, the warm-up activity results in an increase in muscle temperature, which elevates muscle enzyme activity. Third, preliminary exercise affords the athlete an opportunity to perform stretching exercises. The duration of the warm-up may be from 5 to 20 minutes, depending on environmental conditions and the nature of the training activity. Although limited data exist, a recent review concludes that a proper warm-up may reduce the possibility of muscle injury due to pulls or strains (33, 94) and may also improve physical performance (34). Nonetheless, additional research is needed to definitively demonstrate whether a warm-up can deter exercise-induced injuries.

Immediately following the training session, a period of low-intensity "cool-down" exercises should be performed. The principal objective of a cool down is to return "pooled" blood from the exercised skeletal muscles back to the central circulation. Similar to the warm-up, the length of the cool down may vary from 10 to 30 minutes, depending on environmental conditions, the age and fitness level of the individual, and the nature of the training session.

IN SUMMARY

- Every training session should consist of a warm-up period, a workout session, and a cool-down period.
- Although limited data exist, it is believed that a warm-up reduces the risk of muscle and/or tendon injury during exercise.

TRAINING TO IMPROVE AEROBIC POWER

Recall from chapter 13 that endurance training improves $\dot{V}O_2$ max by increasing both maximal cardiac output and the a-$\bar{v}$ O_2 difference (i.e., increasing the muscle's ability to extract O_2). Therefore, a training program designed to improve maximal aerobic power must overload the circulatory system and stress the oxidative capacities of skeletal muscles as well. As in all training regimens, specificity is critical. The athlete should stress the specific muscles to be used in his or her sport. In other words, runners should train by running, cyclists should train on the bicycle, swimmers should swim, and so forth.

There are three principal aerobic training methods used by athletes: (1) interval training, (2) long, slow distance (low-intensity), and (3) high-intensity, continuous exercise. Controversy exists as to which of these training methods results in the greatest improvement in $\dot{V}O_2$ max. Indeed, there does not appear to be a magic training formula for all athletes to follow. However, evidence suggests that training intensity is the most important factor in improving $\dot{V}O_2$ max (50, 76, 77, 81). Nonetheless, from a psychological standpoint, it would appear that a mixing of all three methods would provide the needed variety to prevent the athlete from becoming bored with a single and rather monotonous training program.

Note that improvement of $\dot{V}O_2$ max is only one variable related to endurance. Recall from chapter 20 that although a high $\dot{V}O_2$ max is important for success in endurance events, both movement economy and the lactate threshold are also important variables. Therefore, training to improve endurance performance should not only be geared toward the improvement of $\dot{V}O_2$ max, but should also increase the lactate threshold and improve running economy. A brief discussion of various training methods used to improve endurance performance follows.

Interval Training

Interval training involves the performance of repeated exercise bouts, with brief recovery periods in between. The length and intensity of the **work interval** depends on what the athlete is trying to accomplish. For instance, a longer work interval requires a greater involvement of aerobic energy production, whereas a shorter, more intense interval provides greater participation of anaerobic metabolism. Therefore, interval training that is designed to improve $\dot{V}O_2$ max should generally utilize intervals longer than 60 seconds to maximize the involvement of aerobic ATP production. Further, it is generally believed that high-intensity intervals are more effective in improving aerobic power, and perhaps the lactate threshold, than low-intensity intervals (29, 31, 59). These improvements may be due to the recruitment of fast-twitch (types IIa and IIx) fibers during this type of high-intensity exercise.

One obvious advantage of interval training over continuous running is that this method of training provides a means of performing large amounts of high-intensity exercise in a short time. Further, this training method offers two ways of providing a training overload. For example, the interval training prescription can be modified to provide "overload" in terms of increasing either the total number of exercise intervals performed or the intensity of the work interval. Adjustments to either of these factors allow the coach or athlete to alter the workout plan to accomplish specific training goals. How does one design an interval workout? A complete discussion of the theory and rationale of designing an interval

training program to improve athletic performance is beyond the scope of this chapter; therefore, only an overview of interval training will be provided here. In planning an interval training session, the following variables need to be considered: (1) length of the work interval, (2) intensity of the effort, (3) duration of the rest interval, (4) number of interval sets, and (5) the number of work repetitions. The length of the work interval refers to the distance to be covered during the work effort. In training to improve aerobic power, the work interval should generally last longer than 60 seconds. The intensity of the work effort during interval training can be monitored from a 10-second HR count upon completion of the interval (i.e., 10 sec HR count × 6 = HR per min). In general, exercise HRs should reach 85% to 100% of the maximal HR during interval training. The time between work efforts is termed the **rest interval** and consists of light activity such as walking. The length of the rest interval is generally expressed as a ratio of the duration of the work interval. For example, if the work interval for running 400 meters was 75 seconds, a rest interval of 75 seconds would result in a 1:1 ratio of work to rest. Generally, the rest interval should be at least as long as the work interval (8). In planning an interval training program for athletes who are not already highly trained, a work:rest ratio of 1:3 or 1:2 seems preferable. As a general rule, the HR should drop to approximately 120 beats · min^{-1} near the end of the recovery interval (8).

A **set** is a specified number of work efforts performed as a unit. For instance, a set may consist of 8 × 400-meter runs with a prescribed rest interval between each run. The term **repetition** is the number of work efforts within one set. In the example just given, 8 × 400-meter run repetitions constituted one set. The number of repetitions and sets performed per workout depends on the purpose of the particular training session and the fitness levels of the athletes involved. For more details on interval training, see reference (62).

Long, Slow-Distance Exercise

The use of long, slow-distance (LSD) runs (or cycle rides, long swims, etc.) became a popular means of training for endurance events in the 1970s (21). In general, this method of training involves performing exercise at a low intensity (i.e., 57% $\dot{V}O_2$ max or approximately 70% of max HR) for durations that are generally greater in length than the normal competition distance. Although it seems reasonable that this type of training is a useful means of preparing an athlete to compete in long endurance competitions (marathon running), evidence suggests that short-term, high-intensity exercise is superior to long-term, low-intensity exercise in improving $\dot{V}O_2$ max (50, 51).

One of the historical reasons that researchers have used training sessions of long duration is the common belief that improvements in endurance are proportional to the volume of training performed. Indeed, many coaches and athletes believe that improvements in athletic performance are directly related to how much work was performed during training, and that athletes can reach their potential only by doing long-duration exercise bouts. Evidence by Costill and colleagues (22) contradicts this belief. These workers demonstrated that athletes training 1.5 hours per day performed as well as athletes training 3 hours per day. In fact, the athletes who trained 3 hours per day performed more poorly in some events than the group training 1.5 hours per day. This study illustrates the point that "more" is not always better in endurance training. Therefore, coaches and athletes should carefully consider the volume of training required to reach maximal benefits from long, slow-distance exercise.

High-Intensity, Continuous Exercise

Again, research suggests that continuous, high-intensity exercise is an outstanding means of improving $\dot{V}O_2$ max and the lactate threshold in athletes (25, 27, 30, 40, 50). Although the exercise intensity that promotes the greatest improvement in $\dot{V}O_2$ max may vary from athlete to athlete, it is commonly believed that exercise intensities between 90–100% $\dot{V}O_2$ max are optimal (see figure 21.1) (76). Nonetheless, evidence also indicates that a work rate that is equal to or slightly above the lactate threshold provides improvement in maximum aerobic power (76, 81, 88).

How does the athlete quantify their exercise intensity during a training session? A precise quantification of training intensity during exercise is complicated, but the measurement of exercise heart rate can be used as an estimate of an athlete's relative training

Figure 21.1 Relationship between training intensity and percent improvement in $\dot{V}O_2$ max. Data from references (30, 35, and 59).

intensity. An example of a heart rate-based training intensity scale to prescribe and monitor training of endurance athletes is presented in table 21.2. Obviously, standardizing exercise intensity based on heart rate alone has limitations and fails to account for individual variation among athletes in the relationship between heart rate and blood lactate concentration. Nonetheless, the advantage of this type of intensity scale is the simplicity because athletes can easily measure their heart rates during exercise using electronic heart rate monitors. For more details on using heart rate to monitor training intensity see Seiler (2010) in the Suggested Readings.

Altitude Training Improves Exercise Performance at Sea Level

For many years, endurance athletes believed that living and training at high altitude enhances performance compared to living and training at sea level (69). However, this may not always be true because athletes cannot perform as much high-intensity

---

| TABLE 21.2 | Example of a Five-Zone Intensity Scale to Prescribe and Monitor Exercise |

Training in Athletes

A practical variable to monitor exercise intensity is heart rate expressed as a percent max heart rate. Note that the exercise intensity zones presented in this table are arbitrary, beginning with a relatively low-intensity zone (zone 1) and ending with a high-intensity zone (zone 5). Data are modified from reference (88).

Intensity Zone	% Heart Rate Max	%$\dot{V}O_2$ max	Blood Lactate Levels (mmol · L^{-1})	Typical Training Duration in Zone
1	60–71	50–65	0.8–1.5	1–3 hours
2	72–82	66–80	1.5–2.5	1–2 hours
3	83–87	81–87	2.6–4.0	30–90 min
4	88–92	88–93	4.1–6.0	10–40 min
5	93–100	94–100	>6.1	5–10 min

Dr. Benjamin Levine Is a Pioneer in the Physiology of Training Adaptation

Dr. Benjamin Levine earned his B.S. degree at Brown University and his medical degree from Harvard University. He completed his residency training in internal medicine and cardiology at Stanford University and the University of Texas. Dr. Levine is currently a professor at the University of Texas-Southwestern Medical Center and directs the Institute for Exercise and Environmental Medicine. This institute is a multidisciplinary, integrative physiology research center designed to explore the mechanisms that limit human performance in both health and disease.

Dr. Levine's research has greatly advanced our understanding of the physiology of training adaptation. In this regard, one of Dr. Levine's major contributions is his work on the benefits of altitude training for endurance athletes. Here's the story: For more than 50 years, endurance athletes have used high-altitude training (altitudes >6,000 feet above sea level) in an effort to improve sea-level performance. The rationale for this practice is that both altitude adaptation and hypoxic exercise training have been proposed to improve $\dot{V}O_2$ max and exercise performance. However, hypoxic exercise impairs the athlete's ability to perform high-intensity exercise; therefore, training at altitude may limit exercise-training adaptation. To study this issue, Dr. Levine and his colleague, Dr. James Stray-Gundersen, performed several landmark studies investigating the impact of living and training at high altitude on endurance performance. Their work led to the development of the altitude training modality known as "Live-High, Train-Low." Their studies show that athletes living at high altitudes but performing their training at lower altitudes exhibited improved endurance performance gains compared to athletes who live and train at high altitudes. The Levine/Stray-Gundersen concept of "Live-High, Train-Low" has become the model by which many endurance athletes use altitude training in preparation for major competitions.

In addition to his work on high-altitude training, Dr. Levine has made many other major contributions to our understanding of the physiological adaptations to endurance exercise training. Indeed, his work has greatly improved our knowledge about the cardiovascular adaptation to exercise and the impact of deconditioning (i.e., bed rest and space flight) on the cardiovascular system. Dr. Levine's work has resulted in more than 150 scientific publications, and many of these papers are widely cited in the research literature.

---

exercise training at altitude compared to sea level. Therefore, by performing less training, a form of de-training could actually occur while living and training at altitude. So, how can athletes design a training program to optimize the physiological benefits of living at altitude without the potentially negative de-training effects?

This altitude-training riddle was solved when researchers developed the altitude training modality known as "Live-High, Train-Low" (63) (see A Look Back—Important People in Science). This training program requires the athlete to spend many hours a day resting and sleeping at altitude, but the athlete performs exercise training sessions at a much lower altitude. This approach affords the athlete the benefit of altitude acclimatization, and by training at a low altitude, the athlete's ability to perform intense training sessions is not hampered by high altitude. This type of altitude training program has been shown to provide significant performance gains compared to training and living at sea level (63).

The physiological adaptation responsible for the endurance performance gains achieved from altitude training remains controversial. Nonetheless, it appears that one of the major advantages is that residing at high altitude increases the red blood cell volume, and therefore the oxygen transport capacity of the blood is increased due to a greater hemoglobin concentration (64, 91). For more on altitude adaptation and the Live-High, Train-Low concept, see chapter 24 and Mazzeo (2008) in the References at the end of this chapter (69).

IN SUMMARY

- Historically, training to improve maximal aerobic power has used three methods: (1) interval training, (2) long, slow-distance, and (3) high-intensity, continuous exercise.
- Although controversy exists as to which of the training methods results in the greatest improvement in $\dot{V}O_2$ max, growing evidence suggests that it is intensity and not duration that is the most important factor in improving $\dot{V}O_2$ max.
- The Live-High, Train-Low altitude training program provides significant endurance performance gains compared to training and living at sea level.

INJURIES AND ENDURANCE TRAINING

An important question associated with any type of endurance training is what type of training program presents the lowest risk of injury to the athlete. At present, a clear answer to this question is not available. However, a review of exercise-training-induced injuries suggests that the majority of training injuries are a result of overtraining (e.g., overuse injuries) and occur in the knee (57, 75). The overuse injury can come from either short-term, high-intensity exercise or long-term, low-intensity exercise (75). A commonsense guideline to avoid overuse injuries is to avoid large increases in training volume or intensity. Perhaps the most useful general rule for increasing the training load is the "ten percent rule" (75). In short, the ten percent rule suggests that training intensity or duration should not be increased more than 10% per week to avoid an overtraining injury. For example, a runner running 50 miles per week could increase his/her weekly distance to 55 miles (10% of 50 = 5) the following week.

In addition to overtraining, several other exercise-induced injury risk factors have been identified (75). Among these factors are musculotendonous imbalance of strength and/or flexibility, footwear problems (i.e., excessive wear), anatomical malalignment, poor running surface, and disease (e.g., arthritis, old fracture, etc.) (14).

Note that gender is not an injury risk factor for endurance training (75). Similar to male athletes, it appears that most of the leg injuries in female runners are the result of overtraining (75). This may be especially true for poorly conditioned women beginning training programs.

IN SUMMARY

- The majority of training injuries are a result of overtraining (e.g., overuse injuries) and can come from either short-term, high-intensity exercise or prolonged, low-intensity exercise.
- A useful rule for increasing the training load is the "ten percent rule." The ten percent rule states that training intensity or duration should not be increased more than 10% per week to avoid an overtraining injury.

TRAINING TO IMPROVE ANAEROBIC POWER

Athletic events lasting fewer than 60 seconds depend largely on anaerobic production of the necessary energy. In general, training to improve anaerobic power centers around the need to enhance either the ATP-PC system or anaerobic glycolysis (lactate system) (74). However, some activities require major contributions of both of these anaerobic metabolic pathways to provide the necessary ATP for competition (see table 21.1). Moreover, many activities require ATP production from both aerobic and anaerobic sources. For example, running an 800-meter race is typically performed at a power output that exceeds $\dot{V}O_2$ max by ~30%. Therefore, energy to perform this type of sporting event requires both aerobic and anaerobic energy production.

Anaerobic training is commonly defined as exercise that is performed at intensities above $\dot{V}O_2$ max where the primary aim is to stimulate anaerobic energy production (55). High intensity anaerobic training lasting 2–10 seconds is often termed *speed training*, whereas the term *speed endurance training* is commonly used to describe all forms of anaerobic training lasting longer than 10 seconds (55). Identical to aerobic endurance training, it is critical that the anaerobic training program use the specific muscle groups that are required by the athlete during competition.

Training to Improve the ATP-PC System

Sports such as football, weight lifting, and short dashes in track (100 meters) depend on the ATP-PC system to provide the bulk of the energy needed for competition. Therefore, optimal performance requires a training program that will maximize ATP production via the ATP-PC pathway.

Training to improve the ATP-PC system involves a special type of interval training. To maximally stress the ATP-PC metabolic pathway, short, high-intensity intervals (5 to 10 seconds' duration) using the muscles utilized in competition are ideal. Because of the short durations of this type of interval, limited lactate is produced and recovery is rapid. The rest interval may range between 30 and 60 seconds, depending on the fitness levels of the athletes. For example, a training program for football players might involve repeated 30-yard dashes (with several directional changes), with a 30-second rest period between efforts. The number of repetitions per set would be determined by the athletes' fitness levels, environmental factors, and perhaps other considerations.

Training to Improve the Glycolytic System

After approximately 10 seconds of a maximal effort, there is a growing dependence on energy production from anaerobic glycolysis (32). To improve the capacity of this energy pathway, the athlete must overload

Training to Improve Anaerobic Performance: Questions and Answers with Dr. Michael Hogan

Michael Hogan, Ph.D., *Professor in the Department of Medicine at the University of California–San Diego, is an internationally known exercise physiologist whose research focuses on delivery and utilization of oxygen in skeletal muscle. Dr. Hogan has published more than 100 research articles and his work is widely cited in the scientific literature. Further, he has been a leader in numerous scientific organizations, including the American College of Sports Medicine and the American Physiological Society. In addition to being an internationally known scientist, Dr. Hogan continues to be an active competitor in the pole vault. As a collegiate athlete, Dr. Hogan was a four-year letterman in track and field and a school record holder in the pole vault at the University of Notre Dame. In the years following his graduation from college, Dr. Hogan has continued to train and compete in the pole vault and has recently excelled in both national and international age-group championships in this event. In this box feature, Dr. Hogan answers questions related to training to improve anaerobic power.*

QUESTION: In designing a training program to improve anaerobic power, should weekly training sessions be planned on a "hard-easy" cycle?

ANSWER: Absolutely! This is possibly even more critical in anaerobic power training versus aerobic training. The reason for this is that to improve anaerobic capacity, extremely high-intensity exercise needs to be conducted to totally activate the type IIx fibers within the muscle. Recall from chapter 7 that due to the size principle, type IIx muscle fibers are the last fibers recruited during the muscle activation process. An important component of anaerobic training is to work during the "hard" cycle at an extremely high intensity that subsequently results in increasing muscle fiber size, so that muscle power is increased. A key concern is the duration of the "hard-easy" cycles, as each individual athlete will be very different in how much high-intensity exercise can be endured before the athlete "breaks down" and injury ensues. Knowing the proper balance of "hard-easy" is the difference between an Olympic gold medal and an injured athlete.

QUESTION: In sports or athletic events (e.g., 200-meter dash) that require energy from both the ATP-PC system and glycolysis, is it possible to design a training program to improve energy production from each of these bioenergetic systems?

ANSWER: Yes, these bioenergetic systems can be improved, although not to the degree that adaptation to endurance training (i.e., cardiovascular and oxidative enzyme changes) can be accomplished with aerobic training. The key to anaerobic performance that requires high ATP turnover rates for a short period of time (~30 seconds) is to have as much capacity in the glycolytic and ATP-PC systems and to minimize the factors that lead to fatigue in these short, high-intensity exercise bouts. Studies have demonstrated that glycolytic enzymes can be increased in all fiber-types by high-intensity training, so that more ATP can be generated anaerobically when necessary. Anaerobic training will also slightly improve aerobic capacity of the muscle, which can be important in that any aerobic generation of ATP will result in "sparing" of the ATP-PC and a lower rate of lactate production. Anaerobic training will also improve the speed at which phosphocreatine (PC) can be degraded, so that a faster ATP turnover is possible. It is unclear whether PC levels are affected by training, however creatine supplementation may increase resting levels of PC, thereby potentially improving anaerobic performance.

QUESTION: Recently, much interest has focused upon high-intensity training as a means of improving both anaerobic and aerobic power. Please define high-intensity training and discuss the evidence that this type of training can improve both anaerobic and aerobic bioenergetic systems.

ANSWER: Growing evidence indicates that high-intensity training (HIT), which is characterized by brief repeated bursts of intense exercise (e.g., 30–60 seconds of exercise at 100–120% $\dot{V}O_2$ max), can significantly improve not only anaerobic bioenergetic pathways but maximal aerobic power as well. This has surprised some scientists because, historically, it has been believed that HIT would improve only anaerobic power. Nonetheless, it is now clear that HIT can induce many adaptations in muscle normally associated with traditional endurance exercise training, including increased mitochondrial volume and improved endurance performance.

the "system" via short-term, high-intensity efforts. In general, high-intensity intervals of 20 to 60 seconds' duration are useful in overloading this metabolic pathway.

This type of anaerobic training is both physically and psychologically demanding and thus requires a high commitment on the part of the athlete. Further, this type of training may drastically reduce muscle glycogen stores. For these reasons, athletes often alternate hard-interval training days and light training sessions. For more details on training for improved anaerobic performance, see Ask the Expert 21.1 and Iaia and Bangsbo (2010) in the Suggested Readings.

- Training to improve anaerobic power involves a special type of interval training. In general, the intervals are of short duration and consist of high-intensity exercise (near-maximal effort).

TRAINING TO IMPROVE MUSCULAR STRENGTH

The goal of a strength-training program is to increase the maximum amount of force and power that can be generated by a particular muscle group. In general, any muscle that is regularly exercised at a high intensity (i.e., intensity near its maximum force-generating capacity) will become stronger. Strength-training exercises can be classified into three categories: (1) isometric or static, (2) dynamic or isotonic (includes variable-resistance exercise), and (3) isokinetic. Recall that isometric exercise is the application of force without joint movement, and that dynamic exercise involves force application with joint movement (see chapters 8 and 20). **Variable-resistance exercise** is the term used to describe exercise performed on machines such as Nautilus equipment, which provide a variable amount of resistance during the course of a dynamic contraction. Isokinetic exercise is the exertion of force at a constant speed. Although isometric exercise has been shown to improve strength, isotonic and isokinetic strength training are generally preferred in the preparation of athletes because isometric training does not increase strength over the full range of motion—only at the specific joint angle maintained during training.

What physiological adaptations occur as a result of strength training? This issue was discussed in chapter 13 and will be addressed only briefly here. One of the obvious and perhaps most important physiological changes that occurs following a strength-training program is the increase in muscle mass. Recall from chapter 8 that the amount of force that can be generated by a muscle group is proportional to the cross-sectional area of the muscle (56). Therefore, larger muscles exert greater force than smaller muscles. As discussed in chapter 13, most of the increase in muscle size via resistance training is due to **hypertrophy** (an increase in muscle fiber diameter due to an increase in myofibrils) (2, 3, 87, 89). Nonetheless, research in animals suggests that muscles also increase their size in response to strength training by **hyperplasia** (increase in the number of muscle fibers) (42–44, 58, 87). Although this issue remains controversial, it appears that most of the increase in muscle size due to strength training occurs via hypertrophy (87).

Progressive Resistance Exercise

The most common form of strength training is weight lifting using free weights or various types of weight machines (i.e., dynamic or isokinetic training). To improve strength, weight training must employ the overload principle by periodically increasing the amount of weight (resistance) used in a particular exercise. This method of strength training was first described in 1948 by Delorme and Watkins and is called **progressive resistance exercise (PRE).** Since this early work, numerous other systems of training to improve muscular strength have been proposed, but the concept of PRE is the basis for most weight-training programs.

Resistance training workouts are prescribed around the exercise intensity and the volume of exercise performed. The exercise intensity of resistance training is expressed in terms of the repetitions maximum (RM), where 1 RM is the greatest weight that can be lifted one time using good form. The volume of resistance training is established by the number or repetitions (reps) and sets that are performed. Sets are the number of times a specific exercise is performed, and reps are the number of times a movement is repeated within a set.

General Strength-Training Principles

Muscles increase in strength by being forced to contract at relatively high tensions. If muscles are not overloaded, no improvement in strength occurs. The first application of the overload principle was used by the famous Olympic wrestler, *Milo of Crotona* (500 B.C.). Milo incorporated overload in his training routine by carrying a bull calf on his back each day until the animal reached maturity. Since the days of Milo, athletes have applied the principle of overload to training by lifting heavy objects.

The perfect training regimen for optimal improvement of strength remains controversial. Indeed, there does not appear to be a magic formula for strength training that meets the needs of everyone (1). Therefore, the exercise prescription for strength training should be tailored to the individual. However, a general guideline for a strength-training prescription is as follows: In general, the recommended intensity of training is eight to twelve maximal repetitions (RM) and practiced in multiple sets (1). Rest days between workouts seem critical for optimal strength improvement (1). Therefore, a training schedule of 2–4 days per week is recommended for novice or immediate individuals (1). For advanced weight training, a frequency of 4–6 days per week is recommended when using split routines (i.e., training one to three muscle groups per training session) (1).

A common belief among coaches and athletes is that strength increases in direct proportion to the volume of training (i.e., number of sets performed). Although a physiological link exists between training volume and strength gains, the optimal number of sets to improve strength continues to be debated. Nonetheless, two recent reviews conclude that multiple sets (i.e., 2 or more sets) of resistance exercise results in greater hypertrophy and strength gains compared to one set alone (60, 61). It appears likely that the optimal number of sets for maximal improvement of muscular strength may vary among subjects of different ages and fitness levels (1). Further, it is clear that weight-training programs incorporating extremely high training volumes (e.g., >10 sets) are not required for optimal strength gains (38, 80).

Similar to other training methods, strength training should involve those muscles used in competition.

Indeed, strength-training exercises should stress the muscles in the same movement pattern used during the athletic competition. For instance, a shot-putter should perform exercises that strengthen the specific muscles of the arm, chest, back, and legs that are involved in "putting the shot."

A final concern in the design of strength-training programs for sport performance is that the speed of muscle shortening during training should be similar to those speeds used during the event. For example, many sports require a high velocity of movement. Studies have shown that strength-training programs using high-velocity movements in a sport-specific movement pattern produce superior gains in strength/power-oriented sports. Table 21.3 provides an overview of resistance training guidelines for training programs to

TABLE 21.3 Resistance Training Guidelines for Training Programs That Emphasize Maximal Strength or Muscular Endurance. Data are from reference (1).

Frequency per Week	Number of Sets per Exercise	Number of Repetitions per Set	Intensity (Percentage of 1-RM)	Rest Interval Between Sets
Resistance Training Programs to Maximize Strength Gains				
Novice Trainer				
2–3 total body sessions	1–3	8–12	60–70%	2–3 minutes
Intermediate Trainer				
3 total body sessions 4 split routines	Multiple (>2 sets)	8–12	60–70%	2–3 minutes
Advanced trainer				
4–6 split routines	Multiple (>2 sets)	1–12	80–100% in a periodized program	2–3 minutes
Frequency per Week	Number of Sets per Exercise	Number of Repetitions per Set	Intensity (Percentage of 1-RM)	Rest Interval Between Sets
Resistance Training Programs to Emphasize Muscular Endurance				
Novice trainer				
2–3 total body sessions	Multiple (>2 sets)	10–15	Low (e.g. 30–50%)	1 minute
Intermediate Trainer				
3 total body sessions 4 split routines	Multiple (>2 sets)	10–15	Low (e.g., 30–50%)	1 minute
Advanced Trainer				
4–6 split routines	Multiple (>2 sets)	10–25	Range from 30–60%	1 minute for 10–15 reps 1–2 minutes for 15–25 reps

Note the following definitions: Novice trainer—less than one year of experience with resistance training; Intermediate trainer—2–3 years of experience with resistance training; advanced trainer ≥3 years of experience with resistance training; split routine—body is divided into different areas with each trained in a separate training session.

Periodization of Strength Training

Resistance training workouts are structured around the exercise intensity and "sets" and "reps." Further, when working with athletic populations interested in maximal performance, a strength coach may also specify the rest periods between exercises and sets, the type of muscle action (eccentric or concentric), the number of training sessions per week, and the training volume (the total number of reps done in a workout). Periodized strength training uses these variables (and more) to develop workouts to achieve optimal gains in strength, power, motor performance,

and/or hypertrophy over the course of a season, year, or athletic career (1). Periodization describes a systematic process in which the volume and intensity of training are varied over time. For example, in "linear periodization," the individual is progressed from high volume/low intensity to low volume/high intensity over a specified time period (e.g., months). Are periodized resistance training programs better than nonperiodized programs?

A recent literature review (a meta-analysis) indicates that periodized programs are more effective in promoting

maximal strength than nonperiodized programs for men and women of all age groups and individuals with varying backgrounds in resistance training (i.e., novice or athletes) (84). Consistent with the overload principle, periodization-induced additions to volume, intensity, and frequency resulted in improved strength gains. Several types of periodization have been formulated and are discussed in the American College of Sports Medicine *Position Stand on Progression Models in Resistance Training for Healthy Adults* located in the Suggested Readings.

emphasize gains in maximal strength or muscular endurance. For a complete overview of progression models of strength training see the ACSM position stand (2009) in the Suggested Readings. Further, see the Winning Edge 21.1 for information on Periodization of Strength Training to improve strength gains.

Free Weights Versus Machines

Over the past several years, much controversy has centered around the question of whether training with free weights (barbells) or various types of weight machines (Nautilus, etc.) produces the greater strength gains in athletes. It is clear that both free weights and machines are effective at improving strength. Research shows that free-weight training leads to greater strength improvements in free-weight tests, whereas machine training results in greater strength performance on machine tests (1). When a neutral testing device is used to measure strength, strength improvement from free weights and machines are similar (1, 66). A recent review published by the American College of Sports Medicine concludes that each training mode has some advantages. For example, weight machines are regarded as safer to use, easy to learn, and they allow performance of some exercises that are difficult to achieve with free weights (e.g., knee extension) (1). Advantages of training with free weights include the fact that lifting free weights forces the athlete to control both balance and stabilizing factors. This type of training is useful because most sports require the

athlete to maintain balance and body stability during competition (90). Table 21.4 summarizes some of the advantages and disadvantages of strength training using isometric, dynamic (free weights, Nautilus, etc.), and isokinetic machines.

Concurrent Strength- and Endurance-Training Programs

Strength and endurance training are often done concurrently by athletes and fitness enthusiasts. As discussed in chapter 13, some evidence indicates that performing combined strength- and endurance-training programs may antagonize the strength gains achieved by weight training alone (28, 47, 49, 85). However, whether the combination of weight and endurance training impedes strength gains probably depends on several factors, including the training state of the subjects, the volume and frequency of training, and the way the two training methods are integrated (85). In this regard, Sale (85) has demonstrated that athletes who perform concurrent strength- and endurance-training programs on the same day show a reduction in strength gains compared to athletes performing strength training alone. However, athletes who perform concurrent strength- and endurance-training programs on separate days gain strength as rapidly as athletes performing strength training only (15, 71). Therefore, the current recommendation for the training of power athletes is that the athlete should perform strength- and endurance-training programs on separate days.

Program	Equipment	Advantages	Disadvantages
Isometric	Variety of home-designed devices	Minimal cost; less time required	Not directly applicable to most sport activities; may become boring; progress is difficult to monitor
Dynamic	Free weights	Low cost; specialized exercises may be designed to simulate a particular sport movement; progress easy to monitor	Injury potential due to dropping weights; increase in workout time due to time required to change weights
Dynamic	Commercial weight machines (i.e., Life Fitness®)	Generally safe; progress easy to monitor; small amount of time required to change weight	Does not permit specialized exercise; high cost
Variable resistance	Commercial devices (e.g., Nautilus®)	Has a cam system that provides a variable resistance that changes to match the joint's ability to produce force over the range of motion; progress easy to monitor; safety	High cost; limited specialized exercises
Isokinetic	Commercial isokinetic devices (e.g., Cybex®)	Allows development of maximal resistance over full range of motion; exercises can be performed at a variety of speeds	High cost; limited specialized exercises

TABLE 21.4 Summary of Potential Advantages and Disadvantages of Weight-Training Programs Using Various Types of Equipment

Modified from reference (8).

Gender Differences in Response to Strength Training

It is well established that when absolute strength (i.e., total amount of force applied) is compared in untrained men and women, men are typically stronger. This difference is greatest in the upper body, where men are approximately 50% stronger than women, whereas men are only 30% stronger than women in the lower body (78). This apparent sex difference in strength is eliminated when force production in men and women is compared on the basis of the cross-sectional area of muscle. Figure 21.2 illustrates this point. Notice that as the cross-sectional area of muscle increases (x-axis), the arm flexor strength (y-axis) increases in a linear fashion and is independent of sex. That is, human muscle can generate 3 to 4 kg of force per cm^2 of muscle cross-section regardless of whether the muscle belongs to a male or a female (56).

An often-asked question is "Do women gain strength as rapidly as men when training with weights?" In an effort to answer this question, Wilmore (93) compared the strength change between a group of untrained men and women before and after 10 weeks of isotonic weight training. The results revealed that no differences existed between sexes in the percentage of strength gained during the training period (see figure 21.3). Similar findings have been reported in other studies, and they demonstrate that untrained men and women

Figure 21.2 Arm flexor strength of men and women graphed as a function of muscle cross-sectional area.

Figure 21.3 Strength changes in men and women as a result of a 10-week strength-training program.

respond similarly to weight training (52, 62, 79). However, the aforementioned studies are considered short-term training periods and may not reflect what occurs over long-term training. For instance, it is generally believed that men exhibit a greater degree of muscular hypertrophy than women as a result of long-term weight training. This gender difference in muscular hypertrophy appears to be related to the fact that men have twenty to thirty times higher blood levels of testosterone (52).

Muscle Soreness

It is a common experience for novice weight trainers and sometimes even veteran strength athletes to notice a **delayed-onset muscle soreness (DOMS)** that appears 24 to 48 hours after strenuous exercise. The search for an answer to the question of "What causes DOMS?" has extended over many years. A number of possible explanations have been proposed, including a buildup of lactate in muscle, muscle spasms, and torn muscle and connective tissue. It is clear that lactate does not cause this type of soreness. Based on present evidence, it appears that DOMS is due to tissue injury caused by excessive mechanical force exerted upon muscle and connective tissue (6, 16, 18, 35). Perhaps the strongest data to support this viewpoint come from electron microscopy studies in which electron micrographs taken of muscles suffering from DOMS reveal microscopic tears in these muscle fibers (36).

How does DOMS occur, and what is the physiological explanation for DOMS? Complete answers to these questions are not currently available (for reviews, see references (6, 17, 82)). However, current evidence suggests that DOMS occurs in the following manner (6, 82): (1) strenuous muscular contractions (especially eccentric contractions) result in structural damage in muscle (i.e., disruption of sarcomeres); (2) membrane damage occurs, including damage to the membranes of the sarcoplasmic reticulum; (3) calcium leaks out of the sarcoplasmic reticulum and collects in the mitochondria, which inhibits ATP production; (4) the buildup of calcium also activates enzymes (proteases), which degrade cellular proteins, including contractile proteins (41); (5) membrane damage combines with a breakdown of muscle proteins and results in an inflammatory process, which includes an increase in prostaglandins/histamine production and production of free radicals (19); and finally (6) the accumulation of histamines and edema surrounding muscle fibers stimulates free nerve endings (pain receptors), which results in the sensation of pain in the muscle (see figure 21.4).

How does one avoid being a victim of DOMS following exercise? It appears that DOMS occurs most frequently following intense exercise using muscles that are unaccustomed to being worked (17, 21). Further, eccentric exercise (i.e., lengthening contractions)

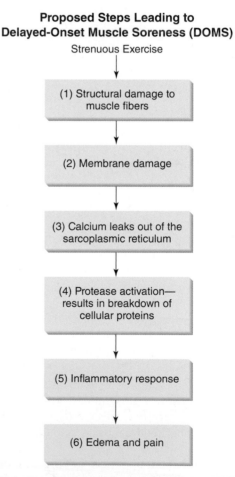

Figure 21.4 Proposed model to explain the occurrence of delayed-onset muscle soreness (DOMS) resulting from strenuous muscular exercise.

appears to cause greater suffering from DOMS than does concentric work. Therefore, a general recommendation for the avoidance of DOMS is to slowly begin a specific exercise during the first five to ten training sessions. This pattern of slow progression allows the exercised muscles to "adapt" to the exercise stress and therefore reduces the incidence or severity of DOMS (see Research Focus 21.1). For more information on DOMS, see Ask the Expert 21.2 and Proske and Allen (2005) in the References (82).

IN SUMMARY

- Improvement in muscular strength can be achieved via progressive overload by using either isometric, isotonic, or isokinetic exercise. Isotonic or isokinetic training seems preferable to isometric exercise in developing strength gains in athletes, because isometric strength gains occur only at the specific joint angles that are held during isometric training.
- Although untrained men exhibit greater absolute strength than untrained females, there do not appear to be gender differences in strength gains during a short-term weight-training program.
- Delayed-onset muscle soreness (DOMS) is thought to occur due to microscopic tears in muscle fibers or connective tissue. This results in cellular degradation and an inflammatory response, which results in pain within 24 to 48 hours after strenuous exercise.

TRAINING TO IMPROVE FLEXIBILITY

Historically, it has been believed that improvement of flexibility via stretching reduces the risk of exercise-induced injury. Nonetheless, at present, limited evidence exists to support the concept that stretching prevents injuries during exercise and participation in many sports (5, 46, 73). Further, a general consensus is that stretching in addition to warm-up does not reduce the risk of overuse injuries(73).

Although improved flexibility may not reduce the risk of exercise-induced injury, the ability to move joints through a full range of motion is important in many sports. Indeed, loss of flexibility can result in a reduction of movement efficiency. Therefore, many athletic trainers and coaches recommend regular stretching exercises to improve flexibility and perhaps optimize the efficiency of movement.

There are two general stretching techniques in use today: (1) **static stretching** (continuously holding a stretch position), and (2) **dynamic stretching** (sometimes referred to as ballistic stretching if movements are not controlled). Although both techniques result in an improvement in flexibility, static stretching is considered to be superior to dynamic stretching because (1) there is less chance of injury (9), (2) static stretching causes less muscle spindle activity when compared to dynamic stretching, and (3) there is less chance of muscle soreness. Stimulation of muscle spindles during dynamic stretching can produce a stretch reflex and therefore result in muscular contraction. This type of muscular contraction counteracts the desired lengthening of the muscle and may increase the chance of injury.

Research has shown that 30 minutes of static stretching exercises performed twice per week will improve flexibility within 5 weeks (26). It is recommended that the stretch position be held for 10 seconds at the beginning of a flexibility program and increased to 60 seconds after several training sessions. Each stretch position should be repeated three to five times, with the number increased up to ten repetitions. Overload is applied by increasing the range of motion during the stretch position and increasing the amount of time the stretch position is held.

Preceding a static stretch with an isometric contraction of the muscle group to be stretched is an effective means of improving muscle relaxation and may enhance the development of flexibility (12, 92). This stretching technique is called **proprioceptive neuromuscular facilitation (PNF).** The procedure generally requires two people and is performed as follows (65): A training partner moves the target limb passively through its range of motion; after reaching the end point of the range of motion, the target muscle is isometrically contracted (against the partner) for 6 to 10 seconds. The target muscle is then relaxed and is again stretched by the partner to a greater range of motion. The physiological rationale for the use of PNF stretching is that muscular relaxation follows an isometric contraction because the contraction stimulates the Golgi tendon organs, which inhibit contraction during the subsequent stretching exercise.

IN SUMMARY

- Limited evidence exists to support the notion that improved joint mobility (flexibility) reduces the incidence of exercise-induced injury.
- Stretching exercises are often recommended to improve flexibility and optimize the efficiency of movement.
- Improvement in flexibility can be achieved via static or dynamic stretching, with static stretching being the preferred technique.

Protection Against Exercise-Induced Muscle Soreness: The Repeated Bout Effect

Performing a bout of unfamiliar exercise often results in muscle injury and delayed-onset muscle soreness (DOMS). This is particularly true when the bout of unfamiliar exercise involves eccentric actions. Interestingly, following recovery from DOMS, a subsequent bout of the same exercise results in minimal symptoms of muscle injury and soreness; this is called the "repeated bout effect" (72). This protective effect of prior exercise has been recognized for more than 40 years. Although many theories have been proposed to explain the repeated bout effect, the specific mechanism responsible for this exercise-induced protection is unknown and continues to be debated. In general, three primary theories have been proposed to explain the repeated bout effect: (1) neural theory, (2) connective tissue theory, and (3) cellular theory (72).

The neural theory proposes that the exercise-induced muscle injury occurs in a relatively small number of active type II (fast) fibers. In the subsequent exercise bout, a change occurs in the pattern of recruitment of muscle fibers to increase motor unit activation to recruit a larger number of muscle fibers. This results in the contractile stress being distributed over a larger number of fibers. Hence, there is a reduction in stress within individual fibers, and no muscle injury occurs during subsequent exercise bouts.

The connective tissue theory argues that muscle damage due to the initial exercise bout results in an increase in connective tissue to provide more protection to the muscle during the stress of exercise. This increased connective tissue is postulated to be responsible for the repeated bout effect.

Finally, the cellular theory predicts that exercise-induced muscle damage results in the synthesis of new proteins (e.g., stress proteins, cytoskeletal proteins, etc.) that improve the integrity of the muscle fiber. The synthesis of these "protective proteins" reduces the strain on the muscle fiber and protects the muscle from exercise-induced injury.

Which of these theories best explains the repeated bout effect is unknown. It seems unlikely that one theory can explain all the various observations associated with the repeated bout effect. Thus, it is possible that the repeated bout effect occurs through the interaction of various neural, connective tissue, and cellular factors that respond to the specific type of exercise-induced muscle injury (72). This idea is summarized in figure 21.5.

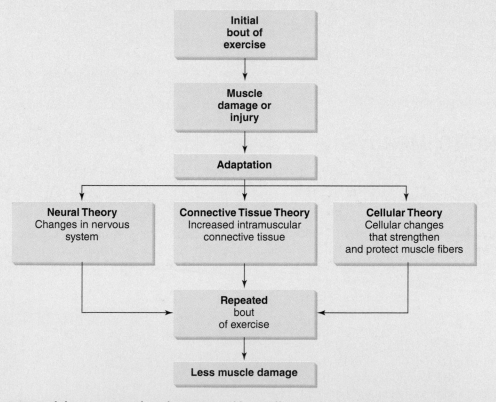

FIGURE 21.5 Proposed theories to explain the "repeated bout effect." Briefly, an initial bout of exercise results in muscle injury. This muscular injury results in a physiological adaptation, which occurs via changes in the nervous system, muscle connective tissue, and/or cellular changes within muscle fibers. One or all of these adaptations serve to protect the muscle from injury during a subsequent bout of exercise. Figure redrawn from McHugh et al. (83).

ASK THE EXPERT 21.2

Exercise-Induced Muscle Soreness:
Questions and Answers with Dr. Priscilla Clarkson

Priscilla M. Clarkson is a Professor of Exercise Science and Associate Dean for the School of Public Health and Health Sciences at the University of Massachusetts–Amherst. She has served as President of the American College of Sports Medicine (ACSM) and has received numerous academic awards, including the National ACSM Citation Award, the New England ACSM Honor Award, the Excellence in Education Award from the Gatorade Sport Science Institute, and the University of Massachusetts Chancellor's Medal.

Professor Clarkson has published more than 100 scientific research articles and has given numerous national and international scientific presentations. The major focus of her research is exercise-induced muscle soreness and damage. In this box feature, she responds to three applied questions related to exercise and muscle soreness.

QUESTION: Several popular fitness publications have suggested that the use of nonsteroidal anti-inflammatory drugs (e.g., ibuprofen) following an intense exercise bout will reduce exercise-induced muscle soreness. Is this concept supported by the research literature?

ANSWER: Studies that have examined the effects of nonsteroidal anti-inflammatory drugs (NSAIDs) on the reduction of muscle soreness after exercise have produced inconsistent results. There are many reasons to explain these inconsistent findings, including the different types and intensities of exercises used to induce soreness, different types of NSAIDs used, and different doses of the NSAID. Another important reason for the lack of consistent results is that the amount of reduction in soreness by the NSAIDs is small, generally less than 15%. On a scale of 1–10 (with 10 being very, very sore), a person who scores an 8 would be expected to see a reduction of soreness to about a 7. This is a small reduction relative to the large inter-

subject variability in the soreness response to the exercise. In other words, some individuals will experience a high degree of soreness while others experience little soreness in response to the same exercise stimulus. Therefore, to detect small differences in soreness due to a treatment, a large population of subjects needs to be tested. Published studies on the effects of NSAIDs on muscle soreness have used sample sizes that are likely too small to provide conclusive evidence.

A key question is whether NSAIDs should even be considered as a treatment to reduce muscle soreness. NSAIDs, like all drugs, have side effects. Given that NSAIDs will only reduce muscle soreness by a small amount and the long-term consequences of NSAID use on muscle recovery are not known, it may be unwise to risk experiencing side effects for so little benefit. Moreover, soreness will dissipate in a couple of days anyway with no intervention. Unless the muscle pain is unbearable, NSAIDs should be used with discretion.

QUESTION: Animal studies suggest that estrogen may protect skeletal muscle from stress-induced injury. This has led to the speculation that women may be protected from exercise-induced muscle injury. Do the studies performed in your laboratory suggest that compared to men, women are less susceptible to exercise-induced muscle damage?

ANSWER: The data from animal models clearly show that estrogen serves a protective role against contraction-induced muscle injury. When these data were first published, it was assumed that women would show less injury in response to eccentric exercise compared with men, because of the higher estrogen levels in women. However, our laboratory examined differences in the development of muscle soreness

and losses in muscle force and range of motion (common indirect indicators of muscle damage) in a large group of men and women both immediately after and during several days following exercise. We found that the men and women experienced a similar degree of soreness and strength loss. However, women actually showed a greater loss in range of motion. Clearly, estrogen does not play the same role in women as has been seen in the animal models of exercise-induced muscle injury.

QUESTION: Some authors have postulated that supplementation with oral creatine could reduce exercise-induced muscle injury by protecting muscle membranes. Research in your laboratory has directly addressed this issue in humans. Based on your data, does creatine supplementation protect skeletal muscle against exercise-induced injury?

ANSWER: To determine whether creatine supplementation would protect against eccentric contraction-induced injury, we had subjects ingest either 20 g creatine or a placebo for 5 days. This dosage has been shown to increase creatine levels in skeletal muscle. After the 5-day supplementation period, subjects performed fifty maximal, eccentric contractions of the elbow flexors. The results indicated that the development of soreness and muscle injury did not differ between the groups. Therefore, these results indicate that creatine supplementation offers no obvious protection against this type of exercise damage to muscle. Any protection offered by an increased amount of creatine in the muscle may be no match for the strain induced by the severe exercise that the subjects performed. Whether using a less-strenuous exercise would have shown any benefits of creatine awaits further study.

YEAR-ROUND CONDITIONING FOR ATHLETES

It is common for today's athletes to engage in year-round conditioning exercises. This is necessary to prevent gain of excessive body fat and to prevent extreme physical detraining between competitive seasons. The training periods of athletes can be divided into three phases: (1) off-season training, (2) preseason training, and (3) in-season training, and can incorporate the periodization techniques discussed earlier in this chapter (see The Winning Edge 21.1). A brief description of each training period follows.

Off-Season Conditioning

In general, the objectives of off-season conditioning programs are to (1) prevent excessive fat weight gain, (2) maintain muscular strength or endurance, (3) maintain ligament and bone integrity, and (4) maintain a reasonable skill level in the athlete's specific sport. Obviously, the exact nature of the off-season conditioning program will vary from sport to sport. For example, a football player would spend considerably more time performing strength-training exercises than would a distance runner. Conversely, the runner would incorporate more running into an off-season conditioning program than would the football player. Hence, specific exercises should be selected on the basis of the sport's demands.

No matter what the sport, it is critical that an off-season conditioning program provide variety for the athlete. Further, off-season conditioning programs generally use a training regimen that is composed of low-intensity, high-volume work. This combination of low-intensity training and variety may prevent the occurrence of "overtraining syndromes" and the development of psychological staleness. Figure 21.6 contains a list of some recommended training activities for off-season conditioning.

Off-season conditioning allows athletes to concentrate on fitness areas where they may be weak.

Therefore, it is important that off-season programs be designed for the individual. For instance, a basketball player may lack leg strength and power and therefore have a limited vertical jump. An off-season conditioning program allows this athlete to engage in specific strength-training activities that will improve leg power and enhance vertical jumping capacity.

Preseason Conditioning

The principal objective of preseason conditioning (e.g., 8 to 12 weeks prior to competition) is to increase to a maximum the capacities of the predominant energy systems used in a particular sport. In the transition from off-season conditioning to preseason conditioning, there is a gradual shift from low-intensity, high-volume exercise to high-intensity, low-volume exercise. As in all phases of a training cycle, the program should be sport specific.

In general, the types of exercise performed during preseason conditioning are similar to those used during off-season conditioning (figure 21.6). The principal difference between off-season and preseason conditioning is the intensity of the conditioning effort. During preseason conditioning, the athlete applies a progressive overload by increasing the intensity of workouts, whereas off-season conditioning involves high-volume, low-intensity workouts.

In-Season Conditioning

The general goal of in-season conditioning for most sports is to maintain the fitness level achieved during the preseason training program. For instance, in a sport such as football, in which there is a relatively long competitive season, the athlete must be able to maintain strength and endurance during the entire season. A complicating factor in planning an in-season conditioning program for many team sports is that the season may not have a clear-cut ending. That is, at the end of the regular season, playoff games may extend the season an additional several weeks. Therefore, it is difficult in these types of sports to plan a climax in the conditioning program, and so there is the need for a maintenance training program.

Suggested Activities for the Various Phases of A Year-Round Training Program

Off-Season	Preseason	In-Season
Weight training	Weight training	Maintenance program
Running	Running	
Skill practice →	Skill practice →	
Participation in other sports	Learning strategies (increased intensity)	

Figure 21.6 Recommended activities for the various phases of year-round training.

IN SUMMARY

- Year-round conditioning programs for athletes include an off-season program, a preseason program, and an in-season program.
- The general objectives of an off-season conditioning program are to prevent excessive fat weight gain, maintain muscular strength and endurance, maintain bone and ligament strength, and preserve a reasonable skill level in the athlete's specific sport.

COMMON TRAINING MISTAKES

Some of the most common training errors include (1) overtraining, (2) undertraining, (3) using exercises and work-rate intensities that are not sport specific, (4) failure to plan long-term training schedules to achieve specific goals, and (5) failure to taper training prior to a competition. Let's discuss each of these training errors briefly.

Overtraining may be a more significant problem than undertraining for several reasons. First, overtraining (workouts that are too long or too strenuous) may result in injury or reduce the athlete's resistance to disease (see chapter 6). Further, overtraining may result in a psychological staleness, which can be identified by a general lack of enthusiasm on the part of the athlete (72). The general symptoms of overtraining include (1) elevated heart rate and blood lactate levels at a fixed submaximal work rate, (2) loss in body weight due to a reduction in appetite, (3) chronic fatigue, (4) psychological staleness, (5) multiple colds or sore throats, and/or (6) a decrease in performance (see figure 21.7). An overtrained athlete may exhibit one or all of these symptoms (11, 37, 53). Therefore, it is critical that coaches and trainers recognize the classic symptoms of overtraining and be prepared to reduce their athletes' workloads when overtraining symptoms appear. Recall that specific training programs should be planned for athletes when possible to compensate for individual differences in genetic potential and fitness levels. This is an important point to remember when planning training programs for athletic conditioning.

For more details on overtraining, see Halson and Jeukendrup (2004) in the References (45).

Another common mistake in the training of athletes is the failure to plan sport-specific training exercises. Often coaches or trainers fail to understand the importance of the law of specificity, and they develop training exercises that do not enhance the energy capacities of the skeletal muscles used in competition. This error can be avoided by achieving a broad understanding of the training principles discussed earlier in this chapter.

Further, coaches, trainers, and athletes should plan and record training schedules designed to achieve specific fitness objectives at various times during the year. Failure to plan a training strategy may result in the misuse of training time and ultimately result in inferior performance.

Finally, failure to reduce the intensity and volume of training prior to competition is also a common training error. Achieving a peak athletic performance requires a healthy blend of proper nutrition, training, and rest. Failure to reduce the training volume and/or intensity prior to competition results in inadequate rest and compromises performance. Therefore, in an effort to achieve peak performance, athletes should reduce their training load for several days prior to competition; this practice is called **tapering.** The goal of tapering is to provide time for muscles to resynthesize glycogen to maximal levels and to allow muscles to heal from training-induced damage. Although the optimum length of a taper period continues to be debated, a reduced training load of 3 to 21 days has been used successfully in both strength and endurance sports (54, 68). Indeed, runners and swimmers can reduce their training load by approximately 60% for up to 21 days without a reduction in performance (20, 39, 54).

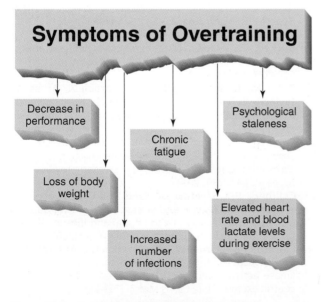

Figure 21.7 Common symptoms of overtraining.

IN SUMMARY

- Common mistakes in training include undertraining, overtraining, performing nonspecific exercises during training sessions, failing to carefully schedule a long-term training plan, and failing to taper training prior to a competition.
- Symptoms of overtraining include (1) elevated heart rate and blood lactate levels at a fixed submaximal work rate, (2) loss in body weight due to a reduction in appetite, (3) chronic fatigue, (4) psychological staleness, (5) increased number of infections, and/or (6) a decrease in performance.
- Tapering is the term applied to short-term reduction in training load prior to competition. Research has shown that tapering prior to a competition is useful in improving performance in both strength and endurance events.

STUDY QUESTIONS

1. Explain how knowledge of the energy systems used in a particular activity or sport might be useful in designing a sport-specific training program.
2. Provide an outline of the general principles of designing a training program for the following sports: (1) football, (2) soccer, (3) basketball, (4) volleyball, (5) distance running (5,000 meters), and (6) 200-meter dash (track).
3. Define the following terms as they relate to interval training: (1) work interval, (2) rest interval, (3) work-to-rest ratio, and (4) set.
4. How can interval training be used to improve both aerobic and anaerobic power?
5. List and discuss the three most common types of training programs used to improve $\dot{V}O_2$ max.
6. Discuss the practical and theoretical differences between an interval training program used to improve the ATP-PC system and a program designed to improve the lactate system.
7. List the general principles of strength development.
8. Define the terms *isometric*, *isotonic*, *dynamic*, and *isokinetic*.
9. Outline the model to explain delayed-onset muscle soreness proposed by Armstrong.
10. Discuss the use of static and dynamic stretching to improve flexibility. Why is a high degree of flexibility not desired in all sports?
11. List and discuss the objectives of (1) off-season conditioning, (2) preseason conditioning, and (3) in-season conditioning.
12. What are some of the more common errors made in the training of athletes?

SUGGESTED READINGS

ACSM. 2009. American College of Sports Medicine position stand. Progression models in resistance training for healthy adults. *Med Sci Sports Exerc* 41:687–708.

Hawley, J. A. 2009. Molecular responses to strength and endurance training: Are they incompatible? *Appl Physiol Nutr Metab* 34:355–61.

Iaia, F. M., and J. Bangsbo. 2010. Speed endurance training is a powerful stimulus for physiological adaptations and performance improvements of athletes. *Scand J Med Sci Sports* 20 Suppl 2:11–23.

Fradkin, A. J., T. R. Zazryn, J. M. Smoglia. 2010. Effects of warming-up on physical performance: A systematic review with meta-analysis. *J Strength Cond Res* 24:140–48.

Krieger, J. W. 2010. Single vs. multiple sets of resistance exercise for muscle hypertrophy: A meta-analysis. *J Strength Cond Res* 24:1150–59.

McHugh, M. P., and C. H. Cosgrave. 2010. To stretch or not to stretch: The role of stretching in injury prevention and performance. *Scand J Med Sci Sports* 20:169–81.

Midgley, A. W., L. R. McNaughton, and A. M. Jones. 2007. Training to enhance the physiological determinants of long-distance running performance: Can valid recommendations be given to runners and coaches based on current scientific knowledge? *Sports Med* 37:857–80.

Midgley, A. W., L. R. McNaughton, and M. Wilkinson. 2006. Is there an optimal training intensity for enhancing the maximal oxygen uptake of distance runners?: Empirical research findings, current opinions, physiological rationale and practical recommendations. *Sports Med* 36:117–32.

Seiler, S. 2010. What is best practice for training intensity and duration distribution in endurance athletes? *Int J Sports Physiol Perform* 5:276–91.

REFERENCES

1. **ACSM.** American College of Sports Medicine position stand. Progression models in resistance training for healthy adults. *Med Sci Sports Exerc* 41: 687–708, 2009.
2. **Alway SE, Sale DG, and MacDougall JD.** Twitch contractile adaptations are not dependent on the intensity of isometric exercise in the human triceps surae. *Eur J Appl Physiol Occup Physiol* 60: 346–352, 1990.
3. **Alway SE, Stray-Gundersen J, Grumbt WH, and Gonyea WJ.** Muscle cross-sectional area and torque in resistance-trained subjects. *Eur J Appl Physiol Occup Physiol* 60: 86–90, 1990.
4. **Amir O, Amir R, Yamin C, Attias E, Eynon N, Sagiv M, Sagiv M, and Meckel Y.** The ACE deletion allele is associated with Israeli elite endurance athletes. *Exp Physiol* 92: 881–886, 2007.
5. **Andersen J.** Stretching before and after exercise: effect on muscle soreness and injury risk. *Journal of Athletic Training* 40: 218–220, 2005.
6. **Armstrong RB.** Mechanisms of exercise-induced delayed onset muscular soreness: a brief review. *Med Sci Sports Exerc* 16: 529–538, 1984.
7. **Astorino TA, Allen RP, Roberson DW, Jurancich M, Lewis R, McCarthy K, and Trost E.** Adaptations to high-intensity training are independent of gender. *Eur J Appl Physiol* 2010.
8. **Åstrand P, and Rodahl K.** *Textbook of Work Physiology.* New York: McGraw-Hill, 1986.
9. **Berger R.** *Applied Exercise Physiology.* Philadelphia: Lea & Febiger, 1982.
10. **Bouchard C, Sarzynski MA, Rice TK, Kraus WE, Church TS, Sung YJ, Rao DC, and Rankinen T.** Genomic predictors of maximal oxygen uptake response to standardized exercise training programs. *J Appl Physiol* 2010.
11. **Bowers R, and Fox E.** *Sports Physiology.* New York: McGraw-Hill, 1992.
12. **Burke E.** Physiological similar effects of similar training programs in males and females. *Research Quarterly* 48: 510–517, 1977.
13. **Calvo M, Rodas G, Vallejo M, Estruch A, Arcas A, Javierre C, Viscor G, and Ventura JL.** Heritability of explosive power and anaerobic capacity in humans. *Eur J Appl Physiol* 86: 218–225, 2002.
14. **Carvalho AC, Junior LC, Costa LO, and Lopes AD.** The association between runners' lower limb alignment with running-related injuries: a systematic review. *Br J Sports Med* 45: 339, 2011.
15. **Chilibeck PD, Syrotuik DG, and Bell GJ.** The effect of concurrent endurance and strength training on quantitative estimates of subsarcolemmal and intermyofibrillar mitochondria. *Int J Sports Med* 23: 33–39, 2002.
16. **Clarkson PM, Byrnes WC, McCormick KM, Turcotte LP, and White JS.** Muscle soreness and serum creatine kinase activity following isometric, eccentric, and concentric exercise. *Int J Sports Med* 7: 152–155, 1986.

17. **Clarkson PM, Nosaka K, and Braun B.** Muscle function after exercise-induced muscle damage and rapid adaptation. *Med Sci Sports Exerc* 24: 512–520, 1992.
18. **Clarkson PM, and Sayers SP.** Etiology of exercise-induced muscle damage. *Can J Appl Physiol* 24: 234–248, 1999.
19. **Close GL, Ashton T, McArdle A, and Maclaren DP.** The emerging role of free radicals in delayed onset muscle soreness and contraction-induced muscle injury. *Comp Biochem Physiol A Mol Integr Physiol* 142: 257–266, 2005.
20. **Costill D.** Effects of reduced training on muscular power in swimmers. *Physician and Sports Medicine* 13: 94–101, 1985.
21. **Costill DL, Coyle EF, Fink WF, Lesmes GR, and Witzmann FA.** Adaptations in skeletal muscle following strength training. *J Appl Physiol* 46: 96–99, 1979.
22. **Costill DL, Thomas R, Roberts RA, Pascoe D, Lambert C, Barr S, and Fink WJ.** Adaptations to swimming training: influence of training volume. *Med Sci Sports Exerc* 23: 371–377, 1991.
23. **Coyle EF, Martin WH, III, Bloomfield SA, Lowry OH, and Holloszy JO.** Effects of detraining on responses to submaximal exercise. *J Appl Physiol* 59: 853–859, 1985.
24. **Coyle EF, Martin WH, III, Sinacore DR, Joyner MJ, Hagberg JM, and Holloszy JO.** Time course of loss of adaptations after stopping prolonged intense endurance training. *J Appl Physiol* 57: 1857–1864, 1984.
25. **Davies CT, and Knibbs AV.** The training stimulus: the effects of intensity, duration and frequency of effort on maximum aerobic power output. *Int Z Angew Physiol* 29: 299–305, 1971.
26. **Deschenes M.** Short review: motor coding and motor unit recruitment pattern. *Journal of Applied Sport Science Research* 3: 33–39, 1989.
27. **Dudley GA, Abraham WM, and Terjung RL.** Influence of exercise intensity and duration on biochemical adaptations in skeletal muscle. *J Appl Physiol* 53: 844–850, 1982.
28. **Dudley GA, and Djamil R.** Incompatibility of endurance-and strength-training modes of exercise. *J Appl Physiol* 59: 1446–1451, 1985.
29. **Fox E, and Mathews D.** *Interval Training: Conditioning for Sports and General Fitness.* Philadelphia: W. B. Saunders, 1974.
30. **Fox EL, Bartels RL, Billings CE, Mathews DK, Bason R, and Webb WM.** Intensity and distance of interval training programs and changes in aerobic power. *Med Sci Sports* 5: 18–22, 1973.
31. **Fox EL, Bartels RL, Billings CE, O'Brien R, Bason R, and Mathews DK.** Frequency and duration of interval training programs and changes in aerobic power. *J Appl Physiol* 38: 481–484, 1975.
32. **Fox EL, Robinson S, and Wiegman DL.** Metabolic energy sources during continuous and interval running. *J Appl Physiol* 27: 174–178, 1969.
33. **Fradkin AJ, Gabbe BJ, and Cameron PA.** Does warming up prevent injury in sport? The evidence from randomised controlled trials? *J Sci Med Sport* 9: 214–220, 2006.
34. **Fradkin AJ, Zazryn TR, and Smoliga JM.** Effects of warming-up on physical performance: a systematic review with meta-analysis. *J Strength Cond Res* 24: 140–148, 2010.
35. **Friden J, and Lieber RL.** Structural and mechanical basis of exercise-induced muscle injury. *Med Sci Sports Exerc* 24: 521–530, 1992.
36. **Friden J, Sjöström M, and Ekblom B.** Myofibrillar damage following intense eccentric exercise in man. *Int J Sports Med* 4: 170–176, 1983.
37. **Fry RW, Grove JR, Morton AR, Zeroni PM, Gaudieri S, and Keast D.** Psychological and immunological correlates of acute overtraining. *Br J Sports Med* 28: 241–246, 1994.
38. **Galvao D, and Taafee D.** Single- vs. multiple-set resistance training: recent developments in the controversy. *Journal of Strength and Conditioning Research* 18: 660–667, 2004.
39. **Gibala MJ, MacDougall JD, and Sale DG.** The effects of tapering on strength performance in trained athletes. *Int J Sports Med* 15: 492–497, 1994.
40. **Gibbons E.** Effects of various training intensity levels on anaerobic threshold and aerobic capacity in females. *Journal of Sports Medicine and Physical Fitness* 23: 315–318, 1983.
41. **Gissel H, and Clausen T.** Excitation-induced Ca^{2+} influx and skeletal muscle cell damage. *Acta Physiol Scand* 171: 327–334, 2001.
42. **Gonyea W, Ericson GC, and Bonde-Petersen F.** Skeletal muscle fiber splitting induced by weight-lifting exercise in cats. *Acta Physiol Scand* 99: 105–109, 1977.
43. **Gonyea WJ.** Role of exercise in inducing increases in skeletal muscle fiber number. *J Appl Physiol* 48: 421–426, 1980.
44. **Gonyea WJ, Sale DG, Gonyea FB, and Mikesky A.** Exercise induced increases in muscle fiber number. *Eur J Appl Physiol Occup Physiol* 55: 137–141, 1986.
45. **Halson SL, and Jeukendrup AE.** Does overtraining exist? An analysis of overreaching and overtraining research. *Sports Med* 34: 967–981, 2004.
46. **Hart L.** Effect of stretching on sport injury risk: a review. *Clin J Sport Med* 15: 113, 2005.
47. **Hawley JA.** Molecular responses to strength and endurance training: are they incompatible? *Appl Physiol Nutr Metab* 34: 355–361, 2009.
48. **Henderson J, Withford-Cave JM, Duffy DL, Cole SJ, Sawyer NA, Gulbin JP, Hahn A, Trent RJ, and Yu B.** The EPAS1 gene influences the aerobic-anaerobic contribution in elite endurance athletes. *Hum Genet* 118: 416–423, 2005.
49. **Hickson RC.** Interference of strength development by simultaneously training for strength and endurance. *Eur J Appl Physiol Occup Physiol* 45: 255–263, 1980.
50. **Hickson RC, Bomze HA, and Holloszy JO.** Linear increase in aerobic power induced by a strenuous program of endurance exercise. *J Appl Physiol* 42: 372–376, 1977.
51. **Hickson RC, Hagberg JM, Ehsani AA, and Holloszy JO.** Time course of the adaptive responses of aerobic power and heart rate to training. *Med Sci Sports Exerc* 13: 17–20, 1981.
52. **Holloway JB, and Baechle TR.** Strength training for female athletes: a review of selected aspects. *Sports Med* 9: 216–228, 1990.
53. **Hooper SL, Mackinnon LT, Howard A, Gordon RD, and Bachmann AW.** Markers for monitoring overtraining and recovery. *Med Sci Sports Exerc* 27: 106–112, 1995.
54. **Houmard JA, Costill DL, Mitchell JB, Park SH, Hickner RC, and Roemmich JN.** Reduced training maintains performance in distance runners. *Int J Sports Med* 11: 46–52, 1990.
55. **Iaia FM, and Bangsbo J.** Speed endurance training is a powerful stimulus for physiological adaptations and performance improvements of athletes. *Scand J Med Sci Sports* 20 Suppl 2: 11–23, 2010.
56. **Ikai M, and Fukunaga T.** Calculation of muscle strength per unit cross-sectional area of human muscle by means of ultrasonic measurement. *Int Z Angew Physiol* 26: 26–32, 1968.

57. **Junior LC, Carvalho AC, Costa LO, and Lopes AD.** The prevalence of musculoskeletal injuries in runners: a systematic review. *Br J Sports Med* 45: 351–352, 2011.

58. **Kelley G.** Mechanical overload and skeletal muscle fiber hyperplasia: a meta-analysis. *J Appl Physiol* 81: 1584–1588, 1996.

59. **Knuttgen HG, Nordesjo LO, Ollander B, and Saltin B.** Physical conditioning through interval training with young male adults. *Med Sci Sports* 5: 220–226, 1973.

60. **Krieger JW.** Single versus multiple sets of resistance exercise: a meta-regression. *J Strength Cond Res* 23: 1890–1901, 2009.

61. **Krieger JW.** Single vs. multiple sets of resistance exercise for muscle hypertrophy: a meta-analysis. *J Strength Cond Res* 24: 1150–1159, 2010.

62. **Laursen PB, and Jenkins DG.** The scientific basis for high-intensity interval training: optimising training programmes and maximising performance in highly trained endurance athletes. *Sports Med* 32: 53–73, 2002.

63. **Levine BD, and Stray-Gundersen J.** Living high-training low: effect of moderate-altitude acclimatization with low-altitude training on performance. *J Appl Physiol* 83: 102–112, 1997.

64. **Levine BD, and Stray-Gundersen J.** Point: positive effects of intermittent hypoxia (live high: train low) on exercise performance are mediated primarily by augmented red cell volume. *J Appl Physiol* 99: 2053–2055, 2005.

65. **Liemohn W, and Sharpe G.** Muscular strength and endurance, flexibility, and low-back function. In: *Health/Fitness Instructor's Handbook*, edited by Howley E, and Frank D. Champaign: Human Kinetics, 1992, p. 179–196.

66. **Manning RJ, Graves JE, Carpenter DM, Leggett SH, and Pollock ML.** Constant vs variable resistance knee extension training. *Med Sci Sports Exerc* 22: 397–401, 1990.

67. **Maridaki M.** Heritability of neuromuscular performance and anaerobic power in preadolescent and adolescent girls. *J Sports Med Phys Fitness* 46: 540–547, 2006.

68. **Martin DT, Scifres JC, Zimmerman SD, and Wilkinson JG.** Effects of interval training and a taper on cycling performance and isokinetic leg strength. *Int J Sports Med* 15: 485–491, 1994.

69. **Mazzeo RS.** Physiological responses to exercise at altitude: an update. *Sports Med* 38: 1–8, 2008.

70. **McArdle W, Katch F, and Katch V.** *Exercise Physiology: Energy, Nutrition, and Human Performance.* Baltimore: Lippincott Williams & Wilkins, 1996.

71. **McCarthy JP, Pozniak MA, and Agre JC.** Neuromuscular adaptations to concurrent strength and endurance training. *Med Sci Sports Exerc* 34: 511–519, 2002.

72. **McHugh MP, Connolly DA, Eston RG, and Gleim GW.** Exercise-induced muscle damage and potential mechanisms for the repeated bout effect. *Sports Med* 27: 157–170, 1999.

73. **McHugh MP, and Cosgrave CH.** To stretch or not to stretch: the role of stretching in injury prevention and performance. *Scand J Med Sci Sports* 20: 169–181, 2010.

74. **Medbo JI, and Burgers S.** Effect of training on the anaerobic capacity. *Med Sci Sports Exerc* 22: 501–507, 1990.

75. **Micheli L.** Injuries and prolonged exercise. In: *Prolonged Exercise*, edited by Lamb D, and Murray R. Indianapolis: Benchmark Press, 1988, p. 393–407.

76. **Midgley AW, McNaughton LR, and Jones AM.** Training to enhance the physiological determinants of long-distance running performance: can valid recommendations be given to runners and coaches based on current scientific knowledge? *Sports Med* 37: 857–880, 2007.

77. **Midgley AW, McNaughton LR, and Wilkinson M.** Is there an optimal training intensity for enhancing the maximal oxygen uptake of distance runners?: empirical research findings, current opinions, physiological rationale and practical recommendations. *Sports Med* 36: 117–132, 2006.

78. **Morrow JR, Jr., and Hosler WW.** Strength comparisons in untrained men and trained women athletes. *Med Sci Sports Exerc* 13: 194–197, 1981.

79. **O'Shea J, and Wegner J.** Power weight training in the female athlete. *Physician and Sports Medicine* 9: 109–114, 1981.

80. **Peterson MD, Rhea MR, and Alvar BA.** Applications of the dose-response for muscular strength development: a review of meta-analytic efficacy and reliability for designing training prescription. *J Strength Cond Res* 19: 950–958, 2005.

81. **Priest JW, and Hagan RD.** The effects of maximum steady state pace training on running performance. *Br J Sports Med* 21: 18–21, 1987.

82. **Proske U, and Allen TJ.** Damage to skeletal muscle from eccentric exercise. *Exerc Sport Sci Rev* 33: 98–104, 2005.

83. **Rankinen T, Bray MS, Hagberg JM, Perusse L, Roth SM, Wolfarth B, and Bouchard C.** The human gene map for performance and health-related fitness phenotypes: the 2005 update. *Med Sci Sports Exerc* 38: 1863–1888, 2006.

84. **Rhea MR, and Alderman BL.** A meta-analysis of periodized versus nonperiodized strength and power training programs. *Res Q Exerc Sport* 75: 413–422, 2004.

85. **Sale DG, Jacobs I, MacDougall JD, and Garner S.** Comparison of two regimens of concurrent strength and endurance training. *Med Sci Sports Exerc* 22: 348–356, 1990.

86. **Saltin B, Blomqvist G, Mitchell JH, Johnson RL, Jr., Wildenthal K, and Chapman CB.** Response to exercise after bed rest and after training. *Circulation* 38: VII 1–78, 1968.

87. **Schoenfeld BJ.** Squatting kinematics and kinetics and their application to exercise performance. *J Strength Cond Res* 24: 3497–3506, 2010.

88. **Seiler S.** What is best practice for training intensity and duration distribution in endurance athletes? *Int J Sports Physiol Perform* 5: 276–291, 2010.

89. **Staron RS, Malicky ES, Leonardi MJ, Falkel JE, Hagerman FC, and Dudley GA.** Muscle hypertrophy and fast fiber type conversions in heavy resistance-trained women. *Eur J Appl Physiol Occup Physiol* 60: 71–79, 1990.

90. **Stone M, and O'Bryant H.** *Weight Training: A Scientific Approach.* Minneapolis: Burgess, 1986.

91. **Wehrlin JP, Zuest P, Hallen J, and Marti B.** Live high-train low for 24 days increases hemoglobin mass and red cell volume in elite endurance athletes. *J Appl Physiol* 100: 1938–1945, 2006.

92. **Wilmore J, and Costill D.** *Training for Sport and Activity.* New York: McGraw-Hill, 1993.

93. **Wilmore JH.** Alterations in strength, body composition and anthropometric measurements consequent to a 10-week weight training program. *Med Sci Sports* 6: 133–138, 1974.

94. **Woods K, Bishop P, and Jones E.** Warm-up and stretching in the prevention of muscular injury. *Sports Med* 37: 1089–1099, 2007.

22

Training for the Female Athlete, Children, Special Populations, and the Masters Athlete

■ Objectives

By studying this chapter, you should be able to do the following:

1. Describe the incidence of amenorrhea in female athletes versus the general population.
2. List those factors thought to contribute to "athletic" amenorrhea.
3. Discuss the general recommendations for training during menstruation.
4. List the general guidelines for exercise during pregnancy.
5. Define the term *female athlete triad*.
6. Discuss the possibility that chronic exercise presents a danger to (1) the cardiopulmonary system or (2) the musculoskeletal system of children.
7. List those conditions in type 1 diabetics that might limit their participation in a vigorous training program.
8. Explain the rationale for the selection of an insulin injection site for type 1 diabetics prior to a training session.
9. List the precautions that asthmatics should take during a training session.
10. Discuss the question "Does exercise promote seizures in epileptics?"
11. Graph the change in muscle mass and muscular strength that occur with age.
12. Discuss the factors that contribute to the age-related changes in muscle mass and muscular strength.
13. Discuss the impact of aging on $\dot{V}O_2$ max in both men and women.
14. Outline the factor(s) that are responsible for the age-related decline in endurance performance.

■ Outline

amenorrhea	bulimia	female athlete triad
anorexia nervosa	dysmenorrhea	growth plate (epiphyseal plate)
articular cartilage	epilepsy	sarcopenia

Certainly the general physiological principles of exercise training to improve performance apply to anyone interested in improving athletic performance (see chapter 21). However, when planning competitive training programs for special populations, several specific issues require individual consideration. For example, special training concerns exist for both the female athlete and children. Also, there are specific guidelines for the training of diabetics, asthmatics, and epileptics. Finally, a growing number of masters athletes are competing in endurance events. How does aging impact their physiological capability and ability to train? This chapter addresses each of these issues. Let's begin our discussion with the topic of exercise training for the female athlete.

FACTORS IMPORTANT TO WOMEN INVOLVED IN VIGOROUS TRAINING

The involvement of women in competitive athletics has increased markedly over the past three decades. Previously, many of the decisions regarding the participation of women in sports and exercise programs was made on the basis of limited, or absent, physiological information. Research concerning women and exercise was scarce until recent years. Although many questions concerning the female athlete remain to be answered, current research indicates that there is no reason to limit the healthy female athlete from active participation in endurance or power sports (13, 68). In fact, the general responses of females to exercise and training are essentially the same as those described for males (68, 70), with the exception that exercise thermoregulation is moderately impaired in female athletes during the luteal phase of the menstrual cycle (76). The fact that men and women respond to exercise training in a similar manner is logical because the cellular mechanisms that regulate most physiological and biochemical responses to exercise are the same for both sexes. However, there are several specific concerns related to female participation in vigorous training. In this section we will discuss four key issues related to the female athlete: (1) exercise and the menstrual cycle, (2) eating disorders, (3) bone mineral disorders, and (4) exercise during pregnancy.

Exercise and Menstrual Disorders

Over the past several years there have been increasing reports concerning the influence of intense exercise training on the length of the menstrual cycle (23). Indeed, there are numerous reports in the literature of female athletes who experience "athletic" amenorrhea. The term **amenorrhea** refers to a cessation of menstruation; it is generally defined as less than four menses per year (61).

How common is athletic amenorrhea? It appears that the incidence of amenorrhea is higher in some activities than in others. For example, the occurrence of irregular menses is rather high in distance running and ballet dancing, whereas much lower incidences are reported for swimming and cycling (2, 61). For example, the incidence of amenorrhea in the general population is approximately 3%, whereas the incidence in distance runners is estimated between 10–24% (24, 27).

What causes menstrual cycle dysfunction in athletes? The current belief is that the cause may vary among individual athletes and is probably due to multiple factors. Although some studies linked a low percentage of body fat with athletic amenorrhea (61), evidence does not fully support the notion that low body fat is the principal cause of amenorrhea (48, 85). Whatever the cause of amenorrhea in athletes, it appears to be related to the total amount of training (21, 45, 62). Figure 22.1 illustrates this point. As the weekly training distance increases, the incidence of

Figure 22.1 The relationship between training distance and the incidence of amenorrhea. Notice that as the training distance increases, there is a direct increase in the incidence of amenorrhea.

athletic amenorrhea increases in proportion to the increase in training stress. This finding can be interpreted to mean that too much training either directly or indirectly influences the incidence of amenorrhea. There are at least two ways in which training might influence normal reproductive function. First, exercise alters blood concentrations of numerous hormones (4, 36, 37), which may result in a modification of feedback to the hypothalamus (see chapter 5). This, in turn, may influence the release of female reproductive hormones and therefore modify the menstrual cycle. A second possibility is that high training mileage may result in increased psychological stress. Psychological stress may disrupt the menstrual cycle by increasing blood levels of catecholamines or endogenous opiates, which play a role in regulating the reproductive system (61). For a review of the reproductive system and exercise in women, see reference (80).

Training and Menstruation

The consensus opinion among physicians is that there is little reason for the healthy female athlete to avoid training or competition during menses (50). Indeed, evidence exists that outstanding performances and world records have been established during all phases of the menstrual cycle (30). Therefore, it is not recommended that the female athlete alter her training or competitive schedule because of menses.

Dysmenorrhea (painful menstruation) can be problematic for female athletes. As mentioned previously, the incidence of dysmenorrhea is higher in athletic populations than in nonathletic groups. The explanation for this observation is unknown. However, it is possible that prostaglandins (a type of naturally occurring fatty acid) are responsible for dysmenorrhea in both athletes and nonathletes. The release of prostaglandins begins just prior to the onset of menstrual flow and may last for 2 to 3 days after menses begin. These prostaglandins cause the smooth muscle in the uterus to contract, which in turn causes ischemia (reduced blood flow) and pain (50).

Although athletes who experience dysmenorrhea can continue to train, this is often difficult because physical activity may increase the discomfort. Athletes who experience severe dysmenorrhea should see a physician for treatment (50). Often, dysmenorrhea pain can be treated with over-the-counter medications, which can be taken without interrupting training schedules.

The Female Athlete and Eating Disorders

The perceived low social acceptance for individuals with a high percentage of body fat and an emphasis on having the "perfect" body have increased the incidence of eating disorders (64). Two of the more common eating disorders that affect both female and male athletes are anorexia nervosa and bulimia (53, 87). Because of the relatively high occurrence of these eating disorders in female athletes, we discuss both the symptoms and health consequences of these abnormal eating behaviors.

Anorexia Nervosa **Anorexia nervosa** is a common eating disorder that is unrelated to any specific physical disease. The end result of extreme anorexia nervosa is a state of starvation in which the individual becomes emaciated due to a refusal to eat. The psychological cause of anorexia nervosa is unclear, but it seems to be linked to an unfounded fear of fatness that may be related to family or societal pressures to be thin (28). The incidence of this eating disorder has grown in recent years. It appears that individuals with the highest probability of developing anorexia nervosa are upper-middle-class, young females who are extremely self-critical. The incidence of anorexia nervosa in the United States is currently estimated to be 2 out of every 300 adolescent girls (46).

The anorexic may use a variety of techniques to remain thin, including starvation, exercise, and laxatives (46, 87). The effects of anorexia include excessive weight loss, cessation of menstruation, and, in extreme cases, death. Because anorexia is a serious mental and physical disorder, medical treatment by a team of professionals (physician, psychologist, nutritionist) is necessary to correct the problem. Treatment may require years of psychological counseling and nutritional guidance. The first step in seeking professional treatment for anorexia nervosa is the recognition that a problem exists. Figure 22.2 illustrates the common symptoms of anorexia.

Figure 22.2 Warning signs for anorexia nervosa.

Figure 22.3 Warning signs for bulimia.

Bulimia **Bulimia** is overeating (called binge eating) followed by vomiting (called purging) (69). The bulimic repeatedly ingests large quantities of food and then forces himself or herself to vomit to prevent weight gain. Bulimia may result in damage to the teeth and the esophagus due to vomiting of stomach acids. Like anorexia nervosa, bulimia is most common in female athletes, has a psychological origin, and requires professional treatment when diagnosed. The incidence of bulimia has been estimated as between 1–3% among U.S. females aged 13 to 23.

Most bulimics look normal and are of normal weight. Even when their bodies are slender, their abdomens may protrude due to being stretched by frequent eating binges. Common symptoms of bulimia are illustrated in figure 22.3.

Eating Disorders: Final Comments

Eating disorders have become a major problem in female athletes. Some experts have estimated that as many as 50% of elite female athletes experience some type of eating disorder. The sports with the highest incidence of eating disorders are distance running, swimming, diving, figure skating, gymnastics, body building, and ballet. Although maintaining an optimal body composition for competition is important to achieve athletic success, eating disorders are not an appropriate means of weight loss. Therefore, trainers, athletes, and coaches need to recognize the warning signals of eating disorders and be prepared to assist the athlete in obtaining the appropriate help.

Although the focus in this chapter is on eating disorders in female athletes, it is important to note that eating disorders are also common in female non-athletes. Interestingly, in the nonathletes, exercise has been suggested as a useful intervention to treat eating disorders (51). Indeed, studies indicate that regular exercise can improve the biological and social outcomes in many patients with eating disorders (51). For a review on this topic, see Hausenblas et al. (2008) in the References (51).

Bone Mineral Disorders and the Female Athlete

A growing concern for the female athlete is the loss of bone mineral content (osteoporosis). In general, there are two major causes of bone loss in the female athlete (1, 32):

1. estrogen deficiency due to amenorrhea and
2. inadequate calcium intake due to eating disorders.

Unfortunately, many female athletes suffer bone loss due to both amenorrhea and the inadequate calcium intake associated with an eating disorder (1, 32, 33). Although exercise training has been shown to reduce the rate of bone loss due to estrogen deficiency and low calcium intake, exercise cannot completely reverse this process (1). Therefore, the only solution to the problem of bone mineral loss in the female athlete is to correct the estrogen deficiency and/or increase the calcium intake to normal levels. In both cases, a physician should be involved in prescribing the correct treatment for the individual athlete (see A Closer Look 22.1).

Exercise During Pregnancy

Chapter 17 provided an overview of the current guidelines for exercising for fitness during pregnancy. As discussed in chapter 17, it is generally agreed that women who are physically fit prior to pregnancy can continue to perform regular exercise during pregnancy (3, 12). Indeed, guidelines by the American College of Obstetricians and Gynecologists state that pregnancy should not be a state of confinement, and pregnant women with uncomplicated pregnancies should be encouraged to engage in regular physical activity (8).

Although pregnant women can safely perform low- to moderate-intensity exercise, can female athletes maintain an active training program during pregnancy? The short answer to this question is yes, but some qualifications exist. First, both recreational and competitive athletes with uncomplicated pregnancies can continue to train during pregnancy, but they should carefully monitor their body temperature during exercise to prevent hyperthermia (8). Specifically, pregnant athletes should avoid high intensity and/or long training sessions that raise body core

The Female Athlete Triad

It is generally accepted that three of the most common health problems facing the young female athlete are (1) amenorrhea, (2) eating disorders, and (3) bone mineral loss. Collectively, these problems are interrelated and are called the **female athlete triad** (63, 74). Growing evidence indicates that these problems are linked and that one problem can promote another (10, 17, 18, 74). For example, an eating disorder can lead to inadequate nutrient intake resulting in a diminished intake of calcium and vitamin D. Further, eating disorders are known to contribute to amenorrhea, and long-term amenorrhea is associated with low blood levels of estrogen (85). Importantly, the combination of inadequate calcium/vitamin D intake and low estrogen levels can result in a loss of bone mineral content.

At present, researchers do not completely understand the cause of the female athlete triad. However, evidence indicates that the three corners of the female athlete triad are interrelated through both psychological and physiological mechanisms. These interactions are illustrated in figure 22.4. For example, psychological pressures to perform well in athletic competition, coupled with the physiological stress of intense exercise training, can lead to eating disorders and an energy imbalance. Although the causes of menstrual disorders are multiple, it seems that the amenorrhea observed in many female athletes is due to a negative energy balance due to both an eating disorder and intense exercise training (17). Collectively, this stress results in disturbances in the hormones that regulate the menstrual cycle, and if energy availability continues to be low over a prolonged period of time, the menstrual cycle is temporarily "switched

FIGURE 22.4 Interrelationships between the three components that compose the female athlete triad. It is believed that a combination of both psychological and physiological stress can lead to eating disorders and energy imbalance in female athletes. This energy imbalance, coupled with other stresses (psychological and physiological), can promote menstrual problems such as amenorrhea. Amenorrhea is associated with lowered blood levels of estrogen, which increases the risk of bone mineral loss. Further, decreased energy intake may lead to deficiencies in both calcium and vitamin D consumption and also contribute to a loss of bone minerals.

off" to conserve energy (17). The ensuing amenorrhea results in reduced production of estrogen by the ovaries and low blood levels of estrogen. Because estrogen protects the skeleton from bone resorption, reduced estrogen increases the risk of bone mineral loss (17, 85). Collectively, low estrogen levels and deficiencies of calcium and vitamin D (due to eating disorders) places the female athlete at great risk for osteopenia (loss of bone mineral density) (17).

What is the incidence of the female athlete triad among athletic women? A recent study involving female athletes from a variety of sports concluded that approximately 4% of all female athletes meet the criteria for the female athlete triad by exhibiting an eating disorder, amenorrhea, and bone mineral loss (83). Further, as many as 26% of these female athletes possessed at least two of the compo-

nents of the female athlete triad. Interestingly, this study also revealed that as many as 3% of nonathletic women (ages 13–29) may also suffer from all three components of the triad (83). Therefore, the health problems associated with the female athlete triad are not limited to athletes.

Growing evidence indicates that each component of the female athlete triad develops on a continuum and the triad may occur in stages (29). If early stages are not treated properly, they can progress toward the extremes of the triad. Therefore, protection of the female athlete's health from the triad is dependent upon early detection of symptoms of one or more of the components of the triad and successful treatment of the problem. For more details on the female athlete triad, see Birch (2005) and Nattiv et al. (2007) in the References (17, 74).

temperature above 1.5° C (8). In this regard, aquatic exercise is considered an excellent form of training for pregnant athletes because it allows cardiovascular conditioning in a medium that facilitates accelerated heat loss.

It is also important that pregnant athletes maintain adequate hydration during training by consuming fluid at regular intervals (e.g., every 15 minutes) during exercise. Fluid balance can be monitored by weighing before and after the exercise session. Any loss of body weight is fluid loss and should be replaced by drinking the appropriate amount of fluid (e.g., 0.5-kg weight loss = 500 ml fluid). Moreover, the energy cost of exercise sessions should be estimated and balanced by appropriate energy intake.

Finally, it is also critical that pregnant athletes apply good judgment when planning exercise programs. Athletes should be aware that it may be necessary to reduce the training intensity and volume as the pregnancy advances (8). Importantly, it is recommended that all physically active women should be examined regularly by their physician to assess the effects of their exercise programs on the developing fetus, and adjustments should be made if appropriate (8).

Risk of Knee Injury in Female Athletes

Knee injuries are common in many sports. Although the risk of knee injuries varies across sports, studies reveal that compared to males, female athletes are at higher risk for knee injury in jumping and cutting sports (e.g., basketball, volleyball, soccer, etc.) (16, 34). In particular, knee injuries such as anterior cruciate ligament (ACL) injuries occur at a higher rate in female athletes compared to male athletes at a similar level of competition (34, 88). For example, in a study of male and female professional basketball players, female athletes suffered 60% more ACL injuries than males (88). This increased risk of knee injury in female athletes is not limited to professional athletes and impacts both collegiate and high school athletes as well (34, 73, 89). For example, National Collegiate Athletic Association statistics reveal that women sustain ACL injuries at a rate that is almost 4 times higher than men in basketball and 2.4 times higher than men in soccer (34).

Why are females at a greater risk for ACL injuries? Unfortunately, a definitive answer to this question is not available. However, it has been speculated that several factors may play a role in placing women at higher risk for knee injuries; these include fluctuation in sex hormones during the menstrual cycle, gender differences in knee anatomy, and dynamic neuromuscular imbalances (34). A discussion of the evidence to support each of these potential risk factors follows.

In reference to sex hormones and knee injuries, studies reveal that the risk of ACL injury is increased in female athletes during the follicular and ovulatory phase of the menstrual cycle (34). However, the direct link between sex hormones and the increased risk of tear of the ACL remains unclear. In this regard, some investigators propose that sex hormones influence the structure of the ACL, perhaps compromising both the strength of the ligament and/or proprioceptive

feedback (34). Nonetheless, direct evidence to support this concept is limited.

Studies investigating gender differences in knee anatomy as a determinant of the risk of knee injuries have failed to provide definitive evidence that anatomical explanations are responsible for gender differences in the rate of knee injuries. For example, although women are more likely to have knee joint laxity (loose joint) than men, this fact has not been correlated to the higher rate of knee injury in women (34). Therefore, it does not appear that gender differences in knee anatomy can explain why females are at higher risk for ACL injuries.

Dynamic neuromuscular imbalance in the knee is an area of research related to ACL tears in women that continues to grow. Dynamic neuromuscular imbalance refers to a combination of imbalanced factors including muscular strength, proprioception, and landing biomechanics. In regard to muscle strength, women have less quadriceps and hamstring strength than men, even when normalizing for body weight (57). This is significant because exercises that strengthen both the quadriceps and hamstring muscles provide protection against knee injury (19, 52). Evidence also exists that the higher incidence of knee injury in women compared to men may be linked to an imbalance in knee proprioceptive and neuromuscular control in female athletes (34). Nonetheless, more detailed studies are required before a firm conclusion can be reached on the role that proprioception plays in gender differences in knee injury. Finally, published reports reveal that women run, jump, and land differently than men when playing sports (34). This is important because the usual mechanism for noncontact ACL injury involves a deceleration in limb speed before changing directions or landing with the knee between full extension and 20 degrees of flexion (34). In this regard, compared to males, female athletes have been shown to land with knee angles that pose a greater risk of ACL injury (34). Therefore, a neuromuscular difference between males and females that impacts landing or other movement strategies may partly explain why female athletes are at greater risk for knee injuries in sports compared to male athletes.

In summary, compared to men, female athletes are at high risk for certain types of knee injuries (e.g., ACL injury). Current evidence suggests that male/female differences in dynamic neuromuscular imbalance (e.g., leg muscle strength, jumping and landing strategies) may contribute to gender differences in the risk of knee injuries. For a discussion of programs aimed at reducing ACL injury in women, please see Bien (2011) in the Suggested Readings.

IN SUMMARY

- The incidence of amenorrhea in female athletes appears to be highest in distance runners and ballet dancers when compared to other sports. Although the cause of amenorrhea in female athletes is not clear, it appears likely that multiple factors (e.g., the amount of training and psychological stress) are involved.

- There appears to be little reason for female athletes to avoid training during menstruation unless they experience severe discomfort due to dysmenorrhea. Athletes who experience severe dysmenorrhea should see a physician for treatment.

- Two of the more common eating disorders are anorexia nervosa and bulimia.

- The three most common health problems facing the young female athlete are amenorrhea, eating disorders, and bone mineral loss; collectively, these problems have been called the *female athlete triad.*

- Short-term, low-intensity exercise does not appear to have negative consequences during pregnancy. However, data suggest that long-duration or high-intensity training should be carefully monitored during pregnancy.

- Female athletes are at greater risk for knee injuries compared to males. Evidence suggests that male/female differences in dynamic neuromuscular imbalance (e.g., differences in leg muscle strength and/or jumping and landing strategies) may contribute to gender differences in the risk of knee injuries.

SPORTS CONDITIONING FOR CHILDREN

There are many unanswered questions about the physiologic responses of the healthy child to various types of exercise. This is due to the limited number of investigators studying children and exercise, and because of ethical considerations in studying children. For instance, few investigators would puncture a child's artery, take a muscle biopsy, or expose a child to harsh environments (e.g., heat, cold, high altitudes) to satisfy scientific curiosity. Because of these ethical constraints, current knowledge concerning training for children is limited primarily to the cardiopulmonary system, with a growing body of information concerning the possibility of musculoskeletal injury as a result of specific types of sports training. The following discussion addresses some of the important issues concerning child participation in vigorous conditioning programs.

Training and the Cardiopulmonary System

As youth sports teams increase in popularity, one of the first questions asked is, "Are the hearts of children strong enough for intensive sports conditioning?" In other words, is there a possibility of "overtraining" young athletes, with the end result being permanent damage to the cardiovascular system? The answer to this question is no. Children involved in endurance sports such as running or swimming improve their maximal aerobic power comparable to adults and show no indices of damage to the cardiopulmonary system (7, 54, 65, 75, 79). Over the past several years, children have safely trained for and completed marathon runs in less than 4 hours. If proper techniques of physical training are employed, with a progressive increase in cardiopulmonary stress, children appear to adapt to endurance training in a fashion similar to adults (6, 79). Further, the risk of a cardiac sudden death in young endurance athletes is small (See Clinical Applications 22.1.).

Training and the Musculoskeletal System

Organized vigorous training in some types of sports (e.g., swimming, basketball, volleyball, track and field) does not adversely affect growth and development in children (67). This is true for both boys (38) and girls (9). In fact, moderate physical training has been shown to augment or optimize growth in children and reduce the risk of obesity and type II diabetes (35, 38). Therefore, many investigators have concluded that a certain amount of physical activity is necessary for normal growth and development. However, is there danger of overtraining and injury to bones and cartilage (11, 39, 42)?

One of the long-standing concerns with intense endurance or resistance training in children is that the growing bones of a child are more susceptible to certain types of mechanical injury than those of the adult, primarily because of the presence of growth cartilage (67). Growth cartilage is present at the **growth plate (epiphyseal plate), articular cartilage** (cartilage at joints), and the sites of major muscle-tendon insertions in the child (67). The location of the growth plate for the knee joint is illustrated in figure 22.5. The growth plate is the site of bone growth in long bones. The time at which bone growth ceases varies from bone to bone, but growth is generally complete by 18 to 20 years of age (67). Upon completion of growth, growth plates ossify (harden with calcium) and disappear, and growth cartilage is replaced by a permanent "adult" cartilage.

CLINICAL APPLICATIONS 22.1

Risk of Sudden Cardiac Death in Young Athletes

Cardiovascular-related sudden death represents 72% of all exercise-related deaths in athletes less than 18 years of age. However, in healthy young athletes, the risk of sudden cardiac injury or death during participation in sports or exercise is relatively small. For example, the incidence of sudden death in young athletes in the United States has been estimated to be 1 death per 45,000 athletes (31). Importantly, almost all of these deaths resulted from congenital heart defects and did not result from exercise per se (31, 78).

Four cardiovascular abnormalities account for the majority of sudden cardiac deaths in young athletes: (1) hypertrophic cardiomyopathy (pathologically enlarged heart); (2) congenital (inherited) abnormalities of the coronary arteries; (3) aortic aneurysms; and (4) congenital stenosis (narrowing) of the aortic valve (31, 78).

Can a medical exam identify athletes at risk for sudden death? In many cases, yes. A medical history and a physical exam from a qualified physician are good tools for detecting heart disease that could pose a risk for the young athlete participating in sports (25). However, some cardiac abnormalities that can cause death during sports participation are difficult to detect during routine medical examination (31, 78). Nonetheless, a medical exam along with a cardiac evaluation can potentially reduce the risk of sudden cardiac death by identifying those young athletes who are predisposed to cardiac injury (31).

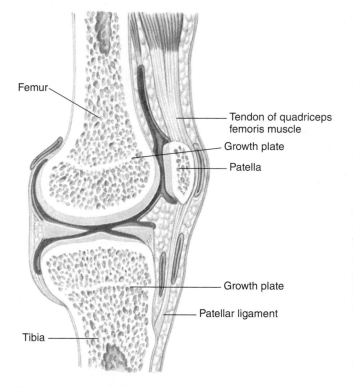

Figure 22.5 Location of the growth plate (epiphyseal plate) associated with the long bones in the leg.

Can children perform heavy endurance training or strength training without long-term musculoskeletal problems? Currently, there are no published reports or case studies indicating that endurance exercise has adverse effects on bone growth in children. Further, studies have investigated the effects of resistance exercise training on children (6–12 years of age) and have concluded that supervised resistance exercise does not damage bone, muscle, or the epiphyseal plate (41, 86). Further, recent reviews on the effects of resistance exercise on children have concluded that under proper supervision, resistance training can be performed safely in youth athletes without bone or cartilage injury (11, 39, 42). In fact, it is well established that resistance training has numerous health benefits in children. For example, weight training has been shown to promote bone health by increasing bone mineral density to prepubertal boys and girls (11). It is also clear that resistance training is effective in promoting muscular strength in prepubertal boys and girls (40, 43). Interestingly, this training induced muscular strength is achieved with limited hypertrophy in prepubertal children (11). Therefore, the resistance training-induced increase in muscular strength in children appears to be achieved primarily by changes in the nervous system alone (e.g., improved motor unit recruitment, etc.).

Progress in Pediatric Exercise Science

As discussed earlier, our knowledge about pediatric exercise science has developed slowly because of ethical concerns of using children in research. Nonetheless, knowledge in this field has expanded during the past several years. One of the pioneers promoting research in pediatric exercise science was Dr. Oded Bar-Or (see A Look Back—Important People in Science). Moreover, the creation of the scientific journal *Pediatric Exercise Science* has stimulated additional research in exercise during childhood. Therefore, it is anticipated that scientific knowledge of pediatric exercise science will grow rapidly during the coming years.

A LOOK BACK—IMPORTANT PEOPLE IN SCIENCE

Oded Bar-Or Was a Pioneer in Pediatric Exercise Physiology

Oded Bar-Or (1937–2005) was born and raised in Jerusalem, Israel. He was trained as a medical doctor at Hadassah Medical School (Israel), and following graduation, he traveled to the United States to begin post-doctoral research training in exercise physiology in the laboratory of Dr. Elsworth Buskirk at Pennsylvania State University. After completing his post-doctoral studies in 1969, Dr. Bar-Or returned to Israel and established the Department of Sports Medicine at the Wingate Institute. During his tenure at the Wingate Institute,

Dr. Bar-Or and his colleagues earned international acclaim in sports science research and his research group developed the Wingate Anaerobic Power Test that remains in use today (chapter 20).

In 1981, Professor Bar-Or left the Wingate Institute to join the faculty at McMaster University in Hamilton, Ontario (Canada). Upon arrival at McMaster, he established the Children's Exercise and Nutrition Center and began a lifelong quest to increase our knowledge about pediatric exercise science. During his tenure at McMaster, his research focused on understanding the physiological dif-

ferences between adults and children in their response to exercise. A major portion of this work was dedicated to resolving how children differ from adults in their cardiorespiratory and thermoregulatory responses to exercise in hot environments. Indeed, Dr. Bar-Or was one of the first investigators to study children's thermoregulatory responses and acclimatization to exercise. Dr. Bar-Or's legacy in pediatric exercise physiology includes more than 180 research publications, and he also authored or coauthored ten books on a variety of topics in pediatric sports medicine and exercise physiology.

IN SUMMARY

- Current evidence indicates that endurance training is not detrimental to the growth and development of the cardiovascular system in children. Further, there is no evidence that endurance exercise training has a negative impact on bone and cartilage health.
- The risk of sudden cardiac death in youth athletes is extremely low (1/145,000 athletes).
- The consensus of current scientific evidence indicates that under proper supervision, resistance training can be performed safely in youth athletes without bone or cartilage injury.
- Resistance training in prepubertal children has been shown to increase both bone density and muscular strength with limited muscle hypertrophy.

COMPETITIVE TRAINING FOR DIABETICS

As discussed in chapter 17, there is a beneficial effect of exercise on diabetes, and physicians often recommend regular exercise for diabetics as a part of their therapeutic regimen (i.e., to help maintain control of blood glucose levels). We will limit our discussion to type 1 diabetics, because type 2 diabetics are less likely to engage in training for performance purposes. Can type 1 diabetics train vigorously and take part in

competitive athletics? The answer to this question is a qualified yes. In long-term diabetic patients with microvascular complications (damage to small blood vessels) or neuropathy (nerve damage), exercise should be limited and extensive training is not generally recommended (15, 67). However, in individuals who maintain good blood glucose control and are free from other medical complications, diabetes in itself should not limit the type of exercise or sporting event (81).

What precautions should the diabetic athlete take to allow safe participation in training programs? An overview of exercise training for fitness in diabetic populations was presented in chapter 17 and will be reviewed here only briefly. The key to safe participation in sport conditioning for the diabetic athlete is to learn to avoid hypoglycemic episodes during training. Because diabetics vary in their response to insulin, each diabetic athlete, in cooperation with his or her personal physician, must determine the appropriate combination of exercise, diet, and insulin for optimal control of blood glucose concentrations. In general, exercise should take place after a meal and should be part of regular routine. It is often recommended that a reduction in the amount of insulin injected be considered on days in which the athlete is engaged in strenuous training (15, 77, 81). A major concern for the diabetic athlete is the site of the insulin injection prior to exercise. Insulin injected subcutaneously in the leg prior to running (or other forms of leg exercise) results in an increased rate of insulin uptake due to elevated leg blood flow. This could result in exercise-induced hypoglycemia and may be avoided by using an insulin injection site in the abdomen or the arm (83). Conversely, if the training regimen requires arm exercise (e.g., rowing), the site of insulin injection should be away from the working muscle (e.g., abdomen). Having a glucose solution or carbohydrate snack available during training sessions may help avoid hypoglycemic incidents during workouts.

Can diabetics obtain the same benefits from training as nondiabetics? The consensus answer to this question is yes. Although untrained, diabetic children tend to be less fit than normal children (58), young diabetics respond to a conditioning program in a manner similar to healthy children (67). Empirical observations suggest that when the diabetic athlete's blood glucose is carefully regulated, he or she can compete and excel in a variety of competitive sports.

IN SUMMARY

- Type 1 diabetics who are free of diabetic complications should not be limited in the type or quantity of exercise.
- The key for safe sports participation for the type 1 diabetic is for the athlete to learn to avoid hypoglycemic episodes.

TRAINING FOR ASTHMATICS

It is generally agreed that most children, adolescents, and adults with asthma can safely participate in all sports with the exception of SCUBA diving, provided they are able to control exercise-induced bronchospasms via medication or careful monitoring of activity levels (71). In fact, evidence suggests that aerobic training can reduce airway inflammation and improve asthmatic symptoms in some asthma patients (66). A prerequisite for planning training programs for asthmatics is that the proper therapeutic regimen for managing the athlete's particular type of asthma be worked out prior to commencement of a vigorous training program (see chapter 17). When the asthma is under control, planning the training schedule for asthmatic athletes is identical to planning for athletes without asthma (see chapter 21). However, as mentioned in chapter 17, it is often recommended that the asthmatic athlete keep an inhaler (containing a bronchodilator) handy during training sessions, and that workouts be conducted with other athletes in case a major attack occurs.

The issue of the safety of an asthmatic participating in SCUBA diving continues to be debated. The controversy centers around the fact that divers who experience an asthma attack while diving are at high risk for pulmonary barotrauma (damage to the lung

due to high pressure) (26). However, a recent review on the subject suggests that asthmatics with normal airway function at rest who do not exhibit exercise-induced asthma have a risk of barotrauma during diving similar to that of healthy individuals (26).

IN SUMMARY

- Asthmatics can safely participate in all sports with the possible exception of SCUBA diving, provided they are able to control exercise-induced bronchospasms via medication or careful monitoring of activity levels.
- The question of the safety of an asthmatic participating in SCUBA diving continues to be unanswered. Nonetheless, evidence suggests that asthmatics who do not exhibit exercise-induced asthma and have normal airways at rest are at no greater risk during diving than are healthy individuals.

EPILEPSY AND PHYSICAL TRAINING

The term **epilepsy** refers to a transient disturbance of brain function, which may be characterized by a loss of consciousness, muscle tremor, and sensory disturbances. Because the occurrence of epileptic seizures is not easily predicted, should epileptics engage in vigorous training programs? Unfortunately, there is little information available to answer this question. Before a clear-cut recommendation for the participation of epileptics in athletics can be made, two fundamental questions must be answered. First, does intense physical activity increase the risk of an epileptic seizure? Second, does the occurrence of a seizure during a particular sports activity expose the athlete to unnecessary risk? Let's examine the available evidence concerning each of these questions.

Does Exercise Promote Seizures?

There is one rare type of epileptic seizure that has been shown to be induced by exercise per se (22). These are tonic (continuous motor activity) seizures, which have been reported to occur during a variety of sports activities. Fortunately, this type of seizure can be controlled in most instances by anticonvulsant drugs.

However, stress is among the most commonly reported causes of seizures in people with epilepsy (5). For example, patients report that the frequency of their seizures increases if they are exposed to an increase in excitement, tension, sadness, or other strong emotions (5). Given that exercise is physical stress, does exercise per se, promote seizures (22)?

As for other types of seizure disorders, physicians remain divided in their opinions as to whether exercise increases the risk of seizure occurrence. A report by Gotze et al. (49) suggests that exercise does not increase the risk of seizures in epileptic children or adolescents. In fact, Gotze (49) argues that exercise appears to reduce the incidence of seizures in epileptics by increasing the threshold for seizures. In support of these claims, reviews on epilepsy and sports have concluded that there is a reduction in the number of seizures during exercise (3, 5, 84). In contrast, Kuijer (59) has suggested that the epileptic is at an increased risk of experiencing a seizure during exercise and during recovery from exercise. In this regard, several factors related to exercise have been hypothesized to increase the risk of seizures (84): (1) physical fatigue, (2) hyperventilation, (3) hypoxia, (4) hyperthermia, (5) hypoglycemia, (6) electrolyte imbalance, and (7) emotional stress associated with competitive sports. In conclusion, division exists in the medical community concerning the risk of exercise and seizures. It seems logical that generalizations about exercise and the epileptic patient cannot be made. Each patient is unique concerning the type, frequency, and severity of epileptic seizures. Therefore, physicians, parents, and coaches must make case-by-case decisions on the wisdom of competitive sports for individual patients.

Another specific concern for the participation of epileptics in contact sports is whether a blow to the head might mediate a seizure. Again, physicians remain divided in their opinions. Some authors believe the risks are high (56), whereas others argue that no studies exist to prove that repeated head trauma in epileptics causes a recurrence of seizures (47, 60). See Arida et al. (2009) in the Suggested Readings for more details.

Risk of Injury Due to Seizures

Clearly, there are many competitive sports activities (e.g., football, boxing) during which the occurrence of a seizure would expose the athlete to a risk of harm. However, the occurrence of a seizure during many types of daily routine activities (e.g., climbing stairs) or recreational sports (e.g., SCUBA diving, mountain climbing) could also pose a threat to the epileptic (47). Whether the epileptic should participate in physical training or sports must be determined on an individual basis by the use of common sense and advice from a sports physician. The benefit-risk ratio of sports participation may vary greatly from case to case and is dependent on the exact nature of the patient's epilepsy and the sport being considered. A child with only a minor seizure problem may, with the aid of medication, experience only a rare seizure with little visible alteration in behavior or consciousness due to the seizure. This type of epileptic could likely participate in most training activities without harm (14, 49). In contrast, an epileptic who experiences frequent and major seizures would not be a candidate for many types of sports. For a detailed discussion of epilepsy and exercise, see Arida et al. (2009) in the Suggested Readings.

IN SUMMARY

- Questions about safe participation for epileptics in training programs must be answered on an individual basis.
- The benefit-risk ratio of sports participation may vary greatly from case to case and depends on the type of epilepsy involved and the sport being considered.

EXERCISE PERFORMANCE AND TRAINING FOR MASTERS ATHLETES

There are a growing number of people over the age of 50 that compete in competitive athletic events. These "masters athletes" represent an interesting subgroup of older adults because they possess unique physiological characteristics that could be termed as "exceptionally successful aging" (82). The masters athlete often trains on a daily basis and strives to maintain athletic performances that he/she achieved at earlier ages. However, a decline in athletic performance at advancing ages is inevitable. In the next two segments we describe the age-related changes in muscular strength and endurance performance and discuss the physiological reasons for the decline in physical capabilities with age.

Age-Related Changes in Muscular Strength

It is well known that aging results in a progressive decrease in muscular strength. Although changes in the nervous system do occur during aging, most of the loss in strength with aging is due to a decline in muscle mass. The age-related loss of muscle mass is termed **sarcopenia** and the rate of muscle loss with age is illustrated in Figure 22.6. Age-related sarcopenia occurs due to both a decrease in fiber size and a decrease in the number of fibers present in the muscle (44). However, most of the age-related loss in muscle mass is due to a loss of muscle fibers (44, 72). The mechanisms responsible for this age-related loss of

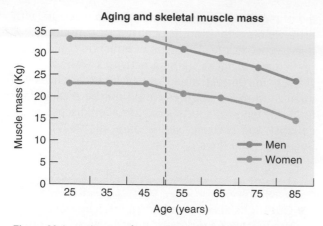

Figure 22.6 Aging results in a loss of muscle mass with aging in both men and women. Data are from reference (57).

muscle remain unclear. Nonetheless, it appears that a number of factors contribute to sarcopenia, including inactivity, free radical-mediated damage (oxidative stress) to muscle fibers, inflammation, and decreases in anabolic hormones such as testosterone (20).

You will note in figure 22.6 that there is little loss of muscle mass before the age of 50. However, after age 50 there is a progressive loss of skeletal muscle mass in both men and women. The rate of muscle loss with aging is variable across individuals but both men and women tend to lose muscle mass at a rate of 1–2% per year after the age of 50 (20). Therefore, men and women can lose 40–60% of their total muscle mass from age 50 to age 80.

Although aging results in a loss of muscle mass and strength in all people, a life-long program of strength training can maintain a relatively high level of muscle strength across the lifespan. For example, figure 22.7 illustrates the age-related change in leg muscle strength in three individuals that differ in exercise habits. In this illustration, the trained individual

has maintained a lifetime of resistance training (2–3 days/week). The active individual is engaged in routine walking exercise (~5,000 steps/3–5 days week) but does not engage in resistance training. The sedentary individual does not participate in regular exercise and is the classic "couch potato." Note that the rate of muscle strength loss with aging does not differ between these individuals. Nonetheless, the resistance-trained individual maintains a higher level of leg muscle strength across the lifespan compared to both the active and sedentary individual. Therefore, while strength training cannot prevent age-related muscle loss, an individual who engages in regular resistance training can maintain a much higher level of muscular strength throughout the lifespan compared to less active individuals.

Aging and Endurance Performance

Similar to the age-related loss of muscular strength, aging also results in a decline in endurance performance and $\dot{V}O_2$ max. For example, figure 22.8 illustrates the changes in men's and women's 10,000 (10K)-meter running times with advancing age. Notice that 10K-performance times increase (i.e., decreased performance) with age in a curvilinear fashion, with the most rapid changes in performance occurring after approximately age 60. Similarly, $\dot{V}O_2$ max also declines with age in trained men and women (figure 22.9). Notice that limited change occurs in $\dot{V}O_2$ max until age 40 (55). However, the age-related decline in $\dot{V}O_2$ max in both men and women is approximately a 1% loss per year after age 40. Although endurance training can increase the $\dot{V}O_2$ of people of all ages, endurance exercise cannot prevent the age-related decline in $\dot{V}O_2$ max. However, individuals that maintain an active program of endurance training throughout the lifespan can sustain a higher $\dot{V}O_2$ max compared to sedentary individuals (figure 22.10).

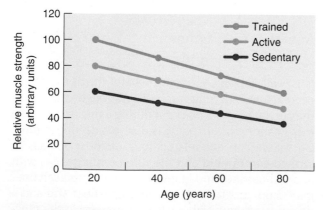

Figure 22.7 Aging is associated with a significant loss of muscular strength. Notice, however, that regular strength training can greatly delay this age-related loss in muscle force production. Modifed from references (18, 78).

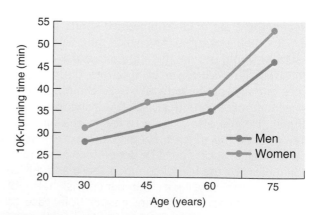

Figure 22.8 Changes in men's and women's 10,000-meter (10K) running times with advancing age. Data are from World Masters Athletics.

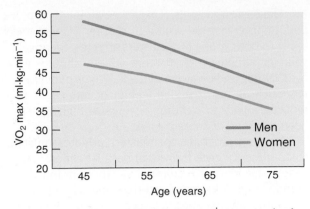

Figure 22.9 The age-related decline in $\dot{V}O_2$ max in both endurance trained men and women. Data are from reference (53).

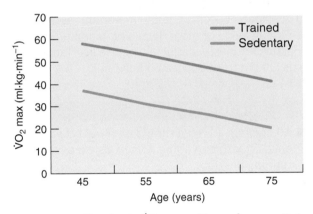

Figure 22.10 Changes in $\dot{V}O_2$ max with age for men. Data are from reference (53).

What factors contribute to the age-related decline in endurance performance and $\dot{V}O_2$ max?

Recall from chapter 20 that the primary determinants of endurance performance are $\dot{V}O_2$ max, exercise economy, and the maximal exercise intensity that is sustained during endurance exercise. Let's discuss the impact of aging on each of these factors.

Maximal aerobic capacity ($\dot{V}O_2$ max) is the upper limit of maximal energy production via oxidative phosphorylation and is a major determinant of endurance exercise performance. Recall that $\dot{V}O_2$ is determined by both cardiac output and the uptake of oxygen by the tissues (i.e., a-$\bar{v}$ O_2 difference) as defined by the Fick equation (chapter 13):

$$\dot{V}O_2 \text{ max} = \text{maximal cardiac output} \times \text{maximal a-}\bar{v}\text{ }O_2 \text{ difference}$$

Studies indicate that the age-related decline in $\dot{V}O_2$ max occurs due to a decrease in both maximal cardiac output and a decline in the maximal a-$\bar{v}$ O_2 difference (82). This point is illustrated in figure 22.11.

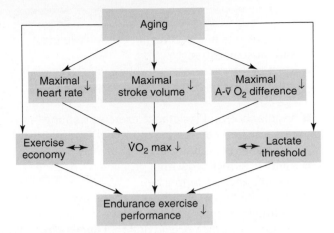

Figure 22.11 Factors and physiological mechanisms responsible for the age-related decline in endurance exercise performance in healthy adults. Figure has been modified from reference (85). Down arrows indicate decreases whereas horizontal arrows indicate no change.

Note that the age-related decline in maximal cardiac output is due to a decrease in both maximal heart rate and the maximal stroke volume. The age-related decay in the maximal oxygen extraction (a-$\bar{v}$ O_2 difference) is likely due to a combination of factors, including a decline capillary density and mitochondrial volume (82).

Exercise economy is measured as the steady-state oxygen consumption while exercising at a submaximal exercise intensity below the lactate threshold. Exercise economy is important for endurance performance because athletes who are more efficient use less energy to perform a given exercise task. Several studies indicate that exercise economy does not change with age; therefore, changes in economy are not a major factor in explaining the age-related decline in endurance performance (figure 22.11).

The ability to work at a high percentage of one's maximal oxygen uptake during submaximal exercise is an important determinant of endurance performance and is often evaluated in the laboratory by measurement of the lactate threshold (chapter 20). The lactate threshold does not change with aging when expressed relative to the $\dot{V}O_2$ max (82). Therefore, age-related changes in the lactate threshold are not a key factor in determining the decline in endurance performance with age (82).

To summarize, success in endurance events is dependent upon $\dot{V}O_2$ max, exercise economy, and the lactate threshold. Aging does not appear to have a negative impact on both the lactate threshold and exercise economy. In contrast, aging results in a progressive decline in $\dot{V}O_2$ max, which is the primary factor that contributes to the age-related decline in endurance performance.

- Aging results in a decline in both muscle mass and muscular strength.
- Most of the age-related decline in both skeletal muscle mass and strength occur following age 50.
- Regular bouts of resistance exercise training can assist in maintaining muscle mass and muscular strength throughout the lifespan.
- Aging is associated with a progressive decline in endurance performance.
- The major factor contributing to the age-related decline in endurance performance is a decrease in $\dot{V}O_2$ max, which occurs due to a decline in both maximal cardiac output and maximal a-$\bar{v}$ O_2 difference.
- Endurance exercise training can protect against age-related decreases in $\dot{V}O_2$ max but cannot completely halt this decline.

Training Guidelines for Masters Athletes

A detailed discussion of exercise training for the masters athlete is beyond the scope of this chapter. Nonetheless, an overview of some of the key considerations for training of masters athletes are presented. First, it is important for any masters athlete to gain medical clearance prior to beginning a rigorous exercise training program. A complete medical exam should include a physical exam along with an exercise stress test to ensure that rigorous exercise does not pose a health risk for the older athlete.

The basic principles of exercise training to improve performance were presented in chapter 21, and these apply to both young and masters athletes. Identical to younger athletes, the masters athlete should avoid overtraining and be aware of the key signs of overtraining, such as an excessive feeling of fatigue at rest, reduced ability to perform a workout, higher resting heart rate, and disrupted sleep.

Training programs for masters athletes must be customized for each individual because differences in genetic capacities for adaptation vary from individual to individual. Add to this fact differences in age, training status, and competitive schedule, and the importance of planning individual training programs for masters athletes becomes obvious. A critical consideration in planning training programs for all masters athletes is to avoid overuse injuries by scheduling adequate recovery periods between rigorous workouts. Indeed, scheduling rest days between challenging workouts becomes more important as athletes increase in age. For more details on planning training programs for masters athletes, please see Tanaka and Seals (2008) in the Suggested Readings.

- All masters athletes should gain medical clearance prior to beginning a rigorous exercise training program.
- The fundamental principles of exercise training apply to people of all ages.
- Training programs for masters athletes must be customized to meet the needs of the individual and consider such factors as age and current training status.

STUDY QUESTIONS

1. Outline several possible causes of "athletic" amenorrhea.
2. What is the current recommendation for training and competition during menstruation?
3. Discuss the role of prostaglandins in mediating dysmenorrhea.
4. Based on present information, what are reasonable guidelines for advising the pregnant athlete concerning the intensity and duration of training?
5. Define the *female athlete triad*.
6. What factors contribute to bone mineral loss in the female athlete?
7. Discuss the notion that intense exercise might result in permanent damage to (a) the cardiovascular system or (b) the musculoskeletal system in children.
8. What is the recommendation for type 1 diabetics with no physical complications for entering a competitive training program?
9. What factors should be considered when advising the diabetic athlete concerning safe participation in athletic

conditioning? Include in your discussion suggestions concerning meal timing, injection sites for insulin, and the availability of glucose drinks during training sessions.
10. What is the current opinion concerning the safe participation of asthmatics in competitive athletics?
11. Define the term *epilepsy*.
12. Discuss the possibility that exercise increases the risk of seizures for epileptics.
13. What factors should be considered in assessing the risk-to-benefit ratio of sports participation for epileptics?
14. Graph the change in both muscle mass and muscular strength with age.
15. What factors contribute to the age-related changes in muscle mass and muscular strength?
16. Discuss the impact of aging on $\dot{V}O_2$ max in both men and women.
17. What factor(s) are responsible for the age-related decline in endurance performance?

SUGGESTED READINGS

Ackerman, K. E., and M. Misra. 2011. Bone health and the female athlete triad in adolescent athletes. *Phys Sportsmed* 39:131–41.

Arida, R. M. et al. 2009. Physical exercise in epilepsy: What kind of stressor is it? *Epilepsy Behav* 16:381–87.

Armstrong, N., and A. R. Barker. 2011. Endurance training and elite young athletes. *Med Sport Sci* 56:59–83.

Armstrong, N., and A. M. McManus. 2011. Physiology of elite young male athletes. *Med Sport Sci* 56:1–22.

Bien, D. P. 2011. Rationale and implementation of anterior cruciate ligament injury prevention warm-up programs in female athletes. *J Strength Cond Res* 25:271–85.

Faigenbaum, A. D. et al. 2009. Youth resistance training: Updated position statement paper from the national strength and conditioning association. *J Strength Cond Res* 23:S60–79.

Manore, M. M., L. C. Kam, and A. B. Loucks. 2007. The female athlete triad: components, nutrition issues, and health consequences. *J Sports Sci* 25 Suppl 1:S61–71.

Morton, A. R., and K. D. Fitch. 2011. Australian association for exercise and sports science position statement on exercise and asthma. *J Sci Med Sport* 14:312–16.

Tanaka, H., and D. R. Seals. 2008. Endurance exercise performance in Masters athletes: Age-associated changes and underlying physiological mechanisms. *J Physiol* 586:55–63.

REFERENCES

1. **Ackerman KE, and Misra M.** Bone health and the female athlete triad in adolescent athletes. *Phys Sportsmed* 39: 131–141, 2011.

2. **Andersen AE.** Anorexia nervosa and bulimia: a spectrum of eating disorders. *J Adolesc Health Care* 4: 15–21, 1983.

3. **Arida RM, Cavalheiro EA, de Albuquerque M, da Silva AC, and Scorza FA.** Physical exercise in epilepsy: the case in favor. *Epilepsy Behav* 11: 478–479, 2007.

4. **Arida RM, Scorza FA, Terra VC, Cysneiros RM, and Cavalheiro EA.** Physical exercise in rats with epilepsy is protective against seizures: evidence of animal studies. *Arq Neuropsiquiatr* 67: 1013–1016, 2009.

5. **Arida RM, Scorza FA, Terra VC, Scorza CA, de Almeida AC, and Cavalheiro EA.** Physical exercise in epilepsy: what kind of stressor is it? *Epilepsy Behav* 16: 381–387, 2009.

6. **Armstrong N, and Barker AR.** Endurance training and elite young athletes. *Med Sport Sci* 56: 59–83, 2011.

7. **Armstrong N, and McManus AM.** Physiology of elite young male athletes. *Med Sport Sci* 56: 1–22, 2011.

8. **Artal R, and O'Toole M.** Guidelines of the American College of Obstetricians and Gynecologists for exercise during pregnancy and the postpartum period. *Br J Sports Med* 37: 6–12; discussion 12, 2003.

9. **Åstrand P.** Girl swimmers. *Acta Paediatric Scandinavica* 147(Suppl.): 1–75, 1963.

10. **Beals KA, and Meyer NL.** Female athlete triad update. *Clin Sports Med* 26: 69–89, 2007.

11. **Behm DG, Faigenbaum AD, Falk B, and Klentrou P.** Canadian Society for Exercise Physiology position paper: resistance training in children and adolescents. *Appl Physiol Nutr Metab* 33: 547–561, 2008.

12. **Beilock SL, Feltz DL, and Pivarnik JM.** Training patterns of athletes during pregnancy and postpartum. *Res Q Exerc Sport* 72: 39–46, 2001.

13. **Benjamin HJ.** The female adolescent athlete: specific concerns. *Pediatr Ann* 36: 719–726, 2007.

14. **Bennett D.** Sports and epilepsy: to play or not to play. *Seminars in Neurology* 1: 345–357, 1981.

15. **Bhaskarabhatla KV, and Birrer R.** Physical activity and diabetes mellitus. *Compr Ther* 31: 291–298, 2005.

16. **Bien DP.** Rationale and implementation of anterior cruciate ligament injury prevention warm-up programs in female athletes. *J Strength Cond Res* 25: 271–285, 2011.

17. **Birch K.** Female athlete triad. *BMJ* 330: 244–246, 2005.

18. **Brooks G, Fahey T, and Baldwin K.** *Exercise Physiology: Human Bioenergetics and Its Applications.* New York: McGraw-Hill, 2005.

19. **Brophy RH, Silvers HJ, and Mandelbaum BR.** Anterior cruciate ligament injuries: etiology and prevention. *Sports Med Arthrosc* 18: 2–11, 2010.

20. **Buford TW, Anton SD, Judge AR, Marzetti E, Wohlgemuth SE, Carter CS, Leeuwenburgh C, Pahor M, and Manini TM.** Models of accelerated sarcopenia: critical pieces for solving the puzzle of age-related muscle atrophy. *Ageing Res Rev* 9: 369–383, 2010.

21. **Bullen BA, Skrinar GS, Beitins IZ, von Mering G, Turnbull BA, and McArthur JW.** Induction of menstrual disorders by strenuous exercise in untrained women. *N Engl J Med* 312: 1349–1353, 1985.

22. **Burger LJ, Lopez RI, and Elliott FA.** Tonic seizures induced by movement. *Neurology* 22: 656–659, 1972.

23. **Castelo-Branco C, Reina F, Montivero AD, Colodron M, and Vanrell JA.** Influence of high-intensity training and of dietetic and anthropometric factors on menstrual cycle disorders in ballet dancers. *Gynecol Endocrinol* 22: 31–35, 2006.

24. **Cobb KL, Bachrach LK, Greendale GA, Marcus R, Neer R, Nieves J, Sowers M, Brown BW, Jr., Gopalakrishnan G, Luetters C, Tanner H, Ward H, and Kelsey JL.** Disordered eating, menstrual irregularity, and bone minerial density in female distance runners. *Medicine in Science in Sports and Exercise* 35: 711–719, 2003.

25. **Corrado D, Basso C, Pavei A, Michieli P, Schiavon M, and Thiene G.** Trends in sudden cardiovascular death in young competitive athletes after implementation of a preparticipation screening program. *JAMA* 296: 1593–1601, 2006.

26. **Cypcar D, and Lemanske RF, Jr.** Asthma and exercise. *Clin Chest Med* 15: 351–368, 1994.

27. **Dale E, Gerlach DH, and Wilhite AL.** Menstrual dysfunction in distance runners. *Obstet Gynecol* 54: 47–53, 1979.

28. **Dalle Grave R.** Eating disorders: progress and challenges. *Eur J Intern Med* 22: 153–160, 2011.

29. **De Souza MJ.** Menstrual disturbances in athletes: a focus on luteal phase defects. *Med Sci Sports Exerc* 35: 1553–1563, 2003.

30. **De Souza MJ, and Metzger DA.** Reproductive dysfunction in amenorrheic athletes and anorexic patients: a review. *Med Sci Sports Exerc* 23: 995–1007, 1991.

31. **Drezner J, and Corrado D.** Is there evidence for recommending electrocardiogram as part of the pre-participation examination? *Clin J Sport Med* 21: 18–24, 2011.

32. **Drinkwater BL, Bruemner B, and Chesnut CH, III.** Menstrual history as a determinant of current bone density in young athletes. *JAMA* 263: 545–548, 1990.

33. **Drinkwater BL, Nilson K, Chesnut CH, III, Bremner WJ, Shainholtz S, and Southworth MB.** Bone mineral content of amenorrheic and eumenorrheic athletes. *N Engl J Med* 311: 277–281, 1984.

34. **Dugan SA.** Sports-related knee injuries in female athletes: what gives? *Am J Phys Med Rehabil* 84: 122–130, 2005.

35. **Ekblom B.** Effect of physical training in adolescent boys. *J Appl Physiol* 27: 350–355, 1969.

36. **Enea C, Boisseau N, Fargeas-Gluck MA, Diaz V, and Dugue B.** Circulating androgens in women: exercise-induced changes. *Sports Med* 41: 1–15, 2011.

37. **Enea C, Boisseau N, Ottavy M, Mulliez J, Millet C, Ingrand I, Diaz V, and Dugue B.** Effects of menstrual cycle, oral contraception, and training on exercise-induced changes in circulating DHEA-sulphate and testosterone in young women. *Eur J Appl Physiol* 106: 365–373, 2009.

38. **Eriksson BO.** Physical training, oxygen supply and muscle metabolism in 11–13-year old boys. *Acta Physiol Scand Suppl* 384: 1–48, 1972.

39. **Faigenbaum AD, Kraemer WJ, Blimkie CJ, Jeffreys I, Micheli LJ, Nitka M, and Rowland TW.** Youth resistance training: updated position statement paper from the national strength and conditioning association. *J Strength Cond Res* 23: S60–79, 2009.

40. **Faigenbaum AD, Loud RL, O'Connell J, Glover S, and Westcott WL.** Effects of different resistance training protocols on upper-body strength and endurance development in children. *J Strength Cond Res* 15: 459–465, 2001.

41. **Faigenbaum AD, Milliken LA, and Westcott WL.** Maximal strength testing in healthy children. *J Strength Cond Res* 17: 162–166, 2003.

42. **Faigenbaum AD, and Myer GD.** Resistance training among young athletes: safety, efficacy and injury prevention effects. *Br J Sports Med* 44: 56–63, 2010.

43. **Faigenbaum AD, Westcott WL, Loud RL, and Long C.** The effects of different resistance training protocols on muscular strength and endurance development in children. *Pediatrics* 104: e5, 1999.

44. **Faulkner JA, Larkin LM, Claflin DR, and Brooks SV.** Age-related changes in the structure and function of skeletal muscles. *Clin Exp Pharmacol Physiol* 34: 1091–1096, 2007.

45. **Feicht CB, Johnson TS, Martin BJ, Sparkes KE, and Wagner WW, Jr.** Secondary amenorrhoea in athletes. *Lancet* 2: 1145–1146, 1978.

46. **Fitzpatrick KK, and Lock J.** Anorexia nervosa. *Clin Evid (Online)* 2011: 2011.

47. **Fountain NB, and May AC.** Epilepsy and athletics. *Clin Sports Med* 22: 605–616, x–xi, 2003.

48. **Galle PC, Freeman EW, Galle MG, Huggins GR, and Sondheimer SJ.** Physiologic and psychologic profiles in a survey of women runners. *Fertil Steril* 39: 633–639, 1983.

49. **Gotze W, Kubicki S, Munter M, and Teichmann J.** Effect of physical exercise on seizure threshold (investigated by electroencephalographic telemetry). *Dis Nerv Syst* 28: 664–667, 1967.

50. **Hale R.** Factors important to women engaged in vigorous physical activity. In: *Sports Medicine*, edited by Strauss R. Philadelphia: W. B. Saunders, 1984.

51. **Hausenblas HA, Cook BJ, and Chittester NI.** Can exercise treat eating disorders? *Exerc Sport Sci Rev* 36: 43–47, 2008.

52. **Hewett TE, Lindenfeld TN, Riccobene JV, and Noyes FR.** The effect of neuromuscular training on the incidence of knee injury in female athletes: a prospective study. *Am J Sports Med* 27: 699–706, 1999.

53. **Holm-Denoma JM, Scaringi V, Gordon KH, Van Orden KA, and Joiner TE, Jr.** Eating disorder symptoms among undergraduate varsity athletes, club athletes, independent exercisers, and nonexercisers. *Int J Eat Disord* 42: 47–53, 2009.

54. **Ingjer F.** Development of maximal oxygen uptake in young elite male cross-country skiers: a longitudinal study. *J Sports Sci* 10: 49–63, 1992.

55. **Jackson AS, Sui X, Hebert JR, Church TS, and Blair SN.** Role of lifestyle and aging on the longitudinal change in cardiorespiratory fitness. *Arch Intern Med* 169: 1781–1787, 2009.

56. **Jennett B.** Early traumatic epilepsy: incidence and significance after nonmissile injuries. *Arch Neurol* 30: 394–398, 1974.

57. **Kanehisa H, Okuyama H, Ikegawa S, and Fukunaga T.** Sex difference in force generation capacity during repeated maximal knee extensions. *Eur J Appl Physiol Occup Physiol* 73: 557–562, 1996.

58. **Komatsu WR, Gabbay MA, Castro ML, Saraiva GL, Chacra AR, de Barros Neto TL, and Dib SA.** Aerobic exercise capacity in normal adolescents and those with type 1 diabetes mellitus. *Pediatr Diabetes* 6: 145–149, 2005.

59. **Kuijer A.** Epilepsy and exercise, electroencephalographical and biochemical studies. In: *Advances in Epileptology: The X Epilepsy International Symposium*, edited by Wada J, and Penry J. New York: Raven Press, 1980.

60. **Livingston S, and Berman W.** Participation of epileptic patients in sports. *JAMA* 224: 236–238, 1973.

61. **Loucks AB, and Horvath SM.** Athletic amenorrhea: a review. *Med Sci Sports Exerc* 17: 56–72, 1985.

62. **Loucks AB, Vaitukaitis J, Cameron JL, Rogol AD, Skrinar G, Warren MP, Kendrick J, and Limacher MC.** The reproductive system and exercise in women. *Med Sci Sports Exerc* 24: S288–293, 1992.

63. **Manore MM, Kam LC, and Loucks AB.** The female athlete triad: components, nutrition issues, and health consequences. *J Sports Sci* 25 Suppl 1: S61–71, 2007.

64. **Martinsen M, Bratland-Sanda S, Eriksson AK, and Sundgot-Borgen J.** Dieting to win or to be thin? A study of dieting and disordered eating among adolescent elite athletes and non-athlete controls. *Br J Sports Med* 44: 70–76, 2010.

65. **McManus AM, and Armstrong N.** Physiology of elite young female athletes. *Med Sport Sci* 56: 23–46, 2011.

66. **Mendes FA, Almeida FM, Cukier A, Stelmach R, Jacob-Filho W, Martins MA, and Carvalho CR.** Effects of aerobic training on airway inflammation in asthmatic patients. *Med Sci Sports Exerc* 43: 197–203, 2011.

67. **Micheli L.** *Pediatric and Adolescent Sports Medicine.* Philadelphia: W. B. Saunders, 1984.

68. **Micheli LJ, Smith A, Biosca F, and Sangenis P.** IOC position statement on girls and women in sport. 2002.

69. **Miller CA, and Golden NH.** An introduction to eating disorders: clinical presentation, epidemiology, and prognosis. *Nutr Clin Pract* 25: 110–115, 2010.

70. **Mitchell JH, Tate C, Raven P, Cobb F, Kraus W, Moreadith R, O'Toole M, Saltin B, and Wenger N.** Acute response and chronic adaptation to exercise in women. *Med Sci Sports Exerc* 24: S258–265, 1992.

71. **Morton AR, and Fitch KD.** Australian association for exercise and sports science position statement on exercise and asthma. *J Sci Med Sport* 2011.

72. **Narici MV, and Maffulli N.** Sarcopenia: characteristics, mechanisms and functional significance. *Br Med Bull* 95: 139–159, 2010.

73. **National Federation of High School Associations.** High school participation survey. Indianapolis 2002.

74. **Nattiv A, Loucks AB, Manore MM, Sanborn CF, Sundgot-Borgen J, and Warren MP.** American College of Sports Medicine position stand. The female athlete triad. *Med Sci Sports Exerc* 39: 1867–1882, 2007.

75. **Nottin S, Vinet A, Stecken F, N'Guyen LD, Ounissi F, Lecoq AM, and Obert P.** Central and peripheral cardiovascular adaptations to exercise in endurance-trained children. *Acta Physiol Scand* 175: 85–92, 2002.

76. **Pivarnik JM, Marichal CJ, Spillman T, and Morrow JR, Jr.** Menstrual cycle phase affects temperature regulation during endurance exercise. *J Appl Physiol* 72: 543–548, 1992.

77. **Pruett E.** Insulin and exercise in the non-diabetic man. In: *Exercise Physiology*, edited by Fotherly K, and Pal S. New York: Walter de Gruyter, 1985.

78. **Rowland T.** Screening for risk of cardiac death in young athletes. *Sports Science Exchange* 12: 1–5, 1999.

79. **Rowland TW.** Trainability of the cardiorespiratory system during childhood. *Can J Sport Sci* 17: 259–263, 1992.

80. **Scheid JL, and De Souza MJ.** Menstrual irregularities and energy deficiency in physically active women: the role of ghrelin, PYY and adipocytokines. *Med Sport Sci* 55: 82–102, 2010.

81. **Sutton J.** Metabolic responses to exercise in normal and diabetic individuals. In: *Sports Medicine*, edited by Strauss R. Philadelphia: W. B. Saunders, 1984.

82. **Tanaka H, and Seals DR.** Endurance exercise performance in Masters athletes: age-associated changes and underlying physiological mechanisms. *J Physiol* 586: 55–63, 2008.

83. **Torstveit MK, and Sundgot-Borgen J.** The female athlete triad exists in both elite athletes and controls. *Med Sci Sports Exerc* 37: 1449–1459, 2005.

84. **Van Linschoten R.** Epilepsy and sports. *Sports Medicine* 10: 9–19, 1990.

85. **Warren MP.** The effects of exercise on pubertal progression and reproductive function in girls. *J Clin Endocrinol Metab* 51: 1150–1157, 1980.

86. **Weltman A, Janney C, Rians CB, Strand K, Berg B, Tippitt S, Wise J, Cahill BR, and Katch FI.** The effects of hydraulic resistance strength training in pre-pubertal males. *Med Sci Sports Exerc* 18: 629–638, 1986.

87. **Yager J, and Andersen AE.** Clinical practice: anorexia nervosa. *N Engl J Med* 353: 1481–1488, 2005.

88. **Zelisko JA, Noble HB, and Porter M.** A comparison of men's and women's professional basketball injuries. *Am J Sports Med* 10: 297–299, 1982.

89. **Zilmer D.** Gender specific injury patterns in high school varsity basketball. *Journal of Women's Health* 1: 69–76, 1992.

23

Nutrition, Body Composition, and Performance

By studying this chapter, you should be able to do the following:

1. Describe the effect of various carbohydrate diets on muscle glycogen and on endurance performance during heavy exercise.

2. Contrast the "classic" method of achieving a supercompensation of the muscle glycogen stores with the "modified" method.

3. Describe some potential problems when glucose is ingested immediately prior to exercise, and how these problems can be avoided.

4. Describe the importance of blood glucose as a fuel in prolonged exercise and the role of carbohydrate supplementation during the performance.

5. Contrast the evidence that protein is oxidized at a faster rate during exercise with the evidence that the use of labeled amino acids may be an inappropriate methodology to study this issue.

6. Describe the need for protein during the adaptation to a new, more strenuous exercise level with the protein need when the adaptation is complete.

7. Defend the recommendation that a protein intake that is 12% to 15% of energy intake is sufficient to meet an athlete's need.

8. Describe the recommended fluid replacement strategies to use before exercise, during exercise of different durations, and following exercise.

9. Describe the salt requirement of the athlete compared to that of the sedentary individual, and the recommended means of maintaining sodium balance.

10. List the steps leading to iron deficiency anemia and the special problem that athletes have in maintaining iron balance.

11. Provide a brief summary of the effects of vitamin supplementation on performance.

12. Characterize the role of the precompetition meal on performance and the rationale for limiting fats and proteins.

13. Explain why one must be careful in recommending specific body fatness values for individual athletes.

■ Outline

This chapter on nutrition, body composition, and performance is an extension of chapter 18 because the primary emphasis must be on achieving health-related goals before performance-related goals are examined. In fact, the information presented here must be examined in light of what the average person needs. Does an athlete need additional protein? What percentage of body fat is a reasonable goal for an athlete? We will address these questions in that order. For a more detailed look at these issues see Suggested Readings for *Clinical Sports Nutrition* by Burke and Deakin, and *Nutrition for Health, Fitness and Sport* by Williams.

In chapter 18 we indicated the recommended range of nutrient intakes:

- Adults should get 45% to 65% of their calories from carbohydrates, 20% to 35% from fat, and 10% to 35% from protein.

This simple statement is important because it sets the stage for a discussion of what athletes should and do eat to support vigorous training programs and provide the fuel for the diverse performances that make up competitive athletics.

CARBOHYDRATE

The recommended range for carbohydrate intake is quite broad to meet the needs of the whole population and allow one to address special needs linked to a reduced capacity for using carbohydrates (e.g., type 2 diabetics). Because carbohydrate oxidation makes up a larger percentage of total energy production as exercise intensity increases, it should be no surprise that most athletes need more carbohydrate than the average person. This section considers the use of carbohydrates in the days prior to a performance, during the performance itself, and post-performance.

Carbohydrate Diets and Performance

In 1967, three studies were published from the same Swedish laboratory that set the stage for our understanding of the role of muscle glycogen in performance (1, 9, 63). Hermansen et al. (63) showed muscle glycogen to be systematically depleted during heavy (77% $\dot{V}O_2$ max) exercise, and when exhaustion occurred, glycogen content was near zero. Ahlborg et al. (1) found that work time to exhaustion was directly related to the initial glycogen store in the working muscles. Bergström et al. (9) confirmed and extended this by showing that by manipulating the

Figure 23.1 Effect of different diets on the muscle glycogen concentration and work time to exhaustion.

quantity of carbohydrate in the diet, the concentration of glycogen in muscle could be altered and, along with it, the time to exhaustion. In their study, subjects consumed 2,800 kcal/d using either a low-CHO (fat and protein) diet, a mixed diet, or a high-carbohydrate diet in which 2,300 kcal came from carbohydrate. Glycogen contents of the quadriceps femoris muscle were, respectively, 0.63 (low), 1.75 (average), and 3.31 (high) g/100 g muscle, and performance time for exercise at 75% $\dot{V}O_2$ max averaged 57, 114, and 167 minutes. Figure 23.1 shows these results. In brief, the muscle glycogen content and performance time could be varied with diet. These laboratory findings were confirmed by Karlsson and Saltin (75), who had trained subjects run a 30-km race twice, once following a high-carbohydrate diet and the other time after a mixed diet. The initial muscle glycogen level was 3.5 g/100 g muscle following the CHO diet and 1.7 g/100 g muscle following the mixed diet. The best performance of all subjects occurred during the high-CHO diet. Interestingly, the pace at the start of the race was not faster; instead, the additional CHO allowed subjects to maintain the pace for a longer period of time. An important finding in this study was that compared to those on the high-CHO diet, pace did not fall off for those on the mixed diet until about halfway through the race (about 1 hour or so). This suggests that the normal mixed diet used in the study would be suitable for run or cycle races lasting less

Jonas Bergström, M.D., Ph.D.—From the Needle Biopsy Technique and Muscle Glycogen to Much, Much More

Dr. Jonas Bergström had a major impact on the field of exercise physiology, even though most of his research work focused on renal function, in which he had an international reputation. A multitalented man, he pursued medicine only after deciding to give up a career as a recognized jazz musician. He studied medicine at the Karolinska Institute in Stockholm, Sweden, and graduated in 1956. He did subsequent training in renal physiology and biochemistry, and his thesis work, *Muscle Electrolytes in Man*, resulted in the development of the percutaneous (needle) muscle biopsy technique. The introduction of that technique allowed numerous investigators around the world to study muscle function and metabolism at rest and during exercise—studies that revolutionized our understanding of exercise physiology, be it in muscle fiber typing, substrate use during exercise, or adaptation to spaceflight. The classic studies on muscle glycogen use during exercise that were just described were made possible because of this technique, and Dr. Bergström was a lead scientist in those studies.

When he started his career as a physician, there was little that could be done for those in renal failure. He was the leading force in securing the funds, space, and support to develop a chronic dialysis program in Sweden. However, his extensive background in biochemistry and metabolism allowed him to have a major impact on nutritional factors related to renal function.

His research led to the development of special low-protein diets that could reduce the buildup of urea in the blood, and its associated symptoms, which postponed the need for dialysis for months and years. His research also addressed issues related to blood pressure and blood volume during dialysis, the make-up of the fluids used in dialysis (to reduce protein breakdown), and the importance of preventing inflammation in renal disease patients through proper diet. His work impacted the care of renal disease patients around the world, and he was recognized with numerous awards throughout his career for his outstanding contributions. Dr. Bergström died in 2001.

Source: Obituary. Jonas Bergström (1929–2001). 2002. *Nephrology Dialysis Transplantation* 17:936–38.

than 1 hour. See A Look Back—Important People in Science for an individual who had a major impact on our understanding of this aspect of exercise physiology, even though it was not his primary research focus.

Given the importance of muscle glycogen in prolonged endurance performance, it is no surprise that investigators have tried to determine what conditions will yield the highest muscle glycogen content. In 1966, Bergström and Hultman (10) had subjects do one-legged exercise to exhaust the glycogen store in the exercised leg while not affecting the resting leg's glycogen store. When this procedure was followed with a high-carbohydrate diet, the glycogen content was more than twice as high in the previously exercised leg, compared to the control leg. Further, they found that in subjects who had the high-carbohydrate diet following the protein/fat diet (plus doing exhausting exercise), the muscle glycogen stores were higher than when the mixed diet preceded the high-carbohydrate treatment (10). This combination of information led to the following *classical method of* achieving a muscle glycogen **supercompensation:**

- prolonged, strenuous exercise to exhaust muscle glycogen store,
- a fat/protein diet for 3 days while continuing to train, and

- a high-carbohydrate diet (90% CHO) for 3 days, with inactivity.

There were some practical problems with this approach to achieving a high muscle glycogen content, given that it required 7 days to prepare for a race. Further, some subjects could not tolerate either the extremely low- (high fat and protein) or high- (90%) carbohydrate diets. Sherman (103) proposed a *modified plan* that causes supercompensation. The plan requires a tapering of the workout from 90 minutes to 40 minutes while eating a 50% CHO diet (350 g/d). This is followed by 2 days of 20-minute workouts while eating a 70% CHO diet (500–600 g/d) and, finally, a day of rest prior to the competition with the 70% CHO diet (or 500–600 g/d). This regimen was shown to be effective in increasing the glycogen stores to *high values* consistent with good performance (see figure 23.2). Studies have shown that when carbohydrate intake is about 10g/kg body weight using foods with a high glycemic index (see chapter 18), only 1 day was needed to achieve very high muscle glycogen levels in all muscle fiber types (13, 44). The elevated muscle glycogen levels can last as long as 5 days, depending on the level of activity and the amount of carbohydrate ingested during that time (6).

Figure 23.2 Modification of the classic glycogen loading technique to achieve high muscle glycogen levels with minimal changes in a training or diet routine. Glycogen levels are in glucose units (gu) per kilogram (kg).

Sedlock identified three factors that determine the efficacy of carbohydrate loading in women (101):

- Total energy intake—there is a need to increase caloric intake while keeping the percentage of carbohydrates in the diet high (e.g., 75%).
- Carbohydrate intake should be ≥ 8 gm per kilogram of body weight.
- Menstrual cycle phase can affect the outcome; women can store more glycogen during the luteal phase.

Given that glycogen is stored with water (3+ grams water per gram of carbohydrate), athletes need to be aware of a potential feeling of fullness and heaviness, especially for those doing weight-bearing exercise (101).

IN SUMMARY

- Performance in endurance events is improved by a diet high in carbohydrates due primarily to the increase in muscle glycogen.
- When workouts are tapered over several days while additional CHO (70% of dietary intake) is consumed, a "supercompensation" of the glycogen store can be achieved.

Carbohydrate Intake Prior to or During a Performance

The focus on muscle glycogen as the primary carbohydrate source in heavy exercise has always diminished the role that blood glucose plays in maintaining carbohydrate oxidation in muscle. In Coggan and Coyle's review (24), they correct this perception for exercises that last 3 to 4 hours, in which blood glucose and muscle glycogen share equally in contributing to carbohydrate oxidation. In fact, as muscle glycogen decreases, the role that blood glucose plays increases until, at the end of 3 to 4 hours of exercise, it may be the sole source of carbohydrate. This is what makes blood glucose an important fuel in prolonged work, and why so much attention has been directed at trying to maintain the blood glucose concentration.

Unfortunately, the liver glycogen supply also decreases with time during prolonged exercise, and because gluconeogenesis can supply glucose at a rate of only 0.2 to 0.4 g/min when the muscles may be consuming it at a rate of 1 to 2 g/min, hypoglycemia is a real possibility. Hypoglycemia (blood glucose concentration <2.5 mmoles/liter) results when the rate of blood glucose uptake is not matched by release from the liver and/or small

What is needed for the day-to-day replenishment of muscle glycogen?

It takes about 24 hours to replenish muscle glycogen following prolonged, strenuous exercise, provided that about 500 to 700 g of carbohydrate are ingested (29, 44, 50, 72). The point that must be emphasized is that a person who is eating 55% to 60% of calories from carbohydrate is already consuming what is needed to replace muscle glycogen on a day-to-day basis. If an athlete requires 4,000 kcal per day for caloric balance and 55% to 60% is derived from carbohydrates, then 2,200 to 2,400 kcal (55%–60% of 4,000 kcal) or 550 to 600 g of carbohydrate will be consumed. This quantity is consistent with what is needed to restore muscle glycogen to normal levels 24 hours after strenuous exercise (4). This is important for training considerations, and this "regular" diet would require little or no change to meet the carbohydrate load (500–600 g/d) described by Sherman to achieve supercompensation (103).

However, concerns have been raised because most of these guidelines have been based on male subjects, who have high or very high caloric intakes. When applied to women, results are not as consistent.

intestine. Hypoglycemia has been shown to occur during exercise at 58% $\dot{V}O_2$ max for 3.5 hours (8) and at 74% $\dot{V}O_2$ max for 2.5 hours (32). However, the number of subjects who demonstrate central nervous system dysfunction varied from none (45) to only 25% of the subjects (32). Although no absolutely clear association exists between hypoglycemia and fatigue, the availability of blood glucose as an energy source is, without question, linked to the performance of prolonged (3 to 4 hours) strenuous exercise (24). How should carbohydrate be taken in before and during exercise to maintain the high rate of carbohydrate oxidation needed for performance?

Carbohydrate Intake Prior to a Performance The timing and the type of carbohydrate are important to top off the body's carbohydrate stores prior to a performance. One of the earliest studies showed that when 75 g of glucose were ingested 30 to 45 minutes before exercise requiring 70% to 75% $\dot{V}O_2$ max, plasma glucose and insulin were elevated at the start of exercise, and muscle glycogen was used at a *faster rate* during the exercise (27). This is counter to the goal of sparing muscle glycogen, and performance was shown to decrease 19% with such a treatment (48). In contrast to this early study, various reviews of this topic indicate that the blood glucose and plasma insulin responses to pre-exercise glucose feedings are quite variable (some will experience a lowering of blood glucose; most will not), and that, in general, performance in prolonged exercise is either improved or not affected (3, 74, 102). The pre-exercise carbohydrate feeding is viewed as a means of topping off both muscle and liver glycogen stores. Generally, such procedures result in carbohydrates being used at a higher rate, but because of the large amount of carbohydrate ingested, the plasma glucose concentration is maintained for a longer period of time. Jeukendrup provides the following observations and recommendations relative to pre-exercise feedings (74):

- The fall in blood glucose during submaximal exercise (62–72% $\dot{V}O_2$ max) following ingestion of 75 g of carbohydrate an hour before the exercise cannot be prevented by ingesting a smaller (~22 g) or larger (>155 g) amount of carbohydrate.
- High glycemic index carbohydrates taken in an hour before exercise lead to a higher blood glucose and insulin responses, compared to moderate or low glycemic index carbohydrates.
- The hypoglycemic response is quite variable, with some athletes being much more susceptible than others. Interestingly, this responsiveness is not linked to insulin sensitivity.

- To minimize the risk of hypoglycemia, carbohydrates can be ingested just prior to the exercise (in last 5 minutes), or during the warm-up.
- The form in which the carbohydrate is ingested does not matter. One can use a solid, gel, or liquid carbohydrate product. Clearly, the type should be left to the athlete.

Athletes who are more responsive to pre-exercise carbohydrate feedings (i.e., experience symptoms of hypoglycemia) should test different types of carbohydrate (low, moderate, high glycemic index), ingest carbohydrates just before the performance or during the warm-up, or if that doesn't work, avoid carbohydrates in the 90 minutes before exercise (74).

Carbohydrate Intake During a Performance In contrast to the pre-exercise feeding studies in which there was some variability in the outcome, there is a great deal of consensus that feeding carbohydrate during exercise delays fatigue and improves performance. Interestingly, the improved performance appears to have nothing to do with sparing the muscle glycogen store. Muscle glycogen is depleted at the same rate during prolonged vigorous (70–75% $\dot{V}O_2$ max) exercise, with or without carbohydrate ingestion; however, liver glycogen is not (22, 24). The ingestion of carbohydrate appears to spare the liver glycogen store by directly contributing carbohydrate for oxidation. If additional carbohydrate is not ingested during prolonged exercise, the blood glucose concentration decreases as the liver stores are depleted, resulting in an inadequate rate of carbohydrate oxidation by muscle. Central nervous system activation of muscle is diminished by hypoglycemia, resulting in a reduced power output (92). Consistent with that, the rating of perceived exertion (RPE) is lower with carbohydrate supplementation during prolonged exercise (19, 110). Figure 23.3 shows Coggan and Coyle's model of how carbohydrate is supplied to muscle during prolonged exercise under fasted and fed conditions. The rate of muscle glycogen depletion is not different; however, when fed carbohydrates, the subjects last longer due to the increased availability of blood glucose. This effect varies with the dose, with a greater rate of ingestion (i.e., 15 g/hr vs. 60 g/hr) leading to better performances (106). When is the best time to consume carbohydrates during exercise?

Coggan and Coyle indicate that carbohydrates can be ingested throughout exercise, or can be taken 30 minutes before the anticipated time of fatigue, with no difference in the outcome (24). This is consistent with their contention that it is the increased availability of glucose late in exercise that delays fatigue. In exercise tests at 75% $\dot{V}O_2$ max, the time to

Figure 23.3 Blood glucose and muscle glycogen use when subjects fasted or were fed carbohydrates (CHO) during prolonged exercise.

fatigue was extended by about 45 minutes with carbohydrate ingestion. Because muscles use blood glucose at the rate of about 1 to 1.3 g/min late in exercise, sufficient carbohydrate should be ingested to provide an additional 45 to 60 g (45 min × 1 to 1.3 g/min) of carbohydrate. There is general agreement that this can be achieved when carbohydrates are taken in at the rate of about 30 to 60 g/hr during exercise (24). The 120 to 240 g of glucose consumed (4 hrs × 30 to 60 g/hr) provides for the 45 to 60 g needed at the end of exercise, but also supports the elevated carbohydrate metabolism throughout exercise. Glucose, sucrose, or **glucose polymer** solutions are all successful in maintaining the blood glucose concentration during exercise, but the palatability of the solution is improved if glucose polymer solutions are used for concentrations above 10%. Is there anything that can be added to these drinks to have a larger impact on performance?

There is evidence that the addition of caffeine (5.3 mg · kg⁻¹) to carbohydrate drinks improves time-trial performance without affecting carbohydrate oxidation during steady state exercise (69). There also is some support for the addition of protein to carbohydrate sports drinks, but not without exception. A recent systematic review of this literature showed that, compared to carbohydrate alone, the coingestion of protein and carbohydrate improved time to exhaustion, but not time-trial performances—so the improvement appeared to depend on the test used to evaluate performance. When the beverages were adjusted to match them in total calories (since, in some, the added protein increased the caloric content compared to the carbohydrate-alone beverage), the improvement in performance was reduced in half, but it was still an improvement (107). Studies published after this review found either an improvement in endurance performance (47) or no change (12). Interestingly, the outcomes followed the performance test

used, as mentioned above. We are sure to hear more about this in the future.

A new question regarding carbohydrate drinks has arisen: Does simply rinsing the mouth with the drink at regular intervals during the performance result in an improved performance? The answer appears to be yes when applied to time-trial performances in both cyclists (21) and runners (99). In one of the studies, brain centers (as observed using MRI) associated with reward were activated with the carbohydrate mouth rinse whether it was sweet (glucose) or not (maltodextrin) (21). In contrast, Beelen et al. (7) found no improvement in time-trial performance with this procedure when performed with well-fed subjects (versus those who fasted overnight).

Carbohydrate delivery from the stomach to the small intestine increases with the concentration of glucose, but fluid delivery slows down when the carbohydrate concentration exceeds 8%. This trade-off in glucose versus fluid delivery can be balanced by drinking 375 to 750 ml/hr of an 8% solution of carbohydrate, which would deliver 30 to 60 grams of glucose per hour to the blood (4, 34). One final point: Even when the blood glucose concentration is maintained by either glucose infusion or ingestion during exercise, the subject will eventually stop; this indicates that fatigue is related to more than the delivery of fuel to muscles (24). For an update on carbohydrate drinks and performance, see Ask the Expert 23.1.

Carbohydrate Intake Post-Performance

The degree of muscle glycogen depletion varies with the duration and intensity of the exercise. The limiting factor in muscle glycogen synthesis is glucose transport across the cell membrane. Following a bout of heavy exercise there is an increase in the muscle cell's permeability to glucose, an increase in

Chapter Twenty-Three   Nutrition, Body Composition, and Performance   **523**

ASK THE EXPERT 23.1

Carbohydrate Drinks and Performance: Questions and Answers with Dr. Ronald J. Maughan

Ron Maughan obtained his B.Sc. (Physiology) and Ph.D. from the University of Aberdeen, and held a lecturing position in Liverpool before returning to Aberdeen where he stayed for more than 20 years. He is now located at the School of Sport, Exercise and Health Sciences at Loughborough University, England. He chairs the Nutrition Working Group of the International Olympic Committee. His research interests are in the physiology, biochemistry, and nutrition of exercise performance, with an interest in both the basic science of exercise and the applied aspects that relate to health and to performance in sport.

QUESTION: Athletes use carbohydrate drinks to improve performance. What type of athlete would benefit most from this strategy?

ANSWER: All athletes will find these drinks useful in some training and competition situations. During exercise, they are especially important when the exercise time exceeds about 30 to 40 minutes. They provide carbohydrate as an energy source and this is especially important if there has not been an opportunity for complete recovery of the body's carbohydrate stores since the last training session or competition. These drinks also promote water absorption and supply some electrolytes, so they are particularly important when sweat losses are high. Athletes should get into the habit of using these drinks in training as well as in competition. Training sessions feel easier, the risk of heat illness is greatly reduced, and the quality of training may be better maintained: this is important for

those who take exercise for fun as well as for the elite athlete. The reduction in the perception of effort is especially important for those who exercise for health; if the exercise feels easier, they are more likely to stick to an exercise program. Strength and power athletes may train for long periods, but often do not have the awareness of the need for rehydration that exists in endurance sports. Of course, the calories need to be taken into account, and those on an energy-restricted diet may limit their use of sport drinks for this reason.

QUESTION: Given the existing research support for this strategy, what are the most important questions remaining to be answered?

ANSWER: Many questions remain to be answered, but these relate mostly to the application of the basic science in practical situations. The basic ingredients of carbohydrate-electrolyte sports drinks (water, sugar, and salt) have not changed substantially, but we need to have a better understanding of the optimum formulation for use in different situations. We now know that a mixture of different carbohydrates, including both glucose and fructose, can increase the availability and oxidation of ingested carbohydrates and can enhance performance compared to drinks that contain only glucose. There are situations in which a higher or a lower carbohydrate content would be better, and athletes have to recognize that different drinks may be better suited to different exercise and environmental conditions. There is also

some debate about the need for electrolyte replacement in different situations. We also need to learn how to communicate current knowledge more effectively to athletes and coaches, and this is perhaps the biggest challenge we face at present.

QUESTION: Are there any differences between these traditional carbohydrate drinks and the new "energy drinks" being advertised to improve performance?

ANSWER: The new energy drinks are mostly very high in sugar, hence, the energy, and they also usually contain caffeine to give a feeling of more energy. These drinks can have disadvantages in some situations. Because of the high carbohydrate content, the osmolality of these drinks is very high, and the body actually secretes water into the small intestine after they have been ingested. This exacerbates any dehydration and can cause gastrointestinal discomfort. Some of the newer energy drinks do not contain energy at all: they contain only caffeine (plus a few flavorings, etc.) to give a feeling of more energy. Although moderate doses of caffeine can help performance, the very high doses in some of these products can increase the risk of dehydration due to increased urine loss and can lead to overarousal that results in poorer performance in some skilled tasks. Some athletes also report that high doses of caffeine make it difficult to sleep at night when they have used high doses of caffeine in competitions held in late afternoon or evening.

glycogen synthase activity, and an increase in the muscle's sensitivity to insulin (72). To take advantage of these factors carbohydrates ($1.0 - 1.5 \text{ g} \cdot \text{kg}^{-1}$) need to be consumed within 30 minutes after exercise and at 2-hour intervals for up to 6 hours if one wants to replace glycogen stores quickly. High

glycemic foods are better in this regard. However, if time is not crucial, eating a balance of carbohydrates, fats, and protein will achieve both carbohydrate replacement and the promotion of an optimal rate of muscle protein synthesis needed for tissue repair and hypertrophy (4).

IN SUMMARY

- Pre-exercise carbohydrate feedings are used to top off the body's carbohydrate stores. Individuals who experience symptoms of hypoglycemia should test different approaches or avoid this procedure.
- Muscle glycogen is depleted at the same rate, whether or not glucose is ingested during prolonged performance.
- The ingestion of glucose solutions during exercise extends performance by providing carbohydrate to the muscle at a time when muscle glycogen is being depleted.
- To restore glycogen stores quickly after exercise, carbohydrates should be consumed ($1.0 - 1.5$ g $\cdot$ kg^{-1}) within the first 30 minutes post-exercise and at 2-hour intervals for 6 hours.

PROTEIN

The adult RDA for protein is 0.8 gm $\cdot$ kg^{-1} $\cdot$ d^{-1} and is easily met by a diet having 12% of its energy (kcal) as protein. For example, if the daily energy requirement for an adult male weighing 72 kg is 2,900 kcal/day, then about 348 kcal are taken in as protein (12% of 2,900 kcal). At 4 kcal/g, this person would consume approximately 87 g protein per day, representing 1.2 g $\cdot$ kg^{-1} $\cdot$ d^{-1} (87 g/70 kg), or 50% more than the RDA standard. Does an athlete have to take in more protein than specified in the RDA, or is the normal diet adequate? Confusing as it may seem, the answer to both questions appears to be yes.

Protein Requirements and Exercise

Adequacy of protein intake has been based primarily on nitrogen(N)-balance studies. Protein is about 16% N by weight, and when N-intake (dietary protein) equals N-excretion, the person is in N-balance. Excretion of less N than one consumes is called positive N-balance, and the excretion of more N than one consumes is called negative N-balance. This latter condition, if maintained, is inconsistent with good health due to the potential loss of lean body mass. Based on these N-balance studies, it was generally believed that the 0.8 g $\cdot$ kg^{-1} $\cdot$ d^{-1} RDA standard was adequate for those engaged in prolonged exercise. In these studies, urinary N excretion was usually used as an index of N-excretion, because about 85% of N is excreted this way (81). However, some experiments suggest this method of measurement may underestimate amino acid utilization in exercise. Lemon and Mullin (82) found that although there was no difference in urinary N excretion compared to rest, the loss of N in sweat increased 60- to 150-fold during exercise, suggesting that as much as 10% of the energy requirement of the exercise was met by the oxidation of amino acids.

Other studies, using different techniques, supported these observations. Muscle has been shown to release the amino acid alanine in proportion to exercise intensity (46), and the alanine is used in gluconeogenesis in the liver to generate new plasma glucose. Several investigators have infused a stable isotope (^{13}C-label) of the amino acid leucine to study the rate at which amino acids are mobilized and oxidized during exercise. In general, the rate of oxidation (measured by the appearance of $^{13}CO_2$) is higher during exercise than at rest in rats and humans (35, 66, 116). Taken as a group, these studies suggest that amino acids are used as a fuel during exercise to a greater extent than previously believed. They also suggest that the protein requirement for those involved in prolonged exercise is higher than the RDA (81). However, there is more to the story.

Oxidation of Amino Acids Part of the justification for a greater protein requirement in those who exercise is based on work using isotopes of amino acids whose metabolism could be traced during exercise. That is, if an amino acid is metabolized, the "labeled" $^{13}CO_2$ is exhaled and can be used as a marker of its rate of use. The essential amino acid leucine has been used as being representative of the amino acid pool. The previously mentioned work showed that leucine oxidation is increased with exercise (35, 66, 116). This implies that the catabolism of protein is higher during exercise compared to rest. Wolfe et al. (123) confirmed this greater rate of leucine oxidation during exercise but failed to show an increase in urea production, a primary index of protein catabolism. It was concluded that the N contained in leucine does not find its way to plasma urea N as a result of exercise (121, 122); instead, the N in leucine is transferred to intermediates (pyruvate) to form alanine, which is later used in the liver in gluconeogenesis.

These results raised additional questions, so another experiment was conducted to see if leucine was, in fact, representative of the amino acid pool. The investigators used the amino acid lysine and found different results for the same experimental procedures. On the basis of their experiments, Wolfe et al. (122, 123) concluded that leucine cannot be used as a model of whole-body protein metabolism during exercise, that changes in (or lack of) urea production during exercise may not reflect an accurate picture of protein breakdown, and finally, that the data provide no rationale for increasing protein intake when exercising (122, 123). A review supports this proposition and indicates that even if the leucine requirement is three times the RDA in individuals who exercise, the mixed diet of a typical athlete is sufficient to meet those needs (14). This takes us back to nitrogen-balance studies as a focal point of determining the protein requirements for athletes.

Whole-Body Nitrogen Balance Studies The ability to maintain N-balance during exercise appears to be dependent on the following (14, 16, 79–81):

- the training state of the subject,
- the quality and quantity of protein consumed,
- total calories consumed,
- the body's carbohydrate store, and
- the intensity, duration, and type (resistance versus endurance) of exercise.

If measurements of protein utilization are made during the first few days of an exercise program, formerly sedentary subjects show a negative N-balance (figure 23.4). However, after about 12 to 14 days of training, this condition disappears and the person can maintain N-balance (55). So, depending on the point into the training program where the measurements are made, one could conclude either that more protein is needed (during the adaptation to exercise) or that protein needs can be met by the RDA (after the adaptation is complete) (16). Butterfield indicates that in N-balance studies the length of time needed to achieve a new steady state depends on the magnitude of the change in the level of N-intake, and the absolute amount of N consumed, and that the recommended minimum of a 10-day adaptation period may be inadequate when N-intake is very large (14).

Another factor influencing the conclusion one would reach about protein needs during exercise is whether the person is in caloric balance—that is, taking in enough kcal to cover the cost of the added exercise. For example, it has been shown that by increasing the energy intake 15% more than that needed to maintain weight, an increase in N-retention occurred during exercise when these subjects consumed only 0.57 g $\cdot$ kg^{-1} $\cdot$ d^{-1} of egg white protein (16). In a parallel study by the same group (109), a 15% deficit in energy intake was created while subjects consumed either 0.57 or 0.8 g $\cdot$ kg^{-1} $\cdot$ d^{-1} egg white protein. When taking in 15% fewer calories than needed, the 0.8 g $\cdot$ kg^{-1} $\cdot$ d^{-1} protein intake was associated with a negative N-balance of 1 g $\cdot$ d^{-1}. However, when the subjects did 1 or 2 hours of exercise, the negative N-balance improved to a loss of only 0.51, or 0.27 g $\cdot$ d^{-1}, respectively. During the treatment in which the subjects were in caloric balance, the RDA of 0.8 g $\cdot$ kg^{-1} $\cdot$ d^{-1} was sufficient to achieve a positive N-balance for both durations of exercise. It is clear, then, that to make proper judgments about the adequacy of the protein intake, the person must be in energy balance.

A final nutritional factor that can influence the rate of amino-acid metabolism during exercise is the availability of carbohydrate. Lemon and Mullin (82) showed that the quantity of urea found in sweat was cut in half when subjects were carbohydrate loaded as opposed to carbohydrate depleted (see figure 23.5). Further, as figure 23.6 shows, the ingestion of glucose during the latter half of a 3-hour exercise test at 50% $\dot{V}O_2$ max reduces the rate of oxidation of the amino acid leucine (35). So, not only is caloric balance important in protein metabolism, but the ability of the diet to provide adequate carbohydrate must also be considered.

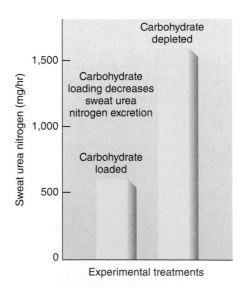

Figure 23.5 Effect of initial muscle glycogen levels on sweat urea nitrogen excretion during exercise. A high muscle glycogen level decreases the excretion of urea nitrogen in sweat during exercise.

Figure 23.4 Effect of exercise on nitrogen balance.

Figure 23.6 Effect of glucose ingestion on the rate of metabolism of the amino acid leucine. Glucose ingestion decreases the rate of amino acid oxidation.

Protein Requirements for Athletes

How much protein does an athlete need? To answer that question, one needs to consider the fact that the RDA for protein varies from country to country (0.8 to $1.2 \text{ g} \cdot \text{kg}^{-1} \cdot \text{d}^{-1}$), and that most of these standards do not consider vigorous exercise done by athletes. The Dutch did, and offered $1.5 \text{ g} \cdot \text{kg}^{-1} \cdot \text{d}^{-1}$ as the standard for athletes (79). So, again, how much protein is needed? It depends on the athletic status of the individual and the intensity and type of exercise. The Institute of Medicine's Food and Nutrition Board stated that there is little or no evidence that more than $0.8 \text{ g} \cdot \text{kg}^{-1} \cdot \text{d}^{-1}$ of protein is needed for healthy adults who engage in resistance or endurance exercise (70). In contrast, for elite athletic populations doing high-intensity endurance exercise, there is general agreement that the requirement appears to be around 1.2 to $1.4 \text{ g} \cdot \text{kg}^{-1} \cdot \text{d}^{-1}$ (14, 78–80), and this was supported in a recent ACSM Position Stand on this topic (4). However, for strength training there has been a history of less agreement. Butterfield (14) felt that $0.9 \text{ g} \cdot \text{kg}^{-1} \cdot \text{d}^{-1}$, close to the RDA, is sufficient for "maintenance" of existing body protein stores in strength trainers. For those strength-training elite athletes who are adding muscle mass, the requirement may be as high as $1.7 \text{ g} \cdot \text{kg}^{-1} \cdot \text{d}^{-1}$ (4). The current recommended range of protein intake for resistance training, 1.2 to $1.7 \text{ g} \cdot \text{kg}^{-1} \cdot \text{d}^{-1}$, has been consistently supported over the past 20 years, and is unlikely to change in the near future (4, 14, 78, 94, 108). It is important for the athlete to remember to maintain caloric balance because of the consequences a negative caloric balance can have on N-balance. The general agreement and stability of these recommendations for protein intake does not mean that there are no more issues to deal with. Current questions revolve around the timing of protein intake for optimal gains in muscle mass, and whether some types of protein are better than others (see The Winning Edge 23.1).

THE WINNING EDGE 23.1

Timing of Protein Intake for Maximum Effect

There is no question that following a resistance training workout, muscle protein synthesis (MPS) is increased. But it is increased even more when amino acids are either ingested or infused, compared to a fasted state. For obvious practical reasons the focus has been on ingestion rather than infusion, and the following observations have been made about how to obtain optimal results (64, 73, 95):

■ MPS is activated most strongly when amino acids are available in the first hour following the workout.
  ● This approach to timing of protein intake is even more important for older adults.
■ Whey protein (20% of milk protein) is digested more rapidly than casein protein (80% of milk protein) or soy protein and yields a higher level of essential amino acids (EAA) in the blood, with the EAA being a driving force for MPS.
  ● Casein protein provides a longer and more sustained EAA response, making milk a good post-exercise drink because it contains both proteins, naturally.
■ There is only limited information on the impact of these post-exercise protein feedings over the course of a full resistance-training program, but the available evidence supports the recommendation.

■ Some recommend that the supplement be composed of both carbohydrate and protein to take advantage of the insulin response (73), whereas others don't see the need for the carbohydrate when protein intake is adequate (95).
■ The amount of high-quality protein needed post-exercise to optimally stimulate MPS is modest (~25 g), containing 8–10 g of EAA (95), though others recommend (for a 70-kg person) 35–40 g protein, plus 70–84 g carbohydrates (73).

This is clearly an exciting area of research, and we are sure to see a more complete picture in the near future.

Another way to approach this question is to consider the protein requirement of a human from childhood to adulthood. The RDA for protein is 1.5 g · $kg^{-1} \cdot d^{-1}$ during the second 6 months of life, decreasing to 0.95 g · $kg^{-1} \cdot d^{-1}$ by ages 4 to 8, and reaching the adult value of 0.8 g · $kg^{-1} \cdot d^{-1}$ by age 18 (see appendix C). During this period of time an individual may increase body weight by a factor of ten (15 lb to 150 lb). This is not unlike what was previously mentioned about the adaptation to exercise. During the initial days of an exercise training program when the muscles are adapting to the new exercise, the protein requirement might be higher than the RDA, and data of Gontzea (55, 56) support this proposition. However, after the person has adapted to the exercise, the requirement would revert to the RDA.

At the beginning of this section on the protein requirements for athletes, a question was raised: Does an athlete have to take in more protein than the RDA, or is the normal diet adequate? During intense endurance training or strength training, the requirement of protein may be higher than the RDA. So the answer is yes to that part of the question. It is also yes to the second part, in that the average person typically takes in 50% more than the RDA for protein. Brotherhood (12) reports that an average athlete's diet is about 16% protein, exceeding 1.5 g · $kg^{-1} \cdot d^{-1}$ (88% more than RDA!). These values exceed the RDA of young children who are in a chronic state of positive nitrogen balance, and approach the upper limit of the recommendations of Lemon (14, 79, 80). In support of dietary protein intake being sufficient, two recent studies found that protein supplements provided no advantage in terms of strength gains in a resistance training program in both young experienced trained athletes (65) and in older individuals experiencing sarcopenia (17). It would appear that while scientists deal with questions of the effect of exercise on the oxidation of amino acids, and to what extent the RDA for athletes is greater than 0.8 g · $kg^{-1} \cdot d^{-1}$, the athlete following a normal dietary pattern will consume more than enough protein to meet the needs associated with exercise, assuming that caloric intake is adequate.

Some concern has been raised about consuming too much dietary protein, especially with regard to amenorrheic athletes (15). High-protein diets lead to an increase in Ca^{++} excretion, and for many years it was believed that the Ca^{++} was of bone origin and of real concern for the amenorrheic athlete (42, 62). Recent studies suggest otherwise. Short-term diets high in protein have been shown to simultaneously increase Ca^{++} absorption from the intestine, and there is no evidence of an impact on net stores of bone Ca^{++}. However, those on a low-protein diet show a reduction in Ca^{++} absorption from the intestine, and long-term use of such diets could seriously compromise skeletal health (76, 77).

In contrast, some concern has been expressed that athletes consuming a vegetarian diet might not be able to meet the protein requirement. A recent review by Venderley and Campbell (113) reported that protein intakes ranged from 10–12%, 12–14%, and 14–18% in vegans, lacto-ovo vegetarians, and omnivores, respectively. The lacto-ovo vegetarians have easy access to high-quality and easily accessed protein in eggs and milk products. On the other hand, athletes who are vegans do not, and they may benefit from careful dietary planning with a sports-related registered dietician to realize performance goals (113). See Suggested Readings for a recent review by Fuhrman and Ferreri, and a position stand by Borrione, Grasso, Quaranta, and Parisi that addresses this issue.

IN SUMMARY

- The protein requirement for those engaged in light-to-moderate endurance exercise is equal to the RDA of 0.8 g · $kg^{-1} \cdot d^{-1}$; however, it is 1.2–1.4 g · $kg^{-1} \cdot d^{-1}$ for athletes who participate in high-intensity endurance exercise.
- For resistance training, the recommended range of protein intake is 1.2 to 1.7 g · $kg^{-1} \cdot d^{-1}$.
- Bottom line: The average protein intake of an athlete exceeds 1.5 g · $kg^{-1} \cdot d^{-1}$, more than enough to cover most protein requirements.

WATER AND ELECTROLYTES

Chapter 12 described in some detail the need to dissipate heat during exercise to minimize the increase in core temperature. The primary mechanism for heat loss at high work rates in a comfortable environment, and at all work rates in a hot environment, is the evaporation of sweat. Sweat rates increase linearly with exercise intensity, and in hot weather sweat rates can reach 2.8 liters per hour (26). In spite of attempts to replace water during marathon races, some runners lose 8% of their body weight (26). Given that water losses in excess of 2% adversely affect endurance performance, especially in hot weather, there is a clear need to maintain water balance (2, 4). Of course, more than water is lost in sweat. An increased sweat rate means that a wide variety of electrolytes, such as Na^+, K^+, Cl^-, and Mg^{++}, are lost as well (26). These electrolytes are needed for normal functioning of excitable tissues, enzymes, and hormones. It should be no surprise then that investigators have been concerned about the optimal way to replace water and electrolytes to reduce the chance of health-related problems and increase the chance of optimal performance (85).

Fluid Replacement—Before Exercise

The goal of prehydrating is to be euhydrated (have a normal body water content) before the exercise or competition begins. In general, with sufficient time (8 to 24 hours) between the end of one exercise (competition) and the next, foods and beverages consumed at meals will be sufficient. If the time frame is too short, the following steps can be taken (2, 4):

■ Slowly drink beverages (e.g., ~5–7 ml · kg^{-1}) at least 4 hours before exercise.

■ If urine is not produced or if it is dark in color, drink more fluid (e.g., ~3–5 ml · kg^{-1}) 2 hours before the exercise.

■ Using beverages with sodium in them (20–50 mEq · L^{-1}) or salted snacks would help retain the fluid.

Some investigators have used large volumes of water or have taken glycerol (86) to create a hyperhydrated state (body water content greater than normal) prior to exercise; in fact, recent studies provide guidelines for an optimal dose of glycerol to accomplish this goal (57, 112). However, there is no clear evidence that better performances will result compared to euhydration (2), and the practice of using glycerol is discouraged (4).

Fluid Replacement—During Exercise

The goal of drinking beverages during exercise is to reduce the chance of becoming excessively dehydrated (2% body weight loss from water deficit) (2). Fortunately, for some sports in which play is intermittent (football, tennis, golf), water replacement during the activity is possible. However, in athletic events such as marathon running, there are no formal breaks in the activity to allow for replacement. In these latter activities, in which a high rate of heat production is coupled with the potential problems of environmental heat and humidity, the athlete is at great risk. Studies confirm the need to replace fluids as they are lost during exercise in order to maintain moderate heart rate and body temperature responses (59, 96). Figure 23.7 shows changes in esophageal temperature, heart rate, and rating of perceived exertion during 2 hours of exercise at 62% to 67% V̇O$_2$ max under four conditions of fluid replacement: (a) no fluid, (b) small fluid (300 ml/hr), (c) moderate fluid (700 ml/hr), and (d) large fluid (1,200 ml/hr). The fluid was a "sport drink" containing 6% carbohydrate and electrolytes (33). As you can see, there were marked differences in the responses over time. The lowest heart rate, body temperature, and rating of perceived exertion were associated with the highest rates of fluid replacement (30, 33). It must be added that although most of the attention on fluid replacement is directed at those who participate in

Figure 23.7 Core temperature (esophageal temperature), heart rate, and perceived exertion during 120 min of exercise when subjects ingested no fluid, or small (300 ml/hr), moderate (700 ml/hr), or large (1,200 ml/hr) volumes of fluid. A rating of 17 for perceived exertion corresponds to "Very Hard," 15 is "Hard," and 13 is "Somewhat Hard." Values are means ±SE.
*Significantly lower than no fluid, P < 0.05.
†Significantly lower than small fluid, P < 0.05.
§Significantly lower than moderate fluid, P < 0.05.

prolonged endurance exercise, it is clear that the same message must reach those who participate in intermittent exercise (104). Given that fluid replacement during exercise is clearly beneficial, how much fluid should be taken at one time? Should it be warm or cold? Should it contain electrolytes and glucose?

Costill and colleagues (28, 31) provided some of the original answers to these questions. One study examined the effects of fluid volume, temperature, glucose concentration, and the intensity of exercise on the rate at which fluid leaves the stomach to the small intestine. They determined this by giving the

Figure 23.8 Effect of fluid volume, glucose concentration, solute temperature, and the intensity of exercise on the rate of fluid absorption from the gastrointestinal tract.

subject the fluid in question and then, 15 minutes later, aspirating the contents of the stomach. Figure 23.8 summarizes the results of that study. A glucose concentration above 139 mM (2.5%) slowed gastric emptying (i.e., increased residue; figure 23.8a). The optimal volume to ingest was 600 ml (figure 23.8b), and colder drinks appeared to be emptied faster (i.e., decreased residue; figure 23.8c). Finally, exercise had no effect on gastric emptying until the intensity exceeded 65% to 70% $\dot{V}O_2$ max (figure 23.8d). Using the same technique, which has been shown to be valid (49), studies have confirmed that intensities below 75% $\dot{V}O_2$ max do not affect the rate of gastric emptying (87), and that there is no difference between running and cycling in the rate of gastric emptying for exercise intensities of 70% to 75% $\dot{V}O_2$ max (67, 87, 98). However, dehydration and/or high body temperature have been shown to delay gastric emptying (88, 97). While most of the later work supports the findings shown in figure 23.8, the one exception is with regard to the carbohydrate content of the drink.

In the original study (28), the effectiveness of a drink was evaluated 15 minutes after ingestion by aspirating the contents of the stomach. Davis and colleagues (38, 39) questioned the use of the aspiration technique, because it simply measures how much fluid leaves the stomach, not how much is actually absorbed into the blood from the small intestine. They used heavy water (D_2O) as a tracer of fluid absorption from the gastrointestinal tract to the blood and found that a 6% glucose-electrolyte solution was absorbed as fast as or faster than water at rest (39) or during exercise (38). Two additional studies that used the aspiration technique (84, 93) found that when either a 10% glucose solution or glucose

polymer solutions containing 5% to 10% carbohydrate were ingested at 15- to 20-minute intervals during prolonged exercise at 65% to 70% $\dot{V}O_2$ max, there was no difference in the gastric emptying rate of either solution compared to water. The improved performance of the carbohydrate drinks in the most recent studies may be related to the experimental procedures, which included the ingestion of small volumes (~200 ml) at regular intervals (15 to 20 minutes) during prolonged exercise, with the aspiration occurring at the end of the entire exercise session (not 15 minutes after ingestion). An additional benefit of these glucose solutions is that the extra carbohydrate helps to maintain the blood glucose during exercise (see earlier discussion). It must be added, however, that drinks containing more than 8% glucose remain in the stomach longer, with subjects complaining of gastrointestinal distress (2, 4). If fluid intake is most important and carbohydrate is secondary, a drink should be fashioned accordingly.

Because sweat rates vary so much among individuals, it is recommended that individuals estimate their sweat rates (measure weight pre- and post-exercise [competition], and account for the volume of fluid ingested) to determine how much to drink. Also, they should "practice" drinking the beverage in routine workouts to determine if it works for them. The following should be considered for a sport beverage (2, 71):

■ temperature should be between 15 and 21°C,
■ beverage should contain ~20 to 30 mEq · L^{-1} sodium and 2 to 5 mEq · L^{-1} potassium, and
■ contain 5% to 10% carbohydrate.

The greatest rates of carbohydrate delivery occur when a mixture of sugars is used (e.g., glucose, sucrose, fructose, maltodextrin) (2). Interestingly, and in contrast to popular beliefs, caffeine consumption does *not* create a water-electrolyte imbalance or hyperthermia, or reduce exercise-heat tolerance (5).

A range of values are given for the electrolyte and carbohydrates to allow drinks to better meet expected demands. Gisolfi and Duchman (53) provide the following guidelines:

- during exercise lasting less than 1 hour (80–130% $\dot{V}O_2$ max), the athlete should drink 500 to 1,000 ml of water;
- for exercise durations between 1 and 3 hours (60–90% $\dot{V}O_2$ max), the drink should contain 10 to 20 mEq of Na^+, and Cl^-, and 6% to 8% carbohydrate, with 500 to 1,000 ml/hr meeting the carbohydrate need, and 800 to 1,600 ml/hr meeting the fluid need; and
- for events of more than 3 hours' duration, the drink should contain 20 to 30 mEq of Na^+, and Cl^-, and 6% to 8% carbohydrate, with 500 to 1,000 ml/hr meeting the carbohydrate and fluid needs of most athletes.

Allowances must be made for the individual differences in the frequency and volume of ingestion. The addition of salt to the drink enhances its palatability, promotes fluid and carbohydrate absorption, and replenishes some of the electrolytes lost during the activity. An additional reason sodium has been added to the drinks is related to concerns that have been raised about the potential for hyponatremia, a dangerously low Na^+ concentration that can occur when a person hydrates only with water or hypotonic drinks during extremely long (>4 hours), ultra-endurance athletic events (2, 4, 90, 114). (See The Winning Edge 23.2.)

Fluid Replacement—After Exercise

Gisolfi and Duchman (53) also provided a drink for recovery that is consistent with the need to replenish electrolytes and muscle glycogen: The drink should contain 30 to 40 mEq of Na^+, and Cl^-, and deliver 50 g of carbohydrate per hour. If an individual has to rehydrate quickly, it is recommended that ~1.5 liters of fluid be ingested for every kilogram of weight lost to compensate for the increased urine output (2). One can use a sport drink or other beverages to rehydrate following exercise. One study compared a carbohydrate-electrolyte (CE) drink to skim milk. The subjects consumed 150% of the body weight lost as a result of doing an exercise bout in the heat. Three hours after they ingested the beverages the subjects achieved euhydration with the CE drink and were slightly hyperhydrated with the skim milk. The milk provided 113 gm of carbohydrate vs. 137 for the CE drink, but the milk also provided 75 gm of protein—allowing the milk to address multiple needs during recovery (115).

Salt (NaCl)

One of the Dietary Guidelines for Americans presented in chapter 18 was to decrease the intake of sodium. Although the point was made that Americans consume two to three times the amount needed for optimal health, is the dietary intake sufficient for an athlete who participates in regular vigorous physical activity? The mass of sodium in the body determines the water content, given the way water is reabsorbed at the kidney. If a person becomes sodium depleted, body water decreases, and the risk of heat injury increases. An untrained and unacclimatized individual (see chapter 24) loses more Na^+ in sweat than a trained and acclimatized person. If the unacclimatized person has 1.9 g Na^+ per liter of sweat and loses 5 liters of sweat (11 pounds), the person would lose 9.5 grams of Na^+ per day. As the person becomes acclimatized to heat, the sodium content in sweat decreases to about half that, and Na^+ loss is about 5 g/day. Given that Na^+ is 40% of NaCl by weight, a person would have to consume 12.5 g of salt per day to meet that demand. It is generally believed that an individual with a high Na^+ loss can stay in sodium/water balance by simply adding salt to food at mealtime, rather than by consuming salt tablets (118). The best single practical test of the success of salt/water replacement procedures is to obtain a nude body weight measure in the morning, after voiding. Additional information about adequate hydration can be obtained by measuring urine specific gravity of the morning urine (2). The general dietary routine followed by athletes must be successful, because early-morning body weight remains relatively constant despite large daily sweat losses. Given what has just been presented, you might think there is no disagreement about whether dehydration impairs exercise performance—but you would be wrong. See the "point-counterpoint" of Noakes and Sawka in Suggested Readings.

IN SUMMARY

- Fluid replacement during exercise reduces the heart rate, body temperature, and perceived exertion responses to exercise, and the greater the rate of fluid intake, the lower the responses.
- Cold drinks are absorbed faster than warm drinks, and when exercise intensity exceeds 65% to 70% $\dot{V}O_2$ max, gastric emptying decreases.
- For exercise lasting less than 1 hour, the focus is on water replacement only. When exercise duration exceeds 1 hour, drinks should contain Na^+, Cl^-, and carbohydrate.
- Salt needs are easily met at mealtime, and salt tablets are not needed. In fact, most Americans take in more salt than is required (see chapter 18).

Hyponatremia

A primary driving force shaping fluid replacement recommendations over the past 60 years was the potential for dehydration during athletic events due to inadequate consumption of fluids. Over the past decade a different problem, hyponatremia, has surfaced—that associated with drinking too much fluid during long-term athletic events and diluting the body's sodium level (4, 89, 90). The normal range of the serum sodium concentration is 135–145 mEq · L^{-1}. The risks associated with hyponatremia vary with the sodium concentration (100):

- *Mild* (Na$^+$ = 131–134 mEq · L^{-1})—generally causes no symptoms
- *Moderate* (Na$^+$ = 126–130 mEq · L^{-1})—can result in bloating, malaise, headache, nausea, vomiting, fatigue, confusion, and persistent and involuntary leg movements
- *Severe* (Na$^+$ <126 mEq · L^{-1})—can cause altered mental status, coma, seizures, and even death

The risk factors associated with hyponatremia include the following (18):

- Individual factors
  - Genetic predisposition for high sodium sweat rates (43)
  - Variation in symptoms at the same sodium concentration (100)
- Overdrinking—drinking too much relative to need
- Exercise duration >4 hr of continuous physical activity
- Low body weight <20 BMI
- Women—smaller stature; slower speeds
- Pre-exercise overhydration
- Insufficient sodium in foods consumed
- Weight gain—fluid retention during race

Given these risk factors it is no surprise that, in marathons, symptomatic hyponatremia is more likely to occur in smaller individuals who run slowly, sweat less, and drink relatively large volumes of water and other hypotonic fluids, before, during, and after the race (2). In response to this problem, the ACSM released recommendations from their Roundtable Series on the topic: hydration and physical activity (20):

- Work to minimize risk of both hyponatremia and dehydration. Athletes are encouraged to neither underhydrate nor overhydrate, because each has significant consequences.

Dehydration, especially during warm/hot weather conditions, occurs more frequently and is also life threatening. The message is to drink intelligently, not maximally.

- Athletes should determine their typical sweat rate during a practice run (e.g., 60 min)
  - Measure weight lost, e.g., 1.9 kg (1.9 L)
  - Add volume of fluid consumed, e.g., +0.5 L
  - Subtract volume of urine excreted, if any, e.g., 0.0 L
  - Sweat rate = 1.9 L + 0.5 L − 0.0 L = 2.4 L/60 min = 0.04 L/min or 40 ml/min
- Drink to match fluid loss and on a schedule. The fluid should be consumed over a set period of time, rather than rapidly in a "catch-up" fashion. If athletes are not sweating much and are not thirsty, fluid replacement should be modest.
- Consume salty foods and beverages. Foods and beverages with sodium help promote fluid retention and stimulate thirst. Those performing long-duration exercise should consume snacks and fluids containing sodium to help prevent hyponatremia.

MINERALS

Iron

A vast majority of the body's iron is found in hemoglobin in the red blood cells (erythrocytes) that are involved in oxygen transport to tissues (see chapter 10). Other iron-containing molecules include myoglobin and the cytochromes in the electron transport chains of mitochondria. The remainder of the body's iron is stored in various tissues, primarily tied to the protein ferritin, with the serum ferritin (SF) levels being a good index of the body's iron store (117). In addition to SF being used to assess iron status, some propose using the serum concentration of soluble transferrin receptor (sTfR) to monitor iron depletion.

Iron is transported in the serum bound to transferrin, which, in turn, binds to a transferrin receptor on the cell's surface in order for the iron to be taken into the cell. A breakdown product of the transferrin receptor (sTfR) circulates in the serum and is a good measure of the number of these receptors on the cells. A recent study of male and female athletes recommends its use in addition to traditional measures to anticipate problems before they become worse (83). The higher the level of sTfR in the serum, the greater is the level of anemia. In addition, the degree to which iron is bound to transferrin (transferrin saturation) also is used as a marker of iron status.

As mentioned in chapter 18, iron deficiency is the most common nutritional deficiency. The stages of iron deficiency are spelled out in table 23.1, as well as the

TABLE 23.1	Population Cut-offs for Hematological Markers Commonly Used to Evaluate Iron Status in Clinical Practice	
Stages of Iron Deficiency	Hematological Markers	Deficiency/Overload State
Stage 1 Depleted iron stores	Stainable iron in bone marrow	Absent
	Total iron binding capacity	>400 μg/dL
	Serum ferritin	<12 μg/L (>15 years)
Stage 2 Early functional iron deficiency	Transferrin saturation	<16% (>10 years)
	Serum transferrin receptor (sTfR)	>8.5 mg/L
Stage 3 Iron deficiency anemia	Hemoglobin	<130 g/L (males >15 years)
		<120 g/L (females >15 years)
	Mean cell volume	<80 fL

From V. Deakin, "Prevention, Detection, and Treatment of Iron Depletion and Deficiency in Athletes." In *Clinical Sports Nutrition*, edited by L. M. Burke and V. Deakin. New York: McGraw-Hill, 2010, pp. 222–267.

tests used to detect deficiencies. The groups of athletes with the highest risk of iron depletion and deficiency include female athletes, distance runners, and vegetarians (and those who eat little red meat) (40). Iron depletion may be as high as 20–35% in women runners, in contrast to 3.5–8% in male runners; however, because some use different cut-off values for SF (<16 to <30 μg/L, rather than <12 μg/L), it is difficult to make comparisons across studies. Anemia is much less common, being about 5–7% in female athletes (60). As iron stores are depleted, the iron containing compounds ferritin, hemoglobin, transferrin, myoglobin, and cytochromes become depleted. Given that hemoglobin is a necessary part of the oxygen-transport process, it is not surprising that in individuals with iron deficiency anemia, endurance and work performance are decreased (52, 54, 60). Interestingly, when the low-hemoglobin condition is corrected in iron-deficient animals by transfusion, $\dot{V}O_2$ max is brought back to normal, but not endurance time. This suggests that while hemoglobin levels may be high enough to achieve a normal $\dot{V}O_2$ max, iron deficiency affects the iron-containing cytochromes (electron transport chain) that are involved in oxidative phosphorylation, and endurance performance is adversely affected (36). In a similar study (37), iron supplementation brought the $\dot{V}O_2$ max back to normal values faster than that of mitochondrial activity (measured by pyruvate oxidase activity) and endurance performance (see figure 23.9).

What causes iron deficiency in athletes? A combination of factors are linked to iron deficiency in athletes (40, 60):

- High iron requirement due to
  - Blood loss in GI tract
  - Greater red blood cell damage due to simple "pounding" on hard surfaces

Figure 23.9 Recovery of various physiological capacities with iron repletion. Note that recovery of endurance lagged behind $\dot{V}O_2$ max.

- Hemoglobin loss in urine and sweat
- Variable blood loss in menses

- Low iron intake linked to
  - Low energy intake
  - Vegetarian diets
  - Diets low in red meat
  - Dieting for weight loss

Consistent with this, Diehl et al. (41) have shown decreases in serum ferritin over the course of a field hockey season, and from one hockey season to the next, in female athletes. The average value at the end of the season in third-year players was 10.5 μg · L^{-1} (below the 12 μg · L^{-1} standard), indicating iron depletion (61). A recent study indicated that even though female athletes may have some iron-status variables in the normal range, they may still be in a state of non-anemic iron depletion. This argues for better tracking of female athletes over their careers (58). Iron deficiency and anemia are also concerns for the military. Two recent studies from Israel indicate that 24% of female recruits were anemic (25), and 4.5% of males had hemoglobin levels below 12 g · dl^{-1} (91).

Generally, when a person has a deficiency in iron stores, there is an increased uptake of dietary iron. Unfortunately, athletes do not appear to follow that pattern. Factors that can affect the absorption of iron include (40):

- Facilitators
  - Amount of heme iron in food (e.g., meat). Heme iron is more readily absorbed than non-heme iron (found in vegetables), but less than 15% of dietary iron is heme iron
  - Vitamins A and C
  - Peptides from partial digestion of meat protein
- Inhibitors
  - Cereal grains, legumes, nuts, peanut butter, bran, soy products
  - Tea, coffee, red wine, some spices
  - Peptides from partial digestion of plant proteins

Given the impact of so many variables on iron status, especially in women, it should be no surprise that supplementation may be needed (40, 60). This is especially the case for those on vegetarian diets (4, 11, 51). Some may choose to take an iron supplement each day as an ounce of prevention, but such a practice is not without problems (e.g., intolerance, overdose, drug interactions) and should not be done indiscriminately (4, 40, 60, 118).

VITAMINS

Chapter 18 provided the details about the RDA for each vitamin. Many of these vitamins are directly involved in energy production, acting as coenzymes in mitochondrial reactions associated with aerobic metabolism. Unfortunately, the old adage that "if a little is good, more will be better" has been applied to the question of whether the RDA for athletes is higher than that for sedentary people, rather than a factual research base. In general, the major reviews of this issue over the past 30 years have systematically concluded that, in general:

- vitamin supplementation is unnecessary for the athlete on a well-balanced diet,
- people who are *clearly deficient* in certain vitamins have improved performance when values return to normal, and

- individuals taking large doses of fat-soluble vitamins or vitamin C should be concerned about toxicity (8, 23, 111, 118).

The central concern raised by these reviewers is for the small athlete on a low-energy diet who may not make wise food selections, a point reinforced in a recent set of recommendations. In these situations a single RDA multivitamin/mineral pill might be appropriate (4). For those who believe the adage and want to take a high-potency multivitamin, one study showed that 90 days on such a pill had no effect on maximal aerobic power, endurance running performance, or strength (105). Additional information on the use of nutritional supplements to improve athletic performance is presented in chapter 25, where ergogenic aids are discussed.

IN SUMMARY

- Iron deficiency in athletes may be related to an inadequate intake of dietary iron as well as a potentially greater loss in sweat and feces. In spite of this deficiency, athletes may absorb less than what a sedentary group of anemic individuals absorbs. Iron supplementation may be recommended for female athletes as a result of an annual clinical assessment of iron status.
- Vitamin supplementation is unnecessary for an athlete on a well-balanced diet. However, for those with a clear deficiency, supplementation is warranted.

PRECOMPETITION MEAL

The two most important nutritional practices associated with optimal performance in endurance exercise are (a) to eat a high-carbohydrate diet in the days preceding competition when the intensity and duration of workouts are reduced, and (b) to drink liquids at regular intervals during the competition. Consistent with our previous discussion, the purposes of the precompetition meal are the following (4, 118):

- to provide adequate hydration,
- to provide carbohydrate to "top off" already high carbohydrate stores in the liver,
- to avoid the sensation of hunger on a relatively empty stomach,
- to minimize GI tract problems (gas, diarrhea), and
- to allow the stomach to be relatively empty at the start of competition.

Unfortunately, the type of precompetition meal served at various universities throughout this country may rely more on tradition than nutrition. The standard rare steak before a boxing match or football game to bring out the animal instinct, or careful planning to make sure that the color of the Jell-O* is the same as it was when the team won last year's championship, are less than rational, but may be useful in pulling the team together to get ready for competition. Problems arise when the precompetition meal is responsible for poor performance because of its own characteristics (high fat and protein) or the inability of the athlete to tolerate the meal without vomiting or experiencing diarrhea due to the emotion associated with competition. These latter events would cause dehydration, a condition inconsistent with optimal performance. It is clear that beyond what is recommended in the nutrient makeup of a precompetition meal, the ability of the athlete to tolerate it must be considered (4, 118).

Nutrients in Precompetition Meal

To achieve the purposes of the precompetition meal, the following general guidelines are provided (4):

- Sufficient fluid should be consumed to maintain hydration
- Carbohydrates should make up the majority of the meal, but large amounts of simple sugars, especially fructose, should be avoided because of the potential for gastrointestinal problems such as diarrhea.
- The meal should be low in fats and fiber to facilitate gastric emptying.
- Protein should make up a small part of the meal because the metabolism of protein increases the acid load that must be buffered and finally excreted by the kidneys.
- The foods should be familiar to and well liked by the athlete.

Table 23.2 presents two precompetition meals that meet these considerations. These meals should be eaten about 3 hours prior to competition (118). Some coaches and athletes prefer one of the commercially available liquid meals as the precompetition meal because of convenience. These liquid meals can also be consumed throughout the day (along with additional water) when events or games are scheduled over long periods of time. Given that some people may not react favorably to any new "food," these liquid meals should be tried on practice days rather than on game day to make sure they are suitable.

*Jell-O is a registered trademark of General Foods, Inc.

TABLE 23.2	Two Examples of Pre-competition Meals Containing 500–600 Kilocalories
Meal A	**Meal B**
Glass of orange juice	One cup low-fat yogurt
One bowl of oatmeal	One banana
Two pieces of toast with jelly	One toasted bagel
Sliced peaches with skim milk	One-half cup raisins

From: Williams MH. *Nutrition for Health, Fitness and Sport.* New York: McGraw-Hill, 2010, p. 77.

IN SUMMARY

- The precompetition meal should provide for hydration and adequate carbohydrate to "top off" stores while minimizing hunger symptoms, gas, and diarrhea.
- Varieties of commercially available liquid meals are consistent with these goals.

BODY COMPOSITION AND PERFORMANCE

In chapter 18 we discussed body composition from a health perspective, with the range of body fatness values, using the two-component system, associated with health and fitness being:

Health	**Fitness**
Males: 8–22% fat	5–15% fat
Females: 20–35% fat	16–28% fat

The question is, are these values optimal for athletic performance?

Table 23.3 lists a summary of body fatness values by sport (120). Many are average values and do not represent the range that might be observed in a study. For example, a study might find an average value of 12% body fat for a group of football players, but the range might be 5% to 19%. In a sport or activity in which body weight must be carried along (e.g., running or jumping), there is a negative correlation between body fatness and performance (119, 120).

There is little question that regular measurements of body composition are useful for athletes to monitor changes during the season as well as over the off-season. In this way the athlete will know whether changes in body weight represent gains or losses of body fatness. What is more difficult is

TABLE 23.3	Percent Body Fat Values for Male and Female Athletes		
Athletic Group or Sport	**Male**	**Female**
Baseball	11.8–14.2	—
Basketball	7.1–10.6	20.8–26.9
Canoeing	12.4	—
Football		
Backs	9.4–12.4	—
Linebackers	13.7	—
Linemen	15.5–19.1	—
Quarterbacks, kickers	14.1	—
Gymnastics	4.6	9.6–23.8
Ice hockey	13–15.1	—
Jockeys	14.1	—
Orienteering	16.3	18.7
Pentathlon	—	11.0
Racquetball	8.3	14.0
Skiing		
Alpine	7.4–14.1	20.6
Cross-country	7.9–12.5	15.7–21.8
Nordic combined	8.9–11.2	—
Ski jumping	14.3	—
Soccer	9.6	—
Speed skating	11.4	—
Swimming	5.0–8.5	20.3
Tennis	15.2–16.3	20.3
Track and field		
Distance runners	3.7–18.0	15.2–19.2
Middle distance runners	12.4	—
Sprinters	16.5	19.3
Discus	16.3	25.0
Jumpers/hurdlers	—	20.7
Shot put	16.5–19.6	28.0
Volleyball	—	21.3–25.3
Wrestling	4.0–14.4	

From J. H. Wilmore, "Body Composition in Sport Medicine: Directions for Future Research," in *Medicine and Science in Sports Medicine* 15:21–31, 1983. Copyright © 1983 American College of Sports Medicine, Indianapolis IN. Reprinted by permission.

careful measurement, percent fat can be estimated with an error of about 2.5% fat. So when an athlete is measured as being 15.0% body fat, the true value may be as high as 17.5% and as low as 12.5% (68). Other techniques have larger errors, which would only complicate one's ability to make a specific absolute body fatness recommendation to an athlete (see discussion in chapter 18).

Another reason caution must be used in making an absolute recommendation for each athlete is that it ignores the normal variation in body fatness found in elite athletes in any particular sport. An elite group of volleyball players may have an average value of 12%, but the range among the team members might be 6% to 16%. No one would think of telling the athlete with 6% body fat to increase body fatness to reach the team average, and the same advice holds true for the one at 16% body fatness who is playing with world-class skill. A recommendation to alter body composition to achieve better performance must be made against the background of present performance and general health status as seen in sleeping patterns, adequate diet, mental outlook, and so on. The implementation of longer workouts or a reduction in caloric intake might change the percent body fat in the appropriate direction, but either one could adversely affect the athlete's ability to tolerate a work-out or to study for exams. Wilmore's (119) observation of one of the best female distance runners who held most of the American middle distance records should be remembered when making such recommendations: The champion was 17% body fat when most of the elite female runners were <12%.

Monitoring body fatness in athletes by skinfold or underwater weighing is a reasonable procedure to follow because it allows a coach or trainer to observe *changes* in body fatness over the course of a season and from one year to the next. The information is also useful to the athletes who, when they finish their competitive careers, must attend to what is a reasonable body weight in order to be within the optimal body fatness range for health and fitness.

providing a fixed absolute recommendation about what body fatness should be for optimal performance for each individual.

One of the main reasons one must be careful in making absolute recommendations, such as "This athlete should reduce her percent body fat from 15.6% to 14.0%," is that the athlete may already be 14% body fat. Each *individual estimate* of body fatness, even done by the underwater weighing technique, has an error in measurement that cannot be ignored. With some methods such as underwater weighing and with

IN SUMMARY

■ The body fat percentage consistent with excellence in performance is different for men and women and varies within gender from sport to sport. Average values for a team should not be applied to any single individual without regard to overall health status as seen in diet, sleep, and mental outlook. Further, it is "natural" for some athletes to have a higher body fatness than others in order to perform optimally.

STUDY QUESTIONS

1. What procedures would you follow to cause a super-compensation of muscle glycogen?
2. To what factors should women attend to enhance glycogen loading?
3. How could glucose ingestion prior to exercise actually increase the rate of glycogen depletion? What could be done to minimize this effect?
4. Does carbohydrate ingestion during exercise slow down muscle glycogen depletion? Does it improve performance?
5. Is the protein requirement of an athlete higher than that of a sedentary person? Should protein intake be increased? Explain.
6. What would you recommend to an athlete to reduce the chance of dehydration during exercise?
7. How does the fluid replacement strategy differ for short and long races?
8. What factors contribute to iron deficiency in female athletes? What can be done to address these factors?
9. Does an athlete need additional vitamins for optimal performance? Explain.
10. What are the primary considerations for a precompetition meal?
11. Given a champion female distance runner with 17% body fat, what should you consider before recommending that she decrease her percent fat to 15%?

SUGGESTED READINGS

American College of Sports Medicine. 2009. Nutrition and athletic performance. *Medicine and Science in Sports and Exercise* 41:709–31.

Borrione, P., L. Grasso, F. Quaranta, and A. Parisi. 2009. FIMS Position Statement 2009: Vegetarian diet and athletes. *International SportMed Journal* 10:53–60.

Burke, L. M, and V. Deakin. 2010. *Clinical Sports Nutrition*. New York: McGraw-Hill.

Fuhrman J., and D. M. Ferreri. 2010. Fueling the vegetarian (vegan) athlete. *Current Sports Medicine Reports* 9:233–41.

Noakes, T. D., and M. N. Sawka. 2007. Point-Counterpoint: Does dehydration impair exercise performance? *Medicine and Science in Sports and Exercise* 39:1209–17.

Williams, M. H. 2010. *Nutrition for Health, Fitness and Sport*. New York: McGraw-Hill.

REFERENCES

1. **Ahlborg B.** Muscle glycogen and muscle electrolytes during prolonged physical exercise. *Acta Physiologica Scandinavica* 70: 129–142, 1967.
2. **American College of Sports Medicine.** Exercise and fluid replacement. *Medicine and Science in Sports and Exercise* 39: 2007.
3. **American College of Sports Medicine.** Joint position statement: nutrition and athletic performance. American College of Sports Medicine, American Dietetic Association, and Dietitians of Canada. *Medicine and Science in Sports and Exercise* 32: 2130–2145, 2000.
4. **American College of Sports Medicine.** Nutrition and athletic performance. *Medicine and Science in Sports and Exercise* 41: 709–731, 2009.
5. **Armstrong LE, Casa DJ, Maresh CM, and Ganio MS.** Caffeine, fluid-electrolyte balance, temperature regulation, and exercise-heat tolerance. *Exercise and Sport Sciences Reviews* 35: 135–140, 2007.
6. **Arnall DA, Nelson AG, Quigley J, Lex S, Dehart T, and Fortune P.** Supercompensated glycogen loads persist 5 days in resting trained cyclists. *European Journal of Applied Physiology* 99: 251–256, 2007.
7. **Beelen M, Berghuis J, Bonoparte B, Ballak SB, Jeukendrup AE, and van Loon LJC.** Carbohydrate mouth rinsing in the fed state: lack of enhancement of time-trial performance. *International Journal of Sport Nutrition and Exercise Metabolism* 19: 2009.
8. **Belko AZ.** Vitamins and exercise: an update. *Medicine and Science in Sports and Exercise* 19: S191–196, 1987.
9. **Bergstrom J, Hermansen L, Hultman E, and Saltin B.** Diet, muscle glycogen and physical performance. *Acta Physiol Scand* 71: 140–150, 1967.
10. **Bergstrom J, and Hultman E.** Muscle glycogen synthesis after exercise: an enhancing factor localized to the muscle cells in man. *Nature* 210: 309–310, 1966.
11. **Borrione P, L. G, Quaranta F, and Parisi A.** FIMS Position Statement 2009: vegetarian diet and athletes. *International SportMed Journal* 10: 53–60, 2009.
12. **Breen L, Tipton KD, and Jeukendrup A.** No effect of carbohydrate-protein on cycling performance and indices of recovery. *Medicine and Science in Sports and Exercise* 42: 1140–1148, 2010.
13. **Bussau VA, Fairchild TJ, Rao A, Steele P, and Fournier PA.** Carbohydrate loading in human muscle: an improved 1 day protocol. *European Journal of Applied Physiology* 87: 290–295, 2002.
14. **Butterfield G.** Amino acids and high protein diets. In: *Ergogenics: Enhancement of Performance in Exercise and Sport*, edited by Lamb D, and Williams M. Carmel: Brown & Benchmark, 1991, p. 87–117.
15. **Butterfield GE.** Whole-body protein utilization in humans. *Medicine and Science in Sports and Exercise* 19: S157–165, 1987.
16. **Butterfield GE, and Calloway DH.** Physical activity improves protein utilization in young men. *The British Journal of Nutrition* 51: 171–184, 1984.
17. **Campbell WW.** Synergistic use of higher-protein diets or nutritional supplements with resistance training to counter sarcopenia. *Nutrition Reviews* 65: 416–422, 2007.
18. **Carter III R.** Exertional heat illness and hyponatremia: an epidemiological prospective. *Current Sports Medicine Reports* 7: S20–S27, 2008.
19. **Carter J, Jeukendrup AE, Mundel T, and Jones DA.** Carbohydrate supplementation improves moderate and high-intensity exercise in the heat. *Pflugers Arch* 446: 211–219, 2003.
20. **Casa DJ, Clarkson PM, and Roberts WO.** American College of Sports Medicine roundtable on hydration and physical activity: consensus statements. *Current Sports Medicine Reports* 4: 115–127, 2005.

21. **Chambers ES, Bridge MW, and Jones DA.** Carbohydrate sensing in the human mouth: effects on exercise performance and brain activity. *Journal of Applied Physiology-London* 587: 1779–1794, 2009.

22. **Chryssanthopoulos C, Williams C, and Nowitz A.** Influence of a carbohydrate-electrolyte solution ingested during running on muscle glycogen utilisation in fed humans. *International Journal of Sports Medicine* 23: 279–284, 2002.

23. **Clarkson P.** Vitamins and trace minerals. In: *Ergogenics: Enhancement of Performance in Exercise and Sport*, edited by Lamb D, and Williams M. Carmel: Brown & Benchmark, 1991, p. 123–182.

24. **Coggan AR, and Coyle EF.** Carbohydrate ingestion during prolonged exercise: effects on metabolism and performance. *Exercise and Sport Sciences Reviews* 19: 1–40, 1991.

25. **Constantini N, Dubnov G, Foldes AJ, Mann G, Magazanik A, and Siderer M.** High prevalence of iron deficiency and anemia in female military recruits. *Military Medicine* 171: 866–869, 2006.

26. **Costill DL.** Sweating: its composition and effects on body fluids. *Annals of the New York Academy of Sciences* 301: 160–174, 1977.

27. **Costill DL, Coyle E, Dalsky G, Evans W, Fink W, and Hoopes D.** Effects of elevated plasma FFA and insulin on muscle glycogen usage during exercise. *Journal of Applied Physiology* 43: 695–699, 1977.

28. **Costill DL, and Saltin B.** Factors limiting gastric emptying during rest and exercise. *Journal of Applied Physiology* 37: 679–683, 1974.

29. **Costill DL, Sherman WM, Fink WJ, Maresh C, Witten M, and Miller JM.** The role of dietary carbohydrates in muscle glycogen resynthesis after strenuous running. *The American Journal of Clinical Nutrition* 34: 1831–1836, 1981.

30. **Coyle E.** Fluid and carbohydrate replacement during exercise: how much and why? Barrington: Gatorade Sports Science Institute, 1994.

31. **Coyle EF, Costill DL, Fink WJ, and Hoopes DG.** Gastric emptying rates for selected athletic drinks. *Research Quarterly* 49: 119–124, 1978.

32. **Coyle EF, Hagberg JM, Hurley BF, Martin WH, Ehsani AA, and Holloszy JO.** Carbohydrate feeding during prolonged strenuous exercise can delay fatigue. *Journal of Applied Physiology* 55: 230–235, 1983.

33. **Coyle EF, and Montain SJ.** Benefits of fluid replacement with carbohydrate during exercise. *Medicine and Science in Sports and Exercise* 24: S324–330, 1992.

34. **Coyle EF, and Montain SJ.** Carbohydrate and fluid ingestion during exercise: are there trade-offs? *Medicine and Science in Sports and Exercise* 24: 671–678, 1992.

35. **Davies C.** Glucose inhibits CO_2 production from leucine during whole body exercise in man. *Journal of Physiology* 332: 40–41, 1982.

36. **Davies KJ, Donovan CM, Refino CJ, Brooks GA, Packer L, and Dallman PR.** Distinguishing effects of anemia and muscle iron deficiency on exercise bioenergetics in the rat. *The American Journal of Physiology* 246: E535–543, 1984.

37. **Davies KJ, Maguire JJ, Brooks GA, Dallman PR, and Packer L.** Muscle mitochondrial bioenergetics, oxygen supply, and work capacity during dietary iron deficiency and repletion. *The American Journal of Physiology* 242: E418–427, 1982.

38. **Davis JM, Burgess WA, Slentz CA, Bartoli WP, and Pate RR.** Effects of ingesting 6% and 12% glucose/electrolyte beverages during prolonged intermittent cycling in the heat. *European Journal of Applied Physiology and Occupational Physiology* 57: 563–569, 1988.

39. **Davis JM, Lamb DR, Burgess WA, and Bartoli WP.** Accumulation of deuterium oxide in body fluids after ingestion of D2O-labeled beverages. *Journal of Applied Physiology* 63: 2060–2066, 1987.

40. **Deakin V.** Prevention, detection and treatment of iron depletion and deficiency in athletes. In: *Clinical Sports Nutrition*, edited by Burke LM, and Deakin V. New York: McGraw-Hill, 2010, p. 222–267.

41. **Diehl DM, Lohman TG, Smith SC, and Kertzer R.** Effects of physical training and competition on the iron status of female field hockey players. *International Journal of Sports Medicine* 7: 264–270, 1986.

42. **Drinkwater BL, Nilson K, Chesnut CH, III, Bremner WJ, Shainholtz S, and Southworth MB.** Bone mineral content of amenorrheic and eumenorrheic athletes. *The New England Journal of Medicine* 311: 277–281, 1984.

43. **Eichner ER.** Genetic and other determinants of sweat rate. *Current Sports Medicine Reports* 7: S36–S40, 2008.

44. **Fairchild TJ, Fletcher S, Steele P, Goodman C, Dawson B, and Fournier PA.** Rapid carbohydrate loading after a short bout of near maximal-intensity exercise. *Medicine and Science in Sports and Exercise* 34: 980–986, 2002.

45. **Felig P, Cherif A, Minagawa A, and Wahren J.** Hypoglycemia during prolonged exercise in normal men. *The New England Journal of Medicine* 306: 895–900, 1982.

46. **Felig P, and Wahren J.** Amino acid metabolism in exercising man. *The Journal of Clinical Investigation* 50: 2703–2714, 1971.

47. **Ferguson-Stegall L, McCleave EL, Ding ZP, Kammer LM, Wang B, Doerner PG, Liu Y, and Ivy JL.** The effect of low carbohydrate beverage with added protein on cycling endurance performance in trained athletes. *Journal of Strength and Conditioning Research* 24: 2577–2586, 2010.

48. **Foster C, Costill DL, and Fink WJ.** Effects of preexercise feedings on endurance performance. *Medicine and Science in Sports* 11: 1–5, 1979.

49. **Foster C, and Thompson NN.** Serial gastric emptying studies: effect of preceding drinks. *Medicine and Science in Sports and Exercise* 22: 484–487, 1990.

50. **Friedman JE, Neufer PD, and Dohm GL.** Regulation of glycogen resynthesis following exercise. Dietary considerations. *Sports Medicine (Auckland, NZ)* 11: 232–243, 1991.

51. **Fuhrman J, and Ferreri DM.** Fueling the vegetarian (vegan) athlete. *Current Sports Medicine Reports* 9: 233–241, 2010.

52. **Gardner GW, Edgerton VR, Senewiratne B, Barnard RJ, and Ohira Y.** Physical work capacity and metabolic stress in subjects with iron deficiency anemia. *The American Journal of Clinical Nutrition* 30: 910–917, 1977.

53. **Gisolfi CV, and Duchman SM.** Guidelines for optimal replacement beverages for different athletic events. *Medicine and Science in Sports and Exercise* 24: 679–687, 1992.

54. **Gledhill N.** The influence of altered blood volume and oxygen transport capacity on aerobic performance. *Exercise and Sport Sciences Reviews* 13: 75–93, 1985.

55. **Gontzea I, Sutzescu P, and Dumitrache S.** The influence of adaptation of physical effort on nitrogen balance in man. *Nutrition Reports International* 11: 231–236, 1975.

56. **Gontzea I, Sutzescu P, and Dumitrache S.** The influence of muscular activity on nitrogen balance, and on the need of man for protein. *Nutrition Reports International* 10: 35–43, 1974.

57. **Goulet EDB.** Glycerol-induced hyperhydration: a method for estimating the optimal load of fluid to be ingested before exercise to maximize endurance performance. *Journal of Strength and Conditioning Research* 24: 74–78, 2010.

58. **Gropper SS, Blessing D, Dunham K, and Barksdale JM.** Iron status of female collegiate athletes involved in different sports. *Biological Trace Element Research* 109: 1–14, 2006.

59. **Hamilton MT, Gonzalez-Alonso J, Montain SJ, and Coyle EF.** Fluid replacement and glucose infusion during exercise prevent cardiovascular drift. *Journal of Applied Physiology* 71: 871–877, 1991.

60. **Haymes EM.** Iron. In: *Sports Nutrition*, edited by Driskell JA, and Wolinsky I. Boca Raton: CRC Taylor & Francis, 2006, p. 203–216.

61. **Haymes EM.** Nutritional concerns: need for iron. *Medicine and Science in Sports and Exercise* 19: S197–200, 1987.

62. **Hegsted M, Schuette SA, Zemel MB, and Linkswiler HM.** Urinary calcium and calcium balance in young men as affected by level of protein and phosphorus intake. *The Journal of Nutrition* 111: 553–562, 1981.

63. **Hermansen L, Hultman E, and Saltin B.** Muscle glycogen during prolonged severe exercise. *Acta Physiol Scand* 71: 129–139, 1967.

64. **Hoffman J.** Protein intake: effect of timing. *Strength and Conditioning Journal* 29: 26–34, 2007.

65. **Hoffman J, Ratamess N, and Kang J.** Effects of protein supplementation on muscular performance and resting hormonal changes in college football players. *Journal of Sports Science and Medicine* 6: 2007.

66. **Hood DA, and Terjung RL.** Amino acid metabolism during exercise and following endurance training. *Sports Medicine (Auckland, NZ)* 9: 23–35, 1990.

67. **Houmard JA, Egan PC, Johns RA, Neufer PD, Chenier TC, and Israel RG.** Gastric emptying during 1 h of cycling and running at 75% $\dot{V}O_2$ max. *Medicine and Science in Sports and Exercise* 23: 320–325, 1991.

68. **Houtkooper L, and Going S.** Body composition: how should it be measured? Does it affect performance? Barrington: Gatorade Sports Science Institute, 1994.

69. **Hulston CJ, and Jeukendrup A.** Substrate metabolism and exercise performance with caffeine and carbohydrate intake. *Medicine and Science in Sports and Exercise* 40: 2096–2104, 2008.

70. **Institute of Medicine.** Water. In: *Dietary Reference Intakes for Energy, Carbohydrate, Fiber, Fat, Protein and Amino Acids (macronutrients)*. Washington DC: National Academy Press, 2002, p. 73–185.

71. **Institute of Medicine.** Water. In: *Dietary Reference Intakes for Energy, Carbohydrate, Fiber, Fat, Protein and Amino Acids (macronutrients)*. Washington, DC: National Academy Press, 2005, p. 73–185.

72. **Ivy JL.** Muscle glycogen synthesis before and after exercise. *Sports Medicine (Auckland, NZ)* 11: 6–19, 1991.

73. **Ivy JL, and Ferguson LM.** Optimizing resistance exercise adaptations through the timing of post-exercise carbohydrate-protein supplementation. *Strength and Conditioning Journal* 32: 30–36, 2010.

74. **Jeukendrup A, and Killer SC.** The myths surrounding pre-exercise carbohydrate feeding. *Ann Nutri Metab* 57: 18–25, 2010.

75. **Karlsson J, and Saltin B.** Diet, muscle glycogen, and endurance performance. *Journal of Applied Physiology* 31: 203–206, 1971.

76. **Kerstetter JE, O'Brien KO, Caseria DM, Wall DE, and Insogna KL.** The impact of dietary protein on calcium absorption and kinetic measures of bone turnover in women. *The Journal of Clinical Endocrinology and Metabolism* 90: 26–31, 2005.

77. **Kerstetter JE, O'Brien KO, and Insogna KL.** Dietary protein, calcium metabolism, and skeletal homeostasis revisited. *The American Journal of Clinical Nutrition* 78: 584S–592S, 2003.

78. **Lemon PW.** Do athletes need more dietary protein and amino acids? *International Journal of Sport Nutrition* 5 Suppl: S39–61, 1995.

79. **Lemon PW.** Effect of exercise on protein requirements. *Journal of Sports Sciences* 9 Spec No: 53–70, 1991.

80. **Lemon PW.** Protein and amino acid needs of the strength athlete. *International Journal of Sport Nutrition* 1: 127–145, 1991.

81. **Lemon PW.** Protein and exercise: update 1987. *Medicine and Science in Sports and Exercise* 19: S179–190, 1987.

82. **Lemon PW, and Mullin JP.** Effect of initial muscle glycogen levels on protein catabolism during exercise. *Journal of Applied Physiology* 48: 624–629, 1980.

83. **Milic R, Martinovic J, Dopsaj M, and Dopsaj V.** Haematological and iron-related parameters in male and female athletes according to different metabolic energy demands. *European Journal of Applied Physiology* 111: 449–458, 2011.

84. **Mitchell JB, Costill DL, Houmard JA, Flynn MG, Fink WJ, and Beltz JD.** Effects of carbohydrate ingestion on gastric emptying and exercise performance. *Medicine and Science in Sports and Exercise* 20: 110–115, 1988.

85. **Murray R.** Fluid needs in hot and cold environments. *International Journal of Sport Nutrition* 5 Suppl: S62–73, 1995.

86. **Nelson JL, and Robergs RA.** Exploring the potential ergogenic effects of glycerol hyperhydration. *Sports Medicine (Auckland, NZ)* 37: 981–1000, 2007.

87. **Neufer PD, Young AJ, and Sawka MN.** Gastric emptying during exercise: effects of heat stress and hypohydration. *European Journal of Applied Physiology and Occupational Physiology* 58: 433–439, 1989.

88. **Neufer PD, Young AJ, and Sawka MN.** Gastric emptying during walking and running: effects of varied exercise intensity. *European Journal of Applied Physiology and Occupational Physiology* 58: 440–445, 1989.

89. **Noakes T.** Hyponatremia in distance runners: fluid and sodium balance during exercise. *Current Sports Medicine Reports* 1: 197–207, 2002.

90. **Noakes TD, Norman RJ, Buck RH, Godlonton J, Stevenson K, and Pittaway D.** The incidence of hyponatremia during prolonged ultraendurance exercise. *Medicine and Science in Sports and Exercise* 22: 165–170, 1990.

91. **Novack V, Finestone AS, Constantini N, Shpilberg O, Weitzman S, and Merkel D.** The prevalence of low hemoglobin values among new infantry recruits and nonlinear relationship between hemoglobin concentration and physical fitness. *American Journal of Hematology* 82: 128–133, 2007.

92. **Nybo L.** CNS fatigue and prolonged exercise: effect of glucose supplementation. *Medicine and Science in Sports and Exercise* 35: 589–594, 2003.

93. **Owen MD, Kregel KC, Wall PT, and Gisolfi CV.** Effects of ingesting carbohydrate beverages during exercise in the heat. *Medicine and Science in Sports and Exercise* 18: 568–575, 1986.

94. **Phillips SM.** Protein requirements and supplementation in strength sports. *Nutrition (Burbank, Los Angeles County, Calif)* 20: 689–695, 2004.

95. **Phillips SM.** The science of muscle hypertrophy: making dietary protein count. *Proceedings of the Nutrition Society* 70: 100–103, 2011.

96. **Pitts G, Johnson R, and Consolazio F.** Work in the heat as affected by intake of water, salt and glucose. *American Journal of Physiology* 142: 353–359, 1944.

97. **Rehrer NJ, Beckers EJ, Brouns F, ten Hoor F, and Saris WH.** Effects of dehydration on gastric emptying and gastrointestinal distress while running. *Medicine and Science in Sports and Exercise* 22: 790–795, 1990.

98. **Rehrer NJ, Brouns F, Beckers EJ, ten Hoor F, and Saris WH.** Gastric emptying with repeated drinking during running and bicycling. *International Journal of Sports Medicine* 11: 238–243, 1990.

99. **Rollo I, Cole M, Miller R, and Williams C.** Influence of mouth rinsing a carbohydrate solution on 1-hr running performance. *Medicine and Science in Sports and Exercise* 42: 798–804, 2010.

100. **Sallis RE.** Fluid balance and dysnatremias in athletes. *Current Sports Medicine Reports* 7: S14–S19β, 2008.

101. **Sedlock DA.** The latest on carbohydrate loading: a practical approach. *Current Sports Medicine Reports* 7: 209–213, 2008.

102. **Sherman W.** Carbohydrate feedings before and after exercise. In: *Perspectives in Exercise Science and Sports Medicine*, edited by Lamb R, and Williams M. New York: McGraw-Hill, 1991.

103. **Sherman W.** Carbohydrates, muscle glycogen, and muscle glycogen supercompensation. In: *Ergogenic Aids in Sports*, edited by Williams M. Champaign: Human Kinetics, 1983, p. 3–26.

104. **Shi X, and Gisolfi CV.** Fluid and carbohydrate replacement during intermittent exercise. *Sports Medicine (Auckland, NZ)* 25: 157–172, 1998.

105. **Singh A, Moses FM, and Deuster PA.** Chronic multivitamin-mineral supplementation does not enhance physical performance. *Medicine and Science in Sports and Exercise* 24: 726–732, 1992.

106. **Smith JW, Zachwieja JJ, Peronnet F, Passe DH, Massicote D, Lavoie C, and Pascoe DD.** Fuel selection and cycling endurance performance with ingestion of [^{13}C] glucose: evidence for a carbohydrate dose response. *Journal of Applied Physiology* 108: 1520–1529, 2010.

107. **Stearns RL, Emmanuel H, Volek JS, and Casa DJ.** Effects of ingesting protein in combination with carbohydrate during exercise on endurance performance: a systematic review with meta-analysis. *Journal of Strength and Conditioning Research* 24: 2192–2202, 2010.

108. **Tarnopolsky M.** Protein requirements for endurance athletes. *Nutrition (Burbank, Los Angeles County, Calif)* 20: 662–668, 2004.

109. **Todd K, Butterfield G, and Calloway D.** Nitrogen balance in men with adequate and deficit energy intake at 3 levels of work. *Journal of Nutrition* 114: 2107–2118, 1984.

110. **Utter AC, Kang J, Nieman DC, Dumke CL, McAnulty SR, Vinci DM, and McAnulty LS.** Carbohydrate supplementation and perceived exertion during prolonged running. *Medicine and Science in Sports and Exercise* 36: 1036–1041, 2004.

111. **Van der Beek EJ.** Vitamins and endurance training: food for running or faddish claims? *Sports Medicine (Auckland, NZ)* 2: 175–197, 1985.

112. **Van Rosendal SP, Osborne MA, Fassett RG, and Coombes JS.** Guidelines for glycerol use in hyperhydration and rehydration associated with exercise. *Sports Medicine* 40: 113–139, 2010.

113. **Venderley AM, and Campbell WW.** Vegetarian diets : nutritional considerations for athletes. *Sports Medicine (Auckland, NZ)* 36: 293–305, 2006.

114. **Vrijens DM, and Rehrer NJ.** Sodium-free fluid ingestion decreases plasma sodium during exercise in the heat. *Journal of Applied Physiology* 86: 1847–1851, 1999.

115. **Watson P, Love TD, Maughan RJ, and Shirreffs SM.** A comparison of the effects of milk and a carbohydrate-electrolyte drink on the restoration of fluide capacity in a hot, humid environment. *European Journal of Applied Physiology* 104: 633–642, 2008.

116. **White TP, and Brooks GA.** [U-14C]glucose, -alanine, and -leucine oxidation in rats at rest and two intensities of running. *The American Journal of Physiology* 240: E155–165, 1981.

117. **Widmaier EP, Raff H, and Strang KT.** *Vander's Human Physiology.* New York: McGraw-Hill, 2008.

118. **Williams MH.** *Nutrition for Health, Fitness and Sport.* New York: McGraw-Hill, 2010.

119. **Wilmore J.** Body composition and sports medicine: research considerations. In: *Report of the Sixth Ross Conference on Medical Research.* Columbus: Ross Laboratories, 1984, p. 78–82.

120. **Wilmore JH.** Body composition in sport and exercise: directions for future research. *Medicine and Science in Sports and Exercise* 15: 21–31, 1983.

121. **Wolfe R.** Does exercise stimulate protein breakdown in humans?: isotopic approaches to the problem. *Medicine and Science in Sports and Exercise* 19: S172–S178, 1987.

122. **Wolfe RR, Goodenough RD, Wolfe MH, Royle GT, and Nadel ER.** Isotopic analysis of leucine and urea metabolism in exercising humans. *Journal of Applied Physiology* 52: 458–466, 1982.

123. **Wolfe RR, Wolfe MH, Nadel ER, and Shaw JH.** Isotopic determination of amino acid-urea interactions in exercise in humans. *Journal of Applied Physiology* 56: 221–229, 1984.

24

Exercise and the Environment

■ Objectives

By studying this chapter, you should be able to do the following:

1. Describe the changes in atmospheric pressure, air temperature, and air density with increasing altitude.
2. Describe how altitude affects sprint performances and explain why that is the case.
3. Explain why distance running performance decreases at altitude.
4. Draw a graph to show the effect of altitude on $\dot{V}O_2$ max and list the reasons for this response.
5. Graphically describe the effect of altitude on the heart rate and ventilation responses to submaximal work, and explain why these changes are appropriate.
6. Describe the process of adaptation to altitude and the degree to which this adaptation can be complete.
7. Explain why such variability exists among athletes in the decrease in $\dot{V}O_2$ max upon exposure to altitude, the degree of improvement in $\dot{V}O_2$ max at altitude, and the gains made upon return to sea level.
8. Describe the potential problems associated with training at high altitude and how one might deal with them.
9. Explain the circumstances that caused physiologists to reevaluate their conclusions that humans could not climb Mount Everest without oxygen.
10. Explain the role that hyperventilation plays in helping to maintain a high oxygen-hemoglobin saturation at extreme altitudes.

11. List and describe the factors influencing the risk of heat injury.
12. Provide suggestions for the fitness participant to follow to minimize the likelihood of heat injury.
13. Describe in general terms the guidelines suggested for running road races in the heat.
14. Describe the three elements in the heat stress index, and explain why one is more important than the other two.
15. List the factors influencing hypothermia.
16. Explain what the wind chill index is relative to heat loss.
17. Explain why exposure to cold water is more dangerous than exposure to air of the same temperature.
18. Describe what the "clo" unit is and how recommendations for insulation change when one does exercise.
19. Describe the role of subcutaneous fat and heat production in the development of hypothermia.
20. List the steps to follow to deal with hypothermia.
21. Explain how carbon monoxide can influence performance, and list the steps that should be taken to reduce the impact of pollution on performance.

By now it should be clear that performance is dependent on more than simply having a high $\dot{V}O_2$ max. In chapter 23, we saw the role of diet and body composition on performance, and in chapter 25 we will formally consider "ergogenic" or work-enhancing aids and performance. Sandwiched between these chapters is a discussion of how the environmental factors of altitude, heat, cold, and pollution can influence performance.

ALTITUDE

In the late 1960s, when the Olympic Games were scheduled to be held in Mexico City, our attention was directed at the question of how altitude (2,300 meters at Mexico City) would affect performance. Previous experience at altitude suggested that many performances would not equal former Olympic standards or, for that matter, the athlete's own personal record (PR) at sea level. On the other hand, some performances were actually expected to be better because they were conducted at altitude. Why? What happens to $\dot{V}O_2$ max with altitude? Can a sea-level resident ever completely adapt to altitude? We will address these and other questions after a brief review of the environmental factors that change with increasing altitude.

Atmospheric Pressure

The **atmospheric pressure** at any spot on earth is a measure of the weight of a column of air directly over that spot. At sea level the weight (and height) of that column of air is greatest. As one climbs to higher and higher altitudes, the height and, of course, the weight of the column are reduced. Consequently, atmospheric pressure decreases with increasing altitude, the air is less dense, and each liter of air contains fewer molecules of gas. Since the *percentages* of O_2,

CO_2, and N_2 are the same at altitude as at sea level, any change in the partial pressure of each gas is due solely to the change in the atmospheric or barometric pressure (see chapter 10). The decrease in the partial pressure of O_2 (PO_2) with increasing altitude has a direct effect on the saturation of hemoglobin and, consequently, oxygen transport. This lower PO_2 is called **hypoxia,** with **normoxia** being the term to describe the PO_2 under sea-level conditions. The term **hyperoxia** describes a condition in which the inspired PO_2 is greater than that at sea level (see chapter 25). In addition to the hypoxic condition at altitude, the air temperature and humidity are lower, adding potential temperature regulation problems to the hypoxic stress of altitude. How do these changes affect performance? To answer that question we will divide performances into short-term anaerobic performances and long-term aerobic performances.

Short-Term Anaerobic Performance

In chapters 3 and 19 we described the importance of the anaerobic sources of ATP in maximal performances lasting 2 minutes or less. If this information is correct, and we think it is, then the short-term anaerobic races shouldn't be affected by the low PO_2 at altitude, because O_2 transport to the muscles is not limiting performance. Table 24.1 shows this to be the case when the sprint performances of the 1968 Mexico City Olympic Games ($\sim$2,300 m) were compared to those in the 1964 Tokyo Olympic Games (sea level) (59). The performances improved in all but one case, in which the time for the 400-meter run for the women was the same. The reasons for the improvements in performance include the "normal" gains made over time from one Olympic Games to the next and the fact that the density of the air at altitude offers less resistance to movements at high speeds. Improvements in the 100-meter and 400-meter races for each increase

TABLE 24.1 **Comparison of Performances in Short Races in the 1964 and 1968 Olympic Games**

Olympic Games	Short Races: Men				Short Races: Women			
	100 m	200 m	400 m	800 m	100 m	200 m	400 m	800 m
1964 (Tokyo)	10.0 s	20.3 s	45.1 s	1 m 45.1 s	11.4 s	23.0 s	52.0 s	2 m 1.1 s
1968 (Mexico City)	9.9 s	19.8 s	43.8 s	1 m 44.3 s	11.0 s	22.5 s	52.0 s	2 m 0.9 s
% change*	+1.0	+2.5	+2.9	+0.8	+3.5	+2.2	0	+0.2

*+ sign indicates improvement over 1964 performance.

From E. T. Howley, "Effect of Altitude on Physical Performance," in G. A. Stull and T. K. Cureton, *Encyclopedia of Physical Education, Fitness and Sports: Training, Environment, Nutrition, and Fitness.* Copyright © 1980 American Alliance for Health, Physical Education, Recreation and Dance, Reston VA. Reprinted by permission.

of 1,000 meters in altitude have been estimated to be about 0.08 s and 0.06 s, respectively (9, 96). The issue of lower air resistance sparked controversy over Bob Beamon's fantastic performance in the long jump in the Mexico City Games (see A Closer Look 24.1).

Long-Term Aerobic Performance

Maximal performances in excess of 2 minutes are primarily dependent on oxygen delivery, and, in contrast to the short-term performances, are clearly affected by the lower PO_2 at altitude. Table 24.2 shows the results of the distance running events from 1,500 meters up through the marathon and the 50,000-meter walk, and as you can see, performance was diminished at all distances but the 1,500-meter run (59). This performance is worthy of special note, given that it was expected to be affected, as were the others. It is more than just of passing interest that the record setter was Kipchoge Keino, who was born and raised in Kenya at an altitude similar to that of Mexico City. Did he possess a special adaptation due to his birthplace? We will come back to this question in a later section. We would like to continue our discussion of

the effect of altitude on performance by asking, "Why did the performance fall off by as much as 6.2% in the long-distance races?"

IN SUMMARY

- The atmospheric pressure, PO_2, air temperature, and air density decrease with altitude.
- The lower air density at altitude offers less resistance to high-speed movement, and sprint performances are either not affected or are improved.

Maximal Aerobic Power and Altitude

The decrease in distance running performance at altitude is similar to what occurs when a trained runner becomes untrained—it would clearly take longer to run a marathon! The similarity in the effect is related to a decrease in maximal aerobic power that occurs with detraining and with increasing altitude. Figure 24.1 shows that $\dot{V}O_2$ max decreases in a linear fashion, being about 12% lower at 2,400 meters (7,400 feet), 20% lower at 3,100 meters (10,200 feet), and 27% lower

A CLOSER LOOK 24.1

Jumping Through Thin Air

In the 1968 Olympic Games in Mexico City, Bob Beamon shattered the world record in the long jump with a leap of 29 feet 2.5 inches (8.90 m), 21.75 in (55 cm) longer than the existing world record. Because the record was achieved at altitude where air density is less than that at sea level, some questions were raised about the true magnitude of the achievement. Recent progress in biomechanics has made it

possible to determine just how much would have been gained by doing the long jump at altitude (124). The calculations had to consider the mass of the jumper, a drag coefficient based on the frontal area exposed to the air while jumping, and the difference in the air density between sea level and Mexico City. The result indicated that approximately 2.4 cm (less than an inch) would have been gained by doing the jump

at altitude where the air density is less. This confirmed the extraordinary nature of Beamon's performance. Scientists have tried to predict the effect of altitude on running performances by considering the opposing factors of lower air density and the reduced availability of oxygen (87). The latter factor is discussed relative to long-distance races.

Olympic Games	Long Races: Men					
	1,500 m	3,000 m	5,000 m	10,000 m	Marathon	50,000 m Walk
1964 (Tokyo)	3 m 38.1 s	8 m 30.8 s	13 m 48.8 s	28 m 24.4 s	2 h 12 m 11.2 s	4 h 11 m 11.2 s
1968 (Mexico City)	3 m 34.9 s	8 m 51.0 s	14 m 05.0 s	29 m 27.4 s	2 h 20 m 24.6 s	4 h 20 m 13.6 s
% change*	+1.5	−3.9	−1.9	−3.7	−6.2	−3.6

*+ sign indicates improvement over 1964 performance.

From E. T. Howley, "Effect of Altitude on Physical Performance," in G. A. Stull and T. K. Cureton, *Encyclopedia of Physical Education, Fitness and Sports: Training, Environment, Nutrition, and Fitness.* Copyright © 1980 American Alliance for Health, Physical Education, Recreation and Dance, Reston VA. Reprinted by permission.

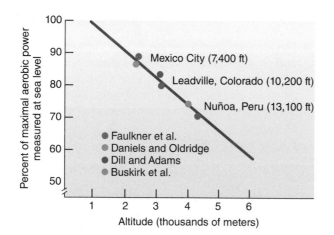

Figure 24.1 Changes in maximal aerobic power with increasing altitude. The sea-level value for maximal aerobic power is set to 100%. From E. T. Howley, "Effect of Altitude on Physical Performance," in G. A. Stull and T. K. Cureton, *Encyclopedia of Physical Education, Fitness and Sports: Training, Environment, Nutrition, and Fitness.* Copyright © 1980 American Alliance for Health, Physical Education, Recreation and Dance, Reston VA. Reprinted by permission.

at about 4,000 meters (13,100 feet) (15, 25, 28, 36). Although it should be no surprise that endurance performance decreases with such changes in $\dot{V}O_2$ max, why does $\dot{V}O_2$ max decrease?

Cardiovascular Function at Altitude Maximal oxygen uptake is equal to the product of the maximal cardiac output and the maximal arteriovenous oxygen difference, $\dot{V}O_2 = CO \times (CaO_2 - C\bar{v}O_2)$. Given this relationship, the decrease in $\dot{V}O_2$ max with increasing altitude could be due to a decrease in cardiac output and/or a decrease in oxygen extraction. It will become clear in the following paragraphs that oxygen extraction is a major factor causing a decrease in $\dot{V}O_2$ max at all altitudes, with decreases in maximal cardiac output contributing primarily at higher altitudes.

Maximal cardiac output is equal to the product of maximal heart rate and maximal stroke volume. In several studies the maximal heart rate was unchanged at altitudes of 2,300 meters (33, 92), 3,100 meters (45), and 4,000 meters (15), while changes in maximal stroke volume were somewhat inconsistent (64). If these two variables, maximal stroke volume and maximal heart rate, do not change much at these altitudes, then the decrease in $\dot{V}O_2$ max must be due to a difference in oxygen extraction.

Although oxygen extraction ($CaO_2 - C\bar{v}O_2$) could decrease due to a decrease in the arterial oxygen content (CaO_2) or an increase in the mixed venous oxygen content ($C\bar{v}O_2$), the primary cause is the desaturation of the arterial blood due to the low PO_2 at altitude. The lower atmospheric PO_2 causes the alveolar PO_2 to be lower. This reduces the pressure gradient for oxygen diffusion between the alveolus and the pulmonary capillary blood, thus lowering the arterial PO_2. As you recall from chapter 10, as the arterial PO_2 falls, there is a reduction in the volume of oxygen bound to hemoglobin. At sea level, hemoglobin is about 96% to 98% saturated with oxygen. However, at 2,300 meters and 4,000 meters, saturation falls to 88% and 71%, respectively. These decreases in the oxygen saturation of hemoglobin are similar to the reductions in $\dot{V}O_2$ max at these altitudes described earlier. Because maximal oxygen transport is the product of the maximal cardiac output and the arterial oxygen content, the capacity to transport oxygen to the working muscles at altitude is reduced due to desaturation, even though maximal cardiac output may be unchanged during acute exposures up to altitudes of 4,000 meters (64). However, it must be added that a variety of studies have shown a decrease in maximal heart rate at altitude. Although some of these decreases have been observed at altitudes of 3,100 meters (28) and 4,300 meters (33), it is more common to find lower maximal heart rates above altitudes of 4,300 meters. For example, compared to maximal HR at sea level, maximal HR was observed to be 24 to 33 beats/minute lower at 4,650 meters (15,300 feet) and 47 beats/minute lower at about 6,100 meters (20,000 feet) (48, 95). This depression in maximal heart rate is reversed by acute restoration of normoxia, or the use of atropine (48). This altitude-induced bradycardia suggests that myocardial hypoxia may trigger the slower heart rate to decrease the work and, therefore, the oxygen demand of the heart muscle.

As mentioned earlier, during an acute exposure to altitude, stroke volume during exercise is only slightly reduced, if at all. However, prolonged exposures to altitude results in a reduction in plasma volume that leads to a lower end diastolic volume and stroke volume (77). This means that $\dot{V}O_2$ max decreases at a faster rate at the higher altitudes due to the combined effects of the desaturation of hemoglobin and the decrease in maximal cardiac output.

This desaturation of arterial blood at altitude affects more than $\dot{V}O_2$ max. The cardiovascular responses to submaximal work are also influenced. Due to the fact that each liter of blood is carrying less oxygen, more liters of blood must be pumped per minute in order to compensate. This is accomplished through an increase in the HR response, since the stroke volume response is at its highest point already, or it is actually lower at altitude due to the hypoxia (2). This elevated HR response is shown in figure 24.2 (45). This has implications for more than the performance-based athlete. The average person who participates in an exercise program will have to decrease the intensity of exercise at altitude in order to stay in the target heart rate zone. Remember, the exercise prescription needed for a cardiovascular training effect includes a proper duration of exercise to achieve an appropriate total caloric expenditure (see chapter 16). If the intensity is too high, the person will have more difficulty achieving that goal.

Respiratory Function at Altitude In the introduction to this section we mentioned that the air is less dense at altitude. This means that there are fewer

Figure 24.3   The effect of altitude on the ventilation response to submaximal exercise.

O_2 molecules per liter of air, and if a person wanted to consume the same number of liters of O_2, pulmonary ventilation would have to increase. At 5,600 meters (18,400 feet), the atmospheric pressure is one-half that at sea level, and the number of molecules of O_2 per liter of air is reduced by one-half; therefore, a person would have to breathe twice as much air to take in the same amount of O_2. The consequences of this are shown in figure 24.3, which presents the ventilation responses of a subject who exercised at work rates demanding about a $\dot{V}O_2$ of 1 to 2 L $\cdot$ min^{-1} at sea level and at three altitudes exceeding 4,000 meters. The pulmonary ventilation is elevated at all altitudes, reaching values of almost 180 L $\cdot$ min^{-1} at 6,400 meters (21,000 feet) (95). This extreme ventilatory response requires the respiratory muscles, primarily the diaphragm, to work so hard that fatigue may occur. We will see more on this in a later section dealing with the assault on Mount Everest.

IN SUMMARY

- Distance-running performances are adversely affected at altitude due to the reduction in the PO_2, which causes a decrease in hemoglobin saturation and $\dot{V}O_2$ max.
- Up to moderate altitudes (~4,000 meters) the decrease in $\dot{V}O_2$ max is due primarily to the decrease in the arterial oxygen content brought about by the decrease in atmospheric PO_2. At higher altitudes, the rate at which $\dot{V}O_2$ max falls is increased due to a reduction in maximal cardiac output.
- Submaximal performances conducted at altitude require higher heart rate and ventilation responses due to the lower oxygen content of arterial blood and the reduction in the number of oxygen molecules per liter of air, respectively

Figure 24.2   The effect of altitude on the heart-rate response to submaximal exercise.

Chapter Twenty-Four   Exercise and the Environment   **545**

Acclimatization to High Altitude

The low PO_2 at altitude triggers an increase in hypoxia inducible factor-1 (HIF-1) that is present in most cells of the body. HIF-1 activates genes associated with erythropoietin (EPO) production that is involved in red blood cell production, vascular endothelial growth factors that are involved in the generation of new blood vessels, and nitric oxide synthase that promotes the synthesis of nitric oxide that is involved in vasodilation (110). In the high altitude populations of the Andes in South America, the acclimatization response to the low PO_2 at altitude is to produce additional red blood cells to compensate for the desaturation of hemoglobin. In the mining community of Morococha, Peru, where people reside at altitudes above 4,540 meters, hemoglobin levels of 211 g $\cdot$ L^{-1} have been measured, in contrast to the normal 156 g$\cdot$ L^{-1} of the sea-level residents in Lima, Peru. This higher hemoglobin compensates rather completely for the low PO_2 at those altitudes (62):

Sea level: 156 g $\cdot$ L^{-1} times 1.34 ml O_2 $\cdot$ g^{-1} at 98% saturation = 206 ml $\cdot$ L^{-1}

4,540 m: 211 g $\cdot$ L^{-1} times 1.34 ml O_2 $\cdot$ g^{-1} at 81% saturation = 224 ml $\cdot$ L^{-1}

One of the best tests of the degree to which these high-altitude residents have adapted is found in the $\dot{V}O_2$ max values measured at altitude. Average values of 46 to 50 ml $\cdot$ kg^{-1} $\cdot$ min^{-1} were measured on the altitude natives (65, 74–76), which compares favorably with sea-level natives in that country and in ours.

There is no question that any sea-level resident who makes a journey to altitude and stays a while will experience an acclimatization process that includes an increase in red blood cell number. However, the adaptation will probably never be as complete as seen in the permanent residents. This conclusion is drawn from a study that compared $\dot{V}O_2$ max values of several different groups: (a) Peruvian lowlanders and Peace Corps volunteers who came to altitude as adults, (b) lowlanders who came to altitude as children and spent their growing years at altitude, and (c) permanent altitude residents (36). The $\dot{V}O_2$ max values were 46 ml $\cdot$ kg^{-1} $\cdot$ min^{-1} for the altitude residents and those who arrived there as children. In contrast, the lowlanders who arrived as adults and spent only 1 to 4 years at altitude had values of 38 ml $\cdot$ kg^{-1} $\cdot$ min^{-1}. This indicates that to have complete acclimatization, one must spend the developmental years at high altitude. This may help explain the surprisingly good performance of Kipchoge Keino's performance in the 1,500-meter run at the Mexico City Olympic Games mentioned earlier, because he spent his childhood at an altitude similar to that of Mexico City.

The elevated hemoglobin concentration of the Peruvian permanent altitude residents was believed to be the primary means by which humans adapted in order to live at high altitudes. That is no longer the case. It has become clear that those who live at high altitudes in Tibet have achieved that level of acclimatization by a different means compared to those who live in the Andes (71, 108, 116, 134). Tibetan residents adapt by increasing the oxygen saturation of hemoglobin, rather than the concentration of hemoglobin, which may be 30 g/L lower than Andeans living at comparable altitudes. Tibetan Sherpas' superior performance at extreme altitudes is linked, not to an exceptional $\dot{V}O_2$ max at altitude, but to better lung function, maximal cardiac output, and level of oxygen saturation of hemoglobin (110). The different types of adaptations observed in these populations is related to the natural selection of those with unique genes that promote either an increase in red blood cell production (e.g., Andean) or an increase in oxygen saturation (Tibetan) that is a result of an increase in nitric oxide in the lungs that promotes an increase in blood flow (116, 134).

IN SUMMARY

- Andeans adapt to high altitude by producing more red blood cells to counter the desaturation caused by the lower PO_2. Andean altitude residents who spent their growing years at altitude show a rather complete adaptation as seen in their arterial oxygen content and $\dot{V}O_2$ max values. Lowlanders who arrive as adults show only a modest adaptation.
- In contrast, Tibetan high altitude residents adapt by increasing the oxygen saturation of the existing hemoglobin, a result of increased blood flow to the lungs due to high nitric oxide levels.

Training for Competition at Altitude

It was clear to many of the middle- and long-distance runners who competed in the Olympic Trials or Games in 1968 that the altitude was going to have a detrimental effect on performance. Using $\dot{V}O_2$ max as an indicator of the impact on performance, scientists studied the effect of immediate exposure to altitude, the rate of recovery in $\dot{V}O_2$ max as the individual stayed at altitude, and whether $\dot{V}O_2$ max was higher than the pre-altitude value upon return to sea level. The results were interesting, not due to the general trends that were expected, but to the extreme variability in response among the athletes. For example, the decrease in $\dot{V}O_2$ max upon ascent to a 2,300-meter altitude ranged from 8.8% to 22.3% (92); at 3,090 meters it ranged from 13.9% to 24.4% (28); and at 4,000 meters the decrease ranged from 24.8% to 34.3% (15). One of the major conclusions that could be drawn from these data is that the best runner at sea level might not be the best at altitude if that person had the largest drop in $\dot{V}O_2$ max. Why such variability? Studies of this phenomenon suggest that the variability in the decrease in $\dot{V}O_2$ max across individuals relates to the degree to which athletes experience desaturation of arterial blood during maximal work (66, 72, 89). Chapter 10 described the effect that arterial desaturation has on $\dot{V}O_2$ max of superior athletes at sea level. If such desaturation can occur under sea-level conditions, then the altitude condition should have an additional impact, with the magnitude of the impact being greater on those who suffer some desaturation at sea level. Consistent with that, exposure to a simulated altitude of 3,000 meters resulted in a 20.8% decrease in $\dot{V}O_2$ max for trained subjects and only a 9.8% decrease for untrained subjects (66).

The decrease in $\dot{V}O_2$ max upon exposure to altitude was not the only physiological response that varied among the athletes. There also was a variable response in the size of the increase in $\dot{V}O_2$ max as the subjects stayed at altitude and continued to train. One study, lasting 28 days at 2,300 meters, found the $\dot{V}O_2$ max to increase from 1% to 8% over that time (94). Some found the $\dot{V}O_2$ max to gradually improve over a period of 10 to 28 days (6, 26, 28, 92), while others (33, 45) did not. In addition, when the subjects returned to sea level and were retested, some found the $\dot{V}O_2$ max to be higher than before they left (6, 26, 28), whereas others found no improvements (15, 36, 43). Why was there such variability in response?

There are several possibilities. If an athlete was not in peak condition before ascending to altitude, the combined stress of the exercise and altitude could increase the $\dot{V}O_2$ max over time while at altitude and show an additional gain upon return to sea level. Evidence exists both for (106) and against (1, 32, 121) the idea that the combination of altitude and exercise stress leads to greater changes in $\dot{V}O_2$ max than exercise stress alone. Another reason for the variability is related to the altitude at which the training was conducted. When runners trained at high (4,000 meters) altitude, the intensity of the runs (relative to sustained sea-level speeds) had to be reduced to complete a workout, due to the reduction in $\dot{V}O_2$ max that occurs at altitude. As a result, the runner might actually "detrain" while at altitude, and subsequent performance at sea level might not be as good as it was before going to altitude (15). Daniels and Oldridge (25) provided a way around this problem by having runners alternate training at altitude (7 to 14 days) and at sea level (5 to 11 days). Using an altitude of only 2,300 meters, the runners were still able to train at "race pace," and detraining did not occur. In fact, thirteen personal records were achieved by the athletes when they raced at sea level. For more on this, see Saunders, Pyne, and Gore's review on endurance training at altitude in Suggested Readings. The focus on gaining the benefits of acclimation to altitude has resulted in a strategy in which the athlete lives at high altitude but trains at low altitude—without ever leaving low altitude. See The Winning Edge 24.1.

IN SUMMARY

- When athletes train at altitude, some experience a greater decline in $\dot{V}O_2$ max than others. This may be due to differences in the degree to which each athlete experiences a desaturation of hemoglobin. Remember, some athletes experience desaturation during maximal work at sea level.
- Some athletes show an increase in $\dot{V}O_2$ max while training at altitude, whereas others do not. This may be due to the degree to which the athlete was trained before going to altitude.
- In addition, some athletes show an improved $\dot{V}O_2$ max upon return to sea level, whereas others do not. Part of the reason may be the altitude at which they train. Those who train at high altitudes may actually "detrain" due to the fact that the quality of their workouts suffers at the high altitudes. To get around this problem, athletes can alternate low-altitude and sea-level exposures, or follow a "live high, train low" program.

The Quest for Everest

The most obvious tie between exercise and altitude is mountain climbing. The climber faces the stress of altitude, cold, radiation, and, of course, the work of climbing up steep slopes or sheer rock walls. A goal of some mountaineers has been to climb Mount Everest, at 8,848 meters, the highest mountain on earth. Figure 24.4 shows various attempts to climb Everest during the twentieth century (131). Special note should be made of Hillary and Tensing, who were the first to do it, and Messner and Habeler, who, to the amazement of all, did it without supplemental oxygen in 1978. See Messner in the Suggested Readings for complete details on how they accomplished this feat. This achievement brought scientists back to Everest in 1981 asking how this was possible. This section provides some background to this fascinating story.

In 1924, Norton's climbing team attempted to scale Everest without O_2 and almost succeeded—they stopped only 300 meters from the summit (84). This 1924 expedition was noteworthy because data were collected on the climbers and porters by physicians and scientists associated with the attempt. In addition, new questions have been raised about two of the climbers who died in their attempt to reach the summit (see A Closer Look 24.2). The story of this assault

Live High, Train Low, or the Reverse!

There is great interest in the "live high, train low" strategy as a way of improving endurance performance. The "live high" refers to being exposed to a low PO_2 to obtain the unique benefits mentioned earlier, and "train low" refers to doing exercise at sea level (or a very low altitude) to not affect the intensity and/or duration of the workouts. However, support for this is mixed due to the influence of a wide variety of factors: subjects, length of study, intensity and volume of training, the altitude (be it simulated or real), and the length of stay at altitude (135). One study tried to shed some light on why there is such variability in response to this training strategy (22). Thirty-nine collegiate runners were divided into "responders" and "nonresponders" on the basis of changes in their 5,000-meter run time following training at a high-altitude training camp. All of the runners had lived "high" (2,500 m), but some had trained at 2,500 to 3,000 m (high-high group), some at 1,200 to 1,400 m (high-low group), and some had done low-intensity training at 2,500 to 3,000 m and interval work at low altitude (high-high-low). The responders were found to have an increase in plasma erythropoietin (EPO), red blood cell volume, and $\dot{V}O_2$ max, which provides a strong physiological connection to the increased performance in the 5,000-m run after altitude training. Interestingly, while the nonresponders had an increase in EPO, they did not have an increase in either red blood cell mass or $\dot{V}O_2$ max. Another difference between the responders and nonresponders was in their ability to maintain the quality of their workouts at altitude: nonresponders demonstrated a 9% reduction in interval-training velocity and a significantly lower $\dot{V}O_2$ during the intervals. There were two take-home messages from this study:

- live at a high enough altitude to elicit an increase in red blood cell mass (due to an acute increase in EPO), and

- train at a low enough altitude to maintain interval-training velocity. For runners who experience a significant desaturation of hemoglobin at sea level, even low-altitude training may be inconsistent with maintaining interval-training velocity.

It would seem that the physiology related to improvements in endurance performance following a live-high, train-low protocol is well described and accepted; however, that is not the case. Since the above study (22) was published, there has been a "point-counterpoint" debate on this issue (67), along with a series of letters to the editor in response to the debate (67), and an explosion of new research. Simply put, in contrast to the above link of altitude exposure to the increase in red blood cell mass, and then $\dot{V}O_2$ max and performance, other studies have shown that 6 weeks of intermittent hypoxia during training improved $\dot{V}O_2$ max and muscle oxidative potential and performance, without a change in red cell mass (30, 88, 139). A summary of potential mechanisms, other than red cell mass, linked to the improved performance following exposure to hypoxia was recently published (41). The focus in this review was on improved mitochondrial function and increased buffering capacity.

Given that intermittent hypobaric hypoxia (3 hrs/day, 5 days/wk at 4,000–5,500 m) for 4 weeks increased EPO, but did not increase red blood cell production or improve performance (42, 103), questions have been raised about what "dose" of altitude exposure is needed to generate a response. On the basis of several studies, it appears that 4 weeks of altitude exposure of ≥ 22 hrs/day at 2,000–2,500 meters is needed to elicit increases in red blood cell mass, $\dot{V}O_2$ max, and performance (125, 133). If a simulated altitude is used for fewer hours per day (12–16 hrs), a higher

elevation (2,500–3,000 m) is needed. Clearly, such changes in $\dot{V}O_2$ max can have a favorable effect on athletic performances such as the marathon (21), so it is no surprise that the World Anti-Doping Agency (WADA) has examined the live-high, train-low approach to improving performance (because it results in changes in red blood cell mass similar to blood doping—see chapter 25). Interestingly, although WADA raised concerns from both an ethical standpoint and a violation of the "spirit of sport" criterion, it has not taken action at this time (132).

Although the live high, train low approach has been widely adopted, there is another school of thought that recommends a "live low, train high" approach, in which subjects train in hypoxia, but remain in normoxia the rest of the time. In this case the hypoxic environment exists only during exercise and is viewed as an option to avoid the negative impacts of prolonged exposure to high altitudes mentioned earlier. In general, $\dot{V}O_2$ max and blood parameters (e.g., hemoglobin concentration) are unchanged with this type of training. Further, Vogt and Hoppeler feel that it is difficult to draw strong conclusions regarding muscle adaptations due to this type of training because of differences in the training state of the subjects, the intensity and duration of the training, and the simulated altitude used (121). However, there is some limited evidence that when an athlete must perform at altitude, this type of training is beneficial. Given the small potential gains (~1%–2%) and the considerable costs, difficulties and potential risks (however small (7)), associated with either living high and training low or the reverse, only elite endurance athletes should consider these types of training strategies (110). See Millet et al. in the Suggested Readings for how the various hypoxic training methods can be combined.

Figure 24.4 The highest altitudes attained by climbers in the twentieth century. In 1924 the climbers ascended within 300 meters of the summit without supplemental oxygen. It took another 54 years to climb those last 300 meters.

is good reading for those interested in mountain climbing and provides evidence of the keen powers of observation of the scientists. Major Hingston noted the respiratory distress associated with climbing to such heights, stating that at 5,800 meters (19,000 feet) "the very slightest exertion, such as the tying of a bootlace, the opening of a ration box, the getting into a sleeping bag, was associated with marked respiratory distress." At 8,200 meters (27,000 feet) one climber "had to take seven, eight, or ten complete respirations for every single step forward. And even at that slow rate of progress he had to rest for a minute or two every twenty or thirty yards" (84). Pugh, who made observations during a 1960–61 expedition to Everest, believed that fatigue of the respiratory muscles may be the primary factor limiting such

endeavors at extreme altitudes (95). Further, Pugh's observations of the decreases in $\dot{V}O_2$ max at the extreme altitudes suggested that $\dot{V}O_2$ max would be just above basal metabolism at the summit, making the task an unlikely one at best. How then did Messner and Habeler climb Everest without supplemental O_2?

This was one of the primary questions addressed by the 1981 expedition to Everest. As mentioned earlier, $\dot{V}O_2$ max decreases with altitude due to the lower barometric pressure, which causes a lower PO_2 and a desaturation of hemoglobin. In effect, the $\dot{V}O_2$ max at the summit of Everest was predicated on the observed rate of decrease in $\dot{V}O_2$ max at lower altitudes and then extrapolated to the barometric pressure at the top of the mountain. One of the first major findings of the 1981 expedition was that the barometric pressure at

A CLOSER LOOK 24.2

Mallory and Irvine—Did They Reach the Summit?

In the 1924 Everest expedition, two of the climbers, Norton and Somervell, left camp at 8,220 m (27,000 feet) to challenge the summit without supplemental oxygen. Somervell had to stop due to the cold air aggravating his frostbitten throat, but Norton continued on until he reached 8,580 m (28,314 feet)—a record for those not using supplemental oxygen that lasted for 54 years. A few days later, George L. Mallory and Andrew C. Irvine made an attempt with oxygen, but they never returned. Given that they were last

seen on the way to the summit, questions were raised about whether they had made it, and died on the way down. The 1999 Mallory and Irvine Research Expedition attempted to answer this question by finding their remains, and perhaps, some evidence that they might have achieved their goal. They knew that both climbers had cameras, and they were hoping to find photographic evidence to put this question to rest. The team did find Mallory's body at 27,000 feet, but unfortunately, could not find a camera.

After burying Mallory, they looked for additional evidence to try to determine where he fell from, to land where he did. One of his oxygen bottles placed him in a position consistent with a move to the summit; however, there was not enough evidence to conclude that the two climbers had achieved their goal. Nor was there enough to prove that they had not. The mystery continues (50). See Johnson, Hemmleb, and Simonson in the Suggested Readings for more on this adventure.

the summit was 17 mm Hg higher than previously believed (127, 130). This higher barometric pressure increased the estimated inspired PO_2 and made a big difference in the predicted $\dot{V}O_2$ max. Figure 24.5 shows that the $\dot{V}O_2$ max predicted from the 1960–61 expedition was near the basal metabolic rate, whereas the value predicted from the 1981 expedition was closer to 15 ml · kg^{-1} · min^{-1} (127, 130). This $\dot{V}O_2$ max value was confirmed in the Operation Everest II project in which subjects did a simulated ascent of Mount Everest over a 40-day period in a decompression chamber (25, 117). This $\dot{V}O_2$ max value of 15 ml · kg^{-1} · min^{-1} helps to explain how the climbers were able to reach the summit without the aid of supplemental oxygen. However, it was not the only reason.

The arterial saturation of hemoglobin is dependent upon the arterial PO_2, PCO_2, and pH (see chapter 10). A low PCO_2 and a high pH cause the oxygen hemoglobin curve to shift to the left, so that hemoglobin is more saturated under these conditions than under normal conditions. A person who can ventilate great volumes in response to hypoxia can exhale more CO_2 and cause the pH to become elevated. It has been shown that those who successfully deal with altitude have strong hypoxic ventilatory drives, allowing them to have a higher arterial PO_2 and oxygen saturation (113). In fact, when alveolar PCO_2 values were obtained at the top of Mount Everest in the 1981 expedition, the climbers had values much lower than expected (128). This ability to hyperventilate, coupled with the barometric pressure being higher than expected, resulted in higher arterial PO_2, and of course, $\dot{V}O_2$ max values. How high must your $\dot{V}O_2$ max be to climb Mount Everest?

Figure 24.5 shows that the climbers in the 1981 expedition had $\dot{V}O_2$ max values at sea level that were higher than those of the 1960–61 expedition. In fact,

Figure 24.5 Plot of maximal oxygen uptake measured at a variety of altitudes, expressed as inspired PO_2 values. The 1964 data of Pugh et al. predicted the $\dot{V}O_2$ max to be equal to basal metabolic rate. The estimation based on the finding that the barometric pressure (and PO_2) was higher than expected at the summit shifts the estimate to about 15 ml · kg^{-1} · min^{-1}.

several of the climbers had been competitive marathon runners (127), and, given the need to transport oxygen at these high altitudes to do work, having such a high $\dot{V}O_2$ max would appear to be a prerequisite to success in climbing without oxygen. Subsequent measurements on other mountaineers who had scaled 8,500 meters or more without oxygen confirmed this by showing them to possess primarily type I muscle fibers and to have an average $\dot{V}O_2$ max of 60 ± 6 ml · kg^{-1} · min^{-1} (85). However, there was one notable exception: One of the subjects in this study was Messner, who had climbed Mount Everest without oxygen; his $\dot{V}O_2$ max was 48.8 ml · kg^{-1} · min^{-1} (85). West et al. (129) provide food for thought in this regard: "It remains for someone to elucidate the evolutionary processes responsible for man being just able to reach the highest point on Earth while breathing ambient air." However, there is more to consider in climbing Mount Everest than a person's $\dot{V}O_2$ max.

It has been a common experience in mountain climbing, especially with prolonged exposure to high altitudes, for climbers to lose weight, secondary to a loss of appetite (63). Clearly, if a large portion of this weight loss were muscle, it would have a negative impact in the climber's ability to scale the mountain. Some research work from both simulated and real ascents of Mount Everest provides some insight into what changes are taking place in muscle and what may be responsible for those changes. In the Operation Everest II 40-day simulation of an ascent to Mount Everest, the subjects experienced a 25% reduction in the cross-sectional area of type I and type II muscle fibers, and a 14% reduction in muscle area (43, 70). These observations were supported by data from a real ascent that combined both heavy exercise and severe hypoxia (54, 58). What could have caused these changes? The Operation Everest II data on nutrition and body composition showed that caloric intake decreased 43% from 3,136 to 1,789 kcal/day over the course of the 40-day exposure to hypoxia. The subjects lost an average of 7.4 kg, with most of the weight from lean body mass, despite the availability of palatable food (105). The hypoxia itself was a sufficient stimulus to suppress the appetite and alter body composition. Whether such changes in muscle mass are linked directly to changes in $\dot{V}O_2$ max, they would clearly affect performance. (See A Closer Look 24.3 for how acute, versus chronic, exposure to altitude can affect the lactate response to exercise.)

IN SUMMARY

- Climbers reached the summit of Mount Everest without oxygen in 1978. This surprised scientists who thought $\dot{V}O_2$ max would be just above resting $\dot{V}O_2$ at that altitude. They later found

The Lactate Paradox

When a submaximal test is conducted at altitude, the heart rate, ventilation, and lactate responses are higher than what are measured at sea level. This is no surprise for the heart rate and ventilation responses, because there is less oxygen per liter of blood and air, respectively. The elevated lactate response is also not unexpected, the assumption being that the hypoxia of altitude provides additional stimulation of glycolysis. What is surprising is that when the same exercise is done after the subject has been acclimated to altitude for 3 or 4 weeks (chronic hypoxia), the lactate response is substantially reduced. This is the lactate paradox—that the same hypoxic stimulus in chronic hypoxia gives rise to a lower lactate response than observed when the subject is first exposed (acute hypoxia) to altitude (101).

A variety of studies have been done to try to uncover the causes of the reduced lactate response to exercise during chronic exposure to altitude. The results from some of these studies have shown that the lower lactate is not due to a greater oxidative capacity of the muscle, an improved capillary-to-fiber ratio, or an improvement in oxygen delivery (44, 101). Instead, the reduction in lactate seems to be associated with a lower plasma epinephrine concentration which, as we know from chapter 5, would provide less stimulation of glycogenolysis via β-adrenergic receptor stimulation (78, 101). Evidence supporting this proposition comes from a study in which propranolol (a β-adrenergic receptor blocking drug) was shown to reduce the lactate response to acute hypoxia to a level

seen only after chronic hypoxia (101). However, the changes in epinephrine with acclimatization to altitude cannot entirely explain the lower lactate response (78). The lower lactate response may also be due to muscular adaptations resulting in tighter metabolic control such that the ADP concentration does not increase as much during exercise; this results in less stimulation of glycolysis (44). Consequently, the lactate paradox may be the result of both hormonal (epinephrine) and intracellular (lower [ADP]) adaptations that occur with chronic exposure to hypoxia. The most recent attempt to explain the lactate paradox is found in a "viewpoint" by Noakes (82), with commentaries by other authors and Noakes' rebuttal (83). This explanation focuses on the brain's need to protect oxygen delivery to itself by limiting muscle recruitment when exercise is done under chronic exposure to hypoxia. If the brain limits the recruitment of muscle fibers, less carbohydrate is metabolized and less lactate will be produced. However, commentaries (23) from various authors, including the authors of the principal paper cited by Noakes, argued against that hypothesis.

In contrast to the above, a study by van Hall et al. (119), published in 2001, suggested that the lactate paradox was simply a time-dependent phenomenon, being present during the early weeks of acclimatization and disappearing thereafter. Two years later, Pronk et al. (91) challenged this conclusion. They measured the lactate response to the same absolute work load on ascent to altitude and at 2, 4, 6, and 8 weeks to track changes in the

response over time at altitude. They observed the expected increase in the blood lactate response to exercise upon ascent to altitude, and the now-classic decrease in the blood lactate response with continued exposure to altitude. They also confirmed the link of the lactate response to changes in plasma catecholamines. They concluded that there was no evidence of a reversal of the lactate paradox with continued altitude exposure. Lundby and van Hall's response (69) to this study, and Pronk's counterresponse (90), make interesting reading, but indicate how much the two are apart.

To further complicate matters, in a 2009 study from van Hall's group (120), lowlanders who were taken to 4,100 m altitude had the same elevated lactate response during exercise upon acute exposure to that altitude, and after 2 weeks and 8 weeks of acclimatization (compared to sea level). They showed that the muscle lactate concentration was the same at exhaustion across all conditions, from sea level to 8 weeks of chronic hypoxia. Further, the epinephrine and norepinephrine concentrations were increased above sea level values in acute hypoxia, and were further increased after weeks of acclimation, signifying a normal sympathetic nervous system response to exercise. Last, the ADP concentration in muscle was not different across conditions. These finding are obviously at odds with the Pronk et al. study (91) and other proponents of the lactate paradox. Although the pros and cons have already been debated (123, 126), we are sure to hear more in the years ahead.

that the barometric pressure was higher than they previously had thought and that the estimated $\dot{V}O_2$ max was about 15 ml $\cdot$ kg^{-1} $\cdot$ min^{-1} at this altitude.

- Those who are successful at these high altitudes have a great capacity to hyperventilate. This drives down the PCO_2 and the [H$^+$] in

blood, and allows more oxygen to bind with hemoglobin at the same arterial PO_2.

- Finally, those who are successful at climbing to extreme altitudes must contend with the loss of appetite that results in a reduction in body weight and in the cross-sectional area of type I and type II muscle fibers.

HEAT

Chapter 12 described the changes in body temperature with exercise, how heat loss mechanisms are activated, and the benefits of acclimation to heat. This section extends that discussion by considering the prevention of thermal injuries during exercise.

Hyperthermia

Our core temperature (37° C) is within a few degrees of a value (45° C) that could lead to death (see chapter 12). Given that, and the fact that distance running races, triathlons, fitness programs, and football games occur during the warmer part of the year, the potential for heat injury, **hyperthermia,** is increased (13, 46, 61). Heat injury is not an all-or-none affair, but includes a series of stages that need to be recognized and attended to in order to prevent a progression from the least to the most serious (60). Table 24.3 summarizes each stage, identifying signs, symptoms, and the immediate care that should be provided (19). The most rapid and preferred way to reduce body temperature of those with heat stroke is by cold water immersion (5, 20). Although it is important to recognize and deal with these problems, it is better to prevent them from happening.

Figure 24.6 shows the major factors related to heat injury. Each one independently influences susceptibility to heat injury:

TABLE 24.3	Heat-Related Problems and Their Treatment	
Heat Illness	**Signs and Symptoms**	**Immediate Care**
Heat syncope—fainting or excessive loss of strength because of excessive heat	Headache Nausea	Normal intake of fluids.
Heat cramps—spasmodic muscular contractions caused by exertion in extreme heat	Muscle cramping (calf is very common location) Multiple cramping (very serious)	Isolated cramps: Apply pressure to the cramp and release, stretch muscle slowly and gently, apply gentle massage, and ice. Hydrate by drinking lots of water. Multiple cramps: Danger of heatstroke; treat as heat exhaustion.
Heat exhaustion—collapse with or without loss of consciousness, suffered in conditions of heat and high humidity, largely resulting from the loss of fluid and salt by sweating	Profuse sweating Cold, clammy skin Normal or slightly elevated temperature Pale Dizzy Weak, rapid pulse Shallow breathing Nausea Headache Loss of consciousness Thirst	Move individual out of the sun to a well-ventilated area. Place in shock position, with feet elevated 12 to 18 in. (31–46 cm); prevent heat loss or gain. Gently massage the extremities. Apply gentle ROM movement to the extremities. Force consumption of fluids. Reassure the individual. Monitor body temperature and other vital signs. Refer to a physician.
Heatstroke—final stage of heat exhaustion in which the thermoregulatory system shuts down to conserve depleted fluid levels	Generally no perspiration Dry skin Very hot Temperature as high as 106 °F (41.1° C) Skin color bright red or flushed (dark-pigmented individuals will have ashen skin) Rapid, strong pulse Labored breathing Change in behavior Unresponsive	Treat as an extreme medical emergency. Transport to hospital quickly. Remove as much clothing as possible without exposing the individual. Cool quickly, starting at the head and continuing down the body; use any means possible (fan, hose down, pack in ice). Wrap in cold, wet sheets for transport. Treat for shock; if breathing is labored, place in a semi-reclining position.

From: Carver S. 2007. Injury prevention and treatment. In: *Fitness Professional's Handbook*, edited by Howley E, and Franks B. Champaign: Human Kinetics, p. 375–397. [Permission needed]

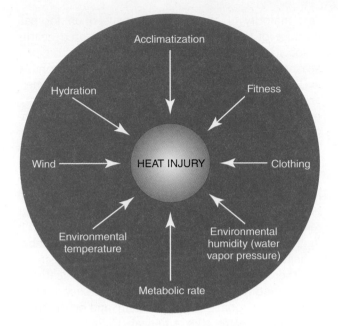

Figure 24.6   Factors affecting heat injury.

Figure 24.7   The effect of different types of uniforms on the body temperature response to treadmill running.

Fitness   A high level of fitness is related to a lower risk of heat injury (40). Fit subjects can tolerate more work in the heat (29), acclimate faster (13), and sweat more (11). However, very fit individuals can still develop exercise-related heat stroke (5).

Acclimation   Exercise in the heat for 10 to 14 days, either at low intensity (<50% $\dot{V}O_2$ max) and long duration (60–100 min) or at moderate intensity (75% $\dot{V}O_2$ max) and short duration (30–35 min), accomplish the following (5, 13, 57, 68).

- increases plasma volume and capacity to sweat,
- increases $\dot{V}O_2$ max, maximal cardiac output, and power output at the LT,
- lowers body temperature and heart rate responses to exercise,
- reduces salt loss in sweat and the chance of sodium depletion, and
- increases aerobic exercise performance.

This acclimation process is the best protection against exercise-related heat stroke and heat exhaustion (5).

Hydration   Inadequate hydration reduces sweat rate and increases the chance of heat injury (109, 111, 112). Chapter 23 discussed the procedures for fluid replacement. Generally, there are no differences among water, electrolyte drinks, or carbohydrate-electrolyte drinks in replacing body water during exercise (18, 24, 136).

Environmental Temperature   Convection and radiation heat-loss mechanisms are dependent on a temperature gradient from skin to environment. Exercising in temperatures greater than skin temperatures

results in a heat gain. Evaporation of sweat must then compensate if body temperature is to remain at a safe value. See the later discussion on the use of the Wet Bulb Globe Temperature as a guide to reducing the risk of heat injury.

Clothing   Expose as much skin surface as possible to encourage evaporation. Choose materials, such as cotton, that will "wick" sweat to the surface for evaporation. Materials impermeable to water will increase the risk of heat injury. Figure 24.7 shows the influence of different uniforms on the body temperature response to treadmill running (73). Because many exercise-related heat injuries occur during the first four days of American football practice, attention to limiting clothing as well as attending to acclimation and hydration is advised (5).

Humidity (Water Vapor Pressure)   Evaporation of sweat is dependent on the water vapor pressure gradient between skin and environment. In warm/hot environments, the relative humidity is a good index of the water vapor pressure, with a lower relative humidity facilitating evaporation. See the later discussion on the use of the Wet Bulb Globe Temperature as a guide to reducing the risk of heat injury.

Metabolic Rate   Given that core temperature is proportional to work rate, metabolic heat production plays an important role in the overall heat load the body experiences during exercise. Decreasing the work rate decreases this heat load, as well as the strain on the physiological systems that must deal with it.

Wind   Wind places more air molecules into contact with the skin and can influence heat loss in two ways. If a temperature gradient for heat loss exists between the skin and the air, wind will increase the rate of heat loss by convection. In a similar manner, wind increases the rate of evaporation, assuming the air can accept moisture.

Even the time of day is a consideration when it comes to exercise performance during heat exposure. With its typical diurnal variation, core temperature is lower and the body's heat storage capacity is higher in the morning, compared to the afternoon, when resting core temperature is elevated (98). When male cyclists rode to exhaustion at 65% $\dot{V}O_2$ max in a warm environment (35° C, 60% RH), time to exhaustion was longer in the morning trial (45.8 min) compared to the afternoon trial (40.5 min). Core temperature was lower in the morning trial for the first 25 minutes, but was not different at exhaustion (52). The results suggested that the greater heat storage capacity contributed to the difference.

For a practical guide on the prevention and treatment of heat-related illness, see Howe and Boden in the Suggested Readings.

Implications for Fitness The person exercising for fitness needs to be educated about all of the previously listed factors. Suggestions might include:

- providing information on heat illness symptoms: cramps, lightheadedness, and so on,
- exercising in the cooler part of the day to avoid heat gain from the sun or structures heated by the sun,
- gradually increasing exposure to high heat/ humidity to safely acclimatize,
- drinking water before, during, and after exercise and weighing in each day to monitor hydration,
- wearing only shorts and a tank top to expose as much skin as possible,
- taking heart rate measurements several times during the activity and reducing exercise intensity to stay in the target heart rate (THR) zone.

The latter recommendation is most important. The heart rate is a sensitive indicator of dehydration, environmental heat load, and acclimation. Variation in any of these factors will modify the heart rate response to any fixed, submaximal exercise. It is therefore important for fitness participants to monitor heart rate on a regular basis and to slow down to stay within the THR zone. Age is sometimes raised as a predisposing factor related to heat injury, but that may not be the case after you account for the factors mentioned previously. We would like to direct the interested reader to a brief and clearly written review of this topic by Kenney and Munce in the Suggested Readings.

Implications for Performance Heat injury has been a concern in athletics for decades. Initially, the vast majority of attention was focused on football because of the large number of heat-related deaths associated with that sport (14). Emphasis on preseason conditioning to improve fitness and promote acclimation, drinking water during practice and games, and weighing in each day to monitor hydration resulted in a steady reduction of heat-related deaths throughout the early 1990s. However, since that time there has been an increase in the number of heat-related deaths in football, especially at the high school level. In fact, among U.S. high school athletes, heat illness is the leading cause of death and disability (39). There is a need to return to the vigilance and practices that resulted in the low death rates of the early 1990s. It might be added that during the time that the number of heat-related deaths in football players was decreasing, there was an increase in the number of deaths in another athletic activity—long-distance road races (46, 62). In response to this problem, and on the basis of sound research, the American College of Sports Medicine developed a Position Stand on the Prevention of Thermal Injuries During Distance Running (3), parts of which have been recently updated (5). The elements recommended in this position statement are consistent with what we previously presented:

Medical Director

- A sports medicine physician should work with the race director to enhance safety and coordinate first-aid measures.

Race Organization

- Minimize environmental heat load by planning races for the cooler months, and at a time of day (before 8:00 A.M. or after 6:00 P.M.) to reduce solar heat gain.
- Use an environmental heat stress index (see the next section, "Environmental Heat Stress") to help make decisions about whether to run a race.
- Have a water station every 2 to 3 km; encourage runners to drink 150 to 300 milliliters of water every 15 minutes.
- Clearly identify the race monitors and have them look for those who might be in trouble due to heat injury.
- Have traffic control for safety.
- Use radio communication throughout the race course.

Medical Support

- Medical director coordinates ambulance service with local hospitals and has the authority to evaluate or stop runners who appear to be in trouble.
- Medical director coordinates medical facilities at race site to provide first aid.

Competitor Education

- Provide information about factors related to heat illness that were discussed previously.
- Encourage the "buddy system" (see chapter 17). The primary focus in these recommendations is on safety.

Environmental Heat Stress The previous discussion mentioned high temperature and relative humidity as factors increasing the risk of heat injuries. To quantify the overall heat stress associated with any environment, a Wet Bulb Globe Temperature (**WBGT**) guide was developed (3). This overall heat stress index is composed of the following measurements:

Dry Bulb Temperature (T_{db})

- Ordinary measure of air temperature taken in the shade

Black Globe Temperature (T_g)

- Measure of the radiant heat load measured in direct sunlight

Wet Bulb Temperature (T_{wb})

- Measurement of air temperature with a thermometer whose mercury bulb is covered with a wet cotton wick. This measure is sensitive to the relative humidity (water vapor pressure) and provides an index of the ability to evaporate sweat.

The formula used to calculate the WBGT index shows the importance of this latter wet bulb temperature in determining heat stress (3):

$$WBGT = 0.7\ T_{wb} + 0.2\ T_g + 0.1\ T_{db}$$

The risk of exertional heat stroke (EHS) is classified as follows (5, 102):

WBGT ≤50.0° F (≤10.0° C)	Risk of hypothermia; EHS can occur
WBGT 50−65° F (10−18.3° C)	Low risk of both hypothermia and hyperthermia; EHS can occur
WBGT 65.1−72.0° F (18.4−22.2° C)	Caution: risk of heat illness increases; high-risk persons monitored or not compete
WBGT 72.1−78.0° F (22.3−25.6° C)	Extreme caution; risk of hyperthermia increased for all
WBGT 78.1−82.0° F (25.7−27.8° C)	Extreme caution; high risk for unfit, non-acclimatized
WBGT ≥82.1° F (≥27.9° C)	Extreme risk of hyperthermia; cancel or postpone

In addition to environmental factors contributing to the risk of heat injury, there is no question about their impact on performance. For example, the fastest marathons are run at environmental temperatures of 10.6–12.8°C for men and 11.6–13.6°C for women; times are systematically slower with higher environmental temperatures (30, 31). Not surprisingly, precooling the body prior to exercise in the heat improves performance; however, practical recommendations on how to do this are just being developed (97). In a recent study, both a standard whole-body immersion in 10°C water for 10 minutes and a new approach using a combination of consuming 14 g/kg of an ice slurry sports drink while wearing iced towels were effective in lowering core temperature prior to a cycling time trial in hot and humid conditions. However, the new approach of doing both internal and external cooling was more effective from a performance standpoint (107).

IN SUMMARY

- Heat injury is influenced by environmental factors such as temperature, water vapor pressure, acclimation, hydration, clothing, and metabolic rate. The fitness participant should be educated about the signs and symptoms of heat injury, the importance of drinking water before, during, and after the activity, gradually becoming acclimated to the heat, exercising in the cooler part of the day, dressing appropriately, and checking the HR on a regular basis.
- Road races conducted in times of elevated heat and humidity need to reflect the coordinated wisdom of the race director and medical director to minimize heat and other injuries. Concerns include running the race at the correct time of the day and season of the year, frequent water stops, traffic control, race monitors to identify and stop those in trouble, and communication between race monitors, medical director, ambulance services, and hospitals.
- The heat stress index includes dry bulb, wet bulb, and globe temperatures. The wet bulb temperature, which is a good indicator of the water vapor pressure, is more important than the other two in determining overall heat stress.

COLD

Altitude and heat stress are not the only environmental factors having an impact on performance. A WBGT of 10° C or less is associated with hypothermia. **Hypothermia** results when heat loss from the body exceeds heat production and is defined, clinically, as a core temperature below 35° C (95° F), which is a drop of about 2° C (3.5° F) below normal body temperature (4).

Cold air facilitates this process in more ways than are readily apparent. First, and most obvious, when air temperature is less than skin temperature, a gradient for heat loss exists for convection, and physiological mechanisms involving peripheral vasoconstriction and shivering come into play to counter this gradient. Second, and less obvious, cold air has a low water vapor pressure, which encourages the evaporation of moisture from the skin to further cool the body. The combined effects can be deadly, as witnessed in Pugh's report of three deaths during a "walking" competition over a 45-mile distance (93).

Hypothermia can range in severity from mild to severe (4):

- Mild hypothermia
  - 35° C (95° F)—maximal shivering
  - 34° C (93.2° F)—amnesia, poor judgment
- Moderate hypothermia
  - 33° C (91.4° F)—ataxia, apathy
  - 31° C (87.8° F)—shivering ceases, pupils dilate
  - 29° C (85.2° F)—unconscious
- Severe hypothermia
  - 28° C (82.4° F)—ventricular fibrillation
  - 26° C (78.8° F)—no response to pain
  - 24° C (75.2° F)—hypotension, bradycardia
  - 19° C (66.2° F)—EEG silence
  - 13.7° C (56.7° F)—lowest temperature for adult survival

Figure 24.8 shows the factors related to hypothermia. These include environmental factors such as temperature, water vapor pressure, wind, and whether air or water is involved; insulating factors such as clothing and subcutaneous fat; the characteristics of the individuals involved (e.g., age and gender); and the capacity for sustained heat production, including fuels available. We will now comment on each of these relative to hypothermia. For a thorough presentation on this topic, see the American College of Sports Medicine's Position Stand (4) and the National Athletic Trainers' Association position statement (17).

Environmental Factors

Heat loss mechanisms introduced in chapter 12 included conduction, convection, radiation, and evaporation. Given that hypothermia is the result of higher heat loss than heat production, understanding how these mechanisms are involved will facilitate a discussion of how to deal with this problem.

Conduction, convection, and radiation are dependent on a temperature gradient between skin and environment; the larger the gradient, the greater the rate of heat loss. What is surprising is that the environmental temperature does not have to be below freezing to cause hypothermia. In effect, other environmental factors interact with temperature to create the dangerous condition by facilitating heat loss—namely, wind and water.

Wind Chill Index   The rate of heat loss at any given temperature is directly influenced by the wind speed. Wind increases the number of cold air molecules coming into contact with the skin so that heat loss is accelerated. The **wind chill index** indicates what the "effective" temperature is for any combination of temperature and wind speed. Siple and Passel (115) developed a formula for predicting how fast heat would be lost at different wind speeds and temperatures:

$$\text{Wind chill (kcal} \cdot \text{m}^{-2} \cdot \text{h}^{-1}) = [\sqrt{WV \times 100} + 10.45 - WV] \times (33 - T_A)$$

where WV = wind velocity (m · sec^{-1}); 10.45 is a constant; 33 is 33° C, which is taken as the skin temperature; and T_A = ambient dry bulb temperature in °C. Siple and Passel estimated how long it would take for exposed flesh to freeze and tabulated the levels of "danger" associated with combinations of wind speed and temperature.

This formula (38), which had been used for many years, was thought to overestimate the effect of increasing wind speed on tissue freezing and underestimated the effect of decreasing temperature (27). The following wind chill formula has been adopted by the National Weather Service (http://www.crh.noaa.gov/dtx/New_Wind_Chill.htm):

$$\text{Wind chill (°F)} = 35.74 + 0.6215\,(T) - 35.75\,(V^{0.16}) + 0.4275T\,(V^{0.16})$$

where wind speed (V) is in mph, and temperature (T) is in °F.

Table 24.4 provides the calculated wind chill temperatures for a variety of wind speeds and temperatures, along with estimates of the time it would take for frostbite to occur. Keep in mind that if you are running, riding, or cross-country skiing into the wind, you

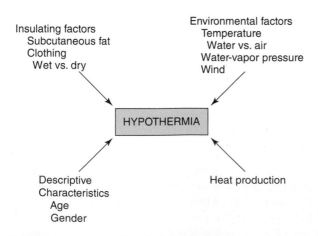

Figure 24.8   Factors affecting hypothermia.

TABLE 24.4 Wind Chill Chart

Wind (MPH)	Temperature (°F)																	
Calm	40	35	30	25	20	15	10	5	0	−5	−10	−15	−20	−25	−30	−35	−40	−45
5	36	31	25	19	13	7	1	−5	−11	−16	−22	−28	−34	−40	−46	−52	−57	−63
10	34	27	21	15	9	3	−4	−10	−16	−22	−28	−35	−41	−47	−53	−59	−66	−72
15	32	25	19	13	6	0	−7	−13	−19	−26	−32	−39	−45	−51	−58	−64	−71	−77
20	30	24	17	11	4	−2	−9	−15	−22	−29	−35	−42	−48	−55	−61	−68	−74	−81
25	29	23	16	9	3	−4	−11	−17	−24	−31	−37	−44	−51	−58	−64	−71	−78	−84
30	28	22	15	8	1	−5	−12	−19	−26	−33	−39	−46	−53	−60	−67	−73	−80	−87
35	28	21	14	7	0	−7	−14	−21	−27	−34	−41	−48	−55	−62	−69	−76	−82	−89
40	27	20	13	6	−1	−8	−15	−22	−29	−36	−43	−50	−57	−64	−71	−78	−84	−91
45	26	19	12	5	−2	−9	−16	−23	−30	−37	−44	−51	−58	−65	−72	−79	−86	−93
50	26	19	12	4	−3	−10	−17	−24	−31	−38	−45	−52	−60	−67	−74	−81	−88	−95
55	25	18	11	4	−3	−11	−18	−25	−32	−39	−46	−54	−61	−68	−75	−82	−89	−97
60	25	17	10	3	−4	−11	−19	−26	−33	−40	−48	−55	−62	−69	−76	−84	−91	−98

Frostbite Times   ▢ 30 minutes   ▢ 10 minutes   ▢ 5 minutes

Wind Chill (°F) = 35.74 + 0.6215T − 35.75 (V$^{0.16}$) + 0.4275 (V$^{0.16}$)

Where T = Air Temperature (°F)   V = Wind Speed (mph)   (Effective 11/01/01)

Figure 24.9 The effect of different water temperatures on survival of shipwrecked individuals.

must add your speed to the wind speed to evaluate the full impact of the wind chill. For example, cycling at 20 mph into calm air at 0° F is equivalent to a wind chill temperature of −22° F. However, it is clear that wind is not the only factor that can increase the rate of heat loss at any given temperature.

Water The thermal conductivity of water is about twenty-five times greater than that of air, so you can lose heat twenty-five times faster in water compared to air of the same temperature (55). Figure 24.9 shows death can occur in only a few hours when a person is shipwrecked in cold water. Unlike air, water offers little or no insulation at the skin-water interface, so heat is rapidly lost from the body. Given that movement in such cold water would increase heat loss from the arms and legs, the recommendation is to stay as still as possible in long-term immersions (4, 55).

IN SUMMARY

- Hypothermia is influenced by natural and added insulation, environmental temperature, vapor pressure, wind, water immersion, and heat production.
- The wind chill index describes how wind lowers the effective temperature at the skin such that convective heat loss is greater than what it would be in calm air at that same temperature.
- Water causes heat to be lost by convection twenty-five times faster than it would be by exposure to air of the same temperature.

Insulating Factors

The rate at which heat is lost from the body is inversely related to the insulation between the body and the environment. The insulating quality is related to the thickness of subcutaneous fat, the ability of clothing to trap air, and whether the clothing is wet or dry.

Subcutaneous Fat An excellent indicator of total body insulation per unit surface area (through which heat is lost) is the average subcutaneous fat thickness (49). Pugh and Edholm's (94) observation that a "fat" man was able to swim for 7 hours in 16° C water with no change in body temperature, whereas a "thin" man had to leave the water in 30 minutes with a core temperature of 34.5° C, supports this statement. Long-distance swimmers tend to be fatter than short-course swimmers. The higher body fatness does more than help maintain body temperature; fatter swimmers are more buoyant, requiring less energy to swim at any set speed (53). In addition, body fatness plays a role in the onset and magnitude of the shivering response to cold exposure (see later discussion in the "Heat Production" section).

Clothing Clothing can extend our natural subcutaneous fat insulation to allow us to sustain very cold environments. The insulation quality of clothing is given in **clo** units, where 1 clo is the insulation needed at rest (1 MET) to maintain core temperature when the environment is 21° C, the RH = 50%, and the air movement is 6 m · min^{-1} (12). Still air next to the body has a clo rating of 0.8. As the air temperature falls, clothing with a higher clo value must be worn to maintain core temperature, because the gradient between skin and environment increases (86). Figure 24.10 shows the insulation needed at different energy expenditures across a broad range of temperatures from −60 to +80° F (12). It is clear that as heat production increases,

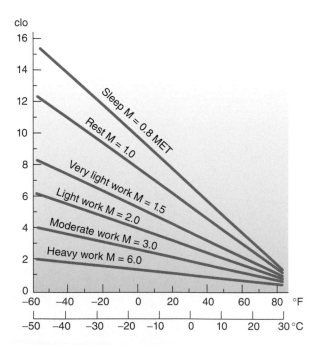

Figure 24.10 Changes in the insulation requirement of clothing (plus air) with increasing rates of energy expenditure over environmental temperatures of −50 to +30° C.

insulation must decrease to maintain core temperature. By wearing clothing in layers, insulation can be removed piece by piece, because less insulation is needed to maintain core temperature. By following these steps, sweating, which can rob the clothing of its insulating value, will be minimized. A practical example of how clothing helps maintain body temperature (and comfort) can be seen in the following study. Heat loss from the head increases linearly from $+32°$ C to $-21°$ C, with about half of the entire heat production being lost through the head when the temperature is $-4°$ C. Wearing a simple "helmet" with a clo rating of 3.5 allows an individual to stay out indefinitely at $0°$ C (37).

Clothing offers insulation by trapping air, a poor conductor of heat. If the clothing becomes wet, the insulating quality decreases because the water can now conduct heat away from the body at a faster rate (55). A primary goal, then, is to avoid wetness, due either to sweat or to weather. This problem is exacerbated by the cold environment's very low water vapor pressure. Recall from chapter 12 that the water vapor pressure in the environment is the primary factor influencing evaporation and that at low environmental temperatures the water vapor pressure is low even when the relative humidity is high. Think of a time when you finished playing a game indoors and stepped outside into cold, damp weather to cool off. You noticed "steam" coming off your body; how is this possible when the RH is near 100%? The water vapor pressure is high at the skin surface, since the skin temperature is elevated; so, a gradient for water vapor pressure exists. You will cool off very fast under these circumstances. This is why cold, wet, windy environments carry an extra risk of hypothermia. The wind not only provides for greater convective heat loss as described in the wind chill chart, but it also accelerates evaporation (47).

Heat Production

Figure 24.10 shows that the amount of insulation needed to maintain core temperature decreases as energy expenditure increases. This is also true for our "natural" insulation, subcutaneous fat. McArdle et al. (79) showed that when fat men (27.6% fat) were immersed for 1 hour in $20°$ C, $24°$ C, and $28°$ C water, the resting $\dot{V}O_2$ and core temperature did not change compared to values measured in air. In thinner men (<16.8% fat), the $\dot{V}O_2$ increased to counter the rapid loss of heat; however, the core temperature still decreased. When these same subjects did exercise in the cold water, requiring a $\dot{V}O_2$ of 1.7 L $\cdot$ min^{-1}, the fall in body temperature was either prevented or retarded (80), showing the importance of high rates of heat production in preventing hypothermia. More recent studies support these observations, showing

an earlier onset and greater magnitude of shivering in lean subjects when exposed to cold air (118). Similar findings have been reported for fit subjects (8).

Fuel Use Shivering can increase oxygen consumption to 1000 ml/min during resting immersion in cold water, and like moderate exercise of the same intensity, fat is a primary fuel to support shivering in well-fed individuals (4). However, it is clear that inadequate carbohydrate stores may lead to hypoglycemia, which can impact one's ability to shiver. Further, bursts of shivering lead to greater muscle glycogen depletion. Consequently, having adequate carbohydrate stores is important to reduce the risk for hypothermia (4). Given the importance of body fatness and body type in the metabolic response to cold exposure, are there differences due to gender and age?

Descriptive Characteristics

Subject characteristics, such as gender and age, influence the metabolic and body temperature responses to cold exposure.

Gender Sex differences in response to cold water exposure are linked to a woman's higher body fatness, thicker subcutaneous layer, less lean mass, and higher surface area-to-mass ratio, compared to men of the same weight and age. At rest, women show a faster reduction in body temperature than do men, even when subcutaneous fat thickness is the same. In contrast, when exercise is done in cold water, women and men of the same body fatness have similar decreases in body temperature. Consequently, any gender differences in core temperature responses to cold exposure can be explained primarily on the basis of differences in body composition and anthropometry. It must be added that amenorrheic women cannot maintain core temperature during exercise in the cold as well as eumenorrheic women can (4).

Age In general, individuals over 60 years may be less tolerant to cold exposures than younger individuals because the ability of older individuals to vasoconstrict skin blood vessels and conserve heat is reduced. They also have less thermal sensitivity. That is, their response to a decrease in temperature is reduced, allowing time for greater heat loss. In contrast to adults, children have a larger surface area-to-mass ratio and less subcutaneous fat. This results in a faster fall in core temperature on cold water exposure and a greater risk of hypothermia. Similar to the gender differences (or lack thereof) mentioned above, 11- to 12-year-old boys with the same subcutaneous fat as men had the same core temperature response when doing exercise in cold air (4). See A Look Back— Important People in Science for an individual who had

L. G. C. E. Pugh Furthered Our Understanding of How to Survive and Function Well in Extreme Environments

In this chapter that deals with the effect of cold, heat, and altitude on performance, we thought it would be appropriate to highlight an individual who had a major impact on our understanding of the physiology involved in adapting to adverse environments: **Lewis Griffith Cresswell Evans (L.G.C.E.) Pugh, M.D.**

L.G.C.E. Pugh was born in 1909 in England. He attended New College, Oxford, and completed his B.A. in 1931. He then studied natural sciences during 1931–33 and medicine until 1938, at which time he received his B.M and M.A. degrees. He was a competitive downhill and cross-country skier and qualified for England's 1936 Winter Olympics. In 1939 he entered the army as a medical officer and served in Europe and the Middle East. In 1943, he was sent to the Mountain Warfare Training Centre in Lebanon to

select, train, and evaluate troops for mountain warfare. There he became involved in the systematic study of the interaction of altitude, environmental temperature, nutrition, clothing, and fitness on human performance, and he developed training manuals based on his work. Following the war he was involved in British navy research expeditions to the Arctic, and in 1950 he accepted a position in the Medical Research Council's Division in Human Physiology to study the effects of extreme environments.

Dr. Pugh was a major participant in several high-altitude expeditions during the 1950s and 1960s. The first, in 1952, gave him insight into what kinds of clothing, nutrition, hydration, and oxygen were required for humans to function at extreme altitudes. His work is recognized as being crucial to the success of the 1953 British expedition to Mt. Everest in which Edmund Hillary and Tenzing Norgay were the first to reach the summit. In the late 1950s he

joined Edmund Hillary for an Antarctic expedition in which he studied human tolerance to extreme cold; it was also during this time that the two planned to return to Everest. Dr. Pugh was the principal scientist in the 1960–61 Scientific and Mountaineering Expedition to Everest that provided ground-breaking, and yet fundamental, information about how humans adapt to chronic exposure to high altitude. In addition, in the late 1960s he was involved in helping athletes prepare for the Olympic Games which were to take place in Mexico City at an altitude of ~2,300 m. His life's work revolved around understanding how humans adapt to exercise in extreme environments and his findings are as relevant today as they were 60 years ago. He died in 1994.

Sources: Peter H. Hansen. Pugh, (Lewis) Griffith Cresswell Evans (1909–1994), physiologist and mountaineer. *Oxford Dictionary of National Biography.* University of California, San Diego. Mandeville Special Collections Library, Geisel Library. *The Register of* L. G. C. E. *Pugh Papers* 1940–1986.

a major impact on our understanding of the physiology of how humans adapt to extreme environments.

IN SUMMARY

- Subcutaneous fat is the primary "natural" insulation and is very effective in preventing rapid heat loss when a person is exposed to cold water.
- Clothing extends this insulation, and the insulation value of clothing is described in clo units, where a value of 1 describes what is needed to maintain core temperature while sitting in a room set at 21° C and 50% RH with an air movement of 6 m · sec^{-1}.
- The amount of insulation needed to maintain core temperature is less when one exercises because the metabolic heat production helps maintain the core temperature. Clothing should be worn in layers when exercising so one can shed one insulating layer at a time as body temperature increases.
- Heat production increases on exposure to cold, with an inverse relationship between the increase in $\dot{V}O_2$ and body fatness. Women cool faster than men when exposed to cold water, exhibiting a longer delay in the onset of shivering and a lower $\dot{V}O_2$, despite a greater stimulus to shiver.

Dealing with Hypothermia

As body temperature falls, the person's ability to carry out coordinated movements is reduced, speech is slurred, and judgment is impaired. As mentioned earlier, people can die from hypothermia, and the condition must be dealt with when it occurs. The following steps on how to do this are taken from the National Athletic Trainers' Association position statement on cold injuries (17):

- **Mild hypothermia**
  - Remove wet or damp clothing.
  - Insulate the person with warm dry clothing or blankets, covering the head.
  - Move person to warm environment with shelter from wind and rain.

- When rewarming, apply heat only to the trunk and other areas of heat transfer (axilla, chest wall, groin).
- Provide warm, nonalcoholic fluids and food containing 6–8% carbohydrate.

■ **Moderate/severe hypothermia**
- Determine if CPR is necessary and activate emergency medical system.
- Remove wet or damp clothing.
- Insulate the person with warm dry clothing or blankets, covering the head.
- Move person to warm environment with shelter from wind and rain.
- When rewarming, apply heat only to the trunk and other areas of heat transfer (axilla, chest wall, groin).
- If physician is not present, initiate rewarming strategies immediately and continue during transport.
- During treatment/transit, continue to monitor vital signs and be prepared for airway management.

IN SUMMARY

■ For mild hypothermia get the person out of the wind, rain, and cold; remove wet clothing and put on dry clothing; for rewarming, apply heat only to the trunk and other areas of heat transfer; and provide warm drinks and food.

■ For moderate/severe hypothermia do as above, check vital signs, activate emergency medical system, and transport.

AIR POLLUTION

Air pollution includes a variety of gases and particulates that are products of the combustion of fossil fuels. The "smog" that results when these pollutants are in high concentration can have a detrimental effect on health and performance. The gases can affect performance by decreasing the capacity to transport oxygen, increasing airway resistance, and altering the perception of effort required when the eyes "burn" and the chest "hurts." A study on traffic policemen, who are routinely exposed to a full range of pollutants throughout their workday, makes the point. Although their physiological responses were normal at rest, during an exercise test about one-third of the policemen experienced ECG changes and elevated blood pressure responses, with the vast majority of those individuals also experiencing a desaturation of hemoglobin (122). In addition, children living in an air-polluted environment had significantly lower $\dot{V}O_2$ max values compared to those living in areas with better air quality (137).

The physiological responses to these pollutants are related to the amount or "dose" received. The major factors determining the dose are the concentration of the pollutant, the duration of the exposure to the pollutant, and the volume of air inhaled. This last factor increases during exercise and is one reason why physical activity should be curtailed during times of peak pollution levels (34). The following discussion focuses on the major air pollutants: particulate matter, ozone, sulfur dioxide, and carbon monoxide.

Particulate Matter

The air is full of microscopic and submicroscopic particles, many of which can be tied to motor vehicles (especially diesels) and industrial sources. Over the past 10 years, more attention has been focused on the very small particles because of their potential to promote pulmonary infection and actually cross the epithelium to enter the circulation (35). Fine particle pollution causes an elevation in blood pressure in those with pre-existing cardiovascular disease and may contribute to an increased risk of cardiac mortality and morbidity (114, 138). The mechanisms by which this occurs include a decreased capacity of the blood vessels to dilate and a reduction in fibrinolytic activity (81). Finally, evidence exists that these particles cause systemic oxidative stress with damage to DNA (9), and that antioxidant supplements may moderate this effect, especially in those with vitamin deficiencies (104).

Ozone

The ozone we breathe is generated by the reaction of UV light and emissions from internal combustion engines. While a single, 2-hour exposure to a high ozone concentration, 0.75 part per million (ppm), decreases $\dot{V}O_2$ max, recent studies show that a 6- to 12-hour exposure to a concentration of only 0.12 ppm (the U.S. air quality standard) decreases lung function and increases respiratory symptoms. Further, in amateur cyclists who practiced and raced in air containing varying concentrations of ozone, the decrease in pulmonary function following activity was directly related to the ozone concentration (10). Interestingly, an adaptation to ozone exposure can occur, with subjects showing a diminished response to subsequent exposures during the "ozone season." However, concern about long-term lung health suggests that it would be prudent to avoid heavy exercise during the time of day when ozone and other pollutants are elevated (34).

Sulfur Dioxide

Sulfur dioxide (SO_2) is produced by smelters, refineries, and electrical utilities that use fossil fuel for energy generation. SO_2 does not affect lung function in normal subjects, but it causes bronchoconstriction in asthmatics. These latter responses are influenced by the temperature and humidity of the inspired air, as mentioned in chapter 17. Nose breathing is encouraged to "scrub" the SO_2, and drugs like cromolyn sodium and β_2-agonists can partially block the asthmatic's response to SO_2 (34).

Carbon Monoxide

Carbon monoxide (CO) is derived from the burning of fossil fuel, coal, oil, gasoline, and wood, as well as from cigarette smoke. Carbon monoxide can bind to hemoglobin to form carboxyhemoglobin (HbCO) and decrease the capacity for oxygen transport. This has the potential to affect the physiological responses to submaximal exercise (51) and $\dot{V}O_2$ max, as does altitude. The carbon monoxide concentration [HbCO] in blood is generally less than 1% in nonsmokers, but may be as high as 10% in smokers (99). Horvath et al. (56) found that the critical concentration of HbCO needed to decrease $\dot{V}O_2$ max was 4.3%. Figure 24.11 shows the relationship between the blood HbCO concentration and the decrease in $\dot{V}O_2$ max; beyond 4.3% HbCO, $\dot{V}O_2$ max decreases 1% for each 1% increase in HbCO (100).

In contrast, when one performs light work, at about 40% $\dot{V}O_2$ max, the [HbCO] can be as high as 15% before endurance is affected. The cardiovascular system has the capacity to compensate with a larger cardiac output when the HbO_2 concentration is reduced during submaximal work (56, 99, 100). Because it takes 2 to 4 hours to remove half the CO from the blood after the exposure has been removed, CO can have a lasting effect on performances (34).

Unfortunately, it is difficult to predict what the actual [HbCO] will be in any given environment. One must consider the previous exposure to the pollutant, as well as the length of time and rate of ventilation associated with the current exposure. As a result, Raven (99) provides the following guidelines for exercising in an area with air pollution:

- Reduce exposure to the pollutant prior to exercise, because the physiological effects are time- and dose-dependent.
- Stay away from areas where you might receive a "bolus" dose of CO: smoking areas, high-traffic areas, urban environments.
- Do not schedule activities around the times when pollutants are at their highest levels (7–10 A.M. and 4–7 P.M.) due to traffic.

The **Air Quality Index (AQI)** is a measure of the quality of the air for five major air pollutants regulated by the Clean Air Act: ground-level ozone, particulate matter, carbon monoxide, sulfur dioxide, and nitrogen dioxide. Figure 24.12 shows a color-coded chart of the AIQ, with the interpretation of what the numerical values mean. Information on the AIQ is generally provided in a local community's weather forecast and should be suited to the individual—some will experience symptoms at lower levels of pollution than others (16).

Figure 24.11 The effect of the concentration of carbon monoxide in the blood on the change in $\dot{V}O_2$ max.

IN SUMMARY

- Air pollution can affect performance. Exposure to ozone decreases $\dot{V}O_2$ max and respiratory function, and sulfur dioxide causes bronchoconstriction in asthmatics.
- Carbon monoxide binds to hemoglobin and reduces oxygen transport.
- To prevent problems associated with pollution of any type, reduce exposure time; stay away from "bolus" amounts of the pollutant; and schedule activity at the least polluted part of the day.
- The Air Quality Index should be monitored to determine if conditions are safe for exercising outdoors.

Air Quality Index Levels of Health Concern	Numerical Value	Meaning
Good	0 to 50	Air quality is considered satisfactory, and air pollution poses little or no risk
Moderate	51 to 100	Air quality is acceptable; however, for some pollutants there may be a moderate health concern for a very small number of people who are unusually sensitive to air pollution.
Unhealthy for Sensitive Groups	101 to 150	Members of sensitive groups may experience health effects. The general public is not likely to be affected.
Unhealthy	151 to 200	Everyone may begin to experience health effects; members of sensitive groups may experience more serious health effects.
Very Unhealthy	201 to 300	Health alert: everyone may experience more serious health effects
Hazardous	301 to 500	Health warnings of emergency conditions. The entire population is more likely to be affected.

Figure 24.12   The Air Quality Index (AQI)—A Guide to Air Quality and Your Health. AIRNow website. Available at: http://www.airnow.gov/index.cfm?action=aqibasics.aqi

STUDY QUESTIONS

1. Describe the changes in barometric pressure, PO_2, and air density with increasing altitude.
2. Why is sprint performance not affected by altitude?
3. Explain why maximal aerobic power decreases at altitude and what effect this has on performance in long-distance races.
4. Graphically describe the effect of altitude on the HR and ventilation responses to submaximal work and provide recommendations for fitness participants who occasionally exercise at altitude.
5. Describe the process by which an individual adapts to altitude, and contrast the adaptation of the permanent residents of high altitude with that of the lowlander who arrives there as an adult.
6. While training at altitude can be beneficial, how could someone "detrain"? How can you work around this problem?
7. It was formerly believed that a person could not climb Mount Everest without oxygen because the estimated

$\dot{V}O_2$ max at altitude was close to basal metabolic rate. When two climbers accomplished the feat in 1978, scientists had to determine how this was possible. What were the primary reasons allowing the climb to take place without oxygen?
8. List and describe the factors related to heat injury.
9. What is the heat stress index, and why is the wet bulb temperature weighed so heavily in the formula?
10. List the factors related to hypothermia.
11. Explain what the wind chill index is relative to convective heat loss.
12. What is a clo unit, and why is the insulation requirement less when you exercise?
13. What would you do if a person had hypothermia?
14. Explain how carbon monoxide can influence $\dot{V}O_2$ max and endurance performance.
15. What steps would you follow to minimize the effect of pollution on performance?

SUGGESTED READINGS

Howe, A. S., and B. P. Boden. 2007. Heat-related illness in athletes. *American Journal of Sports Medicine* 35:1384–95.

Johnson, L., J. Hemmleb, and E. Simonson. 1999. *The Ghosts of Everest.* Seattle, WA: Mountaineers Books. (Detailed account of the expedition that found Mallory's body.)

Kenney, W. L., and T. A. Munce. 2003. Invited review: aging and human temperature regulation. *Journal of Applied Physiology* 95:598–603.

Messner, R. 1999. *Everest: Expedition to the Ultimate.* Seattle, WA: Mountaineers Books. (A story of the first trip to the summit by Messner and Habeler without oxygen.)

Millet, G. P., B. Roels, L. Schmitt, X. Woorons, and J. P. Richalet. 2010. Combining hypoxic methods for peak performance. *Sports Medicine.* 40:1–25.

Saunders, P. U., D. B. Pyne, and C. J. Gore. 2009. Endurance training at altitude. *High Altitude Medicine & Biology* 10:135–48.

REFERENCES

1. **Adams WC, Bernauer EM, Dill DB, and Bomar JB, Jr.** Effects of equivalent sea-level and altitude training on $\dot{V}O_2$ max and running performance. *Journal of Applied Physiology* 39: 262–266, 1975.
2. **Alexander JK, Hartley LH, Modelski M, and Grover RF.** Reduction of stroke volume during

exercise in man following ascent to 3,100 m altitude. *Journal of Applied Physiology* 23: 849–858, 1967.
3. **American College of Sports Medicine.** Position stand: heat and cold illnesses during distance running. *Medicine and Science in Sports and Exercise* 28: i–x, 1996.

4. **American College of Sports Medicine.** Position stand: prevention of cold injuries during exercise. *Medicine and Science in Sports and Exercise* 38: 2012–2029, 2006.

5. **American College of Sports Medicine.** Position stand. Exertional heat illness during training and competition. *Medicine and Science in Sports and Exercise* 39: 556–572, 2007.

6. **Balke B, Nagle FJ, and Daniels J.** Altitude and maximum performance in work and sports activity. *JAMA* 194: 646–649, 1965.

7. **Bassovitch O.** Intermittent hypoxia training: risks versus benefits. A biomedical engineering point of view. *European Journal of Applied Physiology* 110: 659–660, 2010.

8. **Bittel JH, Nonotte-Varly C, Livecchi-Gonnot GH, Savourey GL, and Hanniquet AM.** Physical fitness and thermoregulatory reactions in a cold environment in men. *Journal of Applied Physiology* 65: 1984–1989, 1988.

9. **Brauner EV, Forchhammer L, Moller P, Simonsen J, Glasius M, Wahlin P, Raaschou-Nielsen O, and Loft S.** Exposure to ultrafine particles from ambient air and oxidative stress-induced DNA damage. *Environmental Health Perspectives* 115: 1177–1182, 2007.

10. **Brunekreef B, Hoek G, Breugelmans O, and Leentvaar M.** Respiratory effects of low-level photochemical air pollution in amateur cyclists. *American Journal of Respiratory and Critical Care Medicine* 150: 962–966, 1994.

11. **Buono MJ, and Sjoholm NT.** Effect of physical training on peripheral sweat production. *Journal of Applied Physiology* 65: 811–814, 1988.

12. **Burton A, and Edholm O.** *Man in a Cold Environment.* London: Edward Arnold, 1955.

13. **Buskirk E, and Bass D.** Climate and exercise. In: *Science and Medicine of Exercise and Sport*, edited by Johnson W, and Buskirk E. New York: Harper & Row, 1974, p. 190–205.

14. **Buskirk E, and Grasley W.** Heat injury and conduct of athletics. In: *Science and Medicine of Exercise and Sport*, edited by Johnson W, and Buskirk E. New York: Harper & Row, 1974, p. 206–210.

15. **Buskirk ER, Kollias J, Akers RF, Prokop EK, and Reategui EP.** Maximal performance at altitude and on return from altitude in conditioned runners. *Journal of Applied Physiology* 23: 259–266, 1967.

16. **Campbell ME, Li Q, Gingrich SE, Macfarlane RG, and Cheng S.** Should people be physically active outdoors on smog alert days? *Canadian Journal of Public Health* 96: 24–28, 2005.

17. **Cappaert TA, Stone JA, Castellani JW, Krause BA, Smith D, and Stephens BA.** National Athletic Trainers' Association postion statement: environmental cold injuries. *Journal of Athletic Training* 43: 640–658, 2008.

18. **Carter JE, and Gisolfi CV.** Fluid replacement during and after exercise in the heat. *Medicine and Science in Sports and Exercise* 21: 532–539, 1989.

19. **Carver S.** Injury prevention and treatment. In: *Fitness Professional's Handbook*, edited by Howley E, and Franks B. Champaign: Human Kinetics, 2007, p. 375–397.

20. **Casa DJ, McDermott BP, Lee EC, Yeargin SW, Armstrong LE, and Maresh CM.** Cold water immersion: the gold standard for exertional heatstroke treatment. *Exercise and Sport Sciences Reviews* 35: 141–149, 2007.

21. **Chapman R, and Levine BD.** Altitude training for the marathon. *Sports Medicine (Auckland, NZ)* 37: 392–395, 2007.

22. **Chapman RF, Stray-Gundersen J, and Levine BD.** Individual variation in response to altitude training. *Journal of Applied Physiology* 85: 1448–1456, 1998.

23. **Commentaries on lactate paradox.** Commentaries on viewpoint: evidence that reduced skeletal muscle recruitment explains the lactate paradox during exercise at high altitude. *Journal of Applied Physiology* 106: 739–744, 2009.

24. **Costill DL, Cote R, Miller E, Miller T, and Wynder S.** Water and electrolyte replacement during repeated days of work in the heat. *Aviation, Space, and Environmental Medicine* 46: 795–800, 1975.

25. **Cymerman A, Reeves JT, Sutton JR, Rock PB, Groves BM, Malconian MK, Young PM, Wagner PD, and Houston CS.** Operation Everest II: maximal oxygen uptake at extreme altitude. *Journal of Applied Physiology* 66: 2446–2453, 1989.

26. **Daniels J, and Oldridge N.** The effects of alternate exposure to altitude and sea level on world-class middle-distance runners. *Medicine and Science in Sports* 2: 107–112, 1970.

27. **Danielsson U.** Windchill and the risk of tissue freezing. *Journal of Applied Physiology* 81: 2666–2673, 1996.

28. **Dill DB, and Adams WC.** Maximal oxygen uptake at sea level and at 3,090-m altitude in high school champion runners. *Journal of Applied Physiology* 30: 854–859, 1971.

29. **Drinkwater BL, Denton JE, Kupprat IC, Talag TS, and Horvath SM.** Aerobic power as a factor in women's response to work in hot environments. *Journal of Applied Physiology* 41: 815–821, 1976.

30. **Dufour SP, Ponsot E, Zoll J, Doutreleau S, Lonsdorfer-Wolf E, Geny B, Lampert E, Fluck M, Hoppeler H, Billat V, Mettauer B, Richard R, and Lonsdorfer J.** Exercise training in normobaric hypoxia in endurance runners. I. Improvement in aerobic performance capacity. *Journal of Applied Physiology* 100: 1238–1248, 2006.

31. **Ely MR, Cheuvront SN, and Montain SJ.** Neither cloud cover nor low solar loads are associated with fast marathon performance. *Medicine and Science in Sports and Exercise* 39: 2029–2035, 2007.

32. **Engfred K, Kjaer M, Secher NH, Friedman DB, Hanel B, Nielsen OJ, Bach FW, Galbo H, and Levine BD.** Hypoxia and training-induced adaptation of hormonal responses to exercise in humans. *European Journal of Applied Physiology and Occupational Physiology* 68: 303–309, 1994.

33. **Faulkner JA, Kollias J, Favour CB, Buskirk ER, and Balke B.** Maximum aerobic capacity and running performance at altitude. *Journal of Applied Physiology* 24: 685–691, 1968.

34. **Folinsbee L.** Discussion: exercise and the environment. In: *Exercise, Fitness, and Health*, edited by Bouchard C, Shephard R, Stevens T, Sutton J, and McPherson B. Champaign: Human Kinetics, 1990, p. 179–183.

35. **Frampton M.** Effects of exposure to ultrafine carbon particles in healthy subjects and subjects with asthma. *Research Report–Health Effects Institute* 126: 1–63, 2004.

36. **Frisancho AR, Martinez C, Velasquez T, Sanchez J, and Montoye H.** Influence of developmental adaptation on aerobic capacity at high altitude. *Journal of Applied Physiology* 34: 176–180, 1973.

37. **Froese G, and Burton AC.** Heat losses from the human head. *Journal of Applied Physiology* 10: 235–241, 1957.

38. **Gates D.** *Man and His Environment: Climate.* New York: Harper & Row, 1972.

39. **Gilchrist J, Murphy M, Comstock RD, Collins C, McIlvain N, and Yard E.** Heat illness among high school athletes-United States, 2005–2009. *Morbidity and Mortality Weekly Report* 59: 1009–1013, 2010.

40. **Gisolfi CV, and Cohen JS.** Relationships among training, heat acclimation, and heat tolerance in men and women: the controversy revisited. *Medicine and Science in Sports* 11: 56–59, 1979.

41. **Gore CJ, Clark SA, and Saunders PU.** Nonhematological mechanisms of improved sea-level performance after hypoxic exposure. *Medicine and Science in Sports and Exercise* 39: 1600–1609, 2007.

42. **Gore CJ, Rodriguez FA, Truijens MJ, Townsend NE, Stray-Gundersen J, and Levine BD.** Increased serum erythropoietin but not red cell production after 4 wk of intermittent hypobaric hypoxia (4,000–5,500 m). *Journal of Applied Physiology* 101: 1386–1393, 2006.

43. **Green HJ, Sutton JR, Cymerman A, Young PM, and Houston CS.** Operation Everest II: adaptations in human skeletal muscle. *Journal of Applied Physiology* 66: 2454–2461, 1989.

44. **Green HJ, Sutton JR, Wolfel EE, Reeves JT, Butterfield GE, and Brooks GA.** Altitude acclimatization and energy metabolic adaptations in skeletal muscle during exercise. *Journal of Applied Physiology* 73: 2701–2708, 1992.

45. **Grover RF, Reeves JT, Grover EB, and Leathers JE.** Muscular exercise in young men native to 3,100 m altitude. *Journal of Applied Physiology* 22: 555–564, 1967.

46. **Hanson PG, and Zimmerman SW.** Exertional heatstroke in novice runners. *JAMA* 242: 154–157, 1979.

47. **Hardy J, and Bard P.** Body temperature regulation. In: *Medical Physiology*, edited by Mount-Castle V. St. Louis: C. V. Mosby, 1974, p. 1305–1342.

48. **Hartley LH, Vogel JA, and Cruz JC.** Reduction of maximal exercise heart rate at altitude and its reversal with atropine. *Journal of Applied Physiology* 36: 362–365, 1974.

49. **Hayward MG, and Keatinge WR.** Roles of subcutaneous fat and thermoregulatory reflexes in determining ability to stabilize body temperature in water. *The Journal of Physiology* 320: 229–251, 1981.

50. **Hemmleb J, and Johnson L.** Discovery on Everest. *Climbing* 188: 98–190, 1999.

51. **Hirsch GL, Sue DY, Wasserman K, Robinson TE, and Hansen JE.** Immediate effects of cigarette smoking on cardiorespiratory responses to exercise. *Journal of Applied Physiology* 58: 1975–1981, 1985.

52. **Hobson RM, Clapp EL, Watson P, and Maughan RJ.** Exercise capacity in the heat is greater in the morning than in the evening in man. *Medicine and Science in Sports and Exercise* 41: 174–180, 2009.

53. **Holmer I.** Physiology of swimming man. In: *Exercise and Sport Sciences Reviews*, edited by Hutton R, and Miller D. Salt Lake City: Franklin Institute, 1979.

54. **Hoppeler H, Kleinert E, Schlegel C, Claassen H, Howald H, Kayar SR, and Cerretelli P.** Morphological adaptations of human skeletal muscle to chronic hypoxia. *International Journal of Sports Medicine* 11 Suppl 1: S3–9, 1990.

55. **Horvath SM.** Exercise in a cold environment. In:*Exercise and Sport Sciences Reviews*, edited by Miller D. Salt Lake: Franklin Institute, 1981, p. 221–263.

56. **Horvath SM, Raven PB, Dahms TE, and Gray DJ.** Maximal aerobic capacity at different levels of carboxyhemoglobin. *Journal of Applied Physiology* 38: 300–303, 1975.

57. **Houmard JA, Costill DL, Davis JA, Mitchell JB, Pascoe DD, and Robergs RA.** The influence of exercise intensity on heat acclimation in trained subjects. *Medicine and Science in Sports and Exercise* 22: 615–620, 1990.

58. **Howald H, Pette D, Simoneau JA, Uber A, Hoppeler H, and Cerretelli P.** Effect of chronic hypoxia on muscle enzyme activities. *International Journal of Sports Medicine* 11 Suppl 1: S10–14, 1990.

59. **Howley E.** Effect of altitude on physical performance. In: *Encyclopedia of Physical Education, Fitness, and Sports: Training, Environment, Nutrition, and Fitness*, edited by Stull G, and Cureton T. Salt Lake: Brighton, 1980, p. 177–187.

60. **Hubbard R, and LE A.** Hyperthermia: new thoughts on an old problem. *The Physician and Sportsmedicine* 17: 97–113, 1989.

61. **Hughson RL, Green HJ, Houston ME, Thomson JA, MacLean DR, and Sutton JR.** Heat injuries in Canadian mass participation runs. *Canadian Medical Association Journal* 122: 1141–1144, 1980.

62. **Hurtado A.** Animals in high altitudes: resident man. In: *Handbook of Physiology: Section 4-Adaptation to the Environment*, edited by Dill D. Washington, DC: American Physiological Society, 1964.

63. **Kayser B.** Nutrition and energetics of exercise at altitude. Theory and possible practical implications. *Sports Medicine (Auckland, NZ)* 17: 309–323, 1994.

64. **Kollias J, and Buskirk E.** Exercise and altitude. In: *Science and Medicine of Exercise and Sport*, edited by Johnson W, and Buskirk E. New York: Harper & Row, 1974.

65. **Kollias J, Buskirk ER, Akers RF, Prokop EK, Baker PT, and Picon-Reategui E.** Work capacity of long-time residents and newcomers to altitude. *Journal of Applied Physiology* 24: 792–799, 1968.

66. **Lawler J, Powers SK, and Thompson D.** Linear relationship between $\dot{V}O_2$ max and $\dot{V}O_2$ max decrement during exposure to acute hypoxia. *Journal of Applied Physiology* 64: 1486–1492, 1988.

67. **Levine BD, and Stray-Gundersen J.** Point: positive effects of intermittent hypoxia (live high: train low) on exercise performance are mediated primarily by augmented red cell volume. *Journal of Applied Physiology* 99: 2053–2055, 2005.

68. **Lorenzo S, Halliwill JR, Sawka MN, and Minson CT.** Heat acclimation improves exercise performance. *Journal of Applied Physiology* 109: 1140–1147, 2010.

69. **Lundby C, and van Hall G.** Lactate metabolism at high altitude. *High Altitude Medicine & Biology* 5: 195–196; author reply 197–198, 2004.

70. **MacDougall JD, Green HJ, Sutton JR, Coates G, Cymerman A, Young P, and Houston CS.** Operation Everest II: structural adaptations in skeletal muscle in response to extreme simulated altitude. *Acta Physiologica Scandinavica* 142: 421–427, 1991.

71. **Marconi C, Marzorati M, Grassi B, Basnyat B, Colombini A, Kayser B, and Cerretelli P.** Second generation Tibetan lowlanders acclimatize to high altitude more quickly than Caucasians. *The Journal of Physiology* 556: 661–671, 2004.

72. **Martin D, and O'Kroy J.** Effects of acute hypoxia on the $\dot{V}O_2$ max of trained and untrained subjects. *Journal of Sports Sciences* 11: 37–42, 1993.

73. **Mathews DK, Fox EL, and Tanzi D.** Physiological responses during exercise and recovery in a football uniform. *Journal of Applied Physiology* 26: 611–615, 1969.

74. **Mazess RB.** Cardiorespiratory characteristics and adaptation to high altitudes. *American Journal of Physical Anthropology* 32: 267–278, 1970.

75. **Mazess RB.** Exercise performance at high altitude in Peru. *Federation Proceedings* 28: 1301–1306, 1969.

76. **Mazess RB.** Exercise performance of Indian and white high altitude residents. *Human Biology; an International Record of Research* 41: 494–518, 1969.

77. **Mazzeo RS.** Physiological responses to exercise at altitude—an update. *Sports Medicine* 38: 1–8, 2008.
78. **Mazzeo RS, Brooks GA, Butterfield GE, Cymerman A, Roberts AC, Selland M, Wolfel EE, and Reeves JT.** Beta-adrenergic blockade does not prevent the lactate response to exercise after acclimatization to high altitude. *Journal of Applied Physiology* 76: 610–615, 1994.
79. **McArdle WD, Magel JR, Gergley TJ, Spina RJ, and Toner MM.** Thermal adjustment to cold-water exposure in resting men and women. *Journal of Applied Physiology* 56: 1565–1571, 1984.
80. **McArdle WD, Magel JR, Spina RJ, Gergley TJ, and Toner MM.** Thermal adjustment to cold-water exposure in exercising men and women. *Journal of Applied Physiology* 56: 1572–1577, 1984.
81. **Mills NL, Tornqvist H, Robinson SD, Gonzalez M, Darnley K, MacNec W, Boon NA, Donaldson K, Blomberg A, Sandstrom T, and Newby DE.** Diesel exhaust inhalation causes vascular dysfunction and impaired endogenous fibrinolysis. *Circulation* 112: 3930–3936, 2005.
82. **Noakes TD.** Evidence that reduced skeletal muscle recruitment explains the lactate paradox during exercise at high altitude. *Journal of Applied Physiology* 106: 737–738, 2009.
83. **Noakes TD.** Last word on viewpoint: evidence that reduced skeletal muscle recruitment explains the lactate paradox during exercise at high altitude. *Journal of Applied Physiology* 106: 745, 2009.
84. **Norton E.** *The Fight for Everest: 1924.* New York: Longmans, Green, 1925.
85. **Oelz O, Howald H, Di Prampero PE, Hoppeler H, Claassen H, Jenni R, Buhlmann A, Ferretti G, Bruckner JC, Veicsteinas A, et al.** Physiological profile of world-class high-altitude climbers. *Journal of Applied Physiology* 60: 1734–1742, 1986.
86. **Pascoe DD, Shanley LA, and Smith EW.** Clothing and exercise. I: biophysics of heat transfer between the individual, clothing and environment. *Sports Medicine (Auckland, NZ)* 18: 38–54, 1994.
87. **Peronnet F, Thibault G, and Cousineau DL.** A theoretical analysis of the effect of altitude on running performance. *Journal of Applied Physiology* 70: 399–404, 1991.
88. **Ponsot E, Dufour SP, Zoll J, Doutrelau S, N'Guessan B, Geny B, Hoppeler H, Lampert E, Mettauer B, Ventura-Clapier R, and Richard R.** Exercise training in normobaric hypoxia in endurance runners. II. Improvement of mitochondrial properties in skeletal muscle. *Journal of Applied Physiology* 100: 1249–1257, 2006.
89. **Powers SK, Martin D, and Dodd S.** Exercise-induced hypoxaemia in elite endurance athletes. Incidence, causes and impact on $\dot{V}O_2$ max. *Sports Medicine (Auckland, NZ)* 16: 14–22, 1993.
90. **Pronk M.** Lactate metabolism at high altitude: a reply. *High Altitude Medicine and Biology* 5: 197–198, 2004.
91. **Pronk M, Tiemessen I, Hupperets MD, Kennedy BP, Powell FL, Hopkins SR, and Wagner PD.** Persistence of the lactate paradox over 8 weeks at 3,800 m. *High Altitude Medicine & Biology* 4: 431–443, 2003.
92. **Pugh L.** Athletes at altitude. *Journal of Physiology (London)* 192: 619–646, 1967.
93. **Pugh LG.** Deaths from exposure on Four Inns Walking Competition, March 14–15, 1964. *Lancet* 1: 1210–1212, 1964.
94. **Pugh LG, and Edholm OG.** The physiology of channel swimmers. *Lancet* 269: 761–768, 1955.
95. **Pugh LG, Gill MB, Lahiri S, Milledge JS, Ward MP, and West JB.** Muscular exercise at great altitudes. *Journal of Applied Physiology* 19: 431–440, 1964.
96. **Quinn MD.** The effects of wind and altitude in the 400-m sprint. *Journal of Sports Sciences* 22: 1073–1081, 2004.
97. **Quod MJ, Martin DT, and Laursen PB.** Cooling athletes before competition in the heat: comparison of techniques and practical considerations. *Sports Medicine (Auckland, NZ)* 36: 671–682, 2006.
98. **Racinais S.** Different effects of heat exposure upon exercise performance in the morning and afternoon. *Scandanavian Journal of Medicine & Science in Sports* 20 Suppl. 3: 80–89, 2010.
99. **Raven P.** Effects of air pollution on physical performance. In: *Encyclopedia of Physical Education, Fitness, and Sports: Training, Environment, Nutrition, and Fitness,* edited by Stull G, and Cureton T. Salt Lake: Brighton, 1980, p. 201–216.
100. **Raven PB, Drinkwater BL, Ruhling RO, Bolduan N, Taguchi S, Gliner J, and Horvath SM.** Effect of carbon monoxide and peroxyacetyl nitrate on man's maximal aerobic capacity. *Journal of Applied Physiology* 36: 288–293, 1974.
101. **Reeves JT, Wolfel EE, Green HJ, Mazzeo RS, Young AJ, Sutton JR, and Brooks GA.** Oxygen transport during exercise at altitude and the lactate paradox: lessons from Operation Everest II and Pikes Peak. *Exercise and Sport Sciences Reviews* 20: 275–296, 1992.
102. **Roberts WO.** Heat and cold: what does the environment do to marathon injury? *Sports Medicine (Auckland, NZ)* 37: 400–403, 2007.
103. **Rodriguez FA, Truijens MJ, Townsend NE, Stray-Gundersen J, Gore CJ, and Levine BD.** Performance of runners and swimmers after four weeks of intermittent hypobaric hypoxic exposure plus sea level training. *Journal of Applied Physiology* 103: 1523–1535, 2007.
104. **Romieu I, Castro-Giner F, Kunzli N, and Sunyer J.** Air pollution, oxidative stress and dietary supplementation: a review. *Eur Respir J* 31: 179–197, 2008.
105. **Rose MS, Houston CS, Fulco CS, Coates G, Sutton JR, and Cymerman A.** Operation Everest. II: Nutrition and body composition. *Journal of Applied Physiology* 65: 2545–2551, 1988.
106. **Roskamm H, Landry F, Samek L, Schlager M, Weidemann H, and Reindell H.** Effects of a standardized ergometer training program at three different altitudes. *Journal of Applied Physiology* 27: 840–847, 1969.
107. **Ross MR, Garvican LA, Jeacocke NA, Laursen PB, Abbiss CR, Martin DT, and Burke LM.** Novel precooling strategy enhances time trial cycling in the heat. *Medicine and Science in Sports and Exercise* 43: 123–133, 2011.
108. **Rupert JL, and Hochachka PW.** Genetic approaches to understanding human adaptation to altitude in the Andes. *The Journal of Experimental Biology* 204: 3151–3160, 2001.
109. **Saltin B.** Circulatory response to submaximal and maximal exercise after thermal dehydration. *Journal of Applied Physiology* 19: 1125–1132, 1964.
110. **Saunders PU, Pyne DB, and Gore CJ.** Endurance training at altitude. *High Altitude Medicine & Biology* 10: 135–148, 2009.
111. **Sawka MN, Francesconi RP, Young AJ, and Pandolf KB.** Influence of hydration level and body fluids on exercise performance in the heat. *JAMA* 252: 1165–1169, 1984.

112. **Sawka MN, Young AJ, Francesconi RP, Muza SR, and Pandolf KB.** Thermoregulatory and blood responses during exercise at graded hypohydration levels. *Journal of Applied Physiology* 59: 1394–1401, 1985.

113. **Schoene RB, Lahiri S, Hackett PH, Peters RM, Jr., Milledge JS, Pizzo CJ, Sarnquist FH, Boyer SJ, Graber DJ, Maret KH, et al.** Relationship of hypoxic ventilatory response to exercise performance on Mount Everest. *Journal of Applied Physiology* 56: 1478–1483, 1984.

114. **Sharman JE, Cockcroft JR, and Coombes JS.** Cardiovascular implications of exposure to traffic air pollution during exercise. *QJM* 97: 637–643, 2004.

115. **Siple P, and Passel C.** Measurements of dry atmospheric cooling in subfreezing temperatures. *Proceedings of the American Philosophical Society* 89: 177–199, 1945.

116. **Strohl KP.** Lessons in hypoxic adaptations from high-altitude populations. *Sleep Breath* 12: 115–121, 2008.

117. **Sutton JR, Reeves JT, Wagner PD, Groves BM, Cymerman A, Malconian MK, Rock PB, Young PM, Walter SD, and Houston CS.** Operation Everest II: oxygen transport during exercise at extreme simulated altitude. *Journal of Applied Physiology* 64: 1309–1321, 1988.

118. **Tikuisis P, Bell DG, and Jacobs I.** Shivering onset, metabolic response, and convective heat transfer during cold air exposure. *Journal of Applied Physiology* 70: 1996–2002, 1991.

119. **Van Hall G, Calbet JA, Sondergaard H, and Saltin B.** The re-establishment of the normal blood lactate response to exercise in humans after prolonged acclimatization to altitude. *The Journal of Physiology* 536: 963–975, 2001.

120. **Van Hall G, Lundby C, Araoz M, Calbet JAL, Sander M, and Saltin B.** The lactate paradox revisited in lowlanders during acclimatization to 4100 m and in high-altitude natives. *J Physiol* 587: 1117–1129, 2009.

121. **Vogt M, and Hoppeler H.** Is hypoxia training good for muscles and exercise performance? *Progress in Cardiovascular Diseases* 52: 525–533, 2010.

122. **Volpino P, Tomei F, La Valle C, Tomao E, Rosati MV, Ciarrocca M, De Sio S, Cangemi B, Vigllarolo R, and Fedele F.** Respiratory and cardiovascular function at rest and during exercise testing in a healthy working population: effects of outdoor traffic air pollution. *Occupational Medicine (Oxford, England)* 54: 475–482, 2004.

123. **Wagner PD, and Lundby C.** The lactate paradox: does acclimatization to high altitude affect blood lactate during exercise? *Medicine and Science in Sports and Exercise* 39: 749–755, 2007.

124. **Ward-Smith AJ.** The influence of aerodynamic and biomechanical factors on long jump performance. *Journal of Biomechanics* 16: 655–658, 1983.

125. **Wehrlin JP, Zuest P, Hallen J, and Marti B.** Live high-train low for 24 days increases hemoglobin mass and red cell volume in elite endurance athletes. *Journal of Applied Physiology* 100: 1938–1945, 2006.

126. **West JB.** Point: the lactate paradox does/does not occur during exercise at high altitude. *Journal of Applied Physiology* 102: 2398–2399, 2007.

127. **West JB, Boyer SJ, Graber DJ, Hackett PH, Maret KH, Milledge JS, Peters RM, Jr., Pizzo CJ, Samaja M, Sarnquist FH, et al.** Maximal exercise at extreme altitudes on Mount Everest. *Journal of Applied Physiology* 55: 688–698, 1983.

128. **West JB, Hackett PH, Maret KH, Milledge JS, Peters RM, Jr., Pizzo CJ, and Winslow RM.** Pulmonary gas exchange on the summit of Mount Everest. *Journal of Applied Physiology* 55: 678–687, 1983.

129. **West JB, Lahiri S, Gill MB, Milledge JS, Pugh LG, and Ward MP.** Arterial oxygen saturation during exercise at high altitude. *Journal of Applied Physiology* 17: 617–621, 1962.

130. **West JB, Lahiri S, Maret KH, Peters RM, Jr., and Pizzo CJ.** Barometric pressures at extreme altitudes on Mt. Everest: physiological significance. *Journal of Applied Physiology* 54: 1188–1194, 1983.

131. **West JB, and Wagner PD.** Predicted gas exchange on the summit of Mt. Everest. *Respiration Physiology* 42: 1–16, 1980.

132. **Wilber RL.** Application of altitude/hypoxic training by elite athletes. *Medicine and Science in Sports and Exercise* 39: 1610–1624, 2007.

133. **Wilber RL, Stray-Gundersen J, and Levine BD.** Effect of hypoxic "dose" on physiological responses and sea-level performance. *Medicine and Science in Sports and Exercise* 39: 1590–1599, 2007.

134. **Wilson MJ, Julian CG, and Roach RC.** Genomic analysis of high-altitude adaptation: innovations and implications. *Current Sports Medicine Reports* 10: 59–61, 2011.

135. **Wolski LA, McKenzie DC, and Wenger HA.** Altitude training for improvements in sea level performance. Is the scientific evidence of benefit? *Sports Medicine (Auckland, NZ)* 22: 251–263, 1996.

136. **Yaspelkis BB, III, and Ivy JL.** Effect of carbohydrate supplements and water on exercise metabolism in the heat. *Journal of Applied Physiology* 71: 680–687, 1991.

137. **Yu IT, Wong TW, and Liu HJ.** Impact of air pollution on cardiopulmonary fitness in schoolchildren. *Journal of Occupational and Environmental Medicine / American College of Occupational and Environmental Medicine* 46: 946–952, 2004.

138. **Zanobetti A, Canner MJ, Stone PH, Schwartz J, Sher D, Eagan-Bengston E, Gates KA, Hartley LH, Suh H, and Gold DR.** Ambient pollution and blood pressure in cardiac rehabilitation patients. *Circulation* 110: 2184–2189, 2004.

139. **Zoll J, Ponsot E, Dufour S, Doutreleau S, Ventura-Clapier R, Vogt M, Hoppeler H, Richard R, and Fluck M.** Exercise training in normobaric hypoxia in endurance runners. III. Muscular adjustments of selected gene transcripts. *Journal of Applied Physiology* 100: 1258–1266, 2006.

25

Ergogenic Aids

■ Objectives

By studying this chapter, you should be able to do the following:

1. Define *ergogenic aid*.
2. Explain why a "placebo" treatment in a "double-blind design" is used in research studies involving ergogenic aids.
3. Describe, in general, the effectiveness of nutritional supplements on performance.
4. Describe the effect of additional oxygen on performance; distinguish between hyperbaric oxygenation and that accomplished by breathing oxygen-enriched gas mixtures.
5. Describe blood doping and its potential for improving endurance performance.

6. Explain the mechanism by which ingested buffers might improve anaerobic performances.
7. Explain how amphetamines might improve exercise performance.
8. Describe the various mechanisms by which caffeine might improve performance.
9. Identify the risks associated with using chewing tobacco to obtain nicotine.
10. Describe the physiological and psychological effects of different types of warm-ups.

■ Key Terms

autologous transfusion
blood boosting
blood doping
blood packing
dental caries
double-blind research design
ergogenic aid
erythrocythemia
erythropoietin (EPO)
homologous transfusion
hyperbaric chamber
induced erythrocythemia
normocythemia
placebo
sham reinfusion
sham withdrawal
sympathomimetic

The preceding chapters have described exercise and dietary plans related to performance. However, no presentation of factors affecting performance would be complete without a discussion of ergogenic aids. **Ergogenic aids** are defined as work-producing substances or phenomena believed to increase performance (80).

Ergogenic aids include nutrients, drugs, warm-up exercises, hypnosis, stress management, blood doping, oxygen breathing, music, and extrinsic biomechanical aids. Although we discussed nutritional issues related to performance in chapter 23, we will provide additional detail about the role of dietary supplements as ergogenic aids in this chapter. In addition, we will discuss ergogenic aids related to aerobic performance (oxygen inhalation and blood doping) and anaerobic performance (blood buffers), as well as various drugs (amphetamines, caffeine, and nicotine) and physical warm-up. Note that anabolic steroids and growth hormone were discussed in chapter 5.

Although the attention of the reader will be focused on athletic performance, where an improvement of less than 1% would alter world records, it must be noted that industrial physiologists have long been concerned about the relationship of lighting, environmental temperature, and background noise (music) to performance in the workplace (80). Research work in this area must be done carefully, with special attention to the research design due to the number of factors that can influence the outcome of the study.

RESEARCH DESIGN CONCERNS

It is sometimes difficult to compare the results of one research study on ergogenic aids with another. The reason for this is that the effect of an ergogenic aid depends on a number of variables (80):

- Amount—too little or too much may show no effect
- Subject—the ergogenic aid may be effective in "untrained" subjects but not "trained" subjects, or vice versa
    —the "value" of an ergogenic aid is determined by the subject
- Task—may work in short-term, power-related tasks, but not in endurance tasks, or vice versa
    —may work for gross-motor, large-muscle activities and not with fine-motor activities, or vice versa
- Use—an ergogenic aid used on an acute (short-term) basis may show a positive effect, but in the long run may compromise performance, or vice versa

Given these variables, scientists are careful in designing experiments in order not to be "fooled" by the result. For example, an athlete may improve performance because he or she believes the substance improves performance, so the "belief" is more important than the substance in determining the outcome. Further, an investigator may "believe" in the ergogenic aid and inadvertently offer different levels of encouragement during the testing of athletes under the influence of the ergogenic aid. These problems are controlled for by using a **placebo** as a treatment condition and using a **double-blind research design**, respectively.

A placebo is a "look-alike" substance relative to the ergogenic aid under consideration, but it contains nothing that will influence performance. The need for such a control is seen in figure 25.1, which describes the gain in strength by a group that was taking a placebo but was told it was an anabolic steroid. It is contrasted with the group's performance prior to taking the placebo. The rate and amount of strength gained was higher with the placebo, indicating the need for such a control if one is to isolate the true effect of a substance (3).

A double-blind research design is one in which neither the subject nor the investigator knows who is receiving the placebo or the substance under investigation. The subjects are randomly assigned to receive pill x or pill y. After all data are collected, the "code" is broken to find out which pill (x or y) was the placebo and which was the substance under investigation. These designs are very complex and difficult to carry out, but they reduce the chance of subject or investigator bias (80).

The scientist must also be careful in the selection of subjects. If a substance is tested as a potential aid to sprinters, it would be reasonable to select subjects from that population so the results can be generalized to that

Figure 25.1 Changes in performance when subjects were told they were taking an anabolic steroid, but were really taking a placebo.

group. Further, the tests used by the investigator should be as close as, or actually be, the performance task (e.g., 100-meter dash). In short, results obtained on a proper subject population but under controlled laboratory conditions using conventional physiological tests may not be useful when taken to the "field" (80).

IN SUMMARY

- Ergogenic aids are defined as substances or phenomena that are work-producing and are believed to increase performance.
- Because an athlete's belief in a substance may influence performance, scientists use a placebo or look-alike substance to control for this effect. In addition, scientists use a double-blind research design in which the investigator and subject are both unaware of the treatment.

DIETARY SUPPLEMENTS

We discussed issues related to basic nutrition in chapter 18 and provided additional detail about the role of nutrition in performance in chapter 23. In this section we go a step further and discuss the role that dietary supplements may play in athletic performance—a point of interest to many athletes. A survey of athletes indicated that more than 80% of U.S. Division I athletes and national or international elite athletes use dietary supplements (75). For more detail on dietary supplements and performance, see texts by Burke and Deakin, and Williams in the Suggested Readings.

One has only to open a strength-training magazine to become aware of the incredible number of dietary supplements promoted as improving the effects of a workout, be it size or strength. Table 25.1 provides a summary of a number of dietary supplements used by strength-training athletes to increase strength, muscle mass, and athletic performance. The columns provide information about the claim made for each substance and the evidence for or against that claim. A quick reading of table 25.1 indicates that little or no support exists for any of the supplements, with the exception of creatine. We all know of the role of phosphocreatine (PC) in high-power events or at the onset of endurance exercise (see chapters 3 and 4). Numerous studies show that creatine supplementation can increase the muscle's creatine concentration. Does it affect performance? (See The Winning Edge 25.1 for more on this developing story.)

Carnitine, another dietary supplement listed in table 25.1, is associated with the transport of fatty acids from the cytoplasm into the mitochondria. Table 25.1 indicates that there was no support for its proported

claim to promote fat loss. However, endurance athletes are also interested in carnitine because of its putative effect on fat use, which may spare carbohydrates and reduce the lactate concentration during exercise. However, Heinonen's review (54) suggests that carnitine supplementation does not enhance fat oxidation nor spare glycogen, reduce body fat, affect lactate accumulation, or affect maximal oxygen uptake.

The use of supplements of any kind needs to be approached with a "buyer beware" attitude. When the U.S. Congress passed the Dietary Supplements Health and Education Act in 1994, it opened the door for the manufacture and sale of dietary supplements, including some (e.g., prohormones) that were not originally envisioned (7, 122). The lack of regulation of these products means that supplements may contain contaminants, some of which may elicit a positive drug test. A case in point is a recent study by Baume et al. (8). They examined 103 dietary supplements and found 3 that had an anabolic steroid in very large amounts that would have generated a positive drug test. One creatine product revealed the presence of two anabolic steroids when urine samples were examined. To prevent the problems associated with using contaminated supplements, extensive testing of products by an independent lab may be warranted—or the athlete should only take those nutritional supplements recommended by a nutritionist/registered dietician (27).

For a summary of the effect of herbs on athletic performance, see a review by Kundrat in the Suggested Readings.

IN SUMMARY

- For the most part, little evidence exists that dietary supplements provide a performance advantage to athletes, with the possible exception of creatine.

AEROBIC PERFORMANCE

Chapter 20 detailed the various tests used to evaluate the physiological factors related to endurance performance. Clearly, an increased ability to transport O_2 to the muscles and a delay in the onset of lactate production are related to improved performance. Two ergogenic aids have been used to try to influence O_2 delivery: the breathing of O_2-enriched mixtures and blood doping.

Oxygen

Given the importance of aerobic metabolism in the production of ATP for muscular work, it is not surprising that scientists have been interested in the effect of

TABLE 25.1   Dietary Supplements for Strength Trainers

Supplement	Description	Claim	Evidence	Comment
Antioxidants (e.g., vitamins A, C, and E)	Chemicals that protect cells from oxidative damage caused by free radicals	Reduce muscle damage resulting from severe or eccentric exercise	Little evidence that performance is enhanced, but some evidence that oxidative damage caused by exercise may be lessened	With continued training, antioxidants produced by the body may be sufficient; if diet is inadequate, supplement
Proteins or branched-chain amino acids	High-protein diets or unique amino acid supplements	Meet greater protein needs associated with training	Dietary intake already exceeds upper limit of known protein requirements	Diet adequate
Lysine, arginine, and ornithine	Amino acids	Increase growth hormone secretion; promote muscle growth	May increase growth hormone, but of very limited magnitude; no effect on muscle mass	Costly and ineffective
β-hydroxy–β-methylbutyrate (HMB)	Metabolite of amino acid leucine	Anti-catabolic—decreases muscle protein breakdown	Not much support for athletic performance, but may have application for clinical conditions in which muscle wasting is present	More research needed
Chromium	Plays role in insulin action	Enhances amino acid uptake	No effect on muscle mass or strength	If taken as picolinate salt, may be dangerous
Vanadium	Plays a role in insulin action	Enhances amino acid uptake	No effect on muscle mass or strength	High doses have serious side effects
Boron	Trace element	Enhances testosterone concentration	No effect	Diet adequate for normally nourished individuals
Creatine	Amino acid	Increases anaerobic power	Improves performance in selected tasks (e.g., repeated sprint bouts)	See The Winning Edge 25.1
Dehydroepiandrosterone (DHEA)	Precursor to testosterone	Enhances testosterone concentration and muscle mass	No effect on testosterone, strength, or muscle mass	Increases estrogen levels and decreases HDL cholesterol; could result in a positive drug test for testosterone
Androstenedione (andro)	Precursor to testosterone	Enhances testosterone concentration and muscle mass	No effect on testosterone, strength, or muscle mass	Increases estrogen levels and decreases HDL cholesterol; could result in a positive drug test for testosterone
Carnitine	Used in fat metabolism	Enhances fat use, decreases body fat	No deficiency in athletes; no effect on metabolic response to exercise	Diet adequate

From references: (2, 62, 73, 136, 141).

Creatine Monohydrate

We are all familiar with the importance of phosphocreatine (PC) as an energy source during short-term, explosive exercise, and as the energy source that helps us to make the transition to the steady state of oxygen uptake during submaximal aerobic exercise (see chapters 3 and 4). Because of PC's importance in explosive exercise, there has been a great deal of interest in the potential of the dietary supplement creatine monohydrate to increase the muscle's concentration of PC and, hopefully, performance.

The total creatine concentration in muscle is about 120 mmol $\cdot$ kg^{-1}, and 2 grams are excreted per day. These 2 grams are replaced by diet (1 gram) and by synthesis (1 gram) from amino acids (28, 123). The first step in a typical creatine monohydrate "loading" plan consists of adding 20 to 25 g to the diet per day for 5 to 7 days (64). This results in ~20% increase in muscle creatine, which approaches what is thought to be the upper limit of the muscle's capacity to store creatine. There is evidence that this elevated level can be achieved with doses as low as 2 to 3 g per day—given time (98). Independent of the means used to achieve the higher levels of creatine in muscle, there is great variability among subjects (28, 123):

■ Individuals with lower initial values (e.g., vegetarians) have greater increases, and some individuals with high presupplement values may not respond to the increased creatine. This has

led to the terms *responders* and *nonresponders*.

■ The ingestion of glucose with the creatine reduces this variation and enhances uptake. In general, the short-term loading scheme appears to improve the ability to maintain muscular force and power output during various exhaustive bouts of exercise, including in older individuals (51, 103), but not without exception (123, 131). Studies that controlled for protein and energy intake show convincingly that it is the creatine itself that brings about these effects (25). In addition, creatine does not impact muscle glycogen, either at rest or following exhaustive exercise (108).

In contrast to scientists using a 5-to-7 day loading regime to determine the effect of an elevated muscle creatine concentration, athletes take the creatine supplement for long periods of time to improve performance. The elevated level of creatine in muscle achieved in the loading phase can be maintained by consuming 2 to 5 grams of creatine monohydrate per day. Interestingly, the "mechanism" for any increase in performance may be only indirectly related to the creatine. For example, greater gains in strength achieved in a weight-training program may be mediated by the athlete's ability to increase the intensity of training, which would, in turn, allow for a greater physiological adaptation (i.e., strength gain) to the training (97, 123). However,

it must be noted that creatine supplementation does not reduce muscle damage resulting from severe exercise (96). What about the down side of creatine supplementation?

Creatine supplementation appears to increase body mass, but this is probably due more to water retention than protein synthesis. Consequently, athletes who must "carry" their own body weight (e.g., runners) might have to be careful not to negatively affect performance (28, 131). Use of a low-dose of creatine monohydrate (~2.3 g/d) (98) or of polyethylene glycosylated creatine (1.25–2.5 g/d) (55) avoided the weight gain, but resulted in improved performance. There are reports of gastrointestinal distress, nausea, and muscle cramping associated with the use of creatine; however, recent reports suggest that at least out to 21 months, there are no long-term adverse effects (7, 95). Since an Upper Level of Intake (UL) standard is not yet available for creatine (see chapter 18 for a description of UL), the use of the Observed Safe Level (OSL) has been suggested as a first step. Based on existing research, an amount of 5 g per day appears to be a safe level for chronic consumption (108). Should it be banned? Volek (123) provides an interesting analogy: Creatine supplementation is linked to enhanced performance of high-intensity, repetitive bouts of exercise in the same way that carbohydrate supplementation is linked to improvements in endurance performance (see chapter 23).

---

additional oxygen (hyperoxia) on performance. But to discuss this issue we must ask the following question: How and when was the O_2 administered to achieve a higher PO_2 in the blood? In his insightful review of this topic, Welch (126) stressed the difficulty of comparing results from studies in which hyperoxia is achieved by increasing the percent of O_2 in the inspired air with those that use a **hyperbaric** (high-pressure) **chamber** with 21% or higher O_2 mixtures. Figure 25.2 shows that performance (e.g., longer time to exhaustion) improves throughout the range of inspired oxygen pressures

when O_2-enriched mixtures are used at a normal pressure of 1 atmosphere ("constant pressure"), compared to the use of a hyperbaric chamber ("increasing pressure"). A study using both weight-lifting tasks and an endurance treadmill run confirmed the lack of effect of hyperbaric hyperoxia on performance (106). The second part of the question is related to the time of administration of the supplemental O_2. Results vary depending on whether the O_2 is administered prior to, during, or following exercise. For that latter reason, this section on oxygen is organized by those conditions.

Figure 25.2 The effect of PO_2 on performance. Constant pressure experiments used oxygen-enriched gas mixtures at sea-level pressure, while the increasing pressure experiments used a hyperbaric chamber to increase the PO_2. From H. W. Welch, "Effects of Hypoxia and Hyperpoxia on Human Performance" in Kent B. Pandolf, ed., *Exercise and Sport Sciences Reviews*, vol. 15. Copyright © 1987 McGraw-Hill, Inc., New York. Reprinted by permission.

Prior to Exercise   The rationale for the use of supplemental oxygen prior to exercise is to try to "store" additional oxygen in the blood so that more will be available at the onset of exercise. It has been estimated that the hemoglobin in arterial blood is about 97% saturated with O_2 at rest (200 ml O_2/L blood). Breathing 100% O_2 would increase the O_2 bound to hemoglobin by only 3%, or 6 milliliters. However, the amount of oxygen physically dissolved in solution is proportional to the arterial PO_2, and when the PO_2 increases from about 100 mm Hg (breathing 21% O_2 at sea level) to about 700 mm Hg (breathing 100% O_2), the dissolved oxygen increases from 3 ml/L to 21 ml/L. If a person has a total blood volume of 5 liters, approximately 100 milliliters of additional O_2 can be "stored" prior to exercise. However, if the person takes a few breaths between the time the O_2 breathing stops and the event begins, the O_2 store will return to that associated with air breathing (133).

The focus of attention on the use of oxygen prior to exercise has been on short-term exercise. In general, in runs of 880 yards or less, weight lifting, stair climbing, and swims of 200 yards or less, the O_2 breathing seemed to be beneficial (82, 133). In addition, evidence suggested that the O_2 breathing needed to take place within 2 minutes of the task (133). Some concern has been expressed about these findings due to the fact that in some cases the subjects knew they were breathing O_2, a factor that could have affected the results (133). Overall, considering the fact that O_2 cannot be breathed up to the start of a sprint event in swimming or track, any effect would be lost before the starter's gun is fired. Therefore, unless one participates in a breath-holding event, oxygen breathing prior to exercise will have little effect on performance.

During Exercise   The rationale for the use of oxygen during exercise to improve performance is based on the proposition that muscle is hypoxic during exercise and additional O_2 delivery will alleviate the problem (127). If this is the case, then the additional O_2 in the blood during O_2 breathing should increase the delivery of O_2 to the muscle and improve performance. However, Welch et al. (127) showed that when one breathes hyperoxic gas mixtures, the increase in the O_2 content of arterial blood (CaO_2) is balanced by a decrease in blood flow to the working muscles such that O_2 delivery ($CaO_2 \times$ flow) is not different from normoxic (21% O_2) conditions. $\dot{V}O_2$ max is increased by only 2% to 5% with hyperoxia, which is about what would be expected, since maximal cardiac output doesn't change and the a-$\bar{v}O_2$ difference does not increase more than 5% to 6% (108) [$\dot{V}O_2$ max = $\dot{Q}$ max $\times$ ($CaO_2 - C\bar{v}O_2$)].

In spite of similarities in O_2 delivery during hyperoxia and normoxia, performance has been shown to increase dramatically as a result of an increase in inspired O_2. Figure 25.2 shows time to exhaustion to be improved by 40% while breathing 100% O_2 (PO_2 = 700 mm Hg). How could this be if O_2 delivery to muscles is not substantially different? The increased availability of O_2 has been shown to decrease pulmonary ventilation and reduce the work of breathing, a change that should lead to an increase in performance (126, 134, 135). In addition, those athletes who experience "desaturation" of hemoglobin during maximal work (see chapters 10 and 24) while breathing 21% O_2 could benefit by breathing oxygen-enriched gas mixtures (92). One study found that when sprinters did three repeat 300-meter sprints at different speeds on a treadmill while breathing 40% oxygen (compared to 21%), hemoglobin saturation was maintained and the fall in blood pH was less (85). Finally, the high PO_2 slows glycolysis during heavy exercise, resulting in a slower accumulation of lactate and H^+ in the plasma and extending the time to exhaustion (57, 126). The reduction in lactate formation in hyperoxia appears to be due to a reduction in the rate of glycogen breakdown so that it is better matched with its subsequent oxidation in the Krebs cycle (112). Given the impracticality of trying to provide O_2 mixtures to athletes during performance, this research on hyperoxia is more useful as a tool to answer questions related to the age-old question of what factor, O_2 delivery or the muscle's capacity to consume O_2, limits aerobic performance (126). However, some have used hyperoxia during training in an attempt to improve performance. A recent study had subjects breathe 60% O_2 (versus 21% O_2) during training to see if it would result in larger gains in $\dot{V}O_2$ max and performance. Subjects were able to exercise at an 8% higher work rate using 60% O_2, but changes in $\dot{V}O_2$ max and time to exhaustion were not different between treatments (88).

After Exercise The rationale for the use of supplemental oxygen after exercise is that the subject might recover more quickly following exercise and be ready to go again. Some of the early work showed just that, but because the subjects knew what gas they were breathing, the results have to be interpreted with caution (82, 133). Wilmore (133) summarized the effects of several studies and concluded that there was no benefit of O_2 breathing during recovery on heart rate, ventilation, and post-exercise oxygen uptake. This conclusion was supported by studies showing no effect of O_2 breathing on subsequent performance in all-out exercise (100).

IN SUMMARY

- Oxygen breathing before or after exercise seems to have little or no effect on performance, whereas oxygen breathing during exercise improves endurance performance.

Blood Doping

In chapter 13 we described how $\dot{V}O_2$ max is limited by maximal cardiac output, given the constraint that blood pressure had to be maintained by vasoconstriction of the active muscle mass. Because maximal O_2 transport is equal to the product of maximal cardiac output ($\dot{Q}$ max) and the O_2 content of arterial blood (CaO_2), one way to improve O_2 delivery to tissue when $\dot{Q}$ max cannot change is to increase the quantity of hemoglobin in each liter of blood. **Blood doping** refers to the infusion of red blood cells (RBCs) in an attempt to increase the hemoglobin concentration ([Hb]) and, consequently, O_2 transport (CaO_2 is equal to the [Hb] $\times$ 1.34 ml O_2/gm Hb). Other terms to describe this are **blood boosting** and **blood packing,** with **induced erythrocythemia** being the proper medical term. However, before we get into this topic it must be remembered that an increase in blood volume (independent of an increase in the hemoglobin concentration) would also favorably affect $\dot{V}O_2$ max and aerobic performance (49).

In blood doping, a subject receives a transfusion of blood, which may be his or her own **(autologous transfusion)** or blood from a matched donor **(homologous transfusion).** The latter procedure is acceptable in times of medical emergencies, but carries the risk of infection and blood-type incompatibility (48); it is therefore not recommended in blood-doping procedures. The need to use your own blood to achieve the goal of a higher [Hb] creates some interesting problems that led to confusion in the early days of research in this area. The primary problem was related to the mismatch between the maximum time blood could be refrigerated and the time period needed for the subject to produce new RBCs and bring the [Hb] back to normal before the reinfusion. Maximum storage time with refrigeration is 3 weeks, during which time about 1% of the RBCs are lost per day. In addition, some RBCs adhere to the storage containers or become so fragile that they will not function upon reinfusion. Because of these problems only about 60% of the removed RBCs could be reinfused (48). The normal time period for replacement of the RBCs following a 400-milliliter donation is 3 to 4 weeks, and following a 900-milliliter donation, 5 to 6 weeks or more are required. If the blood were reinfused at the end of the three-week maximal storage time, the investigator might not have been able to achieve the condition of an increased [Hb] due to RBC loss (decreased 40%) and the below-normal (anemic) values in the subjects. Gledhill (48) makes a strong case for this as a primary reason why studies prior to 1978 showed inconsistent changes in $\dot{V}O_2$ max and performance with blood doping. Another major problem encountered in these early studies was the lack of an adequate research design. There was a need to have a group undergoing a **"sham" withdrawal** (needle placed in the arm but no blood is removed) and a **"sham" reinfusion** (needle placed in the arm but blood is not returned) to act as placebo controls.

The central factor allowing a more careful study of blood doping was the introduction of the freezer preservation technique, which allows the blood to be stored frozen for years with only a 15% RBC loss. This allows plenty of time for the subject to become **normocythemic** (achieve normal [Hb]), so that any effect of the reinfusion can be correctly evaluated (48).

The general findings were that reinfusions of single units (~450 milliliters) of blood showed small but insignificant increases in [Hb], $\dot{V}O_2$ max, and performance, whereas the infusion of two units (900 milliliters) significantly increased the [Hb] (8–9%), $\dot{V}O_2$ max (4–5%), and performance (3–34%). The infusion of three units (1,350 milliliters) of blood caused slightly greater increases in [Hb] (10.8%) and $\dot{V}O_2$ max (6.6%). This large reinfusion caused borderline **erythrocythemia** to be approached, so a 1,350-milliliter infusion probably represents the upper limit that can be used. Figure 25.3 shows a gradual reduction in [Hb] toward the normal value following reinfusion, indicating that increased O_2 transport is maintained for 10 to 12 weeks. This is an important point as far as performance gains are concerned (47).

The classic study by Ekblom et al. in 1972 showed the impact of blood doping on $\dot{V}O_2$ max and performance (37). The improvements in performance (3–34%) were much more variable than the changes in [Hb] or $\dot{V}O_2$ max. Part of the reason for this variation was the type of performance test used. The greatest change was observed in a running test to exhaustion that lasted less than 10 minutes, and the smallest change was observed in a 5-mile time trial,

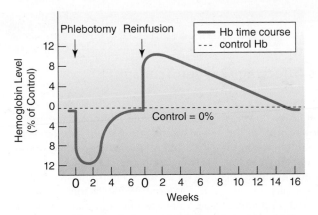

Figure 25.3 Changes in hemoglobin levels in blood following removal (phlebotomy) and reinfusion.

with the improvement being 51 seconds compared to a preinfusion run time of 30:17 (132). Early questions (34) about whether this procedure would "work in the field" were answered in a study on cross-country skiers (12), and judging by the number of cyclists that withdrew from the Tour de France when records of blood doping were uncovered suggests that there is little question of the advantage it provides. See A Look Back—Important People in Science for an individual who got this started.

Although the blood doping issue will always raise a question of ethics, Gledhill presents what amounts to a moral dilemma in the use of blood doping in getting athletes ready for performance at altitude. In chapter 24 we discussed the changes in $\dot{V}O_2$ max and performance at altitude. Those athletes who stay at altitude experience a natural increase in RBC production to deal with the hypoxia. As Gledhill (48) points out, those athletes who can afford to train at altitude accomplish what blood doping does in a manner that is acceptable to the International Olympic Committee. The availability of a recombinant DNA analog of **erythropoietin (EPO)**, the hormone that stimulates red blood cell production, has complicated the picture.

Erythropoietin is used as a part of therapy for those who undergo chemotherapy or dialysis (due to kidney disease). The hormone stimulates red blood cell production to reduce the chance of anemia. This is crucial for a variety of patients, and investigators are trying to optimize the use of EPO (70). Although normal cross-country training does not seem to increase plasma levels of naturally occurring erythropoietin (10), acute exposure to 3,000 and 4,000 meters of simulated altitude has been shown to increase the concentration 1.8- and 3.0-fold, respectively (33). The real concern, of course, is the potential abuse of the DNA-derived analog of this hormone to generate the effects of blood doping, without having to undergo the blood withdrawals and reinfusions. Such abuse is not without its risks, in that RBC production can get

out of hand, as seen in some studies where the increase in the hemoglobin concentration varied from ~4% to ~19% (68). This could lead to extremely high RBC levels in some athletes, which could impair blood flow to the heart and brain, resulting in a myocardial infarction or a stroke.

In fact, within 4 years of its introduction, about twenty top European cyclists died, unexpectedly (36). The EPO causes an increase in the hemoglobin concentration by a simultaneous increase in the red blood cell volume and a decrease in plasma volume, such that blood volume is relatively unchanged (68, 69). Like the blood-doping procedure, the hemoglobin concentration remains elevated for several weeks while the EPO concentration decreases, making detection difficult (68). It should be no surprise that finding those athletes who use blood doping or EPO to gain an advantage is crucial to the "fairness" principle in sport.

In 2002 an organization composed of scientists, pharmaceutical companies, and hematologists was formed to work systematically to prevent abuse of these products and practices by unethical athletes (4). Some progress has been made. For those using a homologous blood transfusion, tests can discriminate between the donor and the recipient by focusing on minor blood group factors (66, 124). For those reinfusing their own packed red blood cells, that same testing procedure will not work because the blood groups are obviously the same. However, systematic progress has been made with an approach that tracks an athlete's blood over years and notes changes in a variety of factors during that time (66). The term "hematological passport" has been applied to this approach, and one group has already made progress in establishing standards or cut-points to use in evaluating an out-of-line response (11). The measurement of hemoglobin mass has been added to that picture, and while it may not be able to detect the impact of EPO on a large percentage of athletes (68), it may be the only option available to catch those using autologous blood transfusions (81, 90). It is clear that as some problems are solved, others appear—for example, artificial oxygen carriers (107). However, there is little evidence of its usefulness at this time (36). Further, use of a hemoglobin-based oxygen carrier (Hemopure™) was also shown to not improve performance (5).

IN SUMMARY

- Blood doping refers to the reinfusion of red blood cells to increase the hemoglobin concentration and oxygen-carrying capacity of the blood.
- Due to improvements in blood storage techniques, blood doping has been shown to be effective in improving $\dot{V}O_2$ max and endurance performance.

A LOOK BACK—IMPORTANT PEOPLE IN SCIENCE

Dr. Björn Ekblom, M.D., Ph.D. Studied Factors Affecting Oxygen Transport, Leading Others to "Blood Doping"

Björn Ekblom received his Ph.D. in 1969 and his M.D. in 1970 from the Karolinska Institute in Stockholm, Sweden, and was appointed Professor of Physiology at the Karolinska Institute in 1977. The focus of his research early in his career was on maximal oxygen uptake ($\dot{V}O_2$ max), the physiological factors linked to $\dot{V}O_2$ max, and the effect of training on $\dot{V}O_2$ max in young and old subjects. Consistent with his interest in the factors affecting $\dot{V}O_2$ max, he examined the role of hemoglobin concentration on oxygen transport and $\dot{V}O_2$ max. In 1972 he published "Responses to Exercise After Blood Loss and Reinfusion," which showed that as you lower or raise the hemoglobin concentration, you can alter $\dot{V}O_2$ max in a systematic manner. This paper set in motion the interest in the use of blood doping to alter oxygen transport, $\dot{V}O_2$ max, and endurance performance, which is currently a major problem in sports (see discussion in this chapter). Dr. Ekblom's studies also investigated the effect of EPO on $\dot{V}O_2$ max and, later, how to detect the presence of EPO in those who might use it in an unethical manner.

Dr. Ekblom made major contributions over the past 40 years in our understanding of $\dot{V}O_2$ max and the various factors that affect it. However, his research interests went well beyond that. He studied temperature regulation during exercise, hemodynamic (i.e., blood pressure, cardiac output) responses to exercise, effects of training on patients with rheumatoid arthritis, and nutritional factors related to performance. In addition to making these important contributions to our understanding of the physiology related to physical training, he also published a number of books and pamphlets related to conditioning and training for different sports. He has published more than 140 peer-reviewed articles, numerous books, eight major review articles, and more than thirty chapters in books. He is currently Professor Emeritus at the Karolinska Institute, where he continues his productive career.

ANAEROBIC PERFORMANCE

Improvements in endurance performance focus on the supply of carbohydrate and oxygen to muscle (see previous sections on oxygen and blood doping in this chapter and on carbohydrate in chapter 23). However, in short-term, all-out performances in which anaerobic energy sources provide the vast majority of energy for muscle contraction, the focus of attention shifts to the buffering of the H^+ released from muscle. This section considers a means by which investigators have tried to buffer the H^+ and improve performance.

Blood Buffers

Elevations in the $[H^+]$ in muscle can decrease the activity of phosphofructokinase (PFK) (118), which may slow glycolysis, interfere with excitation-contraction coupling events by reducing Ca^{++} efflux from the terminal cisternae of the sarcoplasmic reticulum (43), and reduce the binding of Ca^{++} to troponin (83). Decreases in muscle force development have been shown to be linked to increases in muscle $[H^+]$ in both frog muscle (40) and human muscle (116). Finally, when Adams and Welch (1) showed that performance times in heavy exercise (90% $\dot{V}O_2$ max) could be altered by breathing 60% O_2 compared to 21% or 17% O_2, the point of exhaustion was associated with the same arterial $[H^+]$. The mechanisms involved in the regulation of the plasma $[H^+]$ were described in detail in chapter 11. Briefly, the primary means by which H^+ is buffered during exercise is through its reaction with the plasma bicarbonate reserve to form carbonic acid, which subsequently yields CO_2 that is exhaled (respiratory compensation). As the bicarbonate buffer store decreases, the ability to buffer H^+ is reduced and the plasma $[H^+]$ will increase. Knowing this, scientists have explored ways of increasing the plasma buffer store to slow down the rate of H^+ increase during strenuous exercise.

As early as 1932 (29), induced alkalosis (means unknown) was shown to extend run time to exhaustion from (min:sec) 5:22 to 6:04. Since that time, a variety of studies have supported these findings. On the basis of several reviews (16, 58, 65, 86, 93, 99, 129) there appears to be agreement that:

- the optimal dose of bicarbonate used to improve performance was 0.3 g per kilogram of body weight (although 0.2 g/kg may be as effective (110)),
- tasks of a minute or less in duration, even at extremes of intensity, did not seem to benefit from the induced alkalosis, and
- performance gains were shown for tasks of high intensity that lasted about 1 to 10 minutes, or involved repeated bouts of high-intensity exercise with short recovery periods.

However, when bicarbonate is taken over several days (in contrast to just before the test), there appears to be a dose-response effect with $0.5 \text{ g} \cdot \text{kg}^{-1} \cdot \text{d}^{-1}$ being better than $0.3 \text{ g} \cdot \text{kg}^{-1} \cdot \text{d}^{-1}$ (32). Given the potential for blood buffers to have a positive impact on performance, one must be careful to not be fooled by an inadequately designed study, as mentioned at the beginning of this chapter. In the case of blood buffers, McClung and Collins (74) used a research design to help separate out the effect of being told you are getting the buffer (drug) from actually getting the drug. They had four treatments:

1. Told they were going to get the drug/Got the drug
2. Told they were going to get the drug/Did not get the drug
3. Told they were not going to get the drug/Got the drug
4. Told they were not going to get the drug/Did not get the drug

There were several important findings in this study that we need to keep in mind when we deal with ergogenic aids. The "Told drug/Did not get drug treatment (#2)" resulted in a better performance than the "Told they were not going to get the drug/Got the drug treatment (#3)"—in effect, the pure pharmacological effect of the bicarbonate was not as good as the expectation that they were receiving the drug.

The positive impact of the buffers may be related to maintaining the oxygen saturation of hemoglobin during maximal exercise, as well as any improvements at the level of the muscle (84). Sodium citrate has also been shown to be an effective buffer for anaerobic performances of 2 to 4 minutes when taken at 0.5 g/kg (58, 78). However, a recent study comparing the relative benefits of a variety of buffers recommended bicarbonate as the better choice to enhance sprint performance (120). The variability in the effectiveness of the sodium bicarbonate treatment points to inter-individual variation in the response to sodium bicarbonate, and that some short-term anaerobic activities are more dependent on the muscle or plasma $[\text{H}^+]$ as a primary cause of fatigue than others (94). Welch (126) indicates that while subjects may stop at the same $[\text{H}^+]$ within any exercise protocol, the differences that exist among studies in the "terminal" $[\text{H}^+]$ suggest the other factors are more limiting as far as performance is concerned. The use of these agents to cause an alkalosis is not without risks. Large doses of sodium bicarbonate can cause diarrhea and vomiting, both of which are sure to affect performance (46, 65, 129).

IN SUMMARY

- The ingestion of sodium bicarbonate improves the performance of high-intensity exercise of 1 to 10 minutes' duration or repeated bouts of high-intensity exercise.

DRUGS

A variety of drugs have been used to aid performance. Some drugs are as common and "legal" as caffeine and nicotine, whereas others, like amphetamines, are banned from use. We will briefly examine each of these drugs, exploring how they might work to improve performance, as well as the evidence about whether or not they do.

Amphetamines

Amphetamines are stimulants that have been used primarily to recover from fatigue and improve endurance. In 1972, Golding (50) indicated that it was the most abused group of drugs at that time. Amphetamines are readily absorbed in the small intestine, and although the effects reach a peak 2 to 3 hours after ingestion, they persist for 12 to 24 hours (59, 67). Amphetamines are both a **sympathomimetic** drug (simulates catecholamine effects) and a central nervous system stimulant. The drug produces its effects by altering the metabolism and synthesis of catecholamines, or receptor affinity for catecholamines (59, 67).

The most consistent effect of amphetamines is to increase one's arousal or wakefulness, leading to a perception of increased energy and self-confidence (59). The drug affects the redistribution of blood flow, driving it away from the skin and splanchnic areas and delivering more to muscle or brain. This could lead to problems related to a decrease in lactic acid removal (see chapter 3) and an increase in body temperature (see chapter 12). Animal studies show that amphetamines can increase endurance-type performances. However, the dose of the drug was shown to be important, in that smaller doses (1–2 mg/kg) did not have an effect different from control, and large doses (16 mg/kg) appeared to reduce the ability of the rat to swim. Data collected using run tests on rats indicate the same detrimental effect of high doses (7.5–10 mg/kg) of amphetamines (59).

Ivy (59) concluded from an analysis of studies on human subjects that amphetamines extend endurance and hasten recovery from fatigue. Time to exhaustion was increased in spite of no effect on submaximal or maximal $\dot{V}O_2$ (18, 59). Two explanations have been offered. Ivy (59) believes that the endurance aspect of performance can be improved due to amphetamines' catecholamine-like effect in mobilizing FFA and sparing muscle glycogen, similar to that of caffeine (see the caffeine section, next page). Chandler and Blair (18) believe that the amphetamines may simply mask fatigue and interfere with the perception of the normal biological signals that fatigue has occurred. It is this latter conclusion that has raised the most concern about the safety of the athlete, in that during prolonged submaximal work,

β₂-Agonists: Clenbuterol and Salbutamol

Clenbuterol is a drug that was developed to treat airway diseases such as asthma. Its chemical action in the body is to activate beta-2 receptors (β_2-agonists) in tissue (see chapter 5). Although the drug is useful in the treatment of airway diseases, in the early 1980s it was discovered that clenbuterol is a powerful anabolic agent in skeletal muscles. Early studies showed that, in animals, a 14-day treatment with clenbuterol (2 mg/kg/day) resulted in a 10% to 20% increase in muscle mass, converted type I muscle fibers to type II fibers, and caused a selective hypertrophy of type II fibers (26, 139). Further, the time course of clenbuterol-induced muscular hypertrophy was rapid, with muscle growth beginning within 2 days after commencement of treatment.

With the discovery that clenbuterol is a powerful anabolic agent in skeletal muscle, scientific interest in the clinical use of this drug has grown. For example, this compound is potentially useful in the treatment of conditions that result in muscle wasting (i.e.,

aging, spinal cord injury, etc.) (71). Unfortunately, some athletes now use clenbuterol in an effort to increase muscle size and improve performance in power events (e.g., sprinting, football, etc.). What does the research say?

In two recent reviews of this issue, the authors were consistent in finding that inhaled β_2-agonists had no effect on either aerobic or anaerobic performances (21, 89). However, when the β_2-agonists were either ingested or infused, performance was favorably altered, but the two reviews differed in terms of how much:

- Collomp et al. (21) found that in almost all trials, following an acute or short-term administration of the drug at a therapeutic dosage, subjects showed improved performances, whatever the intensity.

- In a meta-analysis of the randomized controlled trials on this issue, Pluim et al. (89) showed that while some performances improved (e.g., endurance time

at 80–85% $\dot{V}O_2$ max), others did not (endurance time at 70% $\dot{V}O_2$ max), even though they were similar in nature. They concluded that while the overall effect of the β_2-agonists on performance was positive, the evidence was weak.

Clearly, this is an area in which additional research is needed to help clarify issues related to the dosage and duration of administration, type of athlete who benefits, and magnitude of change expected in standardized performance tests.

Salbutamol and salmeterol are β_2-agonists used to treat asthma: the former is short-acting (4–6 hours) and the latter is long-acting (~12 hours). The World Anti-Doping Agency (WADA) currently (2011) allows these drugs to be used without the athlete seeking a Therapeutic Use Exemption, a change from previous standards (138). However, if the level of salbutamol in the urine exceeds 1,000 ng/ml, it is presumed not to be due to an intended therapeutic use.

---

especially in a hot and/or humid environment, the decreased blood flow to the skin could cause hyperthermia, leading to death (20, 59, 67).

As mentioned at the beginning of this section, amphetamines' major effect is in increasing wakefulness and producing a state of arousal. However, although amphetamines have restored reaction time in fatigued subjects, the drug does not affect reaction time in alert, motivated, and nonfatigued subjects (23). Given that athletes are usually alert and motivated prior to competition, Golding (50) suggests that amphetamines would be counterproductive, making users hyperirritable and interfering with their sleep. Finally, it is risky to extrapolate from data collected under tightly controlled laboratory conditions using discrete measures related to performance ($\dot{V}O_2$ max, endurance time, reaction time) to the actual performance in a skilled sport in front of a hostile audience for a national championship. That might be excitement enough. Sometimes a drug used for one purpose finds its way into the sporting world because of its unique impact on muscle. See A Closer Look 25.1 for such an example.

IN SUMMARY

- Amphetamines have a catecholamine-like effect that leads to an increased arousal and a perception of increased energy and self-confidence.
- Although amphetamines improve the performance of fatigued subjects, they do not have this effect on alert, motivated, and nonfatigued subjects.

Caffeine

Caffeine is a stimulant that is found in a variety of common foods, drinks, and over-the-counter drugs (see table 25.2). Caffeine has been viewed as an on-again, off-again ergogenic aid. Caffeine was banned by the International Olympic Committee (IOC) in 1962, then removed from the list of banned drugs in 1972. In 1984, the IOC again banned "high levels" in the urine that might have been the result of caffeine injections or suppositories; the standard was set at 12 μg/ml

TABLE 25.2	Caffeine Content of Popular Drinks and Drugs

Popular Beverages (8 oz)	Caffeine (mg)
Coffee, drip	115–175
Coffee, brewed	80–135
Coffee, instant	65–100
Tea, iced	47
Tea, brewed (import)	60
Tea, brewed (domestic)	40
Tea, green	15

Soft Drinks (12 oz)	
Low (e.g., root beer)	23
Most, (e.g., colas)	~45
High (e.g., Mountain Dew)	~55
Jolt	71
Red Bull	80

Non-Prescription Drugs	
NoDoz	200
Vivarin	200
Midol	64

Pain Relievers	
Anacin analgesic	64 mg
Excedrin	130
Tylenol	0

Sources: http://www.holymtn.com/tea/caffeine_content.htm and http://wilstar.com/caffeine.htm

Figure 25.4 Factors influenced by caffeine that might cause an improvement in performance.

(119, 130). Caffeine is again off the list of banned substances. Part of the reason is the availability of caffeine in food and drinks, which makes it a very difficult thing to track and control in an athlete's diet. Since the ban was lifted, analysis of caffeine levels in urine samples from athletes of many different sports show power lifters to have the highest concentration, followed by cyclists and body builders (121). Caffeine is absorbed rapidly from the GI tract, and is significantly elevated in the blood at 15 minutes, with the peak concentration achieved at 60 minutes. Caffeine is diluted by body water, and the physiological response is proportional to the concentration in the body water. There is a natural variability in how people respond to caffeine, with evidence that chronic users are less responsive than abstainers (9, 119).

Although caffeine can affect a wide variety of tissues, figure 25.4 shows that its role as an ergogenic aid is based on its effects on skeletal muscle and the central nervous system, and in the mobilization of fuels for muscular work. The evidence for the enhanced function of skeletal muscle is based primarily on *in vitro* and *in situ* muscle preparations and shows that caffeine can increase tension development (91, 119). This was shown most clearly in fatigued muscle and was believed to be due to increased Ca^{++} release from the ryanodine receptor that mediates the release of Ca^{++} from the sarcoplasmic reticulum (71, 113). In a recent meta-analysis, caffeine ingestion was shown to have a small but positive impact (+7%) on knee extensor maximal strength, with little or no impact on other muscle groups; this is surprising given that the drug obviously reached all muscles. In contrast, muscular endurance was improved by ~148% across muscle groups (125).

Caffeine has long been recognized as a stimulator of the CNS. Caffeine can pass the blood-brain barrier and affect a variety of brain centers, which usually leads to an increased alertness and decreased drowsiness (91, 119). The best evidence supporting caffeine as a CNS stimulant is in the decreased perception of fatigue during prolonged exercise in subjects who took caffeine (24). Recent reviews of the literature supports this proposition with findings that the rating of perceived exertion (RPE) is lower during exercise with caffeine ingestion, accounting for some of the improvement in performance (31, 113).

The role of caffeine in the mobilization of fuel has received considerable attention as the primary means by which it exerts its ergogenic effect. Caffeine has been shown to cause an elevation of glucose and an increase in fatty acid utilization. The elevated glucose could be due to the stimulation of the sympathetic nervous system and the resulting increase in catecholamines, which would increase the mobilization of glucose from the liver. On the other hand, the glucose concentration could be elevated due to a decreased rate of removal related to the suppression of insulin release by catecholamines (see chapter 5) (119). However, some of these metabolic effects are not dependent on catecholamines; instead, they may be related to the products of caffeine breakdown (e.g., theophylline), which are metabolic stimuli in their own right (52). Interestingly, when caffeine is coingested with glucose, the ingested glucose is oxidized at a higher rate than when the glucose is taken without caffeine (140).

Lipid mobilization has been shown to be increased as a result of caffeine ingestion. Figure 25.5 shows that

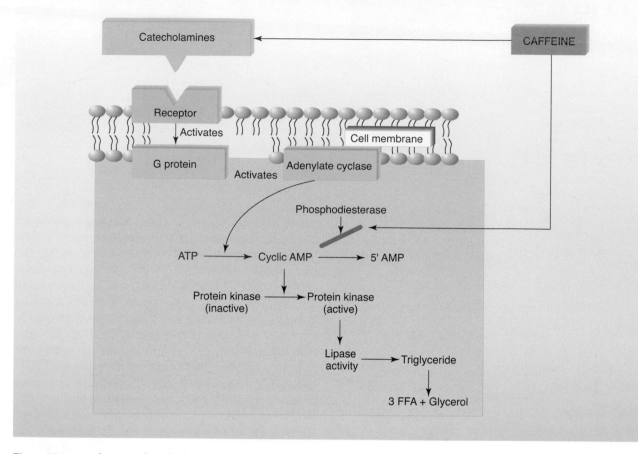

Figure 25.5 Mechanisms by which caffeine might increase free fatty acid mobilization.

the mechanism of action could be related either to the elevated catecholamines increasing the level of cyclic AMP in the adipose cell or to caffeine's blocking of phosphodiesterase activity, which is responsible for breaking down cyclic AMP. Van Handel (119) believes that the latter mechanism is less likely, given the dose of caffeine needed. Plasma free fatty acids increase quickly at rest after ingestion of caffeine (15 minutes) and continue to increase over the next several hours (119). However, during exercise, plasma FFA may (30, 114) or may not (24, 30, 38, 53, 60) be significantly elevated as a result of caffeine ingestion. In addition, while the respiratory exchange ratio may (38, 60) or may not (53, 114) be reduced, both glucose kinetics (105) and the lactate threshold (13, 30, 45) have been shown not to be affected by caffeine ingestion. In addition, there is also variability in the effect of caffeine on improvements in work output or total work time, making it an "ergogenic aid" for some and not for others (30, 31, 38, 45, 53, 60, 111, 130). A recent review confirmed the variability in improvement in endurance performance (range –0.3% to 17.3%, with an average of 3.2%) (44). What causes such variability?

The ergogenic effect appears to be dose dependent and may vary with the type of subject (22);

however, gender and menstrual cycle status do not appear to affect the pharmacokinetics of how caffeine is handled (76). Although some studies show physiological changes with doses as low as 5 to 7 mg/kg (24, 38), others find a 10 mg/kg dose to be inadequate (60). In fact, in other studies, a dose of 15 mg/kg was needed to see an increase in fat metabolism (77, 79). However, when restricted to improvements in sport-specific endurance performance, a dose of 3–6 mg/kg taken prior to or during the performance appears to be sufficient (44). There is also evidence that patterns of caffeine use affect the response to exercise. For example, habitual caffeine users who abstain from caffeine for at least 7 days will optimize the ergogenic effect (44). Further, heavy caffeine users (>300 mg per day) respond differently than those consuming little caffeine (30). Van Handel (119) makes the point that what an investigator observes in a controlled laboratory setting may be masked by a normal sympathetic nervous system response to competition. Given the potential side effects such as insomnia, diarrhea, anxiety, tremulousness, and irritability (119), and the variability among subjects in response to caffeine, one might not see much of an improvement in performance (35, 53, 111). Although caffeine has a diuretic effect, a recent study indicated that rehydration with caffeine-containing beverages during nonexercise periods of two-a-day practices did not hinder hydration status (39). We recommend the review articles by Ganio et al. (44), Tarnopolsky (113), and Warren et al. (125) for more on this topic.

IN SUMMARY

- Caffeine can potentially improve performance through changes in muscle or the central nervous system, or in the delivery of fuel for muscular work. Caffeine can elevate blood glucose and simultaneously increase the utilization of fat.
- Caffeine's ergogenic effect on performance is variable; it appears to be dose-related and less pronounced in subjects who are daily users of caffeine.

Nicotine

Nicotine is a drug with no therapeutic application. However, the fact that it is a part of cigarette and chewing tobacco makes it one of the most abused substances. Nicotine has unpredictable effects due to the fact that it can simultaneously increase sympathetic, parasympathetic, and central nervous system activities (see figure 25.6). Small doses of nicotine increase autonomic activity, while large doses lead to a blocking of the response. The cardiovascular system responds with increases in heart rate and blood pressure due to increased sympathetic nerve activity, and the GI tract responds with an increase in activity via parasympathetic nerve stimulation. There is evidence that both resting metabolic rate and cardiovascular responses to light exercise are increased following nicotine administration (72, 87). Nicotine is easily absorbed through the lungs, mucous membranes, and the skin, and the half-life of nicotine is about 30 to 60 minutes (115).

Nicotine is primarily taken in by either smoking or chewing tobacco. Independent of whether it has a calming or a stimulating effect on an individual, the smoking and chewing of tobacco are associated with major health problems. We already know from chapter 14 that cigarette smoking is linked directly to a variety of cancers and heart and lung diseases. That alone is motivation enough to discourage smoking, independent of the fact that it increases the work of breathing (102), decreases $\dot{V}O_2$ max (63), and lengthens the time needed for $\dot{V}O_2$ to achieve a steady state during submaximal exercise (104). The point is, of course, that cigarette smoke contains more than nicotine—specifically, carbon monoxide and various carcinogens. But what if the nicotine could be obtained without the cigarette smoke?

Smokeless tobacco has become a part of the American sport scene. Smokeless tobacco includes (a) loose leaf tobacco that is placed between the cheek and lower gum and is "chewed," (b) snuff, moist or dry powdered tobacco, that is "dipped" and placed between the cheek or lip and lower gum, and (c) compressed tobacco, a "plug," that is used as loose leaf tobacco.

In the 1990s, the focus of attention was on the use of these products by athletes and the impact that might have on children. Despite media and educational campaigns to inform the public about the risks involved, we have not been as successful as we might like in curbing use of smokeless tobacco. Currently a larger percentage of high school boys use smokeless tobacco (11%) than men (7%) (17).

Although one might be worried about a young person becoming addicted to nicotine through the use of smokeless tobacco, the greatest concern is with regard to damage to teeth (**dental caries**) and gums (periodontal disease), including oral cancer. The increase in dental caries is related, in part, to the sugar content in the pouch and plug tobacco. However, it is more important to focus attention on periodontal disease and cancer. The withdrawal of the gum from a tooth's surface exposes the tooth to greater damage that can lead to the loss of the tooth and potentially to bone loss. The loss of the gum occurs in the area where the tobacco is held in the

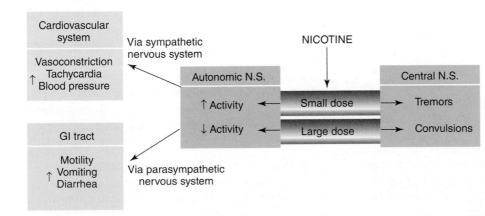

Figure 25.6 Schematic representation of how nicotine can have both relaxing and stimulating effects.

mouth, indicating a clear link. Further, lesions of the mucosa can develop, which can ultimately lead to cancer. While it is known that regular smoking can cause oral cancer, smokeless tobacco users are actually at a greater risk. Independent of any potential beneficial effect of nicotine on performance, the use of smokeless tobacco should be discouraged. Once a person is "hooked," the habit is more difficult to break than that associated with cigarette smoking.

IN SUMMARY

- Nicotine has varied effects depending on whether the parasympathetic or sympathetic nervous system is stimulated. The use of smokeless tobacco can cause dental caries, gum disease, and oral cancer.

PHYSICAL WARM-UP

Warming up prior to moderate or strenuous activity is a general recommendation made for those involved in fitness programs or athletes involved in various types of performance. Most of us accept this as a reasonable recommendation, but is there good scientific support for it? In Franks's original 1972 review (42), he found that 53% of the studies supported the proposition that warm-up was better than no warm-up, 7% the opposite, and 40% found no difference between the two. Concerns were raised about the wide variety of tasks and the methods used to evaluate the effectiveness of warm-up. In his 1983 review, Franks (41) analyzed the role of the participant (trained or untrained), the duration and intensity of the warm-up, and the type of performance as the variables involved in a determination of the effectiveness of warm-up. Before we summarize these findings, a few definitions must be presented.

Warm-up refers to exercise conducted prior to a performance, whether or not muscle or body temperature is elevated. Warm-up activities can be identical to the performance (baseball pitcher throwing with normal form and high speed to a catcher prior to the batter stepping up), directly related to the performance (shot-putter practicing at 75% of normal effort prior to a competition), or indirectly related to a performance (general activities to increase body temperature or arousal) (41). Generally all three are used in a typical warm-up prior to performance, in the reverse order of the above descriptions.

The theoretical benefits of warm-up are physiological, psychological, and safety-related. Physiological benefits would include less muscle resistance and faster enzymatic reactions at high body temperatures. This might lower the oxygen deficit at the onset of work (61, 101), decrease the RER during the subsequent activity (56), or cause a favorable shift in the lactate threshold (19). One review supported most of these effects, but questioned the impact of the warm-up on speeding up rate-limiting enzyme reactions (14). Increases in body temperature as a result of warm-up have been linked to improved performance (41). Skilled performances benefit from identical and direct warm-up, with indirect warm-up sometimes acting in a facilitatory manner. The warm-up procedures can increase arousal, which is good up to a point, and provide the optimal "mental set" for improved performance (14, 41).

Stretching, as a part of warming up, has been recommended as a way to reduce the risk of soft tissue injury. There is no question that such a practice improves joint flexibility, but reviews on this topic provide little support that injury risk is reduced. Weldon and Hill (128) found that most of the available studies were of poor quality, and it was not possible to draw a definitive conclusion regarding stretching and exercise-related injuries. A group of researchers at the Centers for Disease Control and Prevention drew the same conclusion from their review of the literature, and indicated that there was not enough evidence to either endorse or discontinue routine stretching before or after exercise to prevent injuries (117). Witvrouw and colleagues (137) agreed with these general conclusions when applied to most sports. However, for those sports demanding high-intensity stretch-shortening cycles (e.g., soccer, basketball), stretching was viewed as important to keep the muscle-tendon unit compliant enough to store and release energy during explosive movements. Finally, Shrier's comment on the CDC article indicated that there was a need to separate out the effects of stretching outside of periods of exercise from the stretching that precedes exercise. There is evidence that the former approach is associated with injury prevention. Clearly, more research is needed (109). From a safety standpoint, apart from the potential for soft tissue injuries, some evidence suggests that warm-up reduces the "stress" experienced when doing strenuous work. In Barnard et al.'s (6) classic study, six of ten firefighters who did not warm up experienced an ischemic response (reduced myocardial blood flow) as shown by a depressed ST segment on the ECG during strenuous exercise (see chapter 17). All had normal ECG responses when a gradual warm-up preceded the strenuous exercise.

Warming up obviously affects a variety of factors, but is there evidence that it favorably affects performance? The answer is "yes," but with some caveats (15).

- In short-term performances (max effort of ≤10 s) a 3- to 5-minute warm-up improves performance. However, an intense warm-up may result in a decrement in performance due, in part, to a reduction in high-energy phosphates.

- Warm-up improves intermediate-term performances (>10 s, but ≤ 5 min), but not if the intensity is too low ($\leq 40\%$ $\dot{V}O_2$ max) or the recovery time is too long (5–10 minutes). The goal is to begin the performance with a slightly elevated baseline $\dot{V}O_2$, and be sufficiently recovered.

- For long-term performances (fatiguing effort for ≥ 5 minutes), an elevated baseline $\dot{V}O_2$ also improves performance. However, if the warm-up depletes muscle glycogen or increases thermal strain (by elevating body temperature too much), performance may suffer.

So, what is the recommended warm-up? For short-term performances, a warm-up at $\sim 40\%$ to 60% $\dot{V}O_2$ max for 5 to 10 minutes, followed by a 5-minute recovery, is recommended. For intermediate- or long-term performances, the warm-up at $\sim 60\%$ to 70% $\dot{V}O_2$ max for 5 to 10 minutes, with a ≤ 5 minute recovery, is recommended (15). This is very similar to what Franks reported some 25 years ago (41).

IN SUMMARY

- Warm-up activities can be identical to performance, directly related to performance, or indirectly related to performance (general warm-up). Warm-up causes both physiological and psychological changes that are beneficial to performance.

STUDY QUESTIONS

1. What is an ergogenic aid?
2. Why must an investigator use a "placebo" treatment to evaluate the effectiveness of an ergogenic aid?
3. Provide a brief summary of the role that dietary supplements play in improving performance.
4. What is a double-blind research design?
5. Does breathing 100% O_2 improve performance? Recovery?
6. Breathing hyperoxic gas mixtures improves performance without changing O_2 delivery to tissue. How is this possible?
7. What is blood doping and why does it appear to improve performance now when it did not in the earliest investigations?
8. How might ingested buffers improve short-term performances?
9. Although amphetamines improve performance in fatigued individuals, they might not have this effect on motivated subjects. Why?
10. How might caffeine improve long-term performances? Can the results be extrapolated to "real" performances in the field?
11. Chewing tobacco may provide a nicotine "high," but not without risks. What are they?
12. Describe the different types of warm-up activities and the mechanisms by which they may improve performance.

SUGGESTED READINGS

Burke, L. M and V. Deakin. 2010. *Clinical Sports Nutrition*. New York: McGraw-Hill.

Kundrat, S. 2005. Herbs and athletes. *Sport Science Exchange*, no. 96. Gatorade Sport Science Institute.

Williams, M. H. 2010. *Nutrition for Health, Fitness and Sport*. New York: McGraw-Hill.

REFERENCES

1. **Adams RP, and Welch HG.** Oxygen uptake, acid-base status, and performance with varied inspired oxygen fractions. *Journal of Applied Physiology: Respiratory, Environmental and Exercise Physiology* 49: 863–868, 1980.
2. **Alvares TS, Meirelles CM, Bhambhani YN, Paschoalin VMF, and Gomes PSC.** L-arginine as a potential ergogenic aid in healthy subjects. *Sports Medicine* 41: 233–248, 2011.
3. **Ariel G, and Saville W.** Anabolic steroids: the physiological effects of placebos. *Medicine and Science in Sports* 4: 124–126, 1972.
4. **Ashenden MJ.** A strategy to deter blood doping in sport. *Haematologica* 87: 225–232, 2002.
5. **Ashenden MJ, Schumacher YO, Sharpe K, Varlet-Marie E, and Audran M.** Effects of Hemopure on maximal oxygen uptake and endurance performance in healthy humans. *International Journal of Sports Medicine* 28: 381–385, 2007.
6. **Barnard RJ, Gardner GW, Diaco NV, MacAlpin RN, and Kattus AA.** Cardiovascular responses to sudden strenuous exercise—heart rate, blood pressure, and ECG. *Journal of Applied Physiology: Respiratory, Environmental and Exercise Physiology* 34: 833–837, 1973.
7. **Baume N, Hellemans I, and Saugy M.** Guide to over-the-counter sports supplements for athletes. *Int Sport Med J* 8: 2–10, 2007.

8. **Baume N, Mahler N, Kamber M, Mangin P, and Saugy M.** Research of stimulants and anabolic steroids in dietary supplements. *Scandinavian Journal of Medicine & Science in Sports* 16: 41–48, 2006.

9. **Bell DG, and McLellan TM.** Exercise endurance 1, 3, and 6 h after caffeine ingestion in caffeine users and nonusers. *Journal of Applied Physiology: Respiratory, Environmental and Exercise Physiology* 93: 1227–1234, 2002.

10. **Berglund B, Birgegard G, and Hemmingsson P.** Serum erythropoietin in cross-country skiers. *Medicine and Science in Sports and Exercise* 20: 208–209, 1988.

11. **Berglund B, Ekblom B, Ekblom E, Berglund L, Kallner A, Reinebo P, and Lindeberg S.** The Swedish Blood Pass project. *Scandinavian Journal of Medicine & Science in Sports* 17: 292–297, 2007.

12. **Berglund B, and Hemmingson P.** Effect of reinfusion of autologous blood on exercise performance in cross-country skiers. *International Journal of Sports Medicine* 8: 231–233, 1987.

13. **Berry MJ, Stoneman JV, Weyrich AS, and Burney B.** Dissociation of the ventilatory and lactate thresholds following caffeine ingestion. *Medicine and Science in Sports and Exercise* 23: 463–469, 1991.

14. **Bishop D.** Warm up I: potential mechanisms and the effects of passive warm up on exercise performance. *Sports Medicine (Auckland, NZ)* 33: 439–454, 2003.

15. **Bishop D.** Warm up II: performance changes following active warm up and how to structure the warm up. *Sports Medicine (Auckland, NZ)* 33: 483–498, 2003.

16. **Bishop D, Edge J, Davis C, and Goodman C.** Induced metabolic alkalosis affects muscle metabolism and repeated-sprint ability. *Medicine and Science in Sports and Exercise* 36: 807–813, 2004.

17. **Centers for Disease Control and Prevention.** Smokeless tobacco facts. edited by Office on Smoking and Health: Author, 2011.

18. **Chandler JV, and Blair SN.** The effect of amphetamines on selected physiological components related to athletic success. *Medicine and Science in Sports and Exercise* 12: 65–69, 1980.

19. **Chwalbinska-Moneta J, and Hanninen O.** Effect of active warming-up on thermoregulatory, circulatory, and metabolic responses to incremental exercise in endurance-trained athletes. *International Journal of Sports Medicine* 10: 25–29, 1989.

20. **Clarkson PM, and Thompson HS.** Drugs and sport. Research findings and limitations. *Sports Medicine (Auckland, NZ)* 24: 366–384, 1997.

21. **Collomp K, Le Panse B, Candau R, Lecoq AM, and De Ceaurriz J.** Beta-2 agonists and exercise performance. *Science & Sport* 2010.

22. **Conlee R.** Amphetamine, caffeine, and cocaine. In: *Perspectives in Exercise Science and Sports Medicine Vol 4: Ergogenics-Enhancement of Performance in Exercise and Sports*, edited by Lamb D, and Williams M. New York: McGraw-Hill, 1991, p. 285–330.

23. **Conlee RK, Barnett DW, Kelly KP, and Han DH.** Effects of cocaine on plasma catecholamine and muscle glycogen concentrations during exercise in the rat. *Journal of Applied Physiology: Respiratory, Environmental and Exercise Physiology* 70: 1323–1327, 1991.

24. **Costill DL, Dalsky GP, and Fink WJ.** Effects of caffeine ingestion on metabolism and exercise performance. *Med Sci Sports* 10: 155–158, 1978.

25. **Cribb PJ, Williams AD, and Hayes A.** A creatine-protein-carbohydrate supplement enhances responses to resistance training. *Medicine and Science in Sports and Exercise* 39: 1960–1968, 2007.

26. **Criswell DS, Powers SK, and Herb RA.** Clenbuterol-induced fiber type transition in the soleus of adult rats. *European Journal of Applied Physiology and Occupational Physiology* 74: 391–396, 1996.

27. **De Hon O, and Coumans B.** The continuing story of nutritional supplements and doping infractions. *British Journal of Sports Medicine* 41: 800–805; discussion 805, 2007.

28. **Demant TW, and Rhodes EC.** Effects of creatine supplementation on exercise performance. *Sports Medicine (Auckland, NZ)* 28: 49–60, 1999.

29. **Dill D, Edwards H, and Talbot J.** Alkalosis and the capacity for work. *Journal of Biological Chemistry* 97: LVII–LIX, 1932.

30. **Dodd SL, Brooks E, Powers SK, and Tulley R.** The effects of caffeine on graded exercise performance in caffeine naive versus habituated subjects. *European Journal of Applied Physiology and Occupational Physiology* 62: 424–429, 1991.

31. **Doherty M, and Smith PM.** Effects of caffeine ingestion on rating of perceived exertion during and after exercise: a meta-analysis. *Scandinavian Journal of Medicine & Science in Sports* 15: 69–78, 2005.

32. **Douroudos, II, Fatouros IG, Gourgoulis V, Jamurtas AZ, Tsitsios T, Hatzinikolaou A, Margonis K, Mavromatidis K, and Taxildaris K.** Dose-related effects of prolonged $NaHCO_3$ ingestion during high-intensity exercise. *Medicine and Science in Sports and Exercise* 38: 1746–1753, 2006.

33. **Eckardt KU, Boutellier U, Kurtz A, Schopen M, Koller EA, and Bauer C.** Rate of erythropoietin formation in humans in response to acute hypobaric hypoxia. *Journal of Applied Physiology: Respiratory, Environmental and Exercise Physiology* 66: 1785–1788, 1989.

34. **Eichner E.** Blood doping results and consequences from the laboratory and the field. *The Physician and Sportsmedicine* 15: 121–129, 1987.

35. **Eichner E.** The caffeine controversy: effects on endurance and cholesterol. *The Physician and Sportsmedicine* 14: 124–132, 1986.

36. **Eichner ER.** Blood doping: infusions, erythropoietin and artificial blood. *Sports Medicine (Auckland, NZ)* 37: 389–391, 2007.

37. **Ekblom B, Goldbarg AN, and Gullbring B.** Response to exercise after blood loss and reinfusion. *Journal of Applied Physiology: Respiratory, Environmental and Exercise Physiology* 33: 175–180, 1972.

38. **Essig D, Costill D, and Van Handel P.** Effect of caffeine ingestion on utilization of muscle glycogen and lipid during leg ergometer cycling. *International Journal of Sports Medicine* 1: 86–90, 1980.

39. **Fiala KA, Casa DJ, and Roti MW.** Rehydration with a caffeinated beverage during the nonexercise periods of 3 consecutive days of 2-a-day practices. *International Journal of Sport Nutrition and Exercise Metabolism* 14: 419–429, 2004.

40. **Fitts RH, and Holloszy JO.** Lactate and contractile force in frog muscle during development of fatigue and recovery. *The American Journal of Physiology* 231: 430–433, 1976.

41. **Franks B.** Physical warm-up. In: *Ergogenic Aids in Sport*, edited by Williams M. Champaign: Human Kinetics, 1983, p. 340–375.

42. **Franks B.** Physical warm-up. In: *Ergogenic Aids and Muscular Performance*, edited by Morgan W. New York: Academic Press, 1972, p. 160–191.

43. **Fuchs F, Reddy Y, and Briggs FN.** The interaction of cations with the calcium-binding site of troponin. *Biochimica et Biophysica Acta* 221: 407–409, 1970.

44. **Ganio MS, Klau JF, Casa DJ, Armstrong LE, and Maresh CM.** Effect of caffeine on sport-specific endurance-performance: a systematic review. *Journal of Strength and Conditioning Research* 23: 315–324, 2009.

45. **Gastin P, Misner J, Boileau R, and Slaughter M.** Failure of caffeine to enhance exercise performance in incremental treadmill running. *The Australian Journal of Science and Medicine in Sport* 22: 23–27, 1990.

46. **Gledhill N.** Bicarbonate ingestion and anaerobic performance. *Sports Medicine (Auckland, NZ)* 1: 177–180, 1984.

47. **Gledhill N.** Blood doping and related issues: a brief review. *Medicine and Science in Sports and Exercise* 14: 183–189, 1982.

48. **Gledhill N.** The influence of altered blood volume and oxygen transport capacity on aerobic performance. *Exercise and Sport Sciences Reviews* 13: 75–93, 1985.

49. **Gledhill N, Warburton D, and Jamnik V.** Haemoglobin, blood volume, cardiac function, and aerobic power. *Canadian Journal of Applied Physiology = Revue Canadienne de Physiologie Appliquee* 24: 54–65, 1999.

50. **Golding L.** Drugs and hormones. In: *Ergogenic Aids and Muscular Performance*, edited by Morgan W. New York: Academic Press, 1972.

51. **Gotshalk LA, Volek JS, Staron RS, Denegar CR, Hagerman FC, and Kraemer WJ.** Creatine supplementation improves muscular performance in older men. *Medicine and Science in Sports and Exercise* 34: 537–543, 2002.

52. **Graham T, and Spriet L.** Caffeine and exercise performance. Gatorade Sports Science Institute, 1996.

53. **Graham TE, and Spriet LL.** Performance and metabolic responses to a high caffeine dose during prolonged exercise. *Journal of Applied Physiology: Respiratory, Environmental and Exercise Physiology* 71: 2292–2298, 1991.

54. **Heinonen OJ.** Carnitine and physical exercise. *Sports Medicine (Auckland, NZ)* 22: 109–132, 1996.

55. **Herda TJ, Beck TW, Ryan ED, Smith AE, Walter AA, Hartman MJ, Stout JR, and Cramer JT.** Effects of creatine monohydrate and polyethylene glycosylated creatine supplementation on muscular strength, endurance, and power output. *Journal of Strength and Conditioning Research* 23: 818–826, 2009.

56. **Hetzler R.** Effect of warm up on plasma free fatty acid responses and substrate utilization during submaximal exercise. *Research Quarterly for Exercise and Sport* 57: 223–228, 1986.

57. **Hogan MC, Cox RH, and Welch HG.** Lactate accumulation during incremental exercise with varied inspired oxygen fractions. *Journal of Applied Physiology: Respiratory, Environmental and Exercise Physiology* 55: 1134–1140, 1983.

58. **Horswill CA.** Effects of bicarbonate, citrate, and phosphate loading on performance. *International Journal of Sport Nutrition* 5 Suppl: S111–119, 1995.

59. **Ivy J.** Amphetamines. In: *Ergogenic Aids in Sport*. Champaign: Human Kinetics, 1983.

60. **Ivy JL, Costill DL, Fink WJ, and Lower RW.** Influence of caffeine and carbohydrate feedings on endurance performance. *Med Sci Sports* 11: 6–11, 1979.

61. **Jones AM, Koppo K, and Burnley M.** Effects of prior exercise on metabolic and gas exchange responses to exercise. *Sports Medicine (Auckland, NZ)* 33: 949–971, 2003.

62. **Juhn M.** Popular sports supplements and ergogenic aids. *Sports Medicine (Auckland, NZ)* 33: 921–939, 2003.

63. **Klausen K, Andersen C, and Nandrup S.** Acute effects of cigarette smoking and inhalation of carbon monoxide during maximal exercise. *European Journal of Applied Physiology and Occupational Physiology* 51: 371–379, 1983.

64. **Law YLL, Ong WS, GillianYap TL, Lim SCJ, and Von Chia E.** Effects of two and five days of creatine loading on muscular strength and anaerobic power in trained athletes. *Journal of Strength and Conditioning Research* 23: 906–914, 2009.

65. **Linderman J, and Fahey TD.** Sodium bicarbonate ingestion and exercise performance: an update. *Sports Medicine (Auckland, NZ)* 11: 71–77, 1991.

66. **Lippi G, and Banfi G.** Blood transfusions in athletes: old dogmas, new tricks. *Clinical Chemistry and Laboratory Medicine* 44: 1395–1402, 2006.

67. **Lombardo J.** Stimulants and athletic performance (part 1 of 2): amphetamines and caffeine. *The Physician and Sportsmedicine* 14: 128–142, 1986.

68. **Lundby C, and Robach P.** Assessment of total haemoglobin mass: can it detect erythropoietin-induced blood manipulations? *European Journal of Applied Physiology* 108: 197–200, 2010.

69. **Lundby C, Thomsen JJ, Boushel R, Koskolou M, Warberg J, Calbet JA, and Robach P.** Erythropoietin treatment elevates haemoglobin concentration by increasing red cell volume and depressing plasma volume. *The Journal of Physiology* 578: 309–314, 2007.

70. **Macdougall IC.** Meeting the challenges of a new millennium: optimizing the use of recombinant human erythropoietin. *Nephrol Dial Transplant* 13 Suppl 2: 23–27, 1998.

71. **Maltin CA, and Delday MI.** Satellite cells in innervated and denervated muscles treated with clenbuterol. *Muscle & Nerve* 15: 919–925, 1992.

72. **Marks BL, and Perkins KA.** The effects of nicotine on metabolic rate. *Sports Medicine (Auckland, NZ)* 10: 277–285, 1990.

73. **Maughan RJ, King DS, and Lea T.** Dietary supplements. *Journal of Sports Sciences* 22: 95–113, 2004.

74. **McClung M, and Collins D.** "Because I know it will!": placebo effects of an ergogenic aid on athletic performance. *Journal of Sport & Exercise Psychology* 29: 382–394, 2007.

75. **McDowall JA.** Supplement use by young athletes. *Journal of Sport Science & Medicine* 6: 337–342, 2007.

76. **McLean C, and Graham TE.** Effects of exercise and thermal stress on caffeine pharmacokinetics in men and eumenorrheic women. *Journal of Applied Physiology: Respiratory, Environmental and Exercise Physiology* 93: 1471–1478, 2002.

77. **McNaughton L.** Two levels of caffeine ingestion on blood lactate and free fatty acid responses during incremental exercise. *Research Quarterly for Exercise and Sport* 58: 255–259, 1987.

78. **McNaughton L, and Cedaro R.** Sodium citrate ingestion and its effects on maximal anaerobic exercise of different durations. *European Journal of Applied Physiology and Occupational Physiology* 64: 36–41, 1992.

79. **McNaughton LR.** The influence of caffeine ingestion on incremental treadmill running. *British Journal of Sports Medicine* 20: 109–112, 1986.

80. **Morgan W.** Basic considerations. In: *Ergogenic Aids and Muscular Performance*, edited by Morgan W. New York: Academic Press, 1972.

81. **Morkeberg J, Sharpe K, Belhage B, Damsgaard R, Schmidt W, Prommer N, Gore CJ, and Ashenden MJ.** Detecting autologous blood transfusions: a comparison of three passport approaches and four blood markers. *Scandinavian Journal of Medicine & Science in Sports* 21: 235–243, 2011.

82. **Morris A.** Oxygen. In: *Ergogenic Aids in Sports.* Champaign: Human Kinetics, 1983.

83. **Nakamaru Y, and Schwartz A.** The influence of hydrogen ion concentration on calcium binding and release by skeletal muscle sarcoplasmic reticulum. *The Journal of General Physiology* 59: 22–32, 1972.

84. **Nielsen HB, Bredmose PP, Stromstad M, Volianitis S, Quistorff B, and Secher NH.** Bicarbonate attenuates arterial desaturation during maximal exercise in humans. *Journal of Applied Physiology: Respiratory, Environmental and Exercise Physiology* 93: 724–731, 2002.

85. **Nummela A, Hamalainen I, and Rusko H.** Effect of hyperoxia on metabolic responses and recovery in intermittent exercise. *Scandinavian Journal of Medicine & Science in Sports* 12: 309–315, 2002.

86. **Oopik V, Saaremets I, Medijainen L, Karelson K, Janson T, and Timpmann S.** Effects of sodium citrate ingestion before exercise on endurance performance in well trained college runners. *British Journal of Sports Medicine* 37: 485–489, 2003.

87. **Perkins KA, Sexton JE, Solberg-Kassel RD, and Epstein LH.** Effects of nicotine on perceived exertion during low-intensity activity. *Medicine and Science in Sports and Exercise* 23: 1283–1288, 1991.

88. **Perry CG, Talanian JL, Heigenhauser GJ, and Spriet LL.** The effects of training in hyperoxia vs. normoxia on skeletal muscle enzyme activities and exercise performance. *Journal of Applied Physiology: Respiratory, Environmental and Exercise Physiology* 102: 1022–1027, 2007.

89. **Pluim BM, de Hon O, Staal JB, Limpens J, Kuipers H, Overbeek SE, Zwinderman AH, and Scholten RJPM.** β_2-agonists and physcial performance: a systematic review and meta analysis of randomized controlled studies. *Sports Medicine* (Auckland, NZ) 41: 39–57, 2011.

90. **Pottgiesser T, Umhau M, Ahlgrim C, Ruthardt S, Roecker K, and Schumacher YO.** Hb mass measurement suitable to screen for illicit autologous blood transfusions. *Medicine and Science in Sports and Exercise* 39: 1748–1756, 2007.

91. **Powers SK, and Dodd S.** Caffeine and endurance performance. *Sports Medicine* (Auckland, NZ) 2: 165–174, 1985.

92. **Powers SK, Lawler J, Dempsey JA, Dodd S, and Landry G.** Effects of incomplete pulmonary gas exchange on $\dot{V}O_2$ max. *Journal of Applied Physiology: Respiratory, Environmental and Exercise Physiology* 66: 2491–2495, 1989.

93. **Price M, Moss P, and Rance S.** Effects of sodium bicarbonate ingestion on prolonged intermittent exercise. *Medicine and Science in Sports and Exercise* 35: 1303–1308, 2003.

94. **Price MJ, and Simons C.** The effect of sodium bicarbonate ingestion on high-intensity intermittent running and subsequent performance. *Journal of Strength and Conditioning Research* 24: 1834–1842, 2010.

95. **Rawson E, and Clarkson P.** Scientifically debatable: is creatine worth its weight? *Sports Science Exchange,* 2003.

96. **Rawson E, Coni M, and Miles M.** Creatine supplementation does not reduce muscle damage or enhance recovery from resistance exercise. *Journal of Strength and Conditioning Research* 21: 1208–1213, 2007.

97. **Rawson E, and Persky A.** Mechanisms of muscular adaptations to creatine supplementation. *Int Sport Med J* 8: 43–53, 2007.

98. **Rawson ES, Stec MJ, Frederickson SJ, and Miles MP.** Low-dose creatine supplementation enhances fatigue resistance in the absense of weight gain. *Nutrition* 27: 451–455, 2011.

99. **Requena B, Zabala M, and Padial P.** Sodium bicarbonate and sodium citrate: ergogenic aids? *Journal of Strength and Conditioning Research* 19: 213–224, 2005.

100. **Robbins MK, Gleeson K, and Zwillich CW.** Effect of oxygen breathing following submaximal and maximal exercise on recovery and performance. *Medicine and Science in Sports and Exercise* 24: 720–725, 1992.

101. **Robergs RA, Pascoe DD, Costill DL, Fink WJ, Chwalbinska-Moneta J, Davis JA, and Hickner R.** Effects of warm-up on muscle glycogenolysis during intense exercise. *Medicine and Science in Sports and Exercise* 23: 37–43, 1991.

102. **Rode A, and Shepard R.** The influence of cigarette smoking on the oxygen cost of breathing in near-maximal exercise. *Medicine and Science in Sports* 3: 51–55, 1971.

103. **Rogers M, Bohlken R, and Beets M.** Effects of creatine, ginseng, and astragalus supplementation on strength, body composition, mood, and blood lipids during strength-training in older adults. *Journal of Sports Science and Medicine* 5: 60–69, 2006.

104. **Rotstein A, Sagiv M, Yaniv-Tamir A, Fisher N, and Dotan R.** Smoking effect on exercise response kinetics of oxygen uptake and related variables. *International Journal of Sports Medicine* 12: 281–284, 1991.

105. **Roy BD, Bosman MJ, and Tarnopolsky MA.** An acute oral dose of caffeine does not alter glucose kinetics during prolonged dynamic exercise in trained endurance athletes. *European Journal of Applied Physiology* 85: 280–286, 2001.

106. **Rozenek R, Fobel B, and Banks J.** Does hyperbaric oxygen exposure affect high-intensity, short-duration exercise performance? *Journal of Strength and Conditioning Research* 21: 1037–1041, 2007.

107. **Schumacher YO, and Ashenden M.** Doping with artificial oxygen carriers: an update. *Sports Medicine* (Auckland, NZ) 34: 141–150, 2004.

108. **Shao A, and Hathcock JN.** Risk assessment for creatine monohydrate. *Regul Toxicol Pharmacol* 45: 242–251, 2006.

109. **Shrier I.** Special communications: letters to the editor-in-chief. *Medicine and Science in Sports and Exercise* 36: 1832–1833, 2004.

110. **Siegler JC, Midgley AW, Polman RCJ, and Lever R.** Effects of various sodium bicarbonate loading protocols on the time-dependent extracelluar buffering profile. *Journal of Strength and Conditioning Research* 24: 2551–2557, 2010.

111. **Spriet LL.** Caffeine and performance. *International Journal of Sport Nutrition* 5 Suppl: S84–99, 1995.

112. **Stellingwerff T, Glazier L, Watt MJ, LeBlanc PJ, Heigenhauser GJ, and Spriet LL.** Effects of hyperoxia on skeletal muscle carbohydrate metabolism during transient and steady-state exercise. *Journal of Applied Physiology: Respiratory, Environmental and Exercise Physiology* 98: 250–256, 2005.

113. **Tarnopolsky MA.** Effect of caffeine on the neuromuscular system: potential as an ergogenic aid. *Applied Physiology, Nutrition and Metabolism* 33: 1284–1289, 2008.

114. **Tarnopolsky MA, Atkinson SA, MacDougall JD, Sale DG, and Sutton JR.** Physiological responses to caffeine during endurance running in habitual caffeine users. *Medicine and Science in Sports and Exercise* 21: 418–424, 1989.

115. **Taylor P.** Ganglionic stimulating and blocking agents. In: *Goodman and Gilman's The Pharmacological Basis of Therapeutics,* edited by Gilman A, Goodman L, and Gilman A. New York: Macmillan, 1980.

116. **Tesch P, Sjodin B, Thorstensson A, and Karlsson J.** Muscle fatigue and its relation to lactate accumulation and LDH activity in man. *Acta Physiologica Scandinavica* 103: 413–420, 1978.

117. **Thacker SB, Gilchrist J, Stroup DF, and Kimsey CD, Jr.** The impact of stretching on sports injury risk: a systematic review of the literature. *Medicine and Science in Sports and Exercise* 36: 371–378, 2004.

118. **Trivedi B, and Danforth WH.** Effect of pH on the kinetics of frog muscle phosphofructokinase. *The Journal of Biological Chemistry* 241: 4110–4112, 1966.

119. **Van Handel P.** Caffeine. In: *Ergogenic Aids in Sports*, edited by Williams M. Champaign: Human Kinetics, 1983.

120. **Van Montfoort MC, Van Dieren L, Hopkins WG, and Shearman JP.** Effects of ingestion of bicarbonate, citrate, lactate, and chloride on sprint running. *Medicine and Science in Sports and Exercise* 36: 1239–1243, 2004.

121. **Van Thuyne W, and Delbeke FT.** Distribution of caffeine levels in urine in different sports in relation to doping control before and after the removal of caffeine from the WADA doping list. *International Journal of Sports Medicine* 27: 745–750, 2006.

122. **VanThuyne P, VanEenoo P, and Delbeke F.** Nutritional supplements: prevalence of use and contamination with doping agents. *Nutrition Research Reviews* 19: 147–158, 2006.

123. **Volek J.** What we now know about creatine. *ACSM's Health & Fitness Journal* 3: 27–33, 1999.

124. **Voss S, Thevis M, and Schinkothe T.** Detection of homologous blood transfusion. *International Journal of Sports Medicine* 28: 633–637, 2007.

125. **Warren GL, Park ND, Maresca RD, Mckibans KI, and Millard-Stafford ML.** Effect of caffeine ingestion on muscular strength and endurance: a meta-analysis. *Medicine and Science in Sports and Exercise* 42: 1375–1387, 2010.

126. **Welch H.** Effects of hypoxia and hyperoxia on human performance. In: *Exercise and Sports Sciences Reviews*, edited by Pandolf K. New York: Macmillan, 1987, p 191–222.

127. **Welch HG, Bonde-Petersen F, Graham T, Klausen K, and Secher N.** Effects of hyperoxia on leg blood flow and metabolism during exercise. *Journal of Applied Physiology: Respiratory, Environmental and Exercise Physiology* 42: 385–390, 1977.

128. **Weldon SM, and Hill RH.** The efficacy of stretching for prevention of exercise-related injury: a systematic review of the literature. *Manual Therapy* 8: 141–150, 2003.

129. **Wilcox A.** Bicarbonate loading. Gatorade Sports Science Institute, 1992.

130. **Wilcox A.** Caffeine and endurance performance. Gatorade Sports Science Institute, 1990.

131. **Wilcox A.** Nutritional ergogenics and sport performance. In: *The President's Council on Physical Fitness and Sports Research Digest*, edited by Corbin C, and Pangrazi B, Washington: Department of Health and Human Services, 1998.

132. **Williams MH, Wesseldine S, Somma T, and Schuster R.** The effect of induced erythrocythemia upon 5-mile treadmill run time. *Medicine and Science in Sports and Exercise* 13: 169–175, 1981.

133. **Wilmore J.** Oxygen. In: *Ergogenic Aids and Muscular Performance*, edited by Morgan W. New York: Academic Press, 1972, p. 321–342.

134. **Wilson GD, and Welch HG.** Effects of hyperoxic gas mixtures on exercise tolerance in man. *Med Sci Sports* 7: 48–52, 1975.

135. **Wilson GD, and Welch HG.** Effects of varying concentrations of N_2/O_2 and He/O_2 on exercise tolerance in man. *Medicine and Science in Sports and Exercise* 12: 380–384, 1980.

136. **Wilson GJ, Wilson JM, and Manninen AH.** Effects of beta-hydroxy-beta-methylbutyrate (HMB) on exercise performance and ody compostion across levels of age, sex, and training experience: a review. *Nutrition & Metabolism* 5: Article No. 1, 2008.

137. **Witvrouw E, Mahieu N, Danneels L, and McNair P.** Stretching and injury prevention: an obscure relationship. *Sports Medicine (Auckland, NZ)* 34: 443–449, 2004.

138. **World Anti-Doping Agency.** The 2011 Prohibited list: international standard. Switzerland: Author, 2010.

139. **Yang YT, and McElligott MA.** Multiple actions of beta-adrenergic agonists on skeletal muscle and adipose tissue. *The Biochemical Journal* 261: 1–10, 1989.

140. **Yeo SE, Jentjens RL, Wallis GA, and Jeukendrup AE.** Caffeine increases exogenous carbohydrate oxidation during exercise. *Journal of Applied Physiology: Respiratory, Environmental and Exercise Physiology* 99: 844–850, 2005.

141. **Zanchi NE, Gerlinger-Romero F, Guimaraes-Ferreira L, de Siqueira MA, Felitti V, Lira FS, Seelaender M, and Lancha AH.** HMB supplementation: clinical and athletic performance-related effects and mechanisms of action. *Amion Acids* 40: 1015–1025, 2011.

Glossary

absolute $\dot{V}O_2$ the amount of oxygen consumed over a given time period; expressed as liters $\cdot$ min^{-1}.

acclimation the change that occurs in response to repeated environmental stresses and results in the improved function of an existing homeostatic system. In general, acclimation is commonly used to refer to a rapid physiological adaptation that occurs within days to a few weeks.

acclimatization a gradual, long-term adaptation of an organism (e.g., humans) to a change in the environment (e.g., heat exposure). Acclimatization results in the improved function of an existing homeostatic system. Although acclimatization and acclimation are similar terms, acclimatization is often used to describe a gradual physiological adaptation that occurs within months to years of exposure to the environmental stress.

acidosis an abnormal increase in blood hydrogen ion concentration (i.e., arterial pH below 7.35).

acids compounds capable of giving up hydrogen ions into solution.

acromegaly a condition caused by hypersecretion of growth hormone from the pituitary gland; characterized by enlargement of the extremities, such as the jaw, nose, and fingers.

actin a structural protein of muscle that works with myosin in permitting muscular contraction.

action potential the all-or-none electrical event in the neuron or muscle cell in which the polarity of the cell membrane is rapidly reversed and then reestablished.

activation energy Energy required to initiate a chemical reaction. The term *activation energy* is sometimes referred to as the *energy of activation*.

adenosine diphosphate (ADP) a molecule that combines with inorganic phosphate to form ATP.

adenosine triphosphate (ATP) the high-energy phosphate compound synthesized and used by cells to release energy for cellular work.

adenylate cyclase enzyme found in cell membranes that catalyzes the conversion of ATP to cyclic AMP.

adequate intake (AI) recommendations for nutrient intake when insufficient information is available to set an RDA standard.

adrenal cortex the outer portion of the adrenal gland. Synthesizes and secretes corticosteroid hormones, such as cortisol, aldosterone, and androgens.

adrenaline *see* epinephrine.

adrenocorticotrophic hormone (ACTH) a hormone secreted by the anterior pituitary gland that stimulates the adrenal cortex.

aerobic in the presence of oxygen.

afferent fibers nerve fibers (sensory fibers) that carry neural information back to the central nervous system.

afferent neuron sensory neuron carrying information toward the central nervous system.

aldosterone a corticosteroid hormone involved in the regulation of electrolyte balance.

alkalosis an abnormal increase in blood concentration of OH$^-$ ions, resulting in a rise in arterial pH above 7.45.

alpha receptors a subtype of adrenergic receptors located on cell membranes of selected tissues.

alveolar ventilation ($\dot{V}_A$) the volume of gas that reaches the alveolar region of the lung.

alveoli microscopic air sacs located in the lung where gas exchange occurs between respiratory gases and the blood.

amenorrhea the absence of menses.

AMPK (5'adenosine monophosphate activated protein kinase) an important signaling molecule that is activated during exercise due to changes in muscle fiber phosphate/energy levels. AMPK regulates numerous energy producing pathways in muscle by stimulating glucose uptake and fatty acid oxidation during exercise and is also linked to the control of muscle gene expression by activating transcription factors associated with fatty acid

oxidation and mitochondrial biogenesis.

anabolic steroid a prescription drug that has anabolic, or growth-stimulating, characteristics similar to that of the male androgen, testosterone.

anaerobic without oxygen.

anaerobic threshold a commonly used term meant to describe the level of oxygen consumption at which there is a rapid and systematic increase in blood lactate concentration. Also termed the *lactate threshold*.

anatomical dead space the total volume of the lung (i.e., conducting airways) that does not participate in gas exchange.

androgenic steroid a compound that has the qualities of an androgen; associated with masculine characteristics.

androgens male sex hormones. Synthesized in the testes and in limited amounts in the adrenal cortex. Steroids that have masculinizing effects.

angina pectoris chest pain due to a lack of blood flow (ischemia) to the myocardium.

angiotensin I and II these compounds are polypeptides formed from the cleavage of a protein (angiotensinogen) by the action of the enzyme renin produced by the kidneys, and converting enzyme in the lung, respectively.

anorexia nervosa an eating disorder characterized by rapid weight loss due to failure to consume adequate amounts of nutrients.

anterior hypothalamus the anterior portion of the hypothalamus. The hypothalamus is an area of the brain below the thalamus that regulates the autonomic nervous system and the pituitary gland.

anterior pituitary the anterior portion of the pituitary gland that secretes follicle-stimulating hormone, luteinizing hormone, adrenocorticotrophic hormone, thyroid-stimulating hormone, growth hormone, and prolactin.

antidiuretic hormone (ADH) hormone secreted by the posterior pituitary gland that promotes water retention by the kidney.

aortic bodies receptors located in the arch of the aorta that are capable of detecting changes in arterial PO_2.

apophyses sites of muscle-tendon insertion in bones.

arrhythmia abnormal electrical activity in the heart (e.g., a premature ventricular contraction).

arteries large vessels that carry arterialized blood away from the heart.

arterioles a small branch of an artery that communicates with a capillary network.

articular cartilage cartilage that covers the ends of bones in a synovial joint.

atherosclerosis a pathological condition in which fatty substances collect in the layer (intima) of arteries.

atmospheric pressure Downward force exerted in the earth's surface due to the weight of the air above that point.

ATPase enzyme capable of breaking down ATP to ADP + P_i + energy.

ATP-PC system term used to describe the metabolic pathway involving muscle stores of ATP and the use of phosphocreatine to rephosphorylate ADP. This pathway is used at the onset of exercise and during short-term, high-intensity work.

atrioventricular node (AV node) a specialized mass of muscle tissue located in the interventricular septum of the heart; functions in the transmission of cardiac impulses from the atria to the ventricles.

autocrine signaling signaling that occurs when a cell produces and releases a chemical messenger into the extracellular fluid that acts upon the cell producing the signal. The autocrine agent refers to the chemical messenger that is released by the cell.

autologous transfusion blood transfusion whereby the individual receives his or her own blood.

autonomic nervous system portion of the nervous system that controls the actions of visceral organs.

autoregulation mechanism by which an organ regulates blood flow to match the metabolic rate.

axon a nerve fiber that conducts a nerve impulse away from the neuron cell body.

basal metabolic rate (BMR) metabolic rate measured in supine position following a 12-hour fast, and 8 hours of sleep.

bases compounds that ionize in water to release hydroxyl ions (OH^-) or other ions that are capable of combining with hydrogen ions.

beta oxidation breakdown of free fatty acids to form acetyl-CoA.

beta receptor agonist (β-agonist) a molecule that is capable of binding to and activating a beta receptor.

beta receptors adrenergic receptors located on cell membranes. Combine mainly with epinephrine and, to some degree, with norepinephrine.

bioenergetics the chemical processes involved with the production of cellular ATP.

biological control systems a control system capable of maintaining homeostasis within a cell or organ system in a living creature.

blood boosting a term that applies to the increase of the blood's hemoglobin concentration by the infusion of additional red blood cells. Medically termed *induced erythrocythemiu*.

blood doping *see* blood boosting.

blood packing *see* blood boosting.

Bohr effect the right shift of the oxyhemoglobin dissociation curve due to a decrease of blood pH. Results in a decreased affinity for oxygen.

bradycardia a resting heart rate less than 60 beats per minute.

brain stem portion of the brain that includes midbrain, pons, and medulla.

buffer a compound that resists pH change.

bulimia an eating disorder characterized by eating and forced regurgitation.

bulk flow mass movement of molecules from an area of high pressure to an area of lower pressure.

calcitonin hormone, released from the thyroid gland, that plays a minor role in calcium metabolism.

calciuneurin a phosphatase activated by increases in cytosolic calcium; it participates in several adaptive responses in muscle, including fiber growth/regeneration and the fast-to-slow fiber type transition that occurs as a result of exercise training.

calmodulin Calmodulin-dependent kinase (CaMK) is activated during exercise in an intensity-related manner. This important kinase exerts influence on exercise-induced muscle adaptation by contributing to the activation of PCG-1α. The primary upstream signal to activate CaMK is increased cytosolic calcium levels.

capillaries microscopic blood vessels that connect arterioles and venules. Portion of vascular system where blood/tissue gas exchange occurs.

cardiac accelerator nerves part of the sympathetic nervous system that stimulates the SA node to increase heart rate.

cardiac output the amount of blood pumped by the heart per unit of time; equal to product of heart rate and stroke volume.

cardiovascular control center the area of the medulla that regulates the cardiovascular system.

carotid bodies chemoreceptors located in the internal carotid artery; respond to changes in arterial PO_2, PCO_2, and pH.

catecholamines organic compounds, including epinephrine, norepinephrine, and dopamine.

cell body the soma, or major portion of the body of a nerve cell. Contains the nucleus.

cell membrane the lipid-bilayer envelope that encloses cells. Called the *sarcolemma* in muscle cells.

cell signaling a system of communication that governs cellular activities and coordinates cell actions. Cell signaling can occur via numerous signaling pathways, including direct contact of cells.

cellular respiration process of oxygen consumption and carbon dioxide production in cells (i.e., bioenergetics).

central command the control of the cardiovascular or pulmonary system by cortical impulses.

central fatigue factors located prior to the neuromuscular junction that impair the force generating capacity of muscle.

central nervous system (CNS) portion of the nervous system that consists of the brain and spinal cord.

cerebellum portion of the brain that is concerned with fine coordination of skeletal muscles during movement.

cerebrum superior aspect of the brain that occupies the upper cranial cavity. Contains the motor cortex.

chemiosmotic hypothesis the mechanism to explain the aerobic formation of ATP in mitochondria.

cholesterol a 27-carbon lipid that can be synthesized in cells or consumed in the diet. Cholesterol serves as a precursor of steroid hormones, and plays a role in the development of atherosclerosis.

clo unit that describes the insulation quality of clothing.

complement system part of the innate immune system; it forms a second line of defense against infection .The more than twenty proteins that make up the complement system are present in high concentrations in the blood and tissues. When the body is exposed to a foreign agent (e.g. bacterium), the complement system is activated to attack the invader.

concentric action occurs when a muscle is activated and shortens.

conduction transfer of heat from warmer to cooler objects that are in contact with each other. This term may also be used in association with the conveyance of neural impulses.

conduction disturbances refers to a slowing or blockage of the wave of depolarization in the heart, e.g., first-degree AV block, or bundle branch block.

conductivity capacity for conduction.

convection the transmission of heat from one object to another through the circulation of heated molecules.

Cori cycle the cycle of lactate-to-glucose between the muscle and liver.

coronary artery bypass graft surgery (CABGS) the replacement of a blocked coronary artery with another vessel to permit blood flow to the myocardium.

cortisol a glucocorticoid secreted by the adrenal cortex upon stimulation by ACTH.

coupled reactions the linking of energy-liberating chemical reactions to "drive" energy-requiring reactions.

critical power a specific submaximal power output that can be maintained without fatigue.

cromolyn sodium a drug used to stabilize the membranes of mast cells and prevent an asthma attack.

cycle ergometer a stationary exercise cycle that allows accurate measurement of work output.

cyclic AMP a substance produced from ATP through the action of adenylate cyclase that alters several chemical processes in the cell.

cytokines hormone messengers that regulate the immune system by facilitating communication with other cells within the immune system.

cytoplasm the contents of the cell surrounding the nucleus. Called *sarcoplasm* in muscle cells.

Daily Value a standard used in nutritional labeling.

deficiency a shortcoming of some essential nutrient.

degenerative diseases diseases not due to infection that result in a progressive decline in some bodily function.

delayed-onset muscle soreness (DOMS) muscle soreness that occurs 12 to 24 hours after an exercise bout.

dendrites portion of the nerve fiber that transmits action potentials toward a nerve cell body.

dental caries tooth decay; related to sugar content in foods.

deoxyhemoglobin hemoglobin not in combination with oxygen.

diabetes mellitus a condition characterized by high blood glucose levels due to inadequate insulin. Type I diabetics are insulin dependent, whereas Type II diabetics are resistant to insulin.

diabetic coma unconscious state induced by a lack of insulin.

diacylglycerol a molecule derived from a membrane-bound phospholipid, phosphatidylinositol, that activates protein kinase C and alters cellular activity.

diaphragm the major respiratory muscle responsible for inspiration. Dome-shaped—separates the thoracic cavity from the abdominal cavity.

diastole period of filling of the heart between contractions (i.e., resting phase of the heart).

diastolic blood pressure arterial blood pressure during diastole.

Dietary Guidelines for Americans general statements related to food selection that are consistent with achieving and maintaining good health.

Dietary Reference Intakes the framework for nutrient recommendations being made as a part of the revision of the 1989 RDA.

diffusion random movement of molecules from an area of high concentration to an area of low concentration.

direct calorimetry assessment of the body's metabolic rate by direct measurement of the amount of heat produced.

dose the amount of drug or exercise prescribed to have a certain effect (or response).

double-blind research design an experimental design in which the subjects and the principal investigator are not aware of the experimental treatment order.

double product the product of heart rate and systolic blood pressure; estimate of work of the heart.

dynamic refers to an isotonic muscle action.

dynamic stretching stretching that involves controlled movement.

dynamometer device used to measure force production (e.g., used in the measurement of muscular strength).

dysmenorrhea painful menstruation.

dyspnea shortness of breath or labored breathing. May be due to various types of lung or heart diseases.

eccentric action occurs when a muscle is activated and force is produced but the muscle lengthens.

ectomorphy category of somatotype that is rated for linearity of body form.

effect change in variable (e.g., $\dot{V}O_2$ max) due to a dose of exercise (e.g.,

3 days per week, 40 min/day at 70% $\dot{V}O_2$ max).

effector organ or body part that responds to stimulation by an efferent neuron (e.g., skeletal muscle in a withdrawal reflex).

efferent fibers nerve fibers (motor fibers) that carry neural information from the central nervous system to the periphery.

efferent neuron conducts impulses from the CNS to the effector organ (e.g., motor neuron).

ejection fraction the proportion of end-diastolic volume that is ejected during a ventricular contraction.

electrocardiogram (ECG) a recording of the electrical changes that occur in the myocardium during the cardiac cycle.

electron transport chain a series of cytochromes in the mitochondria that are responsible for oxidative phosphorylation.

element a single chemical substance composed of only one type of atom (e.g., calcium or potassium).

endergonic reactions energy-requiring reactions.

endocrine gland a gland that produces and secretes its products directly into the blood or interstitial fluid (ductless glands).

endocrine signaling occurs when cells release chemical signals (hormones) into the blood, which are carried in the blood to all tissues in the body. However, only the cells with a receptor to which the hormone can bind will respond.

endomorphy the somatotype category that is rated for roundness (fatness).

endomysium the inner layer of connective tissue surrounding a muscle fiber.

endorphin a neuropeptide produced by the pituitary gland having pain-suppressing activity.

end-plate potential (EPP) depolarization of a membrane region by a sodium influx.

energy of activation energy required to initiate a chemical reaction.

energy wasteful systems metabolic pathways in which the energy generated in one reaction is used up in another that leads back to the first, creating a futile cycle and requiring a higher resting metabolic rate.

enzymes proteins that lower the energy of activation and, therefore, catalyze chemical reactions. Enzymes regulate the rate of most metabolic pathways.

epidemiology the study of the distribution and determinants of health-related states or events in specified populations, and the application of this study to the control of health problems.

epilepsy a neurological disorder manifested by muscular seizures.

epimysium the outer layer of connective tissue surrounding muscle.

epinephrine a hormone synthesized by the adrenal medulla; also called *adrenaline*.

epiphyseal plate (growth plate) cartilaginous layer between the head and shaft of a long bone where growth takes place.

EPOC an acronym for "excess post-exercise oxygen consumption"; often referred to as the *oxygen debt*.

EPSP excitatory post-synaptic potential. A graded depolarization of a post-synaptic membrane by a neurotransmitter.

ergogenic aid a substance, appliance, or procedure (e.g., blood doping) that improves performance.

ergometer instrument for measuring work.

ergometry measurement of work output.

erythrocythemia an increase in the number of erythrocytes in the blood.

erythropoietin hormone that stimulates red blood cell production.

Estimated Average Requirement (EAR) the average daily nutrient intake level estimated to meet the requirement of half the healthy individuals in a particular group. This value is needed to set the RDA values.

estrogens female sex hormones, including estradiol and estrone. Produced primarily in the ovary and also produced in the adrenal cortex.

evaporation the change of water from a liquid form to a vapor form. Results in the removal of heat.

exercise a subclass of physical activity.

exergonic reactions chemical reactions that release energy.

extensors muscles that extend a limb—that is, increase the angle at a joint.

FAD flavin adenine dinucleotide. Serves as an electron carrier in bioenergetics.

fasciculi a small bundle of muscle fibers.

fast-twitch fibers one of several types of muscle fibers found in skeletal muscle; also called Type II fibers; characterized as having low oxidative capacity but high glycolytic capacity.

female athlete triad a syndrome in which amenorrhea, eating disorders, and bone mineral loss are collectively present.

ferritin the iron-carrying molecule used as an index of whole-body iron status.

field test a test of physical performance performed in the field (outside the laboratory).

flexors muscle groups that cause flexion of limbs—that is, decrease the angle at a joint.

follicle-stimulating hormone (FSH) a hormone secreted by the anterior pituitary gland that stimulates the development of an ovarian follicle in the female and the production of sperm in the male.

food records the practice of keeping dietary food records for determining nutrient intake.

free fatty acid (FFA) a type of fat that combines with glycerol to form triglycerides. Is used as an energy source.

free radicals highly reactive molecules that contain an unpaired electron in their outer orbital.

G protein the link between the hormone-receptor interaction on the surface of the membrane and the subsequent events inside the cell.

gain refers to the amount of correction that a control system is capable of achieving.

General Adaptation Syndrome (GAS) a term defined by Selye in 1936 that describes the organism's response to chronic stress. In response to stress the organism has a three-stage response: (1) alarm reaction; (2) stage of resistance; and (3) readjustment to the stress, or exhaustion.

glucagon a hormone produced by the pancreas that increases blood glucose and free fatty acid levels.

glucocorticoids any one of a group of hormones produced by the adrenal cortex that influences carbohydrate, fat, and protein metabolism.

gluconeogenesis the synthesis of glucose from amino acids, lactate, glycerol, and other short carbon-chain molecules.

glucose a simple sugar that is transported via the blood and metabolized by tissues.

glucose polymer a complex sugar molecule that contains multiple simple sugar molecules linked together.

glycogen a glucose polymer synthesized in cells as a means of storing carbohydrate.

glycogenolysis the breakdown of glycogen into glucose.

glycolysis a metabolic pathway in the cytoplasm of the cell that results in the degradation of glucose into pyruvate or lactate.

Golgi tendon organ (GTOs) a tension receptor located in series with skeletal muscle.

graded exercise test *see* incremental exercise test.

gross efficiency a simple measure of exercise efficiency defined as the ratio of work performed to energy expended, expressed as a percent.

growth hormone hormone synthesized and secreted by the anterior pituitary that stimulates growth of the skeleton and soft tissues during the growing years. It is also involved in the mobilization of the body's energy stores.

HDL cholesterol (high-density lipoprotein cholesterol) cholesterol that is transported in the blood via high-density proteins; related to low risk of heart disease.

heat cramps painful muscle cramps in the abdomen, legs, or arms following strenuous activity in the heat; use direct pressure on cramps, stretch muscles, and gentle ice massage

heat exhaustion symptoms include heavy sweating, rapid pulse, dizziness, and nausea; it is linked to dehydration and can develop into heatstroke. Move to cool or shaded area, place in supine position with legs raised, and provide fluids and cooling.

heat shock proteins an important family of stress proteins that are produced in cells in response to cellular stresses. Following synthesis, heatshock protein can protect cells against disturbances in homeostasis.

heatstroke (also called exertional heatstroke) a life-threatening heat illness in which body temperature is extremely elevated (104 °F or 40 °C); possibility of central nervous system disturbances and organ failure. Rapid whole-body cooling measures should be initiated immediately; treat as medical emergency.

heat syncope sudden dizziness or fainting during or after exercising in the heat related to a drop in blood pressure; may be accompanied by feelings of excessive thirst, fatigue, headache, nausea, and vomiting. Move to cool area and provide fluids.

hemoglobin a heme-containing protein in red blood cells that is responsible for transporting oxygen to tissues. Hemoglobin also serves as a weak buffer within red blood cells.

high-density lipoproteins (HDL) proteins used to transport cholesterol in blood; high levels appear to offer some protection from atherosclerosis.

homeostasis the maintenance of a constant internal environment.

homeotherms animals that maintain a fairly constant internal temperature.

homologous transfusion a blood transfusion using blood of the same type but from another donor.

hormone a chemical substance that is synthesized and released by an endocrine gland and transported to a target organ via the blood.

hydrogen ion (H^+) a free hydrogen ion in solution that results in a decrease in pH of the solution.

hyperbaric chamber chamber where the absolute pressure is increased above atmospheric pressure.

hyperoxia oxygen concentration in an inspired gas that exceeds 21%.

hyperplasia an increase in the number of cells in a tissue.

hyperthermia elevated body temperature due to heat loss not keeping up with heat load from exercise and the environment; linked to heat illnesses.

hypertrophy an increase in cell size.

hypothalamic somatostatin hypothalamic hormone that inhibits growth hormone secretion.

hypothalamus brain structure that integrates many physiological functions to maintain homeostasis; site of secretion of hormones released by the posterior pituitary; also releases hormones that control anterior pituitary secretions.

hypothermia decreased body temperature due to heat loss being greater than heat production; defined clinically as body temperature below 35°C.

hypoxia a relative lack of oxygen (e.g., at altitude).

IGF-1/Akt/mTOR signaling pathway a pathway that plays an important role in the regulation of muscle growth (i.e., protein synthesis) resulting from resistance training. Contractile activity (i.e., muscle stretch) stimulates the secretion of IGF-1 from the active muscle fibers, which acts as an autocrine/paracrine signaling molecule, binding to its membrane receptor and initiating a cascade of molecular events to promote muscle protein synthesis. Binding of IGF-1 to its receptor on the muscle membrane activates the important signaling kinase, Akt. Active Akt then activates another downstream kinase called *mammalian target of rapamycin* (mTOR), which then promotes protein synthesis by improving translational efficiency.

immunity refers to all the mechanisms used in the body to protect against environmental agents that are foreign to the body. Immunity is achieved by a precise coordination of the innate and acquired immune system.

immunotherapy procedure in which the body is exposed to specific substances to elicit an immune response in order to offer better protection upon subsequent exposure.

incremental exercise test an exercise test involving a progressive increase in work rate over time. Often graded exercise tests are used to determine the subject's $\dot{V}O_2$ max or lactate threshold. (Also called *graded exercise test.*)

indirect calorimetry estimation of heat or energy production on the basis of oxygen consumption, carbon dioxide production, and nitrogen excretion.

induced erythrocythemia causing an elevation of the red blood cell (hemoglobin) concentration by infusing blood; also called *blood doping* or *blood boosting.*

infectious diseases diseases due to the presence of pathogenic microorganisms in the body (e.g., viruses, bacteria, fungi, and protozoa).

inflammation part of the complex biological response to harmful stimuli such as bacteria entering the body through a wound in the skin, damaged cells, or other irritants. Clinical signs of local inflammation are redness, swelling, heat, and pain around the injured tissue.

inorganic relating to substances that do not contain carbon (C).

inorganic phosphate (P_i) a stimulator of cellular metabolism; split off, along with ADP, from ATP when energy is released; used with ADP to form ATP in the electron transport chain.

inositol triphosphate a molecule derived from a membrane-bound phospholipid, phosphatidylinositol, that causes calcium release from intracellular stores and alters cellular activity.

insulin hormone released from the beta cells of the islets of Langerhans in response to elevated blood glucose and amino acid concentrations; increases tissue uptake of both.

insulin-like growth factors groups of growth-stimulating peptides released from the liver and other tissues in response to growth hormone.

insulin shock condition brought on by too much insulin, which causes an immediate hypoglycemia; symptoms include tremors, dizziness, and possibly convulsions.

integrating center the portion of a biological control system that processes the information from the receptors and issues an appropriate response relative to its set point.

intercalated discs portion of cardiac muscle cell where one cell connects to the next.

intermediate fibers muscle fiber type that generates high force at a moderately fast speed of contraction, but has a relatively large number of mitochondria (Type IIa).

intracrine signaling a hormone that acts inside a cell. Steroid hormones act through intracellular (mostly nuclear) receptors and, thus, are considered to be intracrines. In contrast, peptide or protein hormones, in general, act as endocrines, autocrines, or paracrines by binding to their receptors present on the cell surface.

ion a single atom or small molecule containing a net positive or negative charge due to an excess of either protons or electrons, respectively (e.g., Na^+, Cl^-).

IPSP inhibitory post-synaptic potential that moves the post-synaptic membrane farther from threshold.

irritability a trait of certain tissues that enables them to respond to stimuli (e.g., nerve and muscle).

isocitrate dehydrogenase rate-limiting enzyme in the Krebs cycle that is inhibited by ATP and stimulated by ADP and P_i.

isokinetic action in which the rate of movement is constantly maintained through a specific range of motion even though maximal force is exerted.

isometric action in which the muscle develops tension, but does not shorten; also called a *static contraction.* No movement occurs.

isotonic contraction in which a muscle shortens against a constant load or tension, resulting in movement.

juxtracrine signaling a type of cell signaling that occurs between two adjacent cells that are in direct contact via a junction across the cell membrane that connects the cytoplasm of the two cells.

ketosis acidosis of the blood caused by the production of ketone bodies (e.g., acetoacetic acid) when fatty acid mobilization is increased, as in uncontrolled diabetes.

kilocalorie (kcal) a measure of energy expenditure equal to the heat needed to raise the temperature of 1 kg of water 1 degree Celsius; also equal to 1,000 calories and sometimes written as calorie rather than kilocalorie.

kilogram-meter   a unit of work in which 1 kg of force (1 kg mass accelerated at 1 G) is moved through a vertical distance of 1 meter; abbreviated as kg-m, kg · m, or kgm.

kinesthesia   a perception of movement obtained from information about the position and rate of movement of the joints.

Krebs cycle   metabolic pathway in the mitochondria in which energy is transferred from carbohydrates, fats, and amino acids to NAD for subsequent production of ATP in the electron transport chain.

lactate   a 3-carbon molecule that is a potential end-product of glucose metabolism.

lactate threshold   a point during a graded exercise test when the blood lactate concentration increases abruptly.

lateral sac   *see* terminal cisternae.

LDL cholesterol   form of low-density lipoprotein responsible for the transport of plasma cholesterol; high levels are indicative of a high risk of coronary heart disease.

lipase   an enzyme responsible for the breakdown of triglycerides to free fatty acids and glycerol.

lipolysis   the breakdown of triglycerides in adipose tissue to free fatty acids and glycerol for subsequent transport to tissues for metabolism.

lipoprotein   protein involved in the transport of cholesterol and triglycerides in the plasma.

low-density lipoproteins (LDL)   form of lipoprotein that transports a majority of the plasma cholesterol; *see* LDL cholesterol.

low-grade chronic inflammation   characterized by a two- to three-fold increase in inflammatory cytokines (e.g., tumor necrosis factor alpha [TNF-α] and Interleukin-6 [IL-6]) and C-reactive protein (CRP).

luteinizing hormone (LH)   also called "interstitial cell stimulating hormone"; a surge of LH stimulates ovulation in middle of menstrual cycle; LH stimulates testosterone production in men.

macrophages   phagocytes that engulf and kill invading bacteria. Macrophages are considered to be a portion of the innate immune system.

major minerals   dietary minerals including calcium, phosphorus, potassium, sulfur, sodium, chloride, and magnesium.

mast cell   connective tissue cell that releases histamine and other

chemicals in response to certain stimuli (e.g., injury).

maximal oxygen uptake ($\dot{V}O_2$ max)   greatest rate of oxygen uptake by the body measured during severe dynamic exercise, usually on a cycle ergometer or a treadmill; dependent on maximal cardiac output and the maximal arteriovenous oxygen difference.

mesomorphy   one component of a somatotype that characterizes the muscular form or lean body mass aspect of the human body.

MET   an expression of the rate of energy expenditure at rest; equal to 3.5 ml · kg^{-1} · min^{-1}, or 1 kcal · kg^{-1} · hr^{-1}.

metabolism   the total of all cellular reactions that occur in cells and includes chemical pathways that result in the synthesis of molecules (anabolic reactions) as well as the breakdown of molecules (catabolic reactions).

mineralocorticoids   steroid hormones released from the adrenal cortex that are responsible for Na^+ and K^+ regulation (e.g., aldosterone).

mitochondrion   the subcellular organelle responsible for the production of ATP with oxygen; contains the enzymes for the Krebs cycle, electron transport chain, and the fatty acid cycle.

mixed venous blood   a mixture of venous blood from both the upper and lower extremities; complete mixing occurs in the right ventricle.

molecular biology   branch of biochemistry involved with the study of gene structure and function.

motor cortex   portion of the cerebral cortex containing large motor neurons whose axons descend to lower brain centers and spinal cord; associated with the voluntary control of movement.

motor neuron   the somatic neuron that innervates skeletal muscle fibers (also called an *alpha motor neuron*).

motor unit   a motor neuron and all the muscle fibers innervated by that single motor neuron; responds in an "all-or-none" manner to a stimulus.

muscle action   term used to describe the muscle movement (e.g., shortening versus lengthening).

muscle spindle   a muscle stretch receptor oriented parallel to skeletal muscle fibers; the capsule portion is surrounded by afferent fibers, and intrafusal muscle fibers can alter the length of the capsule during muscle contraction and relaxation.

muscular strength   the maximal amount of force that can be generated by a muscle or muscle group.

myocardial infarction   death of a portion of heart tissue that no longer conducts electrical activity nor provides force to move blood.

myocardial ischemia   a condition in which the myocardium experiences an inadequate blood flow; sometimes accompanied by irregularities in the electrocardiogram (arrhythmias and ST-segment depression) and chest pain (angina pectoris).

myocardium   cardiac muscle; provides the force of contraction to eject blood; muscle type with many mitochondria that is dependent on a constant supply of oxygen.

myofibrils   the portion of the muscle containing the thick and thin contractile filaments; a series of sarcomeres where the repeating pattern of the contractile proteins gives the striated appearance to skeletal muscle.

myoglobin   protein in muscle that can bind oxygen and release it at low PO_2 values; aids in diffusion of oxygen from capillary to mitochondria.

myosin   contractile protein in the thick filament of a myofibril that contains the cross-bridge that can bind actin and split ATP to cause tension development.

NAD   coenzyme that transfers hydrogen and the energy associated with those hydrogens; in the Krebs cycle, NAD transfers energy from substrates to the electron transport chain.

natural killer cells   an important part of the innate immune system because they are versatile "killers" of foreign agents, including bacteria, viruses, cancer cells, and other unwanted invaders of the body.

negative feedback   describes the response from a control system that reduces the size of the stimulus, e.g., an elevated blood glucose concentration causes the secretion of insulin which, in turn, lowers the blood glucose concentration.

net efficiency   the mathematical ratio of work output divided by the energy expended above rest.

neuroendocrinology   study of the role of the nervous and endocrine systems in the automatic regulation of the internal environment.

neuromuscular junction   synapse between axon terminal of a motor neuron and the motor end plate of a muscle's plasma membrane.

neuron   nerve cell; composed of a cell body with dendrites (projections) that bring information to the cell body, and axons that take information away from the cell body to influence neurons, glands, or muscles.

neutrophils short-lived leukocytes that participate in phagocytosis of bacteria.

NFκB nuclear factor kappa B is a transcriptional activator that promotes the expression of several antioxidant enzymes that protect muscle fibers against free-radical mediated injury.

nitroglycerin drug used to reduce chest pain (angina pectoris) due to lack of blood flow to the myocardium.

norepinephrine a hormone and neurotransmitter; released from postganglionic nerve endings and the adrenal medulla.

normocythemia a normal red blood cell concentration.

normoxia a normal PO_2.

nucleus membrane-bound organelle containing most of the cell's DNA.

nutrient density the degree to which foods contain selected nutrients, e.g., protein, relative to the number of kilocalories.

open-circuit spirometry indirect calorimetry procedure in which either inspired or expired ventilation is measured and oxygen consumption and carbon dioxide production are calculated.

organic describes substances that contain carbon.

osteoporosis a decrease in bone density due to a loss of cortical bone; common in older women and implicated in fractures; estrogen, exercise, and Ca^{++} therapy are used to correct the condition.

overload a principle of training describing the need to increase the load (intensity) of exercise to cause a further adaptation of a system.

overtraining an accumulation of training stress that impairs an athlete's ability to perform training sessions and results in long-term decrements of performance.

oxidative phosphorylation mitochondrial process in which inorganic phosphate (P_i) is coupled to ADP as energy is transferred along the electron transport chain in which oxygen is the final electron acceptor.

oxygen debt the elevated post-exercise oxygen consumption (see EPOC); related to replacement of creatine phosphate, lactate resynthesis to glucose, and elevated body temperature, catecholamines, heart rate, breathing, etc.

oxygen deficit refers to the lag in oxygen uptake at the beginning of exercise.

oxyhemoglobin hemoglobin combined with oxygen; 1.34 ml of oxygen can combine with 1 g Hb.

p38 mitogen activated kinase p38 (p38) is an important signaling molecule that is activated in muscle fibers during endurance exercise. Once activated, p38 can contribute to mitochondrial biogenesis by activating PGC-1α.

pancreas gland containing both exocrine and endocrine portions; exocrine secretions include enzymes and bicarbonate to digest food in the small intestine; endocrine secretions include insulin, glucagon, and somatostatin, which are released into the blood.

paracrine signaling occurs when signals produced by cells act locally on nearby cells to bring about cellular responses.

parasympathetic nervous system portion of the autonomic nervous system that primarily releases acetylcholine from its postganglionic nerve endings.

partial pressure the fractional part of the barometric pressure due to the presence of a single gas, e.g., PO_2, PCO_2, and PN_2.

percent grade a measure of the elevation of the treadmill; calculated as the sine of the angle.

percutaneous transluminal coronary angioplasty (PTCA) a balloon-tipped catheter is inserted into a blocked coronary artery and plaque is pushed back to artery wall to open the blood vessel.

perimysium the connective tissue surrounding the fasciculus of skeletal muscle fibers.

peripheral fatigue factors located after the neuromuscular junctions that impair the force generating capacity of muscle (also called *muscular fatigue*).

peripheral nervous system (PNS) portion of the nervous system located outside the spinal cord and brain.

PGC-1α (peroxisome proliferator-activated receptor-gamma coactivator 1α (PGC-1α) an important signaling molecule activated by endurance exercise and is considered the master regulator of mitochondrial biogenesis in cells.

pH a measure of the acidity of a solution; calculated as the negative $\log_{10}$ of the $[H^+]$ in which 7 is neutral; values that are >7 are basic and <7 are acidic.

phagocytes cells that eat (engulf) foreign agents, such as bacteria.

phosphocreatine a compound found in skeletal muscle and used to resynthesize ATP from ADP.

phosphodiesterase an enzyme that catalyzes the breakdown of cyclic AMP, moderating the effect of the hormonal stimulation of adenylate cyclase.

phosphofructokinase rate-limiting enzyme in glycolysis that is responsive to ADP, P_i, and ATP levels in the cytoplasm of the cell.

phospholipase C membrane-bound enzyme that hydrolyzes phosphatidylinositol into inositol triphosphate and diacylglycerol that, in turn, bring about changes in intracellular activity.

physical activity characterizes all types of human movement; associated with living, work, play, and exercise.

physical fitness a broad term describing healthful levels of cardio-vascular function, strength, and flexibility; fitness is specific to the activities performed.

pituitary gland a gland at the base of the hypothalamus of the brain having an anterior portion that produces and secretes numerous hormones that regulate other endocrine glands and a posterior portion that secretes hormones that are produced in the hypothalamus.

placebo an inert substance that is used in experimental studies, e.g., drug studies, to control for any subjective reaction to the substance being tested.

pleura a thin lining of cells that is attached to the inside of the chest wall and to the lung; the cells secrete a fluid that facilitates the movements of the lungs in the thoracic cavity.

posterior hypothalamus area of the brain responsible for regulation of the body's response to a decrease in temperature.

posterior pituitary gland portion of the pituitary gland secreting oxytocin and antidiuretic hormone (vasopressin) that are produced in the hypothalamus.

power a rate of work; work per unit time; $P = W/t$.

power test a test measuring the quantity of work accomplished in a time period; anaerobic power tests include the Margaria stair climb test and the Wingate test; aerobic power tests include the 1.5-mile run and cycle ergometer and treadmill tests in which power output and oxygen consumption are measured.

primary risk factor a sign (e.g., high blood pressure) or a behavior (e.g., cigarette smoking) that is directly related to the appearance of certain diseases independent of other risk factors.

progressive resistance exercise (PRE) a training program in which the muscles must work against a gradually increasing resistance; an implementation of the overload principle.

prolactin hormone secreted from the anterior pituitary that increases milk production from the breast.

proprioceptive neuromuscular facilitation technique of preceding a static stretch with an isometric contraction.

proprioceptors receptors that provide information about the position and movement of the body; includes muscle and joint receptors as well as the receptors in the semicircular canals of the inner ear.

protein kinase C part of second messenger system that is activated by diacylglycerol and results in the activation of proteins in the cell.

provitamin a precursor of a vitamin.

pulmonary circuit the portion of the cardiovascular system involved in the circulation of blood from the right ventricle to the lungs and back to the left atrium.

pulmonary respiration term that refers to ventilation (breathing) of the lung.

Quebec 10-second test a maximal effort 10-second cycle test designed to assess ultra short-term anaerobic power during cycling.

radiation process of energy exchange from the surface of one object to the surface of another that is dependent on a temperature gradient but does not require contact between the objects; an example is the transfer of heat from the sun to the earth.

receptor in the nervous system, a receptor is a specialized portion of an afferent neuron (or a special cell attached to an afferent neuron) that is sensitive to a form of energy in the environment; *receptor* is also a term that applies to unique proteins on the surface of cells that can bind specific hormones or neurotransmitters.

reciprocal inhibition when extensor muscles (agonists) are contracted, there is a reflex inhibition of the motor neurons to the flexor muscles (antagonists), and vice versa.

Recommended Dietary Allowances (RDA) standards of nutrition associated with good health for the majority of people. Standards exist for protein, vitamins, and minerals for children and adults.

relative V̇O$_2$ oxygen uptake (consumption) expressed per unit body weight (e.g., ml · kg^{-1} · min^{-1}).

releasing hormone hypothalamic hormones released from neurons into the anterior pituitary that control the release of hormones from that gland.

renin enzyme secreted by special cells in the kidney that converts angiotensinogen to angiotensin I.

repetition the number of times an exercise is repeated within a single exercise "set."

residual volume (RV) volume of air in the lungs following a maximal expiration.

respiration external respiration is the exchange of oxygen and carbon dioxide between the lungs and the environment; internal respiration describes the use of oxygen by the cell (mitochondria).

respiratory compensation the buffering of excess H$^+$ in the blood by plasma bicarbonate (HCO$_3^-$), and the associated elevation in ventilation to exhale the resulting CO$_2$.

respiratory exchange ratio (R) the ratio of CO$_2$ production to O$_2$ consumption; indicative of substrate utilization during steady-state exercise in which a value of 1.0 represents 100% carbohydrate metabolism and 0.7 represents 100% fat metabolism.

resting membrane potential the voltage difference measured across a membrane that is related to the concentration of ions on each side of the membrane and the permeability of the membrane to those ions.

resting metabolic rate (RMR) metabolic rate measured in the supine position following a period of fasting (4–12 hours) and rest (4–8 hours).

rest interval the time period between bouts in an interval training program.

reversibility a principle of training that describes the temporary nature of a training effect; adaptations to training are lost when the training stops.

sarcolemma the cell (plasma) membrane surrounding a muscle fiber.

sarcomeres the repeating contractile unit in a myofibril bounded by Z-lines.

sarcopenia the loss of muscle mass associated with aging. Sarcopenia occurs primarily due to muscle atrophy but can also occur due to a loss of muscle fibers.

sarcoplasmic reticulum a membranous structure that surrounds the myofibrils of muscle cells; location of the terminal cisternae or lateral sacs that store the Ca^{++} needed for muscle contraction.

satellite cells undifferentiated cell found adjacent to skeletal muscle fibers. These cells can fuse with existing muscle fibers and contribute

to muscle growth (hypertrophy). It may also be possible that these fibers can differentiate and form a new muscle fiber following muscle injury.

Schwann cell the cell that surrounds peripheral nerve fibers, forming the myelin sheath.

second messenger a molecule (cyclic AMP) or ion (Ca^{++}) that increases in a cell as a result of an interaction between a "first messenger" (e.g., hormone or neurotransmitter) and a receptor that alters cellular activity.

secondary risk factor a characteristic (age, gender, race) or behavior that increases the risk of coronary heart disease when primary risk factors are present.

set a basic unit of a workout containing the number of times (repetitions) a specific exercise is done (e.g., do three sets of five repetitions with 100 pounds).

sex steroids a group of hormones, androgens and estrogens, secreted from the adrenal cortex and the gonads.

sham reinfusion an experimental treatment at the end of a blood doping experiment in which a needle is placed in a vein, but the subject does not receive a reinfusion of blood.

sham withdrawal an experimental treatment at the beginning of a blood doping experiment in which a needle is placed in a vein, but blood is not withdrawn.

sinoatrial node (SA node) specialized tissue located in the right atrium of the heart that generates the electrical impulse to initiate the heartbeat. In a normal, healthy heart, the SA node is the heart's pacemaker.

SI units system used to provide international standardization of units of measure in science.

size principle the progressive recruitment of motor units beginning with the smallest motor neurons and progressing to larger and larger motor neurons.

sliding filament model a theory of muscle contraction describing the sliding of the thin filaments (actin) past the thick filaments (myosin).

slow-twitch fibers muscle fiber type that contracts slowly and develops relatively low tension but displays great endurance to repeated stimulation; contains many mitochondria, capillaries, and myoglobin.

somatostatin hormone produced in the hypothalamus that inhibits growth hormone release from the anterior pituitary gland; secreted from cells in the islet of Langerhans and causes a decrease in intestinal activity.

somatotype body-type (form) classification method used to characterize the degree to which an individual's frame is linear (ectomorphic), muscular (mesomorphic), and round (endomorphic); Sheldon's scale rates each component on 1–7 scale.

spatial summation the additive effect of numerous simultaneous inputs to different sites on a neuron to produce a change in the membrane potential.

specificity a principle of training indicating that the adaptation of a tissue is dependent on the type of training undertaken; for example, muscles hypertrophy with heavy resistance training but show an increase in mitochondria number with endurance training.

spirometry measurement of various lung volumes.

static stretching stretching procedure in which a muscle is stretched and held in the stretched position for 10 to 30 seconds; in contrast to dynamic stretching, which involves motion.

steady state describes the tendency of a control system to achieve a balance between an environmental demand and the response of a physiological system to meet that demand to allow the tissue (body) to function over a period of time.

steroids a class of lipids, derived from cholesterol, that includes the hormones testosterone, estrogen, cortisol, and aldosterone.

stroke volume the amount of blood pumped by the ventricles in a single beat.

strong acids an acid that completely ionizes when dissolved in water to generate H^+ and its anion.

strong bases a base (alkaline substance) that completely ionizes when dissolved in water to generate OH^- and its cation.

ST segment depression an electrocardiographic change reflecting an ischemia (inadequate blood flow) in the heart muscle; indicative of coronary heart disease.

summation repeated stimulation of a muscle that leads to an increase in tension compared to a single twitch.

supercompensation an increase in the muscle glycogen content above normal levels following an exercise-induced muscle glycogen depletion and an increase in carbohydrate intake.

sympathetic nervous system portion of the autonomic nervous system that releases norepinephrine from its postganglionic nerve endings; epinephrine is released from the adrenal medulla.

sympathomimetic substance that mimics the effects of epinephrine or norepinephrine, which are secreted from the sympathetic nervous systems.

synapses junctions between nerve cells (neurons) where the electrical activity of one neuron influences the electrical activity of the other neuron.

systole portion of the cardiac cycle in which the ventricles are contracting.

systolic blood pressure the highest arterial pressure measured during a cardiac cycle.

tapering the process athletes use to reduce their training load for several days prior to competition.

target heart rate (THR) range the range of heart rates describing the optimum intensity of exercise consistent with making gains in maximal aerobic power; equal to 70–85% HR max.

temporal summation a change in the membrane potential produced by the addition of two or more inputs, occurring at different times (i.e., inputs are added together to produce a potential change that is greater than that caused by a single input).

terminal cisternae portion of the sarcoplasmic reticulum near the transverse tubule containing the Ca^{++} that is released upon depolarization of the muscle; also called *lateral sac*.

testosterone the steroid hormone produced in the testes; involved in growth and development of reproductive tissues, sperm, and secondary sex characteristics.

tetanus highest tension developed by a muscle in response to a high frequency of stimulation.

theophylline a drug used as a smooth muscle relaxant in the treatment of asthma.

thermogenesis the generation of heat as a result of metabolic reactions.

thyroid gland endocrine gland located in the neck that secretes triiodothyronine (T_3) and thyroxine (T_4), which increase the metabolic rate.

thyroid-stimulating hormone (TSH) hormone released from the anterior pituitary gland; stimulates the thyroid gland to increase its secretion of thyroxine and triiodothyronine.

thyroxine hormone secreted from the thyroid gland containing four iodine atoms (T_4); stimulates the metabolic rate and facilitates the actions of other hormones.

tidal volume volume of air inhaled or exhaled in a single breath.

Tolerable Upper Intake Level (UL) the highest average daily nutrient intake level that is likely to pose no risk of adverse health effects to almost all individuals in the general population. As intake increases above the UL, the potential risk of adverse effects may increase.

tonus low level of muscle activity at rest.

total lung capacity (TLC) the total volume of air the lung can contain; equal to the sum of the vital capacity and the residual volume.

toxicity a condition resulting from a chronic ingestion of vitamins, especially fat-soluble vitamins, in quantities well above that needed for health.

trace elements dietary minerals including iron, zinc, copper, iodine, manganese, selenium, chromium, molybdenum, cobalt, arsenic, nickel, fluoride, and vanadium.

transferrin plasma protein that binds iron and is representative of the whole body iron store.

transverse tubule an extension, invagination, of the muscle membrane that conducts the action potential into the muscle to depolarize the terminal cisternae, which contain the Ca^{++} needed for muscle contraction.

triiodothyronine hormone secreted from the thyroid gland containing three iodine atoms (T_3); stimulates the metabolic rate and facilitates the actions of other hormones.

tropomyosin protein covering the actin binding sites that prevents the myosin cross-bridge from touching actin.

troponin protein, associated with actin and tropomyosin, that binds Ca^{++} and initiates the movement of tropomyosin on actin to allow the myosin cross-bridge to touch actin and initiate contraction.

twenty-four-hour recall a technique of recording the type and amount of food (nutrients) consumed during a twenty-four-hour period.

twitch the tension-generating response following the application of a single stimulus to muscle.

type I fibers fibers that contain large numbers of oxidative enzymes and are highly fatigue resistant.

type IIa fibers fibers that contain biochemical and fatigue characteristics that are between Type IIb and Type I fibers.

type IIb fibers fibers that have a relatively small number of mitochondria, a limited capacity for aerobic metabolism, and are less resistant to fatigue than slow fibers.

underwater weighing procedure to estimate body volume by the loss of weight in water; result is used to calculate body density and, from that, body fatness.

vagus nerve a major parasympathetic nerve.

variable-resistance exercise strength training in which the resistance varies throughout the range of motion.

veins the blood vessels that accept blood from the venules and bring it back to the heart.

ventilation the movement of air into or out of the lungs (e.g., pulmonary or alveolar ventilation); external respiration.

ventilatory threshold (Tvent) the "breakpoint" at which pulmonary ventilation and carbon dioxide output begin to increase exponentially during an incremental exercise test.

venules small blood vessels carrying capillary blood to veins.

vestibular apparatus sensory organ, consisting of three semicircular canals, that provides needed information about body position to maintain balance.

vital capacity (VC) the volume of air that can be moved into or out of the lungs in one breath; equal to the sum of the inspiratory and expiratory reserve volumes and the tidal volume.

web of causation an epidemiologic model showing the complex interaction of risk factors associated with the development of chronic degenerative diseases.

whole-body density a measure of the weight-to-volume ratio of the entire body; high values are associated with low body fatness.

Wingate test anaerobic power test to evaluate maximal rate at which glycolysis can deliver ATP.

work the product of a force and the distance through which that force moves ($W = F \times D$).

work interval in interval training, the duration of the work phase of each work-to-rest interval.

Credits

Illustrations

CHAPTER 0

Figure 0.1A: Courtesy of Carnegie Institute of Washington, DC. **Figure 0.1B:** Courtesy of COSMED. **Figure 0.2:** Courtesy of W. B. Saunders Company.

CHAPTER 1

Figure 1.9: From J. Coast and H. G. Welch, 1985, "Linear Increase in Optimal Pedal Rate with Increased Power Output in Cycle Ergometry" in *European Journal of Applied Physiology*, 53:339–342. Copyright © Springer-Verlag, Heidelberg, Germany. Reprinted by permission. **Figure 1.10:** From P. Hopkins and S. Powers, 1982, "Oxygen Uptake during Submaximal Running in Highly Trained Men and Women" in *American Corrective Therapy Journal*, 36:130–132 (Now *Clinical Kinesiology: Journal of the American Kinesiotherapy Association*) (formerly the American Corrective Therapy Association). Reprinted by permission.

CHAPTER 2

Figures 2.4, 2.5, and 2.6: From Sylvia S. Mader, *Human Biology*, 9th ed. New York: McGraw-Hill, 2006.

CHAPTER 3

Figure 3.2: From Rod Seeley, Trent Stephens, and Philip Tate, *Anatomy and Physiology*, 8th ed. New York: McGraw-Hill, 2008. **Figures 3.3, 3.4, 3.6, 3.10, 3.16, and 3.20:** From Stuart Ira Fox, *Human Physiology*, 5th ed. Copyright © 1996 Times Mirror Higher Education Group, Inc., Dubuque, IA. All Rights Reserved. Reprinted by permission. **Figures 3.5 and 3.11:** From Stuart Ira Fox, *Human Physiology*, 11th ed., New York: McGraw-Hill, 2011. **Figure 3.7:** From Saladin, *Anatomy & Physiology*, 4th ed. New York: McGraw-Hill, 2007. **Figures 3.13 and 3.17:** From *Biochemistry* by C. K. Mathews and K. E. van Holde. Copyright © 1990 by The Benjamin/Cummings Publishing Company. Reprinted with permission. **Figure 3.15:** From S. Mader, *Human Biology*, 9th ed. New York: McGraw-Hill, 2006. **Figure 3.19:** From Stuart Ira Fox, *Human Physiology*, 10th ed., 2008. New York: McGraw-Hill, 2008. **Figure 3.23:** From S. K. Powers and S. L. Dodd, *Total Fitness: Exercise, Nutrition, and Wellness*, 2nd ed., Copyright © 1999 Allyn & Bacon, Needham Heights, MA. Reprinted by permission.

CHAPTER 4

Figure 4.2: From Bendahan et al., Citrulline/malate promotes aerobic energy production in human exercising muscle. Br J *Sports Med* 36:282–289, 2002. **Figure 4.4:** From S. Dodd, 1984, "Blood Lactate Disappearance at Various Intensities of Recovery Exercise" in *Journal of Applied Physiology*, 57:1462–1465. Copyright © 1984 American Physiological Society, Bethesda, MD. Used by permission. **Figure 4.11:** From G. Brooks and J. Mercier, "Balance of Carbohydrate and Lipid Utilization During Exercise: The 'Crossover Concept'" in *Journal of Applied Physiology*, 76:2253–2261, 1994. Copyright © 1994 American Physiological Society. Reprinted by permission. **Figures 4.14 and 4.15:** From E. Coyle, "Substrate Utilization During Exercise in Active People" in *American Journal of Clinical Nutrition*, 61 (Suppl): 9685–9795, 1995. Copyright © 1995 American Society for Clinical Nutrition, Inc., Bethesda, MD. Reprinted by permission. **Figure 4.16:** From Trudy McKee and James R. McKee, *Biochemistry: The Molecular Basis of Life*, 3rd ed. New York: McGraw-Hill, 2003.

CHAPTER 5

Figure 5.1: From A. J. Vander et al., *Human Physiology: The Mechanisms of Body Function*, 4th ed. Copyright © 1985 McGraw-Hill, Inc., New York. Reprinted with permission. **Figure 5.2:** From Stuart Ira Fox, *Human Physiology*, 11th ed., New York: McGraw-Hill, 2011. Reprinted by permission. **Figure 5.6:** From Stuart Ira Fox, *Human Physiology*, 7th ed., New York: McGraw-Hill, 2002. Reprinted by permission. **Figure 5.7:** Data from V. A. Convertino, L. C. Keil, and J. E. Greenleaf 1983, "Plasma Volume, Renin and Vasopressin Responses to Graded Exercises After Training." American Physiological Association, Bethesda, MD: *Journal of Applied Physiology: Respiration Environment Exercise Physiology*, 54:508–514. **Figure 5.8:** Data from J. T. Maher, et al., 1975, "Aldosterone Dynamics During Graded Exercises at Sea-level and High Altitudes." American Physiological Society, Bethesda, MD: *Journal of Applied Physiology* 39:18–22. **Figure 5.12:** Data from J. E. Turkowski, et al., 1978, "Ovarian Hormonal Responses

to Exercise." American Physiological Society, Bethesda, MD: *Journal of Applied Physiology: Respiration Environment Exercise Physiology*, 44:109–114. **Figure 5.13:** Reprinted with permission from B. Saltin and J. Karlsson, 1971, *Muscle Metabolism During Exercise*, pp. 289–299, edited by B. Pernow and B. Saltin. Copyright © 1971 Plenum Press, New York, NY. **Figure 5.14:** From M. Kjaer, 1989, "Epinephrine and Some Other Hormonal Responses to Exercise in Man: With Special Reference to Physical Training" in *International Journal of Sports Medicine*, 10:2–15. Copyright © 1989 Georg Thieme Verlag, Stuttgart, Germany. Reprinted by permission. **Figure 5.15:** From R. C. Harris, et al., "The Effect of Propranolol on Glycogen Metabolism During Exercise" in *Muscle Metabolism During Exercise*, B. Pernow & B. Saltin, Eds. Copyright © 1971 Plenum Publishing Corporation, New York. Reprinted by permission. **Figure 5.18:** Data from C. T. M. Davies and J. D. Few, 1973, "Effects of Exercise on Adrenocortical Function," American Physiological Society, Bethesda, MD: *Journal of Applied Physiology*, 35:887–891. **Figure 5.20A:** Data from J. Sutton and L. Lazarus, 1976, "Growth Hormone in Exercise: Comparison of Physiological and Pharmacological Stimuli." American Physiological Society, Bethesda, MD: *Journal of Applied Physiology*, 41:523–527. **Figure 5.20B:** Data from J. C. Bunt, et al. 1986, "Sex and Training Differences in Human Growth Hormone Levels During Prolonged Exercise." American Physiological Society, Bethesda, MD: *Journal of Applied Physiology*, 61:1796–1801. **Figure 5.22:** Data from Scott Powers, et al., 1982, "A Different Catecholamine Response during Prolonged Exercise and Passive Heating." American College of Sports Medicine, Indianapolis, IN: *Medicine and Science in Sports and Exercise*, 14:435–439. **Figure 5.23:** From W. W. Winder, et al., 1978, "Time Course of Sympathadrenal Adaptation to Endurance Exercise Training in Man" in *Journal of Applied Physiology: Respiration Environment Exercise Physiology*, 45:370–377. Copyright © 1978 The American Physiological Society, Bethesda, MD. Reprinted with permission. **Figure 5.25A:** Data from L. H. Harley, et al., 1972, "Multiple Hormonal Responses to Graded Exercise in Relation to Physical Training." American Physiological Society, Bethesda, MD: *Journal of Applied Physiology*, 33:602–606. **Figures 5.25B and 5.26:** Data from F. Gyntelberg, et al., 1977, "Effect of Training on the Response of Plasma Glucagon to Exercise." American Physiological Society, Bethesda, MD: *Journal of Applied Physiology: Respiration Environment Exercise Physiology*, 43:302–305. **Figure 5.30A:** From: J. Issekutz and H. Miller, "Plasma-free Fatty Acids During Exercise and the Effect of Lactic Acid." 1962, In *Proceedings of the Society for Experimental Biology and Medicine*, 110:237–239. Copyright © 1962 Society for Experimental Biology and Medicine, New York. Reprinted with permission.

CHAPTER 7

Figure 7.1: From E. Widmaier, H. Raff, and K. Strang, *Vander's Human Physiology*, 10th ed., New York: McGraw-Hill Companies, 2006. **Figures 7.2, 7.10, and 7.19:** From David Shier, Jackie Butler, and Ricki Lewis, *Hole's Human Anatomy & Physiology*, 11th ed. New York: McGraw-Hill, 2007. **Figure 7.3:** From Rod Seeley, Trent Stephens, and Philip Tate, *Anatomy and Physiology*, 8th ed. New York: McGraw-Hill, 2008. **Figure 7.4:** From John W. Hole, Jr., *Human Anatomy and Physiology*, 3rd ed., Copyright © 1984 Times Mirror Higher Education Group, Inc., Dubuque, IA. All rights reserved. Reprinted by permission. **Figures 7.5, 7.6, and 7.7:** From Stuart Ira Fox. *Human Physiology*, 9th ed., New York: McGraw-Hill Companies, 2006. **Figure 7.8:** From S. Mader, *Human Biology*, 9th ed. New York: McGraw-Hill, 2006. **Figures 7.9 and 7.17:** From David Shier, et al., *Hole's Human Anatomy and Physiology*, 7th ed. Copyright © 1996 Times Mirror Higher Education Group, Inc., Dubuque, IA. All rights reserved. Reprinted with permission. **Figure 7.11:** From A.J. Vander et al., *Human Physiology: The Mechanisms of Body Function*, 4th ed. Copyright © 1985 McGraw-Hill, Inc., New York. Reprinted by permission. **Figures 7.12 and 7.13:** From Rod R. Seeley, Trent D. Stephens, and Philip Tate, *Anatomy and Physiology*, 6th ed. New York: McGraw-Hill, 2003. **Figure 7.14:** From John W. Hole, Jr., *Human Anatomy and Physiology*, 5th ed., Copyright © 1990 Times Mirror Higher Education Group, Inc., Dubuque, IA. All rights reserved. Reprinted by permission. **Figure 7.15:** From Stuart Ira Fox, *Human Physiology*. Copyright © 1984 Times Mirror Higher Education Group, Inc., Dubuque, IA. All Rights Reserved. Reprinted with permission.

CHAPTER 8

Figures 8.1, 8.2, and 8.4: From David Shier, et al., *Hole's Human Anatomy and Physiology*, 7th ed. Copyright © 1996 Times Mirror Higher Education Group, Inc., Dubuque, IA. All rights reserved.

Reprinted with permission. **Figures 8.3 and 8.6:** From Stuart Ira Fox, *Human Physiology*, 5th ed. Copyright © 1996 Times Mirror Higher Education Group, Inc., Dubuque, IA. All rights reserved. Reprinted with permission. **Figure 8.5:** From David Shier, Jackie Butler, and Ricki Lewis, *Hole's Human Anatomy & Physiology*, 11th ed. New York: McGraw-Hill, 2007. **Figures 8.7 and 8.8:** From A. J. Vander et al., *Human Physiology: The Mechanisms of Body Function*, 4th ed. Copyright © 1985 McGraw-Hill, Inc., New York. Reprinted with permission. **Figure 8.9:** From Stuart Ira Fox, *Human Physiology*, 11th ed., New York: McGraw-Hill, 2011. Reprinted by permission. **Figure 8.12:** From R. Bottinelli, et al., "Myofibrillar ATPase Activity During Isometric Contractions and Myosin Composition in Rat Single-skinned Muscle Fibers," 1994, in *Journal of Physiology (London)*, 481:633–675. Copyright © 1994 Physiological Society, London. Reprinted by permission. **Figure 8.14:** From S. Fox. *Human Physiology*, 7th ed, New York: McGraw-Hill Companies, 2002. **Figure 8.17:** From Stuart Ira Fox, *Human Physiology*, 2nd ed. Copyright © 1987 Times Mirror Higher Education Group, Inc., Dubuque, IA. All rights reserved. Reprinted with permission.

CHAPTER 9

Figures 9.1, 9.15, and 9.17: From E. Widmaier, H. Raff, and K. Strang, *Vander's Human Physiology*, 10th ed., New York: McGraw-Hill Companies, 2006. **Figures 9.2, 9.11, and 9.12:** From Saladin, *Anatomy & Physiology*, 4th ed. New York: McGraw-Hill, 2007. **Figures 9.7, 9.8, and 9.9:** From Rod Seeley, Trent Stephens, and Philip Tate, *Anatomy and Physiology*, 8th ed. New York: McGraw-Hill, 2008. **Figures 9.10, 9.18, and 9.21:** From Stuart Ira Fox, *Human Physiology*, 5th ed. Copyright © 1996 Times Mirror Higher Education Group, Inc., Dubuque, IA. All rights reserved. Reprinted with permission. **Figure 9.13:** From Stuart Ira Fox. *Human Physiology*, 9th ed., New York: McGraw-Hill Companies, 2006. **Figure 9.14:** From David Shier, Jackie Butler, and Ricki Lewis, *Hole's Human Anatomy & Physiology*, 11th ed. New York: McGraw-Hill, 2007. **Figure 9.16:** From David Shier, et al., *Hole's Human Anatomy and Physiology*, 7th ed. Copyright © 1996 Times Mirror Higher Education Group, Inc., Dubuque, IA. All rights reserved. Reprinted with permission. **Figure 9.19:** From Stuart Ira Fox, *Human Physiology*, 4th ed. Copyright © 1993 Times Mirror Higher Education Group, Inc., Dubuque, IA. All rights reserved. Reprinted with permission. **Figure 9.22:** Data from L. Rowell, 1993, "Human Cardiovascular Adjustments to Exercise and Thermal Stress." American Physiological Society, Bethesda, MD: *Physiological Reviews*, 74:911–915 and L. Rowell, 1986, *Human Circulation Regulation During Physical Stress*. New York, NY: Oxford University Press. **Figure 9.23:** Data from L. Rowell, 1986, *Human Circulation: Regulation During Physical Stress*. New York, NY: Oxford University Press. **Figure 9.24:** From P. Astrand and K. Rodahl, *Textbook of Work Physiology*, 3rd ed. Copyright © 1986 McGraw-Hill Inc., New York. Reprinted by permission of the authors. **Figure 9.25:** Data from L. Rowell, 1974, "Human Cardiovascular Adjustments to Exercise and Thermal Stress." American Physiological Society, Bethesda, MD: *Physiological Reviews*, 54:75–159 and L. Rowell, *Human Circulation: Regulation During Physical Stress*, 1986, New York, NY: Oxford University Press. **Figure 9.26:** Data from P. Astrand, et al., 1965, Intra-arterial Blood Pressure During Exercise with Different Muscle Groups." American Physiological Society, Bethesda, MD: *Journal of Applied Physiology*, 20:253–257. **Figure 9.27:** Data from G. Brenglemann, 1983. "Circulatory Adjustments to Exercise and Heat Stress," Annual Reviews, Inc., Palo Alto, CA: *Annual Review of Physiology*, 45:191–212; E. Fox and D. Costill, 1972, "Estimated Cardiorespiratory Responses during Marathon Running," Heldref Publications, Washington, DC: *Archives of Environmental Health*, 24:315–324; and L. Rowell, 1974, "Human Cardiovascular Adjustments to Exercise and Thermal Stress." American Physiological Society, Bethesda, MD: *Physiological Reviews*, 54:75–159.

CHAPTER 10

Figure 10.1: From David Shier, Jackie Butler, and Ricki Lewis, *Hole's Human Anatomy & Physiology*, 11th ed. New York: McGraw-Hill, 2007. **Figures 10.2, 10.5, 10.6, and 10.7:** From Kent M. Van de Graaff and Stuart Ira Fox, *Concepts of Human Anatomy and Physiology*, 4th ed. Copyright © 1995 Times Mirror Higher Education Group, Inc., Dubuque, IA. All rights reserved. Reprinted by permission. **Figure 10.3:** From E. Widmaier, H. Raff, and K. Strang, *Vander's Human Physiology*, 10th ed., New York: McGraw-Hill Companies, 2006. **Figures 10.4, 10.19, 10.20, 10.24, and 10.25:** From Stuart Ira Fox, *Human Physiology*, 9th ed., New York: McGraw-Hill Companies, 2006. **Figure 10.8:** Courtesy of Sensor-Medics Corporation. **Figures 10.9 and 10.11:** From Saladin, *Anatomy & Physiology*, 4th ed. New York: McGraw-Hill, 2007. **Figure 10.14:** From Stuart Ira Fox, *Human Physiology*, 10th ed., New York: McGraw-Hill, 2008. **Figures 10.15, 10.16, and 10.18:** From Stuart Ira Fox, *Human Physiology*, 5th ed. Copyright © 1996 Times Mirror Higher Education Group, Inc., Dubuque, IA. All

rights reserved. Reprinted with permission. **Figure 10.17:** From Stuart Ira Fox, *Human Physiology*, 3rd ed. Copyright © 1990 Times Mirror Higher Education Group, Inc., Dubuque, IA. All rights reserved. Reprinted with permission. **Figure 10.21:** Data from J. Dempsey and R. Fregosi, 1985, "Adaptability of the Pulmonary System to Changing Metabolic Requirements," Yorke Medical Group, New York, NY: *American Journal of Cardiology*, 55:59D-67D; J. Dempsey, et al., 1986, "Is the Lung Built for Exercise?" American College of Sports Medicine, Indianapolis, IN: *Medicine and Science in Sports and Exercise*, 18:143–155; and S. Powers, et al., 1985, "Caffeine Alters Ventilatory and Gas Exchange Kinetics during Exercise" American College of Sports Medicine, Indianapolis, IN: *Medicine and Science in Sports and Exercise*, 18:101–106. **Figure 10.22:** Data from J. Dempsey, et al., 1986. "Is the Lung Built for Exercise?" American College of Sports Medicine, Indianapolis, IN: *Medicine and Science in Sports and Exercise*, 18:143–155; and S. Powers, et al., 1982, "Ventilatory and Metabolic Reactions to Heat Stress During Prolonged Exercise" International Federation of Sportive Medicine, Turin, Italy: *Journal of Sports Medicine and Physical Fitness*, 22:32–36. **Figure 10.23:** Data from J. Dempsey, et al., 1982, "Limitation to Exercise Capacity and Endurance: Pulmonary System," University of Toronto, Ontario, Canada: *Canadian Journal of Applied Sports Sciences*, 7:4–13; and K. Wasserman, et al., 1973, "Anaerobic Threshold and Respiratory Gas Exchange during Exercise," American Physiological Society, Bethesda, MD, *Journal of Applied Physiology*, 35:236–243.

CHAPTER 11

Figure 11-4: Data from E. Hultman and K. Sahlin, 1980, "Acid-base Balance during Exercise," in R. Hutton and D. Miller, Eds. Franklin Institute Press, Philadelphia, PA: *Exercise and Sport Science Reviews*, 8:41–128; N. Jones, et al., 1977, "Effects of pH on Cardiorespiratory and Metabolic Responses to Exercise," American Physiological Society, Bethesda, MD, *Journal of Applied Physiology*, 43:969–964; and A. Katz, et al., 1984, "Maximum Exercise Tolerance after Induced Alkalosis," Stuttgart, Germany: *International Journal of Sports Medicine*, 5:107–110. **Figure 11.5:** Data from E. Hultman and K. Sahlin, 1986, "Acid-base Balance during Exercise," R. Hutton and D. Miller, Eds. Orlando, FL, Academic Press, Inc.: *Exercise and Sport Science Reviews*, 8:41–128.

CHAPTER 12

Figures 12.7, 12.8, and 12.9: From M. Nelson, 1938, "Die Regulation der Korpertemperatur im Muskelarbeit" in *Scandinavica Archives Physiology*, 79: 193. Copyright © 1938 Blackwell Scientific Publications, Ltd., Oxford, England. Reprinted by permission. **Figure 12.10:** Data from G. Brenglemann, 1977, "Control of Sweating and Skin Flow During Exercise," E. Nadel, Ed. Academic Press, Inc., Orlando, FL: *Problems with Temperature Regulation During Exercise*, and S. Powers, et al., 1982, "Ventilatory and Metabolic Reactions to Heat Stress During Prolonged Exercise," International Federation of Sportive Medicine, Turin, Italy: *Journal of Sports Medicine and Physical Fitness*, 2:32–36.

CHAPTER 13

Figure 13.5: Data from S. Powers, et al., 1994, "Influence of Exercise and Fiber Type on Antioxidant Enzyme Activity in Rat Skeletal Muscle" American Physiological Society, Bethesda, MD: *American Journal of Physiology*, 266:R375–380. **Figure 13.13:** From E. F. Coyle, et al., 1984, "Time Course of Loss of Adaptation after Stopping Prolonged Intense Endurance Training" in *Journal of Applied Physiology*, 57: 1857–1864. Copyright © 1984 American Physiological Society, Bethesda, MD. Reprinted by permission. **Figure 13.14:** From T. J. Terjung, "Muscle Adaptations to Aerobic Training" in *Sports Science Exchange*, Vol. 6, No. 6, 1993. Copyright © 1993 Gatorade Sports Science Institute, Barrington, IL. Reprinted with permission. **Figure 13.15:** From D. G. Sale, 1988, "Neural Adaptations to Resistance Training" in *Medicine and Science in Sports and Exercise*, 20:S135–S143. Copyright © 1988 American College of Sports Medicine, Indianapolis, IN. Reprinted by permission.

CHAPTER 14

Figure 14.1: Source: U.S. Department of Health, Education and Welfare, 1979, *Healthy People: The Surgeon General's Report on Health Promotion and Disease Prevention*. **Figure 14.3:** From C. J. Casperson, "Physical Activity Epidemiology: Concepts, Methods, and Applications to Exercise Science," edited by K. B. Pandolf in *Exercise and Sport Science Reviews*, 17:457, 1989. Copyright © 1989 Williams & Wilkins, Baltimore, MD. Reprinted by permission. **Figure 14.4:** Adapted from P. Libby, Atherosclerosis: the new view. *Scientific American*, November 10, 2002:46–55, 2002. **Figure 14.5:** From P. M. Ridker et al., Rosuvastatin to prevent vascular events in men and women with elevated C-reactive protein. *New England Journal of*

Medicine 359: 2008. **Figure 14.6:** Data from N. M. Kaplan, 1989, "The Deadly Quartet." American Medical Association, Chicago, IL: *Archives of Internal Medicine*, 149:1514–1520; and A. P. Rocchini, 1991, "Insulin Resistance and Blood Pressure Regulation in Obese and Nonobese Subjects." American Heart Association, Dallas, TX: *Hypertension*, 17:837–842. **Figure 14.7:** From J. S. Rana et al., Cardiovascular metabolic syndrome—an interplay of obesity, inflammation, diabetes and coronary heart disease. *Diabetes, Obesity and Metabolism* 9:218–232, 2007. **Figure 14.8:** From T. A. Lakka and D. E. Laaksonen, Physical activity in prevention and treatment of the metabolic syndrome. *Applied Physiology, Nutrition, and Metabolism* 32: 76–88, 2007.

CHAPTER 15

Figure 15.1: From ACSM's Guidelines for Exercise Testing and Prescription. Reprinted by permission. **Figure 15.2:** Copyright © Canadian Society for Exercise Physiology. **Figure 15.3:** From A. D. Martin, "ECG and Medications" in E. T. Howley and B. D. Franks, *Health/Fitness Instructor's Handbook*. Copyright © 1986 Human Kinetics Publishers, Inc., Champaign, IL. Used by permission. **Figures 15.5, 15.7, and 15.9:** From E. T. Howley and B. D. Franks. *Health/Fitness Instructor's Handbook*. Copyright © 1986 Human Kinetics Publishers, Inc., Champaign, IL. Used by permission. **Figure 15.6:** From the YMCA Fitness Testing and Assessment Manual. Copyright © 2000 YMCA of the USA. Reprinted by permission.

CHAPTER 16

Figure 16.1: Data from L. S. Goodman and A. Gilman, eds., 1975, *The Pharmacological Basis of Therapeutics*. New York: Macmillan Publishing Company. **Figure 16.2:** From G. L. Jennings, G. Deakin, P. Komer, T. Meridith, B. Kingwell, and L. Nelson, 1991. "What Is the Dose-Response Relationship between Exercise Training and Blood Pressure?" in *Annals of Medicine*, 23:313–318, Royal Society of Medicine Press, Inc. **Figures 16.3 and 16.4:** From U.S. Department of Health and Human Services. Physical Activity Guidelines Advisory Committee Report 2008, http://www.health.gov/paguidelines/committeereport.aspx. **Figure 16.5:** Data from M. M. Dehn and C. B. Mullins, 1977, "Physiologic Effects and Importance of Exercise in Patients with Coronary Artery Disease," Group Medicine Publications, Inc., New York, NY: *Cardiovascular Medicine*, 2:365; and H. K. Hellerstein and B. A. Franklin, 1984. John Wiley & Sons, Inc., New York, NY: *Rehabilitation of the Coronary Patient*, 2nd ed.

CHAPTER 17

Figure 17.1: From M. Berger, et al., 1977, "Metabolic and Hormonal Effects of Muscular Exercise in Juvenile Type "Diabetics" in *Diabetologia*, 13:355–365. Copyright © 1977 Springer-Verlag, New York, NY. Reprinted by permission. **Figure 17.2:** From E. R. Richter and H. Galbo, 1986, "Diabetes, Insulin and Exercise" in *Sports Medicine*, 3:275–288. Copyright © 1986 Adis Press, Langhorn, PA. Reprinted by permission.

CHAPTER 18

Figure 18.1: From G. M. Wardlaw and A. M. Smith, *Contemporary Nutrition*, 2nd ed. Copyright © 2012 McGraw-Hill, New York, NY. All rights reserved. Reprinted by permission. **Figure 18.3:** Adapted from M. L. Pollock and J. H. Wilmore, *Exercise in Health and Disease*, 2nd ed., 1990. Philadelphia, PA: W. B. Saunders. **Figure 18.4:** From T. G. Lohman, "The Use of Skinfold to Estimate Body Fatness in Children and Youth" in *Journal of Health, Physical Education, Recreation and Dance*, 98:102, November-December 1987. Copyright © 1987 American Alliance for Health, Physical Recreation and Dance, Reston, VA. Reprinted by permission. **Figure 18.7:** From E. Jequier, "Calorie Balance vs Nutrient Balance" in *Energy Metabolism: Tissue Determinants and Cellular Corollaries*, John M. Kinney and Hugh N. Tucker, Eds. Copyright © 1992 Raven Press. Reprinted by permission of Lippincott-Raven Publishers, a Wolters Kluwer Company, New York. **Figure 18.8:** From A. Keys, et al., *The Biology of Human Starvation*, Vol. 1. Copyright © 1950 University of Minnesota Press, Minneapolis, MN. Reprinted by permission. **Figure 18.9:** From L. O. Schulz and D. A. Scholler, "A Compilation of Total Energy Expenditures and Body Weights in Healthy Adults" in *American Journal of Clinical Nutrition*, 60:676–81, 1994. Copyright © 1994 American Society for Clinical Nutrition, Inc., Bethesda, MD. Reprinted by permission. **Figure 18.11:** From J. Mayer, et al., "Exercise, Food Intake, and Body Weight in Normal Rats and Genetically Obese Mice" in *American Journal of Physiology*, 177:544–548. Copyright © 1954 American Physiological Society, Bethesda, MD. Used by permission.

CHAPTER 19

Figure 19.1: From P. Astrand and K. Rodahl, *Textbook of Work Physiology*, 2nd ed. Copyright © 1977 McGraw-Hill, Inc., New York, NY.

Reprinted by permission. **Figure 19.2:** From H. Gibson and R. H. T. Edwards, 1985, "Muscular Exercise and Fatigue" in *Sports Medicine*, 2: 120–132. Copyright © 1985 Adis Press, Langhorn, PA. Reprinted by permission. **Figure 19.3:** From D. G. Sale, "Influence of Exercise and Training in Motor Unit Activation" in Kent B. Pandolf, Ed., *Exercise and Sport Sciences Review*, Vol. 15. Copyright © 1987 McGraw-Hill, Inc., New York. Reprinted by permission.

CHAPTER 20

Figure 20.5: Reprinted with permission from B. Scott and J. Houmard, "Peak Running Velocity Is Highly Related to Distance Running Performance" in *International Journal of Sports Medicine*, 75 (1994): 504–507, Georg Thieme Verlag, Stuttgart, Germany. **Figure 20.9:** From P. Astrand and K. Rodahl, *Textbook of Work Physiology*, 2nd ed. Copyright © 1977 McGraw-Hill, Inc., New York, NY. Reprinted by permission.

CHAPTER 21

Figure 21.2: From M. Ikai and T. Fukunaga, 1968, "Calculation of Muscle Strength per Unit of Cross Sectional Area of a Human Muscle by Means of Ultrasonic Measurement" in *Internationale Zeitschrift fuer Angewanted Physiologie*, 26:26–31. Copyright © 1968 Springer-Verlag, Heidelberg, Germany. Reprinted by permission. **Figure 21.3:** From J. Wilmore, et al., 1974, "Alterations in Strength, Body Composition, and Anthropometric Measurements Consequent to a 10-Week Weight Training Program" in *Medicine and Science in Sports*, 6:133–139. Copyright © 1974 American College of Sports Medicine, Indianapolis, IN. Reprinted by permission.

CHAPTER 22

Figure 22.5: From Kent M. Van de Graaff, *Human Anatomy*, 4th ed. Copyright © 1995 Times Mirror Higher Education Group, Inc., Dubuque, IA. All rights reserved. Reprinted by permission. **Figure 22.6:** Data from F. Ingjer, Development of maximal oxygen uptake in young elite male cross-country skiers: a longitudinal study. *J Sports Sci* 10:49–63, 1992. **Figures 22.9 and 22.10:** Data from S. A. Hawkins, T. J. Marcell, S. Victoria Jaque, and R. A. Wiswell. A longitudinal assessment of change in $\dot{V}O_2$ max and maximal heart rate in master athletes. *Med Sci Sports Exerc* 33:174–1750, 2001.

CHAPTER 23

Figure 23.1: From J. Bergstrom, et al., 1967, "Diet, Muscle Glycogen and Physical Performance" in *Acta Physiologica Scandinavica* 71:140–150. Copyright © 1967 Scandinavian Physiological Society, Stockholm Sweden. Reprinted by permission of Blackwell Scientific Publications, Ltd., Oxford, England. **Figure 23.2:** From W. M. Sherman, 1983, "Carbohydrates, Muscle Glycogen, and Muscle Glycogen Super Compensation" in *Ergogenic Aids in Sports*, pp. 3–26, edited by M. H. Williams. Copyright © 1983 Human Kinetics Publishers, Inc., Champaign, IL. Used with permission. **Figure 23.3:** From John O. Halloszy, Ed., in *Exercise and Sport Science Reviews*, 19:982, 1991. Copyright © 1991 Williams & Wilkins, Baltimore, MD. Reprinted with permission. **Figure 23.5:** Data from P. W. R. Lemon and J. P. Mullin, 1980, "Effect of Initial Muscle Group Glycogen Levels on Protein Catabolism During Exercise," American Physiological Society, Bethesda, MD: *American Journal of Applied Physiology*, 48:624–629. **Figure 23.6:** From C. T. M. Davies, et al., 1982, "Glucose Inhibits CO_2 Production from Leucine during Whole Body Exercise in Man" in *Journal of Physiology*, 332:40–41. Copyright © 1982 Cambridge University Press, Cambridge, England. Reprinted by permission. **Figure 23.7:** From E. F. Coyle and S. J. Montain, 1995, "Benefits of Fluid Replacement with Carbohydrate During Exercise," in *Medicine and Science in Sports and Exercise*, 24:S324-S330. Copyright © 1995 Williams & Wilkins Company, Baltimore, MD. Reprinted by permission. **Figure 23.8:** From D. L. Costill and B. Saltin, 1974, "Factors Limiting Gastric Emptying during Rest and Exercise" in *Journal of Applied Physiology*, 37:679–683. Copyright © 1974 American Physiological Association, Bethesda, MD. Reprinted with permission. **Figure 23.9:** From K. Davies, et al., 1982, "Muscle Mitochondrial Bioenergetics, Oxygen Supply, and Work Capacity during Dietary Iron Deficiency and Repletion" in *Journal of Applied Physiology*, 242:E418–E427. Copyright © 1982 American Physiological Association, Bethesda, MD. Used by permission. **Figure 23.11:** From J. M. Tanner, et al., *The Physique of the Olympic Athlete*. Copyright © 1964 George Allen & Unwin Publishers, Ltd., London England. Reprinted by permission.

CHAPTER 24

Figure 24.1: From E. T. Howley, "Comparison of Performances in Short Races in the 1964 and 1968 Olympic Games," in G. A. Stull and T. K. Cureton, *Encyclopedia of Physical Education, Fitness and Sports: Training, Environment, Nutrition and Fitness*. Copyright © 1980 American Alliance for Health, Physical Education, Recreation and Dance, Reston, VA. Reprinted by permission. **Figure 24.2:** Data from

Grover et al., 1967, "Muscular Exercise in Young Men Native to 3,100 m Altitude," American Physiological Society, Bethesda, MD: *American Journal of Applied Physiology* 22:555–564. **Figure 24.3:** Data from L. G. C. E. Pugh, 1964, "Muscular Exercise at Great Altitudes," American Physiological Society, Bethesda, MD: *Journal of Applied Physiology*, 19:431–440. **Figure 24.4:** From J. B. West and P. D. Wagner, 1980, "Predicted Gas Exchange on the Summit of Mt. Everest" in *Respiration Physiology*, 42:1–16. Copyright © 1980 Elsevier Biomedical Press, Amsterdam, The Netherlands. Reprinted by permission. **Figure 24.5:** From J. B. West, et al., 1983, "Barometric Pressures at Extreme Altitudes on Mt. Everest: Physiological Significance" in *Journal of Applied Physiology*, 54:1188–1194. Copyright © 1983 American Physiological Society, Bethesda, MD. Reprinted by permission. **Figure 24.7:** From D. K. Mathews, et al., 1969, "Physiological Responses during Exercise and Recovery in a Football Uniform" in *Journal of Applied Physiology*, 26: 611–615. Copyright © 1969 American Physiological Society, Bethesda, MD. Reprinted by permission. **Figure 24.9:** Data from G. W. Molnar, 1946. American Medical Association, Chicago, IL: *Journal of the American Medical Association*, 131:1046–1050. **Figure 24.10:** From A. C. Burton and O. G. Edholm, *Man in a Cold Environment*. Copyright © 1955 Edward Arnold Publishers. Reprinted by permission of Edward Arnold Publishers, Division of Hodder & Stoughton Ltd., London, England. **Figure 24.11:** From P. B. Raven, et al., 1974, "Effect of Carbon Monoxide and Peroxyacetyl Nitrate on Man's Maximal Aerobic Capacity" in *Journal of Applied Physiology*, 36: 288–293. Copyright © 1974 American Physiological Society, Bethesda, MD. Reprinted by permission. **Figure 24.12:** "Air Quality Index (AQI) - A Guide to Air Quality and Your Health." AIRNow Web site. Available at: http://airnow.gov/index.cfm ?action=static.aqi. Accessed April 28, 2011.

CHAPTER 25

Figure 25.1: Data from G. Ariel and W. Saville, 1972. "Anabolic Steroids: The Physiological Effects of Placebos," American College of Sports Medicine, Indianapolis, IN: *Medicine and Science in Sports and Exercise*, 4:124–126. **Figure 25.2:** From H. W. Welch, "Effects of Hypoxia and Hyperpoxia on Human Performance" in Kent B. Pandolf, Ed., *Exercise and Sport Sciences Reviews*, vol. 15. Copyright © 1987 McGraw-Hill, Inc., New York. Reprinted by permission. **Figure 25.3:** From N. Gledhill, 1982, "Blood Doping and Related Issues: A Brief Review" in *Medicine and Science in Sports and Exercise*, 14:183–189.

Copyright © 1982 American College of Sports Medicine, Indianapolis, IN. Reprinted by permission.

Photos

Page 1: Action Plus Sports Images/Alamy; **3 (A):** Hulton Archive/Getty Images; **3 (B):** Time & Life Pictures/Getty Images; **4 (left):** Courtesy of The Royal Physiological Society; **4 (right):** Courtesy of The American Physiological Society; **5 (left):** The Carnegie Institution of Washington, D.C.; **5 (right):** Photo courtesy of COSMED USA, Inc.; **6 (top left):** Personal Photo from Horvath Family; **6 (top right):** Courtesy of Michael Sturek Ph.D. Prof and Chair Depart. of Cellular & Integrative Physiology, Indiana University; **6 (bottom):** Library of Congress, Prints & Photographs Division; **7:** Courtesy of W.B. Saunders Company; **10:** Courtesy of the author; **18 (top left):** Ryan McVay/Getty Images; **18 (all others):** Courtesy of the author; **19:** Library of Congress/Photo Researchers; **22:** Photo courtesy of ParvoMedics; **31:** Boyer/Roger Viollet/Getty Images; **55:** Keystone/Getty Images; **73:** AP Images; **101:** Bettmann/Corbis; **131:** Popperfoto/Getty Images; **135:** Photo provided by David C. Nieman; **154:** Photo courtesy of the American Physiological Society; **169:** Hulton-Deutsch Collection/Corbis; **189:** Bettmann/Corbis; **225:** Courtesy of Sensor-Medics Corporation; **242:** Courtesy of The American Physiological Society; **243:** Keisho Katayama; **255:** 2008 acidbase.org/Paul W G Elbers; **262:** Courtesy of The American Physiological Society; **274:** Courtesy of Dr. Michael Sawka; **288 (top):** Joe Angeles/WUSTL; **288 (bottom):** Harry How/Getty Images; **313:** Tim Mantoani/Masterfile; **319 (both):** Courtesy of the author; **343:** Used with permission from the book *Matters of the Heart: Adventures in Sports Medicine*. Healthy Learning. Monterey, California; **359:** Courtesy of American College of Sports Medicine; **385:** Courtesy of Dr. Lindsay Carter; **386:** Courtesy of the author; **413:** Photo provided courtesy of COSMED USA, Inc.; **429:** Digital Collections and Archives, Tufts University; **441:** Digital Vision/Getty Images; **453:** Courtesy of Ball State University Photo Service; **462:** Courtesy of The American Heart Association Journal; **473:** Photo courtesy of Biodex Medical Systems, Inc.; **474 (left):** Photo Courtesy of Lafayette Instrument Company; **474 (right):** Photo courtesy of Biodex Medical Systems, Inc.; **485:** Courtesy of the author; **520:** Courtesy of Dr. Bengt Lindholm; **560:** The Royal Geographical Society; **576:** Courtesy of Arthur Forsberg.

Index

force regulation in, 181–182
involuntary, 175
sliding-filament model, 169,
169b, 170f
steps leading to, 174f
muscular contraction
(cardiac), 191
muscular dystrophy, 183b
muscular endurance, 301
muscular fatigue, 172. See also
exercise-induced fatigue;
fatigue
causes, 173–174
exercise and, 173–174
free radicals and, 447b
heat-related, 273–274
in hot environment,
272–273
space travel and, 449b
muscular force. See force,
muscular
muscular strength, 301. See
also strength training
aging and, 302b, 511–512,
512f
defined, 472
evaluation of, 472–475, 473f,
474f
isokinetic assessment of,
473–474
isometric measurement of,
472–473
resistance training and,
301–302
variable-resistance
measurement of,
474–475
musculoskeletal system,
training and, 507–508
myelin, 141, 143b
myocardial infarction (MI), 191
cardiac rehabilitation,
381–382
enzyme activity in blood,
47b, 47f
heart rate variability and,
202, 203
myocardial ischemia, 198b,
335–336
myocardium, 191–192, 192f
myofibrils, 165f, 166f, 167,
167f, 170
myoglobin, 176, 233
myokines, 111b
myonuclear domain, 166–167
myonuclei, 305–306, 305f
myosin, 169, 303
actin and, 183–184
fast muscle fibers and, 178
muscular contraction and,
169, 170f, 171
resistance training and, 303
in slow fibers, 178
myosin ATPase activity, 177,
178
myosin cross-bridge, 169, 171,
172b, 178, 181
muscle fatigue and, 447b,
449b
myosin isoforms, 176–177,
288
myosing cross-bridge, 169

myotatic reflex, 149–150
MyPlate, 410

N
NA+, fatigue and, 446
NAD (nicotinamide adenine
dinucleotide), 45, 45f, 54,
54b, 54f
NADH, 45, 54b, 54f
aerobic production of ATP
and, 58, 61, 62
endurance training and, 292
Krebs cycle and, 56, 57f
lactate threshold, 77
shuttled into mitochondria,
54, 54b, 58
NADHD, 45, 45f
nasal cavity, 219, 220f
National Academy of
Sciences, Food and
Nutrition Board, 396
National Athletic Training
Association, 273b,
560–561
National Athletic Training
Association's Board of
Certification, 12
National Collegiate Athletic
Association, 507
National Strength and
Conditioning
Association, 12
National Weather Service,
271f, 556
National Weight Control
Registry (NWCR), 430b
natural killer cells, 128, 129,
130, 133
N-balance studies, 525, 526
NE (norepinephrine). See
norepinephrine (NE)
Near Infrared Interactance
(NIR), 412
negative feedback control
system, 34, 35f, 63, 268
negative N-balance, 525, 526,
526f
nerve fiber (axon), 141,
152–153
nervous system, 140–161
anatomical divisions of,
140–148, 140f
autonomic, 159–160
central. See central nervous
system (CNS)
control of voluntary
movement and,
158–159
electrical activity of
neurons, 141–148
equilibrium, 154–155
exercise and brain health,
160–161
functions, 140
homeostasis and, 92
motor control functions of
the brain, 155–158
multiple sclerosis and, 141,
143b
neurons. See neurons
peripheral, 140, 141f,
156–157

resistance training and,
301–302, 302f, 303
sensory information and
reflexes, 148–151
somatic motor functions,
151–154, 152f
spinal cord, 158
vestibular apparatus,
154–155, 155f
net efficiency, 23–27
neural factors to fatigue,
445–446
neural factors to strength and
endurance training, 307
neural input to respiratory
control center, 237–238,
239–240
neural theory, 494b
neural transmission, 141,
169b
neuroendocrine response, 92
neuroendocrinology, 92–96
blood hormone
concentration, 93–94
defined, 92
hormone-receptor
interaction, 94–96
neurohypophysis, 97
neuromuscular cleft, 168
neuromuscular junction, 168,
168f, 445
neurons, 140
action potential, 144, 146f
communication between,
144
electrical activity in,
141–148
irritability, 141
motor. See motor neurons
parts of, 142f
postsynaptic, 142f, 145, 146
preganglionic, 159–160
presynaptic, 142f, 145
resting membrane
potential, 141–142
structure of, 131, 142f
neurotransmitters, 144–145,
156, 159–160, 160f
neutrophils, 128, 128, 129t, 129
Newtons (N), 16–17
NFκB (nuclear factor kappa
B), 295, 296, 297
niacin, 45, 399, 400t–401t
nickel, 399
nicotinamide adenine
dinucleotide (NAD), 45,
45f, 54, 54b, 54f
nicotinamide adenine
dinucleotide, reduced.
See NADH
nicotine, 581–582, 581f
Nielsen, Marius, 4, 4f, 5
Nieman, David, 133, 135b
NIR (near infrared
interactance), 412
nitric oxide, vasodilation and,
209, 210b
nitrogen (N)-balance studies,
525, 526
nitrogen intake, 525, 526, 528
nitroglycerin, 381
Nixon, Richard M., 7

Nobel Prize in Physiology or
Medicine, 3, 4, 19b, 55b,
73b, 169b
nodes of Ranvier, 141
Noll Laboratory, 9
nomogram, 344, 345f
nonbiological control
system, 33f
noncatalyzed reaction, 46
nonshivering thermogenesis,
263, 278, 426
nonsteroidal anti-
inflammatory drugs
(NSAIDs), 495b
norepinephrine (NE), 93, 100,
110t
exercise and, 116, 117f, 118f,
119, 119f
"fight or flight" response
and, 101b
heart rate regulation and,
201–202
hypothalamus and, 268
lactate paradox and, 551b
prolonged exercise and,
75, 81
thermogenesis and, 426
Norgay, Tenzing, 560b
normocythemic, 574
normoxia, 542, 548b
nose, 219
nostril, 220f
nuclear factor kappa B (NFκB),
295, 296
nuclear magnetic resonance
(NMR), 412
nucleus/nuclei
altering activity of DNA in,
94
cell, 42, 42f
in muscle fibers, 166–167
nutrient balance, 422–423,
424
nutrient density, 409–410
nutrients, classes of, 397–409
carbohydrates, 403, 406
fats, 407–409
minerals, 399, 402
protein, 409
vitamins, 399
water, 398–399
nutrition. See also diet
dietary recommendations,
395–396
for exercise-induced
asthma, 378
food group plans, 409–410
food labels, 397, 398f
immune function and, 135b
standards of, 396–397
nutrition and performance,
519–535
carbohydrate intake,
519–524
fluids/electrolytes, 528–531,
532b
minerals, 532–534
precompetition meal,
534–535, 535t
protein, 525–528
salt intake, 531
vitamin, 534

factors influencing, 443, 443f, 459, 459f
fatigue in. *See* fatigue
laboratory assessment. *See* laboratory assessment of performance
long-term. *See* long-term performance
nutrition and. *See* nutrition and performance
short-term. *See* short-term performance
training for. *See* training
perimysium, 165f, 166
periodization, of strength training, 490b
peripheral chemoreceptors, 238, 239f
peripheral fatigue, 445–448
peripheral nerve damage, with type 1 diabetes, 373
peripheral nervous system (PNS)
exercise-induced fatigue and, 156–157
parts of, 140, 140f
relationship between central nervous system and, 141f
somatic portion of, 151–153
permissive hormones, 113
peroxisome proliferator-activated receptor-gamma coactivator 1α (PGC-1α), 298
PFK. *See* phosphofructokinase (PFK) reduction
pH
acid-base balance and, 233–234, 253
blood, endurance training and, 292
changes in arterial blood, 257, 257f
defined, 250
enzyme activity and, 48, 48f
hydrogen ions and, 250
pH scale, 250f
phagocytes, 127, 128–129, 130
pharmacologic stress test, 336, 337b
pharynx, 219, 220f
phosphagen system, 51
phosphates, high-energy, 50. *See also* inorganic phosphate (P$_i$)
phosphocreatine (PC)
fatigue and, 446
supplementation, 570, 572b
phosphocreatine (PC) breakdown, 51, 63
phosphodiesterase, 96
phosphofructokinase (PFK) reduction, 63–64
phospholipids, 49, 407
phosphorus, 404t–405t
phosphorylase, 64, 81b
phosphorylation, 52, 53f, 61. *See also* oxidative phosphorylation
phospolipase C, 96, 96f

photon absorptiometry, 411
phrenic nerves, 222
physical activity (PA). *See also* physical inactivity
caloric intake and, 427–429, 428f
coronary heart disease and, 352
defined, 352
diabetes and, 374
energy expenditure and, 427
epilepsy and, 510
health and, 354–356
heart disease associated with, 318, 319b
lower levels of inflammation with, 322
physical activity pyramid, 366f
recommended guidelines on, 354–356
sequence of, 362–363
warm-up exercises, 582–583
web of causation, 318
Physical Activity Guidelines, 354–356, 358, 430b
physical activity pyramid, 366f
Physical Activity Readiness Questionnaire (PAR-Q), 329, 331f, 334
physical barriers, immunity and, 127–128
physical education
history of, 6
undergraduate academic preparation for, 8–9
physical fitness. *See also* fitness
defined, 352
guidelines for improving, 356, 358
history of concern in, 6–8
Physical Fitness Laboratory, 10b
physical fitness testing. *See* laboratory assessment of performance
physical inactivity
coronary heart disease and, 317b
as public health concern, 7, 8b
as risk factor for coronary heart disease, 318, 319, 352
physical performance assessment. *See* laboratory assessment of performance
physical warm-ups, 582–583
physiological set point, 420, 420f
physiological testing of performance. *See* laboratory assessment of performance
physiologists, 322
physiology
defined, 3
Physiology of Bodily Exercise (Lagrange), 9
P$_i$. *See* inorganic phosphate (P$_i$)

piloerection reflex (goosebumps), 268
pilomotor center, 268
pituitary gland, 97. *See also* anterior pituitary gland
placebo, 569
plasma
defined, 205
hormone concentration in, 93–94
plasma calcium (Ca^{++}), calcitonin and, 100
plasma free fatty acids, 84, 84f, 580
plasma glucose, 84f, 92. *See also* blood glucose
plasma volume, 94, 98
heat acclimation and, 275, 276, 276f
hormone concentration and, 94
training-induced changes in, 286
platelets, 205
pleura, 219
pneumotaxic center, 237
"point-counterpoint" debate, 548b
Pollock, Michael L., 359b
Pollock's Textbook of Cardiovascular Disease and Rehabilitation, 359b
pollution, air, 561–562
polysaccharides, 48
polyunsaturated fats, 408
pons, 155
population attributable risk, 318
Position Stand on Progression Models in Resistance Training for Healthy Adults, 490
positive feedback, in biological control system, 34
positive N-balance, 525
posterior hypothalamus, 267
posterior pituitary gland, 97, 98, 109t, 110t
postganglionic neurons, 159–160
postsynaptic membrane, 146, 147
postsynaptic neuron, 142f, 144, 145, 146
postural tone, brain stem, 156
potassium, 143, 144, 145f, 404t–405t
potassium ions, 143, 144
potassium-40, 411–412
potency, of exercise, 353
power
calculating, 17
defined, 17
measurement of, 18–20
performed on a cycle ergometer, 19–20
terms and units used to express, 17t
power tests, 468–469
cycling, 470–471

jumping, 468
running, 468–469, 469–470, 471
sport-specific, 471–472
preBötzinger Complex, 237
precompetition meal, 534–535
precooling, 274b
pregnancy
exercise during, 387, 389, 504–506
iron intake and, 402
obesity and, 418
thyroxine and, 93–94
prehydrating, 529
prehypertension, 380
preload, 203, 286
prescription of exercise. *See* exercise prescriptions
preseason conditioning, 496
President's Council on Fitness, Sports, and Nutrition, 7
President's Council on Physical Fitness, 7
President's Council on Physical Fitness and Sports, 7
President's Council on Youth Fitness, 7
pressure-sensitive receptors. *See* baroreceptors
presynaptic membrane, 147f
presynaptic neuron, 144, 145
primary amenorrhea, 107
primary bronchus, 221f
primary hypertension, 196
primary risk factors, 317b
primary signal transduction pathways, 295
professional societies, 11
progesterone, 105–107
progression, of exercise program, 356–358
Progressive Aerobic Cardiovascular Endurance Run (PACER), 332b
progressive resistance exercise (PRE), 488
prolactin, 97, 100
prolonged exercise, 75
blood glucose and, 81–84, 82f, 119, 521
cardiovascular response to, 213
energy for, 75, 76f
fuel selection and, 80, 81–82, 82f, 84
homeostasis and, 36
lactate shuttle and, 86b
protein sources and, 85
ventilatory response, 235–236
proprioceptive neuromuscular facilitation (PNF), 493
proprioceptors, 148–151
prostaglandins, 503
proteases, 85
protein kinase C, 96, 111, 112, 119
protein receptor hormone, 92–93

right atrioventricular valve, 190
right atrium, 189, 190f, 191, 197, 202, 228
right ventricle, 189, 190, 190f, 228
risk factors
    cardiorespiratory screening and, 329
    categories of, 315, 315f, 329
    guidelines for determining cause, 318
    for heart disease, 315–317, 316f, 317b
    physical inactivity, 352
    in web of causation, 316, 316f
RNA, messenger (mRNA), 38b, 293, 294, 294f
Robinson, Sid, 5, 6f
Rossiter, Harry, 71b
Rowell, Loring, 11–12
RPE (rating of perceived exertion), 336, 336t, 522, 579
RPE scale, 361, 389
R-R time interval, 202
running. See also distance running; jogging
    estimation of energy expenditure and, 23, 24b
    exercise-induced asthma and, 377
    gastric emptying and, 530
    maximal oxygen uptake and, 451
    net caloric cost per mile for, 431–432, 431t
running economy, 27, 451
running performance
    distance, 451, 452b
    long-distance, 452
running power tests, 468–469
running tests, 332–334, 339
    running anaerobic power tests, 471
    running anaerobic sprint test (RAST), 471
    for soccer, 469–470
RV (residual volume), 226, 226t

S

SA node. See sinoatrial node (SA node)
Salazar, Alberto, 133
Salbutamol, 578b
salt intake, 378, 381, 531. See also sodium
Saltin, Bengt, 287, 288b
same-season repeat concussion, 157b
sarcolemma, 42, 165f, 166, 167f, 168, 445–446
sarcomeres, 166f, 167
sarcopenia, 183b, 385, 511, 512, 528
sarcoplasm, 42, 167, 167f
sarcoplasmic reticulum (SR), 64, 167–168, 167f, 171, 445, 446, 447
Sargent, Dudley, 6–7, 6f
satellite cells, 166

saturated fats, 408
Sawka, Michael, 274b
Schmidt-Nielsen, Bodil, 4
Scholander, Peter F., 5
schools, fitness testing in, 7
Schwann cells, 141
scientists in history, 3, 6
    Andrew F. Huxley, 169b
    August Krogh, 19b
    A. V. Hill, 73b
    Bengt Saltin, 288b
    Benjamin Levine, 485b
    Björn Ekblom, 576b
    Bruno Balke, 343b, 343b
    Claude Bernard, 31b
    David L. Costill, 453b
    D. B. (Bruce) Dill, 262b
    Edward Jenner, 131b
    European, 4
    Fred W. Kasch, 385b
    Hans Krebs, 55b
    Jean Mayer, 429b
    Jeremy N. Morris, 319b
    John O. Holloszy, 288b
    Jonas Bergström, 520b
    Kariman Wasserman, 242b
    L. G. C. E. Pugh, 560b
    Michael L. Pollock, 359b
    Peter Stewart, 255
    Ralph S. Paffenbarger, Jr., 319b
    Robert Bruce, 462b
    Thomas K. Cureton, Jr., 10b
    Walter B. Cannon, 101b
    William Harvey, 189b
screening, 329
    for asthma in children, 378b
    before beginning exercise program, 356
    for cardiorespiratory fitness testing, 329
SCUBA diving, 510
sea level
    altitude and, 542, 544f, 545, 546–547
    hemoglobin at, 544
second messengers, 94–96, 95f, 100
secondary amenorrhea, 107–108
secondary hypertension, 196
secondary messengers in skeletal muscle, 295–296
secondary risk factors, 317b
secondary sex characteristics, 105, 107, 107f
sedentary lifestyle. See physical inactivity
SEE (standard of error of estimates), 411, 412, 413
seizures
    exercise and, 510–511
    risk of injury due to, 511
selenium, 399, 404t–405t
self-renewing stem cell, 128, 128f
Selye, Hans, 103
semilunar valve, 190, 190f
semi-starvation, 425, 425f
sensor(s)
    in biological control system, 33–34

temperature, 35, 262
serotonin, fatigue and, 444
serum cholesterol, 8b, 317, 352, 395, 408
serum ferritin (SF), 532, 533
set, interval training and, 483
set point model, 33
set point, obesity and, 420–421, 420f
set-point temperature, 267–268
settling-point theory, 421
severe hypothermia, 556
sex steroids, 102
    estrogen/progesteron, 105–108
    testosterone, 105
"sham" reinfusion of blood, 574
"sham" withdrawal of blood, 574
shivering, 263, 267, 268, 426, 559
short-term exercise
    energy to perform, 75
    glycogen and, 81–82
short-term performance
    altitude and, 542–543
    factors limiting, 449–450
    fatigue and, 449–450, 450f
SI (system international) units, 16, 16t
    kilocalories converted to, 21
side effects of exercise, 353
signaling events
    leading to endurance training-induced muscle adaptation, 296–297
    leading to resistance training-induced muscle growth, 304–306
    primary signal transduction pathways to skeletal muscle, 295
    secondary messengers in skeletal muscle, 295–296
sinoatrial node (SA node), 197, 197f
    cardiac output and, 201
    heart rate regulation and, 199, 201
Siri equation, 414, 416
size principle, 153, 153b, 154b
skeletal muscle, 165–184. See also muscle fibers (skeletal)
    adaptation to training, 283, 293–297
    in athletes, 179t
    biochemical properties of, 176–177
    cardiac muscle vs., 191
    causes of muscle fatigue, 173–174
    contractile properties of, 177
    contraction, 169, 169b, 170f, 171–172

disease and aging impacting, 183b
exercise performance and, 288
exercise-associated cramps, 175
fiber types, 175–176, 177–179
force regulation in, 181–182
force-velocity/power-velocity relationships, 183–184, 184f
functions, 165
Golgi tendon organs (GTOs), 150–151, 150f
hydrogen ions in working, 252, 252f
length-tension relationship in, 181, 182f
mountain climbing and, 550
muscle action, 179–181
muscle force development, 179–180
muscle spindles, 148, 149–150, 149f
myoglobin in, 233
neuromuscular junction, 168
number of, 165
overload and, 283
oxygen delivery to, during exercise, 207–209
resistance training increasing size of, 303
respiratory, 223b, 223f
secondary messengers in, 295–296
space travel and, 448, 449
speed of muscle action, 180–181
structure of, 165–168, 165f, 166f, 167f
three fiber types, 77
venous return and, 203, 204f
skeletal muscle fibers. See muscle fibers (skeletal)
skin temperature, 263. See also body temperature
skin, the, 127–128
skinfold measurements, 413–414, 416–417, 419, 526
skinfold thickness, 412–413
sleep
    cold acclimation and, 278
    heat production at, 263
sleep apnea, 418
sliding filament model of contraction, 169, 169b
slope of exercise, 353
slow-acting hormones, 113–115
slow-twitch (type I) muscle fibers, 77, 175–178, 176b, 177f, 451
    aging and, 183b, 302b
    endurance training and, 289
    fatigue and, 447–448
    lactate production and, 77–78
    myoglobin in, 233
    resistance training and, 303

T

T cells, 132, 134
T wave, 198, 199f, 200f
talk test, 389
tapering, 497
target heart rate (THR), 360–362, 361f
    jogging and, 362–363
Taylor, Henry Longstreet, 9
temperature. *See also* body temperature; cold environment, exercise and; heat and exercise
    esophageal, 262
    rectal, 262, 268f
    tympanic, 262
temporal summation, 145
"ten percent rule," 486
tendons, 165
tennis, energy expenditure for, 23
tensiometer, 473, 473f
Tepperman, H. M., 101t
Tepperman, J., 101t
terminal bronchioles, 221f
terminal cisternae, 167f, 168, 171
termination criteria, 336
testes, 105, 110t
testing, 329–330. *See also* cardiorespiratory fitness testing; graded exercise tests (GXT); laboratory assessment of performance
    of athletes with asthma, 378
    bicycling, 332
    cardiovascular fitness standards for children, 333b
    of children, 7
    for COPD patients, 379
    coronary heart disease patients, 382
    cycle ergometer, 461
    for estimating cardiorespiratory function (CRF), 332–334
    fitness, 7
    graded exercise tests (GXT), 334–336
    laboratory assessment *vs.*, 459
    procedures, 329–330
    protocols. *See* protocols, testing
    running, 332–334
    of $\dot{V}O_2$, 461–463
    $\dot{V}O_2$ max estimated without, 347b
    walking, 334
testosterone, 105, 105f, 106b, 109t, 110t
tetanus, 181, 182f
Textbook of Cardiovascular Disease and Rehabilitation (Pollock), 359
theophylline, 579
therapeutic dosage of anabolic steroids, 106b

thermic effect of food, 426
thermistors, 262, 263
thermocouples, 262
thermogenesis, 425–426
thiamin, 400t–401t
three-component model of body composition assessment, 413
thymus, 132
thyroid gland, 109t
    calcitonin and, 100
    thyroxine and, 94, 99
thyroid hormones
    cellular activity and, 94
    homeostasis during exercise, 113–114
    thermogenesis and, 426
thyroid-stimulating hormone (TSH), 97, 99
thyroxine (T_4), 93–94, 99–100, 109t, 263
tidal volume (TV), 224–225, 226t
Tipton, C. M., 10t
tobacco. *See* smoking
TOBEC (total body electrical conductivity), 412
Tokyo (1964) Olympic Games, 544t
Tolerable Upper Intake Level (UL), 397
total body electrical conductivity (TOBEC), 412
total body water (TBW), 411, 412, 413
total fiber, 406
total lung capacity (TLC), 226, 226t
Tour de France, 451, 575
toxicity, from vitamins, 399
trace elements, 399
trachea, 219, 220, 220f
training, 282–308. *See also* endurance training; strength training
    altitude and, 484–485, 546–547, 548b
    for asthmatics, 510
    common mistakes, 497
    for competition at altitude, 546–547
    components of, 482
    in cool conditions, 275b
    for COPD patients, 379–380
    for diabetics, 509–510
    for epileptics, 510–511
    factors important to women involved in, 502–507
    for high-intensity, continuous exercise, 484
    to improve aerobic power, 482–485
    to improve anaerobic performance, 486–487, 487b
    to improve flexibility, 493
    improving $\dot{V}O_2$, 285
    injuries and endurance, 486
    interval, 483

for long, slow-distance exercise, 483–484
    lungs adapting to, 242
    for master athlete, 514
    muscle adaptation, 293–297
    physiological effects of strength, 301
    premilitary, 7
    principles of, 283
    responses to, 354
    sports conditioning for children, 507–508
    year-round conditioning, 496
trans fats, 408
transferrin, 532, 533
transport protein, 93–94
transverse tubules, 167f, 168, 171, 445
treadmill, 18f
    computing energy efficiency for, 24–25, 24b
    energy expenditure on, 22
    exercise efficiency estimation, 24b
    for exercise tests, 76
    testing protocols, 341t, 342, 342f
treatment, of chronic obstructive pulmonary disease, 379
tricarboxylic acid cycle, 55b
tricep skinfold measurement, 419
tricuspid valve, 190
"trigger" step in muscular contraction, 171
triglycerides, 49, 407
    aerobic metabolism and, 57
    Krebs cycle and, 57, 58f
triiodothyronine (T_3), 99–100, 109t
tropomyosin, 167, 170f, 171, 172
troponin, 167, 170f, 171, 172
TrueOne metabolic measurement system, 22f
TSH (thyroid-stimulating hormone), 97, 99
t-tubule function, 446
Tvent. *See* ventilatory threshold (Tvent)
twenty-four hour call, 410
twitch, muscle, 180–181, 180f, 182f
two-component body composition system, 413–416
tympanic temperature, 262
type 1 diabetes, 36b
    characteristics, 371
    exercise and, 372–374
    training and, 509–510
    type 2 diabetes *vs.*, 371t
type 1 fibers. *See* slow-twitch (type I) muscle fibers
type 2 diabetes, 36b
    diet and, 375
    exercise and, 374–375

obesity and, 104b
    overview, 371
    prevention or delay of, 375b
    training and, 509
    type 1 diabetes *vs.*, 371t
type II alveolar cells, 221, 221f
type IIa fibers, 178, 448, 483
type IIx fibers. *See* fast-twitch (type II) muscle fibers
tyrosine kinase, 96

U

ultra short-term performances, 448–449, 450f
ultra-endurance events, 453
ultrasounds, 412
undertraining, 497
underwater weighing, 413–416, 415f, 536
units of measure
    calorie, 21
    expressing power, 17t
    expressing work performed, 17, 17t
    metric system, 16, 16t
    SI units, 16, 16t
University of Illinois, 10b
University of Minnesota, Laboratory for Physiological Hygiene, 9
upper-respiratory tract infection (URTI), 133, 136
up-regulation, 94
urea cycle, 55b
U.S. Department of Agriculture, 406b
U.S. *Physical Activity Guidelines*, 8b
USDA food pattern, 409–410
USDA Human Nutrition Research Center on Aging, 429b

V

V (volume), 224
vaccines, smallpox, 131b
vagus nerve, 199
valine, 49, 84
van Slyke apparatus, 4
vanadium, 399, 571t
Vander, A. J., 93f, 98f, 147f
vapor pressure, 264–265, 264t
variability, exercise prescription and, 353
variable-resistance exercise, 488
variable-resistance isokinetic dynamometer, 473–474
variable-resistance measurement of strength, 474–475
vascular resistance, 196, 206
vasoconstriction, 206, 209, 213
vasodilation, 206, 209, 210b
vasomotor control center, 267
vasopressin, 98
VC (vital capacity), 226
VCO_2/VO_2 ratio, 79
V_E (ventilatory threshold), 236, 236f, 239, 240–241